ExpertDDX
Abdomen & Pelvis

SECOND EDITION

Federle | Raman | Tublin

SHAABAN · BORHANI · FURLAN · HELLER

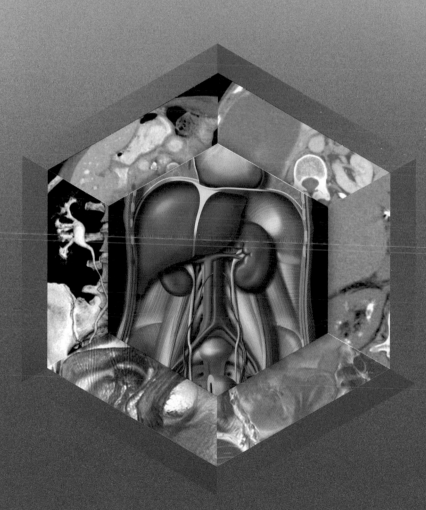

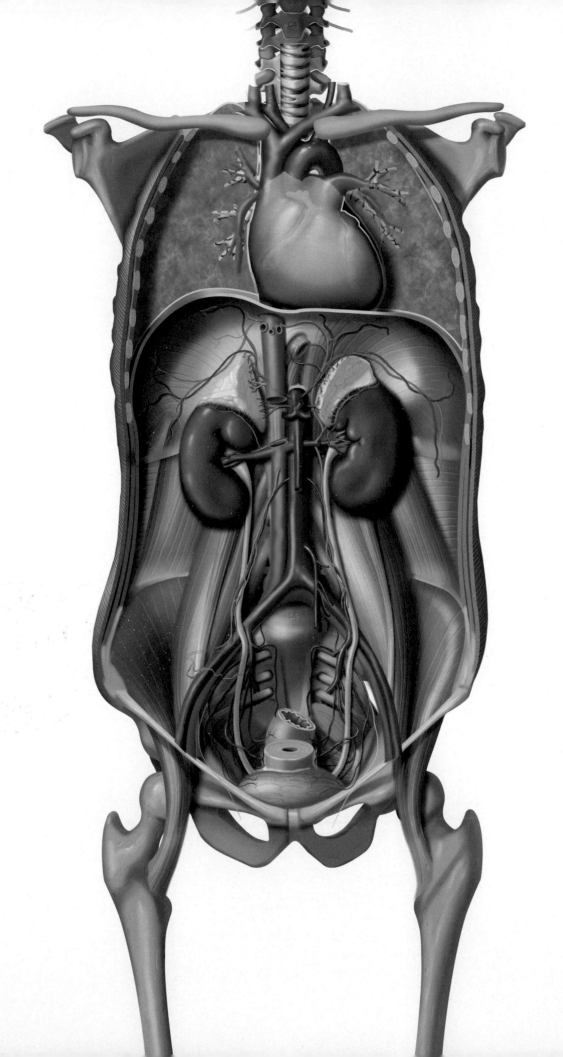

ExpertDDX
Abdomen & Pelvis

SECOND EDITION

Michael P. Federle, MD, FACR
Professor and Associate Chair for Education
Department of Radiology
Stanford University School of Medicine
Stanford, California

Siva P. Raman, MD
Assistant Professor of Radiology
Department of Radiology
Johns Hopkins University School of Medicine
Baltimore, Maryland

Mitchell Tublin, MD
Professor and Vice Chair of Radiology
Chief, Abdominal Imaging Section
University of Pittsburgh School of Medicine
Pittsburgh, Pennsylvania

Akram M. Shaaban, MBBCh
Professor (Clinical)
Department of Radiology and Imaging Sciences
University of Utah School of Medicine
Salt Lake City, Utah

Amir A. Borhani, MD
Abdominal Imaging Fellow
University of Pittsburgh Medical Center
Pittsburgh, Pennsylvania

Alessandro Furlan, MD
Assistant Professor
Department of Radiology, Division of Abdominal Imaging
University of Pittsburgh School of Medicine
Pittsburgh, Pennsylvania

Matthew T. Heller, MD, FSAR
Associate Professor of Radiology
Division of Abdominal Imaging
University of Pittsburgh Medical Center
Pittsburgh, Pennsylvania

ELSEVIER

1600 John F. Kennedy Blvd.
Ste 1800
Philadelphia, PA 19103-2899

EXPERTDDX: ABDOMEN & PELVIS, SECOND EDITION

ISBN: 978-0-323-44287-9

Notices

Publisher Cataloging-in-Publication Data

Names: Federle, Michael P. | Raman, Siva P. | Tublin, Mitchell E.
Title: Expert DDx: Abdomen and pelvis / [edited by] Michael P. Federle, Siva P. Raman, and Mitchell Tublin.
Other titles: Abdomen and pelvis.
Description: Second edition. | Salt Lake City, UT : Elsevier, Inc., [2016] | Includes bibliographical references and index.
Identifiers: ISBN 978-0-323-44287-9
Subjects: LCSH: Abdomen--Anatomy--Handbooks, manuals, etc. | Pelvis--Anatomy--Handbooks, manuals, etc. | MESH: Abdomen--anatomy & histology--Atlases. | Pelvis----anatomy & histology--Atlases.
Classification: LCC RC78.7.D53 D534 2016 | NLM WE 17 | DDC 616.07'54--dc23

International Standard Book Number: 978-0-323-44287-9

Cover Designer: Tom M. Olson, BA

Printed in Canada by Friesens, Altona, Manitoba, Canada

Last digit is the print number: 9 8 7 6 5 4 3 2 1

Dedications

To Lynne, my wife and partner of 45 years.
MPF

To my loving wife, Janani Venkateswaran,
who has been at the heart of all my successes.
To my young son, Jay Raman, who inspires me to do better every day.
To my colleagues at Johns Hopkins, whose support and
guidance have been invaluable.
SPR

To my wife, Mary, and our sons, Daniel, Josh, and Andrew.
Your love and support sustain me.
MT

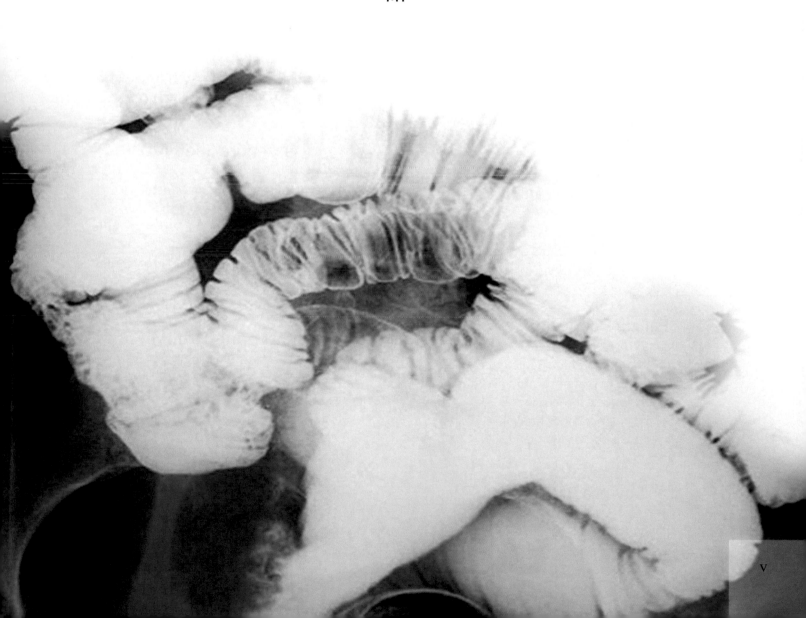

Contributing Authors

Aya Kamaya, MD, FSRU, FSAR
Associate Professor of Radiology
Co-Director, Stanford Body Imaging Fellowship
Stanford University School of Medicine
Stanford, California

Hee Sun Park, MD, PhD
Associate Professor
Department of Radiology
Konkuk University School of Medicine
Seoul, South Korea

**Jade Wong-You-Cheong,
MBChB, MRCP, FRCR**
Professor
Department of Diagnostic Radiology and Nuclear Medicine
University of Maryland School of Medicine
Director of Ultrasound
University of Maryland Medical Center
Baltimore, Maryland

Maryam Rezvani, MD
Associate Professor of Radiology
Department of Radiology
University of Utah School of Medicine
Salt Lake City, Utah

Fauzia Vandermeer, MD
Assistant Professor of Diagnostic Radiology
Associate Program Director, Radiology Residency
Department of Diagnostic Radiology and
Nuclear Medicine
University of Maryland School of Medicine
Baltimore, Maryland

Shweta Bhatt, MD
Associate Professor
Department of Imaging Sciences
University of Rochester Medical Center
Rochester, New York

Gregory E. Antonio, MD, FRANZCR
Clinical Professor (Honorary)
Department of Imaging and Interventional Radiology
The Chinese University of Hong Kong
Hong Kong, People's Republic of China

Eric K.H. Liu, PhD, RDMS
Adjunct Associate Professor
Department of Imaging and Interventional Radiology
The Chinese University of Hong Kong
Hong Kong, People's Republic of China

Ashish P. Wasnik, MD, FSAR
Assistant Professor of Radiology
Director, Medical Student Education
Division of Abdominal Imaging
University of Michigan Health System
Ann Arbor, Michigan

Narendra Shet, MD
Assistant Professor
Assistant Program Director
Radiology Residency Program
Department of Diagnostic Radiology and
Nuclear Medicine
University of Maryland School of Medicine
Baltimore, Maryland

Katherine To'o, MD
Staff Radiologist
Veterans Affairs Palo Alto Health Care System
Palo Alto, California

L. Nayeli Morimoto, MD
Clinical Assistant Professor
Department of Radiology
Stanford University School of Medicine
Stanford, California

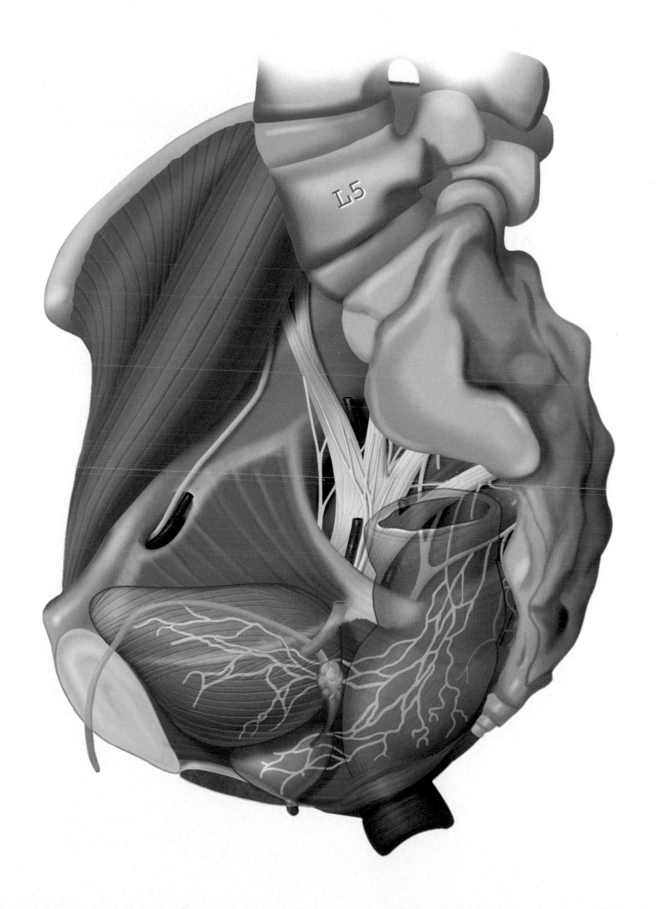

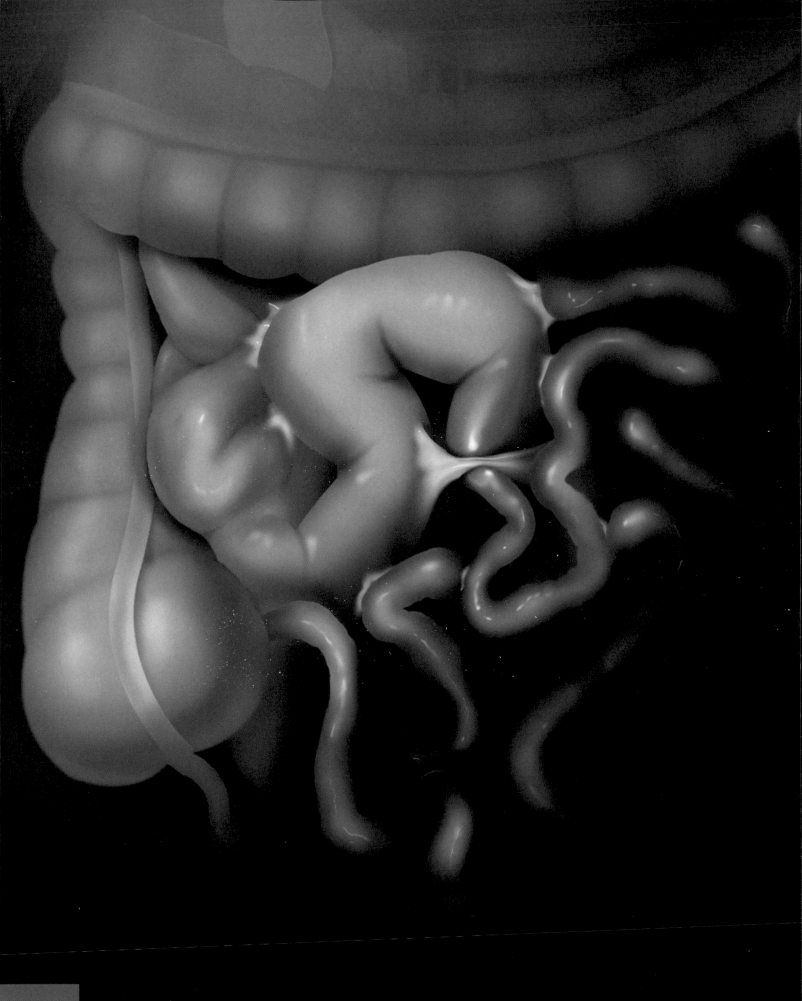

Preface

Radiologists are frequently confronted with challenging imaging interpretations, armed only with knowledge of the patient's clinical presentation (e.g., right upper quadrant pain) or an imaging finding (e.g., a cystic pancreatic mass). In order to narrow the differential diagnosis, the radiologist will attempt to recall information learned during one's training or in more recent venues, such as CME meetings. The diligent may seek assistance with a standard radiology text, but these are often organized by specific diseases or disorders and may not be helpful or efficient in quickly generating a useful differential diagnosis. Internet searches are certainly expedient, but one is likely to wade through numerous unvetted and unreliable sources before coming up with valid content.

Our series of Expert Differential Diagnosis ("DDx") books draw on the accumulated experience and expertise of our Amirsys/Elsevier authors, most of whom have authored and helped edit the encyclopedic *Diagnostic Imaging* books. Our goal is to identify the most common and important clinical and imaging challenges and to provide a list of the common, less common, and rare causes for such challenges. These causes are accompanied by characteristic imaging studies, along with the key clinical and imaging features that allow one to distinguish among the possible etiologies.

The second edition of *Expert DDx: Abdomen* has been substantially expanded to become *Expert DDx: Abdomen & Pelvis*, and we have significantly added to our coverage of the male and female pelvis. In addition to the generic imaging patterns (e.g., "cystic renal mass"), we have added many modality-specific modules, especially focusing on disorders best or typically evaluated by ultrasonography or MR (e.g., "cystic adnexal mass").

We hope that you will find this to be a valuable resource as we seek to add value to our work as radiologists.

Michael P. Federle, MD, FACR
Professor and Associate Chair for Education
Department of Radiology
Stanford University School of Medicine
Stanford, California

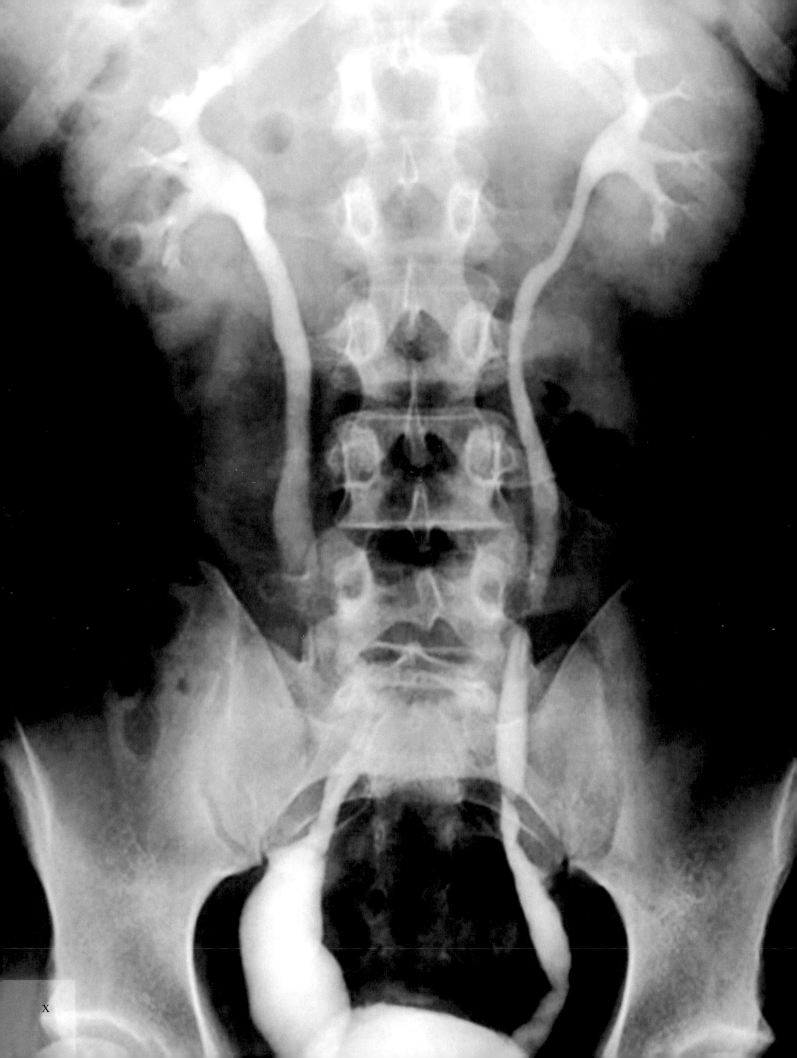

Acknowledgments

Text Editors

Arthur G. Gelsinger, MA
Nina I. Bennett, BA
Terry W. Ferrell, MS
Karen E. Concannon, MA, PhD
Matt W. Hoecherl, BS
Tricia L. Cannon, BA

Image Editors

Jeffrey J. Marmorstone, BS
Lisa A. M. Steadman, BS

Illustrations

Laura C. Sesto, MA
Lane R. Bennion, MS
Richard Coombs, MS

Art Direction and Design

Tom M. Olson, BA
Laura C. Sesto, MA

Lead Editor

Lisa A. Gervais, BS

Production Coordinators

Angela M. G. Terry, BA
Rebecca L. Hutchinson, BA
Emily C. Fassett, BA

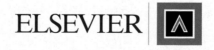

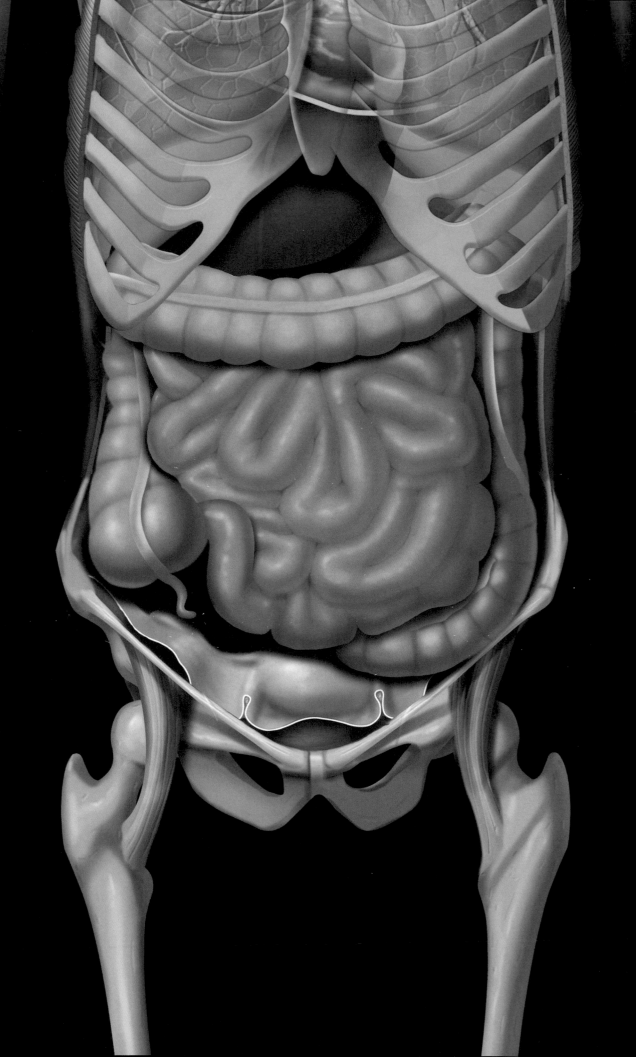

Sections

TABLE OF CONTENTS

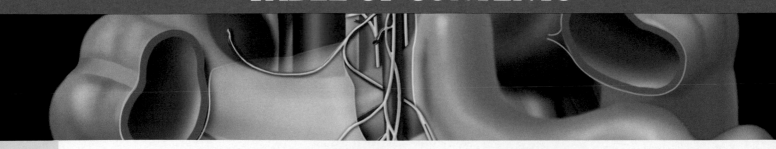

TABLE OF CONTENTS

TABLE OF CONTENTS

TABLE OF CONTENTS

TABLE OF CONTENTS

ExpertDDX

Abdomen & Pelvis

SECOND EDITION

Federle | Raman | Tublin

SHAABAN • BORHANI • FURLAN • HELLER

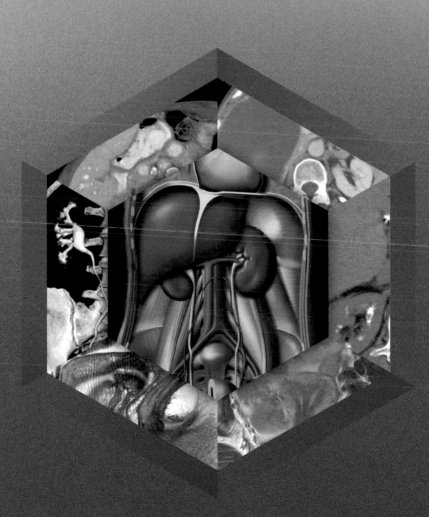

Generic Imaging Patterns

Modality-Specific Imaging Findings

COMPUTED TOMOGRAPHY

DIFFERENTIAL DIAGNOSIS

Common

- Peritoneal Metastases
- Lymphoma
- Mesenteric Lymphadenopathy
- Acute Pancreatitis
- Diaphragmatic Insertions (Mimic)
- Mesenteric Hematoma (Mimic)

Less Common

- Mesothelioma
- Desmoid
- Sclerosing Mesenteritis
- Tuberculous Peritonitis
- Carcinoid Tumor
- Splenosis
- Gastrointestinal Stromal Tumor
- Fat Necrosis
- Primary Papillary Serous Carcinoma

Rare but Important

- Sarcoma of Mesentery or Retroperitoneum
- Leukemia
- Benign Mesenchymal Tumors
- Leiomyomatosis Peritonealis Disseminata
- Other Systemic Diseases

ESSENTIAL INFORMATION

Key Differential Diagnosis Issues

- Peritoneal metastases are, by far, most common cause of solid mass in omentum
- Lymphadenopathy is, by far, most common etiology for solid mesenteric mass

Helpful Clues for Common Diagnoses

- **Peritoneal Metastases**
  - Most common with primary gynecologic (ovary, uterus) and GI malignancies
  - May result in discrete soft tissue masses in omentum and mesentery, usually in conjunction with ascites and peritoneal thickening, nodularity, and enhancement
- **Lymphoma**
  - Very common cause of mesenteric lymphadenopathy, usually in conjunction with lymphadenopathy elsewhere
  - Lymphoma can rarely involve omentum (i.e., peritoneal lymphomatosis), producing confluent soft tissue infiltration that is virtually indistinguishable from carcinomatosis
    - Usually in association with significant lymphadenopathy or extranodal disease elsewhere
    - May be associated with ascites, but less commonly than carcinomatosis
    - Uncommon and most often seen with immunocompromised patients or aggressive forms of lymphoma (such as Burkitt lymphoma)
- **Mesenteric Lymphadenopathy**
  - Many potential infectious, inflammatory, and neoplastic causes (which can manifest as discrete nodes or confluent nodal masses)

- Substantial lymphadenopathy should raise concern for malignancy, but can also be seen with infections or be reactive to inflammatory processes in abdomen
- **Acute Pancreatitis**
  - May produce extrapancreatic necrosis due to leakage of pancreatic enzymes into adjacent mesenteric fat with resultant fat necrosis
    - Can appear very nodular and mass-like, potentially mimicking tumor spread or carcinomatosis
  - Inflammation from pancreatitis may extend into mesentery, creating phlegmon that mimics solid mass
- **Diaphragmatic Insertions (Mimic)**
  - Slips of diaphragm may insert on ribs and costal cartilages, potentially mimicking peritoneal or omental nodularity on axial images
  - Key is to visualize elongated shape of these "masses" and their contiguity with rest of diaphragm
    - Diagnosis easily confirmed on multiplanar reformats
- **Mesenteric Hematoma (Mimic)**
  - Usually seen in patients with history of trauma or coagulopathy, and could mimic hyperdense "mass"

Helpful Clues for Less Common Diagnoses

- **Mesothelioma**
  - Malignant mesothelioma may rarely arise from peritoneum, accounting for 20% of all mesotheliomas
  - Appearance similar to carcinomatosis, including omental/mesenteric nodularity and masses, peritoneal thickening/enhancement, and pleated appearance of mesentery
    - May be associated with ascites, but usually less than is seen with carcinomatosis
    - Can be localized (solitary dominant mass) or diffuse (extensive peritoneal involvement)
  - Presence of pleural plaques can be important clue given relationship between mesothelioma and asbestos
- **Desmoid**
  - Benign, aggressive mesenchymal neoplasm that can involve abdominal wall or mesentery
  - Predisposing risk factors include prior surgery, trauma, Gardner syndrome, or familial polyposis
  - Appears as locally aggressive soft tissue mass, which can compress and invade adjacent structures
  - Variable appearance, but typically hypoenhancing with low signal on T1WI and high signal on T2WI MR
    - Can appear well circumscribed or infiltrative
- **Sclerosing Mesenteritis**
  - Idiopathic inflammatory and fibrotic disorder of mesentery that ranges in appearance from subtle "misty mesentery" to discrete fibrotic mass
  - End-stage disease may result in discrete fibrotic mass (with frequent coarse calcification) that occludes vasculature and produces bowel obstructions
  - Usually located in left upper quadrant, but appearance may be difficult to differentiate from carcinoid tumor
- **Tuberculous Peritonitis**
  - Involvement of peritoneum can result in thickening and nodularity that appears similar to carcinomatosis
  - Results in peritoneal thickening, nodularity, and ascites
  - Frequently associated with tuberculous lymphadenitis, which manifests as necrotic lymphadenopathy

- **Carcinoid Tumor**
  - Spiculated mesenteric mass in RLQ, often with calcification, which is frequently associated with desmoplastic reaction and tethering of adjacent bowel/vasculature
  - Mesenteric mass represents metastasis, with primary tumor most commonly present in terminal ileum
    - Primary ileal tumor may not always be visible on CT, but often is hypervascular on arterial-phase images
- **Splenosis**
  - Traumatic rupture of spleen resulting in implantation of splenic tissue throughout peritoneal cavity
  - Enhancing nodules should have identical enhancement on all phases of imaging to normal spleen
  - Absence of spleen is important clue to diagnosis, but confirmation can be obtained with Tc-99m heat-denatured RBC scan
- **Gastrointestinal Stromal Tumor**
  - Commonly arises from stomach or small bowel, but can be exophytic with extensive mesenteric component
  - Can be massive in size, occupying much of abdomen, making it very difficult to ascertain exact site of origin
    - Should always be strongly considered when confronted by solitary dominant mass occupying sizable portion of abdomen
  - Variable enhancement (can be hypodense or relatively vascular) with frequent internal heterogeneity, ulceration, and necrosis
- **Fat Necrosis**
  - Fat necrosis, including postsurgical fat necrosis, epiploic appendagitis, and omental infarcts, can appear very mass like and simulate malignancy
  - Diagnosis contingent on presence of internal fat and clinical history, although internal fat can be quite insubstantial in some cases
- **Primary Papillary Serous Carcinoma**
  - Rare malignancy seen primarily in postmenopausal women with evidence of diffuse peritoneal tumor spread (e.g., ascites, tumor implants, etc.)
  - Identical in appearance and histology to peritoneal carcinomatosis secondary to ovarian cancer, but without evidence of primary ovarian mass

Helpful Clues for Rare Diagnoses

- **Sarcoma of Mesentery or Retroperitoneum**
  - Primary peritoneal sarcomas are uncommon, although large retroperitoneal sarcomas can grow into peritoneal space
  - Most common primary peritoneal sarcoma is malignant fibrous histiocytoma
  - Usually no specific imaging features for different sarcomas, which appear as nonspecific, large mass
- **Leukemia**
  - Can rarely infiltrate peritoneum with imaging findings similar to carcinomatosis or lymphomatosis
  - Most often seen with acute myeloid leukemia (AML)
- **Benign Mesenchymal Tumors**
  - Encompasses wide variety of benign masses, including hemangiomas, lipomas, and nerve sheath tumors
  - Hemangiomas appear as low-density, poorly marginated masses with characteristic internal phleboliths
  - Lipoma demonstrates uniform fat density without internal complexity to suggest liposarcoma
  - Mesenteric plexiform neurofibromas are most commonly seen in neurofibromatosis type 1
    - Mesenteric low-density mass with branching appearance
- **Leiomyomatosis Peritonealis Disseminata**
  - Dissemination of multiple smooth muscle nodules throughout peritoneum, usually in premenopausal females with history of uterine fibroids
  - Imaging demonstrates multiple peritoneal soft tissue nodules that demonstrate CT attenuation and MR signal characteristics (usually hypointense on T2WI) similar to uterine fibroids
- **Other Systemic Diseases**
  - Amyloidosis, extramedullary hematopoiesis, Erdheim-Chester, and sarcoidosis have had reported cases of mass-like omental/mesenteric involvement

Peritoneal Metastases

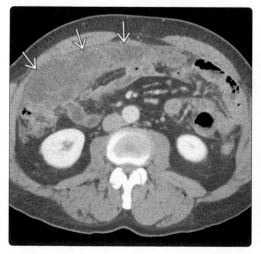

Peritoneal Metastases

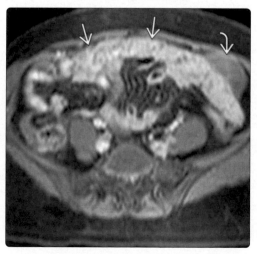

(Left) Axial CECT in a patient with pancreatic cancer demonstrates extensive omental caking ➡ throughout the right anterior omentum, compatible with peritoneal carcinomatosis. (Right) Axial T1WI C+ FS MR demonstrates extensive omental caking ➡ throughout the anterior omentum, along with a small amount of ascites ➡, compatible with peritoneal carcinomatosis.

(Left) *Axial DWI MR in a patient with cholangiocarcinoma demonstrates abnormal restricted diffusion* ➡ *throughout the anterior omentum.* **(Right)** *Axial T1WI C+ FS MR in the same patient demonstrates that the restricted diffusion corresponds to multiple hypoenhancing peritoneal metastases* ➡ *throughout the omentum.*

Peritoneal Metastases

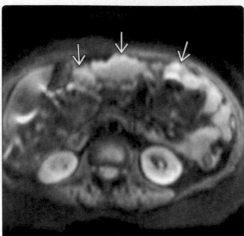

Peritoneal Metastases

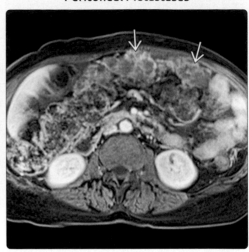

(Left) *Axial CECT demonstrates extensive confluent retroperitoneal* ➡ *and mesenteric* ➡ *lymphadenopathy secondary to non-Hodgkin lymphoma.* **(Right)** *Axial CECT demonstrates a large, confluent mesenteric mass* ➡ *in a patient with non-Hodgkin lymphoma. Notice how the mass surrounds vessels* ➡ *without any appreciable narrowing or attenuation, a classic feature.*

Lymphoma

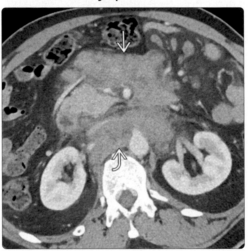

Lymphoma

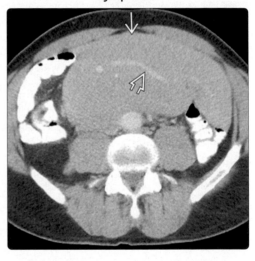

(Left) *Axial CECT in an AIDS patient demonstrates extensive soft tissue infiltration* ➡ *throughout the mesentery and omentum, reflecting lymphomatous involvement (i.e., lymphomatosis).* **(Right)** *Axial CECT demonstrates a large mesenteric soft tissue mass occupying much of the central mesentery* ➡*, as well as extensive soft tissue infiltration of omentum* ➡*, compatible with lymphomatous involvement in this patient with non-Hodgkin lymphoma.*

Lymphoma

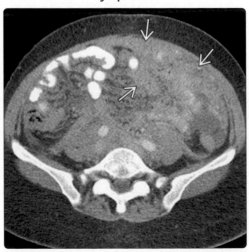

Lymphoma

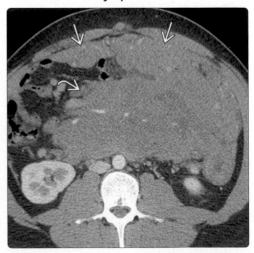

Mesenteric Lymphadenopathy

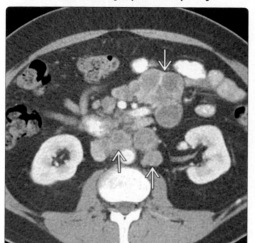

Acute Pancreatitis

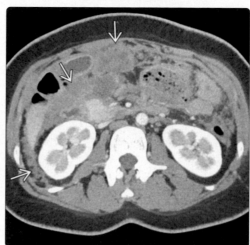

(Left) *Axial CECT demonstrates extensive necrotic lymphadenopathy* ➡️ *in the mesentery and retroperitoneum, representing metastatic lymphadenopathy from the patient's known melanoma.* (Right) *Axial CECT in a patient with severe pancreatitis demonstrates extensive soft tissue density* ➡️ *and nodularity throughout the mesentery and omentum. While almost resembling tumor in its density and texture, these findings reflect extensive extrapancreatic necrosis related to pancreatitis.*

Diaphragmatic Insertions (Mimic)

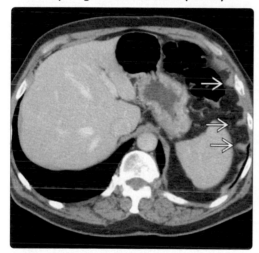

Mesenteric Hematoma (Mimic)

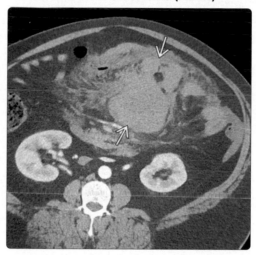

(Left) *Axial CECT shows numerous nodular densities* ➡️ *that mimic peritoneal implants. These "nodules" represent finger-like slips of diaphragm as they near their abdominal wall insertions.* (Right) *Axial CECT demonstrates a large mesenteric hematoma* ➡️. *The hematoma was spontaneous and attributed to a bleeding diathesis.*

Mesothelioma

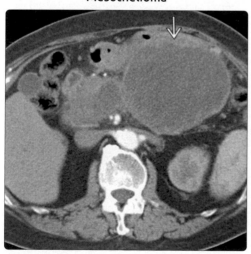

Mesothelioma

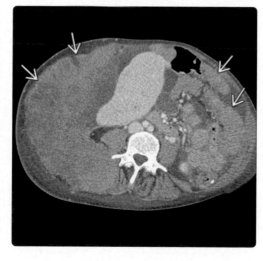

(Left) *Axial CECT demonstrates a large, hypodense, necrotic mass* ➡️ *in the mesentery, found to represent mesothelioma. Focal forms of mesothelioma have a better prognosis than diffuse forms, and can be surgically resected in some instances.* (Right) *Axial CECT demonstrates extensive peritoneal tumor* ➡️ *throughout the upper abdomen, including massive perihepatic tumor fungating into the abdominal wall. These findings are secondary to an aggressive diffuse form of mesothelioma.*

Desmoid

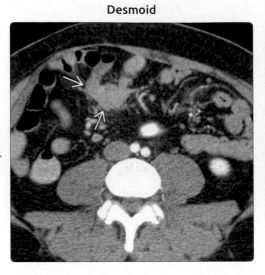

Desmoid

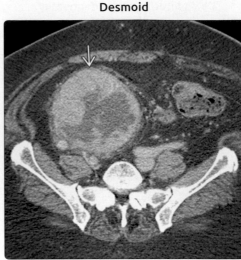

(Left) *Axial CECT demonstrates an infiltrative mesenteric mass* ➡️ *tethering adjacent bowel loops, found to represent a mesenteric desmoid tumor.* (Right) *Axial CECT demonstrates a large, centrally necrotic mass* ➡️ *in the right abdomen, found to be a desmoid tumor in this patient with familial polyposis.*

Sclerosing Mesenteritis

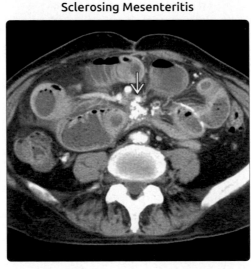

Sclerosing Mesenteritis

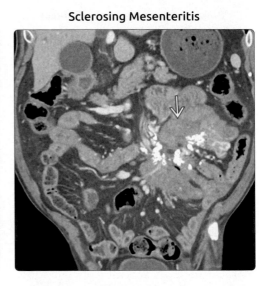

(Left) *Axial CECT demonstrates a calcified mass* ➡️ *in the central mesentery, which tethers multiple surrounding loops of bowel (resulting in a bowel obstruction). This mass was proven to represent sclerosing mesenteritis.* (Right) *Axial CECT demonstrates a dramatic form of sclerosing mesenteritis* ➡️ *in the left upper quadrant with confluent soft tissue and extensive calcification. Notice the manner in which this process tethers and distorts the adjacent bowel and vasculature.*

Carcinoid Tumor

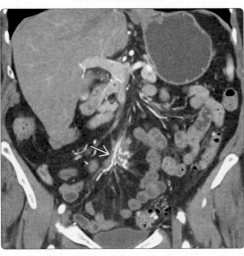

Carcinoid Tumor

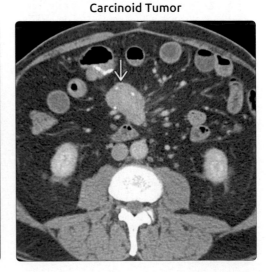

(Left) *Coronal CECT demonstrates spiculated soft tissue* ➡️ *with calcification in the mid-mesentery found to represent a mesenteric metastasis from carcinoid tumor. The primary tumor was found in the ileum at surgery, but was not visible on CT.* (Right) *Axial CECT demonstrates a well-circumscribed mass* ➡️ *in the central mesentery with a few internal punctate calcifications, representing a carcinoid mesenteric metastasis from a primary ileal tumor.*

Splenosis

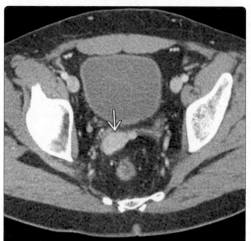

Splenosis

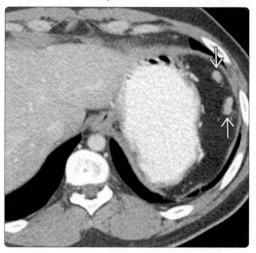

(Left) *Axial CECT demonstrates an enhancing soft tissue nodule* ➡ *in the deep pelvis.* (Right) *Axial CECT in the same patient demonstrates similar-appearing nodules* ➡ *in the left upper quadrant, as well as absence of the spleen, a classic constellation of findings for splenosis.*

Gastrointestinal Stromal Tumor

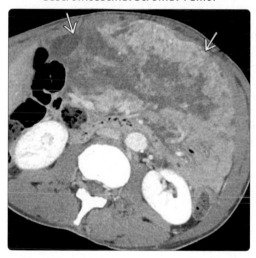

Gastrointestinal Stromal Tumor

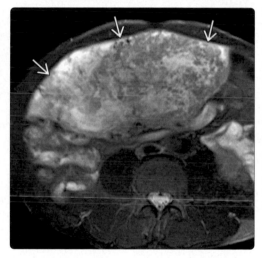

(Left) *Axial CECT demonstrates a huge mass* ➡ *occupying much of the omentum and mesentery. The mass demonstrates very heterogeneous enhancement with areas of necrosis.* (Right) *Axial T2WI FS MR in the same patient once again demonstrates the large mass* ➡*, which is relatively hyperintense with some internal heterogeneity. This mass was found at surgery to represent an exophytic GIST arising from the stomach.*

Benign Mesenchymal Tumors

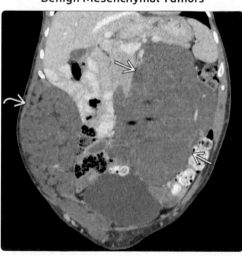

Benign Mesenchymal Tumors

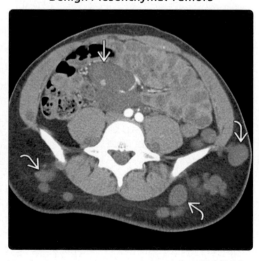

(Left) *Coronal CECT in a patient with neurofibromatosis type 1 demonstrates extensive plexiform neurofibromas occupying a large portion of the mesentery* ➡*, particularly in the left abdomen, with additional lesions seen in the soft tissues* ➡ *on the right.* (Right) *Axial CECT in a patient with NF type 1 demonstrates a large, right-sided mesenteric plexiform neurofibroma* ➡ *surrounding vessels, as well as multiple additional neurofibromas in the subcutaneous fat* ➡*.*

DIFFERENTIAL DIAGNOSIS

Common

- Loculated Ascites
- Abscess, Abdominal
- Pancreatic Pseudocyst
- Peritoneal Metastases
- Cystic Ovarian Neoplasm
- Lymphocele

Less Common

- Pseudomyxoma Peritonei
- Mesenteric Cyst
- Urachal Remnant
- Dermoid (Mature Teratoma)
- Lymphadenopathy, Cystic or Caseated
- Peritoneal Inclusion Cyst
- Hydatid Cyst

ESSENTIAL INFORMATION

Key Differential Diagnosis Issues

- Correctly identifying location and site of origin of cystic mass is critical in generating appropriate differential diagnosis
  - Distinguish cystic lesions of omentum/mesentery from exophytic cysts projecting off visceral organs (i.e., pancreas, kidneys, liver, etc.)
- Any infectious, inflammatory, or neoplastic process in peritoneum may result in loculated ascites and simulate cystic mass

Helpful Clues for Common Diagnoses

- **Loculated Ascites**
  - Ascites may become loculated due to adhesions, peritonitis, or peritoneal malignancy
    - Peritonitis may be infectious (bacterial, viral, fungal, etc.) or inflammatory (e.g., bile peritonitis)
      □ Peritonitis typically associated with smooth, regular thickening and hyperenhancement of peritoneum on CT/MR (± mesenteric fat stranding)
      □ Multiple repetitive bouts of peritonitis can result in severe chronic thickening and calcification of peritoneal lining with loculated ascites, as with chronic peritoneal dialysis (abdominal cocoon)
    - Loculated ascites due to peritoneal carcinomatosis typically associated with irregular, nodular peritoneal thickening and enhancement (± discrete peritoneal soft tissue implants or omental caking)
    - Loculated ascites due to adhesions typically in patients with known history of abdominal surgeries or prior abdominal inflammatory processes
- **Abscess, Abdominal**
  - Loculated collection of fluid (usually fluid density or slightly hyperdense) with peripheral enhancement
    - Ectopic gas within fluid collection, in absence of intervention, highly suspicious for gas-forming infection or hollow-viscus perforation
    - Usually associated with fat stranding and edema in surrounding mesentery (± imaging findings of peritonitis)

  - Innumerable different causes of abscesses, including superinfection of postsurgical fluid collections, bowel perforation, or generalized bacteremia
- **Pancreatic Pseudocyst**
  - Term used to describe fluid collections, in setting of acute edematous pancreatitis, which persist > 4 weeks
  - Loculated fluid collections encapsulated by well-defined wall of granulation tissue
    - Can rarely demonstrate peripheral calcification
  - Pseudocysts can occur almost anywhere in abdomen, including in locations relatively far from pancreas, simulating other intraperitoneal and retroperitoneal cystic masses
    - Most common in lesser sac or near pancreas
  - Most (but not all) pseudocysts decrease in size or resolve over time, helping distinguish them from neoplasms
    - History of pancreatitis important for diagnosis, but some pseudocysts may require aspiration/fluid analysis to differentiate from cystic neoplasm
- **Peritoneal Metastases**
  - Tumors arising from gastrointestinal tract, uterus, or ovaries are most common causes of peritoneal carcinomatosis
  - Loculated ascites is frequent with carcinomatosis, and is usually associated with other signs of peritoneal malignancy, including nodular peritoneal thickening and enhancement, as well as discrete tumor implants
  - Cystic primary tumors (e.g., ovarian cystadenocarcinoma) and their metastases may appear as cystic masses
- **Cystic Ovarian Neoplasm**
  - Most ovarian cystic neoplasms are of epithelial origin (with mucinous and serous subtypes most common)
  - Serous tumors more likely to be truly cystic, while mucinous neoplasms may demonstrate range of densities due to proteinaceous, hemorrhagic, or mucinous constituents
  - Presence of increasing complexity (e.g., thick septations, mural nodularity, papillary projections) should raise concern for malignancy
- **Lymphocele**
  - Simple appearing cyst composed of lymphatic fluid found immediately adjacent to surgical clips, most commonly after lymphadenectomy or other pelvic surgery

Helpful Clues for Less Common Diagnoses

- **Pseudomyxoma Peritonei**
  - Spread of gelatinous mucinous implants throughout peritoneum as result of ruptured appendiceal mucinous neoplasm
    - Term also utilized by some sources to encompass mucinous tumor implants due to other mucinous neoplasms (e.g., ovary or GI tract)
  - Low-density or cystic implants throughout peritoneum, which frequently indent liver and spleen producing scalloped appearance
    - Implants may be associated with curvilinear calcification or other collections of loculated ascites (similar in density to individual mucinous implants)
  - Slowly progressive process frequently associated with bowel obstruction
- **Mesenteric Cyst**

- o Mesenteric cyst is generic term used to described a number of benign congenital cysts (e.g., lymphangioma, enteric cyst, duplication cyst, mesothelial cyst)
- o Lymphangioma appears as a thin-walled cystic lesion with either water density (~ 0 HU) or, rarely, chylous density (~ -20 HU), but no evidence of internal enhancement, soft tissue component, or nodularity
  - – Often demonstrate feathery morphology with multiple loculations and septations
  - – May indent and abut other structures (such as bowel or vessels) without appreciable mass effect
- o GI duplication cysts and enteric cysts appear as simple cysts along antimesenteric border of bowel
- o Mesothelial cysts are simple cysts arising in mesentery
- **Urachal Remnant**
  - o Failure of urachal remnant to close during embryologic development can result in spectrum of abnormalities that can appear as cystic mass
    - – Urachal cyst appears as discrete cyst at midline abdominal wall between bladder dome and umbilicus
    - – Patent urachus appears as channel between bladder dome and umbilicus, with more elongated or tubular morphology
    - – More rare abnormalities include umbilical-urachal sinus (appears as cystic structure near umbilicus) and vesicourachal diverticulum (appears as midline cyst near bladder dome)
  - o Location of cyst between dome of bladder and umbilicus is key to diagnosis, with superinfection and development of urachal adenocarcinoma known complications
    - – Presence of nodularity or soft tissue within remnant should raise concern for tumor
- **Dermoid Cyst (Mature Teratoma)**
  - o Ovarian mass with multiple possible constituents, including fat, soft tissue, and calcification
    - – Internal constituents of dermoid may appear cystic, although measured density is typically less than simple fluid (indicating fat)

- o Multiple possible ultrasound appearances have been described, including diffusely echogenic mass with posterior shadowing (tip-of-iceberg sign), echogenic nodule within larger anechoic lesion (dermoid plug) and dot-dash pattern due to hair in lesion
- o Complications include torsion, superinfection, rupture, and malignant degeneration (very rare)
- **Lymphadenopathy, Cystic or Caseated**
  - o Multiple causes of cystic, caseated, or necrotic lymph nodes include Whipple disease, mycobacterial disease, celiac sprue disease, and necrotic malignant lymphadenopathy (particularly common after treatment)
- **Peritoneal Inclusion Cyst**
  - o Loculated fluid collection in pelvis resulting from peritoneal adhesions
    - – Most often occurs in premenopausal women with prior gynecologic surgery or inflammatory conditions (e.g., endometriosis, pelvic inflammatory disease, etc.) that results in peritoneal scarring
  - o Loculated cystic mass (usually in pelvis) conforming to geographic margins of pelvis
    - – Ovary often located at center of cystic mass due to hormonally active ovaries secreting fluid that becomes loculated
    - – Internal septations within mass are frequent (spiderweb appearance)
  - o Should not demonstrate solid component or mural nodularity
- **Hydatid Cyst**
  - o Peritoneum accounts for 13% of hydatid cysts in abdomen, likely reflecting sequelae of hepatic or splenic hydatid cyst rupture
  - o Appearance is similar to hydatid cysts in liver/spleen, with acute phase characterized by dominant cystic mass with internal daughter cysts or wavy, serpiginous internal densities (water-lily sign)
  - o Chronic hydatid cysts often demonstrate extensive serpiginous internal calcification

Loculated Ascites

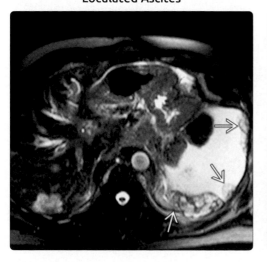

Pancreatic Pseudocyst

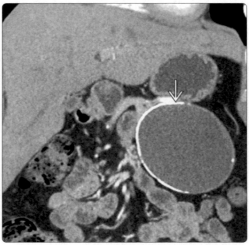

(Left) *Axial T2 FS MR in a patient with metastatic appendiceal adenocarcinoma demonstrates loculated ascites in the left upper quadrant with multiple discrete peritoneal tumor implants ➡ along the margins of the loculated fluid.* **(Right)** *Coronal CECT in a patient with a history of pancreatitis demonstrates a large pseudocyst ➡ arising near the pancreatic tail with extensive peripheral calcification. Although pseudocysts can calcify, as in this case, this is not a common feature.*

Pancreatic Pseudocyst

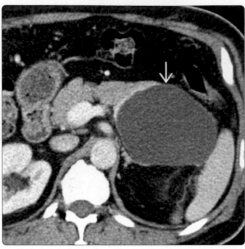

Cystic Ovarian Neoplasm

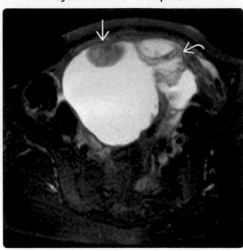

(Left) *Axial CECT in a patient with a known history of pancreatitis demonstrates a large, simple-appearing pseudocyst* ➡ *arising in the vicinity of the pancreatic tail.* (Right) *Axial T2 FS MR demonstrates a large cystic ovarian mass with a large mural nodule* ➡*, as well as additional soft tissue complexity* ➡ *along its left aspect. This was found to represent an aggressive carcinosarcoma at resection.*

Cystic Ovarian Neoplasm

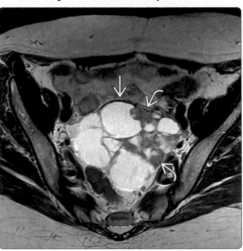

Pseudomyxoma Peritonei

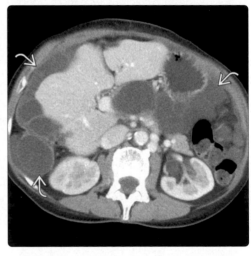

(Left) *Axial T2 FS MR demonstrates a large cystic ovarian mass* ➡ *with multiple internal septations and multiple sites of mural nodularity* ➡*, features strongly suggestive of malignancy. This lesion was found to represent high-grade serous carcinoma at resection.* (Right) *Axial CECT demonstrates multiple low-density gelatinous implants* ➡ *throughout the upper abdomen, including multiple lesions scalloping the surface of the liver, characteristic of pseudomyxoma peritonei.*

Pseudomyxoma Peritonei

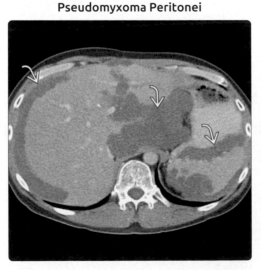

Mesenteric Cyst

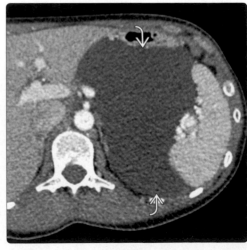

(Left) *Axial CEXT demonstrates a characteristic appearance of pseudomyxoma peritonei, with low-density mucinous implants* ➡ *coating and scalloping the surface of the liver and spleen.* (Right) *Axial CECT demonstrates a large, simple-appearing, low-density cystic mass* ➡ *in the upper abdomen, found to represent a large lymphangioma.*

Mesenteric Cyst

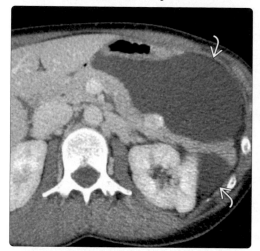

Urachal Remnant

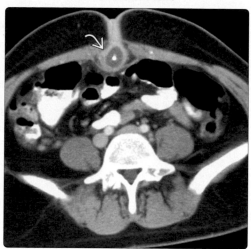

(Left) *Axial CECT demonstrates a large, simple-appearing lymphangioma ⟶ insinuating around multiple structures in the upper abdomen with little mass effect. Note the absence of internal enhancement or other suspicious features.* **(Right)** *Axial CECT demonstrates a midline cystic lesion ⟶ near the umbilicus with a thick wall and internal calcification. This was found to represent an infected urachal cyst at surgical resection.*

Urachal Remnant

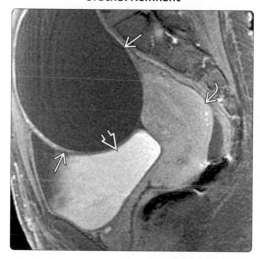

Dermoid (Mature Teratoma)

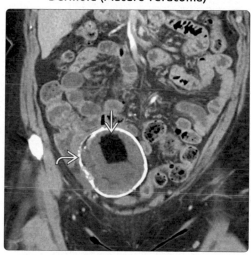

(Left) *Sagittal T1 C+ FS MR shows a large urachal cyst ⟶ that indents the dome of the bladder ⟶ and displaces the uterus ⟶. The bladder urine is opacified due to the IV gadolinium injection.* **(Right)** *Coronal CECT demonstrates a large dermoid ⟶ with thick peripheral calcification and a sizable amount of internal macroscopic fat ⟶. The presence of macroscopic fat within an adnexal mass allows the definitive diagnosis of a dermoid.*

Peritoneal Inclusion Cyst

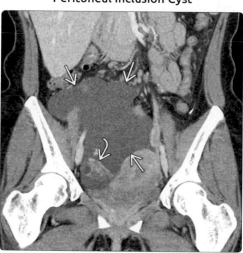

Hydatid Cyst

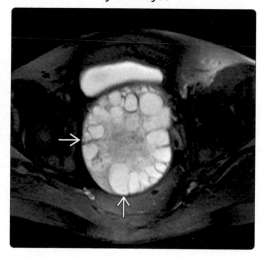

(Left) *Coronal CECT demonstrates a large fluid collection ⟶ in the right pelvis surrounding the right ovary ⟶. The patient had a history of prior pelvic surgery, and this collection had been stable over several examinations, features compatible with a peritoneal inclusion cyst.* **(Right)** *Axial T2 FS MR in a patient from abroad with a known history of a hydatid cyst in the liver demonstrates a classic hydatid cyst ⟶ in the pelvis with multiple internal daughter cysts.*

DIFFERENTIAL DIAGNOSIS

Common

- Sclerosing Mesenteritis
- Omental Infarct
- Epiploic Appendagitis
- Fat Necrosis
- Dermoid Cyst (Mature Teratoma)
- Fibrofatty Mesenteric Proliferation ("Creeping Fat") (Mimic)
- Intussusception (Mimic)

Less Common

- Liposarcoma
- Cystic Fibrosis, Pancreas (Mimic)
- Lipomatous Pseudohypertrophy of Pancreas (Mimic)
- Lipoma, Intestine
- Lipomatous Infiltration, Ileocecal Valve (Mimic)
- Pseudolipoma of Glisson Capsule
- Metastatic Malignant Teratoma
- Peritoneal Lipomatosis

ESSENTIAL INFORMATION

Key Differential Diagnosis Issues

- With rare exceptions, fat-containing lesions in peritoneal space are typically benign entities that can be specifically diagnosed based on imaging appearance
- Fat-containing masses are very common in retroperitoneum (liposarcoma, angiomyolipoma, myelolipoma), and very large retroperitoneal lesions can extend into peritoneal cavity

Helpful Clues for Common Diagnoses

- **Sclerosing Mesenteritis**
  - Idiopathic inflammatory and fibrotic disorder of mesentery (of unknown etiology) that can produce abdominal pain
    - Likely underdiagnosed cause of acute abdominal pain
  - Appearance is variable depending on stage of evolution, but usually located in jejunal mesentery (left upper quadrant)
    - Acute stage appears as subtly increased attenuation of mesenteric fat ("misty mesentery")
    - Can evolve into discrete fat-containing mass with thin pseudocapsule
      - □ Often contains multiple prominent subcentimeter lymph nodes with halo of surrounding spared fat (fat-halo sign)
      - □ Envelops vasculature without narrowing or attenuation
    - Chronic stage can develop into discrete fibrotic mass with calcification and desmoplastic reaction
      - □ Can be associated with bowel obstruction or venous/lymphatic obstruction
      - □ Can be difficult to differentiate from carcinoid tumors at this stage of evolution, although location (jejunal mesentery versus ileal mesentery for carcinoid) can be helpful clue
- **Omental Infarct**
  - Fat necrosis of omentum due to compromised arterial blood supply, which can cause abdominal pain
    - Usually idiopathic, but can also be secondary to prior surgery or trauma
  - Heterogeneous fat-containing mass in omentum with surrounding hyperdense rim (± whorled appearance of vessels leading to infarct)
    - Appears as hyperechoic mass fixed to colon with absent color flow vascularity on US
  - Most often located in right lower quadrant, but can occur anywhere in omentum
  - Typically larger in appearance than epiploic appendagitis without central dot sign
  - Can be extremely large (and simulate tumor) in some cases, particularly when occurring after surgery
    - Unlike tumors, omental infarcts are associated with pain and should become smaller over time
- **Epiploic Appendagitis**
  - Acute inflammation of epiploic appendage of colon, which can cause abdominal pain
  - Small fat-containing mass with hyperdense rim immediately adjacent to colon with mild adjacent fat stranding
    - May demonstrate central dot sign: Thrombosed vein at center of inflamed appendage
  - Can arise anywhere in colon, but usually in left lower quadrant adjacent to descending or sigmoid colon
  - Self-limited process that requires only conservative management
- **Fat Necrosis**
  - Can occur anywhere in body, but typically is result of prior insult (often prior surgery or trauma)
  - Discrete fat-containing mass with weakly enhancing capsule (but no evidence of aggressiveness or local spread) ± calcification
    - Can have variable internal attenuation (with little fat), potentially mimicking fluid collection or soft tissue mass
      - □ Unlike tumor, should (but not always) gradually decrease in size over time
- **Dermoid Cyst (Mature Teratoma)**
  - Most common germ cell neoplasm of ovary
  - Usually asymptomatic, but rare complications include pelvic pain, rupture, torsion, superinfection, or malignant degeneration (very rare)
  - May demonstrate various internal components on CT, including macroscopic fat, calcification, fluid attenuation, or soft tissue density
    - Presence of macroscopic fat within adnexal mass is key to diagnosis, and can be easily confirmed with MR in equivocal cases
  - Multiple possible appearances on US, including tip-of-iceberg sign, dermoid plug, or dot-dash pattern
- **Fibrofatty Mesenteric Proliferation ("Creeping Fat") (Mimic)**
  - Common in longstanding Crohn disease, but can be seen as sequelae of any longstanding or repetitive inflammatory process in abdomen
  - Usually found immediately adjacent to most commonly inflamed segment of bowel (typically right lower quadrant ileocolic mesentery)

- o Manifests as increased amount of mesenteric fat, but does not appear as discrete mass or demonstrate defined borders
- **Intussusception (Mimic)**
  - o Mesenteric fat is drawn into intussuscipiens along with bowel (intussusceptum)
  - o When viewed in cross section, appears as crescent of fat density within intussuscipiens, which might mimic fatty mass or lipoma

Helpful Clues for Less Common Diagnoses

- **Liposarcoma**
  - o Much more common in retroperitoneum, but can very rarely primarily arise in peritoneum or mesentery or extend from retroperitoneal space into peritoneum (particularly when large)
  - o Fat-containing mass with variable attenuation, depending on degree of differentiation
    - Well-differentiated tumors more likely to show predominantly fat attenuation, whereas dedifferentiated tumors more likely to show soft tissue attenuation or other complex components
    - Subtypes based on degree of differentiation include well differentiated, myxoid, dedifferentiated, round cell, and pleomorphic tumors
- **Cystic Fibrosis, Pancreas (Mimic)**
  - o Complete fatty infiltration of pancreas very common in cystic fibrosis and usually seen by end of teenage years
  - o Does not appear mass-like and usually conforms to normal shape of pancreas
  - o Pancreatic insufficiency very common (~ 85%) manifestation of cystic fibrosis
  - o Other manifestations of CF in pancreas include simple pancreatic cysts, scattered punctate calcifications, and stigmata of chronic pancreatitis (due to repeated bouts of acute pancreatitis)
- **Lipomatous Pseudohypertrophy of Pancreas (Mimic)**
  - o Focal or diffuse mass-like enlargement of pancreas with fatty replacement of unknown etiology (possibly related to cirrhosis or viral infection)

- o Pancreas can be severely enlarged and resemble large fat-containing mass
- o Usually benign, incidental finding without patient symptoms
- **Lipoma, Intestine**
  - o Simple lipomas (fat-density spherical mass) may arise in stomach, small bowel, or colon (usually submucosal)
    - Most frequent site is colon (usually right colon)
  - o Uncommon lesions that can be seen anywhere in GI tract and may very rarely cause occult GI bleeding when large and ulcerated
  - o Usually asymptomatic, incidental findings discovered at colonoscopy, surgery, or imaging
- **Lipomatous Infiltration of Ileocecal Valve (Mimic)**
  - o Fatty hypertrophy of ileocecal valve may be confused with intraluminal fatty mass
  - o Typically appears as circumferential fatty proliferation around margins of valve, rather than mass-like
  - o Incidental finding that does not require treatment
- **Pseudolipoma of Glisson Capsule**
  - o Encapsulated fat-containing lesion located within liver capsule (possibly representing degenerated epiploic fat that is trapped by liver capsule during development)
  - o Simple fat-containing nodule along surface of liver
- **Metastatic Malignant Teratoma**
  - o Primary malignant teratomas usually arise in anterior mediastinum or testicle in young patients
  - o Appearance of both primary tumor and metastases is variable depending on degree of differentiation, but metastases can demonstrate internal fat attenuation
- **Peritoneal Lipomatosis**
  - o Fatty proliferation can very rarely occur in peritoneum, similar to more common sites of lipomatosis in pelvis, mediastinum, and epidural space
  - o Exact etiology unknown, but does have strong male predilection and is more common in obese patients
  - o Appears as diffuse fatty proliferation without discrete capsule or mass-like margins

Sclerosing Mesenteritis

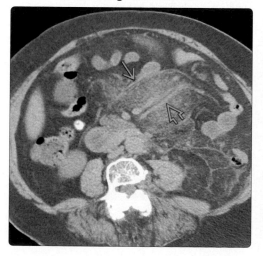

Sclerosing Mesenteritis

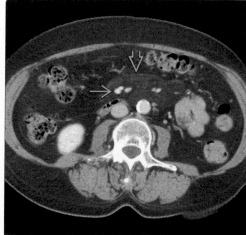

(Left) Axial CECT shows heterogeneous infiltration of the mesenteric fat with a thin capsule ➡ and mesenteric vessels ➡ coursing through without attenuation or narrowing. This is a fairly typical appearance for sclerosing mesenteritis. (Right) Axial CECT demonstrates infiltration of the jejunal mesentery. Note the thin capsule ➡ around the process, as well as the fatty halo around the enlarged nodes ➡, all of which are classic features of sclerosing mesenteritis.

(Left) *Axial CECT shows infiltration of the small bowel mesentery with a thin surrounding pseudocapsule ⊟, as well as multiple enlarged mesenteric nodes ⊟, some of which demonstrate a subtle surrounding halo of spared fat. These findings are characteristic of sclerosing mesenteritis.* (Right) *Sagittal CECT demonstrates a small fat-attenuation mass ⊟ in the anterior omentum with surrounding stranding, compatible with a small omental infarct in this patient with acute abdominal pain.*

Sclerosing Mesenteritis

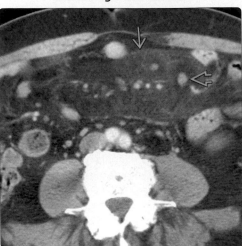

Omental Infarct

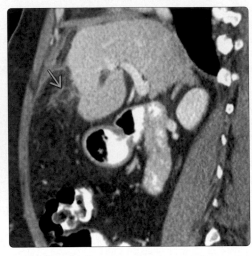

(Left) *Axial CECT in a patient status post laparoscopic distal pancreatectomy demonstrates a large fat-attenuation mass ⊟ in the surgical bed with a surrounding hyperdense rim, representing a large postsurgical omental infarct/fat necrosis.* (Right) *Axial CECT demonstrates a small fat-containing mass ⊟ abutting the left colon with subtle surrounding stranding and edema, compatible with epiploic appendagitis. This is a self-limited abnormality that does not require treatment.*

Omental Infarct

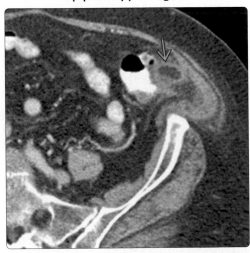

Epiploic Appendagitis

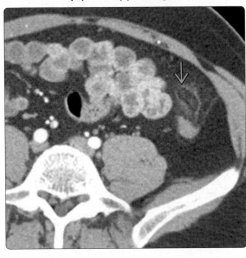

(Left) *Axial CECT demonstrates the characteristic features of epiploic appendagitis, including a small fat-attenuation mass ⊟ abutting the sigmoid colon with a hyperdense rim and surrounding fat stranding.* (Right) *Axial NECT in a female patient demonstrates bilateral fat-containing adnexal masses ⊟ with the larger lesion on the left demonstrating subtle internal calcification ⊟, compatible with bilateral ovarian dermoids.*

Epiploic Appendagitis

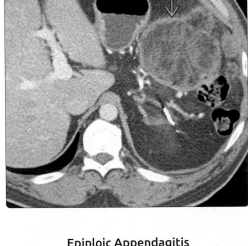

Dermoid Cyst (Mature Teratoma)

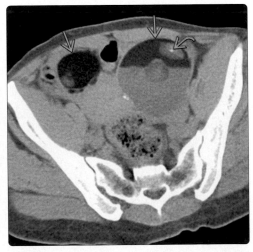

Dermoid Cyst (Mature Teratoma)

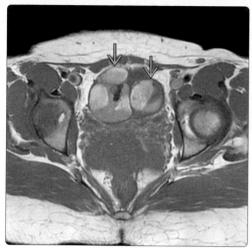

Fibrofatty Mesenteric Proliferation ("Creeping Fat") (Mimic)

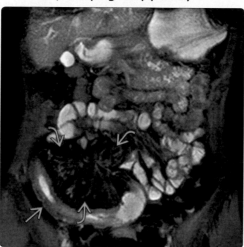

(Left) Axial T1 MR demonstrates bilateral ovarian dermoids ⊡, each of which demonstrates internal T1-hyperintense macroscopic fat, which demonstrated suppression on the fat-suppressed images (not shown). (Right) Coronal T1 C+ MR in a patient with Crohn disease demonstrates diffuse thickening of the terminal ileum ⊡. Note the presence of extensive fibrofatty proliferation ⊡ in the ileocolic mesentery, representing the sequelae of chronic Crohn-related inflammation ("creeping fat").

Liposarcoma

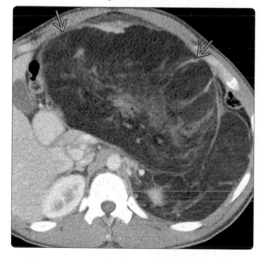

Liposarcoma

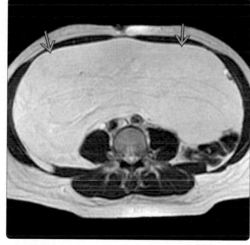

(Left) Axial CECT demonstrates a large, encapsulated, predominantly fat-containing mass ⊡ occupying much of the left and central abdomen, with some internal complexity and soft tissue attenuation. This was found to be a well-differentiated liposarcoma at resection. (Right) Axial T1 MR demonstrates a massive fat-containing, T1-hyperintense mass occupying the entirety of the abdomen ⊡. There is virtually no complexity within this mass, and this was found to be a well-differentiated liposarcoma at resection.

Cystic Fibrosis, Pancreas (Mimic)

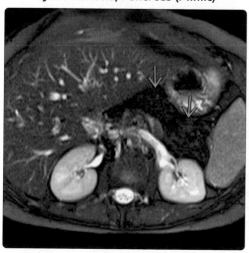

Pseudolipoma of Glisson Capsule

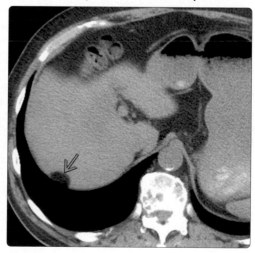

(Left) Axial T2 FS MR in a patient with cystic fibrosis demonstrates the characteristic fatty replacement of the pancreas ⊡ seen commonly in these patients by the end of their teenage years. (Right) Axial NECT demonstrates a small fat-attenuation lesion ⊡ abutting the subcapsular surface of the liver dome, a classic appearance for a small pseudolipoma of Glisson capsule.

DIFFERENTIAL DIAGNOSIS

Common

- Lymphoma
- Metastases
- Reactive Lymphadenopathy due to Localized Inflammation
- Reactive Lymphadenopathy due to Systemic Inflammation
- Postsurgical Lymphadenopathy
- Mesenteric Adenitis
- Sclerosing Mesenteritis
- Mononucleosis
- HIV/AIDS

Less Common

- Sarcoidosis
- Whipple Disease
- Celiac-Sprue Disease

Rare but Important

- Castleman Disease
- Mastocytosis

ESSENTIAL INFORMATION

Key Differential Diagnosis Issues

- No consensus on size threshold for abnormal mesenteric lymph nodes, but normal nodes are typically < 5 mm in short axis
  - There is overlap in size of normal and abnormal nodes, and a few mildly prominent lymph nodes may still be within normal limits
  - Multiplicity of abnormal nodes, nodal calcifications, abnormal node morphology (e.g., irregular margins, adjacent stranding), and abnormal node enhancement (i.e., hyperenhancing, necrotic, etc.) are other features that help determine if nodes are truly abnormal
    - Necrotic lymphadenopathy should raise concern for metastatic disease, tuberculosis, celiac-sprue, or Whipple disease
    - Hypervascular lymphadenopathy should raise concern for Kaposi sarcoma or Castleman disease
    - Calcified lymphadenopathy may be associated with carcinoid tumor or treated/inactive disease (lymphoma or tuberculosis most common)
- **Generalized** mesenteric lymphadenopathy is most likely to be reactive as result of systemic infectious/inflammatory disease or lymphoma
  - Mild generalized lymphadenopathy most likely to be reactive or normal variant
  - Massive generalized mesenteric lymphadenopathy should strongly raise suspicion for lymphoma, or less commonly, metastatic disease
- **Localized** lymphadenopathy should prompt search for adjacent inflammatory process or malignancy
  - For example, right lower quadrant (RLQ) lymphadenopathy should prompt concern for appendicitis, Crohn ileitis, right-sided colon cancer, carcinoid tumor, etc.

Helpful Clues for Common Diagnoses

- **Lymphoma**

  - Non-Hodgkin lymphoma much more commonly involves mesenteric nodes (~ 45% of patients) compared to Hodgkin lymphoma (~ 5-8%), and is most common malignant cause of mesenteric lymphadenopathy
  - Lymph nodes are typically substantially enlarged and may form confluent conglomerate nodal masses
    - Nodes in mesentery are of soft tissue density and often grow around bowel and vessels without causing obstruction or vascular narrowing/occlusion
    - Sandwich sign: Mesenteric nodal mass grows on both sides of vasculature-appearing similar to sandwich
  - Look for evidence of nodal (e.g., chest, abdomen, axilla, and neck) or extranodal disease elsewhere in body
  - Nodes may demonstrate calcification after treatment, but virtually never calcify prior to treatment
- **Metastases**
  - Mesenteric lymphadenopathy most commonly occurs adjacent to primary GI tract malignancy
    - Common abdominal malignancies to produce adjacent mesenteric lymphadenopathy include colon cancer (most common), pancreatic cancer, carcinoid, and small bowel adenocarcinoma
    - Most of these malignancies produce lymphadenopathy of soft tissue density, although carcinoid nodal metastases tend to be hypervascular with frequent central calcification and desmoplastic reaction (spiculation and tethering of adjacent bowel/vasculature)
    - Lymph node metastases may often be first clue as to presence of tumor in bowel as bowel lesion may be relatively subtle on imaging
  - Most common extraabdominal malignancies to produce generalized mesenteric lymphadenopathy are melanoma, lung cancer, and breast cancer
- **Reactive Lymphadenopathy due to Localized Abdominal Inflammation**
  - Abdominal inflammatory disorders often result in reactive lymphadenopathy in adjacent mesentery
  - Appendicitis frequently associated with cluster of mildly enlarged nodes in RLQ mesentery
  - Crohn disease also frequently results in mild lymphadenopathy in RLQ ileocolic mesentery (usually in setting of active inflammation of ileum)
    - Look for evidence of active ileitis, include bowel wall thickening, mucosal hyperemia, fat stranding, etc.
  - Diverticulitis may result in very mild lymphadenopathy in sigmoid mesocolon
    - Significantly enlarged nodes, however, are uncommon, and raise concern for malignancy
    - Colonic wall thickening with regional lymphadenopathy should be considered colon cancer until proven otherwise and should prompt colonoscopy
  - Infectious enteritis or colitis frequently associated with mild localized mesenteric lymphadenopathy
- **Reactive Lymphadenopathy due to Systemic Inflammation**
  - Mesenteric nodes may be mildly enlarged in patients with underlying systemic inflammatory disorders (e.g., lupus, rheumatoid arthritis, systemic sclerosis, vasculitis)
  - Lymphadenopathy in such cases is usually very mild and found in multiple other locations

- **Postsurgical Lymphadenopathy**
  - Mildly enlarged mesenteric lymph nodes are very common finding in immediate postoperative setting after abdominal surgery (especially involving GI tract)
  - Lymphadenopathy usually quite minimal and should resolve in a few weeks
- **Mesenteric Adenitis**
  - Self-limited disorder usually affecting children and young adults which may be related to underlying occult infection of terminal ileum (e.g., viral, *Yersinia*, etc.)
  - Results in cluster of mildly enlarged lymph nodes in RLQ mesentery without evidence of another primary cause for inflammation (e.g., appendicitis, etc.)
- **Sclerosing Mesenteritis**
  - Probably underdiagnosed cause of persistent or recurrent abdominal pain
  - Results in mild hazy infiltration of small bowel mesentery (misty mesentery) with prominent or mildly enlarged internal lymph nodes and halo of spared fat surrounding these lymph nodes and vessels
  - Thin pseudocapsule surrounds infiltrated mesentery
- **Mononucleosis**
  - Typically diagnosed in young adult with fever, malaise, and other mild constitutional symptoms
  - Frequently associated with generalized lymphadenopathy, including mesenteric lymphadenopathy, as well as splenomegaly
- **HIV/AIDS**
  - Direct HIV infection may result in mild mesenteric lymphadenopathy (and nodes elsewhere)
  - Mesenteric lymphadenopathy may be manifestation of opportunistic infection (especially with CD4 < 50/mL)
    - Both *Mycobacterium avium* (MAC) and tuberculosis can result in centrally necrotic or low-density lymph nodes (although soft tissue density nodes are also possible)
    - MAC can result in massive or conglomerate mesenteric lymphadenopathy
  - Also consider malignancies in AIDS patients with low CD4 counts, including lymphoma and Kaposi sarcoma
    - Kaposi sarcoma can involve many different nodal compartments and frequently produces hypervascular lymph nodes

Helpful Clues for Less Common Diagnoses

- **Sarcoidosis**
  - Not infrequently involves upper abdominal organs, including hepatosplenomegaly with small hypoenhancing nodules in liver or spleen
  - Sarcoidosis classically results in thoracic lymphadenopathy, but can also result in retroperitoneal or mesenteric lymphadenopathy
- **Whipple Disease**
  - Results from systemic bacterial infection caused by *Tropheryma whipplei*
  - May result in mesenteric lymphadenopathy, which is characteristically low density (10-20 HU), and small bowel wall thickening
- **Celiac-Sprue Disease**
  - Can result in cavitating mesenteric node syndrome with low-attenuation mesenteric lymphadenopathy
  - Nodes regress once patient placed on gluten-free diet
  - Patients with celiac disease do have higher risk of lymphoma, and persistence of nodes, especially with soft tissue density, should raise concern for malignancy

Helpful Clues for Rare Diagnoses

- **Castleman Disease**
  - Benign lymphoproliferative disorder, which can be either localized or (rarely) diffuse
  - Can result in mesenteric lymphadenopathy, which can be hypervascular
- **Mastocytosis**
  - Rare disorder that may be idiopathic or secondary to underlying hematologic malignancy that results in excessive number of mast cells
  - Patients present with flushing, diarrhea, vomiting, abdominal pain, and skin manifestations
  - May present with hepatosplenomegaly, small bowel wall thickening, omental infiltration, and abdominal lymphadenopathy (mesenteric or retroperitoneal)

Lymphoma

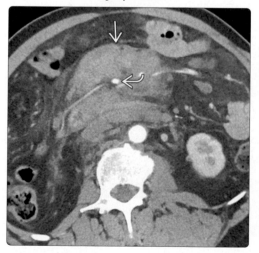

Lymphoma

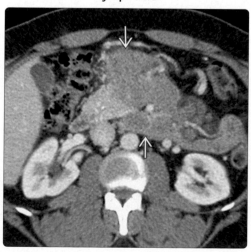

(Left) *Axial CECT demonstrates extensive mesenteric lymphadenopathy* ➜ *that surrounds and sandwiches mesenteric vessels* ➜ *without attenuation or narrowing, classic for lymphoma.* **(Right)** *Axial CECT in a patient with HIV/AIDS demonstrates extensive conglomerate mesenteric lymphadenopathy* ➜*, found to represent diffuse large B-cell lymphoma.*

Metastases

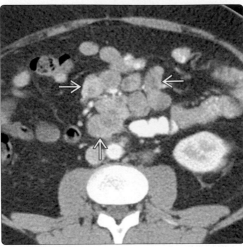

Metastases

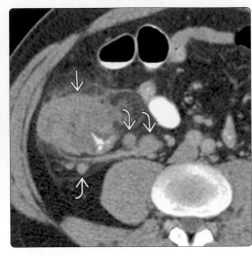

(Left) *Axial CECT demonstrates multiple enlarged central mesenteric lymph nodes ➡, some of which demonstrate subtle internal heterogeneous enhancement or necrosis, found to represent metastatic melanoma.* (Right) *Axial CECT demonstrates marked mass-like wall thickening ➡ of the cecum, compatible with the patient's biopsy-proven colon adenocarcinoma. Multiple prominent or enlarged metastatic lymph nodes ➡ are present around the margins of the cecum.*

Metastases

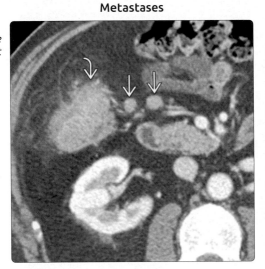

Metastases

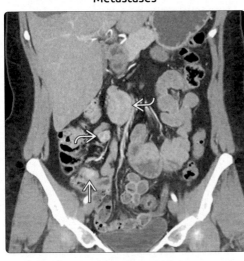

(Left) *Axial CECT demonstrates a mass ➡ in the right colon, found to represent a primary colon adenocarcinoma, with mildly enlarged lymph nodes ➡ in the adjacent ileocolic mesentery.* (Right) *Coronal CECT demonstrates a hypervascular mass ➡ in the terminal ileum, found to be a carcinoid tumor. The primary mass is much less conspicuous compared to extensive hypervascular lymphadenopathy ➡ in the right abdominal mesentery.*

Metastases

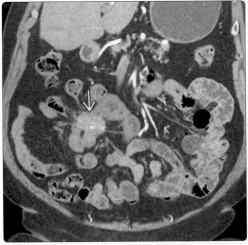

Reactive Lymphadenopathy due to Localized Inflammation

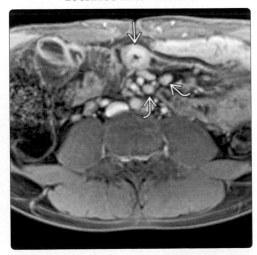

(Left) *Coronal CECT demonstrates a spiculated hypervascular metastasis ➡ to the right lower quadrant (RLQ) mesentery in a patient with carcinoid. Notice the subtle calcification within the mass, as well as the desmoplastic reaction with tethering of adjacent bowel loops.* (Right) *Axial T1 C+ FS MR in a patient with Crohn disease demonstrates thickening and hyperemia of a bowel loop ➡ due to active inflammation, as well as mildly enlarged reactive lymph nodes ➡ clustered in the adjacent mesentery.*

Mesenteric Adenitis

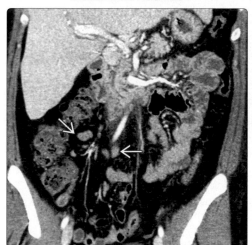

Sclerosing Mesenteritis

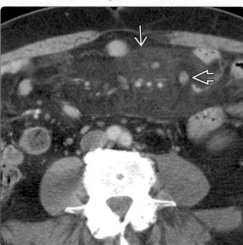

(Left) *Axial CECT in a young person with RLQ pain demonstrates several nonspecific RLQ lymph nodes* ➡. *No appendicitis was found on CT. These findings were thought to be secondary to mesenteric adenitis.* (Right) *Axial CECT demonstrates infiltration of the small bowel mesentery, set off by a pseudocapsule* ➡. *Multiple enlarged mesenteric nodes are present* ➡ *with a halo of surrounding spared fat, classic for sclerosing mesenteritis.*

HIV/AIDS

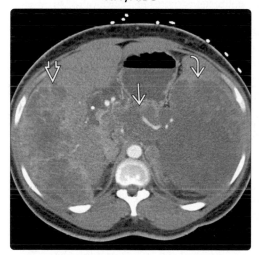

HIV/AIDS

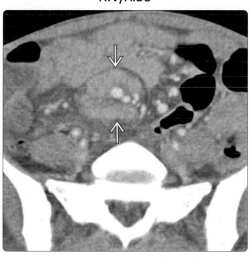

(Left) *Axial CECT in an AIDS patient demonstrates large, heterogeneous masses in the liver* ➡ *and spleen* ➡, *as well as significant conglomerate lymphadenopathy* ➡ *in the upper abdomen, all of which was found to represent Kaposi sarcoma.* (Right) *Axial CECT in an AIDS patient demonstrates enlarged lymph nodes* ➡ *clustered in the central mesentery, found to represent the sequelae of MAI infection.*

HIV/AIDS

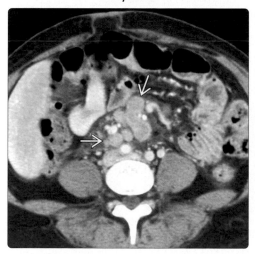

Sarcoidosis

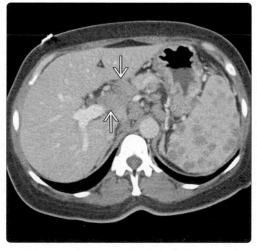

(Left) *Axial CECT shows mesenteric nodes* ➡ *with a peculiar low-density or caseated appearance, characteristic of Mycobacterial infection in this patient with AIDS.* (Right) *Axial CECT demonstrates multiple small, hypodense nodules in the spleen, as well as multiple enlarged upper abdominal lymph nodes* ➡ *in the right upper quadrant, all of which was found to be secondary to sarcoidosis.*

DIFFERENTIAL DIAGNOSIS

Common

- Biliary Tract Calcifications
  - Gallstones
  - Porcelain Gallbladder
- Hepatic and Splenic Calcifications
  - Calcified Hepatic Masses (Primary or Metastatic)
  - Splenic and Hepatic Granulomas
  - Splenic Cysts
  - Echinococcal Cysts
  - Ischemia/Infarct
- Pancreatic Calcifications
  - Chronic Pancreatitis
  - Calcified Pancreatic Masses
- Urinary Tract and Adrenal Calcifications
  - Urolithiasis
  - Calcified Renal Masses
  - Renal Cysts
  - Renal TB
  - Adrenal Parenchymal Calcification
  - Calcified Adrenal Masses
  - Prostatic or Vas Deferens Calcification
  - Bladder Calculi
- Female Reproductive Organ Calcifications
  - Uterine Leiomyoma (Fibroid)
  - Ovarian Neoplasms
- Abdominal Wall or Soft Tissue Calcifications
  - Abdominal Injection Sites
  - Costal Cartilage Calcification (Mimic)
  - Calcified or Ossified Scar
  - Calcinosis Syndromes
- Vascular Calcifications
- Bowel Calcifications
  - Appendicolith (Fecalith)
  - Mucocele of Appendix
- Mesenteric or Peritoneal Calcifications
  - Calcified Lymph Nodes
  - Sclerosing Peritonitis
  - Pseudomyxoma Peritonei
  - Lymphangioma
  - Sclerosing Mesenteritis

ESSENTIAL INFORMATION

Key Differential Diagnosis Issues

- Abdominal calcifications broadly divided into several types
  - **Metastatic calcification** reflects deposition of calcium salts in normal tissue (e.g., renal failure with secondary hyperparathyroidism)
    - Requires hypercalcemia and alkaline pH environment
  - **Dystrophic calcification** reflects deposition of calcium salts in tissue damaged by trauma, ischemia, infarction, infection, or tumor
  - **Ossification** reflects formation of bone in damaged tissue (e.g., ovarian teratoma or ossification within incision scar)
  - **Concretions** occur due to calcified precipitates inside vessel or hollow viscus (e.g., gallstones, renal calculi, phleboliths)

  - **Conduit wall calcifications** are calcifications in wall of fluid-conducting tube (e.g., arterial calcification, aneurysm, vas deferens calcification)
    - Appear as ring-like or tram-track linear calcifications, which are often discontinuous
  - **Cystic calcification** reflects calcified wall of fluid-filled mass
  - **Solid mass calcification** encompasses greatest variety of etiologies and appearances

Helpful Clues for Common Diagnoses

- **Biliary Tract Calcifications**
  - **Gallstones** vary greatly in density depending on their type, ranging from soft tissue density to densely calcified
    - Only ~ 20% of stones are visible on radiographs
    - Calcium bilirubinate stones may be densely calcified and are most likely to be seen on radiographs
    - Cholesterol stones can be isoattenuating to bile and difficult to visualize on radiographs or CT
    - Gallstones can appear laminated or faceted ± internal gas (Mercedes-Benz sign)
  - **Porcelain gallbladder** represents calcification within wall of gallbladder
    - Much easier to perceive on CT, but appears as thin crescentic calcification in RUQ on radiographs
- **Hepatic and Splenic Calcifications**
  - Variety of **hepatic masses** can demonstrate calcification
    - Primary tumors: Hemangioma (central coarse calcification), adenoma (usually eccentric and secondary to prior hemorrhage), fibrolamellar hepatocellular carcinoma (coarse calcification in central scar), and conventional hepatoma
    - Metastases: Consider mucinous tumors (e.g., from colon), which produce stippled or faint calcifications
  - **Splenic and hepatic granulomas** appear as multiple punctate calcifications (easier to appreciate on CT)
    - Occur secondary to old healed granulomatous infection (e.g., histoplasmosis, TB)
  - **Splenic cysts** may demonstrate peripheral wall calcification, which is more common with acquired (rather than congenital) cysts
  - **Echinococcal cysts** can demonstrate extensive internal whorled or serpiginous calcification in chronic phase
  - Dystrophic calcification can occur at sites of parenchymal scarring due to prior **ischemia or infarcts**
- **Pancreatic Calcifications**
  - **Chronic pancreatitis** may be associated with parenchymal/intraductal calcifications (along with dilated pancreatic duct)
  - Several types of cystic and solid **pancreatic masses** may demonstrate calcification
    - Pancreatic neuroendocrine tumor most common solid mass to calcify (usually central and coarse)
    - Mucinous cystic neoplasm (MCN), solid pseudopapillary neoplasms, serous cystadenoma, and pseudocysts are cystic masses with frequent calcification
      - MCNs often have peripheral curvilinear calcification, while serous cystadenomas may have coarse calcifications within central scar
- **Urinary Tract and Adrenal Calcifications**

- **Urolithiasis**: All renal calculi are opaque on CT (except indinavir-induced stones)
  - Only larger and calcified stones are visible on plain radiographs (urate stones are lucent)
  - Stones tend to form and layer dependently within **calyceal diverticula**
- Calcifications can be present in variety of **renal neoplasms**, including renal cell carcinoma, Wilms tumor, and multilocular cystic nephroma
- Calcifications are common in **renal cysts** (typically thin or smooth along periphery or within septa), although Bosniak classification considers thick, irregular, or nodular calcifications as risk factors for malignancy
  - Calcifications are common with polycystic kidney disease due to cyst wall calcifications or stones
- **Renal TB** in chronic setting can result in severe atrophy and parenchymal calcification
- **Adrenal parenchymal calcifications** are usually coarse and typically reflect prior hemorrhage or infection (especially TB or histoplasmosis)
- Calcifications may be present within **adrenal masses**, including myelolipoma (usually coarse calcification in mass with macroscopic fat), adrenocortical carcinoma, pheochromocytoma, and adrenal cyst
- Dense central dystrophic **prostate calcifications** are common in aging men, but can also reflect sequelae of prior prostatitis, malignancy, or BPH
- **Vas deferens calcifications** appear as paired tubular "conduit" calcifications in pelvis extending midline
  - Tend to be present most often in insulin-dependent diabetic patients or in elderly patients
- **Bladder stones** most often due to urinary stasis or migration of stones from upper urinary tract
- **Female Reproductive Organ Calcification**
  - Uterine calcifications usually reflect presence of **fibroids**, with variety of possible appearances (e.g., whorled, flocculent, heterogeneous, popcorn)
  - **Dermoids** frequently contain calcification (representing bone or teeth), often within mural nodule
  - Calcification can also be found in **epithelial ovarian neoplasms**, especially serous malignancies

- **Abdominal Wall or Soft Tissue Calcifications**
  - **Abdominal injection sites** can develop calcification (usually as oval rim), especially common in buttocks
  - **Costal cartilage calcification (mimic)**: Irregular bilateral, symmetrical, cartilaginous calcification is more often seen in older women
  - **Calcified or ossified scar** may develop within midline surgical incision (usually with vertical orientation)
  - **Calcinosis syndromes** may produce calcifications in subcutaneous soft tissues and musculature
    - Associated with connective tissue diseases (e.g., scleroderma, CREST, lupus, dermatomyositis)
- **Vascular Calcifications**
  - Wide variety of different vascular calcifications can be seen, including
    - **Atherosclerotic** (tram-track morphology)
    - **Mönckeberg calcifications** in renal failure (diffuse circumferential arterial calcification)
    - Peripheral calcifications in wall of **aneurysm**
    - Linear venous calcifications due to **chronic deep venous thrombosis**
    - **Phleboliths** (small calcifications within veins which often demonstrate lucent centers)
- **Bowel Calcifications**
  - **Fecalith** is calcification resulting from hardened fecal material and can be associated with appendicitis
  - **Appendiceal mucocele** may demonstrate curvilinear wall calcification
- **Mesenteric or Peritoneal Calcifications**
  - **Calcified lymph nodes** may result from prior TB or other granulomatous infections, or rarely, treated lymphoma
  - **Sclerosing peritonitis** is form of chronic peritonitis often resulting from prior peritoneal dialysis that manifests as extensive peritoneal thickening and calcification
  - Mucinous implants in **pseudomyxoma peritonei** may be associated with curvilinear or punctate calcifications
  - **Lymphangiomas** may demonstrate fine calcifications along their wall or within septations
  - **Sclerosing mesenteritis** in its final stages may result in LUQ calcified mass with tethering of bowel and vessels

Gallstones

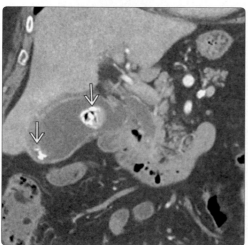

Porcelain Gallbladder

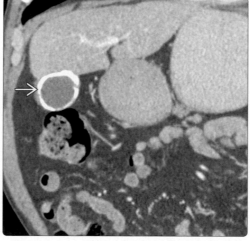

(Left) Coronal CECT demonstrates large, calcified gallstones ➡ in the gallbladder. Gallstones may be of variable attenuation, with calcified gallstones the easiest to appreciate on CT or radiographs. (Right) Coronal CECT demonstrates prominent calcification of the gallbladder wall ➡, compatible with a porcelain gallbladder. The association between porcelain gallbladder and gallbladder carcinoma is now considered somewhat debatable.

Calcified Hepatic Masses (Primary or Metastatic)

Splenic and Hepatic Granulomas

(Left) *Axial CECT demonstrates large, heterogeneously calcified mass lesions* ➡ *in the liver, as well as a similarly calcified lymph node mass* ➡ *in the gastrohepatic ligament. These findings reflect metastases from the patient's primary mucinous colon cancer.* **(Right)** *Axial NECT demonstrates multiple punctate calcifications in the spleen, likely related to old healed granulomatous disease.*

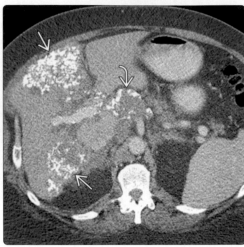

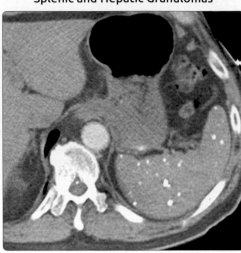

Splenic Cysts

Echinococcal Cysts

(Left) *Axial NECT demonstrates an incidentally discovered benign splenic cyst* ➡ *with prominent peripheral calcification. Acquired splenic cysts are more likely to demonstrate calcification compared to congenital splenic cysts.* **(Right)** *Axial NECT demonstrates a large, heavily calcified mass* ➡ *in the liver, with a characteristically whorled or serpiginous pattern of calcification. This represents a large, chronic echinococcal cyst in a patient who had emigrated from an endemic area.*

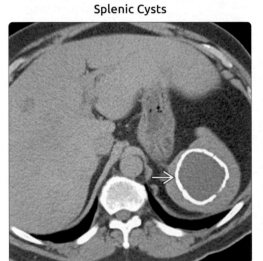

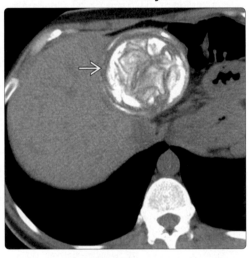

Ischemia/Infarct

Chronic Pancreatitis

(Left) *Axial CECT in a patient status post liver transplant demonstrates patchy areas of calcification throughout the liver parenchyma, which were found on biopsy to represent the sequelae of ischemia and rejection.* **(Right)** *Axial CECT demonstrates an atrophic pancreas* ➡ *with extensive calcification, findings diagnostic of chronic pancreatitis.*

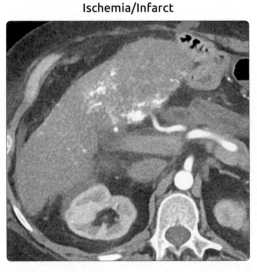

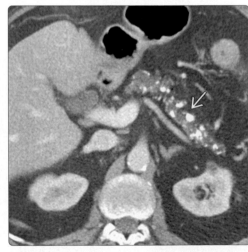

Calcified Pancreatic Masses

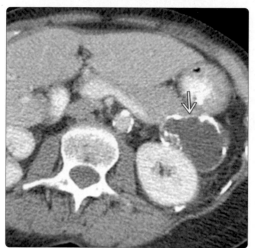

Calcified Pancreatic Masses

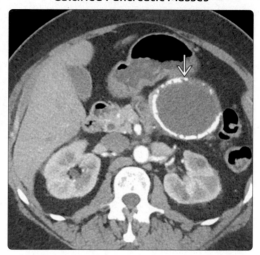

(Left) *Axial CECT demonstrates a cystic mass ➡ with peripheral calcification arising from the pancreatic tail in an older woman, found to represent a mucinous cystic neoplasm.* (Right) *Axial CECT demonstrates a cystic mass ➡ near the pancreatic tail with extensive surrounding rim calcification. The patient had a history of pancreatitis, and this was found to be a pseudocyst.*

Urolithiasis

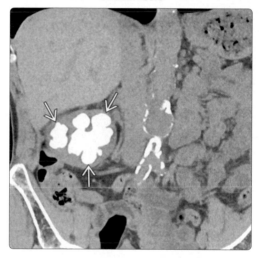

Calcified Renal Masses

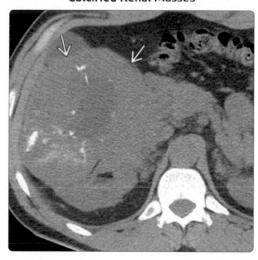

(Left) *Coronal NECT demonstrates a massive staghorn renal calculus ➡ almost completely filling the right intrarenal collecting system.* (Right) *Axial NECT demonstrates a large, right-sided renal mass ➡ with multiple internal calcifications, found to represent a chromophobe renal cell carcinoma at surgical resection.*

Bladder Calculi

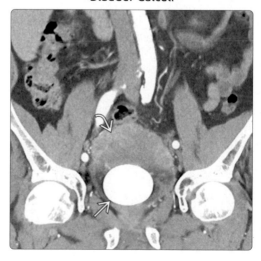

Ovarian Neoplasms

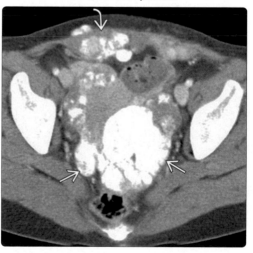

(Left) *Coronal CECT demonstrates a massive, high-density stone ➡ within the bladder. Also note the presence of extensive mass-like thickening ➡ of the bladder wall, compatible with bladder cancer (urothelial carcinoma).* (Right) *Axial CECT in a female patient demonstrates a large pelvic mass ➡ with extensive, large calcification, found to represent an ovarian serous carcinoma. A similar-appearing soft tissue mass with calcification ➡ in the right anterior pelvic wall represents a metastasis.*

Ovarian Neoplasms

Ovarian Neoplasms

(Left) Axial CECT demonstrates a large pelvic mass in a young female patient with extensive internal fat, a discrete fat-fluid level ➡, and internal calcification ➡, compatible with a dermoid cyst. *(Right)* Axial NECT demonstrates a large cystic mass ➡ in the pelvis with extensive internal calcifications ➡, found to represent ovarian cancer in this elderly female patient.

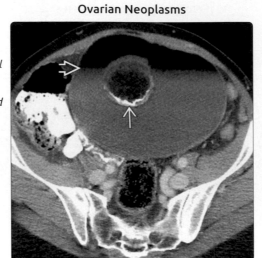

Abdominal Injection Sites

Calcified or Ossified Scar

(Left) Axial NECT shows multiple calcified injection granulomas ➡ in the subcutaneous fat of the buttocks. *(Right)* Coronal CECT shows a linear ossified scar ➡ along a prior midline abdominal incision.

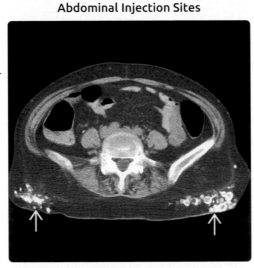

Calcinosis Syndromes

Vascular Calcifications

(Left) Axial NECT demonstrates extensive calcifications ➡ in the subcutaneous soft tissues and musculature of the pelvis in a patient with scleroderma. *(Right)* Axial NECT in a patient with end-stage renal disease demonstrates shrunken end-stage kidneys and extensive upper abdominal arterial vascular tram-track calcifications ➡.

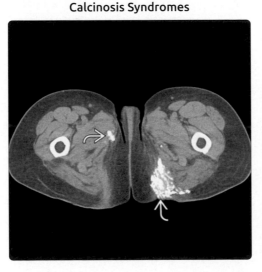
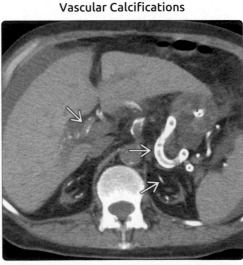

Vascular Calcifications

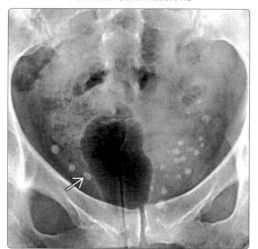

Vascular Calcifications

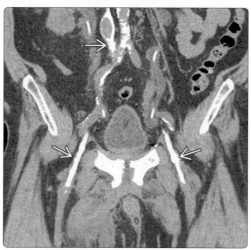

(Left) *Frontal radiograph shows multiple phleboliths in the pelvis (having their typical distribution) mainly below the iliac spines, some with central lucency* ➡. (Right) *Coronal NECT demonstrates an atretic appearance of the IVC and iliac veins, with extensive linear calcification in the IVC and external iliac veins* ➡, *findings compatible with the patient's known history of chronic deep venous thrombosis.*

Mucocele of Appendix

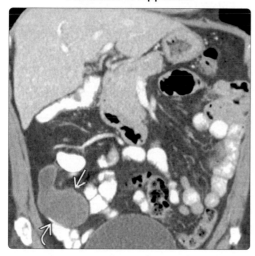

Calcified Lymph Nodes

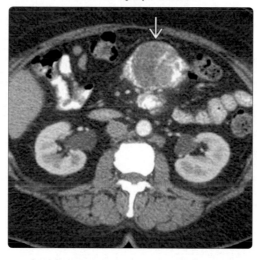

(Left) *Coronal CECT demonstrates a large, tubular-shaped cystic mass* ➡ *with subtle peripheral calcification* ➡. *On close inspection, this cystic mass connected with the cecum, and represents a large appendiceal mucocele.* (Right) *Axial CECT in a patient with a history of treated non-Hodgkin lymphoma demonstrates a residual soft tissue mass* ➡ *with calcification in the mesentery, representing the sequelae of treatment. The mass was stable over several exams and was not metabolically active on PET.*

Sclerosing Peritonitis

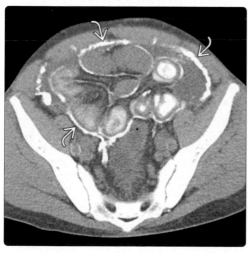

Sclerosing Mesenteritis

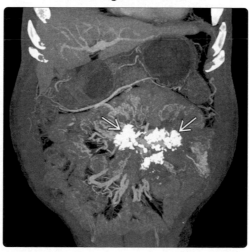

(Left) *Axial NECT demonstrates extensive calcification* ➡ *of the peritoneal lining and along the surface of bowel loops in a patient with sclerosing peritonitis related to a prior history of peritoneal dialysis.* (Right) *Coronal volume-rendered CECT demonstrates extensive calcification* ➡ *in the left upper quadrant mesentery with tethering of adjacent bowel loops and vasculature, representing an end-stage form of sclerosing mesenteritis.*

DIFFERENTIAL DIAGNOSIS

Common

- Normal Postoperative Pneumoperitoneum
- Barotrauma
- Iatrogenic Injuries or Complications
  - Bowel Anastomotic Leak
- Perforated Ulcer
  - Duodenal Ulcer
  - Gastric Ulcer
- Diverticulitis
- Intestinal Trauma
- Appendicitis
- Thoracic Processes (Mimics)
  - Pneumothorax
  - Subsegmental Atelectasis
  - Cystic Lung Disease
- Colonic Interposition (Mimic)
- Subphrenic Fat (Mimic)

Less Common

- Other Causes of Bowel Perforation
- Peritonitis
- Abdominal Abscess
- Pneumatosis Cystoides Intestinalis
- From Female Genital Tract
- Small Bowel Diverticula
- Foreign Body Perforation

ESSENTIAL INFORMATION

Key Differential Diagnosis Issues

- CT is significantly more sensitive than plain radiographs for detection of pneumoperitoneum, and should be test of choice in cases of suspected hollow viscus perforation
- Upright or decubitus radiographs are much more sensitive than supine films for detection of free air
  - Free intraperitoneal gas difficult to detect on supine radiographs as result of subtle radiographic findings and frequent poor image quality of portable films
- In cases with unexplained free intraperitoneal air, amount and location of gas should help guide diagnosis
  - Gas often located in proximity to site of perforation
    - Gastric/duodenal perforations typically result in free air in upper abdomen (above transverse mesocolon)
    - Jejunal, ileal, and colonic perforations result in free air below transverse mesocolon
  - Small bowel perforation usually results in only small amounts of pneumoperitoneum, while gastric and colon perforations can result in massive free air
    - Perforated ulcers and diverticulitis usually result in relatively small amounts of free air
    - Perforation of colon or misplaced feeding tubes may result in massive free air
- While pneumoperitoneum should (justifiably) raise concern for intestinal perforation, also consider benign causes of pneumoperitoneum when free air is incidental finding in asymptomatic patient

Helpful Clues for Common Diagnoses

- **Normal Postoperative Pneumoperitoneum**
  - Small amount of free air is normal finding after laparotomy or other invasive procedures (e.g., peritoneal dialysis, gastrostomy tube placement, etc.)
    - Seen on CT in almost 90% of patients at 3 days after surgery and 50% at 6 days
    - Typically resolves in 7-10 days, but may rarely persist longer in some patients
      - Free air may persist longer in patients with history of prior surgeries or prior bouts of peritonitis
    - Normal postoperative free air should be minimal, as **large or massive pneumoperitoneum is abnormal finding** that should raise concern for anastomotic leak or perforation
- **Barotrauma**
  - Positive pressure ventilation can lead to alveolar rupture that results in pneumothorax, pneumomediastinum, subcutaneous emphysema, pneumatosis, or pneumoperitoneum
  - Gas in pleural or mediastinal spaces may dissect into peritoneum or retroperitoneum
  - Suspect in patient on positive pressure ventilation with both pneumothorax and pneumoperitoneum
- **Iatrogenic Injuries or Complications**
  - Common causes of injury include endoscopy with bowel perforation, complicated feeding tube placement
  - Bowel anastomotic leak can be seen as complication of any intraperitoneal bowel anastomosis, often manifesting as greater than expected postoperative free air ± imaging findings of peritonitis or abscess
- **Perforated Ulcer**
  - Gastroduodenal ulcers represent most common cause of GI tract perforation
    - Gastric and duodenal ulcers have equal risk of perforation, although duodenal ulcers are 3x as common
  - Duodenal ulcer perforation typically results in ectopic gas, fluid, and fat stranding immediately adjacent to duodenal bulb
    - Gas and fluid may be both intraperitoneal and extraperitoneal (anterior pararenal space)
  - Gastric ulcer perforation often occurs into lesser sac, resulting in collection of gas, fluid, or contrast posterior to stomach with subsequent extension into peritoneal cavity through epiploic foramen (of Winslow)
- **Diverticulitis**
  - Very common cause of pneumoperitoneum in pelvis, although amount of free air usually quite minimal, as omentum walls off perforated diverticulum
    - Usually does not cause generalized peritonitis or large free air, and manifests as a few tiny foci of free air adjacent to inflamed colon (usually sigmoid)
  - Patients may rarely develop large pneumoperitoneum and generalized peritonitis, especially elderly patients and those using steroids
- **Intestinal Trauma**
  - Pneumoperitoneum following blunt trauma is indicative of intestinal perforation until proven otherwise, with duodenum and proximal jejunum most common sites
  - Often associated with ancillary signs of bowel injury, including mesenteric hematoma and bowel wall thickening

- Be aware that diagnostic peritoneal lavage (DPL) performing during initial clinical assessment may result in free intraperitoneal air and fluid
- **Appendicitis**
  - Ruptured appendicitis typically produces only small amount of free air, usually in conjunction with significant free fluid (± loculated fluid collection/abscess)
  - Appendicitis complicated by rupture in ~ 25%
- **Thoracic Processes (Mimics)**
  - A variety of lung abnormalities may simulate pneumoperitoneum on plain radiograph due to proximity to diaphragm
    - Thin crescent of pleural air (pneumothorax) near diaphragm may simulate pneumoperitoneum
    - Plate-like, basal atelectasis may result in curvilinear density that parallels diaphragm, with aerated lung below atelectasis mimicking pneumoperitoneum
    - Cystic lung disease, including bullae and other cysts near diaphragm, may simulate free air on radiographs
- **Colonic Interposition (Mimic)**
  - Also known as Chilaiditi syndrome, when hepatic flexure of colon lies above liver, beneath right hemidiaphragm
  - Not uncommonly mistaken for free air on radiographs
- **Subphrenic Fat (Mimic)**
  - Collections of fat in subxiphoid and perihepatic regions may be quite radiolucent and may be misinterpreted as free air on radiography

Helpful Clues for Less Common Diagnoses

- **Other Causes of Bowel Perforation**
  - Multiple other causes of bowel perforation include
    - Severe bowel distension due to severe ileus, volvulus, or obstruction
    - Bowel ischemia
    - Vasculitis (polyarteritis nodosa and Behçet disease most commonly cause small bowel perforation
    - Severe infection or inflammatory bowel disease
    - Malignancy
      - Lymphoma most common malignant cause of perforation in small bowel, while adenocarcinoma most common cause in colon

- Ingested foreign bodies (e.g., bone, toothpick, etc.)
  - Tend to cause perforations in ileum, ileocecal region, or rectosigmoid
- Radiation therapy
- Fecal stool impaction (i.e., stercoral colitis)
- Chemotherapy or other medications (e.g., steroids, NSAIDs)
  - Small bowel perforations are much less common than colonic perforation
- **Peritonitis**
  - Intraperitoneal gas and fluid may result from pyogenic infection with gas-forming organisms (usually enteric)
  - Usually associated with other signs of peritonitis, including abscess or peritoneal thickening/enhancement
- **Abdominal Abscess**
  - Gas-containing subphrenic abscess may simulate free abdominal gas on upright radiograph
- **Pneumatosis Cystoides Intestinalis**
  - Uncommon, benign form of pneumatosis with cystic collections of gas in bowel wall
    - Most often diagnosed in patients with scleroderma and other collagen vascular disease
    - May relate to steroid use or other immunosuppressive medications
  - Cystic intramural gas may rupture, leading to pneumoperitoneum
  - Even though CT may appear highly concerning, patients are asymptomatic
- **From Female Genital Tract**
  - Retrograde passage of ectopic gas into peritoneum through female genital tract may occur in variety of settings [e.g., following sexual intercourse, pelvic examination, or water sports (e.g., water skiing)]
- **Small Bowel Diverticula**
  - Diverticula arising from duodenum or small intestine may perforate spontaneously due to small bowel diverticulitis or as result of feeding tube placement
  - Perforation of small bowel diverticula usually results in very little free air and does not typically result in peritonitis or need for surgery

Normal Postoperative Pneumoperitoneum

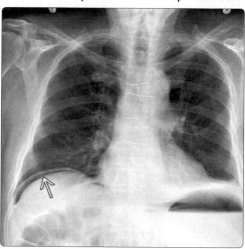

Barotrauma

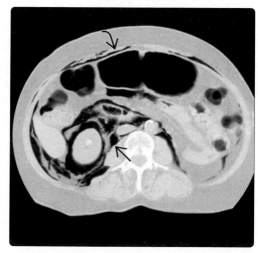

(Left) Frontal chest radiograph acquired after abdominal surgery demonstrates a thin crescent of pneumoperitoneum ➡ under the right hemidiaphragm, a normal finding in the postoperative period. (Right) Axial NECT in a patient on positive pressure ventilation and with known large bilateral pneumothoraces (not shown) demonstrates gas dissecting downward into the abdomen to involve the retroperitoneum ➡ and intraperitoneal space ➡, classic findings for barotrauma.

(Left) *Axial NECT after a low anterior rectal resection demonstrates greater than expected pneumoperitoneum* ➡ *immediately after surgery.* (Right) *Axial NECT in the same patient demonstrates a focal collection of ectopic gas near the rectal anastomosis* ➡. *While small free air is normal after surgery, large free air, as in this case, should suggest the presence of anastomotic leak. This patient required surgical revision of the rectal anastomosis.*

Iatrogenic Injuries or Complications

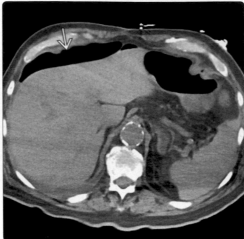

Iatrogenic Injuries or Complications

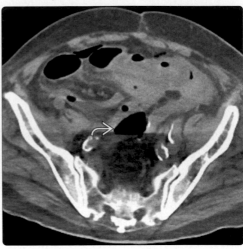

(Left) *Axial NECT after placement of a gastrostomy tube demonstrates subcutaneous emphysema* ➡ *and pneumoperitoneum* ➡, *both of which are expected after the procedure. However, the gastrostomy* ➡ *directly traverses the colon as it enters the stomach, a complication that required open surgery.* (Right) *Axial NECT in a patient with abdominal pain demonstrates foci of small pneumoperitoneum* ➡, *as well as direct extravasation of enteric contrast* ➡ *from the duodenum, compatible with a perforated duodenal ulcer.*

Iatrogenic Injuries or Complications

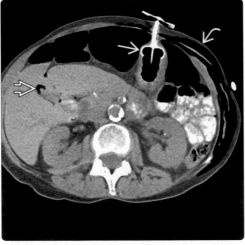

Perforated Ulcer

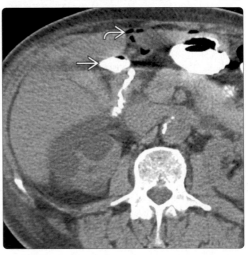

(Left) *Axial CECT in a patient with acute abdominal pain demonstrates irregular thickening of the duodenal bulb* ➡ *with a small amount of immediately adjacent ectopic fluid and gas* ➡. *A perforated duodenal ulcer was found at surgery.* (Right) *Coronal CECT demonstrates a severely thickened and inflamed sigmoid colon due to diverticulitis. The large peridiverticular abscess* ➡ *with internal gas represents the sequelae of perforation.*

Perforated Ulcer

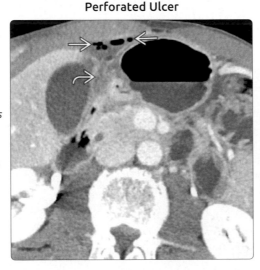

Diverticulitis

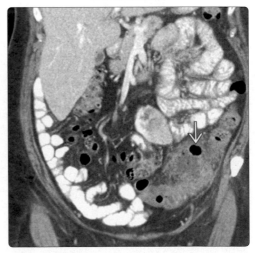

Other Causes of Bowel Perforation

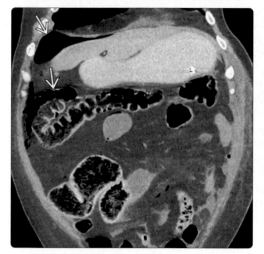

Other Causes of Bowel Perforation

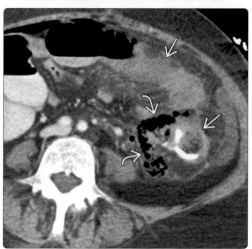

(Left) *Coronal NECT in a critically ill patient demonstrates ectopic gas ➡ immediately adjacent to the hepatic flexure of the colon and under the right hemidiaphragm. The patient was taken to surgery where a perforated colon was found, probably secondary to pseudomembranous colitis.* (Right) *Axial CECT in a patient with ulcerative colitis demonstrates severe thickening and inflammation of the colon ➡ with ectopic gas ➡ directly extending from the colon, compatible with perforation.*

Pneumatosis Cystoides Intestinalis

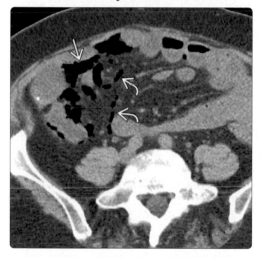

Pneumatosis Cystoides Intestinalis

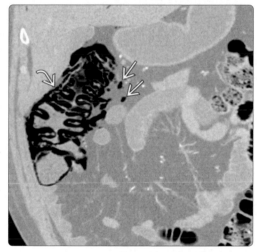

(Left) *Axial NECT in an asymptomatic patient demonstrates bubbly pneumatosis ➡ in the right colon with several foci of adjacent free air ➡. The patient was clinically doing well, and this was thought to represent benign pneumatosis.* (Right) *Coronal CECT in an asymptomatic patient on chronic steroid treatment for autoimmune disease demonstrates extensive benign pneumatosis ➡ throughout the right colon with resultant perforation and small adjacent free air ➡.*

Small Bowel Diverticula

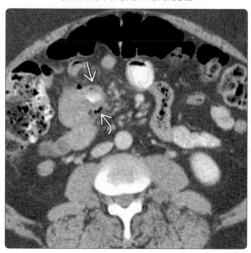

Foreign Body Perforation

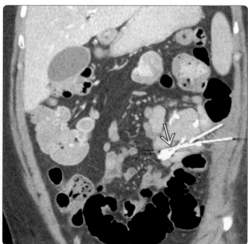

(Left) *Axial CECT in a patient with abdominal pain demonstrates an inflamed contrast-filled diverticulum ➡ arising from a small bowel loop, as well as a tiny focus of adjacent ectopic gas ➡, compatible with small bowel diverticulitis.* (Right) *Coronal CECT in a psychiatric patient demonstrates multiple intentionally ingested pins ➡ perforating through the small bowel into the adjacent abdominal wall. These findings required surgical intervention.*

DIFFERENTIAL DIAGNOSIS

Common

- Abdominal Trauma
- Complication of Surgery
- Coagulopathic Hemorrhage
- Obstetric or Gynecological Source
  - Ruptured Ovarian Cyst
  - Ruptured Ectopic Pregnancy
  - HELLP Syndrome
- Ruptured Aneurysm
- Other Nonhemorrhagic Causes of High-Attenuation Ascites

Less Common

- Neoplastic Hemorrhage
- Ruptured Spleen
- Hemorrhagic Pancreatitis

ESSENTIAL INFORMATION

Key Differential Diagnosis Issues

- Attenuation of blood products will vary depending on age of bleed
  - Acute, unclotted extravascular blood typically demonstrates attenuation of 35-45 HU
    - Blood products may demonstrate slightly lower attenuation in patients with severe anemia
    - Density of blood may also be decreased due to dilution by ascites, urine, bile, or bowel contents
  - Clotted blood is typically higher in attenuation (45-70 HU), explaining why highest density blood is usually found immediately adjacent to site of bleeding (i.e., sentinel clot sign)
    - Sentinel clot sign can be important clue to source of bleeding in difficult cases
    - Blood products distant from site of bleeding usually lower in attenuation
  - Active extravasation of contrast (often easiest to identify on arterial-phase imaging) may be found at sites of active bleeding with attenuation identical to blood pool
    - Identifying active extravasation critical in determining need for urgent embolization or surgery
- Clinical history is key to diagnosis, including recent trauma, recent surgery, anticoagulation, coagulopathy, and pregnancy status
  - In patients without history of trauma, look for evidence of abnormal visceral organ (organomegaly or mass) or vasculature (aneurysm, dissection) that may explain bleeding
  - Unexplained hemoperitoneum in young woman of childbearing age should always prompt correlation with β-hCG levels to exclude ruptured ectopic pregnancy
- CT is critical for diagnosis in cases of large nontraumatic hemoperitoneum, as physical exam can be misleading and hematocrit levels may be normal in acute setting
- Abdominal hemorrhage on MR can be quite variable in signal depending on age of blood products and sequence utilized, and may not follow standard signal characteristics classically described with intracranial hemorrhage

Helpful Clues for Common Diagnoses

- **Abdominal Trauma**
  - Presence of intraabdominal hemorrhage in setting of trauma should prompt careful search for solid organ or bowel injuries, particularly when acute blood seen immediately adjacent to visceral organ or bowel loop
    - Sentinel clot (heterogeneous higher density clot) may be visualized adjacent to source of bleeding
  - Most commonly injured solid organs in abdomen are spleen and liver, with injuries almost always associated with adjacent hematoma
    - Hematoma in such cases usually extends downwards along paracolic gutters into pelvis
  - Duodenum and proximal jejunum most common sites of bowel injury, and presence of mesenteric or interloop blood may be only clue to diagnosis
    - Hematoma in such cases more often centrally located within leaves of mesentery adjacent to bowel loops
- **Complication of Surgery**
  - Diagnosis based on history of recent surgery or other intervention (biopsy, endoscopy, angiography), with blood seen in close proximity to site of intervention
  - Often associated with other postoperative findings, including pneumoperitoneum, subcutaneous gas, and free fluid
- **Coagulopathic Hemorrhage**
  - May result from anticoagulation or bleeding diathesis
  - Most common sites of spontaneous bleeding are iliopsoas compartment and rectus sheath, although hemorrhage can either originate from or track into peritoneal cavity
  - Classically associated with multiple sites of bleeding and frequent internal hematocrit levels (more common with coagulopathic hemorrhage than other causes)
- **Obstetric or Gynecologic Source**
  - Gynecologic causes are most common etiologies for nontraumatic hemoperitoneum in women of child-bearing age, particularly when hemorrhage is located in pelvis
    - Given limitations of CT in female pelvis, correlation with ultrasound and β-hCG levels may be necessary once hemorrhage is identified on CT
    - Ruptured ovarian cyst
      - Common cause of hemorrhage in premenopausal females, with hemorrhage usually localized in pelvis immediately adjacent to adnexa
      - Hemorrhagic cyst may be directly visualized on CT as mixed-attenuation spherical mass arising from adnexa with adjacent hematoma
    - Ruptured ectopic pregnancy
      - Given life-threatening nature of this entity, ectopic pregnancy must be first consideration when confronted with pelvic hemorrhage in woman of child-bearing age
      - CT findings of pelvic hemorrhage in premenopausal female should prompt correlation with β-hCG levels (urine pregnancy test may be falsely negative) and ultrasound
    - HELLP syndrome
      - Peripartum complication of preeclampsia characterized by hemolysis, ↑ liver enzymes, and thrombocytopenia

- □ May be associated with disseminated intravascular coagulation (DIC), hemolysis, hepatic infarction, hepatic rupture, or hemorrhage
- **Ruptured Aneurysm**
  - ○ Bleeding aortic aneurysms usually result in retroperitoneal bleeding, although large hematoma can extend into peritoneal cavity
  - ○ Visceral artery aneurysms usually produce intraperitoneal bleeding, with splenic artery aneurysms most common (60%)
    - – Disproportionately seen in female and pregnant patients with greater risk of rupture
- **Other Nonhemorrhagic Causes of High-Attenuation Ascites**
  - ○ Bladder trauma
    - – Intraperitoneal bladder rupture results in intraperitoneal fluid which may demonstrate variable attenuation
      - □ Unopacified urine is usually of water density, but can appear higher in density due to combination of urine and blood or due to excretion of contrast-opacified urine into bladder
    - – Most definitively diagnosed with CT cystogram after instillation of diluted contrast material into bladder
  - ○ Vicarious excretion
    - – Ascites may be minimally increased in attenuation due to prior administration of IV contrast material, especially when CT performed > 10 minutes after contrast administration
  - ○ Gastrointestinal tract perforation
    - – Ascites may be slightly hyperdense due to presence of extraluminal bowel contents
  - ○ Peritonitis
    - – Often associated with complex, loculated ascites (slightly higher in attenuation than simple fluid) and peritoneal thickening/enhancement
  - ○ Malignant ascites
    - – Often associated with other imaging features of peritoneal carcinomatosis, including peritoneal thickening/nodularity or frank tumor implants

- – Ascites appears complex with slightly higher attenuation than simple fluid (10-25 HU), loculation, and internal septations

Helpful Clues for Less Common Diagnoses

- **Neoplastic Hemorrhage**
  - ○ Any primary or metastatic tumor can bleed, although certain tumors are much more likely to present with significant bleeding
  - ○ Most common hepatic tumors to be associated with bleeding are hepatic adenoma and hepatocellular carcinoma
    - – Tumors near liver capsule most likely to present with large hemoperitoneum
    - – Most other benign (i.e., hemangioma, focal nodular hyperplasia) or malignant liver lesions do not typically present with bleeding
  - ○ Most common pancreatic tumor to present with bleeding is solid pseudopapillary neoplasm (SPEN), a tumor most often seen in young female patients
    - – Bleeding also described with neuroendocrine tumors, acinar cell carcinoma, and metastases (especially melanoma), albeit very uncommonly
  - ○ Angiosarcoma, regardless of location (usually spleen or liver), classically associated with bleeding
  - ○ Lung cancer, renal cell carcinoma, and melanoma most likely metastatic lesions to bleed in abdomen
- **Ruptured Spleen**
  - ○ Enlarged spleen, most often due to infection or tumor (such as lymphoma/leukemia), is at ↑ risk for rupture and can result in massive hemoperitoneum
  - ○ Mononucleosis is most common cause of spontaneous splenic rupture in western societies and may be injured in minor trauma, such as sports activities
- **Hemorrhagic Pancreatitis**
  - ○ Most often seen with severe necrotizing pancreatitis
    - – Bleeding typically due to disruption of small vessels and capillaries by pancreatic enzymes
  - ○ Pseudoaneurysm (most often splenic artery) must be excluded when hemorrhage seen adjacent to pancreas

Abdominal Trauma

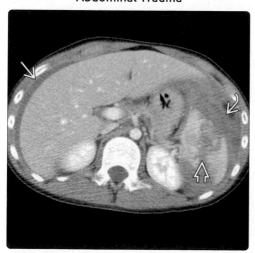

Abdominal Trauma

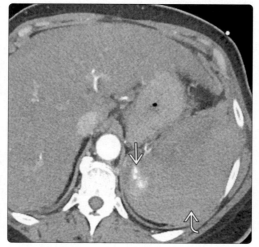

(Left) Axial CECT in a patient with a shattered spleen ➡ after trauma demonstrates a classic sentinel clot sign, with blood around the spleen ➡ higher in density than the blood around the liver ➡. The highest density blood products should be found adjacent to the site of bleeding. (Right) Axial CECT in a trauma patient demonstrates a large left upper quadrant hematoma ➡ with internal active extravasation ➡, a feature that prompted urgent angiographic embolization in this patient.

Abdominal Trauma

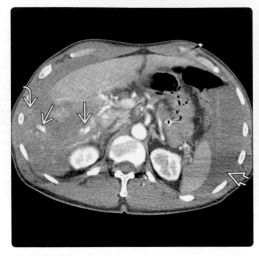

Abdominal Trauma

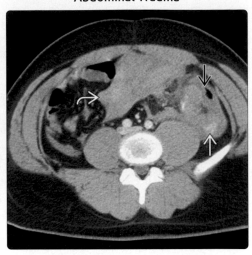

(Left) *Axial CECT after trauma demonstrates a large laceration throughout the right liver with sites of active extravasation ➡ and perihepatic hematoma. Note that the perihepatic hematoma ➡ is subtly denser than the perisplenic hematoma ➡, compatible with the sentinel clot sign.* (Right) *Axial CECT after trauma demonstrates mesenteric hemorrhage ➡ with active extravasation ➡, most of which appears adjacent to the descending colon ➡. Colonic injury was confirmed at surgery.*

Complication of Surgery

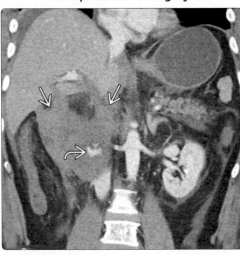

Coagulopathic Hemorrhage

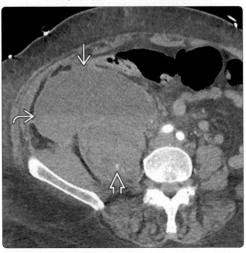

(Left) *Coronal CECT performed after a Whipple procedure demonstrates a hematoma ➡ adjacent to the surgical bed with internal active extravasation ➡, prompting angiographic embolization.* (Right) *Axial CECT in an anticoagulated patient demonstrates a large hematoma ➡ centered in the psoas muscle with extension into the right abdomen and subtle internal active extravasation ➡. Note the presence of a hematocrit level ➡ within the hemorrhage, a common feature with coagulopathic bleeds.*

Ruptured Ovarian Cyst

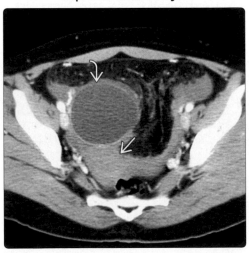

Ruptured Ectopic Pregnancy

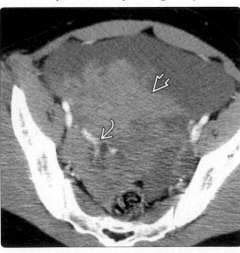

(Left) *Axial CECT shows a large adnexal cyst ➡ with adjacent sentinel clot ➡, compatible with bleeding secondary to a ruptured ovarian cyst.* (Right) *Axial CECT shows a large pelvic hematoma ➡ with evidence of active extravasation ➡ in a young female patient. In the absence of a history of trauma, these findings should prompt correlation with β-HCG levels and ultrasound to exclude a ruptured ectopic pregnancy.*

HELLP Syndrome

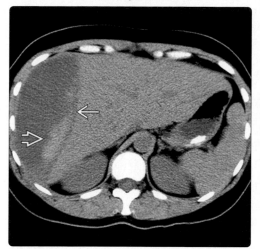

Ruptured Aneurysm

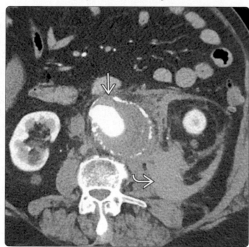

(Left) *Axial NECT in a pregnant patient with HELLP syndrome demonstrates large subcapsular and perihepatic hemorrhage* ➡, *including a portion of which is hyperdense* ➡ *(likely representing clotted blood).* (Right) *Axial CECT demonstrates a large abdominal aortic aneurysm* ➡ *with high-attenuation blood* ➡ *tracking from the aneurysm into the adjacent retroperitoneum, compatible with aneurysm rupture.*

Neoplastic Hemorrhage

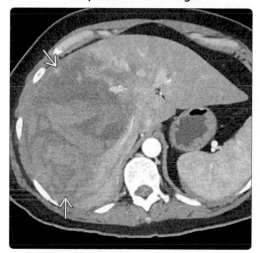

Neoplastic Hemorrhage

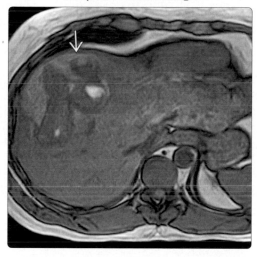

(Left) *Axial CECT demonstrates a large mass* ➡ *in the right liver lobe with extensive internal hemorrhage. This was found to be a large hepatic adenoma in a young female patient using oral contraceptives.* (Right) *Axial T1 MR in a young female patient demonstrates a large right hepatic lobe mass* ➡ *with internal T1-hyperintense hemorrhage, ultimately found to be a hepatic adenoma at resection. Adenoma and hepatocellular carcinoma are the most common liver tumors to present with bleeding.*

Neoplastic Hemorrhage

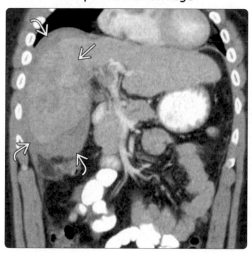

Neoplastic Hemorrhage

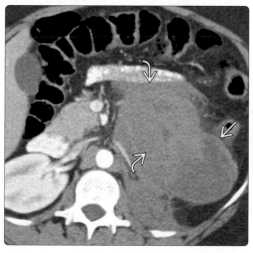

(Left) *Coronal CECT in a cirrhotic patient demonstrates infiltrative tumor* ➡ *throughout the right hepatic lobe, compatible with hepatocellular carcinoma. Note that the tumor has bled into the perihepatic space with hematoma* ➡ *surrounding the right liver lobe.* (Right) *Axial CECT demonstrates a pancreatic mass* ➡ *with internal and surrounding hematoma* ➡, *found to be a solid pseudopapillary neoplasm in this young female patient.*

DIFFERENTIAL DIAGNOSIS

Common

- Cirrhosis and Portal Hypertension
- Heart Failure
- Renal Failure
- Acute Pancreatitis
- Peritonitis
- Lymphoma
- Sclerosing Mesenteritis
- Acute Inflammatory Conditions of Gastrointestinal Tract
  - Diverticulitis
  - Crohn Disease
  - Ischemic Enteritis
- Postsurgical Mesenteric Infiltration
- Carcinoid Tumor

Less Common

- Mesenteric Hemorrhage
- Small Bowel Vasculitis
- Radiation Therapy
- Peritoneal Metastases and Mesothelioma
- Portomesenteric Venous Thrombosis
  - Portal Vein Thrombosis
  - Superior Mesenteric Vein Thrombosis
- Small Bowel Transplantation
- Intestinal Lymphangiectasia
- Leukemic or Lymphomatous Infiltration of Peritoneum
- Liposarcoma

ESSENTIAL INFORMATION

Key Differential Diagnosis Issues

- "Misty mesentery" represents increased attenuation of mesenteric fat as result of infiltration by edema (fluid), inflammation, blood, or tumor
  - Nonspecific finding, significance of which is determined by patient's clinical history, symptoms, and other ancillary imaging findings
- 4 primary etiological categories for "misty mesentery" depending on nature of mesenteric fat infiltration
  - **Edema**: Portal hypertension, heart failure, renal failure, hypoalbuminemia, congenital, postsurgical, radiation therapy, mesenteric vein thrombosis
  - **Inflammation**: Pancreatitis, diverticulitis, Crohn disease, sclerosing mesenteritis, peritonitis, vasculitis
  - **Hemorrhage**: Bowel or mesenteric trauma, anticoagulation, ischemic enteritis
  - **Neoplastic**: Lymphoma, leukemia, peritoneal metastases, mesothelioma

Helpful Clues for Common Diagnoses

- **Cirrhosis and Portal Hypertension**
  - Cirrhosis often results in portal hypertension and hypoproteinemia, both leading to mesenteric edema
  - Mesenteric edema becomes more conspicuous in setting of superimposed mesenteric venous thrombosis
- **Heart Failure**
  - Any form of cardiac dysfunction (e.g., CHF, constrictive pericarditis) may lead to generalized volume overload and edema (including mesenteric edema)

- **Renal Failure**
  - Renal failure resulting in generalized volume overload and edema may cause mesenteric edema
- **Acute Pancreatitis**
  - Most common inflammatory etiology for "misty mesentery"
  - Fluid and inflammation spread from inflamed pancreas both laterally (throughout anterior pararenal space) and ventrally/inferiorly (into leaves of small bowel mesentery and transverse mesocolon)
- **Peritonitis**
  - Inflammation of peritoneal lining may cause edema of adjacent mesenteric fat planes
  - Can result from either infectious (pyogenic, TB) or chemical (bile, peritoneal dialysis) peritonitis
- **Lymphoma**
  - Early Hodgkin or non-Hodgkin lymphoma can, in theory, manifest as only "misty mesentery" with mildly prominent mesenteric nodes
    - Nodes may rarely demonstrate fat-halo sign, potentially leading to misdiagnosis as sclerosing mesenteritis
    - **Almost never** only manifestation of lymphoma, as there are typically legitimately enlarged nodes in mesentery or other lymph node stations
  - Treated lymphoma (radiation or chemotherapy) may result in permanent infiltration of mesenteric fat planes (even though adenopathy may have resolved)
- **Sclerosing Mesenteritis**
  - Exact incidence is unknown but probably more common than conventionally thought
  - "Misty mesentery" with discrete borders (i.e., pseudocapsule measuring < 3 mm) and multiple prominent internal mesenteric lymph nodes
    - Classically "halo" of spared fat with normal density surrounding both lymph nodes and vessels
    - Involved portions of mesentery may demonstrate slightly increased T2 signal on suppressed T2WI
  - Should be diagnosis of exclusion once other causes of "misty mesentery" considered
- **Acute Inflammatory Conditions of Gastrointestinal Tract**
  - Any acute form of bowel inflammation will result in inflammation of adjacent mesentery with increased mesenteric attenuation
  - Increase in mesenteric attenuation tends to be localized near involved segment of bowel
  - Common inflammatory GI causes of mesenteric infiltration include diverticulitis (infiltration of adjacent sigmoid mesocolon), Crohn disease, appendicitis, and bowel ischemia
- **Postsurgical Mesenteric Infiltration**
  - Mild infiltration of mesentery is very common after abdominal surgeries (particularly surgeries of GI tract or mesentery), and this mesenteric infiltration may persist to mild degree long after surgery
- **Carcinoid Tumor**
  - May manifest as spiculated mesenteric mass [usually in right lower quadrant (RLQ)] with internal calcification
    - May result in distortion and narrowing of adjacent vasculature, as well as tethering of small bowel loops (sometimes resulting in obstruction)

– May cause infiltration of RLQ mesentery due to tumor spread or lymphatic/venous obstruction
  ○ Tethered small bowel loops may be thickened as result of chronic venous/lymphatic obstruction
  ○ Primary tumor usually located in terminal ileum

Helpful Clues for Less Common Diagnoses

- **Mesenteric Hemorrhage**
  ○ Acute hemorrhage in mesentery results in high-density hematoma and infiltration of surrounding mesentery with blood products
  ○ Probably most common in setting of trauma, with blood products seen as triangular collections of high-density blood in between bowel loops
    – Though isolated mesenteric injury can occur, presence of mesenteric hemorrhage should prompt careful search for imaging evidence of bowel injury (i.e., bowel wall thickening, pneumoperitoneum)
  ○ Isolated mesenteric or intraperitoneal hemorrhage as result of coagulopathy is quite rare
    – Hemorrhage more often originates from retroperitoneum or abdominal wall musculature and tracks into peritoneal space
    – Largest amount of blood products found outside mesentery/peritoneum
- **Small Bowel Vasculitis**
  ○ Multiple types of vasculitis (Henoch-Schönlein, lupus, etc.) are categorized as small, medium, and large vessel
  ○ Can produce profound small bowel wall thickening and mucosal hyperenhancement, usually in conjunction with extensive mesenteric infiltration and hemorrhage
  ○ May be associated with vascular stigmata of vasculitis depending on size of vessels involved (e.g., arterial wall thickening, vascular "beading," or aneurysms)
- **Radiation Therapy**
  ○ Seen most in pelvic radiation for gynecologic (especially cervical cancer) or rectal malignancies
  ○ May cause permanent infiltration of pelvic fat planes/mesentery, often w/ thickening of pelvic small bowel (radiation enteritis), rectum (radiation proctitis), bladder (radiation cystitis)

- **Peritoneal Metastases and Mesothelioma**
  ○ Earliest signs of peritoneal malignancy may be subtle infiltration of mesentery and omentum, often with evidence of peritoneal thickening and enhancement
    – Infiltration of peritoneal fat may predate development of visible frank soft tissue tumor implants on CT/MR
  ○ Most common causes of peritoneal carcinomatosis are gynecologic and GI malignancies, whereas mesothelioma (very rare tumor) can appear virtually identical
- **Portomesenteric Venous Thrombosis**
  ○ Portal or superior mesenteric vein thrombosis can lead to mesenteric infiltration secondary to leaking of fluid from lymphatics or mesenteric hemorrhage
  ○ Mesenteric infiltration tends to be most conspicuous adjacent to thickened and inflamed loops of small bowel (due to venous ischemia)
  ○ Bowel ischemia related to venous thrombosis tends to result in particularly profound mesenteric infiltration (often with associated mesenteric hemorrhage)
- **Small Bowel Transplantation**
  ○ Mesenteric edema is often striking after small bowel transplant due to transection of lymphatics or rejection of transplanted bowel and its mesentery
- **Intestinal Lymphangiectasia**
  ○ Rare disorder that manifests as dilated lymphatics within small bowel villi, resulting in significant small bowel wall thickening, ascites, and mesenteric edema
- **Leukemic or Lymphomatous Infiltration of Peritoneum**
  ○ May mimic appearance of carcinomatosis, with diffuse infiltration of peritoneal cavity, mass-like thickening of peritoneum, and ascites
- **Liposarcoma**
  ○ Primary peritoneal liposarcomas are rare, but large retroperitoneal liposarcomas can extend into peritoneum
  ○ Large liposarcoma could mimic appearance of sclerosing mesenteritis, as these tumors are encapsulated and demonstrate predominantly fat density with internal stranding and complexity

Cirrhosis and Portal Hypertension

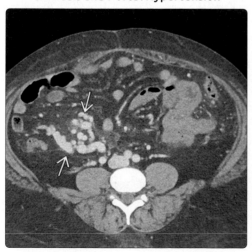

Cirrhosis and Portal Hypertension

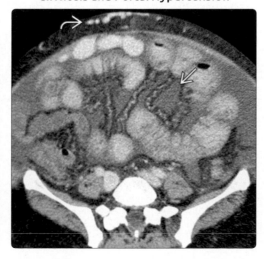

(Left) *Axial CECT in a patient with cirrhosis and portal hypertension demonstrates a cluster of varices* ➡ *in the right aspect of the mesentery. Note the subtle mild infiltration of the mesenteric fat throughout the abdomen, a common feature of portal hypertension.* (Right) *Axial CECT in a patient with cirrhosis and portal hypertension demonstrates mesenteric edema* ➡*, causing the mesenteric vessels and fat to stand out in contrast. Periumbilical varices* ➡ *and ascites are also present.*

Acute Pancreatitis

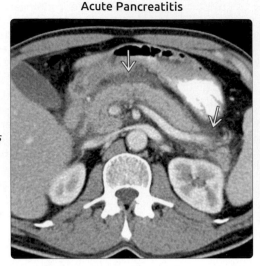

Acute Pancreatitis

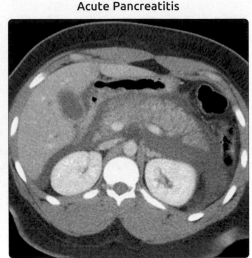

(Left) *Axial CECT in a patient with abdominal pain demonstrates mild pancreatic edema with peripancreatic fluid* ➡️ *tracking along the anterior pararenal space, compatible with acute pancreatitis.* (Right) *Axial CECT demonstrates an enlarged, edematous pancreas with substantial peripancreatic free fluid and blurring of adjacent fat planes, consistent with acute pancreatitis.*

Peritonitis

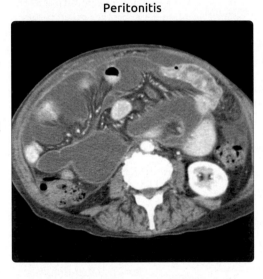

Sclerosing Mesenteritis

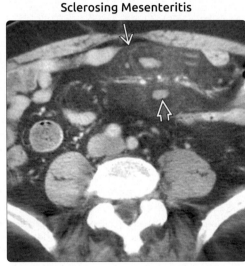

(Left) *Axial CECT shows diffuse infiltration of the mesentery and multiple loculated fluid collections in a patient with bile peritonitis.* (Right) *Axial CECT demonstrates infiltration of the small bowel mesentery, set off by a pseudocapsule* ➡️. *Multiple mildly enlarged mesenteric nodes are present* ➡️ *with a subtle surrounding "halo" of spared fat. These findings are classic for sclerosing mesenteritis.*

Sclerosing Mesenteritis

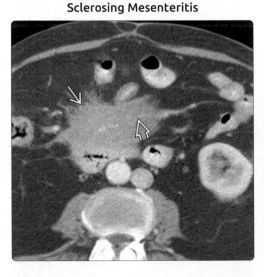

Diverticulitis

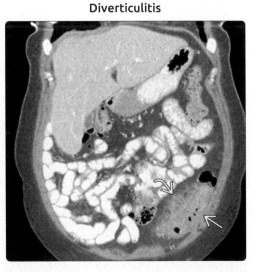

(Left) *Axial CECT shows extensive infiltration of the jejunal mesentery* ➡️ *with encasement of the mesenteric vessels* ➡️ *that results in bowel wall edema. These findings represent an advanced case of sclerosing mesenteritis.* (Right) *Coronal CECT demonstrates a markedly thickened, inflamed sigmoid colon* ➡️ *due to diverticulitis. Note the presence of stranding and infiltration* ➡️ *extending medially into the sigmoid mesocolon.*

Crohn Disease

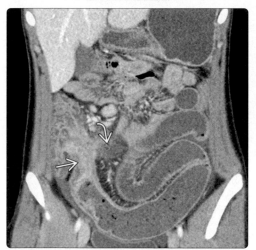

Crohn Disease

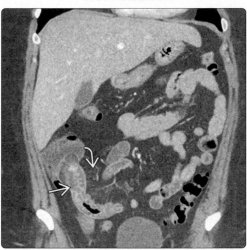

(Left) *Coronal CECT demonstrates thickening and narrowing of the terminal ileum ➡ with resultant proximal small bowel obstruction in a patient with Crohn disease. Note the presence of stranding and infiltration ➡ in the ileocolic mesentery near the terminal ileum.* **(Right)** *Coronal CECT demonstrates thickening and submucosal edema of the distal ileum ➡, compatible Crohn ileitis. There is mild infiltration ➡ of the adjacent right lower quadrant mesentery with fat stranding and inflammation.*

Ischemic Enteritis

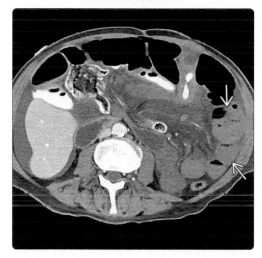

Ischemic Enteritis

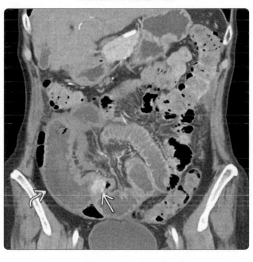

(Left) *Axial CECT demonstrates nonenhancing loops of dilated small bowel ➡ in the left upper quadrant due to bowel ischemia from an internal hernia. Notice the profound infiltration and fat stranding throughout the left upper quadrant mesentery.* **(Right)** *Coronal CECT demonstrates an enhancing carcinoid tumor ➡ in the small bowel, resulting in proximal bowel obstruction. The small bowel ➡ proximal to the mass is dilated, thickened, and hypoenhancing, compatible with ischemia.*

Carcinoid Tumor

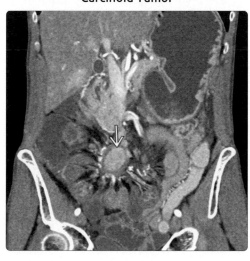

Mesenteric Hemorrhage

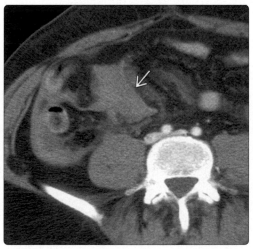

(Left) *Coronal CECT demonstrates an avidly enhancing mesenteric mass ➡, compatible with metastatic carcinoid tumor, resulting in tethering of multiple surrounding bowel loops. There is extensive surrounding infiltration of the mesentery, as well as bowel wall thickening.* **(Right)** *Axial CECT demonstrates the characteristic appearance of a mesenteric injury after trauma, with hematoma ➡ seen between loops of bowel in the mesentery.*

(Left) *Axial CECT in a trauma patient demonstrates mesenteric infiltration and hematoma* ⮞ *with sites of active extravasation* ➡. *Colonic and mesenteric injury were discovered at surgery.* **(Right)** *Coronal CECT demonstrates several markedly thickening, inflamed, poorly enhancing small bowel loops* ⮞ *in the right lower quadrant with adjacent mesenteric infiltration, found to represent small bowel vasculitis due to polyarteritis nodosa.*

Mesenteric Hemorrhage

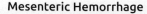
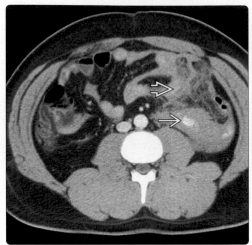

Small Bowel Vasculitis

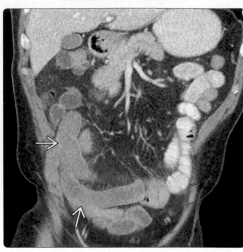

(Left) *Axial CECT demonstrates multiple thick-walled loops of small bowel in the pelvis with submucosal edema, as well as diffuse blurring of pelvic fat planes, reflecting radiation enteritis in a patient receiving treatment for cervical cancer.* **(Right)** *Axial CECT demonstrates multiple thick-walled, hyperenhancing loops of small bowel in the pelvis due to radiation enteritis in a patient receiving radiation therapy for a gynecologic malignancy.*

Radiation Therapy

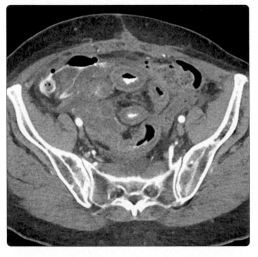

Radiation Therapy

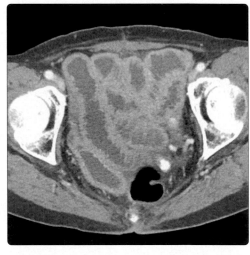

(Left) *Axial CECT in a patient with known gastric cancer demonstrates mild stranding, edema, and nodularity* ➡ *throughout the omentum, compatible with peritoneal carcinomatosis.* **(Right)** *Axial T2 FS MR demonstrates soft tissue* ➡ *throughout the omentum, compatible with "omental caking" due to peritoneal carcinomatosis. Notice the presence of ascites fluid* ⮞ *adjacent to the omental tumor, as well as insinuation among pelvic small bowel loops.*

Peritoneal Metastases and Mesothelioma

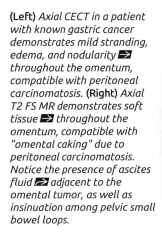

Peritoneal Metastases and Mesothelioma

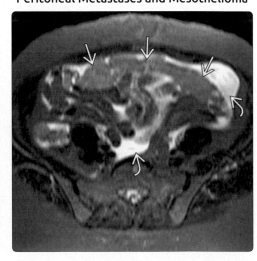

Peritoneal Metastases and Mesothelioma

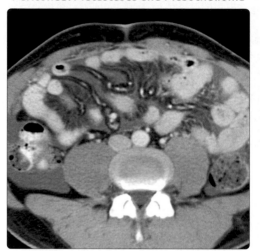

Superior Mesenteric Vein Thrombosis

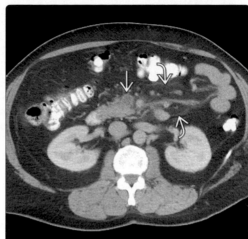

(Left) *Axial CECT shows ascites and a "pleated" appearance of the mesentery, caused by a peritoneal tumor. Peritoneal carcinomatosis could have an identical appearance.* (Right) *Axial CECT demonstrates acute thrombosis of the superior mesenteric vein (SMV) as a result of a hypercoagulability syndrome, with resultant stranding* ➡ *and edema* ⮩ *in the left upper quadrant mesentery.*

Superior Mesenteric Vein Thrombosis

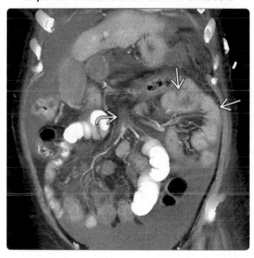

Small Bowel Transplantation

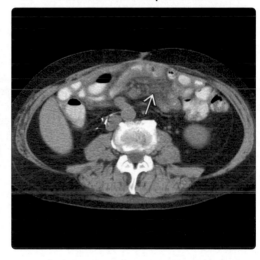

(Left) *Coronal volume-rendered CECT demonstrates thrombus within the SMV* ⮩*, with resultant thickening* ➡ *of multiple small bowel loops due to venous ischemia, as well as diffuse infiltration of the mesentery and moderate ascites.* (Right) *Axial CECT demonstrates extensive infiltration* ➡ *of the small bowel mesenteric allograft along with mural thickening of the bowel wall. Both findings are common and nonspecific in recipients of small bowel transplants and probably indicate some degree of rejection &/or lymphedema.*

Intestinal Lymphangiectasia

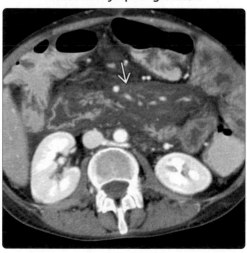

Intestinal Lymphangiectasia

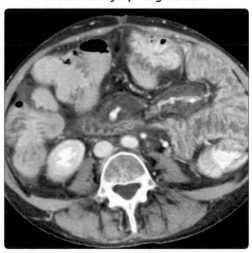

(Left) *Axial CECT shows extensive infiltration of the mesentery* ➡ *and small bowel wall thickening in a young woman with congenital lymphangiectasia of the small bowel.* (Right) *Axial CECT in the same patient with congenital lymphangiectasia once again demonstrates extensive infiltration of the mesentery with diffuse small bowel wall thickening and submucosal edema, classic imaging findings for this rare disorder.*

DIFFERENTIAL DIAGNOSIS

Common

- Hemoperitoneum
  - Traumatic Hemoperitoneum
  - Nontraumatic Causes of Hemoperitoneum
    - Gynecologic or Obstetric Sources
      □ Ruptured Ectopic Pregnancy
      □ Ruptured Ovarian Cyst
      □ Endometriosis
    - Coagulopathic Hemorrhage
      □ Retroperitoneal Hemorrhage
      □ HELLP Syndrome
  - Tumor Associated
  - Ruptured Aneurysm
  - Splenic Rupture
- Vicarious Excretion
- Bladder Trauma
- Perforation of GI Tract

Less Common

- Exudative Ascites
- Pseudomyxoma Peritonei

ESSENTIAL INFORMATION

Key Differential Diagnosis Issues

- Ascites (i.e., intraperitoneal fluid) typically demonstrates water density (0-15 HU) and should be free flowing
  - Free-flowing ascites normally found in subphrenic spaces, Morison pouch, paracolic gutters, pouch of Douglas, and other dependent portions of abdomen
  - Most ascites is transudative (simple), with most common etiologies including liver, heart, or renal dysfunction
    - Transudative ascites almost always demonstrates simple water density
  - Hemorrhage/hemoperitoneum demonstrates higher attenuation on CT, with unclotted blood measuring 30-45 HU and clotted blood measuring 45-70 HU
  - Simple fluid appears anechoic on US, while hemorrhage tends to demonstrate internal echoes

Helpful Clues for Common Diagnoses

- **Traumatic Hemoperitoneum**
  - Probably most common cause of hemorrhagic ascites, with highest density blood products located near site of injury (sentinel clot sign)
    - Blood products further away from site of injury (lysed blood products) usually lower in attenuation
    - Look for evidence of active extravasation (with attenuation similar to blood pool), which can impact decision to undergo angiographic embolization or surgery
    - Hemorrhage may be slightly lower in attenuation than expected in patients with anemia or when hemorrhage is diluted by bile, urine, or bowel contents
  - Most common visceral traumatic injuries (in blunt trauma) causing hemoperitoneum are spleen > liver > bowel/mesentery
- **Nontraumatic Causes of Hemoperitoneum**
  - **Gynecologic or obstetric sources**

- Hemoperitoneum in female of childbearing age (particularly when blood primarily localized in pelvis) should prompt correlation with β-HCG to exclude ruptured ectopic pregnancy
- Other causes include ruptured ovarian hemorrhagic cyst, endometriosis, or rarely, torsion
  □ Ruptured hemorrhagic cyst, in particular, can result in large hemoperitoneum
  - **Coagulopathic hemorrhage**
    - Most often diagnosed in patients on heparin or Coumadin, but also in hemophiliacs and other forms of bleeding diathesis
    - Coagulopathic hemorrhage most often seen in iliopsoas compartment or rectus sheath, but can occur anywhere and may extend into peritoneal cavity (but rarely limited to peritoneal cavity alone)
    - Coagulopathic hemorrhage has particular predisposition for hematocrit levels (fluid-hemorrhage level), as well as multiple sites of bleeding (out of proportion to any history of trauma)
    - HELLP syndrome: Peripartum complication of toxemia, with possible manifestations including hemolysis, thrombocytopenia, hepatic infarction, hepatic rupture, and hemorrhage
  - **Tumor associated**
    - May complicate highly vascular visceral tumors, with hepatic adenoma, hepatocellular carcinoma, angiosarcoma, and vascular metastases (renal cell, neuroendocrine, melanoma, choriocarcinoma) amongst tumors most often associated with bleeding
    - Hepatic tumors most likely to produce hepatic rupture with hemoperitoneum when located in subcapsular position
    - Metastases to solid organs can also rarely bleed, especially lung cancer, renal cell carcinoma, and melanoma
  - **Ruptured aneurysm**
    - Visceral artery aneurysms may rupture and produce intraperitoneal bleeding
      □ Splenic artery aneurysms are most common, particularly in female or pregnant patients
    - Aortic aneurysms produce retroperitoneal hemorrhage, which can rarely extend into peritoneum when particularly massive
  - **Splenic rupture**
    - Spleen can undergo spontaneous rupture, particularly when severely enlarged, usually due to splenic infection, infiltrative processes (such as amyloidosis or Gaucher disease), or neoplastic infiltration
    - Direct correlation between splenic size/weight and risk of rupture
    - Rupture may not be truly spontaneous, as even minor, unnoticed trauma may induce rupture when spleen is massively enlarged
- **Vicarious Excretion**
  - Increased attenuation of ascites fluid due to vicarious excretion occurs in over 50% of patients with ascites
    - Most conspicuous on scans performed more than 10 minutes after intravascular administration of contrast material
    - Occurs regardless of etiology of ascites (benign or malignant)

- Smaller amounts of ascites typically exhibit greater degree of enhancement
- Mild increased attenuation of ascites seen in normal patients and does not necessarily denote renal dysfunction
- May occur more frequently and to greater extent in patients with renal impairment (and less effective renal excretion of contrast)

- **Bladder Trauma**
  - Intraperitoneal rupture of bladder or rupture of urine from ileal conduit or other postoperative bladder diversion can result in intraperitoneal ascites
    - Extravasated urine may be hyperdense when bladder instilled with contrast material (CT cystogram) or contrast excretion into bladder after IV injection

- **Perforation of GI Tract**
  - Can result in hyperdense ascites if enteric fluid contents are mixed with blood products or with oral (enteric) contrast medium

Helpful Clues for Less Common Diagnoses

- **Exudative Ascites**

- Any type of exudative ascites may exhibit slightly higher attenuation (> 15 HU) than simple fluid (but less than hemorrhage)
- Exudative ascites may be seen with variety of causes, including malignant ascites, infection, peritonitis, ischemia, pancreatitis, etc.
- Exudative ascites on US often demonstrates complexity, including internal echoes and septations

- **Pseudomyxoma Peritonei**
  - Accumulation of gelatinous implants throughout abdomen as result of rupture of appendiceal mucinous neoplasm
  - Individual mucinous implants are slightly hyperdense to simple fluid, and can result in scalloping of liver & spleen
  - Often associated with loculated ascites of similar density to mucinous implants (slightly hyperdense to simple fluid)

Traumatic Hemoperitoneum

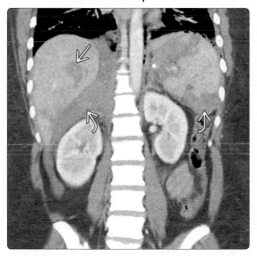

Traumatic Hemoperitoneum

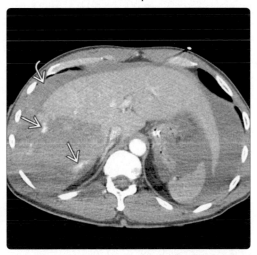

(Left) *Coronal CECT in a trauma patient demonstrates hepatic* ➡ *and splenic lacerations with adjacent hemoperitoneum* ➡. *Spleen and liver injuries are the most common causes of traumatic hemoperitoneum.* (Right) *Axial CECT in a trauma patient demonstrates a large laceration through the right liver with several sites of active extravasation* ➡ *and upper abdominal hemoperitoneum* ➡. *The highest density blood products are found adjacent to the liver injury (sentinel clot sign).*

Traumatic Hemoperitoneum

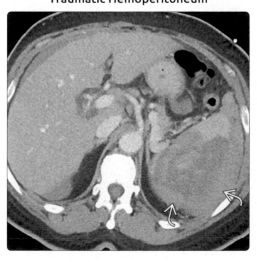

Traumatic Hemoperitoneum

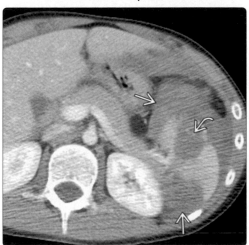

(Left) *Axial CECT in a trauma patient demonstrates a large hematoma* ➡ *surrounding the extensively lacerated spleen.* (Right) *Axial CECT demonstrates extensive lacerations* ➡ *through the spleen with left upper quadrant perisplenic hematoma* ➡.

Ruptured Ovarian Cyst

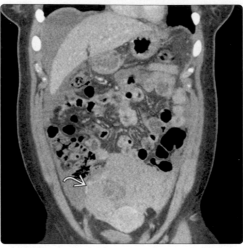

Ruptured Ovarian Cyst

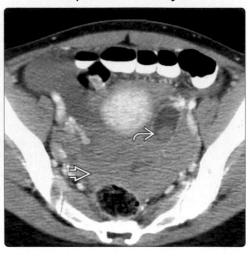

(Left) *Coronal CECT in a young woman with abdominal pain demonstrates a focal hematoma ➡ in the vicinity of the right adnexa, with additional hematoma tracking upward. The patient's β-HCG was negative, and ultrasound showed a right ovarian ruptured hemorrhagic cyst to be the cause of the hemoperitoneum. (Right) Axial CECT shows a high-density focus ➡ within the dependent position of a left adnexal cyst. Surrounding hemoperitoneum ➡ is also noted with a sentinel clot around the ruptured cyst.*

Ruptured Ectopic Pregnancy

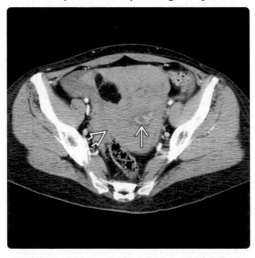

Coagulopathic Hemorrhage

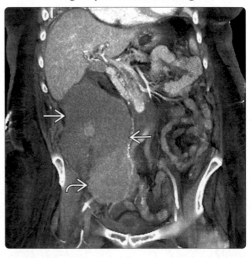

(Left) *Axial CECT shows hemoperitoneum with a sentinel clot ➡ surrounding a focus of ring-like enhancement ➡ in the pelvis. These findings were found to be secondary to a ruptured ectopic pregnancy. (Right) Coronal volume-rendered CECT in an anticoagulated patient demonstrates a large right-sided coagulopathic hemorrhage ➡ centered in the right psoas muscle and adjacent retroperitoneum with higher density blood products ➡ seen within the inferior aspect of the hematoma.*

Coagulopathic Hemorrhage

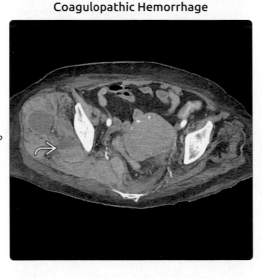

HELLP Syndrome

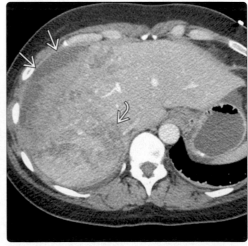

(Left) *Axial CECT in an anticoagulated patient demonstrates right gluteal hematoma with internal hematocrit ➡ levels. Hematocrit levels are particularly common in the setting of coagulopathic bleeding. (Right) Axial CECT in a pregnant patient with HELLP syndrome demonstrate areas of low-density infarction ➡ within the right hepatic lobe, as well as a large mixed-attenuation subcapsular hematoma ➡ along the margin of the right hepatic lobe.*

Tumor Associated

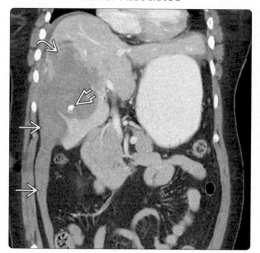

Tumor Associated

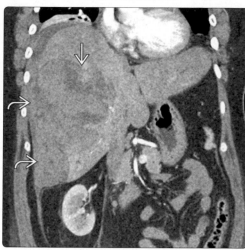

(Left) *Coronal CECT demonstrates a hemorrhagic mass ➡ in the right hepatic lobe with internal active extravasation ➡. The mass has ruptured through the liver capsule with hemorrhage tracking down the right paracolic gutter ➡. This was found at resection to be a bleeding hepatic adenoma.* **(Right)** *Coronal CECT demonstrates a large hemorrhagic mass ➡ in the right hepatic lobe with rupture and perihepatic hematoma ➡. This was ultimately found to represent a bleeding hepatic adenoma at resection.*

Tumor Associated

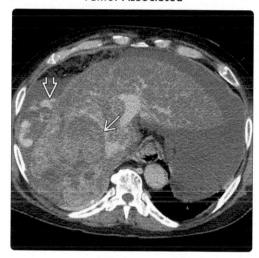

Ruptured Aneurysm

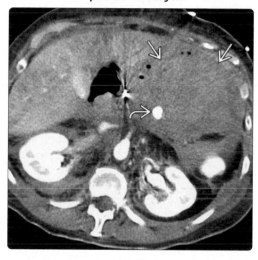

(Left) *Axial CECT demonstrates a large hemorrhagic mass ➡ in the right liver lobe with associated perihepatic hematoma and active extravasation ➡. These findings were found to be secondary to hepatocellular carcinoma with rupture and hemorrhage. Incidentally, the liver is diffusely low density due to alcohol-related steatosis.* **(Right)** *Axial CECT demonstrates large upper abdominal hemoperitoneum ➡ as a result of a ruptured splenic artery aneurysm ➡.*

Bladder Trauma

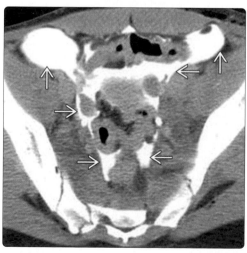

Perforation of GI Tract

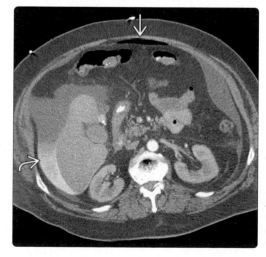

(Left) *Axial CECT in a trauma patient demonstrates intraperitoneal contrast material ➡ surrounding bowel loops and extending up the paracolic gutters. These CT cystogram findings are compatible with intraperitoneal bladder rupture.* **(Right)** *Axial CECT demonstrates extensive free fluid in the upper abdomen, including hyperdense fluid ➡ due to extravasated enteric contrast. Pneumoperitoneum ➡ is also noted in the upper abdomen. These findings were secondary to a perforated duodenal ulcer.*

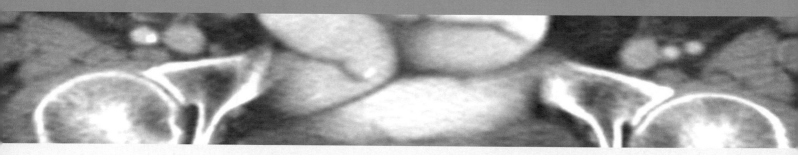

SECTION 2
Abdominal Wall

Anatomically Based Differentials

DIFFERENTIAL DIAGNOSIS

Common

- Abdominal Wall Hernias
  - Inguinal Hernia
  - Ventral Hernia
  - Umbilical Hernia
  - Spigelian Hernia
  - Femoral Hernia
  - Lumbar Hernia
- Abdominal Wall Abscess
- Sebaceous Cyst
- Lipoma
- Keloid
- Hematoma
- Paraumbilical Varices
- Injection Site
- Calcified Scar
- Muscle Asymmetry (Mimic)

Less Common

- Endometriosis
- Calcinosis Syndromes
- Soft Tissue Metastases
- Lymphoma and Leukemia
- Desmoid
- Sarcoma
- Rhabdomyolysis

ESSENTIAL INFORMATION

Key Differential Diagnosis Issues

- Given limitations of clinical examination, imaging plays important role in differentiating true soft tissue masses from hernias, vascular abnormalities, and normal variants
- Most soft tissue masses have nonspecific appearance and may require biopsy or excision for diagnosis

Helpful Clues for Common Diagnoses

- **Abdominal Wall Hernias**
  - **Inguinal hernia**
    - Most common external hernia, which extends into groin anterior to horizontal plane of pubic tubercle
    - Divided into direct (arises anteromedial to inferior epigastric vessels) and indirect (arises superolateral to inferior epigastric vessels) subtypes
  - **Ventral hernia**
    - Broad term describing acquired or congenital hernias through anterior and lateral abdominal wall
    - Midline hernias include epigastric (above umbilicus) and hypogastric (below umbilicus) hernias
    - Incisional hernias occur at prior surgical incision sites
  - **Umbilical hernia**
    - Hernias arising at midline in upper 1/2 of umbilical ring, which can be congenital or acquired
  - **Spigelian hernia**
    - Hernia through defect lateral to rectus sheath (inferior and lateral to umbilicus) often covered by external oblique muscle and aponeurosis
  - **Femoral hernia**
    - Groin hernia extending medial to femoral vessels with frequent compression of femoral vein
    - Most common in elderly female patients with very high risk of strangulation and incarceration
  - **Lumbar hernia**
    - Hernia through defect in lumbar muscle or thoracolumbar fascia
    - Can be congenital or acquired, with many acquired due to incisions in flank region for renal surgery
- **Abdominal Wall Abscess**
  - Loculated fluid collection (± internal gas) with peripheral enhancement and surrounding edema/fat stranding
  - Differentiate drainable abscess from diffuse, nondrainable edema/fluid (cellulitis/phlegmon)
  - Presence of gas-containing abdominal wall abscess in close contiguity with bowel tethered to abdominal wall raises possibility of enterocutaneous fistula
- **Sebaceous Cyst**
  - Common incidental finding, appearing as small, round/oval, well-encapsulated cyst near skin surface
  - Should be low density and nonenhancing without surrounding subcutaneous edema/fat stranding
- **Lipoma**
  - Common incidentally identified mass in subcutaneous tissues and between muscle planes, demonstrating uniform fat density with no internal soft tissue component
  - Differentiate from liposarcoma, which demonstrates internal complexity and soft tissue component (± visible internal blood vessels/vascularity)
  - Confident diagnosis may be difficult on US, although mass should have similar echogenicity to subcutaneous fat
- **Keloid**
  - Benign fibrotic scar tissue or tissue overgrowth at site of soft tissue injury (i.e., surgical incision or trauma)
  - Most often asymptomatic finding, although lesions can be painful or pruritic
  - No clear imaging features to allow differentiation of large keloid from other soft tissue masses
- **Hematoma**
  - Heterogeneous high-density blood products, which gradually evolve and become lower in density over time
  - More diffuse subcutaneous blood products may reflect subcutaneous ecchymosis
- **Paraumbilical Varices**
  - Common portosystemic collaterals in patients with severe cirrhosis and portal hypertension
  - Serpiginous enhancing structures that connect to recanalized paraumbilical vein near falciform ligament
  - May be directly visible or palpable at skin surface (i.e., caput medusae)
- **Injection Site**
  - Extremely common incidental finding in subcutaneous tissues of anterior abdominal wall and buttocks, usually secondary to injection of heparin, insulin, or other medications
  - Small nodular foci associated with ectopic gas, small blood, or fluid

- May chronically evolve into injection granulomas, appearing as rounded or linear foci of soft tissue or calcification (most common in buttocks)
- **Calcified Scar**
  - Heterotopic ossification (myositis ossificans traumatica) can occur at abdominal incision sites and is most common in linear alba after midline abdominal incision
  - Ossified scar in incision can resemble rib (with both cortex and medulla)
- **Muscle Asymmetry (Mimic)**
  - Asymmetric muscles frequently mistaken for mass, and are common secondary to prior surgery, paralysis, myopathy, etc.

Helpful Clues for Less Common Diagnoses

- **Endometriosis**
  - Endometriosis implants may be seen within incision sites after prior C-section or hysterectomy
  - Typically appears as solid, spiculated subcutaneous mass with variable enhancement (usually hypointense on T1WI MR and hyperintense on T2WI)
  - May be associated with clinical history of cyclical pain (corresponding with menstruation) at incision site
- **Calcinosis Syndromes**
  - Dystrophic: Significant calcifications may be seen in setting of response to tissue injury, such as implanted medical device, connective tissue diseases (scleroderma, dermatomyositis, CREST), or severe pancreatitis with fat necrosis (most often in breasts)
  - Metastatic: Seen most often in patients with calcium-phosphate imbalance (renal failure, milk-alkali syndrome)
  - Tumoral calcification: Large globular deposits of calcification near joints
- **Soft Tissue Metastases**
  - Most common malignancies to metastasize to soft tissues are melanoma and renal cell carcinoma
  - Appear as discrete soft tissue nodule or mass(es) in subcutaneous fat or muscle with enhancement similar to primary tumor
  - Easily overlooked on CT if careful survey of soft tissues not undertaken, but often more apparent on PET

- Tumor may also be implanted at site of surgery (probably more common with laparoscopic surgery)
- **Lymphoma and Leukemia**
  - Cutaneous T-cell lymphoma (also known as mycosis fungoides or Sézary syndrome)
    - Skin second most common site of extranodal lymphoma (after GI tract)
    - Skin involvement may be difficult to appreciate on imaging unless unusually nodular or mass-like
  - Subcutaneous panniculitis-like T-cell lymphoma
    - Lymphomatous involvement of subcutaneous soft tissues appearing as site of soft tissue induration/infiltration or as discrete nodules
  - Leukemia cutis (i.e., chloroma or granulocytic sarcoma)
- **Desmoid**
  - Benign, locally aggressive mesenchymal neoplasm which can be intraabdominal or extraabdominal (such as abdominal wall)
  - Abdominal wall lesions most frequently arise from rectus or oblique muscles, especially at incision sites
  - Major risk factors include prior surgery, trauma, Gardner syndrome, and familial adenomatous polyposis
  - Variable appearance, but typically solid, well-defined, hypoenhancing, heterogeneously high signal on T2WI MR, and low signal on T1WI
- **Sarcoma**
  - Malignant mesenchymal soft tissue tumors, which encompass wide range of different histological subtypes
  - May be difficult to differentiate from other soft tissue masses based on imaging alone, although most sarcomas tend to be larger and more heterogeneous with frequent necrosis (± distant metastatic disease)
- **Rhabdomyolysis**
  - Muscle necrosis in response to wide variety of causes, including crush injury, seizures, statin medications, etc.
  - Involved muscles on CT generally appear either normal or abnormally hypodense (due to edema)
  - MR more sensitive, with muscles demonstrating T2 hyperintensity and enlargement, as well as hyperenhancement (can appear ring-like or mass-like)

Inguinal Hernia

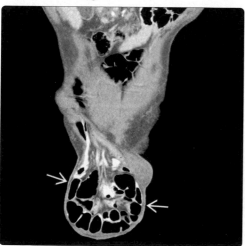

Sebaceous Cyst

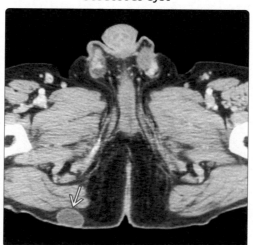

(Left) Coronal CECT demonstrates a massive right inguinal hernia ➡ containing multiple loops of nonobstructed small bowel. (Right) Axial CECT shows an encapsulated, near water density mass ➡ in the left buttock. Sebaceous cysts are a common incidental finding, and when demonstrating a classic appearance, do not require further follow-up or evaluation.

Lipoma

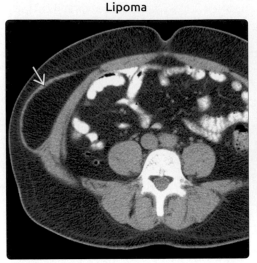

Hematoma

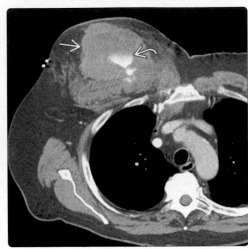

(Left) *Axial CECT demonstrates a large, fat-containing mass ➡ within the right lateral abdominal wall, compatible with a simple lipoma. Note the absence of any complexity or soft tissue component within the mass.* **(Right)** *Axial CECT in a trauma patient demonstrates a large, acute, high-density subcutaneous hematoma ➡ with evidence of considerable internal active extravasation ➡.*

Paraumbilical Varices

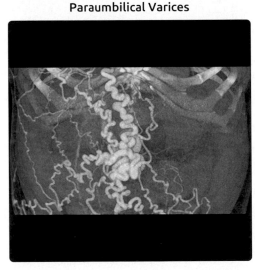

Endometriosis

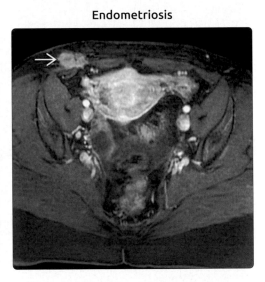

(Left) *Coronal volume-rendered CECT in a patient with cirrhosis and portal hypertension demonstrates massive subcutaneous varices overlying the anterior abdominal wall, representing a caput medusae.* **(Right)** *Axial T1 C+ MR demonstrates an enhancing nodule ➡ in the right anterior pelvic wall, found to represent a scar endometrioma in this patient status post prior laparoscopic pelvic surgery.*

Endometriosis

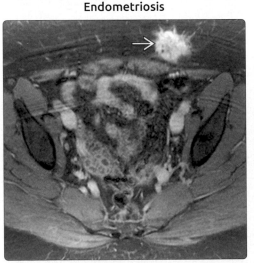

Soft Tissue Metastases

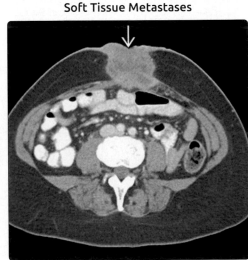

(Left) *Axial T1 C+ MR demonstrates a spiculated, enhancing mass ➡ within the left anterior pelvic wall, found to represent a scar endometrioma in this female patient with cyclical pelvic wall pain in this location.* **(Right)** *Axial CECT demonstrates a large, ill-defined, hypodense mass ➡ in the midline anterior abdominal wall, proven to represent a metastasis from the patient's known primary colon cancer.*

Soft Tissue Metastases

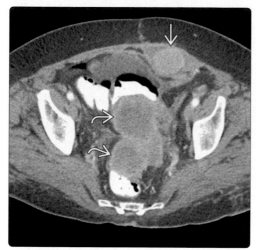

Lymphoma and Leukemia

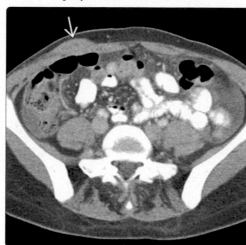

(Left) *Axial CECT in a patient with a history of cervical cancer demonstrates an enhancing metastasis ➡ in the left anterior pelvic wall, as well as additional tumor in the pelvic surgical bed ➡.* (Right) *Axial CECT demonstrates a biopsy-proven chloroma ➡ in the right anterior abdominal wall in a patient with known leukemia.*

Desmoid

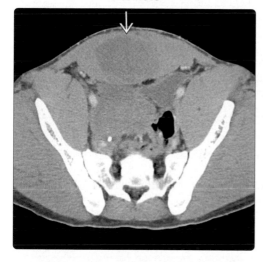

Desmoid

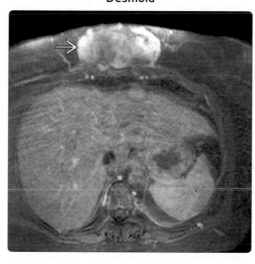

(Left) *Axial CECT demonstrates a large hypodense mass ➡ in the anterior pelvic wall in a patient with known familial polyposis, found to represent a large desmoid tumor.* (Right) *Axial T1 C+ FS MR demonstrates a large, avidly enhancing mass ➡ in the anterior chest wall, found to represent a large desmoid tumor. Desmoid tumors can demonstrate variable enhancement, and in some cases, can be quite avidly enhancing.*

Sarcoma

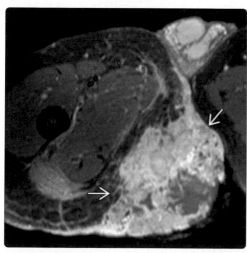

Sarcoma

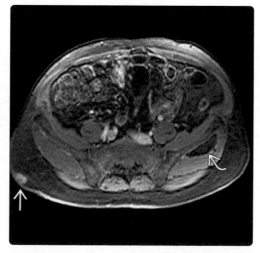

(Left) *Axial T1 C+ FS MR demonstrates a highly invasive, large tumor in the buttock ➡, which enhances significantly. This lesion proved on biopsy to be a high-grade epithelioid sarcoma.* (Right) *Axial T1 C+ FS MR shows a small enhancing lesion ➡ in the superficial gluteal region. This was found to be an extraskeletal soft tissue Ewing sarcoma. Incidentally, a deep left gluteal lipoma ➡ has signal characteristics similar to normal subcutaneous fat.*

DIFFERENTIAL DIAGNOSIS

Common

- Iliopsoas Hematoma
- Asymmetric Musculature (Mimic)
- Secondary Infection/Abscess

Less Common

- Retroperitoneal Fibrosis
- Primary Infection
- Primary Neoplasm
- Secondary Neoplasm

ESSENTIAL INFORMATION

Key Differential Diagnosis Issues

- Iliopsoas compartment masses are much more likely to result from infection or hemorrhage, rather than tumor
- Iliopsoas pathology often due to spread from adjacent infection (such as spine) or adjacent tumor, rather than originating within iliopsoas itself

Helpful Clues for Common Diagnoses

- **Iliopsoas Hematoma**
  - Iliopsoas is most common site for spontaneous retroperitoneal hemorrhage (usually due to bleeding diathesis or anticoagulation)
    - Presence of multiple hematocrit levels within hematoma suggests coagulopathic hemorrhage
  - Other causes include surgery, trauma, or extension of bleeding from adjacent structures (e.g., bleeding renal AML, ruptured abdominal aortic aneurysm, etc.)
  - Appearance variable depending on age of hematoma
    - Acute bleeding may simply appear as homogeneous enlargement of muscle ± hematocrit levels
    - Chronic bleeds may appear hypodense and can be difficult to differentiate from abscess
- **Asymmetric Musculature (Mimic)**
  - Iliopsoas muscles can be asymmetric in size, particularly in patients with unilateral leg amputation, paralysis, or lower extremity/spine arthritis

- **Secondary Infection/Abscess**
  - Infection and abscess formation in iliopsoas typically due to spread of infection from contiguous structures
    - Most commonly infectious spread from bone, kidney, and bowel (including appendix)
      - Paraspinal psoas abscess should prompt careful search for infectious spondylitis (TB or pyogenic)
      - Renal sources of iliopsoas infection include renal/perirenal abscess or xanthogranulomatous pyelonephritis
      - Common bowel sources of iliopsoas infection include appendicitis, diverticulitis, or Crohn disease
    - Often associated with other features of infection (fat stranding, blurring of fat planes, ectopic gas)

Helpful Clues for Less Common Diagnoses

- **Retroperitoneal Fibrosis**
  - Irregular soft tissue mass enveloping aorta, IVC, and ureters, which can involve adjacent psoas muscles
  - Variable enhancement depending on stage, with hyperenhancement in early stages of disease and hypoenhancement in later stages
- **Primary Infection**
  - Iliopsoas compartment is rarely primary site of infection, except in immunocompromised patients (including HIV) and intravenous drug abusers
    - Infection usually due to *Staphylococcus aureus* and mixed gram-negative organisms
- **Primary Neoplasm**
  - Primary mesenchymal tumors (liposarcoma, fibrosarcoma, leiomyosarcoma, hemangiopericytoma, etc.) may rarely originate from iliopsoas compartment
- **Secondary Neoplasm**
  - Hematogenous metastasis (e.g., lymphoma, melanoma) to iliopsoas very rare
  - More commonly directly invaded by adjacent tumors (e.g., retroperitoneal sarcoma, lymphoma, neurogenic tumors, adjacent bone tumor, etc.)
  - Plexiform neurofibroma (in neurofibromatosis) may involve psoas compartment

Iliopsoas Hematoma

Iliopsoas Hematoma

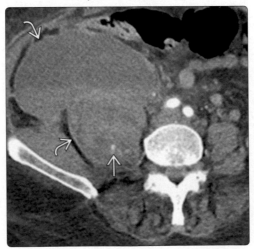

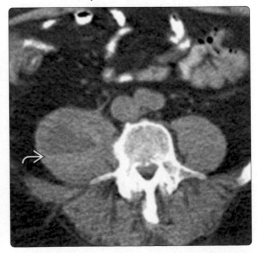

(Left) Axial CECT demonstrates a large hematoma ⇥ extending from the psoas muscle into the adjacent right abdomen. Note the presence of a tiny focus of active extravasation ➡ within the hematoma. (Right) Axial NECT demonstrates enlargement of the right psoas muscle due to coagulopathic hemorrhage. Although the hematoma is partly isodense to the muscle, the presence of a hematocrit level ⇥ makes the bleed more apparent. Hematocrit levels suggest coagulopathy as the underlying cause of the bleed.

Asymmetric Musculature (Mimic)

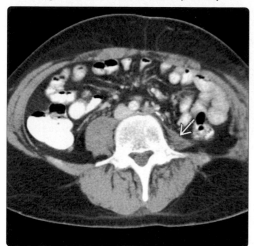

Secondary Infection/Abscess

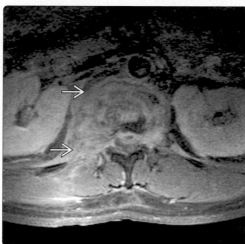

(Left) Axial CECT shows marked asymmetry of the psoas muscles. In this case, the left psoas muscle ➡ is atrophic due to a prior left leg amputation. (Right) Axial T1 C+ FS MR at the level of the renal hilum shows predominantly right-sided enhancing paraspinal and epidural phlegmon ➡, associated with discitis and vertebral osteomyelitis. The presence of psoas infection should always prompt careful appraisal of the spine.

Secondary Infection/Abscess

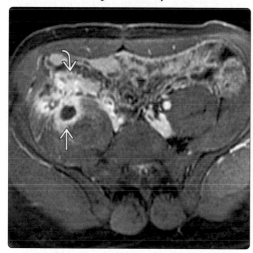

Retroperitoneal Fibrosis

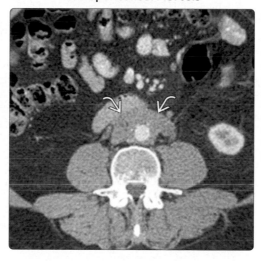

(Left) Axial T1 C+ MR demonstrates an abscess ➡ in the iliopsoas muscle directly contiguous with phlegmonous change ➡ in the right lower quadrant due to the patient's fistulizing Crohn disease. (Right) Axial CECT demonstrates a rind of soft tissue ➡ encasing the aorta and IVC, a classic appearance for retroperitoneal fibrosis.

Primary Neoplasm

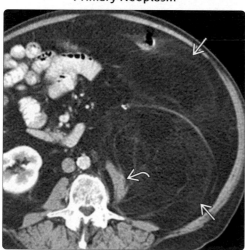

Secondary Neoplasm

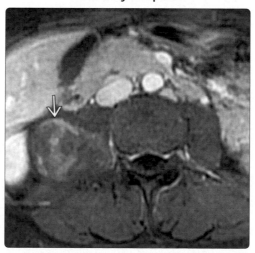

(Left) Axial CECT demonstrates a large, fat-containing mass ➡ occupying much of the left abdomen, with the left psoas muscle ➡ appearing stretched and distorted as a result of the retroperitoneal tumor. This was found to be a well-differentiated liposarcoma at resection. (Right) Axial T1 C+ FS MR demonstrates a heterogeneously enhancing mass ➡ expanding the right psoas muscle, found to be a neurogenic tumor (ganglioneuroma) at resection.

DIFFERENTIAL DIAGNOSIS

Common

- Inguinal Hernia
- Femoral Hernia
- Groin Hematoma
- Groin Pseudoaneurysm
- Inguinal Lymphadenopathy
- Varicocele

Less Common

- Cryptorchidism
- Groin Aneurysm
- Iliopsoas Bursitis
- Bone Tumor
- Inguinal Abscess

ESSENTIAL INFORMATION

Key Differential Diagnosis Issues

- Although clinical exam may diagnose many common groin masses (particularly hernias), imaging often necessary for accurate diagnosis, particularly with atypical masses
  - US 1st-line modality for vascular & male reproductive (e.g., cryptorchidism, varicocele) abnormalities
  - CT and US are best options for diagnosis of groin hernias
  - CT or MR appropriate for suspected musculoskeletal lesions, such as bursitis or bone tumor

Helpful Clues for Common Diagnoses

- **Inguinal Hernia**
  - Divided into **direct** or **indirect** subtypes based on relationship to inferior epigastric vessels
  - Typically located anterior to horizontal plane of pubic tubercle with no significant mass effect on femoral vein
- **Femoral Hernia**
  - Almost always diagnosed in elderly women
  - Extends medial to femoral vein and inferior to inferior epigastric vessels with mass effect on femoral vessels
  - Hernia sac located posterior and lateral to pubic tubercle
  - Highest strangulation rate among groin hernias (25-40%)

- **Groin Hematoma**
  - Most often encountered after groin catheterization, and should prompt search for underlying pseudoaneurysm or active extravasation
- **Groin Pseudoaneurysm**
  - Most often encountered after groin catheterization
  - US demonstrates cystic structure connecting to femoral artery with internal yin-yang biphasic flow
- **Inguinal Lymphadenopathy**
  - Lymph nodes are usually mobile and easily distinguished from hernia based on clinical exam alone, although imaging can easily make distinction in difficult cases
- **Varicocele**
  - Can extend into inguinal canal (as can hydrocele) and may be thought to represent mass on clinical exam
  - US demonstrates tangle of mildly dilated vessels (≥ 3 mm) with slow flow and enlargement during Valsalva

Helpful Clues for Less Common Diagnoses

- **Cryptorchidism**
  - Undescended testicle (which usually are found in vicinity of groin/inguinal canal) can be palpated on physical exam in vast majority of cases
  - US or MR are 1st-line imaging modalities, with MR offering ability to identify intraabdominal testicle
- **Groin Aneurysm**
  - True atherosclerotic aneurysms of common femoral artery are rare and often associated with aneurysms elsewhere (especially aorta and popliteal arteries)
- **Iliopsoas Bursitis**
  - Focal teardrop-shaped collection of fluid immediately anterior to hip joint typically associated with hip joint pathology (such as degeneration, infection, etc.)
- **Bone Tumor**
  - Any benign or malignant primary bone tumor arising from pubic rami or hip can present as groin mass, with CT and MR best initial modalities for evaluation
- **Inguinal Abscess**
  - Focal rim-enhancing fluid collection with surrounding stranding and edema in patient with clinical signs and symptoms of infection

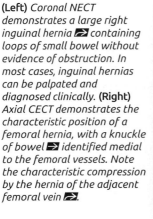

(Left) Coronal NECT demonstrates a large right inguinal hernia ➱ containing loops of small bowel without evidence of obstruction. In most cases, inguinal hernias can be palpated and diagnosed clinically. (Right) Axial CECT demonstrates the characteristic position of a femoral hernia, with a knuckle of bowel ➱ identified medial to the femoral vessels. Note the characteristic compression by the hernia of the adjacent femoral vein ➱.

Inguinal Hernia

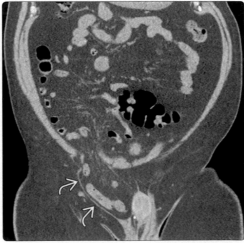

Femoral Hernia

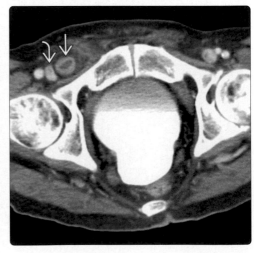

Groin Hematoma

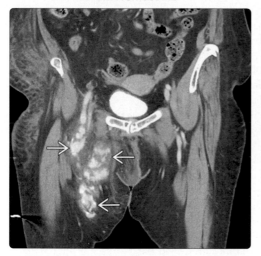

Groin Pseudoaneurysm

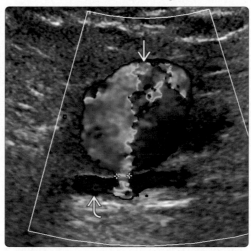

(Left) *Coronal CECT demonstrates a large right groin hematoma with massive active extravasation of contrast* ➡. *This patient had recently undergone a complicated right groin catheterization with subsequent severe blood loss.* (Right) *Color Doppler US in a patient who had undergone recent groin catheterization shows the characteristic features of a pseudoaneurysm* ➡ *with a yin-yang pattern of internal color flow. Notice that the pseudoaneurysm does appear to connect with the adjacent femoral artery* ➡.

Inguinal Lymphadenopathy

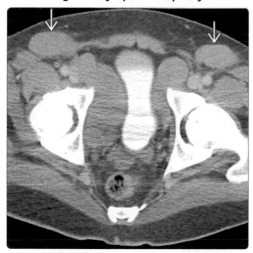

Varicocele

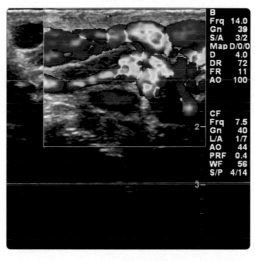

(Left) *Axial NECT in a patient with lymphoma demonstrates extensive pelvic and inguinal lymphadenopathy* ➡, *with resultant compression of the bladder.* (Right) *Sagittal color Doppler ultrasound shows a classic tangle of tortuous vessels within the upper part of the scrotum. Flow and vessel dilation are accentuated by Valsalva maneuver, characteristic of a varicocele.*

Cryptorchidism

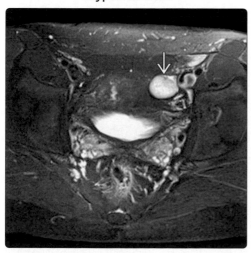

Iliopsoas Bursitis

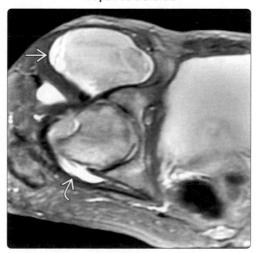

(Left) *Axial T2 FS MR in a patient with an undescended left testicle demonstrates the T2 bright testicle* ➡ *in the left pelvis. MR is the best modality for identifying an undescended testicle, with an advantage over US for identifying testicles in the abdominal/pelvic cavities.* (Right) *Axial T2 FS MR in a patient with rheumatoid arthritis involvement of the right hip demonstrates the classic appearance of iliopsoas bursitis, with a fluid collection* ➡ *containing debris anterior to the right hip. Note the adjacent hip effusion* ➡.

DIFFERENTIAL DIAGNOSIS

Common

- Paralyzed Diaphragm
- Eventration of Diaphragm
- Hiatal Hernia
- Bochdalek Hernia
- Morgagni Hernia
- Traumatic Diaphragmatic Hernia
- Subdiaphragmatic Mass
- Abdominal Abscess
- Unilateral Lung Volume Loss
- Subpulmonic Pleural Effusion (Mimic)

ESSENTIAL INFORMATION

Key Differential Diagnosis Issues

- Axial CT suboptimal for distinguishing diaphragm from spleen, liver, and muscle and identifying many diaphragmatic abnormalities
  - Multiplanar reformations critical for accurate diagnosis
- Diaphragm easier to visualize discretely on MR compared to CT and can demonstrate diaphragm in multiple planes
- Fluoroscopy and ultrasound useful for providing functional information, particularly for paralysis
  - Dynamic MR (not widely utilized) can provide functional information similar to US or fluoroscopy

Helpful Clues for Common Diagnoses

- **Paralyzed Diaphragm**
  - Normal diaphragm that fails to contract secondary to abnormalities of brain, spinal cord, neuromuscular junction, phrenic nerve, or muscle
  - US or fluoroscopy demonstrate no motion or paradoxical (upward) motion during inspiration or sniff test
- **Eventration of Diaphragm**
  - Congenital thinning/weakness of portion of diaphragm, which normally attaches to costal margin
  - Eccentric diaphragmatic contour (usually anteromedial right hemidiaphragm) ± paradoxical motion with large eventrations

- **Hiatal Hernia**
  - Herniation of abdominal contents into thoracic cavity through esophageal hiatus
  - Divided into sliding type (GE junction displaced upward through hiatus) and paraesophageal type (GE junction in normal location with stomach herniating above diaphragm)
- **Bochdalek Hernia**
  - Type of congenital diaphragmatic hernia due to defect in posterolateral diaphragm (usually on left side)
  - Hernia may contain retroperitoneal fat, bowel, kidney, stomach, spleen, or liver
- **Morgagni Hernia**
  - Type of congenital diaphragmatic hernia due to defect in retrosternal diaphragm (usually on right side)
  - Usually located in right cardiophrenic angle and most often contains just omental fat (but can contain colon, liver, small bowel, or stomach)
- **Traumatic Diaphragmatic Hernia**
  - Traumatic injury may be due to blunt or penetrating trauma
  - Multiple imaging signs of injury include dependent viscus sign, collar sign, and dangling diaphragm sign
  - Injuries both above and below diaphragm should raise concern for diaphragmatic injury
- **Subdiaphragmatic Mass**
  - Tumor, hepatomegaly, or splenomegaly can exert mass effect and raise ipsilateral diaphragm
- **Abdominal Abscess**
  - Subphrenic abscess can cause upward displacement of diaphragm due to mass effect, as well as due to splinting (decreased motion of diaphragm due to pain)
- **Unilateral Lung Volume Loss**
  - Diminished unilateral lung volume (lung resection, atelectasis) will cause elevation of ipsilateral diaphragm
- **Subpulmonic Pleural Effusion (Mimic)**
  - Pleural fluid loculated in subpulmonic pleural space will displace lung upward and may simulate elevated diaphragm on radiographs (but not on cross-sectional imaging)

Paralyzed Diaphragm

Eventration of Diaphragm

(Left) Coronal CECT demonstrates marked asymmetric elevation of the left hemidiaphragm. In this case, the left diaphragm 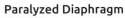 *is paralyzed as a result of phrenic nerve involvement by a mediastinal soft tissue mass* ⟫ *in this patient with metastatic lung cancer.* **(Right)** *Coronal CECT demonstrates the characteristic appearance of diaphragmatic eventration, with focal scalloping of the right anterior hemidiaphragm and superior protrusion of the liver at the site of eventration* ➡.

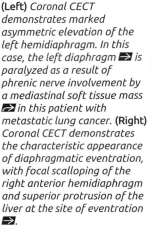
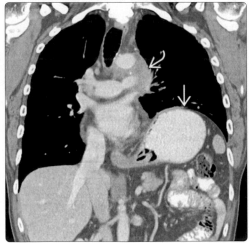
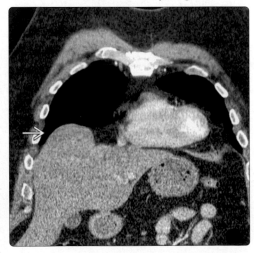

Hiatal Hernia

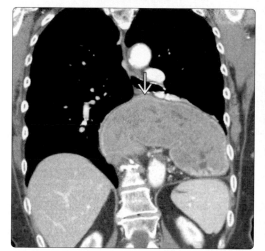

Bochdalek Hernia

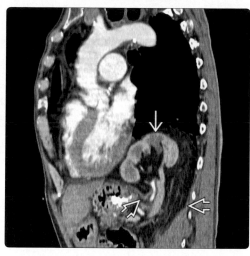

(Left) Coronal CECT demonstrates a large hiatal hernia with the entirety of the stomach ➡ located within the thoracic cavity. (Right) Sagittal CECT demonstrates a large Bochdalek hernia containing bowel and kidney. There is focal interruption of the hemidiaphragm ➡ with herniation of the kidney ➡ into the thorax.

Morgagni Hernia

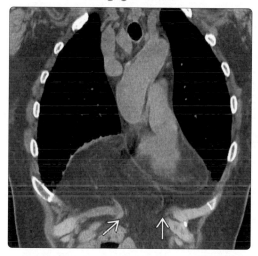

Traumatic Diaphragmatic Hernia

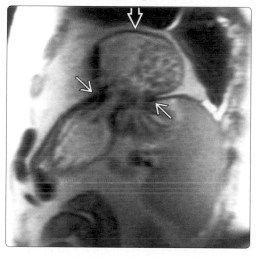

(Left) Coronal NECT shows a characteristic Morgagni hernia, with omental fat herniating into the chest through a defect ➡ in the right anteromedial diaphragm. (Right) Sagittal T2 MR demonstrates a posttraumatic defect ➡ in the left hemidiaphragm with the stomach ➡ herniating into the chest. Note that the diaphragm is identified as a low-signal curvilinear structure. The stomach is pinched as it traverses the defect in the diaphragm.

Traumatic Diaphragmatic Hernia

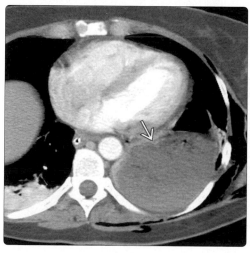

Subpulmonic Pleural Effusion (Mimic)

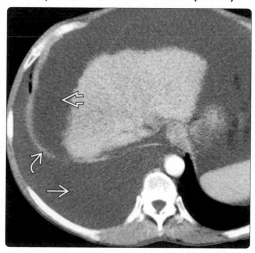

(Left) Axial CECT illustrates the fallen viscus sign associated with traumatic diaphragmatic injury. Note that the stomach ➡ lies in the chest and has fallen medially and posteriorly to lie against the lung and the posteromedial chest wall. (Right) Axial CECT shows a pleural effusion ➡ below the lung and lateral to the diaphragm ➡. Ascites ➡ lies medial to the diaphragm and adjacent to the cirrhotic liver.

DIFFERENTIAL DIAGNOSIS

Common

- Inguinal Hernia
- Femoral Hernia
- Ventral Hernia
  - Incisional Hernia
  - Hypogastric Hernia
  - Epigastric Hernia
- Spigelian Hernia
- Lumbar Hernia
- Umbilical Hernia
- Subcutaneous Abdominal Wall Mass (Mimic)
  - Subcutaneous Hematoma (Mimic)
  - Subcutaneous Abscess (Mimic)
  - Inguinal Lymphadenopathy (Mimic)
  - Soft Tissue Neoplasm (Mimic)
  - Cryptorchidism (Mimic)
- Enterocutaneous Fistula (Mimic)

Less Common

- Obturator Hernia
- Traumatic Abdominal Wall Hernia
- Sciatic Hernia
- Perineal Hernia
- Spermatic Cord Lipoma or Liposarcoma (Mimic)

ESSENTIAL INFORMATION

Key Differential Diagnosis Issues

- CT is most accurate imaging modality for diagnosis of hernias and associated complications
- US can be helpful for determining reducibility of hernias, as well as diagnosis of hernias which are transiently reducible
  - Offers advantage of scanning patient in upright position or with Valsalva maneuver to elicit hernia
  - Efficacy of US for hernias is debatable in literature, and CT should certainly be first-line modality in patients with acute presentation or concerns for hernia-related complications
    - US should be reserved for nonurgent presentation in outpatient setting
- Evaluate any hernia for presence of complications, including bowel involvement, obstruction, and ischemia
  - Different types of hernias are associated with very different risks of complications
- Descriptive terms used to describe abdominal wall hernias
  - **Interparietal** (i.e., interstitial) hernia: Hernia sac is located in fascial planes between abdominal wall muscles without entering subcutaneous soft tissues
  - **Richter** hernia: Entirety of bowel circumference does not herniate (just antimesenteric border of bowel)

Helpful Clues for Common Diagnoses

- **Inguinal Hernia**
  - Most common type of external hernia (~ 80%), with indirect hernias typically congenital (due to weakness of processus vaginalis) and direct hernias usually acquired due to abdominal wall weakness
    - Hernia seen in groin region anterior to horizontal plane of pubic tubercle

- Do not result in compression of femoral vessels (unlike femoral hernia)
  - **Direct** hernias: Hernia sac arises anteromedial to inferior epigastric vessels
  - **Indirect** hernia: Hernia sac arises superomedial to inferior epigastric vessels
    - 5x more common than direct hernias
    - Complications more common with indirect hernias
- **Femoral Hernia**
  - Most commonly seen in elderly female patients (especially > 80 yr), but much less common than inguinal hernias
  - Hernia extends into femoral canal medial to femoral vein and inferior to inferior epigastric vessels, with frequent compression of femoral vein
  - Hernia sac located posterior and lateral to pubic tubercle
  - Very high risk of complications (incarceration, strangulation) and mortality compared to inguinal hernias
- **Ventral Hernia**
  - General term encompassing hernias extending through anterior and lateral abdominal wall
    - Can be acquired or congenital
  - **Epigastric** hernias occur at midline through linea alba above umbilicus, while **hypogastric** hernias occur at midline below umbilicus
  - **Incisional** hernias occur through any prior surgical incision site
    - Most often occur within a few months (usually first 4 months) of surgery, but can occur at later time points as well
    - Parastomal hernias (considered type of incisional hernia) are quite common adjacent to ileostomy or colostomy
  - Even if asymptomatic, most ventral hernias get larger over time with increasing risk of complications, making surgical treatment advisable
- **Spigelian Hernia**
  - Hernia extending through defect in aponeurosis of internal oblique and transverse abdominal muscles
  - Arise along lateral margin of rectus abdominis muscles, at level of arcuate line, inferior and lateral to umbilicus
  - Usually congenital in children and acquired in adults (prior surgery, obesity, pregnancies, etc. are risk factors)
  - High risk of strangulation and incarceration
- **Lumbar Hernia**
  - Hernia extends through defect in lumbar muscle or thoracolumbar fascia (usually below 12th rib and above iliac crest)
    - Can herniate through superior (Grynfeltt-Lesshaft) or inferior (petit) lumbar triangles
  - Most (80%) are acquired, usually due to surgical incisions (especially renal surgery)
  - Complications uncommon due to typically large neck, which makes incarceration/strangulation uncommon
- **Umbilical Hernia**
  - Hernia at midline extends through umbilical ring (usually upper 1/2 of umbilicus)
  - Can be congenital (diagnosed in infancy) or acquired (usually in middle age)

– Congenital type 8x more common in African Americans, but most resolve spontaneously by 4-6 yr of age

– Acquired hernias associated with obesity, multiparity, and ascites

o Very common and usually small/asymptomatic, but larger or symptomatic hernias may require repair

- **Subcutaneous Abdominal Wall Mass (Mimic)**
  o Any subcutaneous or intramuscular mass may be superficially mistaken for hernia on clinical examination, although distinction should be obvious on imaging
  o Consider inguinal lymphadenopathy, abdominal wall tumors, cryptorchidism (especially in children), abscess, hydrocele, varicocele, or hematoma as entities that may be mistaken for hernia on physical examination

- **Enterocutaneous Fistula (Mimic)**
  o Gas- or contrast-filled tract from intraabdominal bowel loop into anterior abdominal wall may be confused for hernia
    – Bowel loops often tethered to anterior abdominal wall at site of fistula
  o Careful examination illustrates lack of true abdominal wall defect

Helpful Clues for Less Common Diagnoses

- **Obturator Hernia**
  o Rare type of hernia extending through obturator foramen into superolateral obturator canal
    – Usually involves loop of ileum but can involve any pelvic viscera
  o Typically seen in elderly female patients (especially older or multiparous females) secondary to either pelvic floor defect or pelvic floor laxity
  o High risk of complications (incarceration, strangulation) and mortality

- **Traumatic Abdominal Wall Hernia**
  o Hernia in anterior abdominal wall developing at site of focal trauma
  o Majority occur in lower abdomen, with iliac crest region very common due to seat belt injuries

o Most commonly seen in young children < 10 yr due to bicycle handlebar injury (e.g., handlebar hernia), but can also be seen in adults after high-energy trauma (e.g., motor vehicle collisions)

- **Sciatic Hernia**
  o Very uncommon hernia involving herniation of bowel loop through greater sciatic foramen laterally into subgluteal region
  o Occurs most often in females, likely as a result of piriformis muscle atrophy

- **Perineal Hernia**
  o Uncommon hernia with hernia sac extending anteriorly through urogenital diaphragm (most common) or posteriorly between levator ani and coccygeus muscles
  o Usually diagnosed in older female patients (> 50 yr) with history of prior surgery in deep pelvis/perineum, prior pregnancies, obesity, or ascites

- **Spermatic Cord Lipoma or Liposarcoma (Mimic)**
  o Uncommon fat-containing mass arising in spermatic cord, which can extend into scrotum inferiorly or inguinal canal/retroperitoneum superiorly
  o When extending into inguinal canal, can mimic inguinal hernia, but lesion typically appears expansile and mass-like
  o Liposarcomas will often demonstrate internal complexity (or even soft tissue component) depending on degree of dedifferentiation
    – Well-differentiated liposarcomas may appear largely fat attenuation and are more apt to be confused for inguinal hernia containing omental fat
    – Usually appear hyperechoic on ultrasound (particularly when well differentiated) with similar echogenicity to subcutaneous fat

Inguinal Hernia

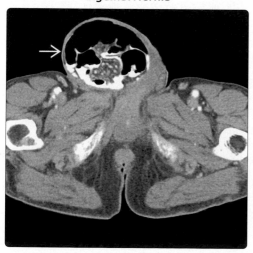

Inguinal Hernia

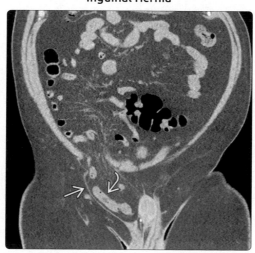

(Left) *Axial CECT demonstrates a large right inguinal hernia ➡ containing multiple loops of small bowel without evidence of obstruction. Inguinal hernias account for the vast majority of external hernias.* **(Right)** *Coronal NECT demonstrates a classic right inguinal hernia ➡ containing loops of small bowel ➡ without evidence of obstruction.*

Femoral Hernia

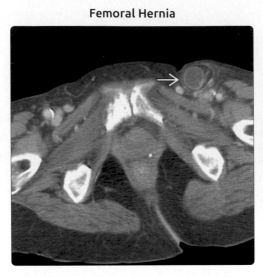

Ventral Hernia

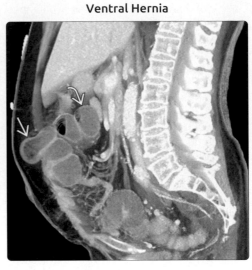

(Left) *Axial CECT demonstrates a herniated bowel loop ➡ in the left groin. Note the close relationship of the hernia to the femoral vessels at the level of the symphysis pubis, characteristic of a femoral hernia.* **(Right)** *Sagittal volume-rendered CECT demonstrates a ventral hernia containing loops of small bowel ➡. The small bowel proximal to the hernia sac is dilated ➡, compatible with small bowel obstruction.*

Epigastric Hernia

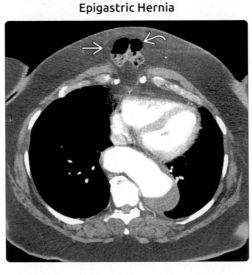

Spigelian Hernia

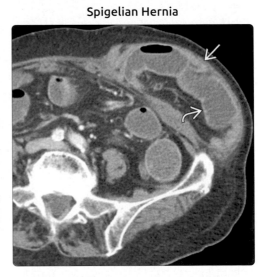

(Left) *Axial CECT in a patient with a history of prior thoracic surgery demonstrates a ventral hernia ➡ arising in the upper abdomen containing a loop of colon ➡. Ventral hernias occurring above the umbilicus, as in this case, are termed epigastric hernias.* **(Right)** *Axial CECT demonstrates a left abdominal spigelian hernia ➡ with multiple dilated loops of small bowel ➡, compatible with small bowel obstruction.*

Lumbar Hernia

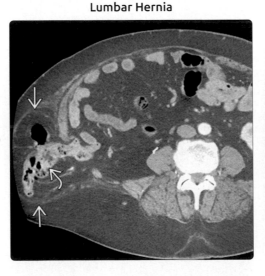

Lumbar Hernia

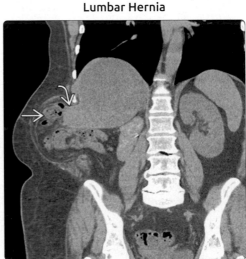

(Left) *Axial CECT demonstrates a large lumbar hernia ➡ in the right flank containing a loop of colon ➡.* **(Right)** *Coronal NECT demonstrates a large lumbar hernia containing colon ➡, as well as a portion of the right hepatic lobe ➡. Lumbar hernias are often secondary to prior surgical incisions and are particularly common after renal surgeries.*

Umbilical Hernia

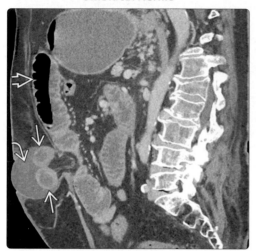

Enterocutaneous Fistula (Mimic)

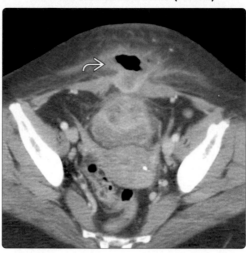

(Left) *Sagittal CECT demonstrates an umbilical hernia containing a thickened loop of small bowel ➡ and ascites ➡. The small bowel ➡ proximal to the hernia sac is dilated and obstructed. The bowel within the hernia sac was found to be ischemic at surgery.* **(Right)** *Axial CECT demonstrates an abdominal wall abscess ➡ due to a fistula (sinus tract) from sigmoid diverticulitis. Prior to imaging, the presumptive diagnosis based on clinical examination was ventral hernia.*

Obturator Hernia

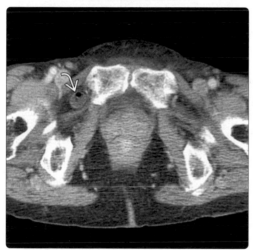

Traumatic Abdominal Wall Hernia

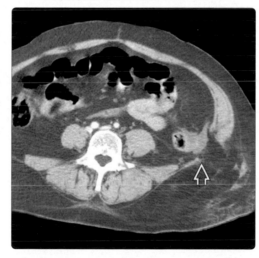

(Left) *Axial CECT demonstrates a loop of small bowel ➡ lying between the obturator externus and pectineus muscles, compatible with an obturator hernia.* **(Right)** *Axial CECT in a trauma patient shows disruption of the musculofascial plane ➡ near the insertion into the iliac crest and thoracolumbar fascia. Note the presence of adjacent subcutaneous hematoma. The spleen was also lacerated (not shown). These findings are compatible with a traumatic hernia.*

Spermatic Cord Lipoma or Liposarcoma (Mimic)

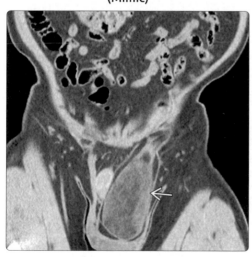

Spermatic Cord Lipoma or Liposarcoma (Mimic)

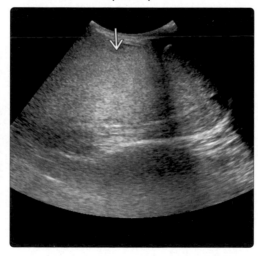

(Left) *Coronal NECT demonstrates a large, mixed-attenuation mass (with a clear fatty component) ➡ extending through the inguinal canal into the left scrotum. This was found to be a spermatic cord liposarcoma at resection.* **(Right)** *Sagittal US in the same patient demonstrates that the mass ➡ is very echogenic as a result of its fatty component, a fairly common appearance for these lesions.*

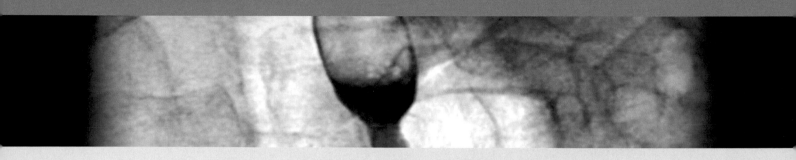

Generic Imaging Patterns

Clinically Based Differentials

DIFFERENTIAL DIAGNOSIS

Common

- Esophageal Carcinoma
- Esophageal Foreign Body
- Intramural Benign Esophageal Tumors

Less Common

- Thrombosed Esophageal Varix
- Inflammatory Polyp, Esophagus
- *Candida* Esophagitis
- Viral Esophagitis
- Papilloma, Esophagus

Rare but Important

- Fibrovascular Polyp
- Esophageal Metastases and Lymphoma
- Esophageal Adenoma
- Esophageal Gastrointestinal Stromal Tumor

ESSENTIAL INFORMATION

Key Differential Diagnosis Issues

- Intraluminal masses usually have irregular surface and acute angles with wall

Helpful Clues for Common Diagnoses

- **Esophageal Carcinoma**
  - Most common tumor of esophagus
  - Luminal narrowing with nodular, ulcerated mucosa
- **Esophageal Foreign Body**
  - Check for history of sudden onset of dysphagia
  - Usually lodges just above point of physiologic or pathologic narrowing
    - e.g., Schatzki ring, web, or carcinoma
  - Repeat barium esophagram or endoscopy after removal or passage of foreign body
- **Intramural Benign Esophageal Tumors**
  - Leiomyoma > lipoma > gastrointestinal stromal tumor > neuroma and others

- Peristalsis may draw mass into esophageal lumen, simulating intraluminal mass
- Overlying mucosa may ulcerate

Helpful Clues for Less Common Diagnoses

- **Thrombosed Esophageal Varix**
  - May be indistinguishable from carcinoma (varicoid carcinoma)
  - Look for confirmatory evidence of cirrhosis and portal hypertension
  - Check medical record for history of attempts at variceal ablation
- **Inflammatory Polyp, Esophagus**
  - Polypoid protuberance just above esophagogastric junction
  - Appears as single, prominent fold or rounded mass
  - Associated with hiatal hernia, reflux
- *Candida* **or Viral Esophagitis**
  - May result in intraluminal sloughed cells, organisms, and debris that appear as mass
  - Usually occurs in immune-suppressed patient
    - Opportunistic infections
- **Papilloma, Esophagus**
  - Benign; small (0.5- to 1.5-cm diameter)

Helpful Clues for Rare Diagnoses

- **Fibrovascular Polyp**
  - Rare benign mass arises from cervical esophagus but grows into giant, sausage-like polypoid mass that may fill much of esophageal lumen
  - CT may show elements of fat and soft tissue within mass
  - Patients may have history of regurgitating sausage-like mass
- **Esophageal Metastases and Lymphoma**
  - Gastric or lung cancer may extend into wall or lumen of esophagus
  - Other metastases and lymphoma are rare
- **Esophageal Gastrointestinal Stromal Tumor**
  - Usual appearance is that of intramural mass

(Left) Spot film from an esophagram shows a mass in the distal esophagus, with the tumor causing a filling defect ➔ and the ulceration a collection of barium ➔ within the mass. (Right) Film from an esophagram shows a filling defect ➔ within the distal esophagus and complete obstruction to distal flow of the barium. Endoscopic finding was a piece of meat stuck above a Schatzki ring.

Esophageal Carcinoma

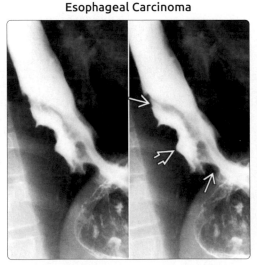

Esophageal Foreign Body

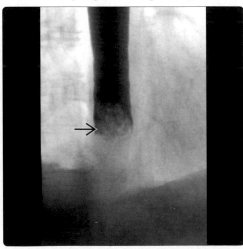

Thrombosed Esophageal Varix

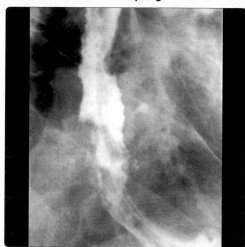

Inflammatory Polyp, Esophagus

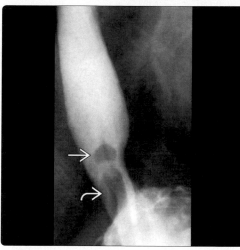

(Left) *Spot film from an esophagram shows fixed irregular luminal narrowing that mimics a large mass. These are thrombosed esophageal varices.* **(Right)** *Spot film from an esophagram shows a polypoid lesion in the distal esophagus ➡ that is contiguous with a nodular, thickened fold ↪ that traverses the esophagogastric junction.*

Candida Esophagitis

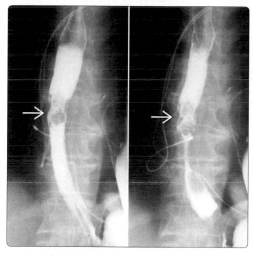

Candida Esophagitis

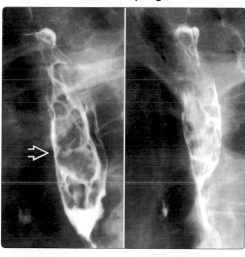

(Left) *Spot film from an esophagram shows an irregular filling defect ➡ closely simulating an esophageal cancer. At endoscopy, this was a mass of inflammatory debris in a patient with Candida esophagitis.* **(Right)** *Oblique esophagram shows a huge mass ➡ that originates in the cervical esophagus and fills most of the lumen.*

Esophageal Metastases and Lymphoma

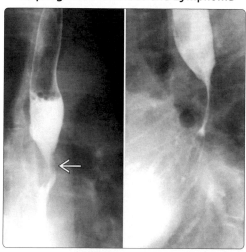

Esophageal Metastases and Lymphoma

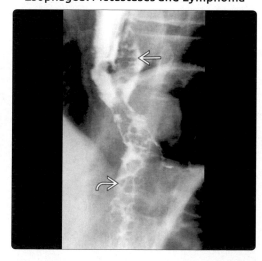

(Left) *Esophagram shows abrupt narrowing of the midesophagus. The tapered margins and intact mucosal folds ➡ correctly suggest an extrinsic process, lung cancer, rather than primary tumor.* **(Right)** *Spot film from an esophagram shows nodular thickened folds in the distal esophagus ➡, simulating a primary esophageal carcinoma. However, nodular folds are also present within the stomach ↪, suggesting the correct diagnosis of gastric fundal carcinoma, with invasion into the esophagus.*

DIFFERENTIAL DIAGNOSIS

Common

- Left Main Bronchus
- Aortic Arch
- Aortic Aneurysm
- Heart
- Cervical or Thoracic Osteophytes
- Hiatal Hernia
- Mediastinal Lymph Nodes
- Aberrant Subclavian Artery
- Enlarged Thyroid

Less Common

- Intramural (Mesenchymal) Esophageal Tumors
- Esophageal Carcinoma (Mimic)
- Gastric Carcinoma (Mimic)
- Esophageal Varices
- Bronchogenic Cyst
- Metastases and Lymphoma, Esophageal

ESSENTIAL INFORMATION

Key Differential Diagnosis Issues

- Extrinsic lesions: Smooth, intact mucosa and obtuse angles at indentation
- Entire lumen may be displaced or compressed
- Extrinsic masses are usually easily recognized on CT
  - Multiplanar reformations are especially helpful

Helpful Clues for Common Diagnoses

- **Left Main Bronchus & Aortic Arch**
  - Normal indentations along left lateral margin
  - Most apparent in left posterior oblique position
- **Aortic Aneurysm**
  - Usually indents distal esophagus obliquely, just above diaphragm
- **Heart**
  - Especially if enlarged
  - Displaces distal 1/3 of esophagus posteriorly

- **Hiatal Hernia**
  - Paraesophageal hernias displace or compress esophagus
- **Mediastinal Lymph Nodes**
  - Enlarged by benign or malignant disease
  - Usually most apparent in midesophagus
- **Aberrant Subclavian Artery**
  - Either aberrant right or left subclavian artery may compress posterior wall of esophagus
  - Easily recognized on CECT
- **Enlarged Thyroid**
  - Goiter may extend into mediastinum
    - Look for cervicothoracic mass with increased attenuation on CT

Helpful Clues for Less Common Diagnoses

- **Intramural (Mesenchymal) Esophageal Tumors**
  - Leiomyoma, gastrointestinal stromal tumor, lipoma, etc.
  - Often difficult on barium esophagram to distinguish extrinsic from intramural mass
    - Classic finding for intramural mass would be smooth mucosal surface; right angle interface with lumen
  - Usually easier with CT
- **Esophageal Carcinoma (Mimic)**
  - Submucosal extension and mediastinal spread may mimic extrinsic lesion
- **Gastric Carcinoma (Mimic)**
  - Spread into submucosal esophagus & thoracic nodes
- **Esophageal Varices**
  - Large or thrombosed varices often simulate mediastinal mass
- **Bronchogenic Cyst**
  - Spherical subcarinal mass; nonenhancing contents
- **Metastases and Lymphoma, Esophagus**
  - Both are much less common than metastases to mediastinal nodes
  - Direct invasion of esophagus from lung cancer is not rare

---

Left Main Bronchus

Aortic Aneurysm

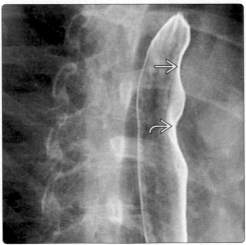
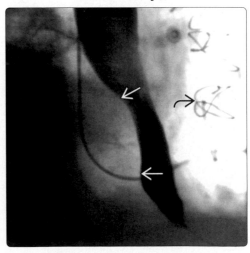

(Left) Spot film from an esophagram shows a normal esophagus with indentations along the left anterolateral wall by the aortic knob ➡ & left main bronchus ➘. (Right) Spot film from an esophagram shows extrinsic indentation ➡ along the posterior wall of the distal esophagus by a dilated, ectatic aorta, in an elderly man. Note sternal wires ➘ from a prior coronary artery graft procedure.

Cervical or Thoracic Osteophytes

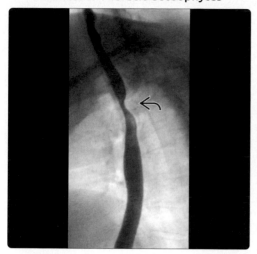

Cervical or Thoracic Osteophytes

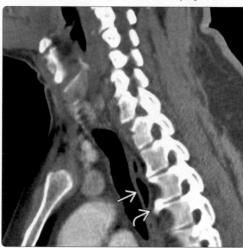

(Left) *In this 49-year-old man, a spot film from an esophagram shows the barium-filled esophagus with a smooth indentation along its posterior wall* ⊟. *A primary, intramural, esophageal tumor was suspected. CT showed no mass but prominent osteophytes at this level.* (Right) *In this 49-year-old man, sagittal CT shows prominent osteophytes at the T3-T4 level* ⊟ *accounting for the indentation & narrowing of the esophagus* ⊟. *Extrinsic indentation by osteophytes more commonly occurs at the lower cervical level.*

Hiatal Hernia

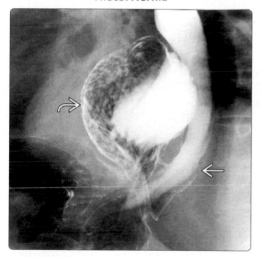

Hiatal Hernia

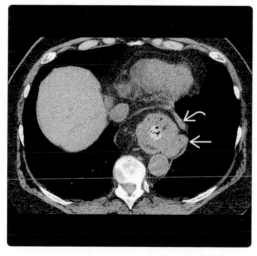

(Left) *Esophagram shows displacement of the distal esophagus by a large, type 3 paraesophageal hernia* ⊟. *The gastroesophageal junction* ⊟ *is in the chest.* (Right) *This patient was found to have a retrocardiac mass on a chest film. CT shows displacement & compression of the esophagus* ⊟ *by a large, type 3 paraesophageal hiatal hernia* ⊟.

Mediastinal Lymph Nodes

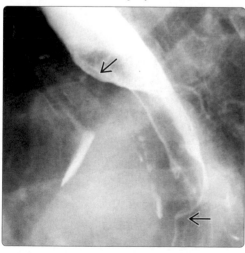

Mediastinal Lymph Nodes

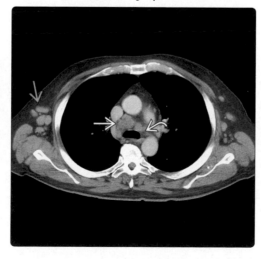

(Left) *A spot film from an esophagram shows a broad indentation* ⊟ *of the anterior wall of the midesophagus by enlarged mediastinal nodes; metastases from primary lung cancer.* (Right) *Axial CECT shows displacement & compression of the esophagus* ⊟ *by mediastinal lymphadenopathy* ⊟. *Other nodal groups were enlarged* ⊟ *in the chest and abdomen, typical of leukemia or lymphoma. Chronic lymphocytic leukemia was confirmed.*

(Left) *Axial CECT shows an aberrant right subclavian artery ➡ arising from the aortic arch and crossing between the spine and the esophagus, within which an enteric feeding tube ➡ is seen. Unrelated mediastinal adenopathy and pleural effusions are also present.* **(Right)** *In this patient with dysphagia & a mediastinal mass, CT shows aneurysmal dilation of an aberrant right subclavian artery ➡ that compressed and displaced the esophagus. The aneurysm lumen contains thrombus ➡.*

Aberrant Subclavian Artery

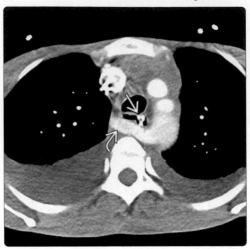

Aberrant Subclavian Artery

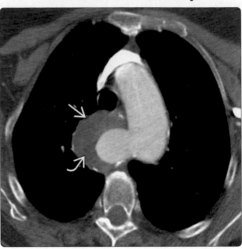

(Left) *A spot film from an esophagram shows persistent dilation of the pharynx ➡ even after passage of the barium bolus. The proximal esophagus is narrowed ➡. CT showed an enlarged thyroid gland.* **(Right)** *In this patient with dysphagia & mass effect on the esophagus seen on esophagram, NECT confirms an enlarged thyroid ➡ that surrounds the proximal esophagus.*

Enlarged Thyroid

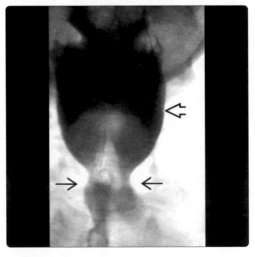

Enlarged Thyroid

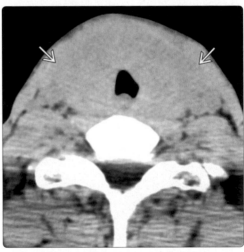

(Left) *Spot film from a barium esophagram demonstrates a mass causing eccentric narrowing of the distal lumen. The mass forms obtuse angles with the wall, and the esophageal folds and mucosa are intact ➡. An esophageal leiomyoma was removed thoracoscopically.* **(Right)** *Axial CECT shows a soft tissue density mass ➡ displacing but not obstructing the esophageal lumen ➡. A benign esophageal leiomyoma was confirmed at resection.*

Intramural (Mesenchymal) Esophageal Tumors

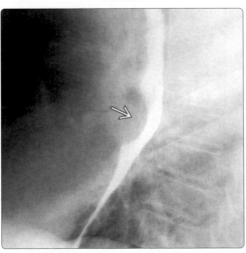

Intramural (Mesenchymal) Esophageal Tumors

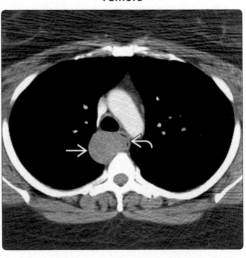

Intramural (Mesenchymal) Esophageal Tumors

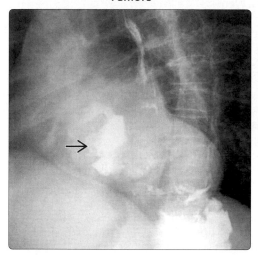

Intramural (Mesenchymal) Esophageal Tumors

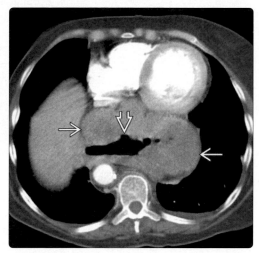

(Left) *In this young man with dysphagia, a spot film from an esophagram shows an irregular collection of barium ➡ within the ulcerated cavity of a mass (an esophageal gastrointestinal stromal tumor).* (Right) *In this young man with dysphagia, CT shows a huge esophageal mass ➡ with a large central ulceration ➡ that contains gas due to communication with the esophageal lumen. This was a GIST of the esophagus.*

Esophageal Varices

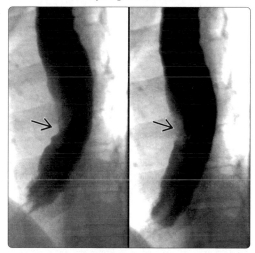

Metastases and Lymphoma, Esophageal

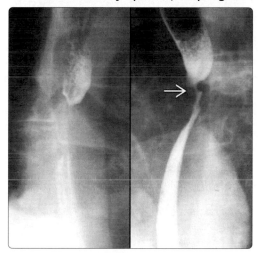

(Left) *Two views from a barium esophagram show fixed serpiginous intramural filling defects ➡ in the esophagus due to sclerosed varices.* (Right) *Two films from an esophagram show abrupt but smooth tapering ➡ of the esophagus at the carinal level, with intact mucosal folds, indicating extrinsic involvement, direct invasion from lung cancer.*

Bronchogenic Cyst

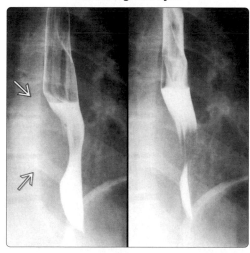

Bronchogenic Cyst

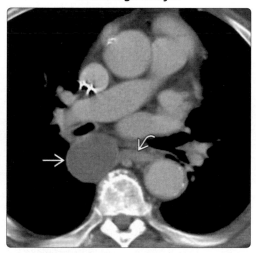

(Left) *Two films from a barium esophagram demonstrate eccentric narrowing of the distal esophageal lumen by a mass ➡ that forms obtuse angles as it meets the barium-filled lumen. The overlying esophageal mucosa and folds are intact (bronchogenic cyst).* (Right) *Axial CECT shows a water density mediastinal mass ➡ arising just below the tracheal carina and indenting the esophagus ➡.*

DIFFERENTIAL DIAGNOSIS

Common

- Achalasia, Cricopharyngeal
- Cervical Osteophytes

Less Common

- Esophageal Webs
- Esophageal Carcinoma
- Esophagitis, Drug-Induced
- Neck Mass

ESSENTIAL INFORMATION

Key Differential Diagnosis Issues

- Determine which side(s) of lumen are indented
  - Cricopharyngeal muscle indents posterior wall
  - Webs usually arise from anterolateral walls
  - Thyroid masses usually encircle anterior & lateral walls

Helpful Clues for Common Diagnoses

- **Achalasia, Cricopharyngeal**
  - Smooth indentation of posterior wall at C5-C6 vertebral level
  - May be intermittent or persistent finding
  - Prominent or persistent contraction may result in dilated pharynx with retained barium
  - Usually associated with various forms of esophageal dysmotility
- **Cervical Osteophytes**
  - May or may not be ossified
  - Indent posterior wall of esophagus, often at several levels
  - Usually asymptomatic, but may be large enough to cause dysphagia
  - Postoperative changes (**cervical laminectomy, fusion**) may have similar effects on esophagus
    - Patients with metallic plate at site of fusion often have symptomatic dysphagia
    - Even in absence of marked mass effect upon esophageal lumen

Helpful Clues for Less Common Diagnoses

- **Esophageal Webs**
  - Thin, shelf-like indentation of lumen
  - May be congenital or acquired
    - e.g., as result of scarring from epidermolysis bullosa
  - May be associated with glossitis and iron-deficiency anemia (Plummer-Vinson syndrome)
  - Arise from anterolateral wall, unlike more common causes of posterior wall indentation
- **Esophageal Carcinoma**
  - Irregular mucosal surface
  - Eccentric or concentric narrowing of lumen
- **Esophagitis, Drug-Induced**
  - Oral medications may have impaired passage through pharyngoesophageal junction
  - May result in esophageal spasm, ulceration, stricture
  - Ask about medications (especially tetracycline and cardiac drugs)
  - Patients usually have abrupt onset of odynophagia (painful swallowing)
- **Neck Mass**
  - Any paraesophageal mass may indent esophagus
  - Near pharyngoesophageal junction, most common are thyroid and parathyroid masses
  - Others to consider include aneurysms, retropharyngeal abscess
  - US, CT, & MR can narrow or establish diagnosis

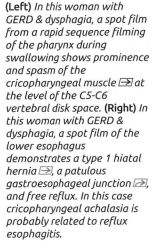

(Left) In this woman with GERD & dysphagia, a spot film from a rapid sequence filming of the pharynx during swallowing shows prominence and spasm of the cricopharyngeal muscle ⇨ at the level of the C5-C6 vertebral disk space. (Right) In this woman with GERD & dysphagia, a spot film of the lower esophagus demonstrates a type 1 hiatal hernia ⇨, a patulous gastroesophageal junction ⇗, and free reflux. In this case cricopharyngeal achalasia is probably related to reflux esophagitis.

Achalasia, Cricopharyngeal

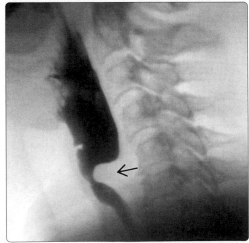

Achalasia, Cricopharyngeal

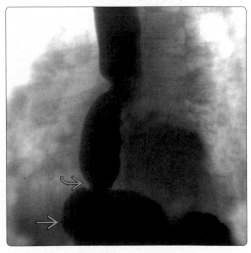

Cervical Osteophytes

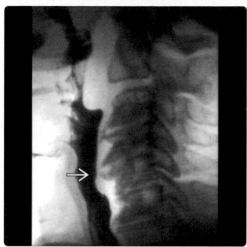

Esophageal Webs

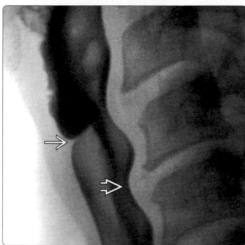

(Left) *A spot film from an esophagram shows indentation of the posterior wall of the pharyngoesophageal junction by cervical osteophytes ➡.* (Right) *Lateral esophagram shows a thin, shelf-like indentation ➡ of anterolateral wall of the pharyngoesophageal junction. The pharynx is mildly dilated above this web. Posterior osteophytes are also noted ➡.*

Esophageal Carcinoma

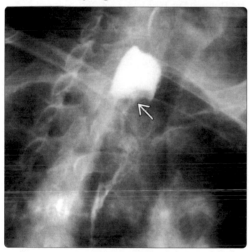

Esophagitis, Drug-Induced

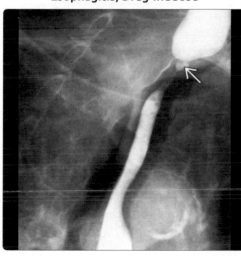

(Left) *A spot film from an esophagram shows an apple core, abrupt, high-grade obstructing lesion ➡ at the thoracic inlet.* (Right) *A spot film from an esophagram shows a tight stricture and ulceration ➡ at the pharyngoesophageal junction, caused by oral medication. Pills more commonly stick at points of physiological narrowing, such as the aortic knob.*

Neck Mass

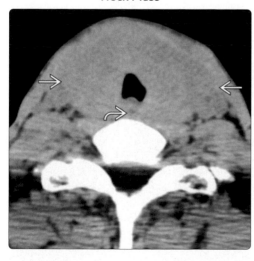

Neck Mass

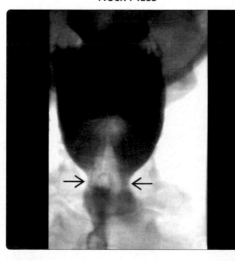

(Left) *In this patient with thyromegaly due to autoimmune thyroiditis, axial NECT shows a markedly enlarged thyroid ➡ that compresses the pharyngoesophageal junction ➡ from all sides.* (Right) *In this patient with thyromegaly due to autoimmune thyroiditis, a spot film from an esophagram shows distention of the pharynx and compression of the proximal esophagus ➡.*

DIFFERENTIAL DIAGNOSIS

Common

- Reflux Esophagitis
- *Candida* Esophagitis
- Drug-Induced Esophagitis
- Viral Esophagitis

Less Common

- Caustic Esophagitis
- Radiation Esophagitis
- Nasogastric Intubation
- Crohn Disease

Rare but Important

- Behçet Disease
- Epidermolysis Bullosa Dystrophica and Pemphigoid

ESSENTIAL INFORMATION

Key Differential Diagnosis Issues

- History is often key (e.g., AIDS, caustic ingestion, other known diseases)

Helpful Clues for Common Diagnoses

- **Reflux Esophagitis**
  - Most common etiology
  - Shallow, punctate, or linear ulcers
  - Check for gastroesophageal reflux
  - Hiatal hernia is common
  - Peptic stricture is common in those with ulceration
- *Candida* **Esophagitis**
  - Ulcers and diffuse raised plaques (shaggy)
  - Odynophagia in immunocompromised patients
  - Often have oral thrush (*Candida*)
- **Drug-Induced Esophagitis**
  - Discrete, superficial ulcers
  - Usually near aortic arch or left main bronchus
  - Odynophagia in patients taking oral medications (tetracycline, KCl, heart medications)
  - Abrupt onset of symptoms

- **Viral Esophagitis**
  - Herpes, CMV, HIV
  - Superficial, often large, flat ulcers
  - Odynophagia in immunocompromised patient

Helpful Clues for Less Common Diagnoses

- **Caustic Esophagitis**
  - Immediate ulceration and spasm
  - Often leads to long stricture of esophagus
- **Nasogastric Intubation**
  - Long-term NG tube leads to reflux and direct trauma to esophagus
  - May cause shallow or long ulcers ± stricture
- **Crohn Disease**
  - Usually in patients with advanced disease
  - Aphthous ulcers (as in stomach and bowel)

Helpful Clues for Rare Diagnoses

- **Behçet Disease**
  - Ulceration of oral, esophageal, and genital mucosa
  - Associated vasculitis
- **Epidermolysis Bullosa Dystrophica and Pemphigoid**
  - Fragile skin and mucous membranes
  - Easily blister, ulcerate, scar
  - Long history of disease
    - Diagnosis is already known

(Left) *Esophagram shows a stricture & large ulcer* ➡ *at the gastroesophageal junction, with shortened esophagus & hiatal hernia.* **(Right)** *Esophagram shows a shaggy or tree bark surface of the esophagus due to diffuse ulceration & raised plaques, typical of severe Candida esophagitis.*

Reflux Esophagitis

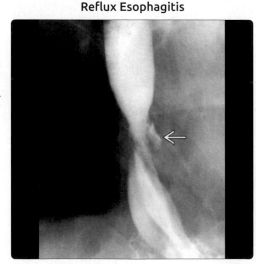

Candida Esophagitis

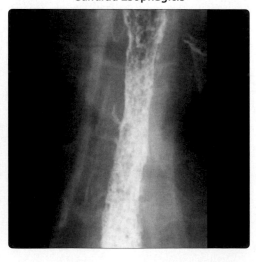

Drug-Induced Esophagitis

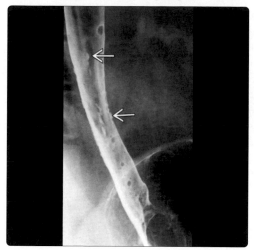

Viral Esophagitis

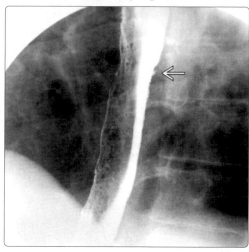

(Left) *Esophagram shows multiple shallow ulcerations ➡, due to tetracycline-induced esophagitis.* (Right) *Esophagram shows multiple small, superficial ulcers ➡, due to herpes esophagitis.*

Caustic Esophagitis

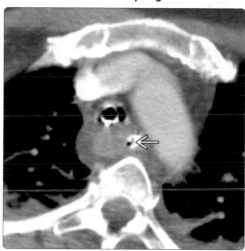

Radiation Esophagitis

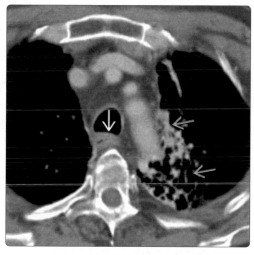

(Left) *In this patient with recent ingestion of lye as a suicide attempt, axial CECT shows massive thickening of the esophageal wall, with its lumen marked by an NG tube ➡. An endotracheal tube is also noted with widespread pulmonary infiltrates.* (Right) *In this patient who had external beam radiation therapy for a left upper lobe lung cancer, axial CECT shows damage to the lungs ➡ along the radiation port. The esophageal wall is thick & the lumen narrowed ➡, also due to radiation-induced injury.*

Radiation Esophagitis

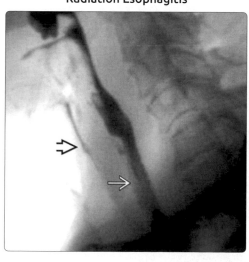

Epidermolysis Bullosa Dystrophica and Pemphigoid

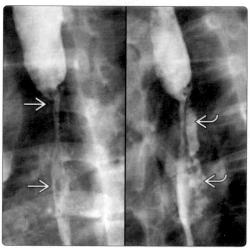

(Left) *In this patient with lung cancer & radiation-induced esophagitis, a spot film from an esophagram shows luminal narrowing ➡ & mucosal ulceration of the proximal esophagus, along with aspiration of barium ➡ into the trachea.* (Right) *Oblique esophagram shows an ulcerated stricture of the midesophagus ➡ due to epidermolysis. Following balloon dilation of the stricture, the esophagus was perforated, with extraluminal contrast extravasation noted ➡.*

DIFFERENTIAL DIAGNOSIS

Common

- Reflux Esophagitis
- *Candida* Esophagitis
- Viral Esophagitis
- Glycogenic Acanthosis
- Undissolved Gas Granules, Bubbles (Mimics)

Less Common

- Barrett Esophagus
- Esophageal Carcinoma

Rare but Important

- Papillomatosis, Esophageal
- Acanthosis Nigricans
- Cowden Disease
- Leukoplakia

ESSENTIAL INFORMATION

Key Differential Diagnosis Issues

- Consider clinical setting
  - Symptoms, age of patient, AIDS, etc.

Helpful Clues for Common Diagnoses

- **Reflux Esophagitis**
  - Poorly defined nodules; granular mucosa
  - Usually affects distal 1/3 of esophagus
  - Gastroesophageal reflux, hiatal hernia
- ***Candida* Esophagitis**
  - Discrete plaques & ulcers; shaggy mucosa
  - May be localized or diffuse
  - Odynophagia in immunocompromised patient
    - May look like tree bark
- **Glycogenic Acanthosis**
  - Numerous small nodules or plaques
  - Less well-defined than candidiasis
  - Asymptomatic lesions of no clinical importance
- **Undissolved Gas Granules, Bubbles (Mimics)**

- Transient finding, usually with 1st swallows during air-contrast esophagram

Helpful Clues for Less Common Diagnoses

- **Barrett Esophagus**
  - Fine surface nodularity is characteristic but difficult to distinguish from other causes
  - Associated esophageal ulceration, stricture
    - Especially in midesophagus
  - Usually distal 1/3 of esophagus
    - Difficult or impossible to distinguish this location & appearance from peptic stricture
  - Associated GE reflux and hiatal hernia
- **Esophageal Carcinoma**
  - Superficial spreading carcinoma can appear as poorly defined, coalescent nodules or plaques
  - Localized more often than diffuse
  - Often asymptomatic

Helpful Clues for Rare Diagnoses

- **Papillomatosis, Esophageal**
  - More commonly affects larynx
  - Related to HPV infection
- **Cowden Disease**
  - Tiny nodules = hamartomatous polyps
  - Hereditary with associated tumors of skin, GI tract, and thyroid
- **Leukoplakia**
  - Common in mouth, rare in esophagus
  - Hyperkeratosis, dysplasia on biopsy

Reflux Esophagitis

Reflux Esophagitis

(Left) *Spot film from an esophagram shows a stricture at the esophagogastric junction ➡, a small hiatal hernia ⇨, and nodular mucosal surface ➡ of the esophagus, all due to GERD.* (Right) *Spot film from an esophagram shows a peptic stricture ➡ of the esophagus along with a small hiatal hernia ⇨. Nodularity of the esophageal mucosa is less evident with full distention of the lumen.*

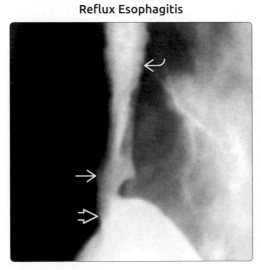
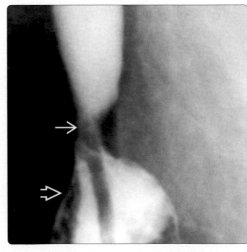

Candida Esophagitis

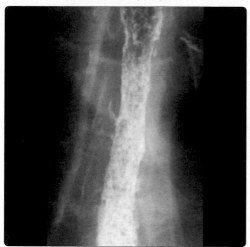

Viral Esophagitis

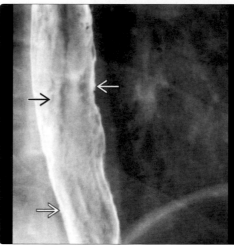

(Left) *Esophagram shows a shaggy tree bark appearance of the esophagus due to ulcerations and plaques from Candida esophagitis.* (Right) *Spot film from an esophagram shows multiple superficial ulcerations ➡ and raised plaques ⇨ in a patient with AIDS. This is viral esophagitis but is indistinguishable from Candida esophagitis by imaging alone.*

Undissolved Gas Granules, Bubbles (Mimics)

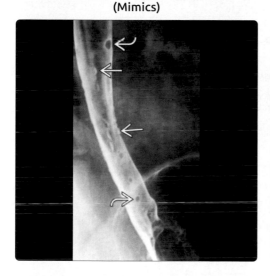

Barrett Esophagus

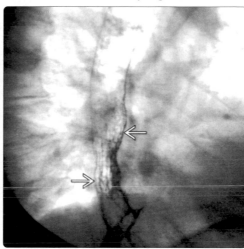

(Left) *Spot film from an esophagram shows multiple radiolucent filling defects ➡ that represent gas bubbles that are adherent to the esophageal surface. Also present are multiple ulcerations ➡ due to tetracycline-induced esophagitis.* (Right) *Spot film from an esophagram shows nodular distal esophageal mucosa ➡ due to Barrett esophagus. A hiatal hernia and reflux were also demonstrated.*

Esophageal Carcinoma

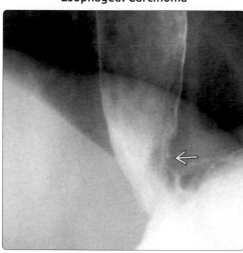

Papillomatosis, Esophageal

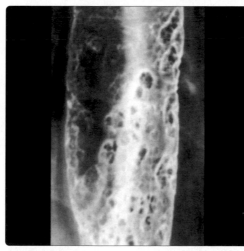

(Left) *Spot film from an esophagram shows nodular thickened folds ➡ in the distal esophagus and fundus of stomach. These nodules are much larger than those seen in most infectious conditions.* (Right) *Esophagram shows clusters of small, irregular nodules that represent biopsy-proven squamous papillomas.*

DIFFERENTIAL DIAGNOSIS

Common

- Reflux Esophagitis
- Barrett Esophagus
- Esophageal Carcinoma
- Scleroderma, Esophagus

Less Common

- Esophageal Metastases and Lymphoma
- Radiation Esophagitis
- Caustic Esophagitis
- Drug-Induced Esophagitis
- *Candida* Esophagitis
- Nasogastric Intubation

Rare but Important

- Crohn Disease
- Graft-vs.-Host Disease
- Glutaraldehyde-Induced Injury
- Epidermolysis and Pemphigoid
- Esophagitis, Eosinophilic

ESSENTIAL INFORMATION

Key Differential Diagnosis Issues

- History is key (e.g., radiation therapy, caustic or drug ingestion, bone marrow transplant)

Helpful Clues for Common Diagnoses

- **Reflux Esophagitis**
  - Peptic stricture of distal 3rd
  - Hiatal hernia, reflux, short esophagus
  - Often with ulceration
  - Short, tapered, symmetric or asymmetric
- **Barrett Esophagus**
  - Distal or midesophagus
  - Often with ulceration
  - Short or moderate length, symmetric or asymmetric
- **Esophageal Carcinoma**
  - Middle 3rd (50%), lower 3rd (30%), upper 3rd (20%)

  - Abrupt narrowing, apple core
  - Irregular nodular surface; ulceration
  - Moderate length; asymmetric
  - Absent peristalsis through length of tumor
- **Scleroderma, Esophagus**
  - Distal 3rd
  - Short or moderate length; symmetric taper
  - Diminished or absent peristalsis
  - Correlate with pulmonary and skin findings

Helpful Clues for Less Common Diagnoses

- **Esophageal Metastases and Lymphoma**
  - Lung or gastric cancer may invade esophagus
  - Hematogenous mets and lymphoma are rare
  - Nodal metastases in mediastinum may compress esophagus
- **Radiation Esophagitis**
  - Long stricture of midesophagus
  - Check for history of radiation therapy (lymphoma, lung, or breast cancer)
- **Caustic Esophagitis**
  - Long, high-grade stricture
- **Nasogastric Intubation**
  - Mimics caustic ingestion stricture

Helpful Clues for Rare Diagnoses

- **Glutaraldehyde-Induced Injury**
  - Agent used to sterilize endoscopes is very caustic if not thoroughly removed

(Left) *Spot film from an esophagram shows a small hiatal hernia, shortened esophagus, and a stricture of the distal esophagus with ulceration* ➡. **(Right)** *Spot film from an esophagram shows a stricture and ulceration* ➡ *of the distal 3rd of the esophagus.*

Reflux Esophagitis

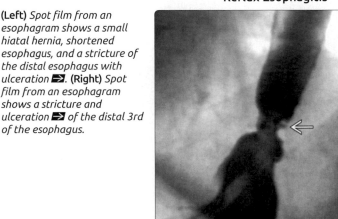

Barrett Esophagus

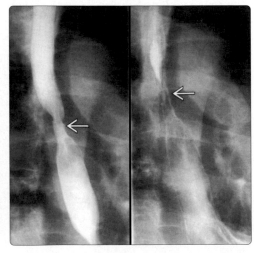

Esophageal Carcinoma

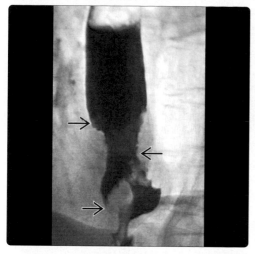

Scleroderma, Esophagus

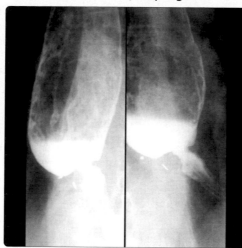

(Left) *Spot film from an esophagram shows an apple core narrowing* ➡ *of the distal esophagus, with nodular, destroyed mucosal surface.* (Right) *Spot film from an esophagram shows a tight stricture of the distal esophagus with a markedly dilated, atonic esophagus. The appearance mimics achalasia, but the stricture is more abrupt and irregular.*

Esophageal Metastases and Lymphoma

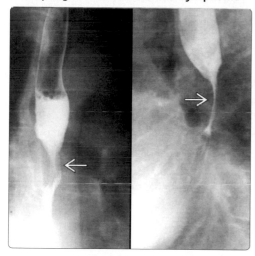

Radiation Esophagitis

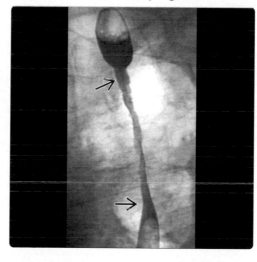

(Left) *Spot film from an esophagram shows a tight but smoothly tapered stricture* ➡ *of the midesophagus, due to direct invasion by lung cancer.* (Right) *Spot film from an esophagram shows a long stricture* ➡ *of midesophagus, 8 months after radiation therapy for right lung cancer and mediastinal lymph node metastases.*

Caustic Esophagitis

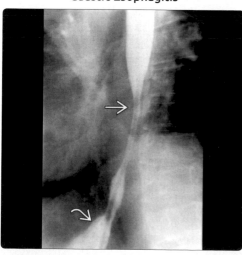

Drug-Induced Esophagitis

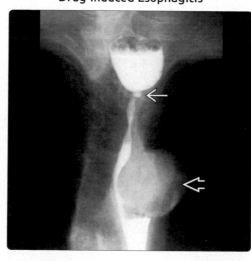

(Left) *Spot film from an esophagram shows a long smooth stricture* ➡ *of the distal 1/2 of the esophagus, with a shortened esophagus causing hiatal hernia* ➡. (Right) *Spot film from an esophagram shows a high-grade stricture and ulceration* ➡ *of the proximal esophagus, just above the aortic knob* ➡, *in this elderly woman with odynophagia.*

DIFFERENTIAL DIAGNOSIS

Common

- Achalasia, Esophagus
- Scleroderma, Esophagus
- Postvagotomy State
- Fundoplication Complications
- Reflux Esophagitis
- Esophageal Carcinoma
- Hiatal Hernia (Mimic)
- Postesophagectomy (Mimic)

Less Common

- Gastric Carcinoma
- Metastases and Lymphoma, Esophageal
- Chagas Disease

ESSENTIAL INFORMATION

Key Differential Diagnosis Issues

- Check for history of prior surgery
  - Esophagectomy (Ivor-Lewis and variations)
  - Fundoplication
  - Vagotomy

Helpful Clues for Common Diagnoses

- **Achalasia, Esophagus**
  - Primary motility disorder; aperistaltic
  - Grossly dilated esophagus; often elongated
  - Ends in smooth taper; "bird beak"
  - Onset in younger patients (20-40 years), progresses with age
- **Scleroderma, Esophagus**
  - Collagen vascular disorder of skin, smooth muscle
    - Commonly affects esophagus, duodenum, and small bowel
  - Diminished or absent peristalsis
  - Stricture and esophageal dilation are late findings
  - More common in women
- **Postvagotomy State**

- Vagotomy often performed for acid peptic disease
- Reflux (peptic) stricture may contribute to dilation
  - But lumen is rarely significantly dilated
- **Fundoplication Complications**
  - Fundoplication wrap may be excessively tight, impairing esophageal emptying
  - Especially common in elderly, who also have presbyesophagus (nonspecific esophageal dysmotility)
- **Reflux Esophagitis**
  - Esophagitis may cause diminished peristalsis
  - Peptic stricture contributes to dilation
- **Esophageal Carcinoma**
  - Narrowed lumen may cause dilation of esophagus upstream
- **Hiatal Hernia (Mimic)**
  - Intrathoracic part of stomach may be mistaken for dilated esophagus
    - More likely to be mistaken on axial CT imaging
    - Coronal reformation can help to clarify
- **Postesophagectomy (Mimic)**
  - Ivor-Lewis or similar operations
  - Stomach may be pulled into thorax, anastomosed to proximal esophagus
  - May be mistaken for dilated esophagus on esophagram, CT, etc.

Helpful Clues for Less Common Diagnoses

- **Gastric Carcinoma**
  - Cancer arising in gastric cardia or fundus may invade distal esophagus submucosa
  - Involvement of intramural nerves may result in diminished peristalsis
  - Tumor may also narrow lumen of distal esophagus
- **Chagas Disease**
  - Parasitic disease common in South America and Mexico

(Left) Upright spot film from an esophagram shows a markedly dilated esophagus with very delayed emptying, indicated by the persistent air-fluid-contrast levels ➡. The esophagus narrows at the esophagogastric junction to a tapered bird beak appearance ➡. (Right) Upright spot film from an esophagram shows marked dilation and atony of the esophagus with stasis of barium & a tight stricture ➡ at the gastroesophageal junction. The appearance mimics achalasia, but clinical features are usually very different.

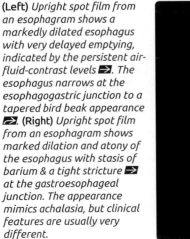
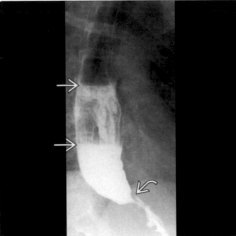

Achalasia, Esophagus

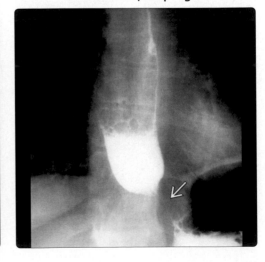

Scleroderma, Esophagus

Postvagotomy State

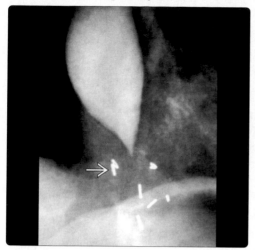

Fundoplication Complications

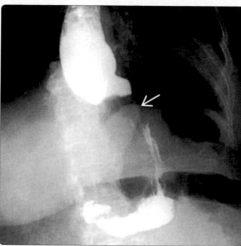

(Left) *Spot film from an esophagram shows a dilated esophagus with a smooth-tapered stricture just above the esophagogastric junction. Note the clips from vagotomy* ➡. **(Right)** *In this elderly woman, an upright spot film from a esophagram shows a dilated esophagus with stasis of food and barium. The esophageal lumen is tightly compressed at the site of the fundoplication* ➡.

Esophageal Carcinoma

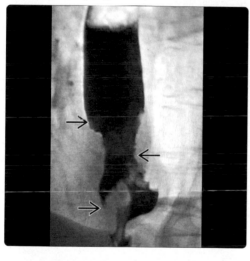

Hiatal Hernia (Mimic)

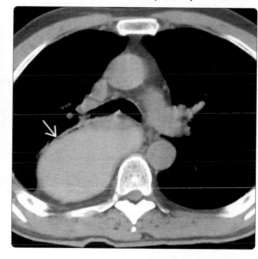

(Left) *Esophagram shows a dilated atonic esophagus with abrupt transition to a narrowed lumen with an apple core, nodular surface pattern* ➡. **(Right)** *Axial NECT shows a dilated tubular structure* ➡ *in the thorax containing oral contrast. On axial CT, it would be difficult to recognize this as a hiatal hernia and not a dilated esophagus.*

Postesophagectomy (Mimic)

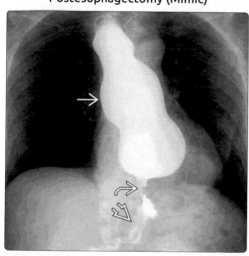

Gastric Carcinoma

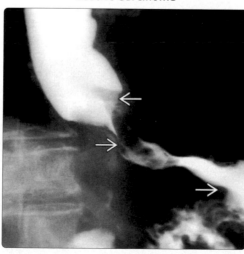

(Left) *Upright film from esophagram shows massive dilation of the gastric conduit* ➡ *that was pulled into the chest to replace resected portion of esophagus. Conduit is not redundant, but it is mechanically obstructed by narrowing as it traverses the diaphragmatic hiatus* ➡. *Subdiaphragmatic stomach* ➡ *is collapsed & normal.* **(Right)** *Spot film from an esophagram shows a dilated esophagus with abrupt narrowing at the GE junction. A mass causes constriction of the gastric cardia & fundus* ➡ *& extends into submucosa of esophagus.*

DIFFERENTIAL DIAGNOSIS

Common

- Zenker Diverticulum
- Traction Diverticulum
- Pulsion Diverticulum
- Hiatal Hernia (Mimic)
- Postesophagectomy (Mimic)
- Fundoplication Complications (Mimic)

Less Common

- Killian-Jamieson Diverticulum
- Intramural Pseudodiverticulosis
- Boerhaave Syndrome (Mimic)

ESSENTIAL INFORMATION

Key Differential Diagnosis Issues

- Most diverticula are pulsion & are associated with abnormalities of esophageal peristalsis

Helpful Clues for Common Diagnoses

- **Zenker Diverticulum**
  - Outpouching from posterior wall of pharyngoesophageal junction; just above cricopharyngeus muscle
  - Usually starts at C5-C6 vertebral level
    - May extend caudally into upper mediastinum
  - Increased prevalence with aging & dysmotility conditions
- **Traction Diverticulum**
  - Usually midesophagus near carina
  - Acquired due to adherence to subcarinal or perihilar granulomatous lymph nodes
  - Look for calcified nodes and granulomas in lungs
- **Pulsion Diverticulum**
  - Saccular, often large, outpouching
  - Distal (epiphrenic) is most common
    - Often has wide mouth from side of distal esophagus
  - Strongly associated with esophageal motility disturbances (e.g., presbyesophagus, diffuse esophageal spasm)

- Easily mistaken for hiatal hernia and vice versa
- **Postesophagectomy (Mimic)**
  - Ivor-Lewis and other procedures for distal esophagectomy & gastric pull-through
  - Gastric conduit pulled into chest and anastomosed to stump of esophagus
    - Anastomosis is usually above carina
  - Outpouching at anastomosis or dilation of gastric conduit may mimic diverticulum or dilated esophagus
    - Look for rugae to distinguish stomach from esophagus
- **Fundoplication Complications (Mimic)**
  - Barium may fill portions of fundal wrap, resembling diverticulum
    - Rugae within collection identify it as stomach

Helpful Clues for Less Common Diagnoses

- **Killian-Jamieson Diverticulum**
  - Originate from anterolateral wall of cervical esophagus
  - Higher, more anterior and usually smaller than Zenker diverticulum
- **Intramural Pseudodiverticulosis**
  - Barium trapped in dilated excretory ducts of deep mucous glands
  - Multiple, tiny (1- to 4-mm depth), flask-like outpouchings
- **Boerhaave Syndrome (Mimic)**
  - Or any cause of esophageal perforation
  - May result in a paraesophageal collection of gas, fluid, or contrast medium

(Left) *Spot film from an esophagram shows a moderate-sized diverticulum ⇥ originating at the pharyngoesophageal junction that extends into the upper mediastinum.* **(Right)** *Spot film from an esophagram shows an outpouching ⇥ from the midesophagus (carinal level). Note the calcified perihilar lymph nodes ⇥.*

Zenker Diverticulum

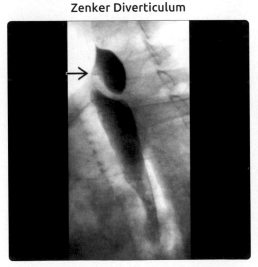

Traction Diverticulum

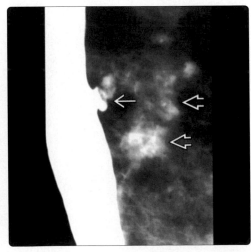

Pulsion Diverticulum

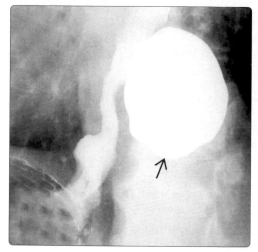

Hiatal Hernia (Mimic)

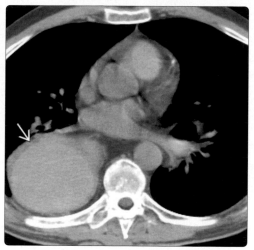

(Left) *Spot film from a barium esophagram demonstrates an unusually large pulsion diverticulum ⊟ projecting from the middistal esophagus. Primary esophageal peristalsis was markedly diminished, and deep tertiary contractions were noted.* (Right) *Axial NECT shows a structure containing oral contrast in the distal thorax, a hiatal hernia ➡. A pulsion diverticulum, gastric conduit, or achalasia could have a similar appearance on CT.*

Fundoplication Complications (Mimic)

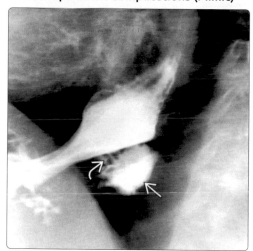

Killian-Jamieson Diverticulum

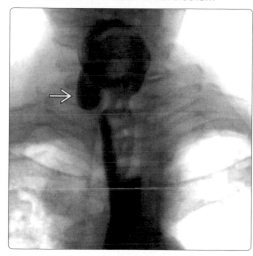

(Left) *Spot film from an esophagram shows a collection of barium ➡ within the fundoplication wrap, which has slipped into the thorax. Note the rugal folds ➡, identifying it as stomach, rather than a leak.* (Right) *Frontal esophagram shows an outpouching ➡ from the anterolateral wall of the cervical esophagus, a Killian-Jamison diverticulum.*

Intramural Pseudodiverticulosis

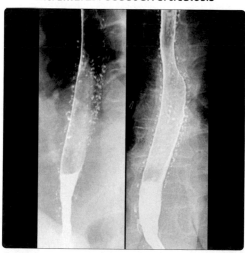

Boerhaave Syndrome (Mimic)

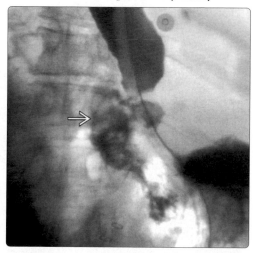

(Left) *Oblique esophagram shows innumerable tiny, flask-shaped outpouchings of barium within the wall of the esophagus.* (Right) *Oblique esophagram shows an irregular collection of contrast (& gas) ➡ in the lower mediastinum, which has leaked out of the perforated distal esophagus.*

DIFFERENTIAL DIAGNOSIS

Common

- Presbyesophagus
- Diffuse Esophageal Spasm
- Achalasia, Esophagus
- Scleroderma, Esophagus
- Reflux Esophagitis
- Surgical Complications
  - Fundoplication Complications
  - Postvagotomy State

Less Common

- Neuromuscular Disorders
- Esophageal Carcinoma
- Gastric Carcinoma

ESSENTIAL INFORMATION

Key Differential Diagnosis Issues

- Manometry and barium esophagram are complementary

Helpful Clues for Common Diagnoses

- **Presbyesophagus**
  - Nonspecific esophageal motility disorder
  - Increased prevalence with aging
  - Decreased primary peristalsis; frequent tertiary (nonpropulsive) contractions
- **Diffuse Esophageal Spasm**
  - Intermittent disruption of primary peristalsis with focally obliterative secondary or tertiary contractions
  - May impart corkscrew appearance to esophagram
  - May cause chest pain simulating angina
- **Achalasia, Esophagus**
  - Absent primary peristalsis
  - May have tertiary contractions early in disease
  - Dilated esophagus ending in tapered bird beak deformity
- **Scleroderma, Esophagus**
  - Multisystem collagen vascular disease

- Early disease: Nonperistaltic esophagus with patulous gastroesophageal (GE) junction
- Late disease: Dilated esophagus with peptic stricture at GE junction; simulates achalasia
- **Reflux Esophagitis**
  - Esophagus is often foreshortened (spasm of longitudinal muscles)
    - Esophageal lumen is usually not very dilated
  - Distal peptic stricture; possible ulcerations and nodular mucosa
  - Esophagitis itself impairs normal peristalsis
- **Surgical Complications**
  - Fundoplication or vagotomy may result in narrowed distal esophagus and poor esophageal emptying

Helpful Clues for Less Common Diagnoses

- **Neuromuscular Disorders**
  - Diseases, such as multiple sclerosis, ALS, myasthenia gravis, may impair esophageal motility
- **Esophageal and Gastric Carcinoma**
  - Combination of luminal narrowing & submucosal nerve plexus destruction
  - Carcinoma of gastric fundus may invade esophageal submucosa
    - Look for nodular, fixed folds in fundus on UGI or CT
    - Endoscopy is mandatory to evaluate for this possibility

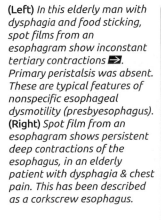

(Left) *In this elderly man with dysphagia and food sticking, spot films from an esophagram show inconstant tertiary contractions ➡. Primary peristalsis was absent. These are typical features of nonspecific esophageal dysmotility (presbyesophagus).* (Right) *Spot film from an esophagram shows persistent deep contractions of the esophagus, in an elderly patient with dysphagia & chest pain. This has been described as a corkscrew esophagus.*

Presbyesophagus

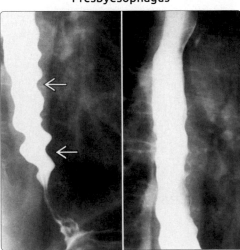

Diffuse Esophageal Spasm

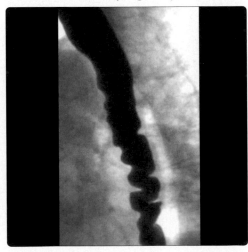

Achalasia, Esophagus

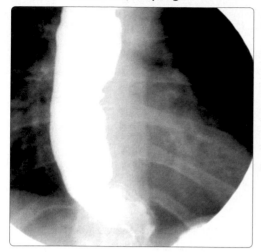

Achalasia, Esophagus

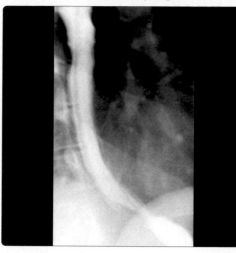

(Left) In this 28-year-old woman with chronic & progressive dysphagia, a spot film from an esophagram shows a very dilated and atonic esophagus terminating in a bird beak narrowing at the gastroesophageal (GE) junction. (Right) In the same 28-year-old-woman, who had been treated with Heller myotomy, a spot film from an esophagram shows a normal caliber esophagus that emptied readily in the upright position. Upright positioning is inadequate to evaluate esophageal dysmotility.

Scleroderma, Esophagus

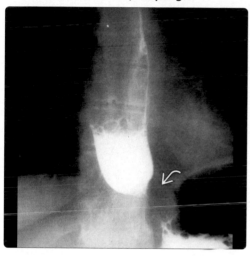

Reflux Esophagitis

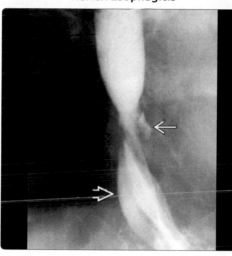

(Left) A single film from a barium esophagram shows a dilated, atonic esophagus with a tight stricture at the GE junction ➧. The esophagus was slow to empty, even in this upright position. This patient also had typical skin & intestinal features of scleroderma. (Right) Spot film from an esophagram shows a deep ulcer ➧ at the GE junction, and a shortened esophagus with hiatal hernia ➧. Primary peristalsis was minimal.

Fundoplication Complications

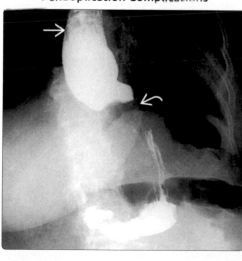

Postvagotomy State

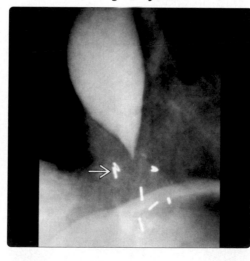

(Left) In this elderly woman who had fundoplication for GERD, a subsequent esophagram shows a markedly dilated esophagus with retention of food ➧ and a very tight lumen at the site of the fundoplication ➧. Esophageal peristalsis was minimal. (Right) Spot film from an esophagram shows a dilated esophagus with a smooth, distal, tapered obstruction. Esophageal peristalsis was minimal. Note the clips ➧ from vagotomy.

DIFFERENTIAL DIAGNOSIS

Common

- Pharyngitis
- Reflux Esophagitis
- *Candida* Esophagitis
- Viral Esophagitis
- Drug-Induced Esophagitis
- Esophageal Foreign Body

Less Common

- Caustic Esophagitis
- Radiation Esophagitis

ESSENTIAL INFORMATION

Key Differential Diagnosis Issues

- Odynophagia: Pain on swallowing
  o Almost always indicates mucosal irritation or ulceration
- Clinical setting & history are key elements in differential diagnosis

Helpful Clues for Common Diagnoses

- **Pharyngitis**
  o Inflammation of pharyngeal mucosa, associated with several common viral and bacterial infections
  o This is clinical, not radiographic, diagnosis
- **Reflux Esophagitis**
  o Distal ulcers/erosions, hiatal hernia, reflux
- *Candida* **Esophagitis**
  o Common cause of odynophagia in immunocompromised patients (can occur in immunocompetent as well)
  o Usually associated with oral thrush
  o Shaggy esophageal surface; raised plaques & shallow ulcers
- **Viral Esophagitis**
  o Usually causes shallow ulcers on otherwise normal esophageal mucosal surface
  o Occurs in immunocompromised patients
- **Drug-Induced Esophagitis**
  o Causes sudden onset of severe odynophagia

  – More common in elderly patients
  – Often caused by antibiotics and cardiac medications
  o Ulceration, spasm, stricture at sites of normal luminal narrowing (aortic arch, left main bronchus, retrocardiac region)
- **Esophageal Foreign Body**
  o Fish or chicken bones often scratch pharynx (e.g., pyriform sinuses) or esophagus when swallowed
  o May be sufficiently radiopaque to visualize in radiography
  o May need to have patient swallow cotton swab soaked in barium to identify luminal projection of foreign body

Helpful Clues for Less Common Diagnoses

- **Caustic Esophagitis**
  o Odynophagia is severe and immediate following ingestion of strong acid or alkaline material
  o May prevent immediate evaluation by barium esophagram
  o CT is good alternative to demonstrate esophageal wall thickening, any evidence of perforation, aspiration pneumonitis

Reflux Esophagitis

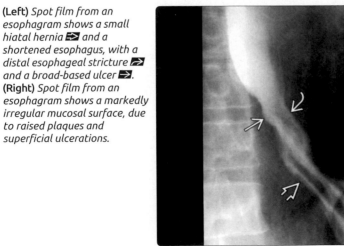

Candida **Esophagitis**

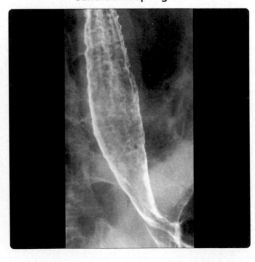

(Left) *Spot film from an esophagram shows a small hiatal hernia ➡ and a shortened esophagus, with a distal esophageal stricture ➡ and a broad-based ulcer ➡.* (Right) *Spot film from an esophagram shows a markedly irregular mucosal surface, due to raised plaques and superficial ulcerations.*

Viral Esophagitis

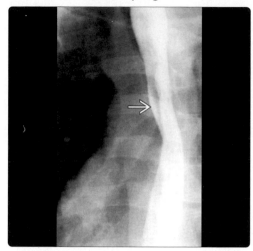

Viral Esophagitis

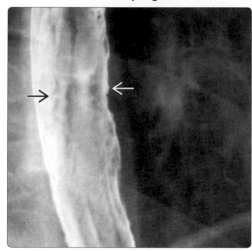

(Left) *Spot film from an esophagram shows a large, shallow ulcer* ➡ *in an otherwise normal esophagus in a patient with AIDS, HIV-induced ulceration.* (Right) *Spot film from an esophagram shows both superficial ulcerations* ➡ *and raised plaques* ➡, *proven to be due to viral (herpes) esophagitis but indistinguishable from Candida esophagitis by imaging.*

Drug-Induced Esophagitis

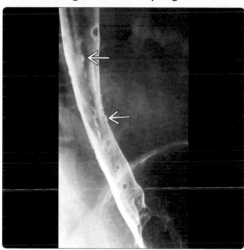

Esophageal Foreign Body

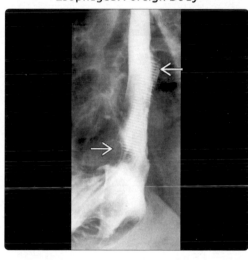

(Left) *Spot film from an esophagram shows multiple ulcerations* ➡ *due to tetracycline in a middle-aged woman with severe odynophagia.* (Right) *Spot film from an esophagram shows a comb* ➡ *within the distal esophagus. This mentally disturbed patient complained of odynophagia and dysphagia, and the foreign body had not been anticipated.*

Caustic Esophagitis

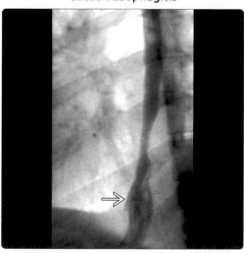

Radiation Esophagitis

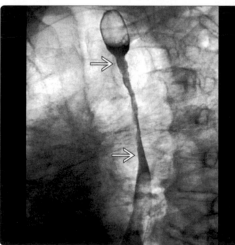

(Left) *Spot film from an esophagram shows a long stricture & shortening of the distal 2/3 of the esophagus, the result of lye ingestion several days before. The stomach* ➡ *is pulled up into the chest as a result of spasm of the longitudinal esophageal muscles.* (Right) *Spot film from an esophagram shows a long stricture* ➡ *of the midesophagus, due to radiation injury, following treatment for lung cancer with mediastinal lymphadenopathy.*

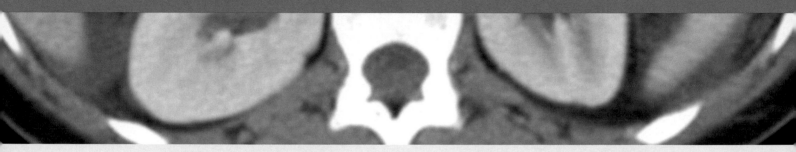

SECTION 4
Stomach

Generic Imaging Patterns

Clinically Based Differentials

DIFFERENTIAL DIAGNOSIS

Common

- Gastric Carcinoma
- Hyperplastic Polyps
- Artifacts
  - Air (Gas) Bubbles
  - Apposed Walls of Stomach
- Adenomatous Polyp
- Bezoar (Mimic)
- Perigastric Mass (Mimic)
  - Splenomegaly and Hypersplenism
  - Renal Cell Carcinoma
  - Hepatocellular Carcinoma
  - Splenosis
- Gastric Varices

Less Common

- Gastrointestinal Stromal Tumor, Gastric
- Intramural Gastric Tumors
- Gastric Metastases and Lymphoma
- Gardner Syndrome
- Hamartomatous Polyposis Syndromes
- Other Mesenchymal Tumors
- Ectopic Pancreatic Tissue
- Hematoma, Gastric
- Duplication Cyst, Stomach

ESSENTIAL INFORMATION

Key Differential Diagnosis Issues

- Primary gastric mucosal lesion
  - Irregular surface; acute angles with inner wall of stomach
- Intramural mass lesion
  - Smooth mucosal surface; sharp obtuse angle with inner wall
- Extrinsic mass lesion
  - Smooth mucosal surface; shallow obtuse angles with gastric wall

Helpful Clues for Common Diagnoses

- **Gastric Carcinoma**
  - Variable morphological features
  - Nodular folds, polypoid mass, ulceration are common in advanced disease
  - Lack of peristalsis and limited distensibility of affected part of stomach are key features on fluoroscopy (upper GI, UGI, series)
  - CT usually shows extension outside stomach (lymphatic, direct invasion, liver metastasis)
- **Hyperplastic Polyps**
  - Round, small, sessile polyps; most common polyps
  - Usually multiple in fundus and body
  - Not premalignant
- **Artifacts**
  - **Air (gas) bubbles**
    - Swallowed air or dissolving gas granules may simulate small polypoid lesions on UGI series
  - **Apposed walls of stomach**
    - On air contrast UGI series, anterior and posterior walls of stomach may temporarily "stick together"

  - May mimic mass lesion in barium pool or mass coated with barium
- **Adenomatous Polyp**
  - Usually solitary, lobulated, or on stalk
  - Usually in antrum
  - Considered premalignant
- **Bezoar (Mimic)**
  - History of prior surgery (e.g., partial gastrectomy), psychiatric disease
  - Adolescent girls may chew on ends of their hair; results in trichobezoar
  - Movable large mass that fills stomach
- **Perigastric Mass (Mimic)**
  - Mass arising from any adjacent structure may simulate gastric mass
  - On upper GI series, extrinsic masses are especially likely to simulate intramural masses of stomach
  - On CT or MR, look for fat plane separating stomach from extrinsic mass
    - Multiplanar imaging is often useful
    - Look for claw sign indicating origin from extragastric organ
- **Gastric Varices**
  - In patient with portal hypertension or splenic vein occlusion
  - Easy to recognize on CECT; may mimic tumor on NECT or UGI series

Helpful Clues for Less Common Diagnoses

- **Gastrointestinal Stromal Tumor, Gastric**
  - Most common cause of large exophytic mass arising from gastric wall
  - Mucosa stretched over mass, may ulcerate
  - CT: Large exophytic mass with central necrosis; may contain gas, oral contrast medium
  - May be benign or malignant
- **Intramural Gastric Tumors**
  - Any component of gastric wall may give rise to benign or malignant tumor
    - Schwannoma, hemangioma, neuroendocrine, etc.
  - Gastric lipoma is most common lesion, recognized by fat content
  - May arise in gastric antrum; may prolapse through pylorus, causing intermittent obstruction
- **Gastric Metastases and Lymphoma**
  - Metastases may be nodular (e.g., melanoma, Kaposi sarcoma) or infiltrative (e.g., breast)
  - Lymphoma: Usually massive, confluent thickening of gastric wall
    - Wall thickening from lymphoma usually exceeds that caused by carcinoma
    - Gastric outlet from lymphoma is uncommon to rare
- **Gardner Syndrome**
  - Familial adenomatous polyposis of colon plus osteomas, desmoid tumors, adrenal, thyroid, and liver carcinomas, etc.
  - May also have adenomatous polyps in stomach
    - Less common than colonic and small bowel polyps
- **Hamartomatous Polyposis Syndromes**
  - Peutz-Jeghers syndrome, Cronkite-Canada, Cowden, etc.

- o Hamartomatous polyps more common in small bowel and colon
  - – Usually multiple, small, broad-based masses
  - – Usually not carpeting bowel (unlike familial polyposis)
- o Polyps are not premalignant, but patients are at increased risk for carcinomas of GI tract (as well as of pancreas, breast, reproductive tract)
- **Ectopic Pancreatic Tissue**
  - o Typical appearance is small mass along greater curvature of antrum
  - o May have central umbilication (opening of primitive pancreatic duct)
- **Hematoma, Gastric**
  - o From blunt or penetrating trauma
  - o Prior placement of percutaneous gastrostomy tube should be considered
- **Duplication Cyst, Stomach**
  - o May or may not communicate with stomach
  - o May have water density or more proteinaceous contents
  - o No enhancement of contents after contrast administration

Alternative Differential Approaches

- Causes of multiple gastric masses
  - o Hyperplastic polyps
  - o Gastric metastases and lymphoma
  - o Gardner syndrome
  - o Hamartomatous polyposis syndromes

SELECTED REFERENCES

1. Ba-Ssalamah A et al: Dedicated multidetector CT of the stomach: spectrum of diseases. Radiographics. 23(3):625-44, 2003
2. Horton KM et al: Current role of CT in imaging of the stomach. Radiographics. 23(1):75-87, 2003
3. Fishman EK et al: CT of the stomach: spectrum of disease. Radiographics. 16(5):1035-54, 1996

Gastric Carcinoma

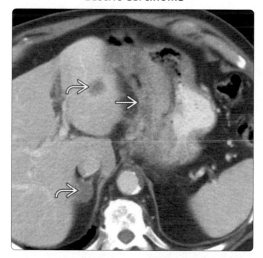

Gastric Carcinoma

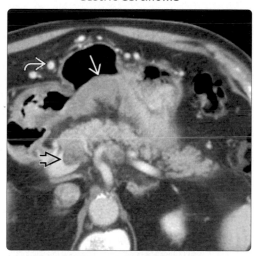

(Left) In this 72-year-old man, axial CECT shows an eccentric, soft tissue density mass ➡ growing along the lesser curve of the stomach. Note the hepatic and adrenal metastases ➡. (Right) In this 72-year-old man, axial CECT shows extension of the mass ➡ along the posterior wall of the stomach to the pylorus. Extension into the splenic vein ➡ results in perigastric varices ➡.

Gastric Carcinoma

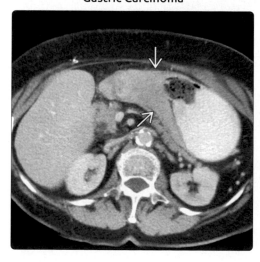

Gastric Carcinoma

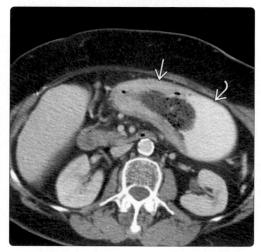

(Left) In this elderly woman, CT shows soft tissue density infiltration of the wall of the distal stomach ➡ with gastric outlet obstruction suggested by the presence of retained food within the stomach. (Right) In this elderly woman, CT shows soft tissue density thickening of the wall of the distal stomach ➡. Note the normal thin gastric wall ➡ for comparison. These are typical findings indicating the scirrhous, fibrotic character of many gastric carcinomas.

Hyperplastic Polyps

Air (Gas) Bubbles

(Left) *Upper GI shows multiple, sharply defined polyps ➡ of similar small size, typical of hyperplastic polyps.* **(Right)** *Frontal upper GI shows what seem to be multiple barium-lined polyps ➡, but these were mobile and transient, representing air bubbles. Upper endoscopy results were normal.*

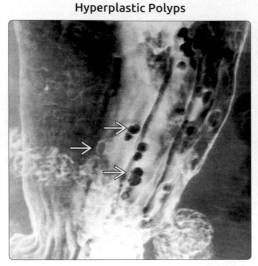

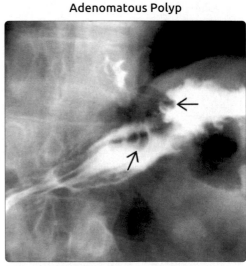

Adenomatous Polyp

Adenomatous Polyp

(Left) *Spot film from an upper GI shows a well-defined, sessile polyp ➡ just caudal to the esophagogastric junction, proven to be an adenomatous polyp on endoscopy and resection.* **(Right)** *Spot film from an upper GI shows several sessile and pedunculated gastric polyps ➡ in an elderly woman that proved to be adenomatous polyps with villous architecture.*

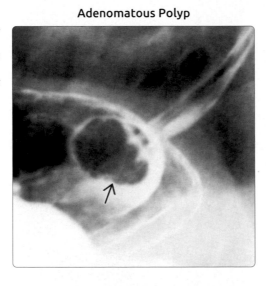

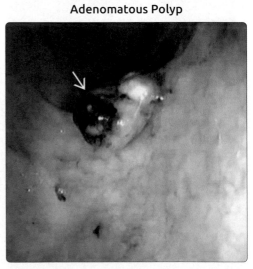

Adenomatous Polyp

Adenomatous Polyp

(Left) *In this 65-year-old woman, a spot film from an upper GI shows a well-defined sessile polyp ➡ with acute angles at its interface with the gastric wall.* **(Right)** *In this 65-year-old woman, endoscopy shows an ulcerated mass ➡ that was a benign adenoma. A band was placed around the base of the polyp, and it was resected at endoscopy.*

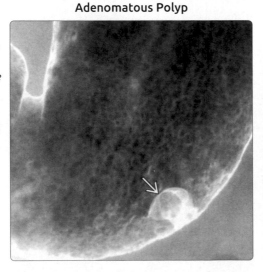

Bezoar (Mimic)

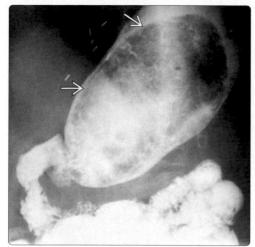

Bezoar (Mimic)

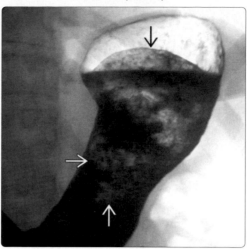

(Left) *Upper GI shows a large mobile filling defect or mass* ➡ *within the stomach. This patient had a prior vagotomy and distal antrectomy (Billroth 1 procedure) for peptic ulcer disease.* (Right) *Upper GI shows a large mass* ➡ *within the distended stomach that seems to conform to the shape of the stomach. Note the rounded superior margin of the mass* ➡ *on this upright film.*

Splenomegaly and Hypersplenism

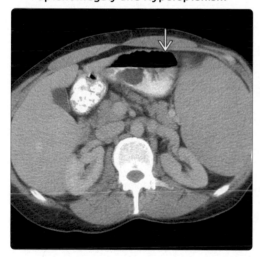

Renal Cell Carcinoma

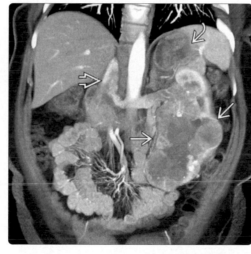

(Left) *Axial CECT shows massive enlargement of the spleen due to chronic lymphocytic leukemia. Note displacement and mass effect on the stomach* ➡. (Right) *Coronal CECT shows a huge mass* ➡ *arising from the left kidney with invasion of the renal vein and inferior vena cava* ➡. *Large masses like this may extrinsically compress the stomach* ➡ *and mimic intramural gastric masses.*

Splenosis

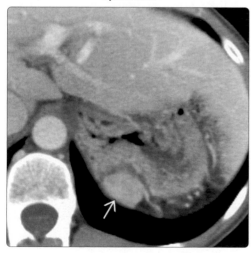

Gastric Varices

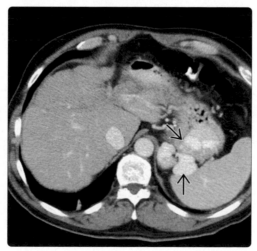

(Left) *Axial CECT shows an intramural mass* ➡ *(splenosis) in a patient who had splenectomy for traumatic splenic rupture some years previously.* (Right) *Axial CECT shows large varices* ➡ *that distort the fundus of the stomach, in a patient with cirrhosis and portal hypertension. On an unenhanced CT or an upper GI series, these could mimic a neoplastic mass.*

(Left) *Axial CECT shows classic intramural mass* ➡ *with obtuse angles & intact gastric mucosa. Central necrosis in mass is clue as to its etiology, a gastric GI stromal tumor.* **(Right)** *In this young woman with upper GI bleeding, axial CT shows an encapsulated spherical mass* ➡ *within wall of stomach, which appears to be draped or stretched around it. Mass is soft tissue in attenuation with a necrotic focus* ➡. *Collection of gas is noted within a surface defect of the mass* ➡ *& overlying gastric mucosa, representing site of ulceration & bleeding.*

Gastrointestinal Stromal Tumor, Gastric

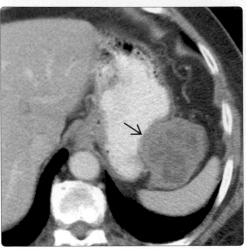

Gastrointestinal Stromal Tumor, Gastric

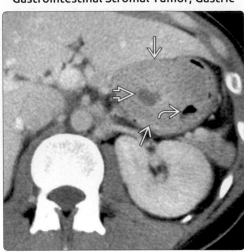

(Left) *In this young woman, coronal CT shows the large intramural gastric mass, with its central necrosis* ➡ *and ulceration* ➡. **(Right)** *Axial NECT shows 1* ➡ *of several fat-density masses (lipomas) within the stomach but actually arising from the gastric wall. Intramural masses of the stomach and GI tract are frequently drawn into the gut lumen by peristalsis.*

Gastrointestinal Stromal Tumor, Gastric

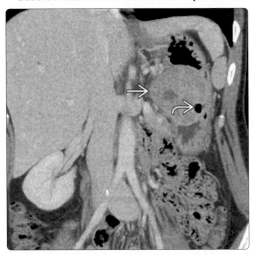

Intramural Gastric Tumors

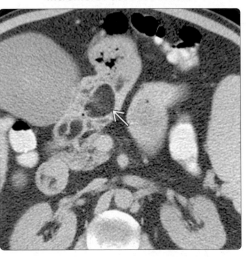

(Left) *In this patient with melanoma, CECT shows several intramural gastric masses* ➡, *along with metastases to nodes* ➡ *and the peritoneal surface* ➡. **(Right)** *Axial CECT shows circumferential, marked, soft tissue density thickening of the gastric wall* ➡ *and extensive perigastric lymphadenopathy* ➡, *typical features of gastric lymphoma.*

Gastric Metastases and Lymphoma

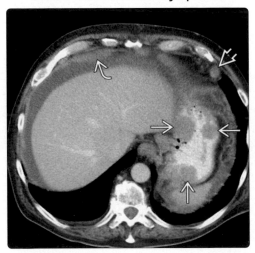

Gastric Metastases and Lymphoma

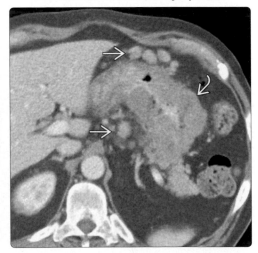

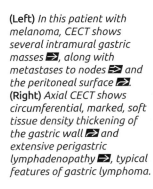

Gastric Metastases and Lymphoma

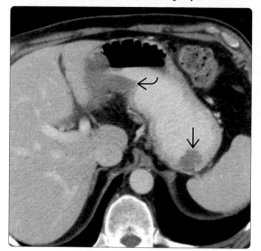

Gastric Metastases and Lymphoma

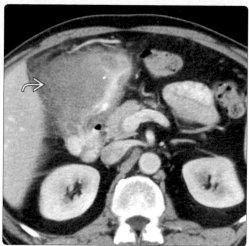

(Left) *Axial CECT shows 2 soft tissue density masses in the stomach representing gastric lymphoma. One is a sessile polyp ⇨, and the other is a bulky, circumferential antral mass ⇨. (Right) Axial CECT shows a bulky, circumferential antral mass ⇨ that is due to gastric lymphoma. There was no gastric outlet obstruction due to the soft nature of lymphomatous masses.*

Gardner Syndrome

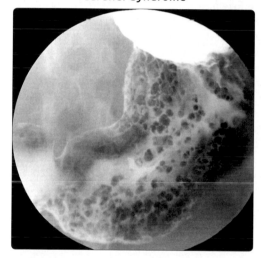

Hamartomatous Polyposis Syndromes

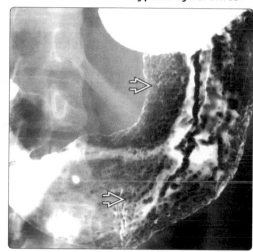

(Left) *Upper GI shows innumerable small polyps that are larger and more irregular than usually seen with hyperplastic polyps. These are adenomatous (premalignant) polyps in a patient with familial polyposis (Gardner syndrome). (Right) Film from an upper GI shows innumerable small gastric polyps ⇨ of similar size. In the general population, these would probably be hyperplastic polyps, but this patient has Peutz-Jeghers syndrome and these are hamartomatous polyps.*

Other Mesenchymal Tumors

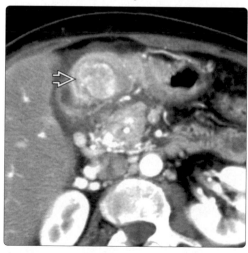

Ectopic Pancreatic Tissue

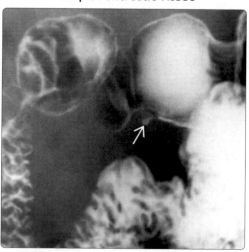

(Left) *Axial CECT shows a highly vascular mass ⇨ in the posterior wall of the stomach as an incidental finding in a patient who had CT evaluation for chronic pancreatitis. This is surgically proven neurolemmoma. (Right) Upper GI shows a classic appearance with a small intramural mass in the greater curve antrum, with a central umbilication ⇨, representing the orifice of a primitive pancreatic duct.*

DIFFERENTIAL DIAGNOSIS

Common

- Gastric Varices
- Pancreatic Pseudocyst
- Gastric Stromal Tumor
- Metastases and Lymphoma, Gastric

Less Common

- Intramural Gastric Tumors
  - Lipoma
  - Neuroendocrine Tumor
  - Glomus Tumor
  - Hemangioma
  - Schwannoma
- Gastric Intramural Hematoma
- Heterotopic (Ectopic) Pancreatic Tissue
- Accessory Spleen or Splenosis
- Gastric Duplication Cyst

ESSENTIAL INFORMATION

Key Differential Diagnosis Issues

- It is often difficult to distinguish intramural from extrinsic masses
  - Even mucosal lesions (e.g., gastric carcinoma) may have overlapping features

Helpful Clues for Common Diagnoses

- **Gastric Varices**
  - CECT: Tortuous, tubular enhancing vessels
  - Seen in portal hypertension or splenic vein occlusion
- **Pancreatic Pseudocyst**
  - Indents posterior wall of stomach
  - Nonenhancing cyst contents
  - Thin wall
  - Gastric mucosal folds overlying pseudocyst are often thickened due to inflammation
- **Gastric Stromal Tumor**
  - GI stromal tumor; well-circumscribed subepithelial mass with large exophytic component

- Often hypervascular with central necrosis
- May have mucosal ulceration
- **Metastases and Lymphoma, Gastric**
  - May be nodular and multiple (melanoma, Kaposi sarcoma) or diffuse (breast cancer)
    - May spread to stomach by direct extension (e.g., from pancreas), hematogenous (melanoma & breast), or via peritoneal seeding of gastric serosal surface (ovarian, uterine, GI primaries)
  - Lymphoma: Usually large, homogeneous tumor that does not obstruct stomach

Helpful Clues for Less Common Diagnoses

- **Intramural Gastric Tumors**
  - Lipoma; characteristic fat density
  - Other mesenchymal tumors (neuroma, fibroma, hemangioma, etc.)
    - Any component of gastric wall may give rise to benign or malignant tumor
    - Except for lipoma, have overlapping & nonspecific imaging features
    - Neuroendocrine tumor, glomus tumors, & hemangiomas are often hypervascular
- **Gastric Intramural Hematoma**
  - Following endoscopy, biopsy, PEG tube placement, or blunt trauma
- **Heterotopic (Ectopic) Pancreatic Tissue**
  - Small mural nodule along greater curvature of antrum with central umbilication
- **Accessory Spleen or Splenosis**
  - May indent or implant on gastric wall
  - Splenosis, following traumatic rupture of spleen, may implant anywhere on peritoneal surface
  - Multiphasic CECT or MR show same enhancement as spleen
  - Focal uptake on Tc heat-damaged RBC radionuclide scan is diagnostic
- **Gastric Duplication Cyst**
  - Rare; may or may not communicate with gastric lumen

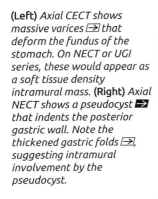

(Left) *Axial CECT shows massive varices ⇥ that deform the fundus of the stomach. On NECT or UGI series, these would appear as a soft tissue density intramural mass.* **(Right)** *Axial NECT shows a pseudocyst ⇥ that indents the posterior gastric wall. Note the thickened gastric folds ⇥, suggesting intramural involvement by the pseudocyst.*

Gastric Varices

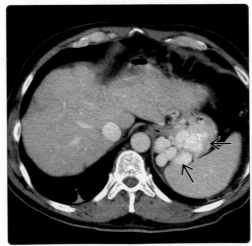

Pancreatic Pseudocyst

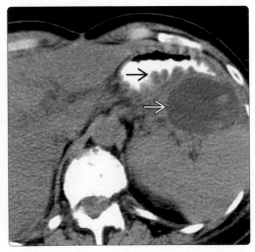

Intramural Mass, Stomach

Gastric Stromal Tumor

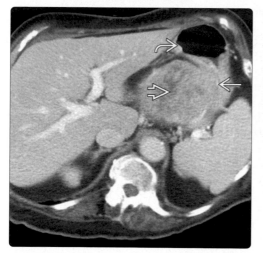

Intramural Gastric Tumors

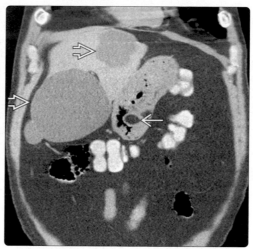

(Left) *CT shows a large, exophytic mass ➡ arising from the lesser curve of the stomach ➡. It is relatively vascular with central areas of necrosis ➡.* **(Right)** *Coronal NECT shows a fat density mass ➡, a lipoma, within the gastric wall. There are 2 large benign cysts ➡ in the liver as unrelated lesions.*

Metastases and Lymphoma, Gastric

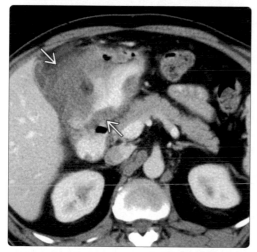

Metastases and Lymphoma, Gastric

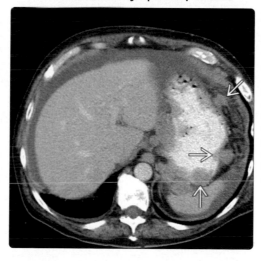

(Left) *Axial CECT shows a large soft tissue density mass ➡ that envelopes the gastric antrum but does not cause gastric outlet obstruction. These are typical findings for gastric lymphoma.* **(Right)** *Axial CECT shows peritoneal and gastric wall metastases as discrete nodules ➡ in this patient with metastatic melanoma. Omental metastases and malignant ascites were also evident.*

Metastases and Lymphoma, Gastric

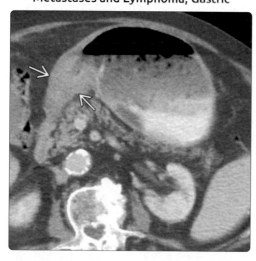

Heterotopic (Ectopic) Pancreatic Tissue

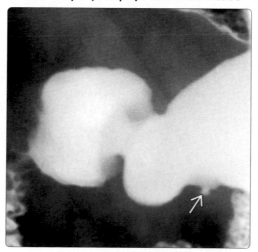

(Left) *Axial CECT shows a circumferential soft tissue density mass ➡ that envelopes and obstructs the gastric antrum. Note the retained food and debris within the proximal stomach. This is metastatic breast cancer (but is indistinguishable from primary gastric cancer by imaging).* **(Right)** *Spot film from an upper GI shows a small intramural mass along the greater curve at the antrum, with a central umbilication ➡, representing the opening of a primitive pancreatic duct.*

DIFFERENTIAL DIAGNOSIS

Common

- Gastric Metastases
- Gastric Lymphoma
- Kaposi Sarcoma

Less Common

- Gastric Carcinoma
- Ectopic Pancreatic Tissue
- Carcinoid, Stomach
- Gastric Stromal Tumor

ESSENTIAL INFORMATION

Key Differential Diagnosis Issues

- Target or bull's-eye lesions are raised nodules or masses with central ulceration
  - Etiology is submucosal mass with ulceration of overlying mucosa
  - Highly suggestive of malignant gastric lesion (or ectopic pancreas)
    - Multiple lesions are almost always malignant
  - Target lesions are different from aphthous lesions (shallow erosions with small edematous mound; seen in gastritis)

Helpful Clues for Common Diagnoses

- **Gastric Metastases**
  - Most common cause of bull's-eye pattern of metastases is malignant melanoma
- **Gastric Lymphoma**
  - GI tract lymphoma can also cause bull's-eye lesions
    - Stomach is most common site
- **Kaposi Sarcoma**
  - Usually in homosexual men with AIDS
  - Stomach is most common site of GI tract involvement

Helpful Clues for Less Common Diagnoses

- **Gastric Carcinoma**
  - Rarely appears as single target lesion

- Central ulceration is common, but surrounding tissue is more irregular and nodular than with other etiologies
- **Ectopic Pancreatic Tissue**
  - Usually single umbilicated lesion in gastric antrum
  - Does not result in multiple bull's-eye lesions
- **Carcinoid, Stomach**
  - From chromograffin cells in gastric mucosa
  - Does not produce carcinoid syndrome
  - Increased frequency in Zollinger-Ellison syndrome and atrophic gastritis
- **Gastric Stromal Tumor**
  - Stomach is most common site of GI stromal tumor
  - Usual appearance: Large exophytic mass arising from gastric wall
  - Erosion of overlying mucosa can result in bull's-eye appearance
    - Gas, fluid, and oral contrast medium may enter central necrotic area of GI stromal tumor

Gastric Metastases

Gastric Metastases

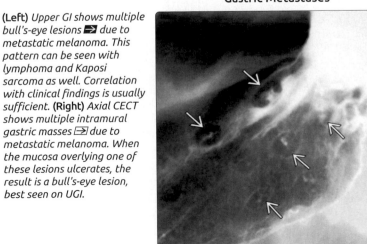

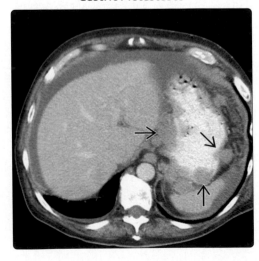

(Left) Upper GI shows multiple bull's-eye lesions ➡ due to metastatic melanoma. This pattern can be seen with lymphoma and Kaposi sarcoma as well. Correlation with clinical findings is usually sufficient. (Right) Axial CECT shows multiple intramural gastric masses ➡ due to metastatic melanoma. When the mucosa overlying one of these lesions ulcerates, the result is a bull's-eye lesion, best seen on UGI.

Gastric Lymphoma

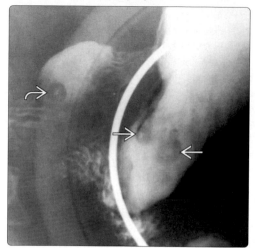

Gastric Lymphoma

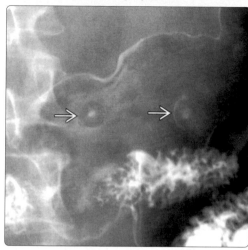

(Left) Upper GI shows multiple classic bull's-eye lesions in the stomach ➡ and duodenum ➡ of this patient with lymphoma. (Right) Upper GI shows classic bull's-eye lesions ➡ in the stomach on this air-contrast study, with small masses and central umbilication.

Gastric Carcinoma

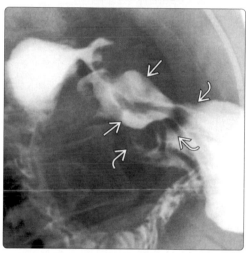

Ectopic Pancreatic Tissue

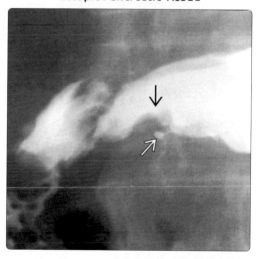

(Left) Upper GI shows a large ulcer ➡ (persistent collection of barium) within a larger mass ➡. This is not what is usually referred to as a bull's-eye lesion, but it is very suggestive of gastric carcinoma. (Right) Upper GI shows a pathognomonic appearance of ectopic pancreas with a small mural mass ➡ in the antrum with an umbilication ➡, representing the orifice of a primitive pancreatic duct, in this 36-year-old man.

Ectopic Pancreatic Tissue

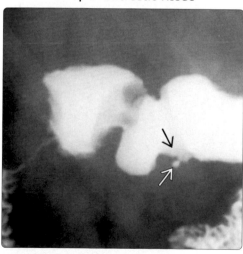

Gastric Stromal Tumor

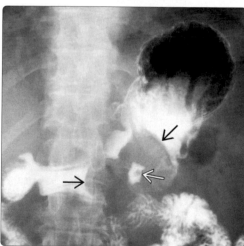

(Left) Upper GI shows a typical small intramural mass ➡ along the greater curve of the antrum with a central umbilication ➡, representing filling of a rudimentary pancreatic duct in a 60-year-old woman. (Right) Upper GI shows a large intramural mass ➡ with a central ulceration ➡, a typical appearance for a gastric GIST. This lesion would be considered by many to be too large to constitute a bull's-eye lesion.

DIFFERENTIAL DIAGNOSIS

Common

- NSAID-Induced Gastritis
- Gastritis (Other Causes)
- Gastric Ulcer

Less Common

- Gastric Carcinoma
- Zollinger-Ellison Syndrome
- Crohn Disease
- Caustic Gastroduodenal Injury

ESSENTIAL INFORMATION

Key Differential Diagnosis Issues

- Gastritis is, by far, most common cause of gastric erosions or ulcerations

Helpful Clues for Common Diagnoses

- **NSAID-Induced Gastritis**
  - Nonsteroidal antiinflammatory drugs, including aspirin
  - Gastric erosion may be varioliform, linear, or serpiginous
  - Erosions may be clustered along dependent surface of stomach, distal body, or antrum
- **Gastritis (Other Causes)**
  - Other medications, alcohol, uremia, idiopathic
  - Appearance similar to NSAID-induced gastritis, regardless of etiology
  - CT shows thick gastric wall, submucosal edema
- **Gastric Ulcer**
  - Deeper erosion, into submucosa or even through wall of stomach
  - Often associated with *Helicobacter pylori* infection
  - Ulcers are usually found along lesser curvature or posterior wall of antrum or body
  - May cause perforation, often through posterior gastric wall into lesser sac
    - Look for enteric contrast medium, gas, blood within lesser sac
    - Usually much more evident on CT than on UGI series

Helpful Clues for Less Common Diagnoses

- **Gastric Carcinoma**
  - Often causes ulceration; usually mass with irregular nodular folds around ulcer crater
  - Superficial or early cancer may have no visible mass
    - This form is rarely ulcerated
  - CT: Soft tissue density, nodular thickening of gastric wall
    - Infiltration of omentum, nodal, peritoneal, or liver mets are often seen
- **Zollinger-Ellison Syndrome**
  - Gastrin-producing islet call (neuroendocrine) tumor of pancreas
  - Intractable, multiple ulcers in stomach, duodenum, even proximal jejunum
  - CT: Hypervascular pancreatic mass (arterial phase), thick gastric folds, metastases
- **Crohn Disease**
  - May induce aphthoid erosions in stomach
  - Chronic involvement: Ram's horn contraction of distal body and antrum

(Left) Spot film from an upper GI shows thickened antral folds with linear erosions ➡ *along the peaks of the folds, diagnostic of some form of gastritis. (Right) Spot film from an upper GI shows superficial rounded and linear erosions* ➡ *(superficial ulcerations). On endoscopy these were interpreted as erosive gastritis, cause not specified.*

NSAID-Induced Gastritis

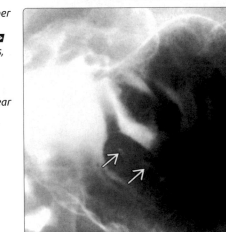

Gastritis (Other Causes)

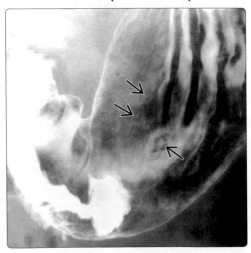

Gastric Ulcer

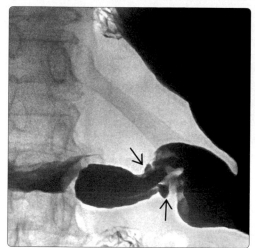

Gastric Ulcer

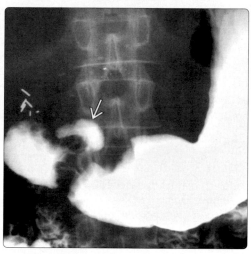

(Left) *Spot film from an upper GI shows contraction of the antrum and thickened folds that extend to the edges of 2 discrete ulcers* ➡. (Right) *Spot film from an upper GI shows a fixed collection of barium* ➡ *extending beyond the confines of the gastric wall. This was a perforated prepyloric ulcer. Note spasm and distortion of the antrum.*

Gastric Ulcer

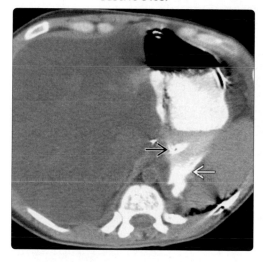

Gastric Carcinoma

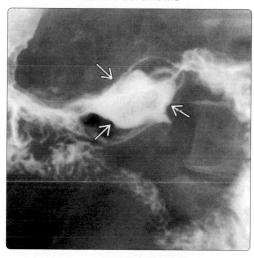

(Left) *Axial NECT shows oral (enteric) contrast medium extravasated into the lesser sac* ➡ *through a perforated gastric ulcer. A nasogastric tube* ➡ *marks the dependent surface of the stomach.* (Right) *Prone oblique spot film from an upper GI shows a large antral ulcer* ➡ *(fixed collection of barium). The surrounding mass is less evident, although fluoroscopy showed a stiff, nonperistaltic distal body and antrum that was found to be a large carcinoma at surgery.*

Zollinger-Ellison Syndrome

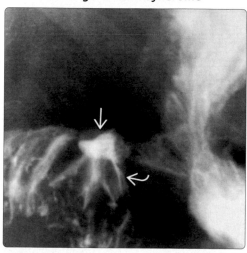

Crohn Disease

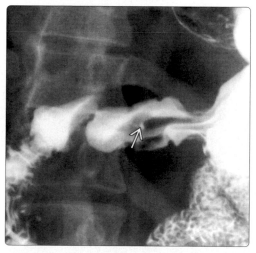

(Left) *Spot film from an upper GI shows an ulcer* ➡ *at the site of a gastroenteric anastomosis following partial gastrectomy & vagotomy for ulcers. Note the folds* ➡ *radiating to edge of ulcer. Recurrent ulcers were a common feature of Zollinger-Ellison syndrome prior to improved diagnosis & therapy.* (Right) *Upper GI shows an aphthous erosion* ➡ *of a thickened antral fold in a young man with proven Crohn gastritis who also had small bowel involvement.*

DIFFERENTIAL DIAGNOSIS

Common

- Hiatal Hernia
- Postesophagectomy
- Achalasia, Esophagus (Mimic)

Less Common

- Postoperative Fluid Collection (Mimic)
- Pulsion Diverticulum, Esophagus (Mimic)

ESSENTIAL INFORMATION

Key Differential Diagnosis Issues

- Dilated esophagus from any etiology may be mistaken for intrathoracic stomach (or vice versa)
  - Look for evidence of surgery (suture lines; portions of stomach missing from abdomen)
- Postoperative conditions can mimic or cause intrathoracic stomach
  - Ivor-Lewis or other type of esophagectomy with gastric pull-through
  - Gastric conduit (intrathoracic stomach) mimics dilated esophagus
- Epiphrenic esophageal diverticulum can mimic stomach on upper GI series, CT or MR

Helpful Clues for Common Diagnoses

- **Hiatal Hernia**
  - Paraesophageal hernias may result in much or all of stomach lying in thorax
  - Type III: Paraesophageal hernia with GE junction & large portion of stomach in thorax
  - Type IV hernia: Intrathoracic stomach that may or may not undergo volvulus & gastric outlet obstruction
    - Gastric volvulus with obstruction demands immediate decompression
- **Postesophagectomy**
  - Common surgical procedure for esophageal carcinoma
  - Much of stomach is pulled into thorax to replace resected portion of esophagus

  - Stomach is usually divided longitudinally 1st, to reduce volume of gastric conduit
  - Distention & slow emptying of conduit are relatively common complications of procedure
  - Esophagogastric anastomosis is usually near thoracic inlet or carina
- **Achalasia, Esophagus (Mimic)**
  - May result in marked dilation of esophagus
  - Distended lumen with air-fluid levels may simulate intrathoracic stomach, especially on axial CT

Helpful Clues for Less Common Diagnoses

- **Postoperative Fluid Collection (Mimic)**
  - Following esophagectomy, fundoplication, or repair of large hiatal hernia
  - May result in large collection of fluid ± gas that may simulate intrathoracic stomach
- **Pulsion Diverticulum, Esophagus (Mimic)**
  - Epiphrenic diverticula may be large
  - Retention of food, fluid, and gas simulates stomach
  - Associated with elderly; esophageal dysmotility syndromes

(Left) Coronal CT shows massive dilation of the herniated stomach ➡, a large type 3 or even 4 paraesophageal hernia with gastric volvulus. (Right) In this elderly woman with chest pain and retching, axial CECT shows a large type IV paraesophageal hernia ➡ (intrathoracic stomach). Note the compressed, atelectatic lung ➡.

Hiatal Hernia

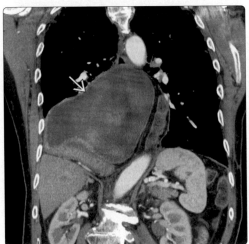

Hiatal Hernia

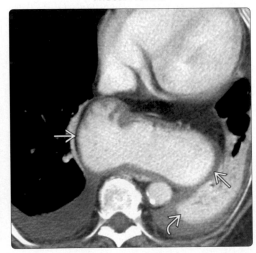

Postesophagectomy

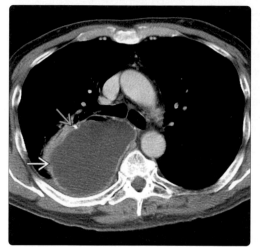

Postesophagectomy

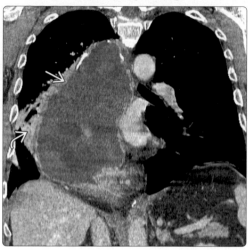

(Left) *In this 66-year-old man who has had an Ivor-Lewis esophagectomy, axial CT shows a dilated gastric conduit* ➡️. *Note the staple line* ➡️ *along the margin of the conduit.* (Right) *In this 66-year-old man who has had an Ivor-lewis esophagectomy, a coronal CT section shows massive dilation of the gastric conduit (intrathoracic stomach)* ➡️ *along with aspiration pneumonitis in the right lower lobe* ➡️.

Postoperative Fluid Collection (Mimic)

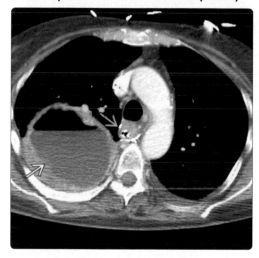

Achalasia, Esophagus (Mimic)

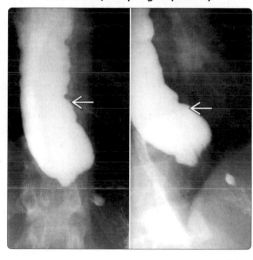

(Left) *In this patient who has had an Ivor Lewis esophagectomy, a loculated collection of gas & fluid* ➡️ *represents a large empyema due to an anastomotic leak but could be easily mistaken for a dilated gastric conduit. The nondilated conduit* ➡️ *is in its expected position.* (Right) *Spot films from an esophagram shows massive dilation of the esophagus* ➡️ *with a tapered, constricting distal segment, classic appearance of achalasia in a 23-year-old woman with progressive dysphagia.*

Postoperative Fluid Collection (Mimic)

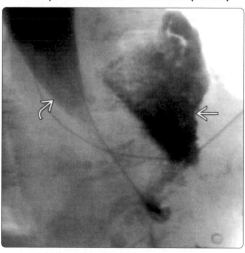

Pulsion Diverticulum, Esophagus (Mimic)

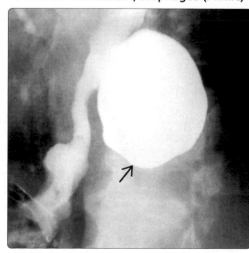

(Left) *Spot film from an esophagram shows extravasation* ➡️ *of water-soluble contrast material from the distal esophagus* ➡️ *or proximal stomach into the mediastinum, following surgical fundoplication for hiatal hernia and reflux.* (Right) *Esophagram shows a large epiphrenic pulsion diverticulum* ➡️ *and signs of esophageal dysmotility in this elderly man with dysphagia.*

DIFFERENTIAL DIAGNOSIS

Common

- Gastritis
- Gastric Ulcer
- Portal Hypertension, Varices
- Gastric Carcinoma
- Pancreatitis, Acute
  - Pancreatic Pseudocyst
- Portal Hypertensive Gastropathy

Less Common

- Gastric Metastases and Lymphoma
- Ménétrier Disease
- Zollinger-Ellison Syndrome
- Caustic Gastroduodenal Injury
- Crohn Disease

Rare but Important

- Tuberculosis
- Radiation Gastritis
- Amyloidosis
- Eosinophilic Gastritis
- Chemotherapy-Induced Gastritis
- Sarcoidosis

ESSENTIAL INFORMATION

Key Differential Diagnosis Issues

- CT helps to narrow differential diagnosis by showing disease beyond stomach
  - Examples: Metastatic tumor; signs of pancreatitis
- CT can show nature of submucosal thickening that is usual source of thick folds
  - Edema: Near water attenuation = inflammatory or infectious
  - Soft tissue density = more likely to be neoplastic
    - Carcinoma, lymphoma, or metastases
- Correlation with history is important
  - Examples: History of pancreatitis, Crohn disease, extragastric malignancy

Helpful Clues for Common Diagnoses

- **Gastritis**
  - Symptomatic with abdominal pain
  - Antrum affected most commonly
  - Look for erosions, especially along rugal folds; limited distensibility
  - Causes: NSAIDs, alcohol, *Helicobacter pylori*
- **Gastric Ulcer**
  - Folds of uniform thickness radiate from edge of ulcer crater
  - Look for extraluminal gas or enteric contrast medium
- **Portal Hypertension, Varices**
  - Varices mostly in fundus
    - Portal hypertensive gastropathy can affect entire stomach
  - Associated with portal hypertension (cirrhosis, splenomegaly, ascites)
  - Also caused by splenic vein occlusion (pancreatic carcinoma, chronic pancreatitis)

- CECT: Usually distinguishes varices from other etiologies of thickened folds; shows underlying cause
  - Varices enhance like vessels on portal venous-phase CECT
  - Thick folds enhance like wall of stomach
- **Gastric Carcinoma**
  - Irregular, nodular, thickened folds
  - Limited distensibility and peristalsis
    - These findings are more evident on UGI series (fluoroscopy) than on CT
  - CT usually shows extragastric spread of tumor
    - Enlarged nodes, liver metastases, omental seeding
- **Pancreatitis, Acute**
  - Fold thickening of posterior wall of stomach, adjacent to pancreas
  - CT signs of pancreatitis: Enlarged gland, peripancreatic infiltration, fluid collections
  - **Pancreatic pseudocyst**
    - Back wall of stomach is often draped over pseudocyst
    - Gastric folds in contact with pseudocyst are thickened

Helpful Clues for Less Common Diagnoses

- **Gastric Metastases and Lymphoma**
  - Lymphoma
    - Massive nodular thickening of folds but usually normal distensibility
  - Metastases may cause nodular intramural masses, ± ulceration, ± limited distensibility
    - Breast cancer especially likely to result in thick folds, limited distensibility
- **Ménétrier Disease**
  - Massive fold thickening in fundus and body
    - Antrum is usually spared
  - Hypersecretion of protein; hyposecretion of acid
    - May result in dilution and poor coating of barium on UGI
- **Zollinger-Ellison Syndrome**
  - Hypersecretion of acid & thick folds, multiple & recurrent ulcers
  - Gastrin-secreting neuroendocrine (islet cell) tumor of pancreas
    - CECT often shows hypervascular pancreatic tumor
  - May be part of multiple endocrine neoplasia syndrome
- **Caustic Gastroduodenal Injury**
  - Ingestion of strong alkali or acid
  - Acute findings = massive wall edema ± ulceration of mucosa
    - Difficult & potentially dangerous to perform UGI series; CT shows pertinent findings in esophagus & stomach, including wall injury & possible perforation
  - End result is often perforation or linitis plastica appearance of stomach
- **Crohn Disease**
  - May cause gastritis with erosions and thickened folds
  - Long-standing involvement may cause ram's horn appearance
    - Nondistensible distal body and antrum with tapered curve toward pylorus

Helpful Clues for Rare Diagnoses

- **Tuberculosis**

- Classic appearance is thickened folds & limited distensibility of stomach & duodenum
- Relatively common in some populations (e.g., Native Americans)
- **Radiation Gastritis**
  - Nonspecific fold thickening & limited distensibility
  - History of upper abdominal radiation therapy is essential to diagnosis
- **Amyloidosis**
  - Look for evidence of systemic amyloid
  - Usually involves antrum
- **Eosinophilic Gastritis**
  - Mostly affects antrum
  - Check for peripheral blood eosinophilia
  - History of allergic diseases
- **Chemotherapy-Induced Gastritis**
  - Usually due to inadvertent perfusion of stomach during hepatic arterial infusion of floxuridine
- **Sarcoidosis**
  - Usually affects antrum
  - Check for pulmonary & hepatic involvement

Gastritis

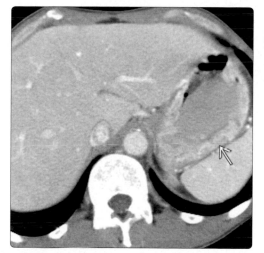

Gastritis

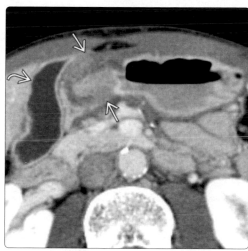

(Left) In this 54-year-old man with acute gastritis, CT shows a thickened and hyperemic gastric wall ➡. (Right) In this 54-year-old man with acute gastritis, CT shows the antrum is contracted with a particularly thickened and edematous wall ➡. The gallbladder is noted for reference ➡.

Gastritis

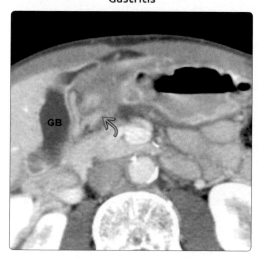

Gastritis

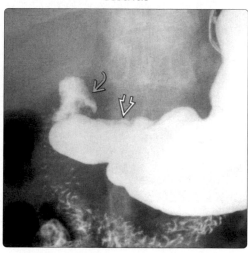

(Left) In this man with acute gastritis, CT shows the base of the duodenal bulb ➡ is indented, and edematous gastric folds are herniating into the bulb. (Right) A spot film in a man with acute gastritis from an upper GI series shows a nondistensible antrum with thickened, nodular folds ➡, and herniation of gastric folds into the duodenal bulb ➡.

Gastric Ulcer

Gastric Ulcer

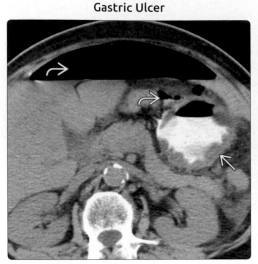

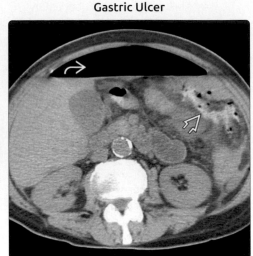

(Left) *In this 64-year-old man with acute abdominal pain, axial NECT shows thick gastric folds ➡ and extraluminal gas ➡ due to a perforated gastric ulcer.* **(Right)** *In this 64-year-old man axial NECT shows free intraperitoneal gas ➡ and extravasation of gastric contrast medium ➡, indicating a perforated gastric ulcer.*

Portal Hypertension, Varices

Portal Hypertension, Varices

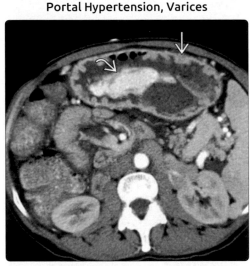

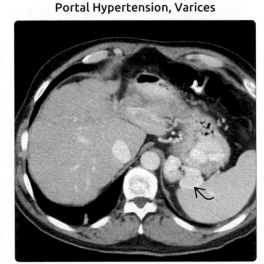

(Left) *Axial CECT shows active bleeding ➡ (extravasation of IV contrast) into stomach due to portal hypertensive gastropathy from cirrhosis. Note the thick folds ➡.* **(Right)** *Axial CECT shows massive gastric wall varices ➡ in the fundus due to cirrhosis. On UGI series or NECT, these may simulate a gastric mass or nonspecific fold thickening.*

Gastric Carcinoma

Gastric Carcinoma

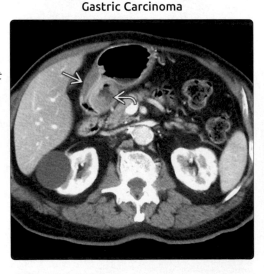

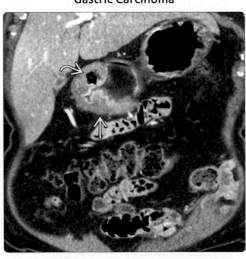

(Left) *CT in an elderly Asian man shows a circumferential soft tissue density mass ➡ that narrows the lumen of the gastric antrum, with an abrupt transition from the distended, thin-walled proximal stomach. An irregular collection of gas and particulate material ➡ is noted within the antral mass.* **(Right)** *Coronal CT in an elderly Asian man shows the antral carcinoma ➡ with an ulcerated surface ➡.*

Gastric Carcinoma

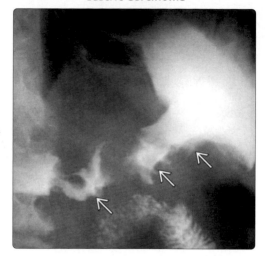

Gastric Carcinoma

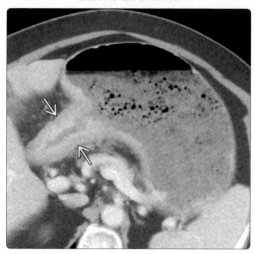

(Left) *In this elderly woman with early satiety & weight loss, a spot film from an UGI shows markedly thickened, nodular folds* ➡️ *in the gastric body & antrum with lack of distensibility. No peristalsis was seen at fluoroscopy through the affected area.* (Right) *In this elderly woman with early satiety, axial CECT shows gastric wall thickening* ➡️ *of soft tissue density through the distal body and antrum. Note signs of gastric outlet obstruction.*

Pancreatitis, Acute

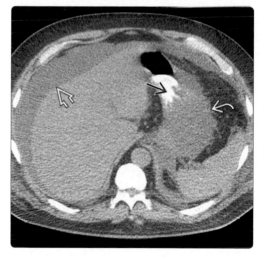

Pancreatitis, Acute

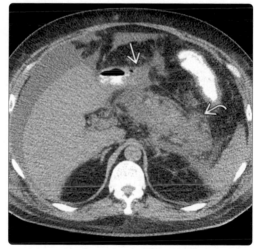

(Left) *In this elderly man with acute pancreatitis, NECT shows ascites* ➡️, *a lesser sac fluid collection* ➡️, *and thickened gastric folds along the greater curvature* ➡️. (Right) *In this elderly man with acute pancreatitis, NECT shows the characteristic infiltration of the peripancreatic fat planes* ➡️. *Those parts of the stomach that abut the inflamed pancreas show thickened folds* ➡️.

Pancreatic Pseudocyst

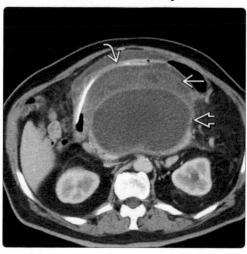

Pancreatic Pseudocyst

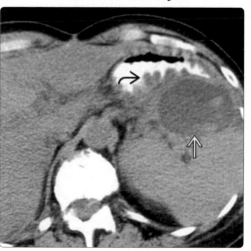

(Left) *Axial CECT shows a large midline pancreatic pseudocyst* ➡️ *with the stomach draped over it. Note the NG tube* ➡️ *within the stomach and the marked gastric wall thickening* ➡️. (Right) *Axial NECT in a 65-year-old woman shows a pancreatic pseudocyst* ➡️ *that displaces the posterior wall of the stomach and results in thickened gastric folds* ➡️.

Stomach

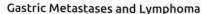

Gastric Metastases and Lymphoma

Gastric Metastases and Lymphoma

(Left) *In this elderly woman with fever and weight loss due to gastric lymphoma, a spot film from a UGI demonstrates marked thickening and blunting of the gastric folds but nearly normal distensibility and no obstruction.* (Right) *In this elderly woman with gastric lymphoma, CT shows a soft tissue density mass ⇨ that diffusely infiltrates the gastric wall. There was no sign of outlet obstruction.*

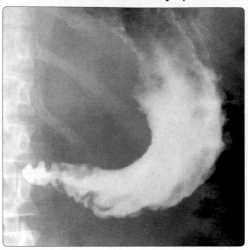

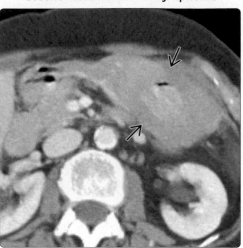

Gastric Metastases and Lymphoma

Gastric Metastases and Lymphoma

(Left) *In this elderly woman with metastatic breast cancer and early satiety, a spot film from an upper GI series shows a scirrhous lesion of the gastric antrum ⇨ that delays gastric emptying.* (Right) *In this elderly woman with breast cancer, CT shows gastric distention and retention of food. The antrum is nondistensible and is infiltrated with a soft tissue density mass ⇨ due to metastasis, though the imaging findings are indistinguishable from primary gastric carcinoma.*

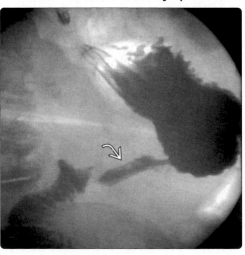

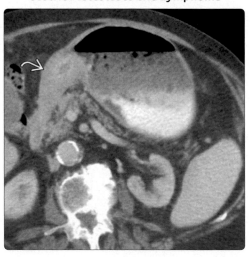

Ménétrier Disease

Ménétrier Disease

(Left) *Upper GI shows massive fold thickening ⇨ limited to the gastric fundus and body, with sparing of the antrum. There are indirect signs of excess fluid secretion with poor coating of the gastric mucosa by the barium.* (Right) *Axial CECT shows massive fold thickening ⇨ that was limited to the gastric fundus and body, mimicking the appearance of cerebral folds. Note the absence of a tumor mass in this 71-year-old woman.*

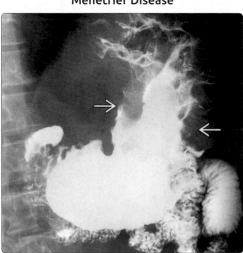

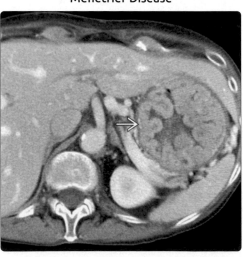

Zollinger-Ellison Syndrome

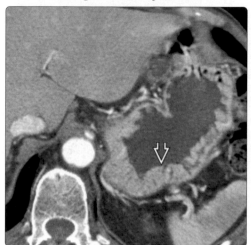

Zollinger-Ellison Syndrome

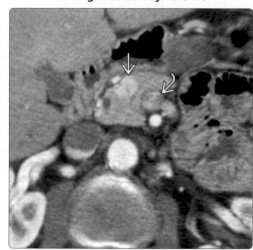

(Left) *In this man with intractable ulcer symptoms, CT shows hyperemia and fold thickening of the stomach* ⇒. **(Right)** *In this man with intractable ulcer symptoms, CT shows small hypervascular mass* ⇒ *in the neck of the pancreas, the gastrinoma responsible for the Zollinger-Ellison syndrome. It is important to distinguish this tumor from the adjacent superior mesenteric vein* ⇒.

Caustic Gastroduodenal Injury

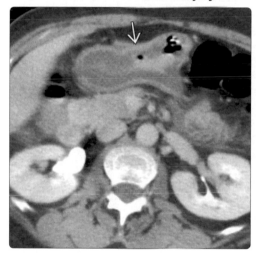

Amyloidosis

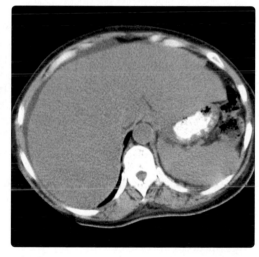

(Left) *In this young woman who drank lye in a suicide attempt, CT shows marked fold thickening, submucosal edema, and luminal narrowing of the stomach* ⇒. *Similar findings were present in the esophagus, along with aspiration pneumonitis.* **(Right)** *Axial NECT shows hepatosplenomegaly and thickened gastric folds due to amyloidosis. Liver biopsy and endoscopy were used to confirm the histologic diagnoses.*

Crohn Disease

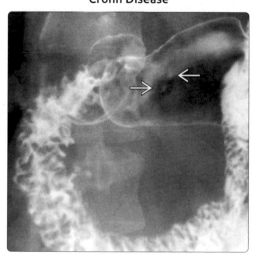

Crohn Disease

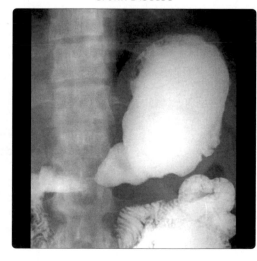

(Left) *In this young woman with Crohn gastritis, a spot film from an UGI shows incomplete distensibility of the antrum, thickened folds, and several shallow ulcerations (aphthous erosions)* ⇒. *Endoscopic biopsy and correlation with clinical findings indicated that these were due to Crohn disease.* **(Right)** *An upper GI series in a 24-year-old man with chronic Crohn disease of stomach & bowel shows decreased distensibility of the stomach with a ram's horn shape of the contracted body and antrum. Also note thickened folds.*

DIFFERENTIAL DIAGNOSIS

Common

- Gastric or Duodenal Ulcer
  - Gastritis
- Gastric Carcinoma
- Gastroparesis
- Postoperative State, Stomach
  - Gastric Bezoar
  - Fundoplication Complications
- Gastric Volvulus
- Hypertrophic Pyloric Stenosis
- Gastric Ileus

Less Common

- Pancreatitis, Acute
- Pancreatitis, Chronic
- Metastases, Gastric
- Duodenal Mass or Stricture
  - Duodenal Carcinoma
  - Annular Pancreas
  - Metastases, Duodenal
- Gastric Polyps
- Superior Mesenteric Artery Syndrome

Rare but Important

- Infiltrating Lesions
  - Crohn Disease (Gastric)
  - Sarcoidosis, Gastric
  - Tuberculosis, Gastroduodenal
  - Syphilis, Stomach
  - Amyloidosis

ESSENTIAL INFORMATION

Key Differential Diagnosis Issues

- Look for mass or stricture in stomach or proximal bowel
- Recent onset of gastric outlet obstruction without long preceding history of "ulcer pain" should suggest malignant etiology
  - Inquire about
    - Recent or chronic symptoms
    - Any known malignancy
    - Recent weight loss

Helpful Clues for Common Diagnoses

- **Gastric or Duodenal Ulcer**
  - Peptic ulcers account for 2/3 of cases of gastric outlet obstruction
  - Prepyloric or duodenal ulcer may cause spasm, edema, and scarring that obstruct gastric outlet
    - Gastritis (many etiologies) is uncommon cause of outlet obstruction
    - Distinguished from ulcer by shallow mucosal erosions
  - Outlet obstruction is late finding
    - Should be preceded by long history of pain attributable to peptic ulcer disease
- **Gastric Carcinoma**
  - 2nd most common cause of gastric outlet obstruction
    - Accounts for almost 1/3 of cases of gastric outlet obstruction

- Involvement of antrum may obstruct outlet
- Gastric carcinoma is often scirrhous
  - "Hard" inflexible mass that limits distensibility and peristalsis
  - Lack of peristalsis is most evident at fluoroscopic UGI series
- **Gastroparesis**
  - Common sequela of diabetes, narcotic analgesics
  - Flaccid stomach without peristalsis
  - Radionuclide gastric emptying study is best diagnostic tool
- **Postoperative State, Stomach**
  - **Gastric bezoar**
    - Increased prevalence following vagotomy and partial gastric resection
    - Look for large heterogeneous mass that fills stomach but is freely movable
      - Mass conforms to shape of stomach
      - May be difficult to distinguish from food from recent meal
  - **Fundoplication complications**
    - Limits ability to belch
    - May result in distention of stomach with swallowed air
      - "Gas bloat" syndrome
- **Gastric Volvulus**
  - Intrathoracic stomach (paraesophageal hernia, type IV)
  - May twist on itself
    - Organoaxial or mesenteroaxial volvulus
  - More important to determine if gastric outlet is obstructed
    - Obstruction may constitute surgical emergency or require endoscopic decompression
- **Hypertrophic Pyloric Stenosis**
  - Common cause in baby boys
  - Rare in adults
  - May be same disease process with delayed diagnosis
  - Over 50% of adults with pyloric stenosis also have gastric ulcers
    - Thought to be due to outlet obstruction and hyperacidity
- **Gastric Ileus**
  - Usually accompanied by dilation of small and large bowel
  - Common sequela of
    - Trauma
    - Postoperative state (usually abdominal surgery)
    - Electrolyte disorder
    - Narcotic analgesic use

Helpful Clues for Less Common Diagnoses

- **Pancreatitis, Acute**
  - Gastric dilatation from several possible etiologies
    - Duodenal inflammation
    - Pain (ileus)
    - Narcotics
- **Pancreatitis, Chronic**
  - May result in stricture of 2nd portion of duodenum
  - Pancreatic pseudocysts can also contribute to functional gastric outlet obstruction
- **Metastases, Gastric**
  - Metastases to stomach may cause scirrhous reaction

- Breast cancer is most common etiology
- Lymphoma of stomach (or duodenum) rarely causes outlet obstruction
- **Duodenal Mass or Stricture**
  - Any process that narrows lumen of duodenum may result in "gastric outlet obstruction" and distention
  - Examples
    - Duodenal carcinoma: Scirrhous circumferential or intraluminal mass
    - Annular pancreas: Characteristic appearance of pancreatic tissue encircling 2nd portion of duodenum
    - Metastases: Carcinomatous metastases or direct invasion from adjacent tumor (e.g., pancreatic carcinoma)
- **Gastric Polyps**
  - Antral polyp may prolapse through and obstruct pylorus
  - Leads to intermittent outlet obstruction
- **Superior Mesenteric Artery Syndrome**
  - Lumen of 3rd portion of duodenum may be compressed as it passes between aorta (and lumbar spine) and superior mesenteric root

- Any condition that narrows aortomesenteric angle will accentuate compression
  - Recent weight loss
  - Prolonged bed rest
  - Immobilization in supine position
  - Collagen vascular diseases (scleroderma, lupus, etc.) that may also cause decreased duodenal peristalsis

Helpful Clues for Rare Diagnoses

- **Infiltrating Lesions**
  - May cause narrowing of gastric antrum and subsequent outlet obstruction
  - Multiple possible etiologies
    - Crohn disease
    - Sarcoidosis
    - Tuberculosis
    - Syphilis
    - Amyloidosis

Gastric or Duodenal Ulcer

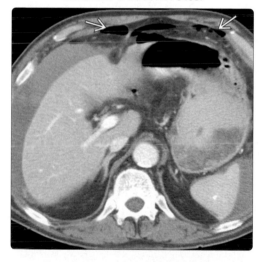

Gastric or Duodenal Ulcer

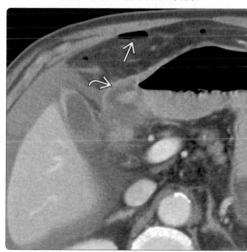

(Left) *In this elderly man, CT shows ascites and free intraperitoneal gas ➡. The stomach is distended.* (Right) *In this elderly man, CT shows free intraperitoneal gas ➡, prepyloric antral wall thickening ➡, and luminal narrowing accounting for gastric outlet obstruction. At surgery, a perforated prepyloric ulcer was found and "patched."*

Gastric Carcinoma

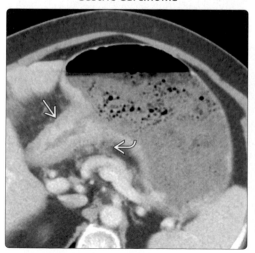

Gastroparesis

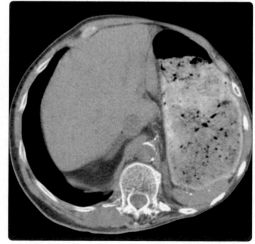

(Left) *Axial CECT shows circumferential thickening of the gastric antrum ➡ of soft tissue attenuation. Note the distended stomach with food debris and perigastric nodes ➡.* (Right) *In this man with gastroparesis due to diabetes, axial NECT shows massive distention of the stomach and retained food debris, with no obstructing mass or ulcer.*

Gastric Dilation or Outlet Obstruction

Fundoplication Complications

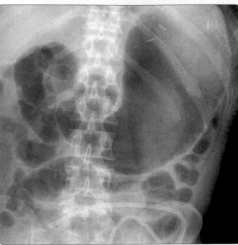

Fundoplication Complications

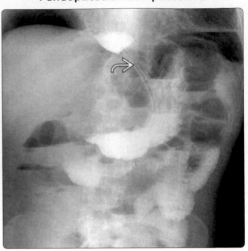

(Left) *In this young man who had recent fundoplication, a supine radiograph demonstrates marked distention of the stomach and moderate distention of bowel.* (Right) *In this young man who had recent fundoplication, an upright film from a UGI series was obtained following placement of an NG tube ➔ & shows less gastric distention but a persistent ileus. The combination of an ileus & the prevention of reflux of gas into the esophagus due to the fundoplication can result in marked distention of the stomach.*

Gastric Volvulus

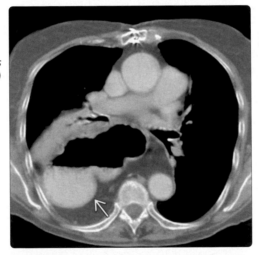

Gastric Volvulus

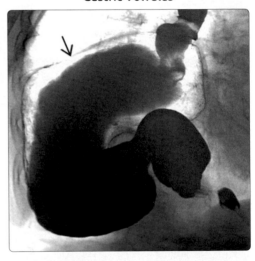

(Left) *In this elderly woman with chest pain and vomiting, CT shows the distended stomach ➔ within a hernia sac in the right thorax, and it is rotated on its long axis.* (Right) *In this elderly woman with chest pain, an upper GI series confirms the organoaxial volvulus of the stomach ➔. The stomach is distended and rotated along its long axis.*

Pancreatitis, Chronic

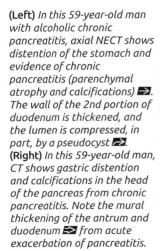
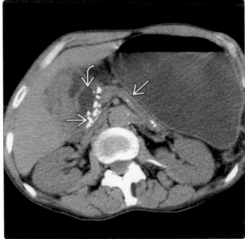

Pancreatitis, Chronic

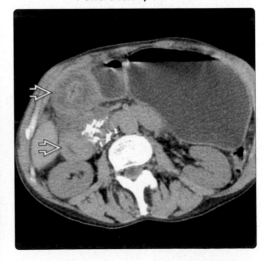

(Left) *In this 59-year-old man with alcoholic chronic pancreatitis, axial NECT shows distention of the stomach and evidence of chronic pancreatitis (parenchymal atrophy and calcifications) ➔. The wall of the 2nd portion of duodenum is thickened, and the lumen is compressed, in part, by a pseudocyst ➔.* (Right) *In this 59-year-old man, CT shows gastric distention and calcifications in the head of the pancreas from chronic pancreatitis. Note the mural thickening of the antrum and duodenum ➔ from acute exacerbation of pancreatitis.*

Metastases, Gastric

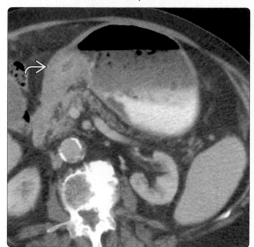

Duodenal Mass or Stricture

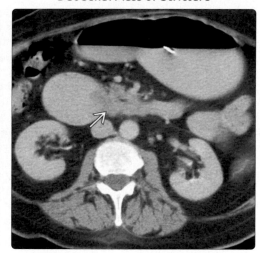

(Left) *Axial CECT shows gastric distention and food debris from outlet obstruction. The antral wall is thickened and the lumen narrowed* ➡ *due to metastatic breast cancer.* (Right) *Axial CT shows dilation of the stomach and duodenum, with abrupt narrowing of the 3rd portion of the duodenum* ➡. *There is an intramural mass that constricts the lumen of the duodenum. At surgery, metastatic breast cancer was confirmed.*

Annular Pancreas

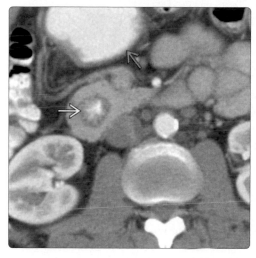

Gastric Polyps

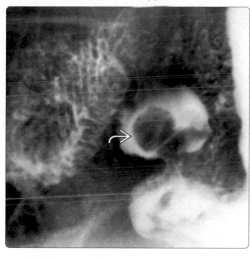

(Left) *Axial CECT shows the 2nd portion of duodenum* ➡ *completely encircled and compressed by pancreatic tissue. Note the distended stomach* ➡. (Right) *Spot film from an upper GI series shows a polyp* ➡ *within the duodenal bulb that has its base in the prepyloric antrum. It periodically herniated through the pylorus, causing partial gastric outlet obstruction.*

Superior Mesenteric Artery Syndrome

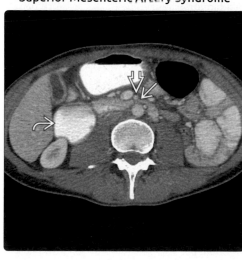

Superior Mesenteric Artery Syndrome

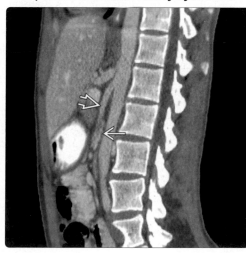

(Left) *In this thin young woman, axial CT shows distention of the stomach and 2nd portion of duodenum* ➡. *The 3rd portion of duodenum* ➡ *is markedly narrowed as it passes between the aorta and the superior mesenteric artery* ➡. (Right) *In this thin young woman, the 3rd portion of the duodenum* ➡ *is markedly compressed between the superior mesenteric artery* ➡ *and the aorta.*

DIFFERENTIAL DIAGNOSIS

Common

- Gastric Carcinoma
- Metastases and Lymphoma, Gastric

Less Common

- Gastritis
- Caustic Gastroduodenal Injury
- Peritoneal Metastases
- Opportunistic Infection, Gastric

Rare but Important

- Crohn Disease, Gastric
- Following Gastric Freezing
- Syphilis, Stomach
- Radiation-Induced Gastritis
- Infiltrative Granulomatous Diseases
  - Tuberculosis
  - Sarcoidosis
  - Amyloidosis

ESSENTIAL INFORMATION

Key Differential Diagnosis Issues

- Linitis plastica is descriptive term, not pathologic diagnosis
  - Refers to rigid, nondistensible, "leather bottle" stomach
  - **Usually due to 1 of 3 etiologies**
    - **Gastric carcinoma**
    - **Metastases** to stomach
      - □ Especially breast cancer
    - **Caustic gastric injury**
  - Many more etiologies for mild to moderate nondistensibility of stomach
    - Malignant neoplasm
      - □ Primary carcinoma or lymphoma, or metastatic to stomach or peritoneal surfaces
    - Gastritis
      - □ Many infectious and inflammatory types
    - Iatrogenic
      - □ Radiation therapy or gastric freezing for control of variceal bleeding
    - Diffuse infiltrative, granulomatous diseases
      - □ TB, sarcoid, syphilis, amyloidosis

Helpful Clues for Common Diagnoses

- **Gastric Carcinoma**
  - Most common cause worldwide
  - May invade and diffusely infiltrate submucosal layer
    - Often produces scirrhous, fibrotic response
  - May have minimal mucosal or intraluminal component
    - Can be missed on endoscopy and biopsy
  - Gastric wall is usually only moderately thickened (1-2 cm)
  - Peristalsis and distensibility are markedly diminished
    - Often most striking finding
    - Best recognized on fluoroscopic UGI series
    - Gastric outlet obstruction may also occur
      - □ Look for distention of proximal portions of stomach
      - □ Retention of food from prior meals
    - Patients complain of early satiety & weight loss, rather than pain
- **Metastases and Lymphoma, Gastric**
  - Some metastases cause scirrhous infiltration of gastric wall and fibrotic reaction
  - May cause linitis plastica appearance indistinguishable from gastric carcinoma
  - **Breast cancer** is most common primary source for this pattern
    - In North America, breast mets may be more common cause of linitis plastica than gastric carcinoma
  - Lymphoma often diffusely infiltrates gastric wall but only causes mild limitation of gastric distention, usually
    - Gastric outlet obstruction is rare occurrence with lymphoma
    - Gastric wall is typically more diffusely thickened & to greater degree > 3 cm with lymphoma

Helpful Clues for Less Common Diagnoses

- **Gastritis**
  - Many etiologies
    - Use of NSAID analgesics
    - Infestation by *Helicobacter pylori* bacteria
    - Alcohol
    - Tobacco
    - Opportunistic infections (viral, mycobacterial, protozoan, etc.) in patients with AIDS or transplant recipients
    - Radiation therapy
  - Limited ability to suggest specific etiology based on imaging findings
  - May have superficial erosions or ulceration of mucosa
  - Gastric folds are thickened, especially in antrum with incomplete distensibility
    - Folds may prolapse through pylorus into duodenal bulb
  - CT shows low-density edematous submucosa
    - Distinguished from soft tissue density seen with malignant infiltration of gastric wall
    - Mucosal hyperenhancement also suggests gastritis
- **Caustic Gastroduodenal Injury**
  - Often accompanied by similar injury to esophagus
  - Accidental or intentional ingestion of strong alkali (lye), acid, or formaldehyde
  - Acute findings
    - Gastric atony and delayed emptying
    - Striking wall thickening and edema
  - Subacute or chronic findings
    - Perforation of stomach
    - Marked loss of gastric, size, distensibility, and peristalsis
      - □ Classic linitis plastica appearance
- **Peritoneal Metastases**
  - Serosal surface of stomach may be coated with peritoneal metastases, limiting distensibility
  - Peritoneal & omental mets and malignant ascites can compress stomach
  - Usual sources: Ovarian, endometrial, GI tract cancers
  - CT is much better than radiography or UGI series in detecting and characterizing these findings

Helpful Clues for Rare Diagnoses

- **Crohn Disease, Gastric**
  - Uncommonly affects stomach, usually in patients with small bowel &/or colon involvement as well
  - Acute
    - Gastric fold thickening and erosions
    - Similar appearance as other causes of gastritis
  - Chronic
    - Limited distensibility of stomach
    - Conical contraction of antrum with ram's horn configuration
- **Following Gastric Freezing**
  - Gastric infusion of iced saline may be used to control GI bleeding
  - If used excessively, can freeze stomach and lead to scarring
- **Infiltrative Granulomatous Diseases**
  - All are rare and probably indistinguishable by imaging alone
    - Syphilis
    - Sarcoidosis
    - TB
    - Amyloidosis
  - All tend to cause fold thickening and limited distention without gastric erosions or ulceration

Gastric Carcinoma

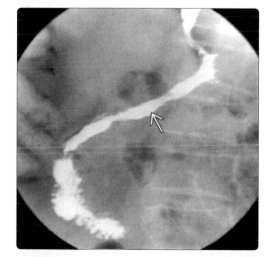

Gastric Carcinoma

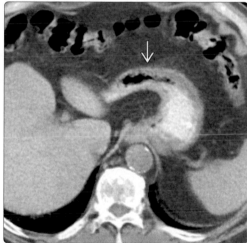

(Left) *Spot film from an upper GI shows a remarkably contracted and nondistensible stomach ➡ due to diffusely infiltrative gastric carcinoma, a classic linitis plastica appearance in an 82-year-old man.* **(Right)** *In this 82-year-old man, axial NECT shows the contracted stomach ➡ due to diffusely infiltrative gastric carcinoma. As depicted by CT, there was no spread beyond the stomach at gastric resection.*

Gastric Carcinoma

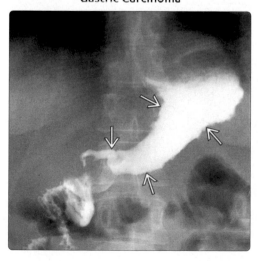

Gastric Carcinoma

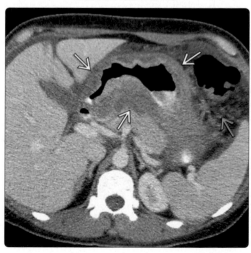

(Left) *In this 40-year-old woman with early satiety & weight loss, a spot film from an upper GI series shows fixed narrowing ➡ of the lumen of the gastric body & antrum. There was no peristalsis & very delayed emptying.* **(Right)** *In this 40-year-old woman, axial CT shows circumferential, soft tissue density thickening of the gastric wall ➡, causing fixed narrowing of the gastric lumen. Peritoneal metastases are also evident ➡.*

Gastric Carcinoma

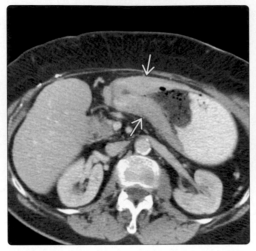

Gastric Carcinoma

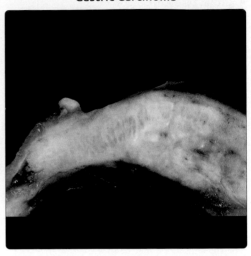

(Left) In this 81-year-old woman, axial CECT shows diffuse tumor infiltration ➡ and lack of distensibility of the gastric antrum and distal body. Retained food debris and distention of the proximal stomach indicate gastric outlet obstruction. (Right) In this 81-year-old woman, the surgical photograph shows the gross appearance of the resected stomach with extensive pale-colored tumor infiltration and fibrosis throughout the gastric wall that accounts for the scirrhous nature of this tumor.

Metastases and Lymphoma, Gastric

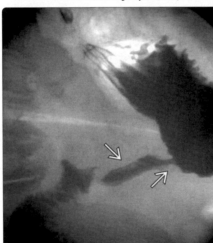

Metastases and Lymphoma, Gastric

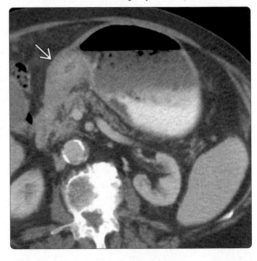

(Left) Spot film from an upper GI in an 84-year-old woman with metastatic breast cancer shows a markedly contracted distal body and antrum of the stomach ➡, that was also very slow to empty (outlet obstruction). (Right) In this 84-year-old woman with metastatic breast cancer, a CECT shows a markedly contracted and nondistensible distal body and antrum of the stomach ➡ with soft tissue density of the submucosa. The retained food and distended proximal stomach indicate outlet obstruction.

Metastases and Lymphoma, Gastric

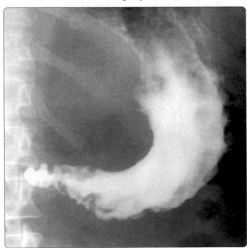

Metastases and Lymphoma, Gastric

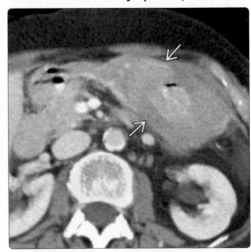

(Left) This spot film from an upper GI in an 75-year-old man with gastric lymphoma series shows diffusely thickened and nodular folds and mildly reduced distention of the stomach but no gastric outlet obstruction. (Right) In this 75-year-old-man with gastric lymphoma, axial CECT shows diffuse, marked, soft tissue density thickening of the gastric wall ➡ due to lymphoma. There was no clinical or radiographic evidence of gastric outlet obstruction.

Gastritis

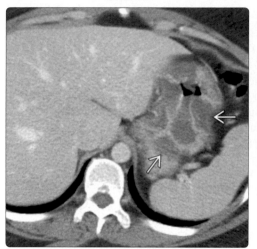

Crohn Disease, Gastric

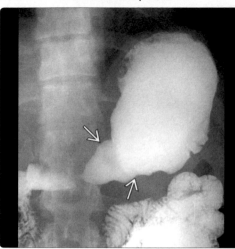

(Left) Axial CECT shows striking gastric intramural edema ➡, causing wall thickening and luminal narrowing of the entire stomach in a 30-year-old man with NSAID-induced gastritis that resolved with antacids & cessation of analgesic use. (Right) Frontal upper GI shows a conical antrum ➡ and reduced distensibility of the stomach due to chronic Crohn gastritis.

Caustic Gastroduodenal Injury

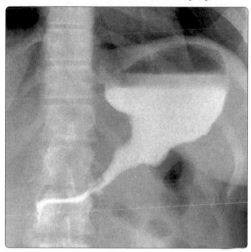

Caustic Gastroduodenal Injury

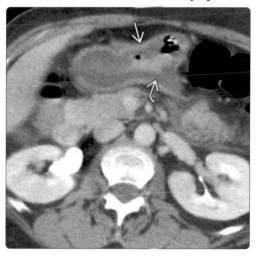

(Left) This upright film from an upper GI shows a shrunken, nondistensible stomach with evidence of gastric outlet obstruction, in a 24-year-old man 2 weeks after ingestion of lye (strong alkali) in a suicide attempt. (Right) Axial CECT shows wall thickening and nondistensibility of the body and antrum ➡, with an edematous submucosal layer ➡, in a 67-year-old woman who ingested lye a few days prior to this CT scan.

Peritoneal Metastases

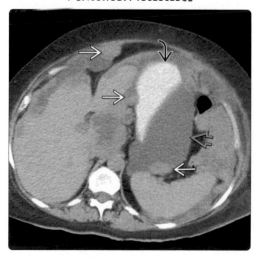

Peritoneal Metastases

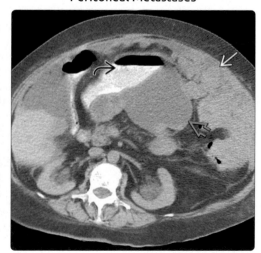

(Left) In this woman with metastatic endometrial carcinoma, axial CECT shows compression of the stomach ➡ by nodular peritoneal metastases ➡ and malignant ascites, involving the lesser sac ➡ and general peritoneal cavity. (Right) In this woman with endometrial cancer, axial CECT shows a large omental cake of tumor ➡ and malignant lesser sac ascites ➡ that compress the stomach ➡.

DIFFERENTIAL DIAGNOSIS

Common

- Functional Dyspepsia
- Acute Esophageal Inflammation or Obstruction
  - Reflux Esophagitis
  - Drug-Induced Esophagitis
  - Esophageal Foreign Body
  - Esophageal Carcinoma
- Acute Gastroduodenal Inflammation or Obstruction
  - Duodenal Ulcer
  - Gastric Ulcer
  - Gastritis
  - Gastric Carcinoma
  - Gastric Metastases
  - Gastrointestinal Stromal Tumor, Stomach
- Acute Biliary Inflammation or Obstruction
  - Acute Cholecystitis
  - Chronic Cholecystitis
  - Choledocholithiasis
  - Ascending Cholangitis
  - Sphincter of Oddi Dysfunction
- Pancreatic Inflammation or Tumor
  - Acute Pancreatitis
  - Chronic Pancreatitis
  - Autoimmune (IgG4) Pancreatitis
  - Pancreatic Pseudocyst
  - Pancreatic Ductal Carcinoma
  - Pancreatic Serous (Microcystic) Adenoma
  - Solid and Pseudopapillary Neoplasm, Pancreas
- Bowel Inflammation or Obstruction
  - Acute Appendicitis
  - Small Bowel Obstruction
  - Crohn Disease
- Hepatic Inflammation or Tumor
  - Viral and Alcoholic Hepatitis
  - Steatosis/Steatohepatitis
  - Hepatic Abscess
  - Hepatic Cysts and Polycystic Liver
  - Hepatic Metastases
  - Hepatocellular Carcinoma
  - Hepatic Adenoma
- Abdominal Hernia (External and Internal)
  - Hiatal Hernia
  - Ventral Hernia
  - Transmesenteric Internal Hernia
  - Paraduodenal Hernia
- Coronary Artery Disease
- Psychosomatic Disorders

ESSENTIAL INFORMATION

Key Differential Diagnosis Issues

- Choice of initial imaging study should be on basis of clinical judgment
  - Barium upper gastrointestinal (UGI) series: Best for GERD, peptic ulcer disease
  - US: Good choice when acute biliary abnormality is considered likely
  - CT: Best for most other considerations

- Some etiologies are clinically apparent (trauma, postoperative, HELLP syndrome, etc.)
  - Not included on this list of differential diagnoses

Helpful Clues for Common Diagnoses

- **Functional Dyspepsia**
  - Pain or discomfort in absence of demonstrable structural or physiologic abnormalities
  - Probably due to abnormal motility, sensation, perception
- **Acute Esophageal Inflammation or Obstruction**
  - **Reflux esophagitis**
    - Irregular ulcerated mucosa of distal esophagus on barium esophagram
    - Often associated with hiatal hernia
  - **Drug-induced esophagitis**
    - Acute onset of odynophagia due to erosive effect of pill within esophagus
  - **Esophageal foreign body**
    - Abrupt onset of chest and epigastric pain, inability to swallow food
    - Food bolus stuck above Schatzki ring or other type of stricture
  - **Esophageal carcinoma**
    - May cause symptomatic esophageal stricture
- **Acute Gastroduodenal Inflammation or Obstruction**
  - **Duodenal or gastric ulcer**
    - Wall thickening, extraluminal gas or contrast medium
    - Complications: Perforation, hemorrhage, gastric outlet obstruction
  - **Gastritis**
    - Heterogeneous group of disorders causing inflammation of gastric mucosa
    - UGI: Antral fold thickening, erosions, limited distensibility
    - CECT: Mucosal enhancement, submucosal edema
  - **Gastric carcinoma**
    - May be symptomatic due to ulcerated surface or gastric outlet obstruction
    - Soft tissue density thickening of wall, narrowing of lumen
      - ± nodal, peritoneal, hepatic metastases
  - **Gastric metastases**
    - Carcinomatous metastases (e.g., from breast, lung) may cause linitis plastica or gastric outlet obstruction similar to primary gastric cancer
  - **Gastrointestinal stromal tumor, stomach**
    - Usually exophytic submucosal mass with central necrosis
    - May contain gas and oral contrast medium if eroded into lumen
- **Acute Biliary Inflammation or Obstruction**
  - **Acute cholecystitis**
    - 95% caused by stone obstructing cystic duct
    - US: Gallstone(s), distended gallbladder with thick wall; positive Murphy sign
    - CT: Same, plus pericholecystic inflammation ± signs of perforation
  - **Choledocholithiasis**
    - 95% of bile duct stones are due to passage from gallbladder into common bile duct (CBD)

□ Imaging: Discrete, low-signal filling defect within bile duct on MRCP

□ MRCP superior to US or CT for visualizing stones

o **Ascending cholangitis**
  – Due to gallstones or biliary-enteric communication
  – Irregular contour, branching pattern, dilation of bile ducts
  – Pneumobilia, hyperenhancement of biliary mucosa

o **Sphincter of Oddi dysfunction**
  – Due to papillary stenosis or sphincter of Oddi dyskinesia
  – Opioids may cause spasm of sphincter of Oddi
  – Diagnosis by ERCP, Tc-HIDA, or MR cholangiography

• **Pancreatic Inflammation or Tumor**

o **Acute pancreatitis**
  – Enlarged pancreas, peripancreatic fluid or infiltrated fat planes, and thickened fascia
  – Heterogeneous enhancement on CECT, nonenhancing necrotic areas

o **Chronic pancreatitis**
  – Atrophy of gland, dilated main duct, intraductal calculi

o **Autoimmune (IgG4) pancreatitis**
  – Part of spectrum of IgG4-related sclerosing diseases (including sclerosing cholangitis)

o **Pancreatic pseudocyst**
  – Collection of pancreatic fluid & inflammatory exudate encapsulated by fibrous & granulation tissue

o **Pancreatic ductal carcinoma**
  – 75% of all pancreatic tumors; usually in pancreatic head
  – Irregular, heterogeneous, poorly enhancing mass with abrupt obstruction of pancreatic duct ± CBD (double duct sign)
  – Extensive local invasion and regional metastases

• **Bowel Inflammation or Obstruction**

o **Acute appendicitis**
  – Early inflammation may cause nausea, epigastric pain, followed by RLQ pain and tenderness
  Thick-walled appendix with inflamed periappendiceal fat, ± ileal mesenteric lymphadenopathy

o **Small bowel obstruction**
  – Many causes (adhesions, hernias, cancer, etc.)
  – Infectious or inflammatory enteritis

o **Crohn disease**
  – Segmental involvement, skip areas
  – Favors distal small bowel
  – Mucosal and mesenteric hyperemia, submucosal edema, lymphadenopathy

• **Hepatic Inflammation or Tumor**

o **Viral and alcoholic hepatitis**
  – Starry-sky appearance: ↑ echogenicity of portal venous walls
  – Hepatomegaly, gallbladder wall thickening, periportal lucency

o **Steatosis and steatohepatitis**
  – Are common causes for epigastric/RUQ discomfort and abnormal liver function tests

o **Hepatic abscess (pyogenic, amebic, hydatid)**
  – Each has characteristic appearance on imaging and unique demographic features
  – Pyogenic
    □ Cluster of grapes, multiseptate
  – Amebic
    □ Usually solitary, thick capsule
  – Hydatid
    □ Spherical outer cyst, with daughter cysts inside
    □ Cyst wall or contents (hydatid sand) may be calcified or echogenic

o **Hepatic metastases, adenoma, primary carcinoma**
  – Any large mass may be symptomatic (epigastric or RUQ pain)
  – Especially those that break through hepatic capsule or cause hemorrhage

• **Abdominal Hernias (External and Internal)**
  o Have characteristic clinical and imaging features

• **Coronary Artery Disease**
  o Inferior wall ischemia/infarction may present by epigastric pain in absence of chest pain

• **Psychosomatic Disorders**
  o More commonly seen in children with anxiety disorders

Reflux Esophagitis

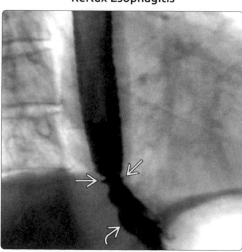

Gastritis

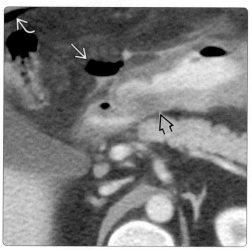

(Left) Esophagram shows a type 1 hiatal hernia ➜ *with a stricture at the esophagogastric junction. Two outpouchings* ➜ *indicate ulcerations of the mucosa. (Right) CT shows free intraperitoneal gas* ➜. *The gastric wall is thickened* ➜, *probably due to gastritis. Just ventral to the duodenal bulb and antrum are small collections of extraluminal gas and oral contrast medium* ➜, *confirming the source of perforation.*

Gastric Ulcer

Gastritis

(Left) *CT shows a thick-walled stomach* ⇨ *and massive free intraperitoneal gas* ⇨*. Extraluminal contrast material and gas are present near the anterior surface of the stomach at the site of the perforated ulcer* ⇨*. (Right) In this young athlete taking large doses of NSAIDs, CT shows marked gastric wall thickening due to submucosal edema* ⇨ *and mucosal hyperemia* ⇨*.*

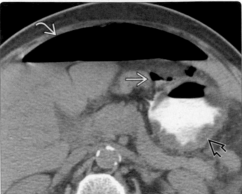
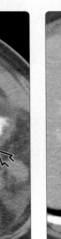

Gastric Carcinoma

Gastric Metastases

(Left) *CT shows a circumferential mass* ⇨ *that narrows the lumen of the gastric antrum. An irregular collection of gas & fluid* ⇨ *is noted within the antral mass, representing an ulcerated portion of the tumor. (Right) CT shows soft tissue density and circumferential thickening of the gastric antrum* ⇨*, resulting in gastric outlet obstruction. The appearance is indistinguishable from primary gastric carcinoma, but this obstruction was due to metastatic breast cancer.*

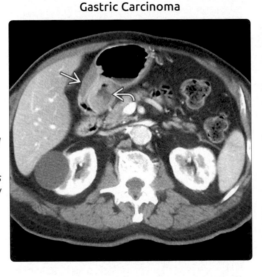
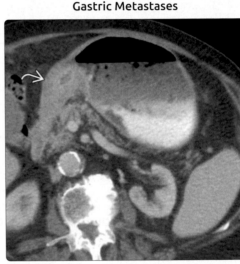

Gastrointestinal Stromal Tumor, Stomach

Acute Cholecystitis

(Left) *Axial CECT shows a large exophytic mass* ⇨ *arising from the posterior wall of the stomach. The center of the tumor is necrotic with an air-fluid level* ⇨*, indicating communication with the gastric lumen. (Right) Sonography shows a distended gallbladder* ⇨ *with diffuse wall thickening* ⇨*, multiple gallstones* ⇨*, and pericholecystic fluid* ⇨*. Sonographic Murphy sign was positive.*

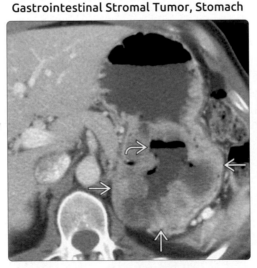
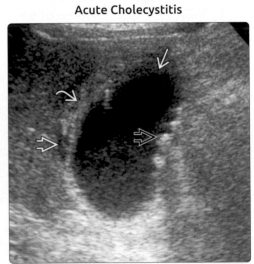

Acute Pancreatitis

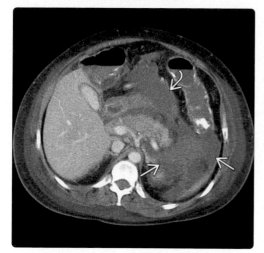

Chronic Pancreatitis

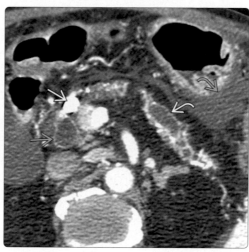

(Left) *CT shows extensive inflammation and exudation of fluid throughout the mesentery ➜ and anterior pararenal space ➜, essentially diagnostic of acute pancreatitis.* **(Right)** *CT shows marked dilation of the pancreatic duct ➜ with parenchymal atrophy and calcifications ➜. The common bile duct is also dilated ➨. Peripancreatic fluid ➨ suggests acute inflammation as well.*

Autoimmune (IgG4) Pancreatitis

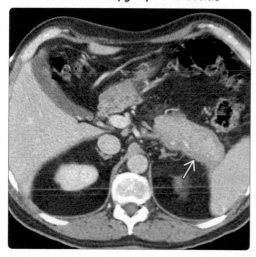

Pancreatic Ductal Carcinoma

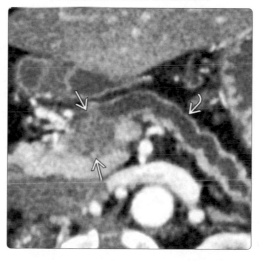

(Left) *In this man with weight loss and epigastric pain, CT shows diffuse infiltration and enlargement of the pancreas ➜ with loss of its normal fatty lobulation. There is a halo or capsule of edematous tissue around the pancreas, with relatively little spread into adjacent tissues.* **(Right)** *This elderly man presented with weight loss & epigastric & back pain. Curved planar reformatted CT shows marked pancreatic parenchymal atrophy and dilation of the pancreatic duct ➜ ending abruptly at a hypodense mass ➜ in the pancreatic head.*

Pancreatic Serous (Microcystic) Adenoma

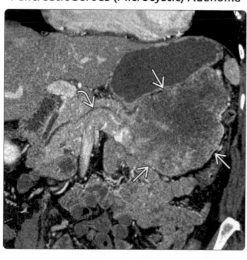

Solid and Pseudopapillary Neoplasm, Pancreas

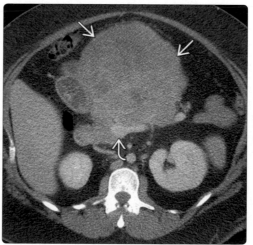

(Left) *In this elderly woman with epigastric discomfort, coronal CT shows a large, encapsulated low-density mass ➜ arising from the pancreatic body and consisting of innumerable tiny cysts. The pancreatic duct ➜ is normal, and no "invasive" features are evident.* **(Right)** *In this young woman with epigastric pain and a palpable mass, CT shows an abdominal mass ➜ that lies ventral to the splenic-portal venous confluence ➜. The mass is well encapsulated and mostly solid but has large foci of central low density, likely representing necrosis.*

Small Bowel Obstruction

(Left) *Coronal CT shows small bowel (SB) segments* ➡ *that are dilated out of proportion to other segments, typical of a closed-loop obstruction. The mesenteric vessels are twisted and dilated* ➡ *with extensive infiltration of the mesentery and ascites* ➡, *indicative of bowel ischemia.* (Right) *The SB series shows marked angulation of segments of SB, with partial obstruction* ➡. *The bowel loops seem to be drawn toward a central point in the mesentery. This patient has chronic Crohn disease with extensive mesenteric and bowel scarring.*

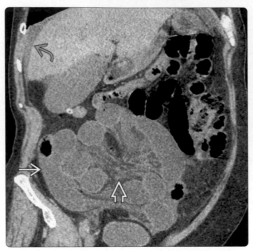

Crohn Disease

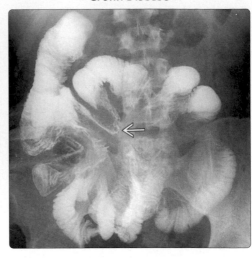

Viral and Alcoholic Hepatitis

(Left) *In this young man with epigastric and RUQ pain due to viral and alcoholic hepatitis, CT shows periportal edema as a collar of low density surrounding the vessels* ➡. (Right) *In this young man with epigastric and RUQ pain due to viral and alcoholic hepatitis, CT shows striking thickening of the gallbladder wall with the lumen almost completely collapsed* ➡. *A small amount of ascites is noted* ➡. *Any cause of acute hepatic engorgement, including steatohepatitis, may cause pain and abnormal liver function.*

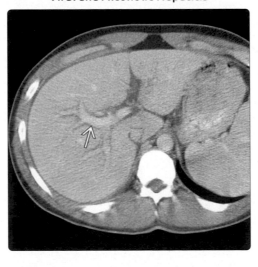

Viral and Alcoholic Hepatitis

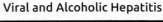

Hepatic Abscess

(Left) *In a man with fever and upper abdominal pain, axial CECT shows a multiloculated mass* ➡ *typical of a pyogenic abscess. The abscess was caused by subacute diverticulitis with portal venous septic thrombophlebitis.* (Right) *In this woman with a history of breast cancer, now with epigastric pain, CT shows hepatomegaly and innumerable poorly defined, coalescent, perivascular, and perihepatic, low-attenuation metastases. The right hepatic vein* ➡ *is compressed.*

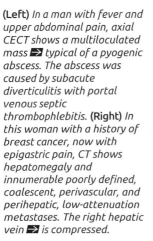
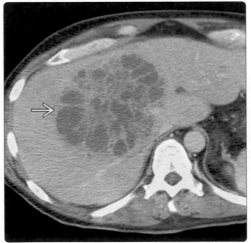

Hepatic Metastases

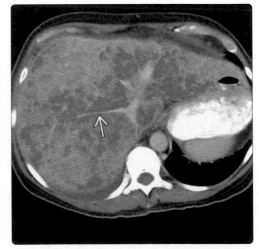

Hepatocellular Carcinoma

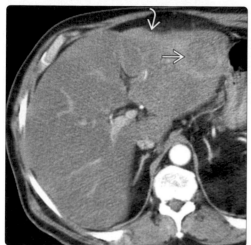

Hepatic Adenoma

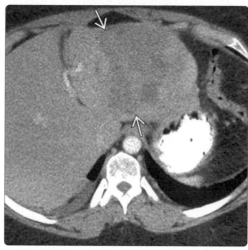

(Left) This man presented with acute epigastric pain. CT shows a heterogeneous, enhancing, encapsulated left lobe hepatic mass ➡. High-attenuation fluid ➡ surrounding the mass and extending through the hepatic capsule represents spontaneous rupture with bleeding. (Right) In this young woman with acute onset of epigastric pain, CT shows a large, heterogeneous, hepatic mass ➡. NECT (not shown) demonstrated foci of hemorrhage within the mass.

Hiatal Hernia

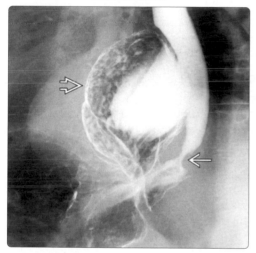

Hiatal Hernia

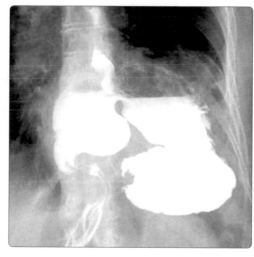

(Left) Spot film from an upper GI series demonstrates a type 3 paraesophageal hiatal hernia, in which the gastroesophageal junction ➡ and fundus ➡ lie within the thorax. (Right) Spot film from an upper GI series shows an "upside down" stomach, located entirely within the thorax, an organoaxial volvulus.

Ventral Hernia

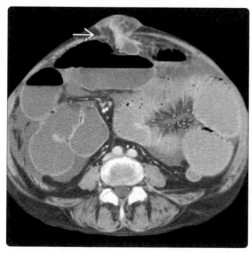

Transmesenteric Internal Hernia

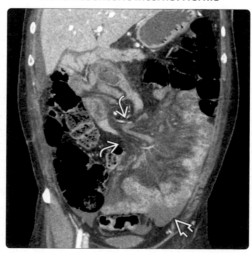

(Left) Axial CECT shows a ventral hernia ➡ that contains a strangulated segment of bowel, resulting in small bowel obstruction. (Right) This patient developed crampy epigastric pain months after a Whipple procedure. Coronal CT shows infiltration of the jejunal mesentery, localized ascites ➡, and abnormally positioned, thick-walled jejunum. The mesenteric vessels are crowded and distorted ➡ where they enter the internal hernia.

Left Upper Quadrant Mass

DIFFERENTIAL DIAGNOSIS

Common

- Splenomegaly and Splenic Masses
- Hepatomegaly and Hepatic Masses
- Gastric Masses and Distention
  - Gastroparesis
  - Gastric Carcinoma
  - Metastases and Lymphoma, Gastric
  - Gastrointestinal Stromal Tumor
  - Gastric Bezoar
- Pancreatic Masses
  - Pancreatic Pseudocyst
  - Mucinous Cystic Pancreatic Tumor
  - Solid and Papillary Neoplasm, Pancreas
- Adrenal Masses
  - Adrenal Carcinoma
  - Adrenal Metastases and Lymphoma
  - Adrenal Cyst
  - Pheochromocytoma
- Abdominal Abscess
- Peritoneal Metastases
- Ascites (Loculated)
- Renal Masses
  - Renal Cyst
  - Renal Cell Carcinoma
  - Renal Angiomyolipoma

Less Common

- Gastric Diverticulum
- Retroperitoneal Sarcoma
- Pseudomyxoma Peritonei
- Abdominal Wall Masses
  - Abdominal Wall Hernia (Mimic)
  - Abdominal Wall Hematoma (Mimic)
- Gastric Volvulus

ESSENTIAL INFORMATION

Key Differential Diagnosis Issues

- Determine whether mass arises from abdominal wall (e.g., hematoma or hernia) or within abdomen
- Distention, enlargement, or mass of any upper abdominal viscus may be perceived as left upper quadrant (LUQ) mass
- Look for claw sign
  - Mass arising from solid organ will replace and distort part of its contour

Helpful Clues for Common Diagnoses

- **Splenomegaly and Splenic Masses**
  - Any cause of splenomegaly may result in palpable or radiographically evident LUQ mass
  - Consider accessory spleen and splenosis, which may cause enlarging mass(es) after splenectomy
    - These should have same attenuation and enhancement pattern as normal spleen
    - Tc-99m-labeled heat-damaged RBC scan is definitive imaging study
  - Also consider splenic masses, metastases, and lymphoma
- **Hepatomegaly and Hepatic Masses**

- Enlarged left lobe of liver is often perceived or palpated as epigastric or LUQ mass
- On axial CT images, may appear to be separated from remainder of liver, as heart indents cephalic surface of liver
- Any mass in left lobe of liver may be a palpable LUQ mass
  - Common: Metastases, HCC, FNH, hemangioma
- **Gastric Masses and Distention**
  - Any gastric tumor [carcinoma, lymphoma, gastrointestinal stromal tumor (GIST), metastases] may result in LUQ mass
    - Exophytic masses (e.g., GIST) may not have obvious gastric origin
    - View multiplanar reformations
  - Also consider gastric distension (gastroparesis, volvulus, gastric outlet obstruction) and gastric bezoar
- **Pancreatic Masses**
  - Pancreatic masses usually displace splenic vein posteriorly and may obstruct it (ductal cancer and chronic pancreatitis)
  - Pseudocyst is most common symptomatic large cystic mass
    - Check for history of pain, elevated pancreatic enzymes
    - Will typically change size over short-term follow-up (days to weeks), unlike cystic tumors
  - Mucinous cystic pancreatic tumor most common large neoplasm in adults
  - Solid and papillary neoplasm in young women
  - Consider serous (microcystic) cystadenoma in older adult
  - Pancreatic ductal cancer usually does not cause palpable mass
    - Hypovascular lesion causing pancreatic ± biliary ductal obstruction is more common
  - Pancreatic metastases and lymphoma are not rare
- **Adrenal Masses**
  - Usually displace splenic vein ventrally
  - Cyst, adenoma, carcinoma, myelolipoma, metastases, pheochromocytoma
  - Most have characteristic appearance but must consider clinical and laboratory findings
    - Cyst: Water density, no enhancement
    - Adenoma: Near water attenuation on NECT; loses signal on opposed phase GRE images
    - Enhances with IV contrast administration
    - Pheochromocytoma: Heterogeneous, brightly enhancing; may be bright on T2WI
- **Abdominal Abscess**
  - Left subphrenic space is common location for seroma or pus after trauma or surgery (e.g., splenectomy)
  - Seroma or abscess in left subphrenic space can be mistaken for spleen
- **Ascites (Loculated)**
  - Loculated collection of fluid may simulate LUQ mass
  - Malignant ascites, especially pseudomyxoma peritonei, may appear heterogeneous and exert mass effect
    - May cause scalloped surface of liver and spleen; displace other organs
- **Renal Masses**
  - Most have characteristic appearance on imaging
  - Look for claw sign of expansile renal mass

- Focal loss of renal parenchyma, with other parenchyma draped around mass
- Includes cysts, renal cell carcinoma, oncocytoma, angiomyolipoma, metastases (plus renal abscess)
- Cyst: Water density, no enhancement, sonolucent, acoustic enhancement deep to cyst
- Renal cell carcinoma: Heterogeneous enhancing lesion
- Angiomyolipoma: Foci of fat, prominent blood vessels
○ Infiltrating renal masses
- Transitional cell carcinoma, lymphoma, renal infections (pyelonephritis and xanthogranulomatous pyelonephritis)
- Renal vein thrombosis may simulate infiltrative mass

Helpful Clues for Less Common Diagnoses

- **Retroperitoneal Sarcoma**
  ○ Rarely localized to LUQ
  ○ Most common is liposarcoma
    - Usually has foci of variable attenuation, including some of near fat density

○ Distinguishing liposarcoma from renal angiomyolipoma or adrenal myelolipoma
  - Liposarcoma is less vascular and displaces retroperitoneal organs, but does not arise from them (e.g., no claw sign in kidney)
- **Abdominal Wall Masses**
  ○ External hernias and hematomas may be mistaken for LUQ mass
  ○ Most hernias have characteristic features allowing easy diagnosis

Splenomegaly and Splenic Masses

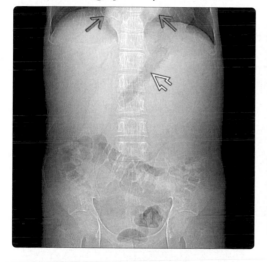

Splenomegaly and Splenic Masses

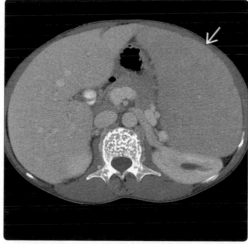

(Left) *This young man with thalassemia major has a palpable, painful LUQ mass. A supine plain film shows the stomach* ➡ *being compressed by an enlarged spleen and liver. Also note the paraspinal masses* ➡, *representing extramedullary hematopoiesis.* (Right) *In this young man with thalassemia, CT shows compression of the stomach by a massively enlarged spleen* ➡ *and liver.*

Splenomegaly and Splenic Masses

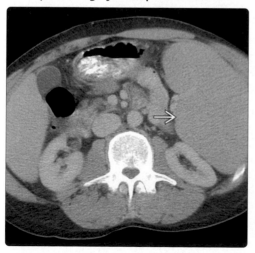

Splenomegaly and Splenic Masses

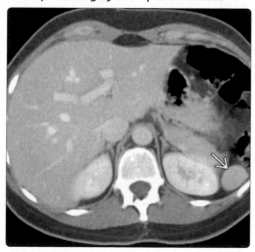

(Left) *Axial CECT shows a markedly enlarged spleen* ➡, *the presenting sign and only imaging abnormality in a 54-year-old man with chronic myelogenous leukemia.* (Right) *In this woman who has breast cancer, a PET/CT scan showed multiple FDG-avid LUQ masses concerning for metastases. On CECT, the lesions* ➡ *had the appearance of spleen, confirmed on heat-damaged RBC scan. She had splenic trauma as a child.*

(Left) *In this patient with a palpable LUQ mass, CT in the portal venous phase shows centripetal, discontinuous enhancement of the mass ➡ with the enhanced portions of the mass ➡ remaining isodense with blood pool.* **(Right)** *In this 62-year-old man with diabetes, CT shows a massively enlarged stomach ➡ filled with particulate debris, fluid, and gas, typical signs of gastroparesis.*

Hepatomegaly and Hepatic Masses

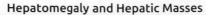

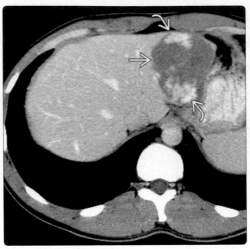

Gastroparesis

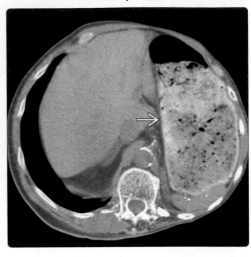

(Left) *Axial CECT shows classic gastric lymphoma as a bulky, infiltrating mass ➡ that does not cause gastric outlet obstruction.* **(Right)** *Axial CECT shows a large exophytic mass ➡ arising from the posterior gastric wall. The gastric origin is suggested by the presence of an air-fluid level ➡ within the necrotic center of the mass, indicating communication with the gastric lumen.*

Metastases and Lymphoma, Gastric

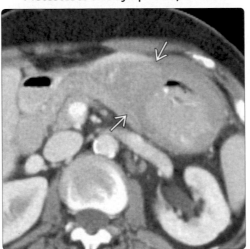

Gastrointestinal Stromal Tumor

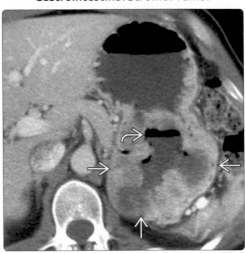

(Left) *Axial T2WI MR shows a large lesser sac pseudocyst ➡ that displaces the stomach ➡ (and later spontaneously decompressed into the stomach).* **(Right)** *In this young woman, axial CECT shows a well-defined, multiseptate, cystic mass ➡ in the pancreatic tail. The individual cysts within the mass are few (~ 6), and relatively large (~ 2 cm diameter). Note dorsal displacement of the splenic vein ➡.*

Pancreatic Pseudocyst

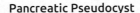

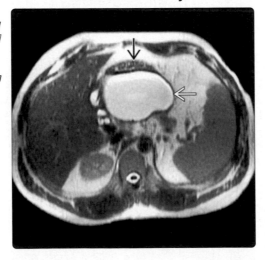

Mucinous Cystic Pancreatic Tumor

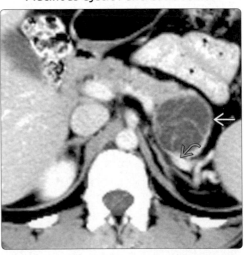

Solid and Papillary Neoplasm, Pancreas

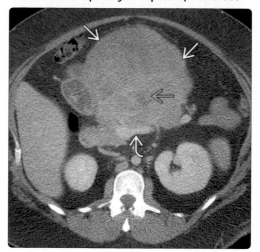

Adrenal Carcinoma

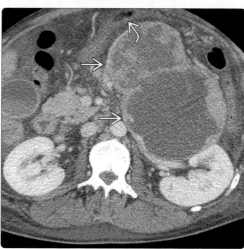

(Left) CT shows a mass ➡ that lies ventral to the splenic-portal venous confluence ➡ that is well encapsulated & mostly solid but has large foci of necrosis ➡. The mass had an intact fat plane separating it from the stomach. (Right) In this woman with Cushing syndrome, CT shows a large hypervascular mass ➡ with extensive necrosis that displaces the stomach ➡ and kidney, without seeming to arise from either. The splenic vein & pancreas were displaced ventrally, helping to distinguish this from a pancreatic mass.

Abdominal Abscess

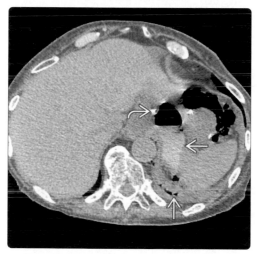

Peritoneal Metastases

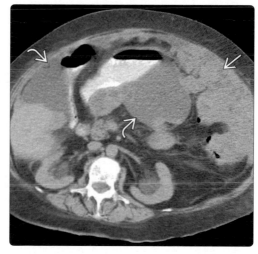

(Left) In this woman who is febrile following gastric bypass surgery, axial CECT shows a complex LUQ mass. Near the pouch-enteric anastomosis ➡ is a large collection of gas, fluid, and enteric contrast medium ➡ that fills much of the left subphrenic space, including that posterior to the spleen. (Right) Axial CECT shows a classic omental cake ➡ and malignant, loculated ascites ➡ due to metastatic endometrial carcinoma.

Pseudomyxoma Peritonei

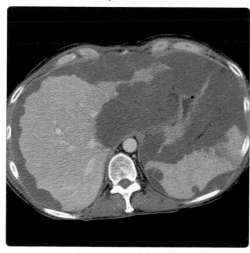

Abdominal Wall Hematoma (Mimic)

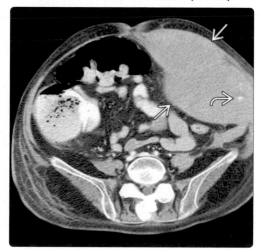

(Left) Axial CECT shows a classic scalloped surface of the liver and spleen and complex ascites filling the abdomen, and presenting as a doughy LUQ mass, metastatic appendiceal mucinous carcinoma. (Right) Axial CT shows a massive rectus sheath hematoma ➡ with foci of active extravasation ➡, representing spontaneous hemorrhage due to anticoagulation medication.

SECTION 5
Duodenum

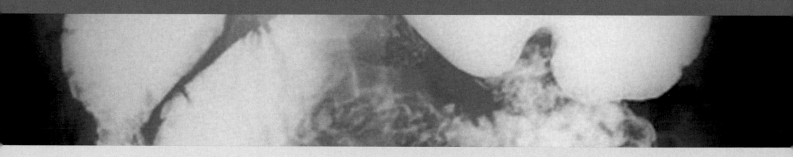

Generic Imaging Patterns

DIFFERENTIAL DIAGNOSIS

Less Common

- Intraluminal Duodenal Lesions
  - Duodenal Polyps
  - Duodenal Carcinoma
- Intramural Duodenal Lesions
  - Mesenchymal Tumors
  - Carcinoid Tumor
  - Metastases and Lymphoma
  - Duodenal Hematoma
  - Duplication Cyst
  - Choledochal Cyst
- Extrinsic Pancreatic Masses
  - Pancreatic Pseudocyst
  - Pancreatic Ductal Carcinoma
  - Annular Pancreas
  - Ampullary Tumor
  - Pancreatic Serous Adenoma
  - Pancreatic Intraductal Papillary Mucinous Neoplasm
  - Pancreatic Endocrine Tumor (Islet Cell)
  - Groove Pancreatitis
  - Autoimmune Pancreatitis
- Extrinsic Gallbladder Lesion
  - Acute Cholecystitis
  - Gallbladder Carcinoma
  - Hydrops or Empyema of Gallbladder
- Extrinsic Renal Mass
  - Renal Cell Carcinoma
  - Renal Cyst
  - Renal Angiomyolipoma
- Extrinsic Colon Mass
  - Colon Carcinoma
  - Infectious Colitis
- Extrinsic Hepatic Mass
  - Hepatomegaly
  - Hepatic Metastases
  - Hepatocellular Carcinoma

ESSENTIAL INFORMATION

Key Differential Diagnosis Issues

- Barium upper gastrointestinal (UGI) series may suggest diagnosis or indicate finding
  - Barium UGI and endoscopy are best for mucosal/intrinsic duodenal lesions
- CT, MR, or US (including endoscopic US) are essential to characterize nature of intramural or extrinsic lesions
- Terminology
  - "2nd duodenum" is 2nd or descending portion of duodenum

Helpful Clues for Less Common Diagnoses

- **Intraluminal Duodenal Lesions**
  - e.g., Brunner gland, hamartomatous, and adenomatous polyps
    - Best evaluated by UGI or endoscopy
  - **Duodenal carcinoma**
    - Usually causes luminal obstruction
  - Some intramural lesions

- e.g., lipomas, duodenal diverticula
- May be drawn into lumen by peristalsis

- **Intramural Duodenal Lesions**
  - **Mesenchymal tumors**
    - Arising from any component of wall (fat, muscle, nerve, etc.)
    - GI stromal tumors (GIST) commonly arise in duodenum
      - Hyperenhancing solid component; necrotic center
      - May erode into lumen of duodenum (gas and enteric contents within GIST)
  - **Metastases and lymphoma**
    - Soft tissue density mass thickening wall, ± luminal obstruction
    - Metastatic carcinomas usually cause obstruction
    - Lymphomas usually do not
      - May actually have aneurysmal dilation of bowel lumen
  - **Duodenal hematoma**
    - Following trauma or anticoagulant therapy
    - High attenuation (> 60 HU) thickens wall, narrows lumen
  - **Duplication cyst**
    - Quite rare in adults
    - Often water attenuation
    - May compress &/or communicate with lumen
  - **Choledochal cyst**
    - Choledochocele (type III or IV) (fusiform dilation) may appear as mass-deforming medial wall of 2nd duodenum
- **Extrinsic Pancreatic Masses**
  - **Pancreatic pseudocyst**
    - In patient with history of pancreatitis and pain, consider pseudocyst
  - **Ampullary tumor**
    - Small mass usually causing obstruction of common bile and pancreatic ducts
  - **Pancreatic serous adenoma**
    - Encapsulated mass in older adult with innumerable tiny cystic components
    - Sponge or honeycomb appearance
    - No invasive features
  - **Pancreatic intraductal papillary mucinous neoplasm**
    - Dilation of main ± side branch pancreatic ducts
    - Usually causes bulging of ampulla of Vater
  - **Pancreatic endocrine tumor (islet cell)**
    - Usually small and hypervascular; rarely cause mass effect on duodenum
    - Gastrinomas may lie within duodenal wall
  - **Groove pancreatitis**
    - Often associated with small cysts in medial wall of duodenum
    - Mimics pancreatic ductal carcinoma clinically and on imaging
- **Extrinsic Gallbladder Lesion**
  - **Acute cholecystitis**
    - Distended gallbladder often compresses lateral wall of 2nd duodenum
  - **Gallbladder carcinoma**
    - Tumor may displace or encase 2nd duodenum

- Invasion of liver, obstruction of bile ducts often evident on US, CT, or MR
- **Extrinsic Renal Mass**
  - Any benign or malignant mass may displace 2nd duodenum
- **Extrinsic Colon Mass**
  - Infectious or neoplastic mass may displace 2nd duodenum
  - Diagnosis is usually evident by combination of CT and clinical findings
- **Extrinsic Hepatic Mass**
  - Hepatomegaly or hepatic mass (especially exophytic)
  - May displace 2nd duodenum

SELECTED REFERENCES

1. Mortelé KJ et al: Multimodality imaging of pancreatic and biliary congenital anomalies. Radiographics. 26(3):715-31, 2006
2. Kim YH et al: Imaging diagnosis of cystic pancreatic lesions: pseudocyst versus nonpseudocyst. Radiographics. 25(3):671-85, 2005
3. Jayaraman MV et al: CT of the duodenum: an overlooked segment gets its due. Radiographics. 21 Spec No:S147-60, 2001
4. Levy AD et al: Gallbladder carcinoma: radiologic-pathologic correlation. Radiographics. 21(2):295-314; questionnaire, 549-55, 2001
5. Hahn PF et al: Duodenal hematoma: the ring sign in MR imaging. Radiology. 159(2):379-82, 1986

Duodenal Polyps
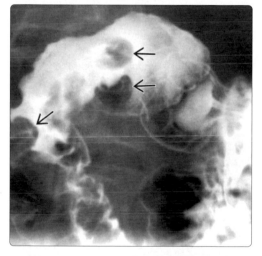

Duodenal Polyps
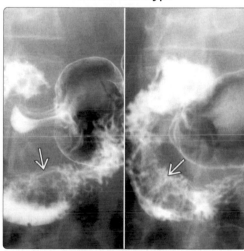

(Left) *Upper gastrointestinal (UGI) shows multiple polypoid filling defects ➡ in the duodenal bulb and 2nd portion of duodenum. Endoscopy and biopsy revealed Brunner gland hyperplasia and hamartomatous change in a patient with hyperacidity.* **(Right)** *Two films from a UGI series show a long polypoid filling defect ➡ within the lumen of the 2nd and 3rd portions of the duodenum. Surgical resection confirmed a benign adenomatous polyp.*

Duodenal Carcinoma
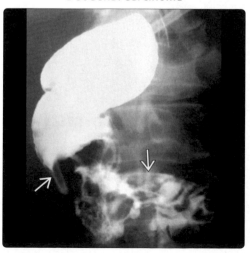

Duodenal Carcinoma
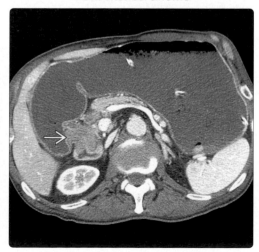

(Left) *In this patient with familial adenomatous polyposis syndrome, a spot film from a UGI shows an apple core appearance of a mass ➡ in the 2nd and 3rd portions of duodenum with irregular, destroyed mucosal pattern.* **(Right)** *CECT shows massive dilation of the stomach, indicating gastric outlet obstruction. A mass ➡ in the proximal duodenum is causing the obstruction. The tumor invades the head of the pancreas, but the bile duct and pancreatic duct were not obstructed.*

Duodenal Mass

Mesenchymal Tumors

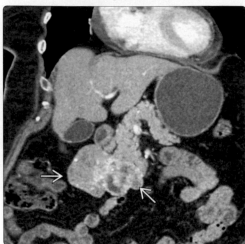

Mesenchymal Tumors

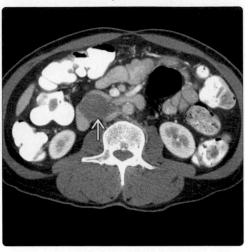

(Left) *Coronal CECT shows a lobulated, heterogeneous mass ➡ arising from the 2nd portion of the duodenum. Portions of the mass are hypervascular while others appear necrotic, which are all typical features of a duodenal GI stromal tumor.* (Right) *Axial CT shows a homogeneous, soft tissue density mass ➡ within the wall of the duodenum, a proven leiomyoma. The wall of the duodenum seems wrapped around the mass, but the duodenal lumen is not obstructed.*

Mesenchymal Tumors

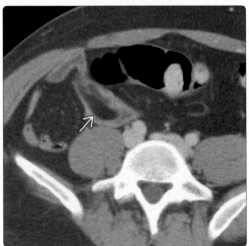

Mesenchymal Tumors

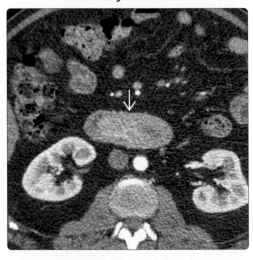

(Left) *CT shows a fat-density mass ➡ within the lumen of the duodenum, even though this lipoma arose from the duodenal wall.* (Right) *CT shows a cylindrical, enhancing mass ➡ within the lumen of the 3rd portion of duodenum, without signs of bowel obstruction. This was a paraganglioma, arising from the duodenal wall.*

Metastases and Lymphoma

Metastases and Lymphoma

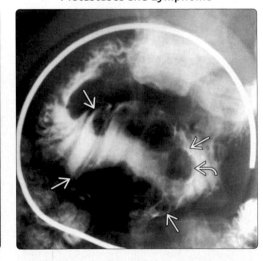

(Left) *Axial CECT shows classic aneurysmal dilation of the 4th portion of the duodenum ➡ with a huge, soft tissue density mass ➡ (lymphoma) with central necrosis ➡, communicating with the duodenal lumen. Note the absence of bowel obstruction or gastric distention.* (Right) *UGI shows aneurysmal dilation ➡ of the 3rd portion of the duodenum with a large intraluminal component ➡, due to malignant melanoma. Lymphoma can appear identical.*

Duodenal Hematoma

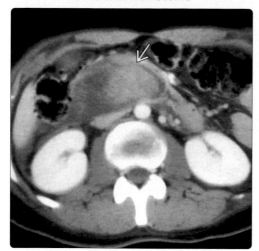

Duplication Cyst

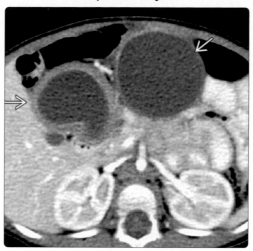

(Left) *In this adolescent boy injured by blunt trauma, CT shows a heterogeneously high-attenuation mass* ➡ *within the wall of the duodenum, representing intramural hematoma. This resolved within 1 week with nonoperative management.* (Right) *In this 9-month-old infant, CECT shows 2 thick-walled cystic masses* ➡, *proven to represent duplication cysts.*

Pancreatic Pseudocyst

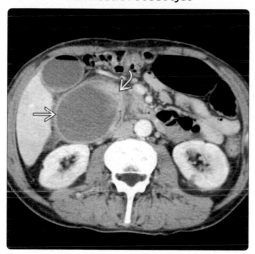

Pancreatic Ductal Carcinoma

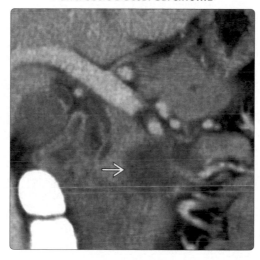

(Left) *In this man with recurrent pancreatitis, axial CECT shows a cystic mass* ➡ *that lies lateral to, and distorts the lumen of, the 2nd portion of the duodenum* ➡, *characteristic of an intramural pseudocyst.* (Right) *In this 46-year-old woman with early satiety and weight loss, coronal CECT shows a hypodense mass* ➡ *arising from the uncinate process that encased the superior mesenteric vein and 3rd portion of duodenum, characteristic of pancreatic ductal carcinoma.*

Annular Pancreas

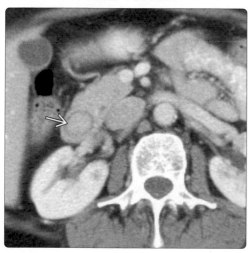

Ampullary Tumor

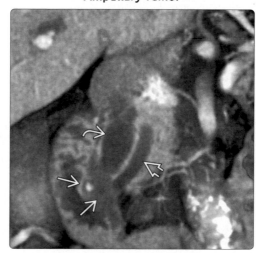

(Left) *In this young man with early satiety, axial CECT shows that the 2nd portion of the duodenum* ➡ *is completely encircled by pancreatic tissue with narrowing of its lumen.* (Right) *In this elderly woman with painless jaundice, coronal CECT shows an ampullary mass* ➡ *causing obstruction of both the pancreatic* ➡ *and common bile* ➡ *ducts, classic findings of ampullary carcinoma.*

Pancreatic Serous Adenoma

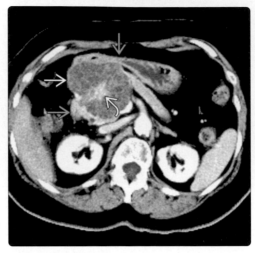

Pancreatic Intraductal Papillary Mucinous Neoplasm

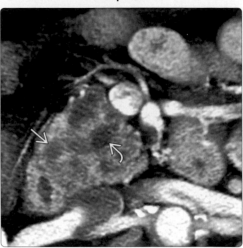

(Left) *In this elderly asymptomatic woman, CT shows a mass* ➡ *in the pancreatic head that displaces the stomach and duodenum* ➡. *The mass is comprised of small cysts separated by thin fibrous septa with a "scar"* ➡ *in the center of the mass.*
(Right) *In this man with jaundice, CT showed dilation of the main & side branches of the pancreatic duct* ➡, *typical of intraductal papillary mucinous neoplasm. In addition, there is a hypodense solid mass* ➡ *that obstructed common bile duct, found to be pancreatic ductal carcinoma.*

Groove Pancreatitis

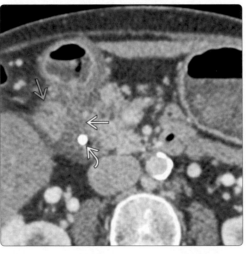

Acute Cholecystitis

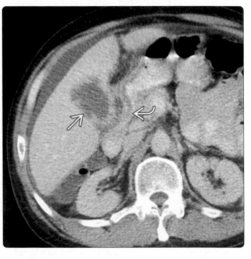

(Left) *In this man with early satiety and jaundice, CT shows a low-density "mass"* ➡ *between the pancreatic head and 2nd duodenum* ➡. *Biliary obstruction was treated with a stent* ➡. *Surgery confirmed groove pancreatitis, though pancreatic carcinoma may have a similar appearance.*
(Right) *Axial CECT shows medial deviation of the 2nd portion of duodenum* ➡ *and a crescentic fluid density paralleling its lateral wall. Note the irregular gallbladder wall thickening* ➡ *and ascites, due to gangrenous, perforated cholecystitis.*

Gallbladder Carcinoma

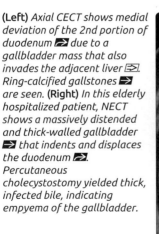

Hydrops or Empyema of Gallbladder

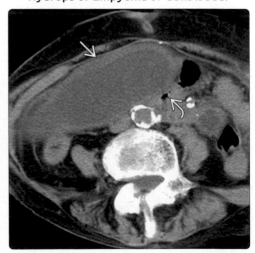

(Left) *Axial CECT shows medial deviation of the 2nd portion of duodenum* ➡ *due to a gallbladder mass that also invades the adjacent liver* ➡. *Ring-calcified gallstones* ➡ *are seen.* (Right) *In this elderly hospitalized patient, NECT shows a massively distended and thick-walled gallbladder* ➡ *that indents and displaces the duodenum* ➡. *Percutaneous cholecystostomy yielded thick, infected bile, indicating empyema of the gallbladder.*

Renal Cell Carcinoma

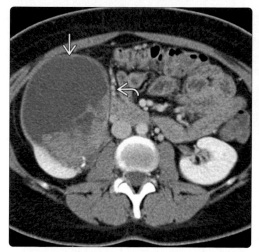

Renal Angiomyolipoma

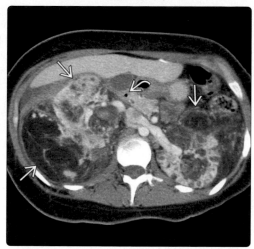

(Left) *Axial CECT shows a large, mixed cystic and solid mass ➡ arising from the right kidney, which is indenting and displacing the 2nd portion of the duodenum ➡. (Right) In this young woman with tuberous sclerosis, CECT shows bilateral cysts and large renal masses ➡ that contain fat and large blood vessels, characteristic of angiomyolipomas (AMLs). The duodenum ➡ is compressed and displaced by the right-sided AMLs.*

Infectious Colitis

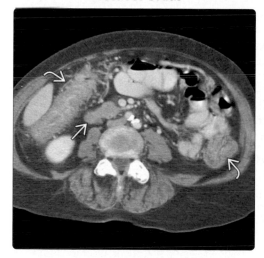

Hepatomegaly

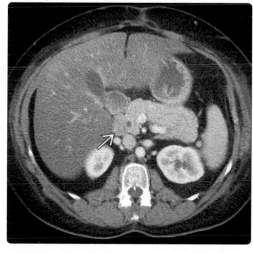

(Left) *In this previously healthy woman, CECT shows pancolitis with hyperemic mucosa and mesentery and submucosal edema ➡. The 2nd portion of the duodenum ➡ was secondarily affected by the adjacent colonic inflammation. (Right) This woman has an enlarged and fatty liver due to chemotherapy-induced steatohepatitis. Note displacement and compression of the 2nd portion of the duodenum ➡.*

Hepatic Metastases

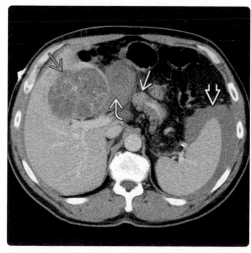

Hepatocellular Carcinoma

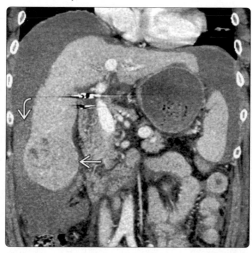

(Left) *In this patient with metastatic melanoma and acute abdominal pain, CT shows one of several liver metastases ➡ with adjacent sentinel clot ➡, indicating rupture. Blood is present throughout the peritoneal cavity ➡. The duodenum ➡ is displaced by tumor and clot. (Right) In this woman presenting with RUQ pain and hypotension, coronal CT shows a spherical, encapsulated mass ➡ with sentinel clot ➡ and ascites. The mass abutted the 2nd duodenum. Surgery confirmed a ruptured hepatocellular carcinoma.*

DIFFERENTIAL DIAGNOSIS

Common

- Ileus
- Small Bowel Obstruction
- Pancreatitis, Acute
- Superior Mesenteric Artery Syndrome
- Postvagotomy
- Scleroderma, Intestinal
- Celiac-Sprue Disease

Less Common

- Strongyloides
- Zollinger-Ellison Syndrome

ESSENTIAL INFORMATION

Key Differential Diagnosis Issues

- Fluoroscopy and CT/MR have complementary roles in evaluation of duodenal dilation
  - Fluoroscopy is better at assessing dynamic changes, peristalsis, effect of positioning
  - Also better at identifying mucosal or constricting lesions
- CT better at showing extrinsic compression and disease beyond duodenum

Helpful Clues for Common Diagnoses

- **Ileus**
  - Duodenum dilated along with small bowel (SB) & colon
  - No transition from dilated to nondilated bowel (in general)
    - It is not uncommon for descending colon to be less dilated than remaining colon or SB in cases of ileus
  - Common etiologies
    - Postoperative, metabolic imbalance, medication
- **Small Bowel Obstruction**
  - Dilation of small bowel "downstream" from duodenum, "upstream" from obstructing lesion
- **Pancreatitis, Acute**
  - Often causes focal ileus of adjacent bowel with dilated lumen

  - May narrow lumen of 2nd and 3rd portion of duodenum
    - Spasm and wall edema
    - Dilation of duodenal lumen upstream from narrowed lumen
- **Superior Mesenteric Artery Syndrome**
  - 3rd duodenum becomes compressed as it passes between aorta and superior mesenteric artery
  - Common in thin, bedridden patients, especially with recent weight loss
  - Look for linear crossing defect on 3rd duodenum (barium upper gastrointestinal study)
    - Narrow angle between aorta and superior mesenteric artery (SMA) on CT, MR angiography
    - Best seen in sagittal plane
- **Postvagotomy**
  - Stomach and duodenum become dilated, atonic
  - Result of loss of parasympathetic innervation
- **Scleroderma, Intestinal**
  - Dilated, decreased peristalsis; "megaduodenum"
  - Look for characteristic changes in esophagus, small bowel, skin
    - Hidebound appearance of small bowel folds
      - Thin and closely spaced
    - Esophagus: Dilated, atonic, ± distal stricture
- **Celiac-Sprue Disease**
  - Look for dilated small bowel with decreased folds in jejunum and signs of malabsorption
  - May also have transient intussusceptions, "conformation" of SB flaccid, dilated segments
  - Correlate with clinical evidence of gluten intolerance

Helpful Clues for Less Common Diagnoses

- **Strongyloides**
  - Causes thickened or effaced folds in duodenum and small bowel
  - May cause lead-pipe appearance of same segments
- **Zollinger-Ellison Syndrome**
  - Thickened folds, increased secretions, ulcerations in stomach and duodenum
  - Gastrin-producing islet cell tumor

(Left) Coronal CECT shows dilated proximal small bowel segments, including duodenum and jejunum ➡, while distal small bowel ➡ is collapsed; obstruction due to adhesions ➡ also seen. (Right) Axial CECT shows dilation of the stomach and second portion of duodenum ➡. Peripancreatic inflammation is evident, and there is a collection of gas and fluid, an abscess ➡. Common duct stent ➡ is also seen.

Small Bowel Obstruction

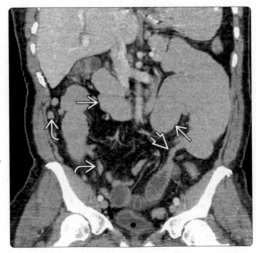

Pancreatitis, Acute

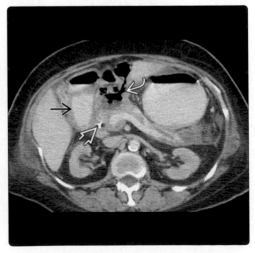

Superior Mesenteric Artery Syndrome

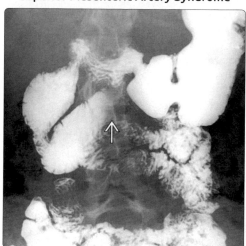

Superior Mesenteric Artery Syndrome

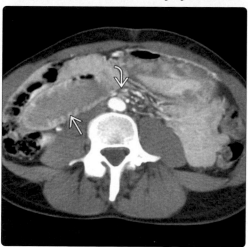

(Left) *Frontal small bowel follow-through shows marked dilation of the 2nd and 3rd portions of duodenum with abrupt narrowing as it crosses the spine, with a vertical straight line demarcation ➡.* (Right) *Axial CECT shows marked dilation of the duodenum ➡, which is compressed with luminal narrowing as it passes between the aorta and the root of the mesenteric vessels ➡.*

Scleroderma, Intestinal

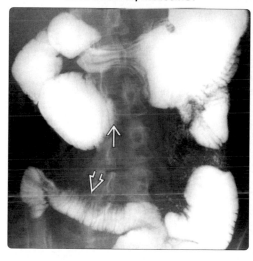

Scleroderma, Intestinal

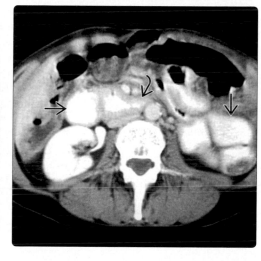

(Left) *Small bowel follow-through shows marked dilation of the duodenum up to where it crosses the spine ➡. The appearance is similar to superior mesenteric artery syndrome, but the abnormal, closely spaced fold pattern of the small bowel ➡ helps to confirm the diagnosis of scleroderma.* (Right) *Axial CECT shows a dilated lumen ➡ of the duodenum and small bowel with fold thickening of the duodenal wall ➡, proven to be scleroderma.*

Celiac-Sprue Disease

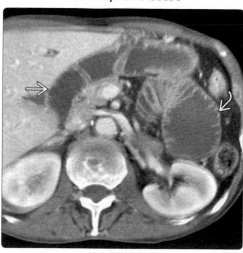

Zollinger-Ellison Syndrome

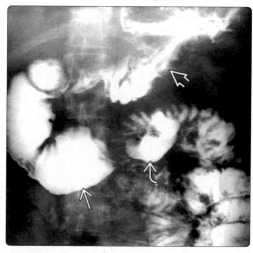

(Left) *Axial CECT shows fluid distention of dilated duodenum ➡ and jejunum, and some atrophy of the jejunal folds ➡. (Right) Spot film from an upper GI shows a dilated duodenum ➡ and thick gastric folds ➡ with dilution of the barium, due to excess fluid (acid). A large jejunal ulcer is seen ➡. A pancreatic neuroendocrine tumor (gastrinoma) was subsequently found.*

Duodenum

DIFFERENTIAL DIAGNOSIS

Common
- Duodenitis
- Duodenal Ulcer
- Brunner Gland Hyperplasia
- Acute Pancreatitis
- Duodenal Hematoma and Laceration
- Chronic Renal Failure

Less Common
- Zollinger-Ellison Syndrome
- Opportunistic Intestinal Infections
- Caustic Gastroduodenal Injury
- Crohn Disease
- Celiac-Sprue Disease
- Metastases and Lymphoma, Duodenal
- Duodenal Varices

ESSENTIAL INFORMATION

Key Differential Diagnosis Issues
- Barium UGI & CT: Complementary studies
  - Fluoroscopic studies are often better for intrinsic duodenal disease
  - CT excels at showing paraduodenal etiologies (e.g., pancreatitis)
- Imaging findings are uncommonly pathognomonic (e.g., duodenal varices); need clinical correlation

Helpful Clues for Common Diagnoses
- **Duodenitis**
  - Inflammation without frank ulceration
  - Same etiologies as gastritis, often coexisting gastritis & duodenitis
  - Occasionally see aphthous erosions on barium UGI
- **Duodenal Ulcer**
  - Discrete ulcer crater with marked spasm of wall and distortion of lumen
  - ± extraluminal gas, fluid, enteric contrast medium
- **Brunner Gland Hyperplasia**

- Thick, nodular folds in duodenal bulb
- Usually associated with duodenitis
- **Acute Pancreatitis**
  - Thick folds, widening of C loop
  - Signs of pancreatitis are usually evident on CT
- **Duodenal Hematoma and Laceration**
  - Thick spiculated folds
  - Etiologies: Focal, epigastric trauma or anticoagulation
- **Chronic Renal Failure**
  - Thick, nodular folds

Helpful Clues for Less Common Diagnoses
- **Zollinger-Ellison Syndrome**
  - Gastrin-producing islet cell tumor often evident on CECT
  - Thick folds & ulcers of stomach & duodenum
- **Opportunistic Intestinal Infections**
  - Giardiasis, strongyloides, cryptosporidiosis
  - More common in immunosuppressed patients
  - Thickened and nodular or effaced folds plus spasm, excess fluid, diarrhea
- **Caustic Gastroduodenal Injury**
  - Esophagus and stomach are usually more affected
- **Crohn Disease**
  - Thickened folds, ulceration, spasm
  - Usually with known disease in small bowel
- **Celiac-Sprue Disease**
  - Usually with small bowel disease
  - Reversed fold pattern: Effaced jejunal folds; prominent ileal folds
- **Duodenal Varices**
  - Portal hypertension &/or portal vein occlusion
  - Duodenal (& gastroesophageal) varices are evident on CECT

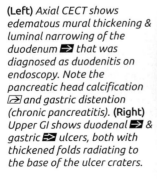

(Left) Axial CECT shows edematous mural thickening & luminal narrowing of the duodenum ➡ that was diagnosed as duodenitis on endoscopy. Note the pancreatic head calcification ⬈ and gastric distention (chronic pancreatitis). (Right) Upper GI shows duodenal ➡ & gastric ➡ ulcers, both with thickened folds radiating to the base of the ulcer craters.

Duodenitis

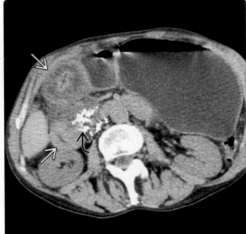

Duodenal Ulcer

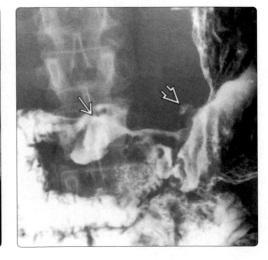

Brunner Gland Hyperplasia

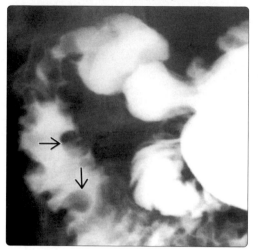

Acute Pancreatitis

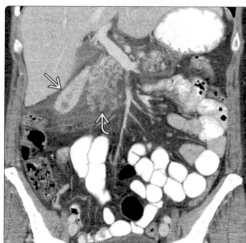

(Left) *Upper GI shows nodular, thickened, and polypoid folds ⇨ in the bulb and 2nd portion of duodenum, proven to represent Brunner gland hyperplasia with some foci of hamartomatous change in some of the nodules.* (Right) *Coronal CECT shows infiltrative changes around the pancreatic head ⇨ with mural thickening and luminal narrowing of the 2nd portion of duodenum ⇨, which shares the anterior pararenal space with the pancreas.*

Duodenal Hematoma and Laceration

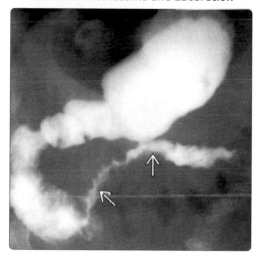

Zollinger-Ellison Syndrome

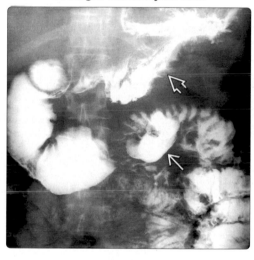

(Left) *Upper GI shows thickened folds and narrowed lumen ⇨ of the distal duodenum, due to spontaneous coagulopathic hemorrhage into the duodenal wall in this 70-year-old woman on Coumadin therapy.* (Right) *Upper GI shows a large distal duodenal or jejunal ulcer ⇨, along with a dilated, partially obstructed 2nd duodenum, & thickened folds with excess fluid (acid) in the stomach ⇨.*

Metastases and Lymphoma, Duodenal

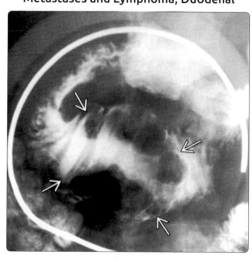

Duodenal Varices

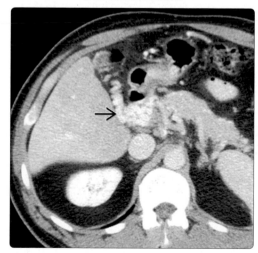

(Left) *Upper GI shows aneurysmal dilation of the lumen and thickening of the folds of the 3rd portion of duodenum, due to an intramural mass ⇨ (metastatic melanoma).* (Right) *Axial CECT shows a collection of varices ⇨ around the 2nd duodenum and pancreatic head in this man with cirrhosis and portal vein thrombosis with cavernous transformation of the portal vein.*

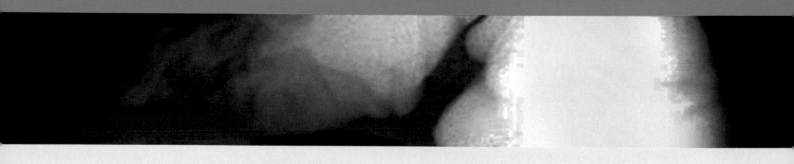

SECTION 6
Small Intestine

Generic Imaging Patterns

Clinically Based Differentials

DIFFERENTIAL DIAGNOSIS

Common

- Food, Pills
- Lymphoid Follicles, Small Bowel
- Intestinal Parasitic Disease

Less Common

- Intestinal Metastases and Lymphoma
- Intramural Benign Intestinal Tumors
- Hamartomatous Polyposis Syndromes
- Gardner Syndrome
- Familial Polyposis

ESSENTIAL INFORMATION

Key Differential Diagnosis Issues

- Most filling defects are food or pills

Helpful Clues for Common Diagnoses

- **Food, Pills**
  - Pills usually have recognizable round or oval shape
  - Corn and other vegetables are common sources of filling defects
  - Especially common in elderly, edentulous patients
- **Lymphoid Follicles, Small Bowel**
  - Prevalent in distal small bowel (SB), especially in children
  - Uniform size (2-4 mm), ill-defined borders due to submucosal location
- **Intestinal Parasitic Disease**
  - Common in some developing countries
  - Ascariasis: Curvilinear filling defects up to 35 cm long

Helpful Clues for Less Common Diagnoses

- **Intestinal Metastases and Lymphoma**
  - Both can lead to multiple polyps, may ulcerate → bull's eye (target) lesions
  - Melanoma most common etiology of SB metastases
- **Intramural Benign Intestinal Tumors**
  - Any mesenchymal component of SB wall

- Lipoma is most commonly recognized due to fat density on CT
  - Multiple neurofibromas in neurofibromatosis
- **Hamartomatous Polyposis Syndromes**
  - Peutz-Jeghers syndrome: Jejunum & ileum > duodenum > colon > stomach
    - Mucocutaneous pigments lesions, lips and skin
  - Cowden disease: Colonic polyps > SB
  - Cronkhite-Canada syndrome: Stomach & colon > SB
- **Gardner Syndrome**
  - Adenomatous polyps in colon, SB, stomach
  - Extracolonic neoplasms (osteomas, ampullary tumors, desmoids, adrenal, thyroid, liver carcinomas)
- **Familial Polyposis**
  - Adenomas in colon > stomach > duodenum > SB

(Left) Spot film of the cecum & terminal ileum from an air-contrast enema shows multiple, small, small bowel (SB) nodules ➡ of uniform size and appearance that represent lymphoid follicles. (Right) Small bowel follow-through shows a long vermiform filling defect ➡ within the SB lumen, a typical appearance for ascaris infestation.

Lymphoid Follicles, Small Bowel

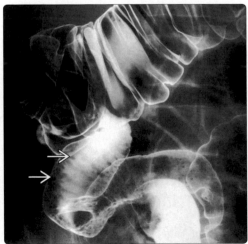

Intestinal Parasitic Disease

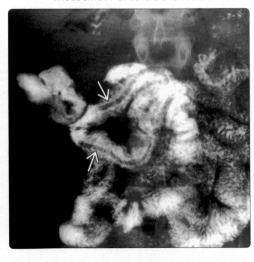

Intestinal Metastases and Lymphoma

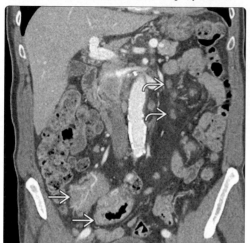

Intestinal Metastases and Lymphoma

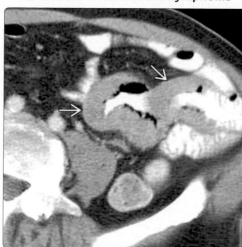

(Left) *Coronal CT shows multiple mesenteric and SB masses ➡ that encase, but do not obstruct, vessels or bowel, typical features of non-Hodgkin lymphoma. Also noted is mesenteric lymphadenopathy ⬈.* (Right) *Axial CECT shows 2 of many SB metastases ➡ from melanoma, with intramural masses and mucosal ulceration.*

Intramural Benign Intestinal Tumors

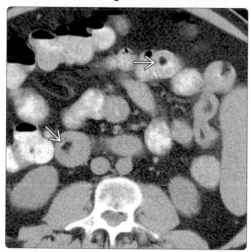

Intramural Benign Intestinal Tumors

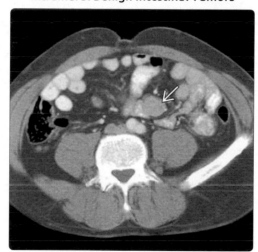

(Left) *Axial NECT shows 2 of several fat density lesions ➡ within the SB, diagnostic of lipomas. These appear to be intraluminal, though they arise in the bowel wall, subsequently being drawn into the lumen by peristalsis.* (Right) *Axial CECT shows one of several soft tissue density nodules ➡ within the SB wall, representing neurofibromas, in a patient with neurofibromatosis*

Hamartomatous Polyposis Syndromes

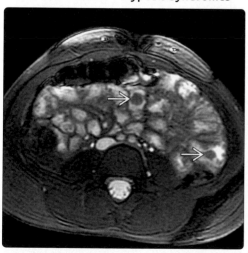

Gardner Syndrome

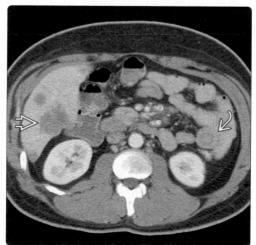

(Left) *MR enterography in this 12-year-old boy with Peutz-Jeghers syndrome shows 2 ➡ of many SB hamartomatous polyps.* (Right) *In this patient with Gardner syndrome, axial CECT shows a small bowel intussusception ⬈, but not the adenomatous polyp that was the likely cause. Liver metastases ➡ are present from a colon carcinoma (not shown on this section).*

DIFFERENTIAL DIAGNOSIS

Common

- Simple Small Bowel Obstruction
- Closed Loop Small Bowel Obstruction
- External Hernia

Less Common

- Peritoneal Metastases
- Sclerosing Peritonitis
- Transmesenteric Postoperative Hernia
- Paraduodenal Hernia
- Transplantation, Small Intestine
- Other Types of Internal Hernia

ESSENTIAL INFORMATION

Key Differential Diagnosis Issues

- Check for internal or external hernia
  - Ask about predisposing conditions
  - e.g., prior Roux-en-Y gastric bypass or liver transplantation
- Check for peritoneal infection or tumor

Helpful Clues for Common Diagnoses

- **Simple Small Bowel Obstruction**
  - Gas and fluid-distended small bowel (SB) loops (> 3 cm) proximal to collapsed loops
  - Transition zone, but no mass, hernia, or other visible cause = adhesive SB obstruction
  - Dilated SB leading into hernia; collapsed SB coming out of hernia = hernia as etiology of SB
- **Closed Loop Small Bowel Obstruction**
  - Markedly distended segment of fluid-filled SB
  - Bowel proximal and distal to closed loop usually not dilated
  - Stretched mesenteric vessels converging toward site of obstruction
  - Distended SB loops appear as balloons on strings
    - This may be most apparent on axial, coronal or sagittal image plan

- **External Hernia**
  - Gas and fluid-filled bowel loops, omental fat, and vessels in ventral, inguinal, or other external hernia sac

Helpful Clues for Less Common Diagnoses

- **Peritoneal Metastases**
  - Serosal metastases encase and obstruct SB
  - Look for soft tissue density thickening of SB walls &/or mesenteric leaves
- **Sclerosing Peritonitis**
  - Results from chronic peritoneal dialysis (uncommonly)
    - Even more rarely as result of infected ascites (bacterial, TB, or fungal peritonitis)
  - Fibrotic and often calcified serosal encasement of SB (cocoon)
- **Transmesenteric Postoperative Hernia**
  - Protrusion of SB loops through congenital or acquired defect of mesentery
  - Most cases are postoperative
    - e.g., liver transplant, gastric bypass procedure
  - Cluster of dilated SB loops with distorted mesenteric vessels, hernia usually not encapsulated
- **Paraduodenal Hernia**
  - Protrusion of bowel loops through congenital paraduodenal fossae
  - Left paraduodenal hernia (75%): Lateral to 4th part of duodenum, between pancreas and stomach
  - Right paraduodenal hernia (25%): Via jejunal mesentericoparietal fossa of Waldeyer
  - Cluster of dilated bowel loops in abnormal location, with crowded, distorted mesenteric vessels
- **Transplantation, Small Intestine**
  - Usually accompanied by considerable mesenteric infiltration and scarring

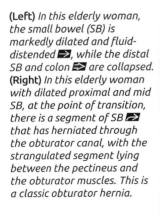

(Left) In this elderly woman, the small bowel (SB) is markedly dilated and fluid-distended ➡, while the distal SB and colon ⇨ are collapsed. (Right) In this elderly woman with dilated proximal and mid SB, at the point of transition, there is a segment of SB ➡ that has herniated through the obturator canal, with the strangulated segment lying between the pectineus and the obturator muscles. This is a classic obturator hernia.

Simple Small Bowel Obstruction

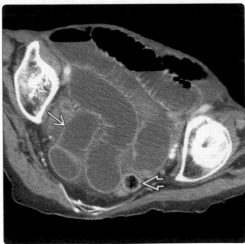

Simple Small Bowel Obstruction

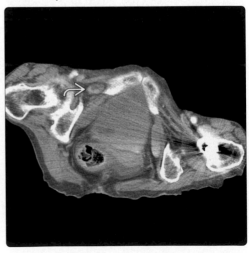

External Hernia

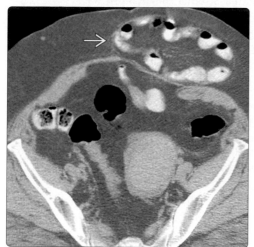

Peritoneal Metastases

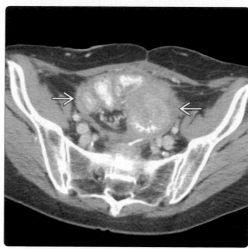

(Left) *Axial CECT shows a cluster of SB ➜ within a large ventral hernia.* **(Right)** *Axial CECT shows a tight cluster of SB ➜ that produced a functional SB obstruction, due to peritoneal (serosal) metastases from ovarian carcinoma that encased the bowel.*

Sclerosing Peritonitis

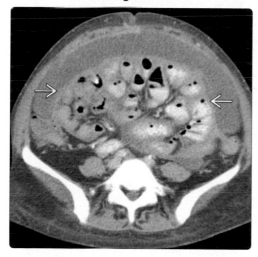

Transmesenteric Postoperative Hernia

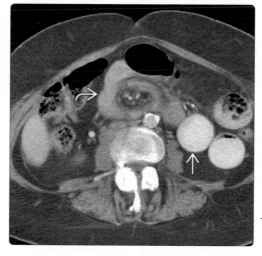

(Left) *Axial CECT shows cluster of SB that produced chronic symptoms of SB obstruction in patient with renal failure on chronic ambulatory peritoneal dialysis, who developed sclerosing peritonitis. Note peritoneal thickening ➜, encasing SB.* **(Right)** *In this patient who had had a Roux-en-Y gastric bypass procedure, the Roux limb and proximal SB ➜ are dilated while the distal SB and colon are collapsed. Note the twisting of the SB mesenteric root ➜. The jejunal anastomotic staple line was displaced, and mesenteric vessels were distorted.*

Paraduodenal Hernia

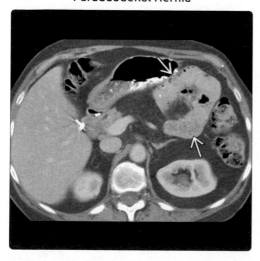

Transplantation, Small Intestine

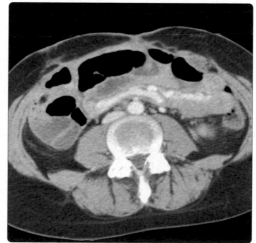

(Left) *Axial CECT shows a sac-of-bowel appearance ➜ of proximal bowel segments to the left of the ligament of Treitz, displacing the stomach forward. Their mesenteric vessels are displaced toward the center of the hernia.* **(Right)** *Axial CECT shows mild dilation of the SB allograft, along with infiltration of its mesentery, both common and nonspecific findings.*

DIFFERENTIAL DIAGNOSIS

Common

- Lymphoma, Small Bowel
- Metastases, Small Bowel
- Bowel-Bowel Anastomosis

Less Common

- Gastrointestinal Stromal Tumor, Intestinal
- Small Bowel Obstruction
- Diverticula, Small Bowel
- Meckel Diverticulum

Rare but Important

- Duplication Cyst, GI Tract

ESSENTIAL INFORMATION

Key Differential Diagnosis Issues

- Luminal dilation plus intramural mass = lymphoma, metastases, or GI stromal tumor

Helpful Clues for Common Diagnoses

- **Lymphoma, Small Bowel**
  - Classic etiology of aneurysmal dilation
  - Destroys myenteric plexus &/or wall of small bowel (SB)
    - Necrotic tumor may form cavity in communication with bowel lumen
    - Destruction of nerves in bowel wall allows dilation of lumen
  - Danger of free perforation into peritoneal cavity if tumor is treated with chemo- or radiation therapy
- **Metastases, Small Bowel**
  - Malignant melanoma is especially likely to cause aneurysmal dilation, similar to lymphoma
  - Usually see other metastases to bowel, mesentery, etc.
- **Bowel-Bowel Anastomosis**
  - Common after prior SB resection, creation of Roux loop, or to bypass stricture
  - Look for staple line at anastomosis

Helpful Clues for Less Common Diagnoses

- **Gastrointestinal Stromal Tumor, Intestinal**
  - Duodenum is 2nd most common site (after stomach)
  - Large, exophyte mass arising from duodenal wall
  - Ulceration of mucosa and central necrosis of tumor are common
  - May result in intratumoral gas and contrast media, resembling aneurysmal dilation
- **Small Bowel Obstruction**
  - Chronically dilated SB may attain large diameter (> 6 cm)
  - Preservation of normal SB folds distinguishes this from aneurysmal dilation related to neoplastic infiltration
- **Diverticula, Small Bowel**
  - Outpouchings from duodenum are very common
  - These are uncommon, but not rare, throughout remainder of SB
  - Perforation of SB diverticula can result in "SB diverticulitis," with abscess cavity
- **Meckel Diverticulum**
  - Arise from distal small bowel
  - Sac-like opening, often containing enteroliths
  - May ulcerate, perforate, intussuscept or obstruct

Helpful Clues for Rare Diagnoses

- **Duplication Cyst**
  - Can arise from SB or any portion of GI tract
  - May communicate with SB lumen, rarely simulating dilated lumen or aneurysmal dilation

---

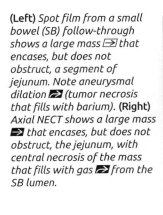

(Left) *Spot film from a small bowel (SB) follow-through shows a large mass ⊋ that encases, but does not obstruct, a segment of jejunum. Note aneurysmal dilation ⊅ (tumor necrosis that fills with barium).* **(Right)** *Axial NECT shows a large mass ⊋ that encases, but does not obstruct, the jejunum, with central necrosis of the mass that fills with gas ⊅ from the SB lumen.*

Lymphoma, Small Bowel

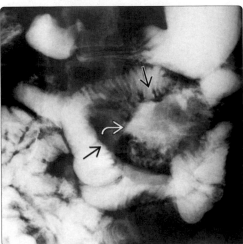

Lymphoma, Small Bowel

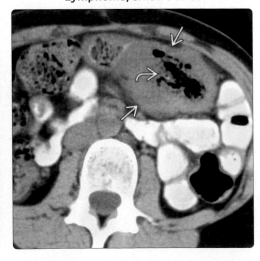

Metastases, Small Bowel

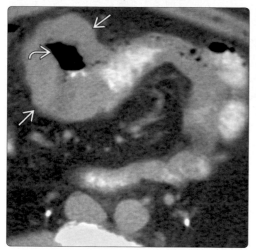

Bowel-Bowel Anastomosis

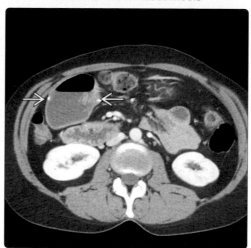

(Left) *In this patient with melanoma metastatic to SB, axial NECT shows a soft tissue mass* ➡ *that encases, but does not obstruct, the SB, with a central necrotic cavity* ➡ *that fills with gas and enteric contrast.* **(Right)** *Axial CECT shows focal dilation of SB without evidence of obstruction. The metallic staple line* ➡ *helps to identify this as the site of a side-to-side SB anastomosis.*

Diverticula, Small Bowel

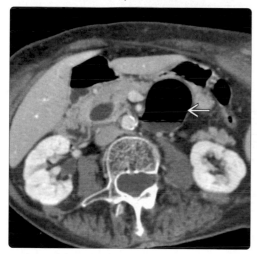

Diverticula, Small Bowel

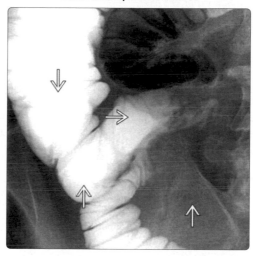

(Left) *Axial CECT shows one of several duodenal and jejunal diverticula* ➡ *with a thin wall and an air-fluid level present.* **(Right)** *Spot film from an upper GI series shows several duodenal and small bowel diverticula* ➡.

Meckel Diverticulum

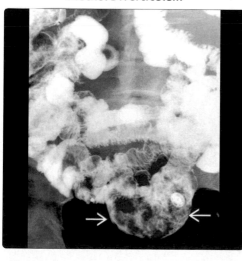

Duplication Cyst, GI Tract

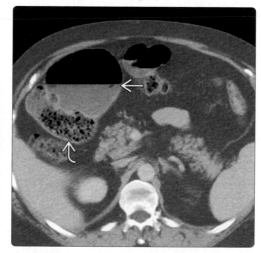

(Left) *Small bowel follow-through shows an unusually large Meckel diverticulum* ➡ *as a blind-ending pouch arising from the distal ileum, filled with a mixture of barium and food debris.* **(Right)** *Axial CECT shows a cystic structure that communicates with the SB lumen (air-fluid level)* ➡ *and causes partial SB obstruction (note SB feces sign)* ➡. *This was a duplication cyst of the ileum.*

DIFFERENTIAL DIAGNOSIS

Common

- Crohn Disease
- Infectious Enteritis
- Acute Appendicitis

Less Common

- Abdominal Abscess
- Cecal Carcinoma
- Carcinoid Tumor
- Tuberculosis
- Metastases and Lymphoma, Intestinal
- Radiation Enteritis
- Small Bowel Carcinoma

ESSENTIAL INFORMATION

Key Differential Diagnosis Issues

- Stenosis (stricture) of terminal ileum is much less common than simple wall thickening, but may be difficult to distinguish between these on single imaging study

Helpful Clues for Common Diagnoses

- **Crohn Disease**
  - Terminal ileum usually initial site of involvement
  - Small bowel follow-through (SBFT): Longitudinal & transverse ulcerations, aphthous lesions in (small bowel) SB & colon
  - CT: Wall thickening, luminal narrowing, mesenteric lymphadenopathy & fibrofatty proliferation
    - Mucosal & mesenteric hyperemia = acute inflammation
    - CT (or MR) is better suited to distinguishing acute from chronic changes related to Crohn disease
- **Infectious Enteritis**
  - Yersinia (gram-negative bacterium) produces radiographic findings similar to Crohn disease
    - Usually resolves quickly, without stricture
  - Other bacterial & viral organisms can cause enteritis, often with cluster of mildly enlarged mesenteric nodes

- **Acute Appendicitis**
  - SB & colon adjacent to inflamed appendix often have wall thickening & luminal narrowing
    - Usually not true stricture
    - May result in functional SB obstruction
  - Key is to identify abnormal appendix on CT, US, or MR

Helpful Clues for Less Common Diagnoses

- **Abdominal Abscess**
  - Pus from any abdominal or pelvic source (appendicitis, diverticulitis, adnexal abscess)
    - May bathe distal ileum, causing wall thickening & spasm
  - Fold thickening & luminal narrowing simulates primary SB inflammation
- **Cecal Carcinoma**
  - May extend into distal SB wall, serosa
  - CT may shows peritoneal & liver metastases
- **Carcinoid Tumor**
  - Common in appendix, distal SB
  - CT: Mesenteric mass (± calcification) usually more evident than primary tumor
    - Primary tumor and metastases are usually hypervascular
  - Marked desmoplastic infiltration of SB mesentery
- **Tuberculosis**
  - May involve cecum & terminal ileum
  - Look for signs of peritonitis & caseated nodes on CT
- **Radiation Enteritis**
  - Usually pelvic SB loops, not terminal ileum
- **Small Bowel Carcinoma**
  - Short segment stricture with overhanging edges (apple core)
  - Mass is soft tissue density
    - Not hypervascular (unlike carcinoid)
  - Typically results in SB obstruction
  - Regional nodal & liver metastases

Crohn Disease

Crohn Disease

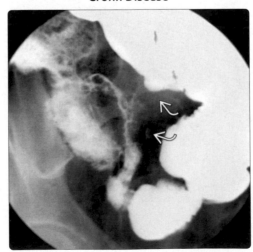
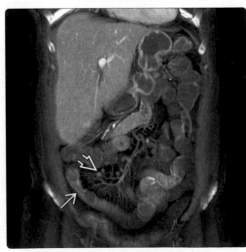

(Left) Small bowel follow-through shows luminal narrowing and mucosal ulceration of the distal ileum and ascending colon. Also noted are mass effect and fistulas ⇗ in the mesenteric fat. (Right) Coronal CECT shows evidence of acute & chronic Crohn disease, including a distal ileal stricture, mucosal hyperenhancement ⇒, mesenteric vascular engorgement and adenopathy ⇒.

Infectious Enteritis

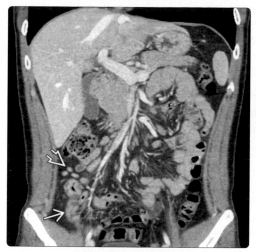

Acute Appendicitis

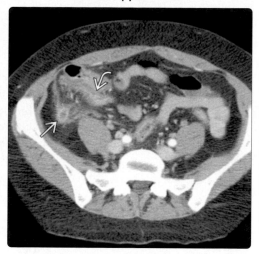

(Left) In this young woman with acute RLQ pain & fever, coronal CECT shows luminal narrowing, mucosal hyperenhancement & submucosal edema in the terminal ileum ➡ & cecum, along with mesenteric lymphadenopathy ➡. The appendix was normal. All signs & symptoms resolved without treatment. (Right) Axial CECT shows a dilated lumen and thickened wall of the appendix ➡, with inflammatory infiltration of the mesenteric fat & secondary inflammation of the terminal ileum ➡.

Abdominal Abscess

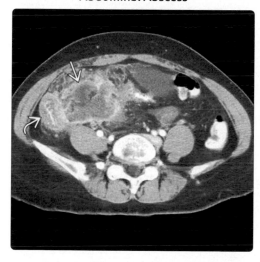

Cecal Carcinoma

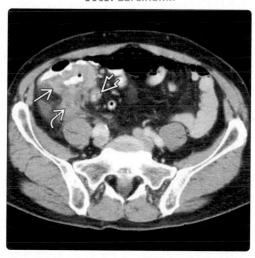

(Left) Axial CECT shows a right lower quadrant abscess ➡ with mural thickening & luminal narrowing of the cecum ➡ and terminal ileum. A perforated appendix was found at surgery. (Right) Axial CECT shows a soft tissue density mass that causes circumferential thickening of the cecal wall ➡ and obstruction of the base of the appendix ➡. There is infiltration of adjacent fat planes and the wall of the terminal ileum ➡.

Carcinoid Tumor

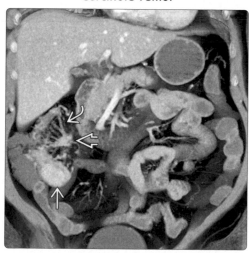

Tuberculosis

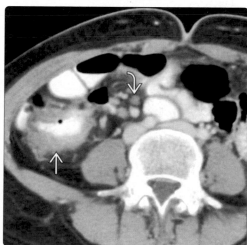

(Left) Coronal CECT shows a hypervascular distal ileal mass ➡ that narrows the lumen. Mesenteric metastases ➡ are also hypervascular and result in a desmoplastic response in the mesentery ➡. (Right) Axial CECT shows mural thickening and luminal narrowing of the cecum ➡ and terminal ileum, with mesenteric adenopathy ➡. Proven ileocecal TB in a young woman who was a Southeast Asian immigrant.

DIFFERENTIAL DIAGNOSIS

Common

- Crohn Disease
- Shock Bowel (Systemic Hypotension)
- Portal Hypertension
- Ischemic Enteritis
- Infectious Enteritis
- Mesenteric Adenitis/Enteritis
- Celiac-Sprue Disease

Less Common

- Opportunistic Intestinal Infections
- Graft-vs.-Host Disease
- Vasculitis, Small Intestine
- Angioedema, Intestinal
- Carcinoid Tumor
- Intramural Hemorrhage
- Hypoalbuminemia
- Radiation Enteritis
- Metastases and Lymphoma, Intestinal
- Endometriosis

Rare but Important

- Lymphangiectasia, Intestinal
- Whipple Disease
- Mastocytosis

ESSENTIAL INFORMATION

Key Differential Diagnosis Issues

- Characterize wall thickening by
  - **Length & degree of involvement**
    - Focal (< 10 cm length of involvement)
      - □ Neoplasm, endometriosis, Crohn disease)
    - Segmental (< 40 cm length)
      - □ Most common; least specific
    - Diffuse (> 40 cm length of involvement)
      - □ Systemic processes (shock, portal hypertension, vasculitis)
  - **Attenuation of submucosal layer**
    - Air: Pneumatosis (ischemic or other causes)
    - Fat: Normal variant, inactive Crohn; cytoreductive chemotherapy
    - Edema/water: Infection, inflammation, or ischemia (not neoplasm)
    - Soft tissue: Least specific
    - Blood (> 60 HU): Intramural hemorrhage
  - **Pattern of enhancement** (homo- or heterogeneous)
    - Heterogeneous suggests neoplastic
  - **Associated findings**
    - Vessel engorgement or thrombosis
    - Lymphadenopathy; edema, ascites
    - Extraintestinal sites of tumor
    - History or signs of shock, portal hypertension, immunosuppression
  - **Degree of mucosal enhancement**
    - Normal [similar to remainder of small bowel (SB)]
    - Increased and often thickened
      - □ Infection (e.g., opportunistic)

- □ Inflammation (e.g., Crohn disease, vasculitis, angioedema)
    - Decreased = ischemia
- **Optimal CT technique**
  - Distend SB lumen by water or neutral contrast agent
  - Rapid IV contrast medium administration (> 2 mL/sec)
  - Multiplanar viewing (especially coronal)

Helpful Clues for Common Diagnoses

- **Crohn Disease**
  - Segmental distribution with skip lesions
  - Submucosal attenuation: Edema in acute; fat density in chronic
  - Mucosal enhancement: Marked in sites of active inflammation
  - Associated findings: Mesenteric hyperemia, fibrofatty proliferation, lymphadenopathy
- **Shock Bowel (Systemic Hypotension)**
  - Diffuse distribution with marked wall thickening
  - Submucosal attenuation: Water density
  - Mucosal enhancement: Intense
  - Associated findings: Mesenteric edema
    - Visceral &/or cerebral traumatic injuries
    - "Collapsed cava" (flattened IVC)
- **Portal Hypertension**
  - Diffuse distribution
  - Submucosal attenuation: Edema (water density)
  - Associated findings: Cirrhosis, ascites, splenomegaly
- **Ischemic Enteritis**
  - Segmental with marked wall thickening in venous obstruction
  - Attenuation: Air (infarction) to edema to blood density
  - Enhancement: Intense mucosal in venous thrombosis; absent in arterial thrombosis
  - Associated findings: Thrombosis of mesenteric vessels, ascites, ileus
    - Minimal wall thickening in arterial occlusion
- **Infectious Enteritis**
  - In previously healthy individuals, usually self-limited
    - Variety of pathogens (bacteria, protozoa, viruses, etc.)
  - Distribution: Long segmental
    - *Giardia*: Duodenum and jejunum
    - *Yersinia, Campylobacter*: Distal ileum and cecum
  - Mucosal hyperenhancement & submucosal edema
  - Associated: Mesenteric adenopathy & diarrhea (liquid bowel contents)
- **Mesenteric Adenitis/Enteritis**
  - Form of infectious enteritis
  - Occurs in children and young adults, presenting with acute RLQ pain
  - Cluster of enlarged ileac mesenteric nodes may be only finding
  - Terminal ileum and cecum may appear inflamed
- **Celiac-Sprue Disease**
  - Most common disease causing malabsorption pattern
    - Dilated, fluid-distended SB, appearing flaccid
    - SB segments indent and conform to each other
    - Decreased fold height in jejunum; increased in ileum (reversed fold pattern)
    - Short segment intussusceptions

Helpful Clues for Less Common Diagnoses

- **Opportunistic Intestinal Infections**
  - Segmental with moderate thickening
  - Submucosal attenuation: Water to soft tissue
  - Associated findings
    - History of AIDS or transplantation
    - Lymphadenopathy (low density in mycobacterial disease)
- **Graft-vs.-Host Disease**
  - Usually diffuse
  - Attenuation: Water to soft tissue
  - Associated findings: Patients have skin and liver involvement
  - By imaging alone, it is difficult or impossible to distinguish graft-vs.-host disease (GVHD) from opportunistic SB infection
- **Vasculitis, Small Intestine**
  - Segmental or diffuse with moderate to marked thickening
  - Attenuation: Air to water to soft tissue to blood
    - Pneumatosis may be due to ischemia or from medications (steroids)
  - Associated findings: Skin and subcutaneous purpura (Henoch-Schönlein), visceral ischemic lesions (lupus, polyarteritis)
- **Angioedema, Intestinal**
  - Congenital or associated with medications (e.g., ACE inhibitors), hepatitis, etc.
  - Segmental distribution
  - Attenuation: Edema (water density)
  - Associated findings: Ascites (almost always)
- **Carcinoid Tumor**
  - Segmental, usually distal ileum
  - Mural mass and mesenteric metastases are hyperenhancing (distinctive feature)
  - Associated findings: Liver metastases
    - Mesenteric mass with calcification
    - Desmoplastic effect on adjacent SB loops
- **Intramural Hemorrhage**

- Segmental with marked thickening
- Attenuation: Blood density (> 60 HU)
- Associated findings: Signs of trauma or coagulopathic bleeding
  - e.g., hematocrit sign: Cellular/fluid levels
- **Radiation Enteritis**
  - Segmental in pelvis
  - Attenuation: Water to soft tissue
  - Associated findings: Evidence of surgery &/or brachytherapy beads in pelvis
- **Metastases and Lymphoma, Intestinal**
  - Segmental or diffuse (lymphoma)
  - Multifocal discrete (metastases, e.g., melanoma)
    - Marked thickening at sites of tumor
  - Attenuation: Soft tissue (not edema)
  - Enhancement: Heterogeneous, nodular (in mass itself)
  - Associated findings: Other metastatic foci (e.g., liver, spleen); lymphadenopathy, splenomegaly (lymphoma)
- **Endometriosis**
  - Focal to segmental with skip areas
  - Attenuation: Soft tissue or blood density
  - Associated findings: Pelvic mass; characteristic features of blood on MR scanning

Helpful Clues for Rare Diagnoses

- **Lymphangiectasia, Intestinal**
  - Diffuse distribution
  - Submucosal and mesenteric edema (marked)
  - Ascites and lower extremity edema
  - Diarrhea (fluid distention of SB and colon)
- **Whipple Disease**
  - Associated: Low-density mesenteric nodes
  - Clinical: Arthralgias, weight loss
- **Mastocytosis**
  - Systemic proliferation of mast cells
  - In gut, abdominal viscera, bones, skin
  - Thickened folds throughout SB with fluid-distended lumen
  - Associated: Dense bones

Crohn Disease

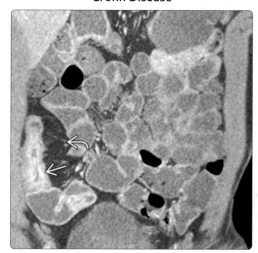

Shock Bowel (Systemic Hypotension)

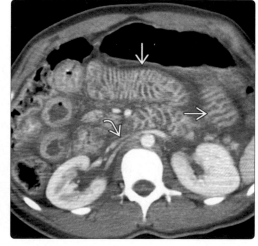

(Left) *Coronal CT shows a thick-walled terminal ileum ➡ with intensely enhancing mucosa and a narrowed lumen. Within the ileal mesentery there are engorged blood vessels and a proliferation of fibrofatty tissue ➢. (Right) Note the intense enhancement of the small bowel mucosa ➡ and kidneys, along with marked edema/infiltration of the mesentery. Also note the "collapsed cava" ➢ and renal veins due to hypovolemia.*

Small Intestine

Portal Hypertension

Portal Hypertension

Ischemic Enteritis

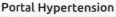

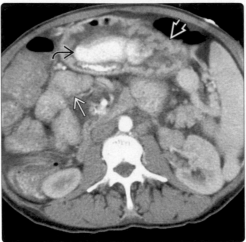

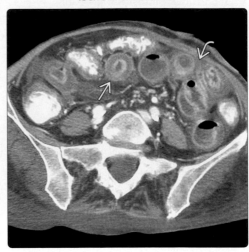

(Left) *CT shows diffuse small bowel (SB) wall edema ➡ due to cirrhosis and portal hypertension. Associated findings include gastric varices ➡, causing active bleeding into the gastric lumen ➡.*
(Right) *Axial CECT shows marked mural thickening ➡ of a long segment of small bowel due to ischemia following a hypotensive episode. Interloop ascites is also noted ➡.*

Infectious Enteritis

Infectious Enteritis

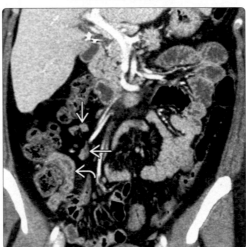

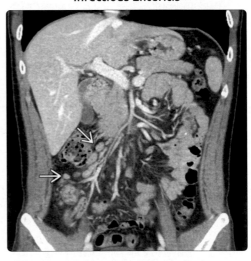

(Left) *This 25-year-old woman had acute RLQ pain and fever. Coronal CT shows a cluster of mildly enlarged lymph nodes ➡ and subtle mucosal hyperenhancement of the terminal ileum ➡. Symptoms resolved spontaneously.*
(Right) *In this 25-year-old woman, coronal CT also shows a cluster of mildly enlarged mesenteric nodes ➡. This finding may be the most evident on imaging, leading to the alternative diagnosis of mesenteric adenitis/enteritis.*

Mesenteric Adenitis/Enteritis

Mesenteric Adenitis/Enteritis

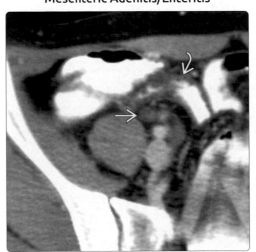

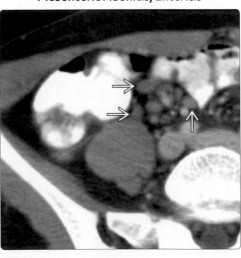

(Left) *In this young woman with RLQ pain, CECT shows a cluster of mildly enlarged mesenteric nodes ➡ in the right lower quadrant and mild thickening of the wall of the terminal ileum ➡. The appendix was normal.* (Right) *In this young woman with acute RLQ pain, CT shows a cluster of mildly enlarged mesenteric nodes ➡, which may be the only or dominant finding, leading to the inconsistent naming of this entity as mesenteric adenitis or infectious enteritis. Symptoms resolved spontaneously.*

Celiac-Sprue Disease

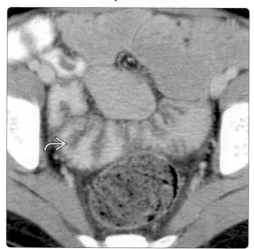

Celiac-Sprue Disease

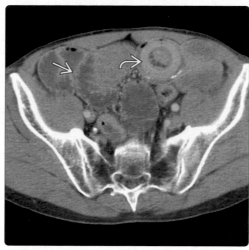

(Left) *In this young man, CT shows fluid distention of the SB. The fold pattern of the jejunum is abnormally effaced, resembling the expected pattern of the ileum. Conversely, the ileal fold pattern is abnormally prominent ➦. Endoscopic biopsy and response to a gluten-free diet confirmed the diagnosis of celiac disease.* (Right) *In this 69-year-old man, CT shows fluid distention of the SB and prominent ileal folds ➥. A short segment, intussusception ➥ is noted.*

Opportunistic Intestinal Infections

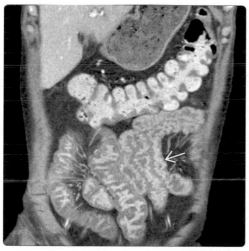

Graft-vs.-Host Disease

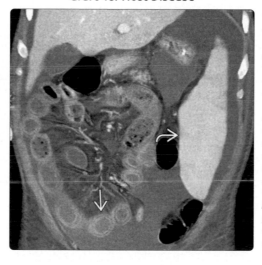

(Left) *This woman had acute severe diarrhea following lung transplantation for cystic fibrosis. Coronal CT shows diffuse SB mucosal hyperenhancement and submucosal edema ➥, proven CMV enteritis.* (Right) *This man had bone marrow transplantation for myelofibrosis and developed a rash and abdominal pain with diarrhea. CT shows diffuse SB submucosal edema ➥ along with ascites and splenomegaly ➥. It is difficult to distinguish graft-vs.-host disease from opportunistic infection by CT alone.*

Vasculitis, Small Intestine

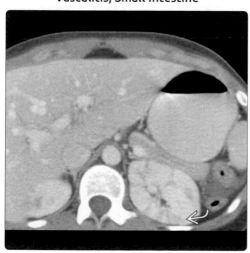

Vasculitis, Small Intestine

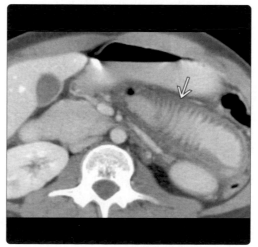

(Left) *In this young woman with abdominal pain, CT shows wedge-shaped and striated zones of decreased attenuation ➥ within the kidneys, and ascites.* (Right) *In this young woman with abdominal pain, CT shows long segmental wall thickening of the jejunum ➥. The combination of the patient's young age, renal and SB involvement suggested vasculitis, and polyarteritis was confirmed.*

Angioedema, Intestinal

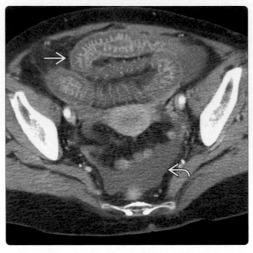

Angioedema, Intestinal

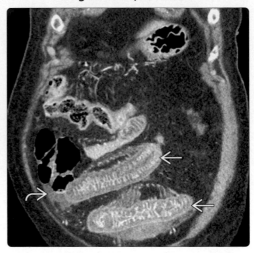

(Left) *In this elderly woman with repeated bouts of laryngeal edema and severe abdominal pain, CT shows long segmental SB wall edema ➡ and ascites ➡. (Right) In this elderly woman with laryngeal edema and abdominal pain, coronal CT shows long segmental SB submucosal edema ➡ and ascites ➡. This was attributed to the use of ACE inhibitor medication, and symptoms and signs resolved with withdrawal of this medication.*

Carcinoid Tumor

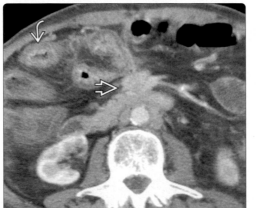

Carcinoid Tumor

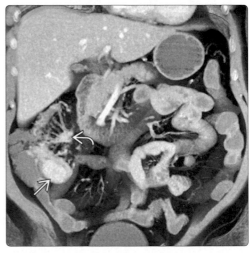

(Left) *In this 64-year-old man, CT shows a hypervascular mesenteric mass ➡ due to nodal metastases. Note the SB wall edema ➡ and tethering due to the desmoplastic effect of the tumor on mesenteric veins and lymphatics. (Right) In this 54-year-old man, coronal CECT shows a hypervascular mass ➡ in the distal ileum, with associated mesenteric metastasis ➡ having a characteristic desmoplastic effect on adjacent bowel.*

Intramural Hemorrhage

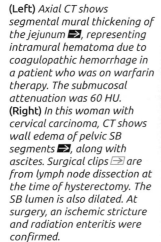
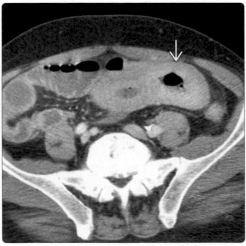

Radiation Enteritis

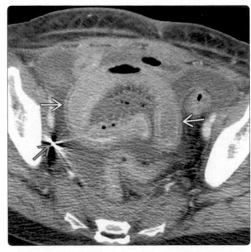

(Left) *Axial CT shows segmental mural thickening of the jejunum ➡, representing intramural hematoma due to coagulopathic hemorrhage in a patient who was on warfarin therapy. The submucosal attenuation was 60 HU. (Right) In this woman with cervical carcinoma, CT shows wall edema of pelvic SB segments ➡, along with ascites. Surgical clips ➡ are from lymph node dissection at the time of hysterectomy. The SB lumen is also dilated. At surgery, an ischemic stricture and radiation enteritis were confirmed.*

Metastases and Lymphoma, Intestinal

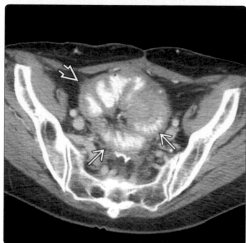

Metastases and Lymphoma, Intestinal

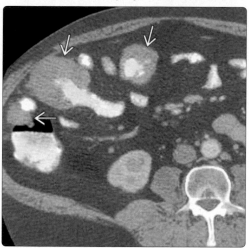

(Left) *In this woman with metastatic ovarian cancer, CT shows loculated, malignant ascites ⮕ and a cluster of SB loops with thickened folds due to serosal metastases ⮕.* (Right) *Axial CECT shows marked soft tissue density wall thickening in several segments of small bowel ⮕. In spite of the large masses, there is no luminal obstruction, typical findings of small bowel lymphoma.*

Lymphangiectasia, Intestinal

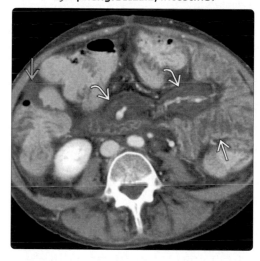

Lymphangiectasia, Intestinal

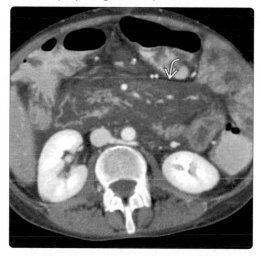

(Left) *In this 36-year-old woman with chronic diarrhea, CT shows ascites ⮕ and submucosal edema throughout much of the small intestine ⮕. More striking is the edema in the root and leaves of mesentery ⮕.* (Right) *In this young woman with chronic diarrhea, CT shows diffuse SB wall edema and striking infiltration of the SB mesentery ⮕.*

Mastocytosis

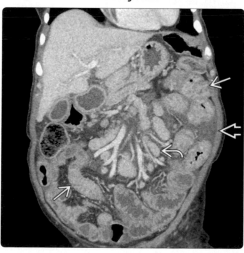

Mastocytosis

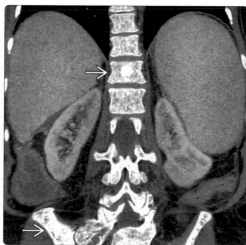

(Left) *In this 64-year-old woman, coronal CT shows widespread abdominal lymphadenopathy ⮕, ascites ⮕, and diffuse SB submucosal edema ⮕.* (Right) *In this 64-year-old woman, CT shows hepatosplenomegaly and multifocal sclerosis of the axial skeleton ⮕, all due to systemic mastocytosis.*

DIFFERENTIAL DIAGNOSIS

Common

- Ischemic Enteritis
- Ischemic Colitis
- Medication-Induced Pneumatosis
- Postoperative State, Bowel
- Postendoscopy
- Pseudopneumatosis (Mimic)
- Pulmonary Causes
  - Barotrauma, Abdominal Manifestations
    - Asthma
    - Chronic Obstructive Pulmonary Disease
    - Cystic Fibrosis
- Small Bowel Obstruction
- Scleroderma
- Necrotizing Enterocolitis

Less Common

- Pneumatosis Cystoides Intestinalis
- Intestinal Trauma
- Small Bowel Transplantation
- Inflammatory Bowel Disease
- Toxic Megacolon
- Graft-vs.-Host Disease
- Caustic Gastroduodenal Injury
- Gas in Wall of Ileal Conduit

ESSENTIAL INFORMATION

Key Differential Diagnosis Issues

- Pneumatosis is radiographic finding, not disease process
  - To determine its significance, must correlate with
    - Patient history
    - Clinical signs and symptoms
  - If pneumatosis is due to ischemia, patient will be very ill
    - Check for laboratory abnormalities (acidosis, leukocytosis, elevated serum amylase)
  - Patients with benign (nonischemic) pneumatosis are usually asymptomatic

Helpful Clues for Common Diagnoses

- **Ischemic Enteritis and Colitis**
  - Spherical or linear collections of gas in submucosa of affected bowel
  - Often associated with portal venous gas
  - Small bowel (SB) ischemia is usually due to occlusion of superior mesenteric artery or superior mesenteric vein
    - Colonic ischemia more often due to hypoperfusion; not thrombotic
- **Medication-Induced Pneumatosis**
  - Corticosteroids, chemotherapy, antirejection medications
  - Any organ or bone marrow transplant recipient
  - Medications may cause tiny perforations of mucosa by inducing atrophy of submucosal lymphoid follicles
- **Postoperative State, Bowel**
  - Bowel-to-bowel anastomosis
  - Gastrostomy, jejunostomy tubes
  - Either may cause gas to leak from bowel lumen into wall

- Patients are usually asymptomatic unless there is leak of other bowel contents or associated SB obstruction
- **Postendoscopy**
  - Upper or lower endoscopy
  - Also after barium or hydrogen peroxide enema
  - Mucosal tear may allow gas leak into wall
- **Pseudopneumatosis (Mimic)**
  - Gas may be trapped against inner wall of bowel, simulating pneumatosis
  - Very common in cecum, ascending colon
    - Usually not seen above air-feces level within colon
  - SB feces sign (in SB obstruction or cystic fibrosis)
    - Gas may be trapped within lumen, up against inner wall of SB
- **Pulmonary Causes**
  - Barotrauma
    - Asthma
    - Chronic obstructive pulmonary disease
    - Pulmonary fibrosis
    - Cystic fibrosis
    - Ventilator
  - Gas dissects down mediastinum, into retroperitoneum, out mesentery, into bowel wall
- **Small Bowel Obstruction**
  - Gas may enter wall of SB, especially if there has been prior SB surgery or intrinsic SB disease (e.g., Crohn disease)
  - Check for signs of closed loop obstruction
    - Disproportionate dilation of cluster of SB loops, engorged vessels, ascites, infiltrated mesentery
    - Pneumatosis with these signs = bowel infarction
  - Correlate with clinical and laboratory evidence of bowel ischemia
- **Scleroderma**
  - And other forms of mixed connective tissue disease
  - Intramural gas may result from bowel disease itself, associated medications (e.g., corticosteroids), or ischemia
    - Must correlate with clinical and laboratory evidence of disease exacerbation or ischemia
- **Necrotizing Enterocolitis**
  - Common cause of pneumatosis in neonates

Helpful Clues for Less Common Diagnoses

- **Pneumatosis Cystoides Intestinalis**
  - Idiopathic, asymptomatic, usually colonic
  - Usually appears as large gas cysts in wall of colon
    - May be mistaken for polyps, if gas density is not appreciated
- **Intestinal Trauma**
  - Serosa of bowel may be avulsed (degloving injury)
  - Leads to devascularization and ischemia of bowel
  - Rarely, may be transient finding not indicative of bowel injury
- **Small Bowel Transplantation**
  - These patients frequently develop benign pneumatosis
  - Many potential causes
    - Medications
    - Bowel-to-bowel anastomoses
    - Rejection
    - Infarction

- o Often requires endoscopic evaluation to distinguish from ischemia
- **Inflammatory Bowel Disease**
  - o Crohn disease, ulcerative colitis, others
  - o Any disease that causes ulceration of bowel mucosa can cause pneumatosis
  - o Patients are often on steroid medications that may also cause pneumatosis
- **Graft-vs.-Host Disease**
  - o Bone marrow transplant recipients
  - o Clinical triad: Damage to gut, skin, liver
  - o Pneumatosis does not necessarily indicate ischemia
    - Patients are receiving medications (steroids, immunosuppression) associated with benign pneumatosis
- **Caustic Gastroduodenal Injury**
  - o Usually limited to esophagus and stomach
  - o Duodenum may also be injured
  - o Mucosal or transmural necrosis may cause pneumatosis &/or perforation of bowel
- **Gas in Wall of Ileal Conduit**
  - o Following cystectomy
  - o Ureters may be anastomosed to ileal conduit
  - o Nonischemic gas may collect transiently within bowel wall
  - o Check for gas-forming infection of urine (may release gas into lumen, or, rarely, into wall of conduit)

SELECTED REFERENCES

1. Rha SE et al: CT and MR imaging findings of bowel ischemia from various primary causes. Radiographics. 20(1):29-42, 2000
2. Feczko PJ et al: Clinical significance of pneumatosis of the bowel wall. Radiographics. 12(6):1069-78, 1992

Ischemic Enteritis

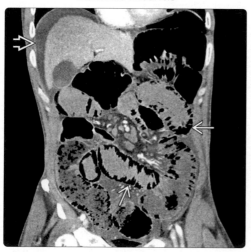

Ischemic Enteritis

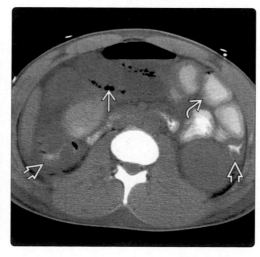

(Left) *Coronal CT shows extensive pneumatosis ➡ throughout the small bowel. Also note dilation of the bowel lumen & ascites ➡, findings that help to confirm that pneumatosis is likely due to bowel ischemia.* **(Right)** *In this patient who had cardiac arrest from near-drowning, CT shows signs of bowel ischemia including generalized ileus. The wall of the colon is thickened ➡. The wall of the small intestine is also thickened ➡, and there is focal pneumatosis ➡.*

Medication-Induced Pneumatosis

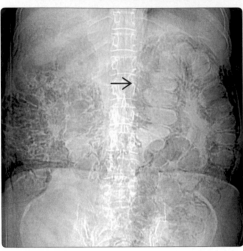

Medication-Induced Pneumatosis

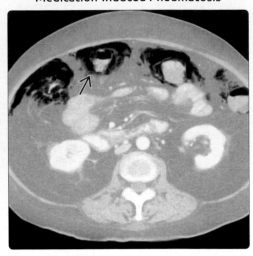

(Left) *In this patient who has had a bone-marrow transplant, a supine radiograph shows extensive colonic pneumatosis ➡, but no small bowel dilation. He remained essentially asymptomatic, & the pneumatosis was attributed to his immunosuppressive medications.* (Right) *In this patient who has had a bone marrow transplantation, CT shows extensive colonic pneumatosis ➡ but no ascites nor ileus. The patient remained well and the pneumatosis slowly resolved without other intervention.*

Postoperative State, Bowel

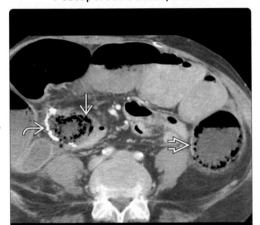

Pseudopneumatosis (Mimic)

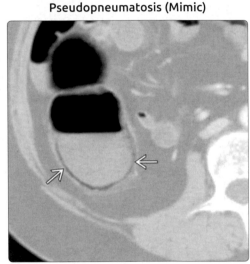

(Left) *Axial CECT shows pneumatosis ➡ near the site of prior bowel resection ➡, but also within bowel some distance removed from the operative site ➡. The patient had signs of sepsis and ischemia was confirmed at surgery.* (Right) *Axial CECT shows gas trapped against the wall of the ascending colon ➡, simulating pneumatosis. Note that this finding is not present in the nondependent colon, where the fluid stool is not in contact with the bowel wall.*

Barotrauma, Abdominal Manifestations

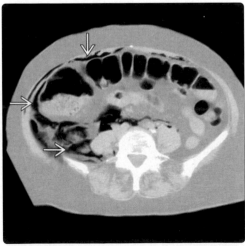

Small Bowel Obstruction

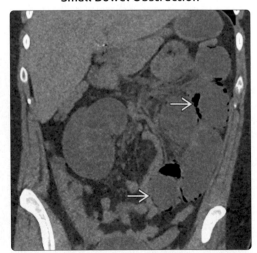

(Left) *Axial CECT shows extensive gas dissecting throughout the abdomen ➡, some of which may be in bowel wall, due to barotrauma in this patient on positive pressure ventilation.* (Right) *In this young woman with an adhesive small bowel (SB) obstruction, coronal CT shows marked luminal dilation and pneumatosis ➡ within proximal SB segments. At surgery the dilated bowel returned to normal appearance following release of adhesions & was not resected.*

Pneumatosis Cystoides Intestinalis

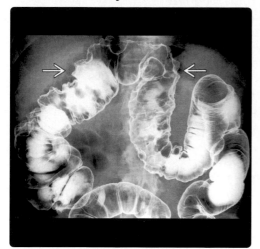

Small Bowel Transplantation

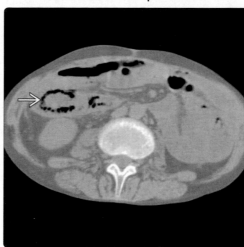

(Left) *This film from an air-contrast enema shows gas cysts* ➡ *within the wall of otherwise normal colon in an asymptomatic man with idiopathic primary colonic pneumatosis.* **(Right)** *The SB allograft is dilated with a thickened wall and with pneumatosis* ➡, *raising concern for infarction. At endoscopy (through the ileostomy), the small bowel mucosa appeared normal.*

Inflammatory Bowel Disease

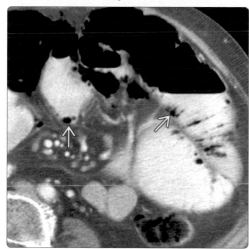

Toxic Megacolon

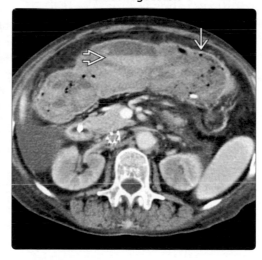

(Left) *In this patient with prior bowel resection for Crohn disease, gas is seen in wall of dilated loops of small intestine* ➡ *in the upper abdomen. In this patient, pneumatosis could be due to ischemia, medication, Crohn disease, or bowel obstruction. At surgery the bowel was determined to be ischemic but not infarcted.* **(Right)** *Axial CECT shows a grossly dilated transverse colon with loss of haustration. There is gas within the wall of the colon* ➡, *hemorrhagic debris within the lumen* ➡, *and ascites. All findings confirmed at colectomy.*

Graft-vs.-Host Disease

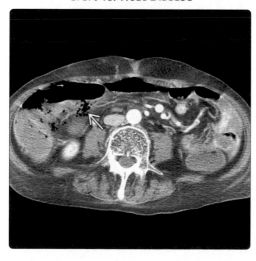

Graft-vs.-Host Disease

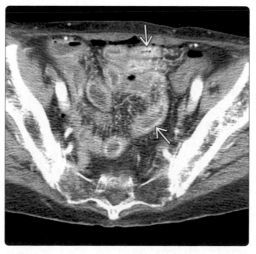

(Left) *In this 64-year-old man who had a bone marrow transplant for leukemia, CT shows pneumatosis* ➡ *within segments of SB and colon. This patient had both graft-vs.-host disease (GVHD) and cytomegalovirus (CMV) infection of the SB.* **(Right)** *In this 64-year-old man who had a bone marrow transplant, CT shows mucosal hyperenhancement* ➡ *and engorged mesenteric vessels. SB biopsy proved both GVHD and infection by CMV. It is often difficult or impossible to distinguish these 2 entities by imaging.*

DIFFERENTIAL DIAGNOSIS

Common

- Vascular Ectasia, Intestinal
- Crohn Disease

Less Common

- Carcinoid Tumor
- Gastrointestinal Stromal Tumor
- Metastases and Lymphoma, Intestinal
- Small Bowel Carcinoma
- Aortoenteric Fistula
- Ischemic Enteritis
- Vasculitis, Small Intestine
- Mesenteric Varices
- Intramural Benign Tumor, Intestinal
- Radiation Enteritis

ESSENTIAL INFORMATION

Key Differential Diagnosis Issues

- **Occult gastrointestinal bleeding** = loss of blood with no source identified by endoscopy
  - Small intestine is most common site
  - CT and capsule endoscopy are complementary for diagnosis
- **Overt gastrointestinal bleeding** = hematemesis, melena, or hematochezia
  - Bleeding site is usually detectable by endoscopy
  - Common sources: Gastric & duodenal ulcers, esophageal varices, tumors of esophagus, stomach, or colon
- Optimal CT technique = CT enterography
  - Distend bowel with water or Volumen
  - Rapid (3-5 mL/s) bolus of IV contrast
  - Multiplanar reformations and multiphasic imaging
    - Nonenhanced phase is useful for baseline
    - Arterial phase (~ 20- to 30-second delay) is mandatory
    - Delayed phase is useful to see pooling of intraluminal opacified blood

Helpful Clues for Common Diagnoses

- **Vascular Ectasia, Intestinal**
  - AVMs are common cause of chronic, obscure GI bleeding
  - Accounting for 40-80% in some series
- **Crohn Disease**
  - Usually presents with abdominal symptoms (pain, diarrhea) unlike most other causes of obscure GI bleeding

Helpful Clues for Less Common Diagnoses

- **Carcinoid Tumor**
  - Hypervascular mass in ileum with mesenteric metastasis and desmoplasia
- **Gastrointestinal Stromal Tumor**
  - Bulky mass, exophytic [small bowel (SB) < duodenum < stomach]
  - Central ulceration in communication with lumen
- **Metastases and Lymphoma, Intestinal**
  - Bull's eye (target) or circumferential mass
  - May cause aneurysmal dilation of lumen (melanoma & lymphoma)
  - Uncommonly cause luminal obstruction
- **Small Bowel Carcinoma**
  - Constricting lesion, usually causes obstruction
- **Aortoenteric Fistula**
  - Complication of graft repair of aortic aneurysm
  - CTA: Focal wall thickening of 3rd portion of duodenum
  - Appears adherent to proximal portion of aortic graft
  - With or without extraluminal gas bubbles, active bleeding into lumen
- **Ischemic Enteritis**
  - SMA or SMV; closed-loop SB obstruction
  - Abnormal enhancement & thickening of SB wall
  - Infiltrated mesentery, ascites, especially with venous thrombosis
- **Vasculitis, Small Intestine**
  - Segmental involvement, thick SB folds
- **Mesenteric Varices**
  - In portal hypertension
  - Usually at site of prior bowel surgery

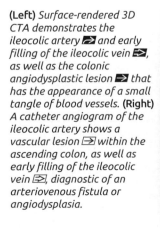

(Left) Surface-rendered 3D CTA demonstrates the ileocolic artery ➡ and early filling of the ileocolic vein ➡, as well as the colonic angiodysplastic lesion ➡ that has the appearance of a small tangle of blood vessels. (Right) A catheter angiogram of the ileocolic artery shows a vascular lesion ➡ within the ascending colon, as well as early filling of the ileocolic vein ➡, diagnostic of an arteriovenous fistula or angiodysplasia.

Vascular Ectasia, Intestinal

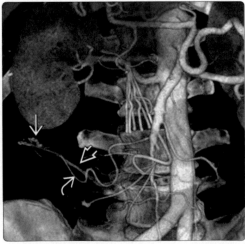

Vascular Ectasia, Intestinal

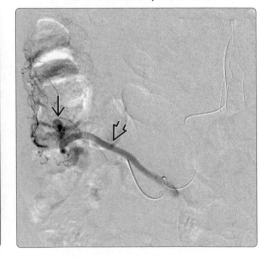

Crohn Disease

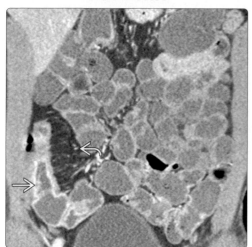

Carcinoid Tumor

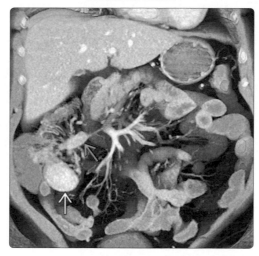

(Left) *Coronal image from a CT enterography study shows mucosal hyperenhancement* ➡ *and wall thickening of the terminal ileum with engorged feeding vessels* ➡ *and fibrofatty proliferation of the adjacent mesenteric fat, diagnostic of acute or chronic Crohn disease.* (Right) *Coronal-plane 3D reformation shows a distal ileal mass* ➡*, a hypervascular mesenteric metastasis* ➡*, and desmoplastic response within the mesentery.*

Gastrointestinal Stromal Tumor

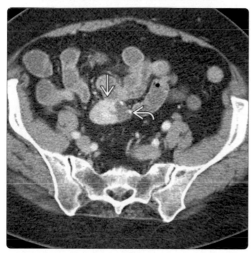

Gastrointestinal Stromal Tumor

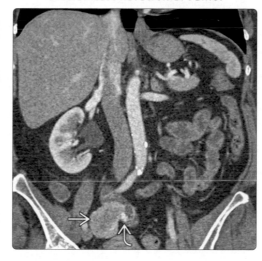

(Left) *CECT enterography shows a brightly enhancing mass* ➡ *arising from the ileum. Within the lumen of the affected segment of bowel, there are high-density foci of extravasated contrast material* ➡*, indicating active bleeding from the mass.* (Right) *Coronal CT shows a partially exophytic, hypervascular mass* ➡ *arising from the small bowel wall, with active bleeding into the bowel lumen* ➡*.*

Metastases and Lymphoma, Intestinal

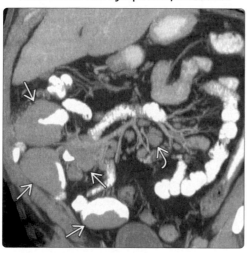

Metastases and Lymphoma, Intestinal

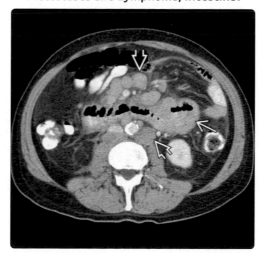

(Left) *Coronal CT shows multifocal small bowel wall masses* ➡ *without bowel obstruction. Also noted is extensive mesenteric lymphadenopathy* ➡*, classic features of intestinal non-Hodgkin lymphoma, though metastatic melanoma could have a similar appearance.* (Right) *In this woman with metastatic melanoma, CT shows extensive lymph node metastases* ➡ *throughout the retroperitoneum and mesentery. Metastasis to the bowel* ➡ *thickens and distorts the wall but does not obstruct the lumen in this case.*

Small Bowel Carcinoma

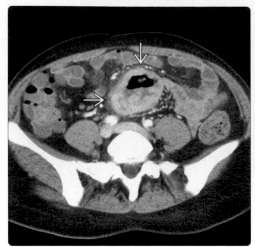

Small Bowel Carcinoma

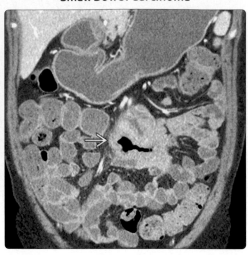

(Left) *Axial CT shows a complex mass ⇨ arising from the bowel wall and invading the surrounding mesentery. An unusual feature of this primary small bowel carcinoma is the lack of luminal obstruction.* (Right) *Coronal CT shows a mass ⇨ arising from the bowel wall and invading adjacent tissues. Hypovascularity of the mass is a typical feature of a primary adenocarcinoma, but the absence of bowel obstruction is an unusual feature.*

Aortoenteric Fistula

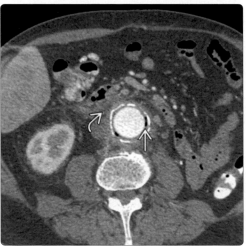

Aortoenteric Fistula

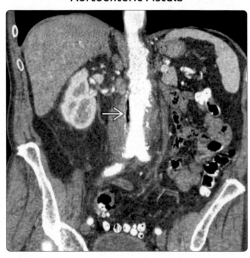

(Left) *In this patient who presented with fever and occult GI bleeding months after surgical repair of an abdominal aortic aneurysm (AAA), CT shows the native, calcified aortic wall wrapped around the synthetic graft. Between the graft and the aortic wall are collections of gas ⇨, indicating infection &/or fistula to gut. There is a rind of soft tissue density surrounding the aorta and 3rd portion of duodenum ⇨.* (Right) *Coronal CT shows soft tissue and gas ⇨ surrounding an aortic graft months after surgical repair of an AAA.*

Ischemic Enteritis

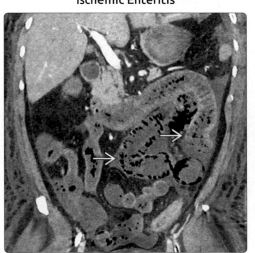

Ischemic Enteritis

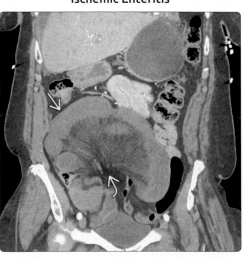

(Left) *CT from man with acute abdominal pain, acidosis, & hematochezia shows dilated small bowel segments with pneumatosis ⇨ & ascites, suggesting bowel infarction.* (Right) *CT from elderly man with crampy abdominal pain & hematochezia shows segmental dilation of fluid-distended small bowel & pinching of mesenteric vessels & bowel ⇨, lacking mucosal enhancement of the dilated small bowel segments ⇨ & infiltration of the mesentery, all findings indicating closed-loop small bowel obstruction with bowel ischemia.*

Vasculitis, Small Intestine

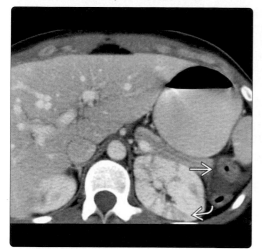

Vasculitis, Small Intestine

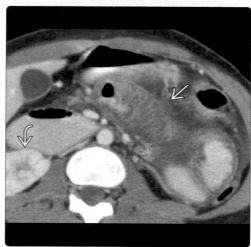

(Left) *In this young woman with severe abdominal pain, CT shows wedge-shaped and striated zones of decreased attenuation ➡ within the kidneys. Small bowel wall thickening and ascites are also noted ➡.* (Right) *In this young woman, CT shows a striated nephrogram ➡, ascites, & marked thickening of the wall of the jejunum ➡. The finding of "inflammatory" or hemorrhagic injury to the bowel wall and kidneys in a young patient is strongly suggestive of vasculitis (polyarteritis nodosa in this case).*

Mesenteric Varices

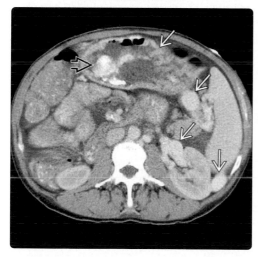

Mesenteric Varices

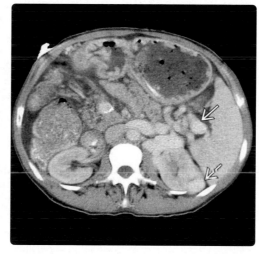

(Left) *In this patient with cirrhosis & portal vein thrombosis, CT shows ascites and extensive varices ➡. Also noted is a hyperdense collection ➡ within the stomach representing active bleeding from gastric varices.* (Right) *In this patient with cirrhosis and portal vein thrombosis, CT shows extensive mesenteric & perirenal varices ➡, any of which can be a site of spontaneous hemorrhage.*

Intramural Benign Tumor, Intestinal

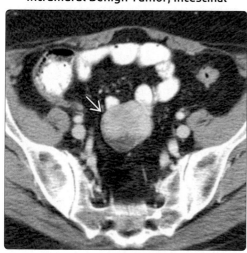

Radiation Enteritis

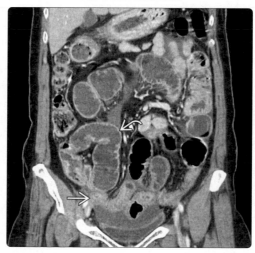

(Left) *Axial CECT shows a heterogeneous mass ➡ in the wall of distal small bowel. The mass, a leiomyoma, caused chronic GI bleeding but not obstruction.* (Right) *In this woman with radiation enteritis following treatment for endometrial carcinoma, coronal CT shows ascites & dilation of the mid small bowel ➡. The small bowel segments within the pelvis have a narrowed lumen and a thickened wall, characterized by submucosal edema ➡.*

DIFFERENTIAL DIAGNOSIS

Common

- Adhesions
- External Hernias
  - Femoral Hernia
  - Inguinal Hernia
  - Obturator Hernia
  - Ventral Hernia
- Peritoneal Metastases
- Crohn Disease
- Congenital Stenosis or Atresia
- Malrotation, Bands
- Cystic Fibrosis

Less Common

- Intestinal Metastases and Lymphoma
- Carcinoid Tumor
- Small Bowel Carcinoma
- Iatrogenic; Small Bowel Intubation
  - Iatrogenic Injury: Feeding Tubes
- Internal Hernias
  - Transmesenteric Internal Hernia
  - Paraduodenal Hernia
- Intussusception
- Intestinal Trauma
- Gallstone Ileus
- Vasculitis
- Radiation Enteritis
- Ischemic Enteritis

Rare but Important

- Intestinal Parasitic Disease
- Meckel Diverticulum

ESSENTIAL INFORMATION

Key Differential Diagnosis Issues

- **3 most common causes**
  - **Adhesions, hernias, cancer**
  - Metastasis to bowel serosa (peritoneal carcinomatosis) is more common cause of small bowel obstruction (SBO) than primary bowel neoplasm
- Obstruction vs. ileus
  - Obstruction: Abrupt transition from dilated to nondilated bowel
    - Air-fluid levels at varying heights
    - Obstructing process is usually evident on CT (except for adhesions)
  - Ileus: No or gradual transition from dilated to nondilated bowel
    - Descending colon often collapsed in ileus; do not mistake for obstruction if there is no pathologic process in proximal descending colon
    - **Ileus plus ascites is especially likely to mimic bowel obstruction**
      - Retroperitoneal colonic segments (ascending, descending colon & rectum) will be collapsed
      - Bowel segments on a mesentery (SB transverse & sigmoid colon) are dilated disproportionately

- **Important to distinguish simple from closed loop obstruction**
- Signs of closed loop SBO
  - Segmental dilation of fluid-distended small bowel (SB) out of proportion to more proximal or distal SB
  - Pinching of SB and mesentery to point or whirl
  - Balloons-on-strings appearance of affected SB
  - Mesenteric infiltration, diminished mucosal enhancement, & ascites suggest ischemia & indicate urgent need for surgery

Helpful Clues for Common Diagnoses

- **Adhesions**
  - Most common cause of SBO in adults
    - Usually result of prior abdominal surgery
  - Sharp transition, acute angulation of bowel
  - Often diagnosis of exclusion
    - No obstructing mass or other cause identified
- **External Hernias**
  - Any defect in abdominal or pelvic muscles or fascial boundary (inguinal, ventral, obturator, etc.)
    - Most can be identified & distinguished by CT criteria
  - Many patients have hernias that are not etiology of bowel obstruction
    - Key to diagnosing hernia as etiology of SB obstruction
      - Dilated bowel enters hernia; collapsed bowel leaves hernia
- **Peritoneal Metastases**
  - Peritoneal-serosal metastases are most common malignant cause of SBO
  - Primary sites in GI and GYN tracts are most common
    - Almost any malignancy may metastasize to peritoneum and serosa
- **Crohn Disease**
  - Favors terminal ileum, may have skip lesions
  - Mesenteric fatty proliferation & cluster of small nodes
- **Congenital Stenosis or Atresia**
  - Diagnosed in infancy
  - Gasless bowel distal to stenotic or atretic segment
    - Double bubble on upright film
- **Malrotation, Bands**
  - Usually diagnosed in childhood
  - Midgut volvulus may occur in adults
    - SB loops are often twisted with whirl sign in volvulus
    - Volvulus may also occur in transmesenteric internal hernia & adhesive closed loop obstruction
- **Cystic Fibrosis**
  - Children or adults may develop SBO due to thick secretions in SB
  - **Distal intestinal obstruction syndrome**
    - Stool distended distal SB
    - Almost unique to cystic fibrosis
    - Optimally managed by aggressive laxatives and enemas, avoiding surgery

Helpful Clues for Less Common Diagnoses

- **Intestinal Metastases and Lymphoma**
  - Metastasis to the bowel itself; intra- or retroperitoneal segments
  - From any primary, especially melanoma, lung, breast, lung cancer

- Lymphoma is less likely to cause SBO than carcinoma (primary or metastatic)
  - Any tumor may cause intussusception & obstruction
- **Carcinoid Tumor**
  - SBO due to tumor itself or mesenteric metastases & desmoplasia
  - Primary tumor and metastases are hypervascular
  - Ileum is most common site
- **Small Bowel Carcinoma**
  - Apple core lesion: Short, circumferential soft tissue density thickening of wall, narrowing of lumen
- **Iatrogenic; Small Bowel Intubation**
  - If balloon-tipped catheter is used for enteral feeding, it may lead to intussusception &/or obstruction
- **Internal Hernias**
  - Transmesenteric internal hernia
    - Protrusion of small bowel through congenital or acquired defect in mesentery
    - Usually follows surgery in which Roux limb has been created
      - Examples: Liver transplantation; Roux-en-Y gastric bypass
    - Cluster of dilated SB loops with distorted mesenteric vessels
      - Dilated bowel lies adjacent to abdominal wall, displacing colon medially
  - Paraduodenal hernia
    - Protrusion of SB loops through congenital or acquired defect in mesentery
      - Left side more common (75%) than right (25%)
      - Look for spherical or ovoid cluster of dilated SB between pancreatic body and posterior gastric wall
      - Mesenteric vessels are crowded and distorted
- **Intussusception**
  - Short, transient, nonobstructing, intussusception is of no clinical concern, usually idiopathic
  - Longer, obstructing intussusception in an adult is usually associated with lead mass
- **Intestinal Trauma**

- Blunt injury of bowel &/or hematoma in bowel wall may cause luminal narrowing and obstruction
- Check for evidence of anticoagulation
- Children more prone to duodenal & SB intramural hematomas than are adults
- **Gallstone Ileus**
  - Triad of intraluminal stone, SB obstruction, biliary gas
  - Almost always in elderly women
- **Vasculitis**
  - Henoch-Schönlein purpura & others
  - Cause bowel wall hemorrhage &/or edema, luminal narrowing or dilation (upstream)
  - Angioedema can produce identical findings
    - Check for C1 esterase deficiency, use of ACE inhibitors
- **Radiation Enteritis**
  - Irregular fold thickening & luminal narrowing, usually in pelvic SB loops
  - Ask about history of prior radiation for pelvic malignancy
- **Ischemic Enteritis**
  - Causes: SMA or SMV thrombosis; closed loop SBO
  - Acute: Fold thickening, submucosal edema, hemorrhage, pneumatosis
  - Chronic: Stricture with tapered margins

Helpful Clues for Rare Diagnoses

- **Intestinal Parasitic Disease**
  - Ascariasis is common cause of SB obstruction in some developing countries
  - Mass of tangled worms may obstruct SB lumen
- **Meckel Diverticulum**
  - Inverted Meckel diverticulum may cause distal SB intussusception and obstruction
  - Inflammation due to perforated Meckel diverticulum may cause SBO

Adhesions

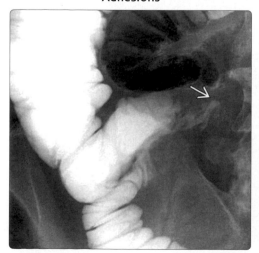

Adhesions

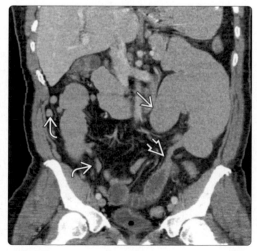

(Left) Spot film from a contrast enema shows angulation & distortion of small bowel (SB) folds directed toward the point of obstruction ➡. There is an abrupt change in caliber of the SB. Retrograde injection of barium showed prior colectomy. (Right) Coronal CECT shows dilated proximal SB loops ➡ with collapsed distal SB ➡ & colon. At the point of transition ➡ there is no mass, hernia, etc.

(Left) *In this elderly woman, CT shows fluid- distended small bowel segments* ➡ *in the pelvis. The distended bowel could be followed into a femoral hernia, while collapsed SB* ➡ *returns from this site.* (Right) *In this elderly woman with small bowel obstruction (SBO) due to a femoral hernia, note the close relationship of the hernia* ➡ *to the femoral vessels at the level of the symphysis pubis, and the compression of the femoral vein* ➡.

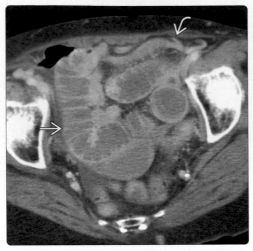
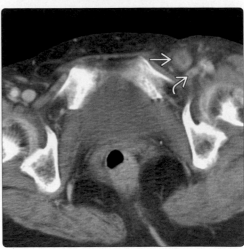

Inguinal Hernia

Ventral Hernia

(Left) *Axial CECT shows a right inguinal hernia* ➡ *containing SB with mild dilation of bowel upstream from the hernia. Note that the hernia contents extend anterior to the femoral vessels.* (Right) *Axial CECT shows a ventral hernia* ➡ *with markedly dilated bowel leading into the hernia and collapsed bowel* ➡ *leaving it. Also note ascites* ➡. *A segment of ischemic bowel was resected as the hernia was repaired.*

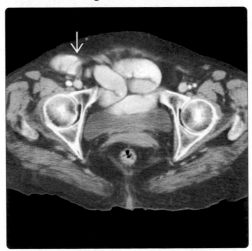
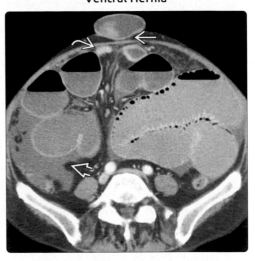

Obturator Hernia

Obturator Hernia

(Left) *In this elderly woman, axial CECT shows dilated proximal* ➡ *and collapsed distal* ➡ *SB loops, with an obturator hernia as the point of obstruction (not shown).* (Right) *In this elderly woman axial CECT shows a segment of distal SB* ➡ *herniated between the obturator externus* ➡ *and pectineus* ➡ *muscles, resulting in an SBO.*

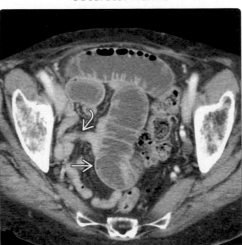
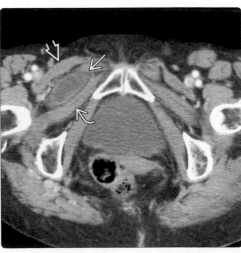

Peritoneal Metastases

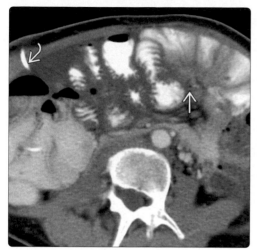

Crohn Disease

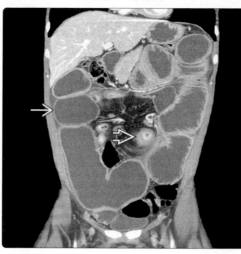

(Left) *In this woman with functional SBO due to ovarian carcinoma metastatic to the peritoneum, CT shows abnormal clustering and angulation of small bowel segments ➡ with wall thickening. A peritoneal drainage catheter ➡ was inserted to drain ascites.* (Right) *Coronal CECT shows marked dilation of SB ➡ proximal to SB loops that have active and chronic Crohn disease, marked by mucosal enhancement, wall thickening, and luminal narrowing ➡.*

Cystic Fibrosis

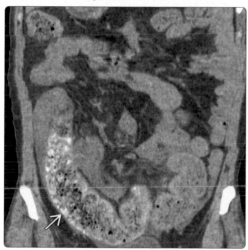

Intestinal Metastases and Lymphoma

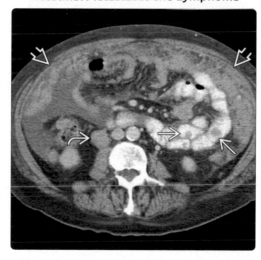

(Left) *Coronal CT shows relatively collapsed proximal SB and colon. The distal ileum is dilated and distended with feces-like inspissated material ➡. These are classic features of distal intestinal obstruction syndrome, which is almost unique to patients with cystic fibrosis.* (Right) *CT shows classic widespread metastases from melanoma, including to the SB ➡, lymph nodes ➡, and omentum with both nodular and diffuse metastases seen ➡.*

Intestinal Metastases and Lymphoma

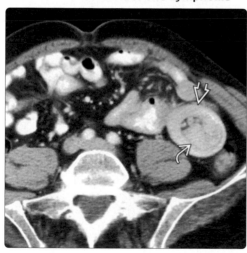

Carcinoid Tumor

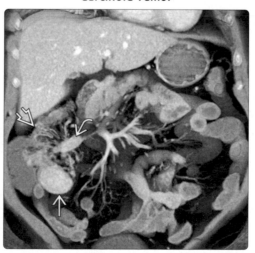

(Left) *Axial CECT shows a small bowel intussusception ➡ causing a partial SBO. The lead mass was a metastatic melanoma ➡ deposit in the bowel wall.* (Right) *CT shows mild dilation of SB upstream from a hypervascular mass ➡ in the ileum. The hypervascular metastasis ➡ & desmoplastic changes in the mesentery ➡ are characteristic of carcinoid tumor.*

(Left) *CT shows a mass in the 3rd portion of the duodenum ⇨, causing partial obstruction. Also evident is regional lymphadenopathy ⇨.* **(Right)** *Axial CECT shows the balloon of an enteric feeding tube ⇨ inflated inappropriately within the SB, causing SBO.*

Small Bowel Carcinoma

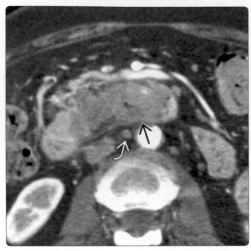

Iatrogenic; Small Bowel Intubation

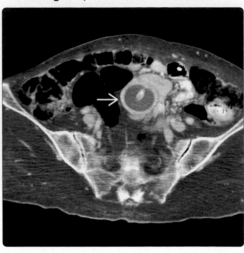

(Left) *In this patient who had a Roux-en-Y gastric bypass procedure, CT shows displacement of the jejunal anastomotic suture line ⇨ from its expected left midabdominal location. The Roux limb & proximal SB are dilated ⇨, displaced, & twisted around their mesentery ⇨ at the site of the mesenteric hernia.* **(Right)** *CT shows a cluster of SB segments that are not dilated, but appear to be confined within a sac ⇨. Note the crowding and displacement of the mesenteric vessels ⇨ in the center of this cluster.*

Transmesenteric Internal Hernia

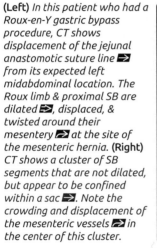
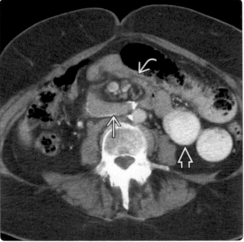

Paraduodenal Hernia

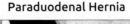

(Left) *Axial CECT shows a distal small bowel intussusception ⇨ due to an inverted or intraluminal Meckel diverticulum.* **(Right)** *CT shows a long segment intussusception ⇨ involving the terminal ileum, with functional SBO. Note the bowel-within-bowel appearance & the presence of mesenteric fat within the lumen of the intussuscipiens. The lead mass was an inverted or intraluminal Meckel diverticulum.*

Meckel Diverticulum

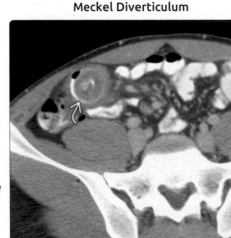

Intussusception

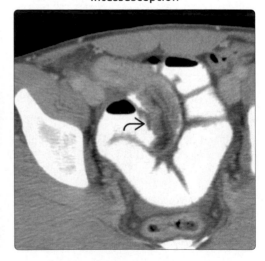
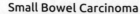

Gallstone Ileus

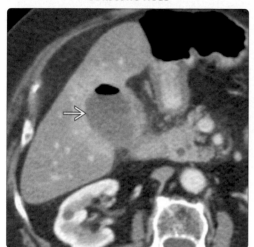

Gallstone Ileus

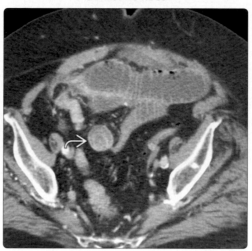

(Left) *Axial CECT shows gas within a thick-walled gallbladder ➜ and enhancement of the adjacent liver due to inflammation. SBO was also present in this elderly woman.* **(Right)** *Axial CECT shows a large laminated gallstone ➔ at the point of SBO in the distal small bowel. Gas was present in the gallbladder of this elderly woman.*

Vasculitis

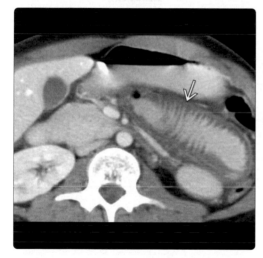

Radiation Enteritis

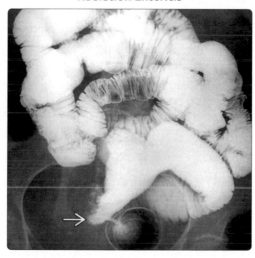

(Left) *Axial CECT shows luminal dilation and wall thickening ➜ of the jejunum, due to polyarteritis nodosa.* **(Right)** *A spot film from a small bowel follow-through shows an abrupt angulation and stricture ➜ of the distal small bowel, simulating an adhesive SBO. At surgery, a radiation-induced stricture was found, due to prior therapy for uterine carcinoma.*

Radiation Enteritis

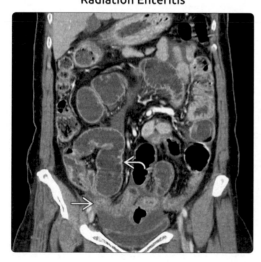

Ischemic Enteritis

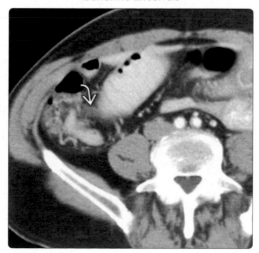

(Left) *In this woman with radiation enteritis following treatment for endometrial carcinoma, coronal CT shows dilation of the proximal and mid SB ➜. In contrast, the SB segments within the pelvis have a narrowed lumen and a thickened wall ➜, characterized by submucosal edema.* **(Right)** *Axial CECT shows a distal SB stricture ➜ with SBO, due to acute and chronic bowel ischemia, proved at surgery.*

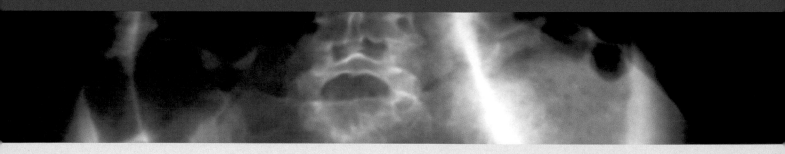

SECTION 7
Colon

Generic Imaging Patterns

Clinically Based Differentials

DIFFERENTIAL DIAGNOSIS

Common

- Colonic Polyps
- Colon or Rectal Carcinoma
- Villous Adenoma
- Feces

Less Common

- Inverted Appendical Stump
- Endometrioma
- Abdominal Abscess
- Metastases and Lymphoma, Colonic
- Tuberculoma
- Ameboma
- Intramural Hematoma
- Solitary Rectal Ulcer Syndrome
- Foreign Body
- Varix, Hemorrhoidal
- Diverticulitis
- Mesenchymal Tumor

ESSENTIAL INFORMATION

Key Differential Diagnosis Issues

- Determine if intraluminal or mucosal lesion
  - Or if intramural or extrinsic mass

Helpful Clues for Common Diagnoses

- **Colonic Polyps**
  - Adenomatous > hyperplastic > hamartomatous
  - Adenomas are more likely to present as solitary filling defect than are other types
- **Colon or Rectal Carcinoma**
  - Sessile or pedunculated polyp, or apple core lesion
- **Villous Adenoma**
  - Frond-like surface; bulky mass
    - Without causing obstruction

Helpful Clues for Less Common Diagnoses

- **Inverted Appendiceal Stump**
  - May appear as discrete polyp in cecal tip
  - Often indistinguishable from other polyps by imaging alone
- **Endometrioma**
  - Implants may cause intramural mass in sigmoid or any part of colon
  - May appear as apple core lesion, closely simulating colon cancer
    - Consider this in any woman of reproductive age
    - CT shows eccentric, extraluminal component better than barium enema
- **Abdominal Abscess**
  - Perforated appendix, diverticulitis, other
  - May cause mass effect & spasm simulating colorectal cancer
  - Diagnosis usually evident with CT and clinical correlation
- **Metastases and Lymphoma, Colonic**
  - Usually drop mets or direct invasion
  - Usually eccentric mural mass, anterior wall of rectum
- **Tuberculoma and Ameboma**
  - Either can cause apple core lesion indistinguishable from colon carcinoma
- **Intramural Hematoma**
  - From blunt or penetrating trauma
- **Foreign Body**
  - May cause intramural hematoma, perforation
  - History is key
- **Varix, Hemorrhoidal**
  - May simulate rectal carcinoma, especially if thrombosed
- **Mesenchymal Tumor**
  - Lipoma, neuroma, fibroma, hemangioma, GIST
  - Neoplasms arising from colonic wall
    - Usually benign
    - Rectal GIST is being recognized more frequently
    - Rectal hemangiomas may demonstrate phleboliths

Colonic Polyps

Colonic Polyps

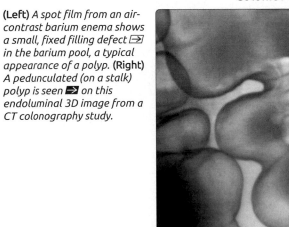

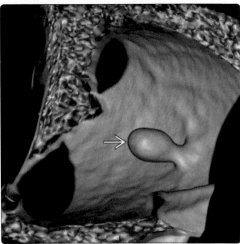

(Left) A spot film from an air-contrast barium enema shows a small, fixed filling defect ➡ in the barium pool, a typical appearance of a polyp. (Right) A pedunculated (on a stalk) polyp is seen ➡ on this endoluminal 3D image from a CT colonography study.

Colon or Rectal Carcinoma

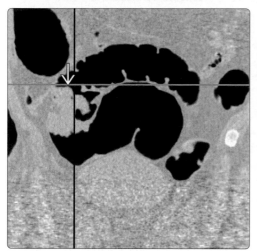

Colon or Rectal Carcinoma

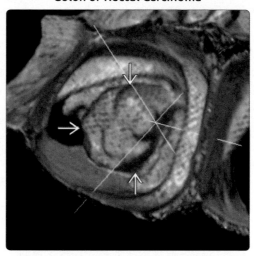

(Left) *Coronal CT colonography shows a large irregular mass* ➡ *in the sigmoid colon.* (Right) *3D endoluminal CT colonography shows a large irregular mass* ➡ *in the sigmoid colon, a typical appearance for carcinoma.*

Villous Adenoma

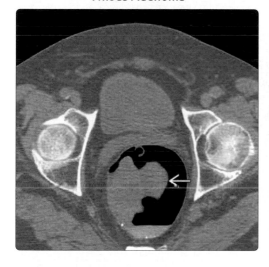

Inverted Appendical Stump

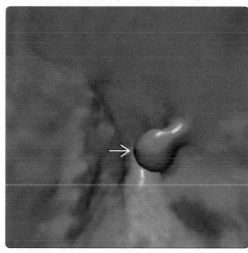

(Left) *Axial NECT shows a large mass* ➡ *arising from the right lateral wall of the rectum. There was no sign of luminal obstruction, a typical feature of these soft, villous tumors.* (Right) *This 3D surface-rendered image from CT colonography shows a small, polypoid lesion* ➡ *in the cecal tip. Other than by its typical location, this inverted appendiceal stump is indistinguishable from other benign polyps.*

Tuberculoma

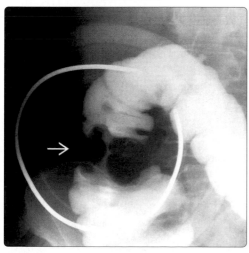

Mesenchymal Tumor

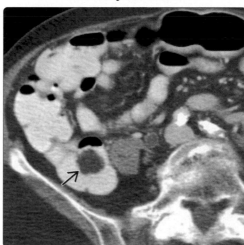

(Left) *A spot film from a barium enema shows a classic apple core constricting lesion* ➡ *in the ascending colon that is indistinguishable from that often seen with a primary colon carcinoma. At surgical resection the lesion proved to be due to tuberculous infection of the colon.* (Right) *Axial CECT shows a spherical fat density mass* ➡ *within the cecum, a typical lipoma.*

DIFFERENTIAL DIAGNOSIS

Common

- Feces
- Air Bubbles
- Colonic Polyps
- Colon Carcinoma
- Ulcerative Colitis

Less Common

- Familial Polyposis
- Gardner Syndrome
- Metastases and Lymphoma, Colonic
- Pseudomembranous Colitis, Diverticulitis
- Lymphoid Follicles (Mimic)
- Hemorrhoids
- Diverticulosis (Mimic)
- Mesenchymal Tumor, Colon
- Pneumatosis (Mimic)
- Endometriosis
- Colonic Varices
- Urticaria, Colon
- Colonic Parasites

ESSENTIAL INFORMATION

Key Differential Diagnosis Issues

- Check if defects are movable (gas or feces)

Helpful Clues for Common Diagnoses

- **Feces**
  - Usually more irregular in shape and size
  - Usually well-coated by barium
- **Air Bubbles**
  - On barium enema
    - Usually not problem on CT colonography
  - Key is change in shape, size, location with positioning
- **Colonic Polyps**
  - Small polyps of uniform size in younger patients are often hyperplastic

- Usually small (< 5 mm), often multiple
- Can be safely disregarded
  - May be sessile or on a stalk (pedunculated)
    - Polyps > 1 cm are often neoplastic (benign or malignant) adenomas
      - Should be resected
- **Colon Carcinoma**
  - Rarely multifocal, but commonly found with other polyps
- **Ulcerative Colitis**
  - Along with granulomatous colitis (Crohn) may result in inflammatory polyps
  - May grow into filiform, pedunculated appearance
  - Associated with increased risk of colon cancer

Helpful Clues for Less Common Diagnoses

- **Familial Polyposis and Gardner Syndrome**
  - Often innumerable adenomatous polyps, may carpet colon
  - Other syndromes may result in multiple adenomatous hamartomatous or hyperplastic polyps
- **Pseudomembranous Colitis**, **Diverticulitis**
  - Any infectious or inflammatory colitis may result in thickened folds that might be mistaken for polypoid lesions
- **Lymphoid Follicles (Mimic)**
  - Small (2-4 mm), submucosal, numerous; more in right colon
- **Diverticulosis (Mimic)**
  - On air-contrast enema, barium-lined diverticulum may simulate barium-coated polyp

---

Feces

Colonic Polyps

(Left) Contrast enema shows innumerable filling defects of varying size in the ascending colon, which is the typical appearance of stool in an unprepped colon. (Right) Contrast enema shows a pedunculated polyp ⊡ on a long stalk ⊡. Also note diverticula ⊿, some filled with barium & some with air that might be mistaken for polyps.

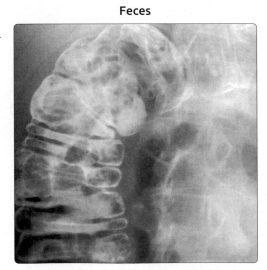

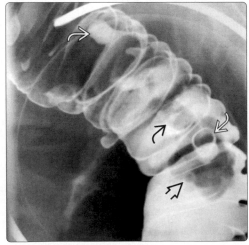

Colonic Polyps

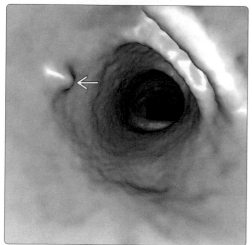

Colonic Polyps

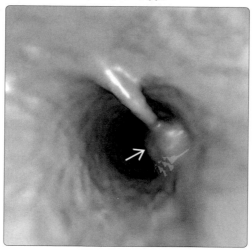

(Left) *Endoscopic image from a CT colonography (CTC) study in a 74-year-old man shows a small, probably hyperplastic, polyp ➡, of no clinical concern.* (Right) *In this 74-year-old man, CTC shows a pedunculated polyp ➡ that was removed at colonoscopy and proved to be benign.*

Colon Carcinoma

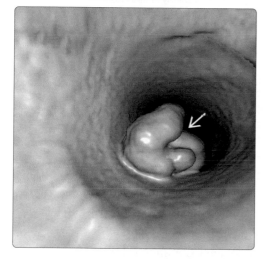

Ulcerative Colitis

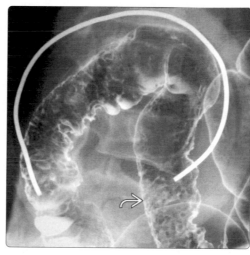

(Left) *CTC in this 74-year-old man shows a large, sessile, polypoid mass ➡. This was removed at left hemicolectomy and proved to be primary colon carcinoma.* (Right) *Spot film from a contrast enema shows multiple filiform polyps ➡ within the colon, in a patient with chronic but quiescent ulcerative colitis.*

Familial Polyposis

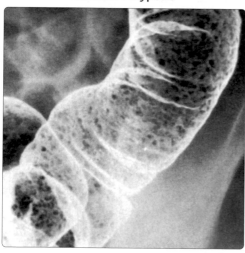

Pneumatosis (Mimic)

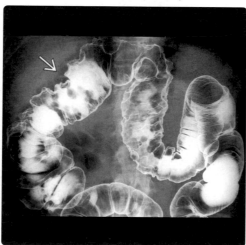

(Left) *Spot film from a contrast enema shows thousands of small polyps that carpet the surface of the colon.* (Right) *Contrast enema shows what appear to be numerous polyps throughout the colon. These are due to intramural blebs of gas ➡ from idiopathic pneumatosis in this asymptomatic patient.*

DIFFERENTIAL DIAGNOSIS

Common

- Crohn Disease
- Appendicitis
- Prominent Ileocecal Valve
  - Lipomatous Infiltration of IC Valve
  - Lipoma of IC Valve
- Colon Carcinoma
- Mesenteric Adenitis
- Infectious Ileocolitis

Less Common

- Carcinoid Tumor
- Cecal Diverticulitis
- Metastases and Lymphoma, Intestinal
- Appendiceal Carcinoma
- Intussusception
- Mucocele of Appendix
- Typhlitis (Neutropenic Colitis)
- Tuberculosis, Colon
- Cecal Volvulus
- Endometriosis
- Ischemic Colitis

ESSENTIAL INFORMATION

Key Differential Diagnosis Issues

- CT: Optimal for evaluation of intra- and extramural disease in RLQ
  - Try to characterize distribution of disease, nature of wall thickening, and associated findings
  - Fat density mural thickening
    - Normal variant or quiescent inflammatory bowel disease
  - Water density
    - Acute inflammation or ischemia
  - Soft tissue density: Least specific
    - Infection
    - Ischemia
    - Inflammation
    - Tumor
- Barium studies: Optimal for mucosal detail
  - e.g., early inflammatory changes of Crohn disease

Helpful Clues for Common Diagnoses

- **Crohn Disease**
  - Most common inflammatory process of terminal ileum and cecum
  - Homogeneous attenuation of thickened bowel wall on CECT
  - Mural stratification lost: Indistinct mucosa, submucosa, muscularis propria
  - Mesenteric fibrofatty proliferation
  - Enlarged mesenteric lymph nodes
  - Mucosal and mesenteric hyperemia
    - Comb or caterpillar sign of engorged mesenteric vessels = active inflammation
- **Appendicitis**
  - Medial wall of cecum and terminal ileum may be thickened by inflammation starting in appendix

- Appendiceal wall is thickened and lumen usually distended
- Often have cluster of mildly enlarged nodes, especially with subacute inflammation
- May have associated abscess following perforation of appendix
- **Prominent Ileocecal Valve**
  - Often normal variant
  - Submucosal fat is usually evident on CT within lips of valve
  - Lipoma is benign neoplasm common in this area
    - Spherical mass of fat
    - Usually seen as eccentric mass near ileocecal valve
- **Colon Carcinoma**
  - Cecum accounts for 25% of colon adenocarcinomas
  - Usually bulky mass without obstruction
    - Surface irregularity identifies mucosal origin
  - May occlude base of appendix
    - May simulate appendicitis clinically and on imaging (dilated lumen of appendix)
  - Adjacent lymphadenopathy is common
    - Also look for peritoneal and hepatic metastases
- **Mesenteric Adenitis**
  - Idiopathic, self-limited inflammation, cluster of enlarged nodes in RLQ
  - Common in children and adolescents
- **Infectious Ileocolitis**
  - Causes acute diarrhea
  - Common causative agents
    - *Yersinia*
    - *Campylobacter*
    - *Salmonella*
  - Mural thickening of cecum and terminal ileum
  - RLQ adenopathy
  - Imaging findings indistinguishable from mesenteric adenitis (may be same disease)

Helpful Clues for Less Common Diagnoses

- **Carcinoid Tumor**
  - Thickening of distal ileal wall and mesenteric mass
    - Mesenteric mass often has focus of calcification
    - Desmoplastic response in mesentery
      - □ Small bowel loops and mesenteric vessels may have stellate configuration and distorted course
    - Primary mass and metastases are hypervascular
- **Cecal Diverticulitis**
  - Can usually identify other diverticula and normal appendix
  - Cecal wall thickened with adjacent inflammatory changes
  - No mucosal hyperemia or submucosal edema
    - Distinguishes this from colitis
- **Metastases and Lymphoma, Intestinal**
  - Lymphoma may cause dramatic bowel wall thickening
    - Often circumferential, multifocal
    - Rarely obstructs bowel lumen or vessels (unlike carcinoma)
  - May have significant adenopathy or involvement of other organs
- **Intussusception**

- Due to tumor or inflammation of ileum or ileocecal valve
- May identify mass within lumen
- Intraluminal crescent of intussuscepted ileal mesenteric fat
- Ileocecal intussusceptions in adults are usually obstructive and due to lead mass (neoplastic, benign or malignant)

- **Mucocele of Appendix**
  - Round or oval, thin-walled, cystic mass near tip of cecum
  - May have curvilinear calcifications in wall
- **Typhlitis (Neutropenic Colitis)**
  - Massive mural thickening of cecal ± ascending colon wall
  - Presents as fever, RLQ tenderness in immunosuppressed patient
- **Tuberculosis, Colon**
  - GI infection generally follows pulmonary infection
    - Obtain chest x-ray in suspected cases
  - Symptoms more chronic than in other causes of infectious colitis
  - Involvement varies from mild thickening to apple core lesion

- Mesenteric adenopathy common

SELECTED REFERENCES

1. Iafrate F et al: Spectrum of normal findings, anatomic variants and pathology of ileocecal valve: CT colonography appearances and endoscopic correlation. Abdom Imaging. 32(5):589-95, 2007
2. Silva AC et al: Spectrum of normal and abnormal CT appearances of the ileocecal valve and cecum with endoscopic and surgical correlation. Radiographics. 27(4):1039-54, 2007
3. Singh A et al: MR imaging of the acute abdomen and pelvis: acute appendicitis and beyond. Radiographics. 27(5):1419-31, 2007
4. Hoeffel C et al: Multi-detector row CT: spectrum of diseases involving the ileocecal area. Radiographics. 26(5):1373-90, 2006
5. Harris A et al: Appendicitis imaging. Radiol Technol. 77(2):111-7; quiz 118-20, 2005
6. Pinto Leite N et al: CT evaluation of appendicitis and its complications: imaging techniques and key diagnostic findings. AJR Am J Roentgenol. 185(2):406-17, 2005

Crohn Disease

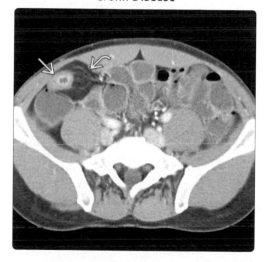

Crohn Disease

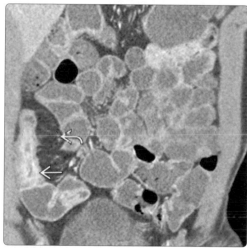

(Left) *In this young man with acute & chronic Crohn disease, CT shows good distention of the small bowel and colon with near water density contrast medium. Terminal ileum ➡ has mucosal hyperenhancement and wall thickening, with adjacent fibrofatty proliferation and mesenteric hyperemia ➡.* (Right) *CT shows mucosal hyperenhancement, wall thickening, and luminal narrowing of terminal ileum ➡. Note mesenteric fatty proliferation and hyperemia ➡.*

Crohn Disease

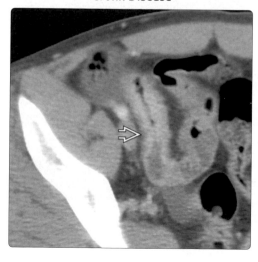

Crohn Disease

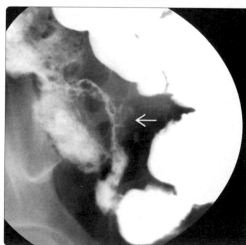

(Left) *Axial CECT shows classic findings in a 19-year-old man with a long segment of terminal ileum wall thickening, luminal narrowing, and mucosal inflammation ➡.* (Right) *Small bowel follow-through shows classic findings in a 19-year-old man with luminal narrowing and wall thickening of the terminal ileum and cecum, cobblestone mucosal ulcerations, and sinus tracks ➡ into the thickened mesenteric fat.*

(Left) *This 34-year-old woman has acute RLQ pain. Coronal CT shows generalized infiltration of the fat planes around the cecal tip and terminal ileum. An appendicolith ➡ is noted within the base of a thickened appendix.* **(Right)** *In this 34-year-old woman with acute appendicitis, the dilated appendix is seen ➡ along with regional adenopathy ⇨.*

Appendicitis

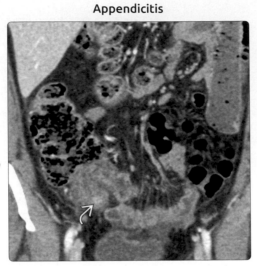

Appendicitis

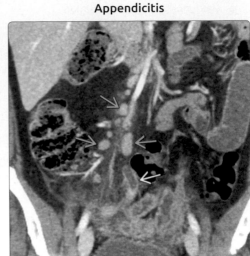

(Left) *Axial CECT shows a dilated lumen and thickened wall of the retrocecal appendix ➡, with infiltration of its mesenteric fat.* **(Right)** *Coronal CECT shows the thick-walled retrocecal appendix ➡ ascending medial to the colon.*

Appendicitis

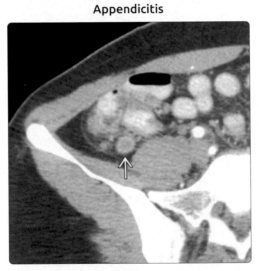

Appendicitis

(Left) *Axial CECT shows an abscess ➡ medial to a thick-walled cecum ➡, both the result of appendiceal perforation.* **(Right)** *Axial CECT shows lipomatous infiltration of both lips of the ileocecal valve ➡, as the terminal ileum ➡ enters the colon.*

Appendicitis

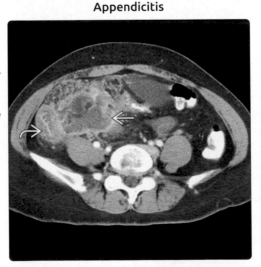

Lipomatous Infiltration of IC Valve

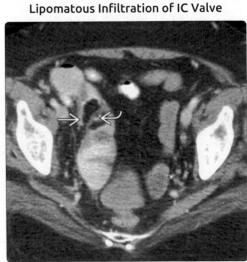

Lipoma of IC Valve

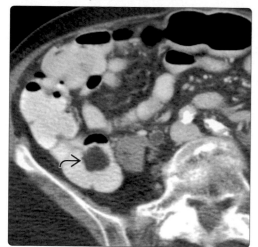

Lipoma of IC Valve

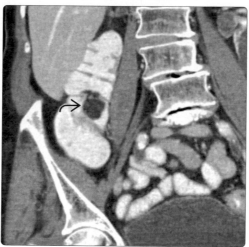

(Left) *Axial CECT shows a spherical fat density mass* → *in the ascending colon in this patient with lipoma.* (Right) *Coronal CECT shows a spherical fat density mass* → *in the ascending colon in this patient with lipoma.*

Colon Carcinoma

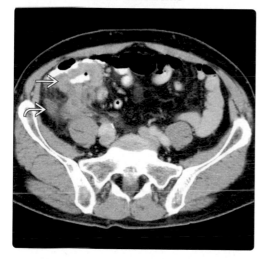

Colon Carcinoma

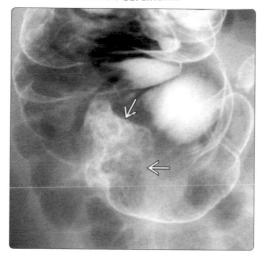

(Left) *Axial CECT shows circumferential thickening of the wall of the cecum* →. *A dilated appendix was seen, along with local lymphadenopathy* → *and omental metastases. This patient presented with signs and symptoms of appendicis.* (Right) *A spot film from a contrast enema shows a polypoid mass* → *in the cecum that has an irregular surface, characteristic of carcinoma.*

Mesenteric Adenitis

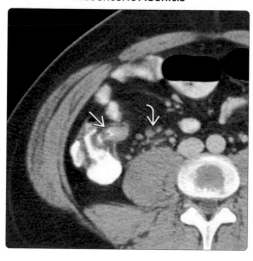

Carcinoid Tumor

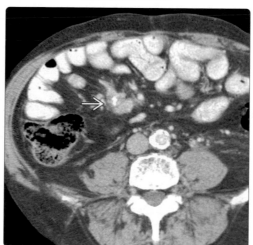

(Left) *Axial CECT shows mild thickening of the wall of the terminal ileum* → *and a cluster of slightly enlarged nodes* →. *The appendix was normal.* (Right) *Axial CECT shows a partially calcified mesenteric mass* → *and a tethered appearance of distal small bowel segments, with mesenteric stranding pointing toward the metastasis.*

Cecal Diverticulitis

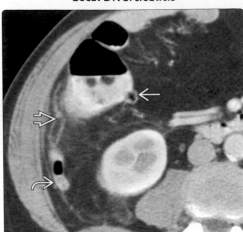

Cecal Diverticulitis

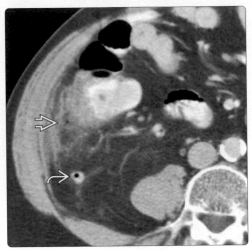

(Left) *Axial CECT shows a normal appendix* ➡ *and a cecal diverticulum* ➡*, with pericolonic inflammatory changes* ➡*. (Right) Axial CECT shows a normal appendix* ➡ *and extensive pericecal inflammatory infiltrates* ➡*. Unlike colitis, most of the inflammation is outside the colonic lumen.*

Metastases and Lymphoma, Intestinal

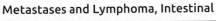
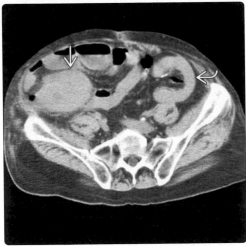

Intussusception

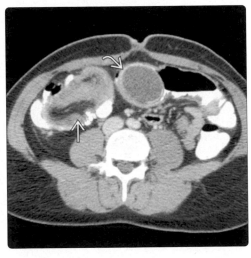

(Left) *Axial NECT shows a soft tissue mass* ➡ *in the ileocecal region in this renal transplant* ➡ *recipient with lymphoma (PTLD) of the appendix.* (Right) *Axial CECT shows an ileocolic intussusception* ➡ *and the lead mass, an appendiceal mucocele* ➡ *(in the transverse colon).*

Intussusception

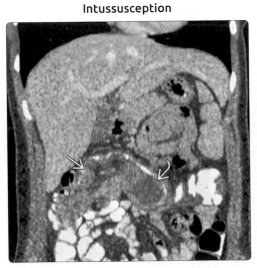

Intussusception

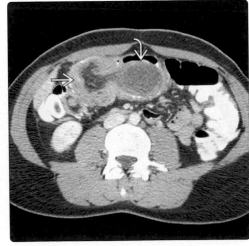

(Left) *Coronal CECT shows an ileocolic intussusception* ➡ *with a mucocele* ➡ *as the lead mass.* (Right) *Axial CECT shows an ileocolic intussusception* ➡ *with the lead mass in the transverse colon, a mucocele* ➡*.*

Mucocele of Appendix

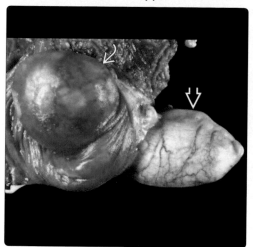

Mucocele of Appendix

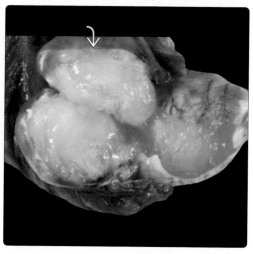

(Left) Gross pathology shows an intussuscepting mass (a mucocele) ➡ within the colon, causing obstruction of the small intestine ➡. (Right) Gross pathology shows a bivalved mucin-filled mucocele ➡ that was the lead mass causing intussusception.

Typhlitis (Neutropenic Colitis)

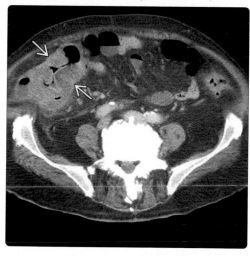

Ischemic Colitis

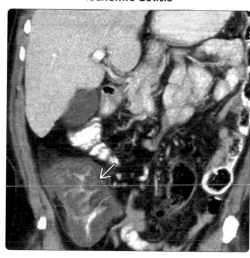

(Left) In this elderly man with leukemia, axial CT shows mesenteric and massive submucosal edema ➡ limited to the wall of the ascending colon and cecum. (Right) Coronal CECT shows marked mural thickening ("thumbprinting") ➡ of the cecum and ascending colon. Note the compressed lumen, submucosal edema, and intense mucosal enhancement. These findings indicate ischemia or inflammation.

Tuberculosis, Colon

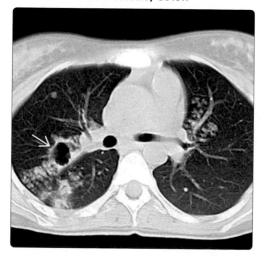

Tuberculosis, Colon

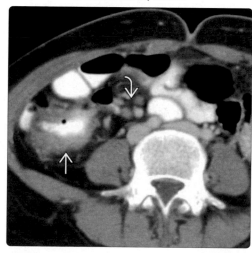

(Left) Axial CECT shows active cavitary pulmonary tuberculosis ➡ in a young woman with ileocecal TB. (Right) Axial CECT shows a thick-walled cecum and terminal ileum ➡ with mesenteric lymphadenopathy ➡ in this young female immigrant from India with tuberculosis (enteric and pulmonary).

DIFFERENTIAL DIAGNOSIS

Common

- Ileus
  - Ogilvie Syndrome
- Colorectal Carcinoma
- Sigmoid Volvulus
- Cecal Volvulus
- Diverticulitis
- Fecal Impaction, Stercoral Colitis

Less Common

- Ischemic Colitis
- Toxic Megacolon
- Endocrine Disorders
- Neuromuscular Disorders

ESSENTIAL INFORMATION

Key Differential Diagnosis Issues

- Do not assume colonic dilation is ileus, without considering rectal or distal colonic obstruction
- Use prone or decubitus film to visualize gas through rectum

Helpful Clues for Common Diagnoses

- **Ileus**
  - Most common cause of colonic distention
  - Usually accompanied by small bowel dilation
  - Many potential causes, including postoperative state, electrolyte or endocrine imbalance, and medications
  - Ogilvie syndrome
    - Disproportionate dilation of cecum and ascending colon
    - Typically occurs acutely in postoperative period
- **Colorectal Carcinoma**
  - Most common cause of colonic obstruction in adults
  - Soft tissue density mass; short segment obstruction
    - Obstruction more common in distal colon
- **Sigmoid Volvulus**
  - Very elongated, dilated sigmoid, folded back on itself

- Coffee bean, football shape
  - Entire colon is dilated, but less than sigmoid
- **Cecal Volvulus**
  - Ascending colon twists on mesentery; becomes obstructed, dilated, displaced toward left upper quadrant
  - Distal colon is not dilated
- **Diverticulitis**
  - Inflammation narrows lumen
  - Long segment involvement with pericolonic infiltration
- **Fecal Impaction, Stercoral Colitis**
  - Common in elderly
  - Look for stercoral colitis
    - Large impacted mass of stool in rectosigmoid colon
    - Can lead to mucosal ulceration and wall perforation
    - Gas or discontinuity in colorectal wall, perirectal infiltration

Helpful Clues for Less Common Diagnoses

- **Ischemic Colitis**
  - May result in stricture (chronically) or spasm (acutely)
    - Colon dilated up to ischemic segment
  - Most common form is hypoperfusion affecting left side of colon ("watershed areas")
- **Toxic Megacolon**
  - Mucosal ulceration, often transmural necrosis
  - Loss of haustral pattern, sloughed mucosa, perforation
  - Infectious colitis probably has surpassed ulcerative colitis as leading cause
    - Specific organisms include *Clostridium difficile*, *Escherichia coli*, *Campylobacter*, amebic, and typhoid
  - Requires urgent discussion with referring physician
    - Patients with toxic megacolon are extremely ill and often require urgent colectomy
- **Endocrine Disorders**
  - Hypothyroidism, diabetes, other endocrine and metabolic disorders
  - May cause ileus or colonic inertia
- **Neuromuscular Disorders**
  - Spinal cord injury, multiple sclerosis, Parkinson, etc.

Ileus

Ogilvie Syndrome

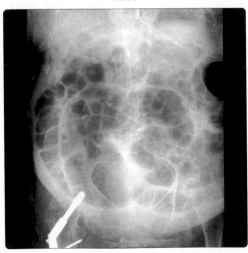 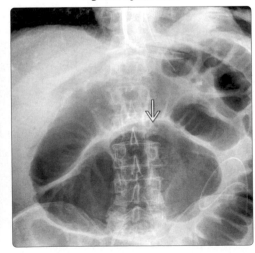

(Left) *Supine radiograph shows diffuse dilation of large and small bowel without transition in an elderly woman recently postoperative for hip fracture stabilization.* (Right) *A supine abdominal film taken 1 day after surgery shows a medially displaced, dilated cecum and ascending colon* ➡️*, with generalized distention of the colon. The cecum measures 15 cm in diameter and is folded upon itself, without apparent volvulus.*

Colorectal Carcinoma

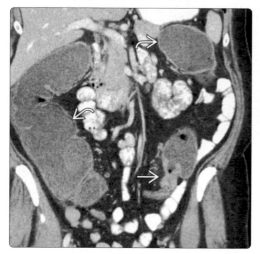

Colorectal Carcinoma

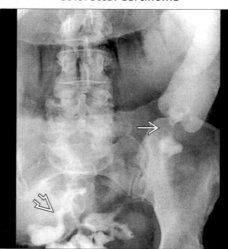

(Left) *In this man with abdominal distention and hematochezia, coronal CECT shows a classic apple core lesion* ➡ *causing obstruction of the descending colon and distention of the more proximal colon* ➡. **(Right)** *In this man with abdominal distention and hematochezia, a spot film from a contrast enema shows a classic apple core lesion* ➡ *of the descending colon, causing high-grade obstruction. The sigmoid colon* ➡ *and small bowel are collapsed.*

Sigmoid Volvulus

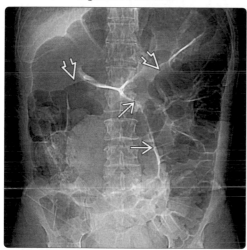

Sigmoid Volvulus

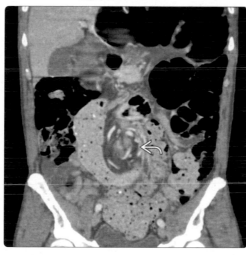

(Left) *In this 59-year-old man, a supine film shows marked dilation of the colon, especially the sigmoid colon. The sigmoid is folded back upon itself, and the apposed walls of the sigmoid colon* ➡ *form the "seam" of the football shape. The sigmoid extends into the upper abdomen above the transverse colon* ➡, *another useful sign in identifying colonic segments.* **(Right)** *In this 59-year-old man, coronal CT shows twisting and engorgement of the sigmoid mesocolon and its vessels* ➡.

Sigmoid Volvulus

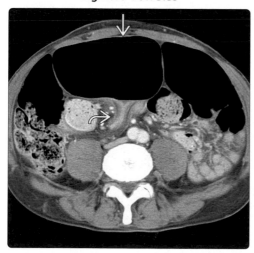

Sigmoid Volvulus

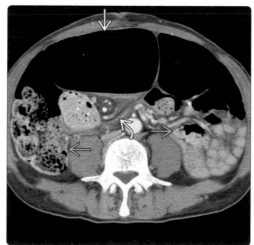

(Left) *In this 59-year-old man, axial CT confirms the massively dilated and redundant sigmoid* ➡, *along with twisting and displacement of the inferior mesenteric vessels supplying this segment of bowel* ➡. **(Right)** *Axial CT shows the massively dilated sigmoid colon* ➡, *which is pinched and twisted at the base of its mesocolon* ➡. *The colon upstream from the volvulus is moderately distended* ➡.

Cecal Volvulus

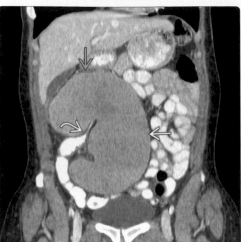

(Left) *In this woman, a coronal CT shows a markedly distended cecum ➡ and contrast-filled terminal ileum entering the ileocecal valve ➡. The base of the cecum ➡ is directed upward.* **(Right)** *In this woman, coronal CT shows that the ileocolic mesentery is twisted (whorled) within the right lower quadrant ➡, confirming the diagnosis of cecal volvulus.*

Cecal Volvulus

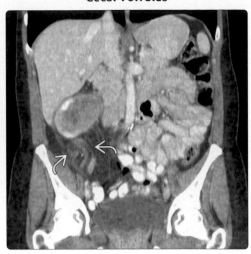

Diverticulitis

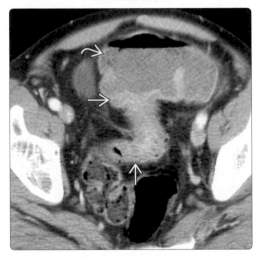

(Left) *CT shows marked dilation of the colon ➡ with abrupt transition to a short segment of luminal narrowing and wall thickening in the sigmoid colon ➡. Neither diverticula nor pericolonic inflammatory changes are evident, but diverticulitis was confirmed as the cause of the obstructing mass.* **(Right)** *This elderly woman had chronic constipation with acute, severe abdominal pain. A supine film shows colonic distention and fecal impaction in the rectum ➡.*

Fecal Impaction, Stercoral Colitis

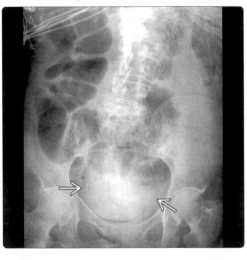

Fecal Impaction, Stercoral Colitis

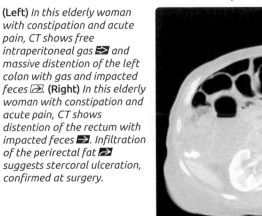

(Left) *In this elderly woman with constipation and acute pain, CT shows free intraperitoneal gas ➡ and massive distention of the left colon with gas and impacted feces ➡.* **(Right)** *In this elderly woman with constipation and acute pain, CT shows distention of the rectum with impacted feces ➡. Infiltration of the perirectal fat ➡ suggests stercoral ulceration, confirmed at surgery.*

Fecal Impaction, Stercoral Colitis

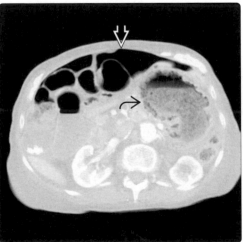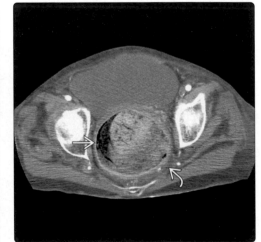

Ischemic Colitis

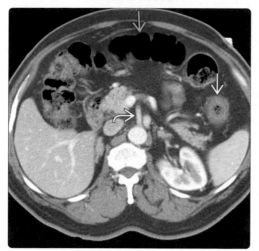

Ischemic Colitis

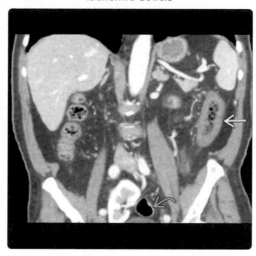

(Left) *This elderly man developed acute abdominal pain and distention after recent hip replacement surgery. Axial CT shows distended colon ⇥ that narrowed abruptly at splenic flexure. Descending colon ⇥ is thick-walled with submucosal edema. Mesenteric vessels ⇥ are patent.* (Right) *In this man with abdominal pain following hip replacement, coronal CT shows wall thickening and luminal narrowing of descending colon ⇥ with sparing of rectum ⇥, typical features of ischemic colitis.*

Toxic Megacolon

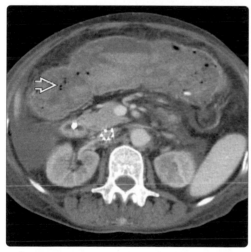

Toxic Megacolon

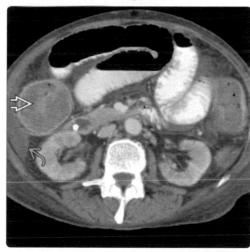

(Left) *In this woman with acute abdominal pain and bloody diarrhea due to Clostridium difficile colitis, CT shows massive dilation of the colon with loss of haustration and intraluminal high-density material representing hemorrhage and sloughed mucosa ⇥.* (Right) *In this woman with toxic megacolon due to C. difficile colitis, CT shows generalized ileus with intracolonic hemorrhage ⇥ and ascites ⇥. Urgent colectomy was required.*

Toxic Megacolon

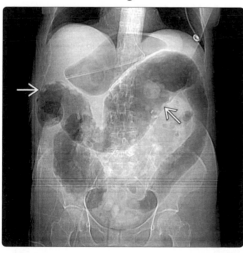

Toxic Megacolon

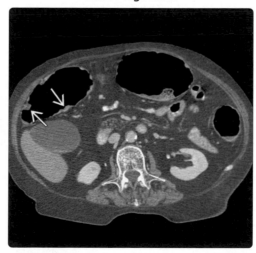

(Left) *In this woman with chronic Crohn colitis, a supine film shows marked dilation of the transverse colon, with a featureless, ahaustral appearance. There is some irregularity of the luminal surface ⇥, suggesting mucosal sloughing or pseudopolyps.* (Right) *In this woman with Crohn colitis not responsive to medical therapy, CT shows the colonic dilation and ahaustral appearance with marked thinning of the wall, which suggests the risk of perforation. Note the tags of inflamed mucosa or pseudopolyps ⇥.*

DIFFERENTIAL DIAGNOSIS

Common

- Ulcerative Colitis
- Infectious Colitis
- Crohn Disease
- Colonic Ileus

Less Common

- Ischemic Colitis

ESSENTIAL INFORMATION

Key Differential Diagnosis Issues

- Any etiology of severe colitis may result in toxic megacolon
  - Infectious colitis is likely more common cause than ulcerative colitis
- Diagnosis of toxic megacolon is based on imaging & clinical features
- **CT is best imaging tool (contrast enema is contraindicated)**
  - Dilated colonic lumen (> 6 cm) is always present
  - Degree of colonic distention is not critical factor in diagnosis
  - Loss of normal colonic folds & mucosal pattern is characteristic
  - Colonic wall may be thickened or abnormally thin
  - May show hemorrhage within colonic lumen; no formed stool
  - Presence of ascites &/or pneumoperitoneum are critical prognostic signs
  - Urgent colectomy is usually mandatory
- Clinical findings
  - Patient appears toxic
    - Fever, tachycardia, hyperpnea, hypotensive
  - Patients with ulcerative colitis usually have known diagnosis
    - May have become refractory to medical therapy
  - Patients with infectious or ischemic colitis may develop toxic megacolon without preceding history of bowel disease

Helpful Clues for Common Diagnoses

- **Ulcerative or Crohn Colitis**
  - May see shortened lead pipe colon
  - Colonic wall is usually not markedly thickened; may be paper thin
  - Crohn (granulomatous) colitis usually occurs with long-standing Crohn involvement of small bowel as well
- **Infectious Colitis**
  - *Clostridium difficile* (pseudomembranous) or others
    - Colonic wall is usually markedly thickened with submucosal edema
    - Mucosal hyperenhancement may evolve to lack of enhancement & mucosal sloughing
  - *Escherichia coli*, *Campylobacter*, typhoid, & amebic colitis are among other reported causes of infectious colitis with toxic megacolon
- **Colonic Ileus (Mimic)**
  - Colonic ileus may occur ± SB involvement
  - Causes include
    - Postoperative
    - Electrolyte disturbances
    - Medications
  - Normal fold & mucosal pattern are preserved
    - Distinguishes ileus from toxic megacolon
  - Acute & severe dilation (> 12 cm on radiography; 10 cm on CT) increases risk of ischemic & perforation
    - Colonic obstruction is not necessary

Helpful Clues for Less Common Diagnoses

- **Ischemic Colitis**
  - Uncommon to rare etiology of toxic megacolon
  - Most common form of ischemic colitis is hypoperfusion
    - Typically results in colonic wall thickening in splenic flexure or sigmoid distribution
      - Watershed zones of overlapping SMA-IMA arterial supply
  - Thromboembolic arterial occlusion more often in SMA distribution
    - More likely to result in colonic infarction, but uncommonly preceded by toxic megacolon

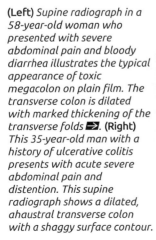

(Left) *Supine radiograph in a 58-year-old woman who presented with severe abdominal pain and bloody diarrhea illustrates the typical appearance of toxic megacolon on plain film. The transverse colon is dilated with marked thickening of the transverse folds ➔. (Right) This 35-year-old man with a history of ulcerative colitis presents with acute severe abdominal pain and distention. This supine radiograph shows a dilated, ahaustral transverse colon with a shaggy surface contour.*

Ulcerative Colitis

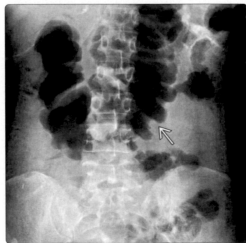

Ulcerative Colitis

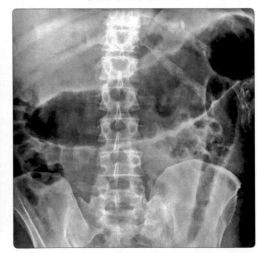

Infectious Colitis

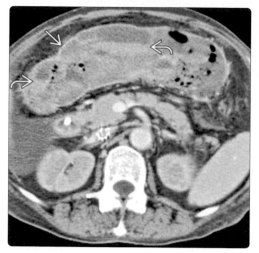

Infectious Colitis

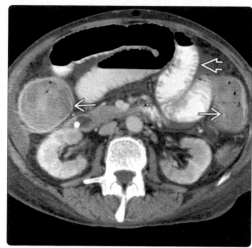

(Left) *In this patient with C. difficile colitis, CT shows a dilated transverse colon* ➡ *with pneumatosis, intraluminal bleeding* ➡*, and sloughed mucosa. The colonic wall is thin; ascites is present.* (Right) *In this patient with C. difficile colitis, axial CECT shows a generalized ileus* ➡*. The colon* ➡ *is massively distended with blood and debris, and its wall is relatively thin. Soon after this scan, the colon perforated and a total colectomy was required.*

Crohn Disease

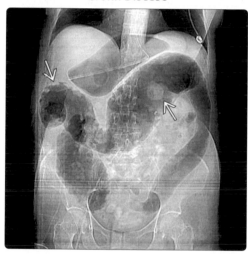

Crohn Disease

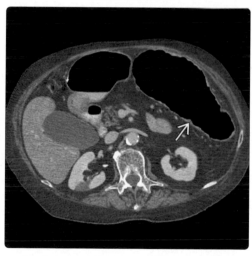

(Left) *In this woman with chronic Crohn (granulomatous) colitis, a supine film shows marked dilation of the transverse colon with a featureless ahaustral appearance. There is some irregularity of the luminal surface* ➡*, suggesting mucosal sloughing or pseudopolyps.* (Right) *In this woman with Crohn colitis, CT shows the colonic dilation and ahaustral appearance with marked thinning of the wall, which suggests the risk of perforation. Note the tags of inflamed mucosa or pseudopolyps* ➡*.*

Crohn Disease

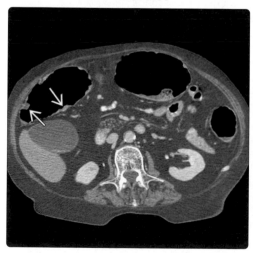

Crohn Disease

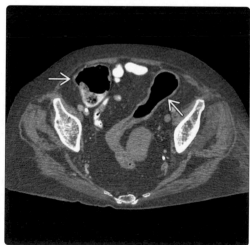

(Left) *In this woman with chronic Crohn colitis CT shows severe dilation of the colon with a thin wall and inflammatory pseudopolyps* ➡*.* (Right) *In this woman with toxic megacolon from Crohn colitis, CT shows the ahaustral, thin-walled segments* ➡ *of nearly the entire colon.*

DIFFERENTIAL DIAGNOSIS

Common

- Diverticulitis
- Crohn Disease
- Postoperative State, Bowel
- Pelvic Malignancy
  - Colon Carcinoma
  - Cervical and Uterine Carcinoma
  - Endometrial Carcinoma
  - Ovarian Cancer
  - Bladder Carcinoma
  - Prostate Carcinoma
- Bladder Instrumentation (Mimic)

Less Common

- Cystitis (Mimic)
  - Emphysematous Cystitis
- Abdominal or Pelvic Abscess
- Infectious Colitis
- Trauma, Colorectal or Vaginal
- Foreign Body

ESSENTIAL INFORMATION

Key Differential Diagnosis Issues

- Gas in urinary bladder may be due to
  - Colovesical or enterovesical fistula
  - Gas-forming infection within bladder or its wall (emphysematous cystitis)
  - Instrumentation that introduces gas into bladder (e.g., catheterization)
  - Check for extensive coliform bacterial infection of urine, pneumaturia
- Surgical resection of any pelvic mass predisposes to fistulas
  - Especially if followed or preceded by radiation therapy
  - Even resection of benign process (e.g., uterine fibroids, endometrioma)
  - Fistulas may develop years later, often due to diverticulitis
- All low rectal anastomoses are prone to leak
  - Resulting perianastomotic abscess can fistulize into any pelvic space, organ, or skin
  - Perianastomotic collection of gas and fluid is presumptive evidence of anastomotic leak
  - Rectal administration of contrast material at fluoroscopy or CT should be considered to document or exclude fistula
    - Generally much more successful than oral administration of contrast
    - Alternatives
      - Contrast injection into cutaneous fistula opening
      - Contrast injection into bladder (cystogram) with fluoroscopic or CT evaluation
- Abdominal or pelvic abscesses of any etiology may erode into gut, bladder, vagina, or skin

Helpful Clues for Common Diagnoses

- **Diverticulitis**
  - Most common etiology for colonic fistulas in industrialized nations
  - Infection can spread to any pelvic structure
    - Examples
      - Fistula to skin
      - Bladder
      - Vagina
      - Hip joint
  - Diverticulitis may cause infection of pelvic scar (e.g., from hysterectomy) leading to colovaginal fistula
- **Crohn Disease**
  - Most common cause of enteric (small bowel) fistulas
    - Can also cause colonic fistulas in setting of Crohn (granulomatous) colitis
  - Often causes perianal fistulas to skin
- **Postoperative State, Bowel**
  - Any pelvic surgery or resection (e.g., rectal, hysterectomy, cesarean section)
    - Examples
      - Rectal
      - Hysterectomy
      - Cesarean section
    - Low anterior resection or sigmoid resection for rectosigmoid carcinoma
    - Creation of ileal pouch with ileoanal anastomosis following colectomy
  - Infection of scar by diverticulitis may cause fistula
  - Leak at rectal or colonic anastomosis may lead to abscess and then fistula
    - This is quite common in patients who have anastomotic leaks from low rectal anastomoses
- **Colon Carcinoma**
  - Usually from sigmoid or rectum
  - Fistula may be spontaneous or follow surgery, radiation, or chemotherapy
  - Especially likely in elderly, diabetic, and debilitated patients
- **Cervical and Uterine Carcinoma**
  - Advanced stage may invade bladder, rectum, or colon
  - Fistula usually follows surgery or therapy
  - Tumor may "bridge" or connect 2 pelvic viscera
    - Subsequent necrosis of tumor may open the connection
  - Benign scar results from resection of cervical/uterine carcinoma
    - Scar may become infected (e.g., from diverticulitis)
    - May result in a colovaginal fistula
- **Bladder Carcinoma**
  - Fistula from local invasion by tumor itself or following therapy
  - Same mechanisms as for gynecologic tumors
    - Tumor or benign scar tissue may form bridge to bowel or other organs
- **Bladder Instrumentation (Mimic)**
  - Foley catheter, cystoscopy, etc.

Helpful Clues for Less Common Diagnoses

- **Cystitis**
  - Can cause or mimic fistula
  - Gas-forming infection in urine or bladder may be mistaken for colovesical fistula
- **Abdominal or Pelvic Abscess**

- ○ Abdominal or pelvic abscess may erode into bladder, vagina, colon, &/or skin
- ○ Postoperative abscesses are most common cause
- ○ Reported as etiologies
  - – Tubo-ovarian
  - – Appendiceal
  - – Other pelvic abscesses
- **Trauma, Colorectal or Vaginal**
  - ○ May create communication between pelvic viscera directly
  - ○ Or may lead to infection with subsequent fistula
    - – Examples
      - □ Foreign body insertion into rectum or vagina
      - □ Complex pelvic fractures
      - □ Stab wounds to pelvis
- **Foreign Body**
  - ○ In bladder, vagina, or rectum, can lead to fistula
    - – Chronic inflammation and infection cause adherence between viscera and tissue breakdown

Diverticulitis

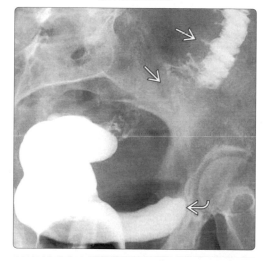

Diverticulitis

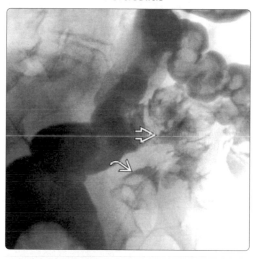

(Left) *In this middle-aged woman with recurrent urinary tract infections, a spot film from a contrast enema shows extensive sigmoid diverticulitis* ➡ *with filling of the urinary bladder* ➡ *via a fistulous track.* (Right) *In this middle-aged woman with recurrent UTIs, a spot film from a contrast enema shows contrast extravasation* ➡ *from the sigmoid colon and a fistula to the bladder, represented by contrast opacification of urine surrounding the Foley catheter balloon* ➡.

Diverticulitis

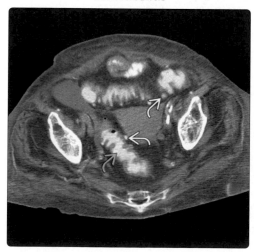

Diverticulitis

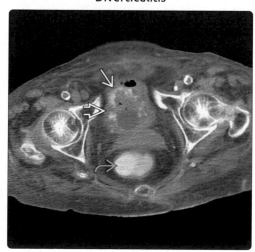

(Left) *In this elderly woman with urosepsis, NECT shows extensive sigmoid diverticular disease* ➡. *Contrast medium had been instilled into the rectosigmoid colon* ➡. (Right) *In this elderly woman with urosepsis, CT shows the contrast-opacified rectum* ➡. *Within the bladder* ➡ *is some of the rectal contrast medium* ➡, *along with gas, debris, and the Foley balloon. Diverticulitis was the source of the colovesical fistula.*

Diverticulitis

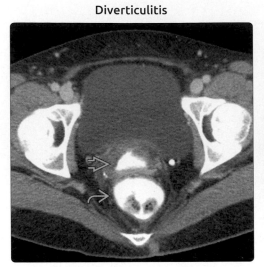

Diverticulitis

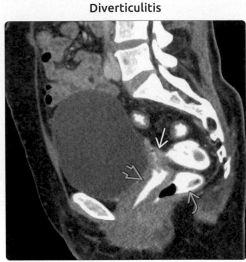

(Left) *This 50-year-old woman developed a foul vaginal discharge years after a hysterectomy for benign uterine fibroids. Contrast material injected by tube into the rectum* ➡ *opacifies the vagina* ➡, *indicating a fistula.* (Right) *In this woman with a colovaginal fistula due to diverticulitis, sagittal CT shows contrast administered into the rectum* ➡, *filling the vagina* ➡ *via a fistulous tract* ➡.

Diverticulitis

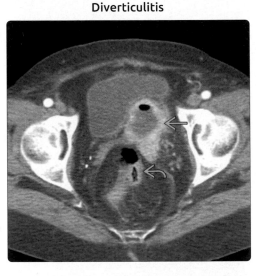

Diverticulitis

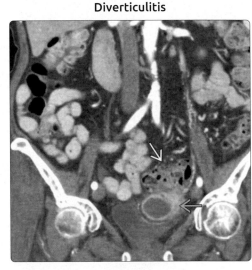

(Left) *In this elderly woman with foul vaginal discharge, CT was performed after rectal administration of contrast medium, showing gas, fluid, and contrast medium within the rectum* ➡ *and uterine lumen* ➡, *indicating a colouterine fistula.* (Right) *In this elderly woman with vaginal discharge, coronal CT shows extensive sigmoid diverticulitis* ➡ *and an adjacent collection of gas and fluid that is within the lumen of the uterus* ➡. *Surgery confirmed a colouterine fistula caused by diverticulitis.*

Diverticulitis

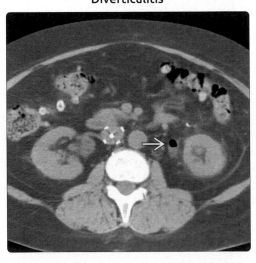

Diverticulitis

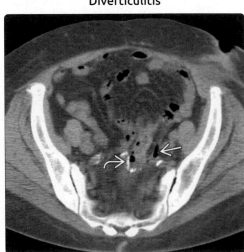

(Left) *This 47-year-old woman had recurrent urinary tract infections following sigmoid resection for diverticulitis. NECT shows gas within the left ureter* ➡ *and renal collecting system.* (Right) *In this woman with recurrent urinary tract infections, CT shows gas in the distal ureter* ➡, *which appears adherent to the site of the stapled anastomosis* ➡ *of the sigmoid colon. Diverticulitis with col;oureteral fistula was confirmed.*

Diverticulitis

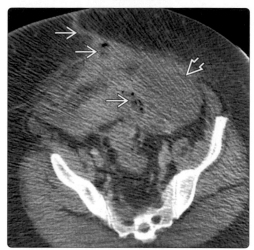

Diverticulitis

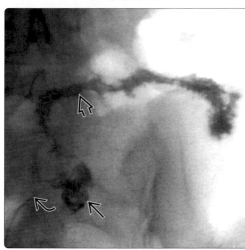

(Left) *This obese young woman has a tender, warm lesion in her abdominal wall, with a foul-smelling discharge. NECT shows a walled-off abscess ⧨ adjacent to the sigmoid colon. There is a tract of gas and fluid ⧨ leading to the anterior abdominal wall defect.* (Right) *In this obese young woman with a tender abdominal wall lesion, injection of a catheter ⧨ inserted into the abdominal wall defect opacifies an abscess cavity ⧨ and the sigmoid colon lumen ⧨, confirming a colocutaneous fistula from diverticulitis.*

Crohn Disease

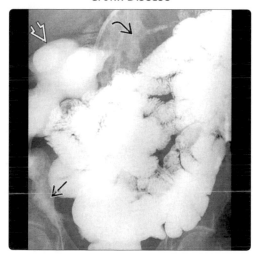

Crohn Disease

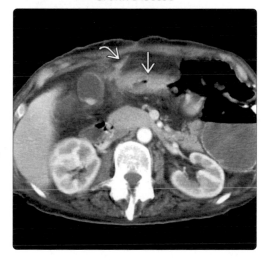

(Left) *This 64-year-old man with Crohn disease developed a feculent fistula to the skin of his anterior abdominal wall. A barium small bowel follow-through shows strictures ⧨ of the transverse colon and terminal ileum ⧨ with a dilated segment of colon ⧨ in between.* (Right) *In this man with Crohn disease and feculent discharge from his abdominal wall, CT shows a stricture and inflammation of the transverse colon ⧨, but also shows the fistula ⧨ to the anterior abdominal wall.*

Crohn Disease

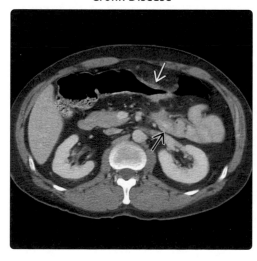

Crohn Disease

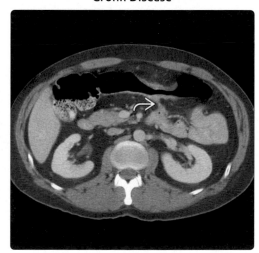

(Left) *In this patient with chronic Crohn disease and recent exacerbation of diarrhea, CT shows inflammation of segments of colon ⧨ and small bowel ⧨.* (Right) *In this patient with chronic Crohn disease, CT shows a fistula ⧨ connecting inflamed small bowel to the colon. This "short circuit" between the mid-small bowel and the transverse colon resulted in massive loss of fluid and electrolytes.*

Crohn Disease

Crohn Disease

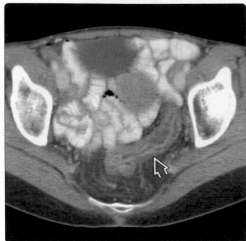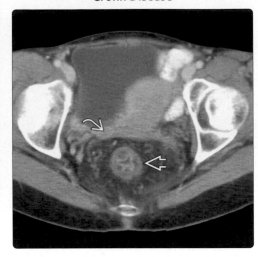

(Left) *In this 54-year-old woman with Crohn disease and a foul-smelling vaginal discharge, CT shows marked inflammation of the wall of the rectosigmoid colon* ➡. (Right) *In this 54-year-old woman, CT shows marked inflammation of the rectum* ➡ *and perirectal tissue, extending to the vagina* ➡.

Crohn Disease

Crohn Disease

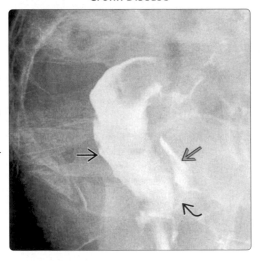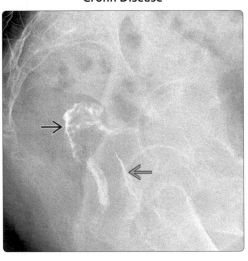

(Left) *In this 54-year-old woman with Crohn colitis, a lateral spot film from a contrast enema shows opacification of the rectosigmoid colon* ➡ *and the vagina* ➡ *through a fistulous tract* ➡ *starting low in the rectum. The image is obscured by contrast spilling onto sheets.* (Right) *In this 54-year-old woman, a repeat film after removal of the stained sheets clearly shows contrast medium in the rectum* ➡ *and vagina* ➡.

Postoperative State, Bowel

Postoperative State, Bowel

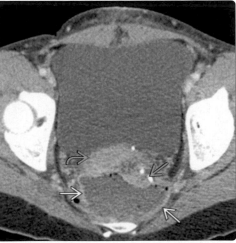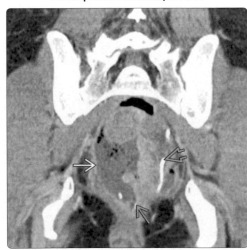

(Left) *This young woman had a colectomy with ileoanal anastomosis for ulcerative colitis. CT shows an encapsulated collection of gas and fluid (abscess)* ➡ *at the anal anastomotic staple line* ➡, *presumptive evidence of an anastomotic leak. The vagina* ➡ *abuts the abscess.* (Right) *Coronal CT in this young woman shows the abscess* ➡ *and anal* ➡ *and pouch anastomotic* ➡ *staple lines. She subsequently developed a colovaginal fistula.*

Cervical and Uterine Carcinoma

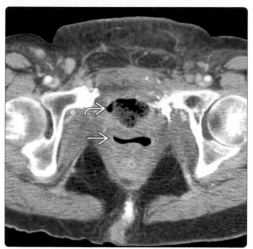

Cervical and Uterine Carcinoma

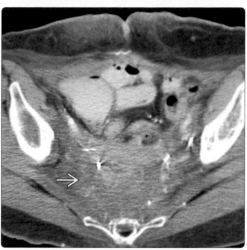

(Left) *Axial CECT shows gas in the vagina* ➔ *and bladder* ➔ *due to rectovaginal and rectovesical fistulas due to cervical carcinoma, status post resection and radiation therapy.* (Right) *Axial CECT shows a large, recurrent malignant and inflammatory pelvic mass* ➔ *following resection and radiation therapy for cervical carcinoma in a woman with rectovaginal and rectovesical fistulas.*

Ovarian Cancer

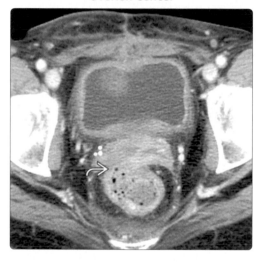

Cystitis (Mimic)

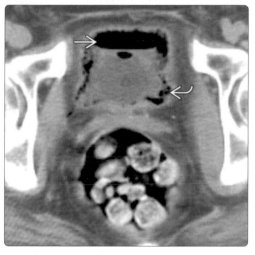

(Left) *Axial CECT shows loss of the fat plane between the rectum and vagina* ➔ *in this woman with history of ovarian cancer with surgery and radiation therapy causing rectovaginal fistula. The urinary bladder wall is also thickened.* (Right) *Axial NECT shows gas within the lumen* ➔ *and wall of the bladder* ➔ *due to emphysematous cystitis. This might be mistaken for a fistula to the colon.*

Trauma, Colorectal or Vaginal

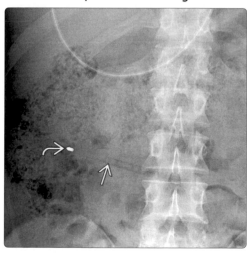

Trauma, Colorectal or Vaginal

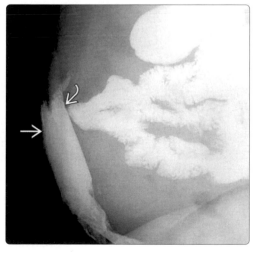

(Left) *This young man developed a cutaneous fistula after stabbing himself in the abdomen with a Bic pen, which he pushed into the abdomen. A radiograph shows the faint outline of the plastic pen* ➔ *and its metal tip* ➔. (Right) *In this man with a self-inflicted stab wound, a lateral view from the SBFT shows a segment of small bowel that is tethered to the anterior abdominal wall* ➔ *with extravasation of barium into a bag* ➔ *that overlies the anterior abdominal wall wound, confirming the enterocutaneous fistula.*

DIFFERENTIAL DIAGNOSIS

Common

- Colon Carcinoma
- Diverticulitis or Diverticulosis
- Ischemic Colitis
- Colonic Metastases and Lymphoma
- Colonic Spasm
- Infectious Colitis
- Ulcerative Colitis
- Crohn (Granulomatous) Colitis

Less Common

- Pancreatitis
- Extrinsic or Intramural Masses
  - Endometriosis
  - Uterine Fibroid
  - Pericolic Abscess
- Postoperative Stricture
- Cathartic Abuse
- Typhlitis (Neutropenic Colitis)
- Rectal Mucosal Prolapse
- Tuberculosis, Colon
- Amebic Colitis
- Radiation Colitis
- Intramural Hematoma, Colon

ESSENTIAL INFORMATION

Key Differential Diagnosis Issues

- Important to describe length, site, and nature of narrowed segment
  - Abrupt narrowing with shoulders or apple-core appearance = carcinoma until proven otherwise
    - May rarely result from infectious or ischemic etiology
  - Longer strictures with smooth, tapered margins are usually benign
- Colon may be narrowed by extrinsic inflammatory process, such as pancreatitis, cholecystitis, abscess, endometriosis
  - Also by extrinsic mass (e.g., uterine fibroid) or even distended urinary bladder
- Barium enema shows strictures and mucosal lesions better than CT
  - CT shows extracolonic processes better

Helpful Clues for Common Diagnoses

- **Colon Carcinoma**
  - Most common cause of colonic stricture and obstruction in adults
  - Short segment of narrowing (< 10 cm)
    - Usually little pericolonic infiltration
  - Regional lymphadenopathy suggests carcinoma (or infection)
- **Diverticulitis or Diverticulosis**
  - Usually causes longer segment (> 10 cm) narrowing, more pericolonic inflammation, no lymphadenopathy
  - Luminal narrowing is often due to circular muscle hypertrophy
    - Best seen on contrast enema as irregular indentation of lumen (cog wheel)
    - Does not imply active inflammation or spasm

- – Is not relieved by administration of glucagon
- **Ischemic Colitis**
  - May be acute, subacute, or chronic
  - Might follow hypoperfusion episode or arterial or venous occlusion
    - Imaging findings vary according to etiology and acuity of ischemia
    - Arterial thrombosis/embolism usually causes small bowel ischemic injury limited to distribution of superior mesenteric artery, with limited bowel wall/mesenteric edema
    - Hypoperfusion is most common etiology for colonic ischemia
      - Usual manifestation is wall thickening and luminal narrowing of watershed segments of colon
      - Splenic flexure > sigmoid colon
- **Colonic Metastases and Lymphoma**
  - Can be hematogenous or lymphatic spread, or direct invasion
    - e.g., from duodenum, stomach, kidneys, gallbladder, uterus, prostate
  - Most common is direct invasion from primary pelvic malignancy
    - e.g., cervical, endometrial, prostatic
  - Drop metastases = intraperitoneal spread of tumor
    - Common site is to pouch of Douglas (rectovesical or rectouterine recess)
      - Mass indents anterior wall of rectum and can be palpated on physical exam
- **Colonic Spasm**
  - May exactly simulate carcinoma on imaging
  - Give IV glucagon to relieve spasm; repeat imaging
- **Infectious Colitis**
  - Tuberculosis and amebic colitis can cause apple core lesion exactly like carcinoma
  - Lymphogranuloma venereum
    - Caused by *Chlamydia trachomatis*
    - Rectosigmoid involvement due to anal intercourse
    - Luminal narrowing, mucosal ulceration, perirectal abscess, rectal fistula
  - Other infectious colitides
    - *Clostridium difficile* and *Campylobacter colitis* usually involve entire colon, but may be segmental
- **Ulcerative or Granulomatous Colitis**
  - May result in diffuse or segmental stricture of colon
    - Short, focal stricture should raise concern for colon carcinoma as complication of chronic colitis

Helpful Clues for Less Common Diagnoses

- **Pancreatitis**
  - Inflammation often spreads laterally within anterior pararenal space to contact proximal descending colon
  - Colon cutoff sign = proximal descending colon is narrowed due to spasm and inflammation caused by pancreatitis
    - Transverse colon is gas distended
- **Endometriosis**
  - Endometrial tissue may implant on any part of intraperitoneal bowel
    - Involves rectosigmoid area in 75-95% of cases

- Typical findings: Extrinsic mass effect on anterior wall of rectosigmoid junction
  - Less common: Polypoid mass, annular constricting lesion
    - Indistinguishable for primary colonic carcinoma
- **Postoperative Stricture**
  - Usually web-like short strictured segment with smooth edges
  - Anastomosis often marked by surgical staple line
- **Cathartic Abuse**
  - Due to chronic use of stimulant laxatives
  - Results in neuromuscular damage of colon
  - Ahaustral colon (simulates chronic ulcerative colitis)
    - Irregular and transient segmental narrowing, primarily in ascending and transverse colon
- **Typhlitis (Neutropenic Colitis)**
  - Luminal narrowing and wall thickening of cecum and ascending colon
  - Due to polymicrobial infiltration of colonic wall
  - Encountered only in severely neutropenic patients
    - Leukemia, bone marrow transplant recipient
- **Rectal Mucosal Prolapse**
  - Solitary rectal ulcer syndrome
  - Usually in women with pelvic floor laxity
  - Repeated episodes of rectal prolapse injure antero-lateral walls of rectum, leading to edema and ulceration
  - May also cause spasm, mural thickening (colitis cystica profunda), stricture
- **Radiation Colitis**
  - Usually follows radiation therapy for pelvic primary malignancy (e.g., cervical or prostate carcinoma)
  - Leads to long stricture of rectosigmoid colon with tapered margins

Colon Carcinoma

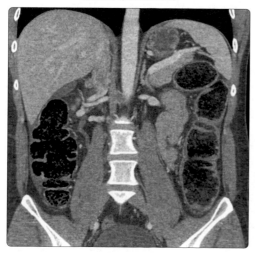

Colon Carcinoma

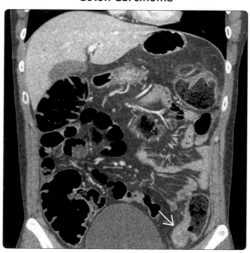

(Left) Coronal CECT shows the colon is grossly dilated with stool and gas. (Right) Coronal CT in the same case shows the colonic obstructing lesion ➡ as a classic apple core carcinoma, with a short segment, soft tissue density thickening of the colonic wall.

Diverticulitis or Diverticulosis

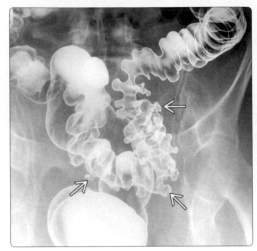

Diverticulitis or Diverticulosis

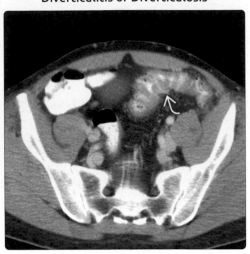

(Left) *Spot film from a BE shows distortion of the lumen of the sigmoid colon. Diverticula* ➡ *project off the surface of the colon. The folds of the sigmoid colon are irregularly spaced, of variable thickness, and markedly distort and narrow the lumen. The distortion of the sigmoid colonic lumen is due to hypertrophy of the circular muscle and shortening of the longitudinal muscle (taenia) layers.* **(Right)** *CECT shows luminal narrowing & wall thickening of the sigmoid colon* ➡ *due to circular muscle hypertrophy.*

Ischemic Colitis

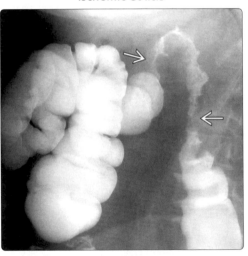

Colonic Spasm

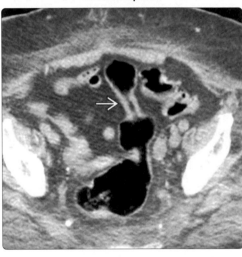

(Left) *Spot film from a contrast enema shows luminal narrowing and fold thickening of the splenic flexure region of colon* ➡. *This is a characteristic location and appearance for hypoperfusion etiology ischemic colitis.* **(Right)** *Axial CECT shows an apparent stricture* ➡ *of the sigmoid colon. This was normal at colonoscopy and probably represented simple spasm. Note normal wall thickness and no infiltration of adjacent fat.*

Infectious Colitis

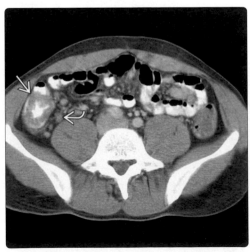

Infectious Colitis

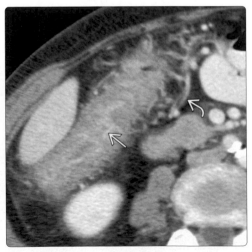

(Left) *Axial CECT shows luminal narrowing and wall thickening of the ascending colon* ➡ *due to Yersinia colitis. Also note some mesocolic lymphadenopathy* ➡. **(Right)** *In this elderly patient with bloody diarrhea, CT showed pancolitis. The colonic lumen is narrowed* ➡ *with submucosal edema and mucosal & mesenteric hyperemia* ➡. *Campylobacter was the responsible organism.*

Ulcerative Colitis

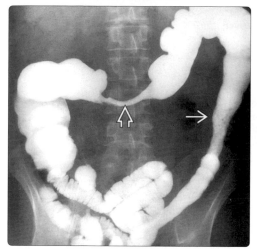

Pancreatitis

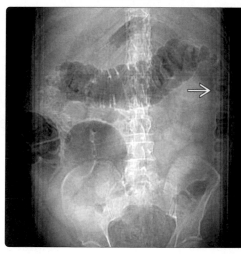

(Left) *A frontal film from a contrast enema shows a shortened ahaustral left colon* ➡ *due to chronic ulcerative colitis. The short, focal stricture in the transverse colon is a carcinoma* ➡. *Note the abrupt proximal margin.* (Right) *A supine radiograph shows dilation of the transverse colon with abrupt narrowing of the anatomic splenic flexure* ➡ *due to pancreatitis that had spread to the colon. This is a classic plain film finding of pancreatitis, called the colon cutoff sign.*

Uterine Fibroid

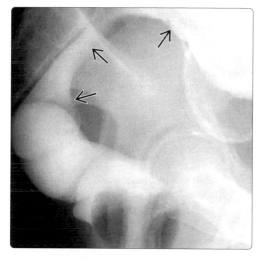

Cathartic Abuse

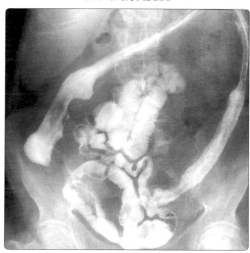

(Left) *Spot film from a contrast enema shows narrowing of the rectosigmoid colon* ➡ *due to extrinsic mass. This proved to be a large uterine fibroid (leiomyoma).* (Right) *A supine film from a contrast enema shows focal and long strictures of the colon due to chronic laxative abuse.*

Tuberculosis, Colon

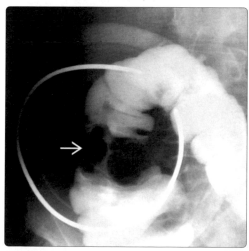

Radiation Colitis

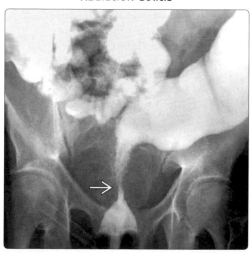

(Left) *Contrast enema shows a classic apple core lesion of the ascending colon, indistinguishable from carcinoma. Proven at surgery to be due to tuberculous infection of the colon* ➡. (Right) *A spot film from a contrast enema shows a high-grade stricture* ➡ *of the rectum that resulted from radiation therapy for a sacral metastatic focus.*

DIFFERENTIAL DIAGNOSIS

Common

- Infectious Colitis
  - Pseudomembranous Colitis
- Ischemic Colitis
- Portal Hypertension, Varices
- Ulcerative Colitis

Less Common

- Typhlitis (Neutropenic Colitis)
- Chemical Proctocolitis
- Diverticulitis
- Intramural Hematoma, Colon
- Metastases and Lymphoma, Colonic
- Pneumatosis

ESSENTIAL INFORMATION

Key Differential Diagnosis Issues

- Thumbprinting describes rounded thickening of transverse colonic folds; usually due to edema
- Basically same differential diagnosis as for submucosal edema, as seen on CT
  - But generally requires more extensive thickening to cause thumbprinting
- **Neoplasm (primary or metastatic) rarely causes thumbprinting**

Helpful Clues for Common Diagnoses

- **Infectious Colitis**
  - **Infectious (including *Clostridium difficile*) colitis is most common cause of marked submucosal edema (thumbprinting)**
  - *Campylobacter*, *Escherichia coli*, staphylococcal, amebic, *Strongyloides*, etc. in general population
  - Cytomegalovirus & others in immune suppressed
  - **Pseudomembranous Colitis**
    - Caused by *C. difficile* infection of colon
    - Has become most common cause of thumbprinting

- Endemic in hospitalized patients, usually those on antibiotic therapy
- **Ischemic Colitis**
  - Often due to hypoperfusion (favors splenic flexure & sigmoid)
  - May be due to venous thrombosis
    - Arterial embolism or thrombosis rarely causes thumbprinting
- **Portal Hypertension, Varices**
  - Cirrhosis ± portal vein thrombosis
  - Often leads to marked colonic edema
  - Usually favors right side of colon
- **Ulcerative Colitis**
  - Or Crohn (granulomatous) colitis
  - Look for ulceration of mucosa
  - Usually causes less submucosal edema than infectious colitis

Helpful Clues for Less Common Diagnoses

- **Typhlitis (Neutropenic Colitis)**
  - Neutropenic colitis, in severely neutropenic patients
  - Usually limited to cecum & ascending colon
- **Chemical Proctocolitis**
  - From glutaraldehyde, used to clean colonoscopes
- **Diverticulitis**
  - Wall thickening may be due to infection, pericolonic abscess, &/or circular muscle hypertrophy
  - Not truly thumbprinting, nor submucosal edema
- **Intramural Hematoma, Colon**
  - Following trauma or anticoagulation
- **Metastases and Lymphoma, Colonic**
  - Rare cause of thumbprinting
  - Lymphoma more likely than metastases to cause multifocal sites of wall thickening
    - Will be soft tissue (not water) density on CT
- **Pneumatosis**
  - Rare variant is pneumatosis cystoides
  - Usually benign, idiopathic, entity limited to rectosigmoid colon
  - Presence of gas cysts in wall of colon is diagnostic

(Left) *Supine radiograph shows classic thumbprinting of the ascending colon* ➡️ *due to cytomegalovirus colitis in a young man with AIDS.* **(Right)** *In this previously healthy young woman, CT shows massive, pancolonic, submucosal edema, imparting a thumbprinting appearance to the transverse colon* ➡️. *Campylobacter was the responsible organism.*

Infectious Colitis

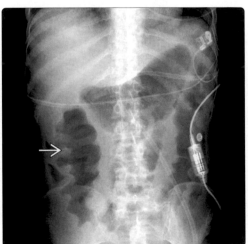

Infectious Colitis

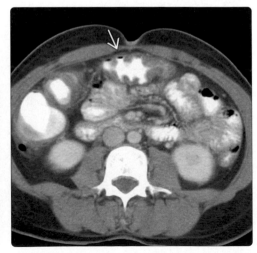

Pseudomembranous Colitis

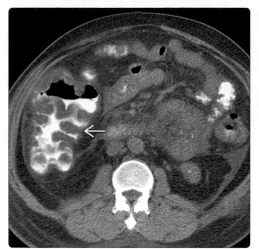

Ischemic Colitis

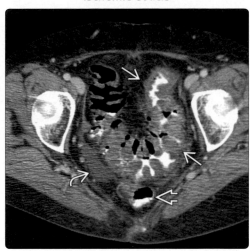

(Left) *In this renal transplant recipient with acute C. difficile colitis, CT shows massive thickening of the wall of the entire colon (pancolitis), with some segments having a thumbprinted appearance ➡. In spite of prompt diagnosis & treatment, toxic megacolon developed & resulted in total colectomy.* (Right) *This elderly patient had acute onset of hematochezia & abdominal pain after a hypotensive episode. CT shows ascites ➡ & thumbprinting of the sigmoid colon ➡ but sparing of the rectum ➡, typical features of hypoperfusion ischemic colitis.*

Portal Hypertension, Varices

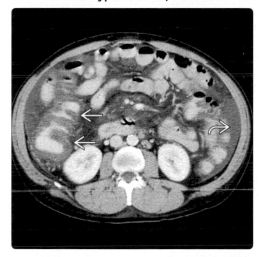

Ulcerative Colitis

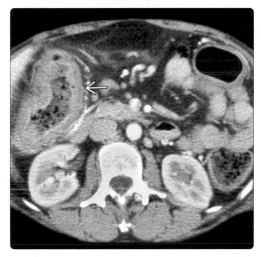

(Left) *Axial CECT shows ascites ➡ and thumbprinting ➡ of the ascending colon, due to cirrhosis and portal hypertension, not colitis.* (Right) *Axial CECT shows marked thickening of the colonic wall, especially the ascending colon, with intense mucosal enhancement ➡. This degree of wall thickening is unusual for ulcerative colitis.*

Typhlitis (Neutropenic Colitis)

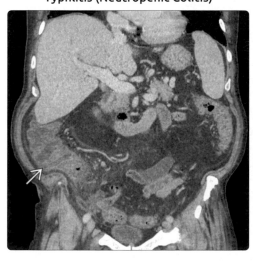

Pneumatosis

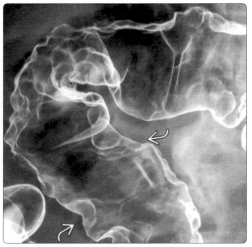

(Left) *In this elderly man with acute leukemia, coronal CT shows massive submucosal edema ➡ limited to the wall of the ascending colon and cecum. These are typical features of typhlitis or neutropenic colitis.* (Right) *Spot film from an air-contrast barium enema shows thumbprinted pattern. The presence of gas blebs ➡ in the colonic wall indicates benign colonic pneumatosis in this asymptomatic patient.*

DIFFERENTIAL DIAGNOSIS

Common

- Diverticulitis
- Infectious Colitis
  - Pseudomembranous Colitis
- Ischemic Colitis
- Ulcerative and Crohn Colitis
- Colon Carcinoma
- Portal Hypertension
- Endometriosis

Less Common

- Obesity (Mimic)
- Typhlitis (Neutropenic Colitis)
- Chemical Proctocolitis
- Colonic Metastases and Lymphoma
- Intramural Hemorrhage
- Pneumatosis of Colon
- Hemolytic Uremic Syndrome
- Angioedema, Intestinal

ESSENTIAL INFORMATION

Key Differential Diagnosis Issues

- **Characterize length & site of involvement**
  - Focal (< 10 cm): Neoplasm, endometriosis, rarely amebic or TB
  - Segmental (10-15 cm length): Diverticulitis most common
  - Right colon & small intestine: Crohn disease, embolic or thrombotic ischemic, portal hypertension, infectious
  - Watershed areas (splenic flexure &/or sigmoid): Hypoperfusion, ischemia
  - Pancolonic with sparing of small intestine: Infectious or ulcerative colitis (not ischemic)
  - Pancolonic sparing rectum: Infectious (not ischemic or ulcerative)
- **Characterize attenuation of submucosal layer**
  - Air density: Pneumatosis (various causes, including ischemia)
  - Fat density: Chronic ulcerative or granulomatous colitis, obesity
  - Near water density: Inflammation or ischemia (not neoplastic)
  - Soft tissue density: Diverticulitis, inflammation, ischemia, tumor
  - High attenuation (> 60 H): Hemorrhage

Helpful Clues for Common Diagnoses

- **Diverticulitis**
  - Wall is thickened over 10-15 cm length by edema & smooth muscle hypertrophy
    - Usually no distinct submucosal layer of low density
  - See diverticula, pericolonic infiltration, ± gas & fluid
- **Infectious Colitis**
  - Long segmental or pancolitis
    - Mucosal hyperemia & marked submucosal edema
  - Difficult to distinguish among etiologies from imaging alone
  - **Pseudomembranous colitis**

- Most impressive wall thickening among colitides
  - Submucosal edema with compressed lumen & intense mucosal enhancement may result in accordion sign or thumbprinting
- Segmental or pancolitis
- Caused by *Clostridium difficile* toxin, endemic in health care facilities
  - No longer confined to hospitalized patients who have received broad spectrum antibiotics
- **Ischemic Colitis**
  - Most common in watershed regions when caused by hypoperfusion
    - Splenic flexure > sigmoid colon
  - Embolic or thrombotic arterial occlusion more commonly affects small intestine and right side of colon
    - Arterial occlusive ischemia usually does not cause much wall thickening
- **Ulcerative and Crohn Colitis**
  - Acute: Wall edema, pericolonic infiltration, mesenteric hyperemia (comb or caterpillar sign)
    - Submucosal edema usually less marked than with infectious colitis
  - Chronic: Submucosal layer is fat density
  - Ulcerative colitis favors rectum & distal colon
  - Granulomatous (Crohn) colitis favors distal ileum with skip areas in SB & colon; perianal involvement
- **Colon Carcinoma**
  - Wall thickening is soft tissue attenuation
  - Usually short segment involvement (< 10 cm)
    - Apple core lesion
    - Right-side colon cancers often bulkier; less likely to obstruct
  - Often with regional adenopathy (strong predictor of cancer with lymphatic spread)
  - Look for hepatic & peritoneal metastases
- **Portal Hypertension**
  - Edema of colonic wall ± small bowel
    - Portal hypertensive colopathy, not inflammatory
  - Look for signs of cirrhosis, ascites
  - (May occur with heart & renal failure)
- **Endometriosis**
  - Implants on colonic wall closely mimic primary colon cancer
    - Short segment, soft tissue density
    - Narrowing, possibly obstructing, colonic lumen
    - May be multifocal, especially in sigmoid colon
  - Correlate with periodic symptoms in young woman

Helpful Clues for Less Common Diagnoses

- **Obesity (Mimic)**
  - Fatty infiltration of submucosal layer may be an asymptomatic finding of no significance
  - Ask about history of prior colitis
- **Typhlitis (Neutropenic Colitis)**
  - Neutropenic colitis
  - Leukemia & bone marrow transplant patients
  - Limited to cecum & ascending colon
  - Wall thickening is marked; wall may perforate
    - Extraluminal gas &/or fluid is ominous sign; usually requires surgery

- **Chemical Proctocolitis**
  - Glutaraldehyde used to sterilize endoscopes
  - If not thoroughly washed from surface of scope, can damage colonic mucosa
- **Colonic Metastases and Lymphoma**
  - Wall thickening is soft tissue density
  - Quite rare; less common than small bowel involvement
- **Intramural Hemorrhage**
  - Uncommon in colon
  - Etiologies: Trauma (including endoscopy), anticoagulation
  - Attenuation is greater than soft tissue (may be apparent only on NECT)
- **Pneumatosis of Colon**
  - Spherical or linear air density
  - From infarction, idiopathic pneumatosis cystoides, or other causes of "benign" pneumatosis
    - Steroid and immunosuppressive medications are common etiology
- **Hemolytic Uremic Syndrome**
  - Primarily a disease of infants & small children

- Caused by toxin of *Escherichia coli* (or other organisms)
- Diarrhea, hemolytic anemia, thrombocytopenia, acute renal failure
- **Angioedema, Intestinal**
  - Inherited deficiency of inhibitor of C1 esterase (part of complement cascade)
  - Similar pathology can be induced by reactions to medications (e.g., ACE inhibitors), and in some patients with viral hepatitis
  - Small bowel involvement more common than colonic

SELECTED REFERENCES

1. Wittenberg J et al: Algorithmic approach to CT diagnosis of the abnormal bowel wall. Radiographics. 22(5):1093-107; discussion 1107-9, 2002
2. Horton KM et al: CT evaluation of the colon: inflammatory disease. Radiographics. 20(2):399-418, 2000

Diverticulitis

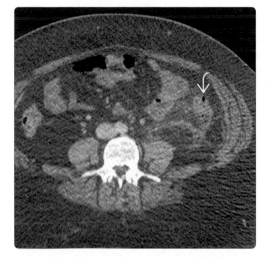

Diverticulitis

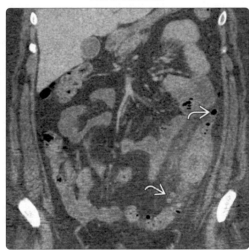

(Left) *In this obese young woman, axial CECT shows extensive infiltration of fat planes surrounding the descending colon, with at least one diverticulum noted* ➡. **(Right)** *In this obese young woman, coronal CECT shows a long segment of descending colon with a thickened wall, pericolonic infiltration, and multiple diverticula* ➡.

Diverticulitis

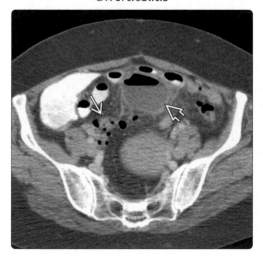

Diverticulitis

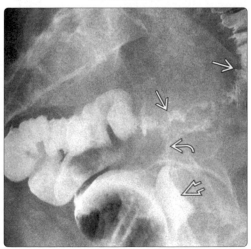

(Left) *In this 60-year-old woman, CT shows extensive sigmoid diverticulosis* ➡ *and a loculated, pericolonic abscess* ➡ *due to diverticulitis.* **(Right)** *In this 63-year-old woman who had a temporary colostomy for diverticulitis, a contrast enema was performed 6 months later in anticipation of reanastomosing her colon. This shows extensive diverticulosis of the sigmoid colon* ➡ *and a fistulous track* ➡ *to the vagina* ➡.

(Left) *In this previously healthy elderly woman, CT shows pancolitis with mucosal and mesenteric hyperemia ➡️ and submucosal edema ➡️. This was Campylobacter colitis. **(Right)** In this 18-year-old woman with acute bloody diarrhea, coronal CECT shows panproctocolitis with marked submucosal edema ➡️. Fluid within the left side of the colon ➡️ indicates a diarrheal state. This was E. coli colitis due to ingestion of contaminated hamburger.*

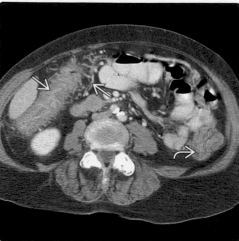

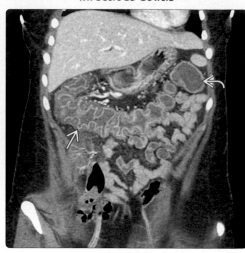

Pseudomembranous Colitis

Ischemic Colitis

(Left) *In this 15-year-old boy hospitalized with pancreatitis, CT shows C. difficile pancolitis with an accordion sign caused by submucosal edema ➡️ compressing and separating the enhanced mucosal folds ➡️. **(Right)** In this woman who recently had cardiac arrest, a contrast enema shows a stricture ➡️ of the proximal descending colon, the classic watershed distribution of the hypoperfusion ischemic colitis.*

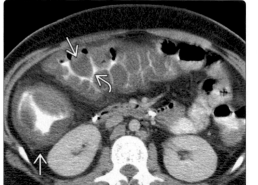

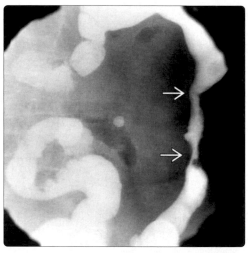

Ischemic Colitis

Ischemic Colitis

(Left) *This 69-year-old woman with cardiac disease developed acute pain and hematochezia following a hypotensive episode. CT shows submucosal edema that was limited to the descending and sigmoid colon ➡️ and ascites ➡️. **(Right)** In this 69-year-old woman with cardiac disease and hematochezia, coronal CT shows wall thickening of the descending and sigmoid colon ➡️, classic for the hypoperfusion etiology of ischemic colitis.*

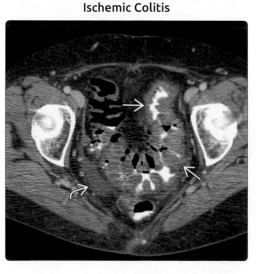

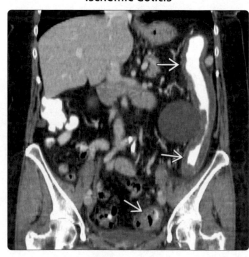

Ulcerative and Crohn Colitis

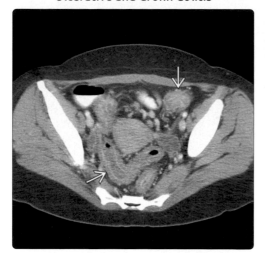

Ulcerative and Crohn Colitis

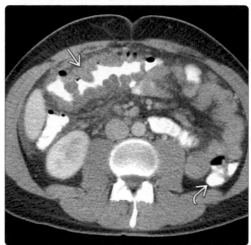

(Left) *In this young woman with recurrent bouts of pain and diarrhea, CT shows marked inflammation of the rectosigmoid colon* ➡, *characterized by mucosal hyperemia and moderate submucosal edema. Endoscopy confirmed ulcerative colitis.* **(Right)** *In this young man with recurrent pain and diarrhea, CT shows massive thickening of the wall of the right side of the colon* ➡ *with relative sparing of the descending colon* ⮡ *and rectum (not shown). Endoscopic biopsy revealed granulomatous (Crohn) colitis.*

Colon Carcinoma

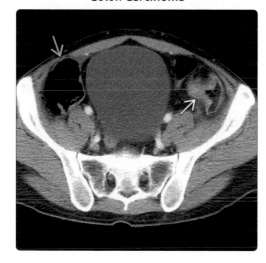

Colon Carcinoma

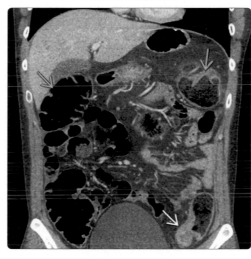

(Left) *This 31-year-old man had symptoms of colonic obstruction. Axial CT shows a grossly dilated colon* ➡ *with stool and gas, ending abruptly at an apple core lesion* ➡ *at the junction of the descending and sigmoid colon.* **(Right)** *In this 31 year old man with constipation and hematochezia, coronal CT shows a grossly dilated colon* ➡ *ending abruptly at an apple core lesion* ➡ *at the junction of the descending and sigmoid colon, a typical appearance for primary colon carcinoma.*

Colon Carcinoma

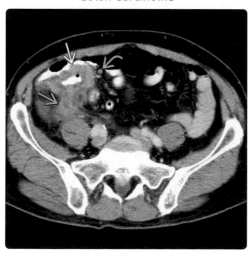

Colon Carcinoma

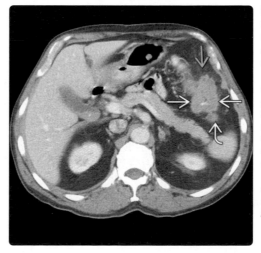

(Left) *In this patient with acute RLQ pain, CT shows a circumferential, bulky, cecal mass* ➡ *that had obstructed the base of the appendix. Transmural invasion* ➡, *lymphadenopathy* ➡, *and peritoneal metastases (not shown) were evident.* **(Right)** *In this man with weight loss, CECT shows a focal, circumferential, colonic soft tissue density mass* ➡. *Transmural infiltration is evident* ➡ *along with omental or mesenteric tumor* ➡.

Portal Hypertension

Portal Hypertension

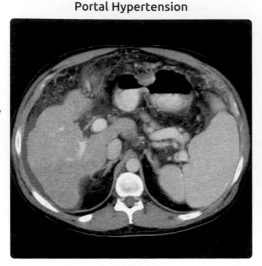

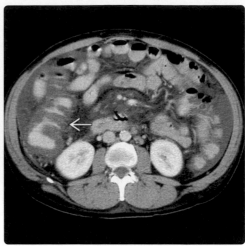

(Left) *In this 60-year-old man with diarrhea, CT shows typical signs of cirrhosis and portal hypertension, including splenomegaly and ascites.* (Right) *In this 60-year-old man with cirrhosis, axial CT shows colonic wall thickening ➡ due to portal hypertensive colopathy.*

Endometriosis

Endometriosis

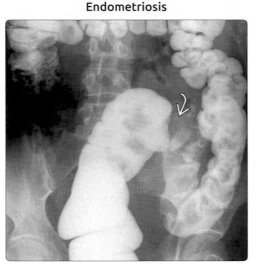

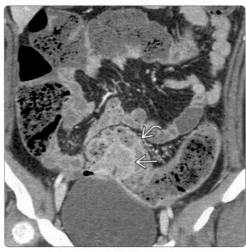

(Left) *This young woman had symptoms of colonic obstruction. A spot film from a contrast enema shows partial obstruction to retrograde filling and a tight, short stricture ➡. The more proximal colon is distended with stool and gas. Colon carcinoma was the primary concern, but endometriosis was confirmed.* (Right) *This young woman had symptoms of colonic obstruction. Coronal CECT shows a colonic stricture ➡ with an eccentric, soft tissue density mass ➡ representing endometriosis.*

Obesity (Mimic)

Colonic Metastases and Lymphoma

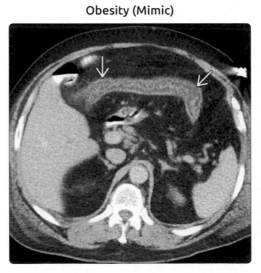

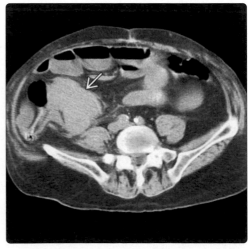

(Left) *Axial CECT shows apparent thickening of the wall of the transverse colon ➡ with submucosal fat density proliferation. There was no history of colitis in this patient; this is a normal variant in obese and some elderly patients.* (Right) *Axial NECT shows a soft tissue density mass ➡ in the cecum and appendix, representing lymphoma (posttransplant lymphoproliferative disorder) in a renal transplant recipient.*

Typhlitis (Neutropenic Colitis)

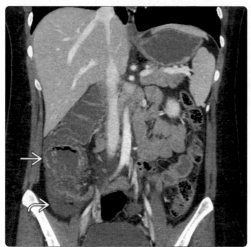

Typhlitis (Neutropenic Colitis)

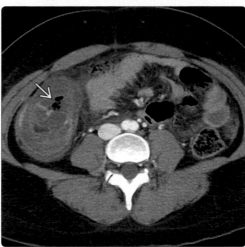

(Left) *In this woman with neutropenia, fever, and RLQ pain due to chemotherapy, coronal CT shows mucosal enhancement and marked submucosal edema* ➡ *limited to the cecum and ascending colon. Ascites* ➡ *raised concern for perforation, confirmed at surgery.* (Right) *In this woman with chemotherapy-induced neutropenic colitis, axial CECT shows marked submucosal edema and pneumatosis* ➡ *in the ascending colon.*

Typhlitis (Neutropenic Colitis)

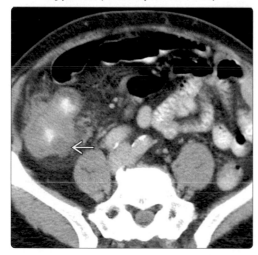

Typhlitis (Neutropenic Colitis)

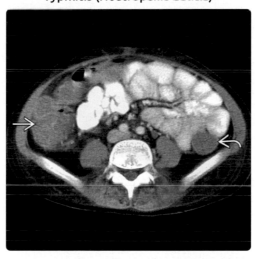

(Left) *Axial CECT shows submucosal edema and luminal narrowing* ➡, *limited to the ascending colon and cecum.* (Right) *In this 11-year-old boy with acute leukemia, CECT shows marked submucosal edema in the wall of the cecum* ➡. *The descending colon* ➡ *is filled with fluid but otherwise normal.*

Pneumatosis of Colon

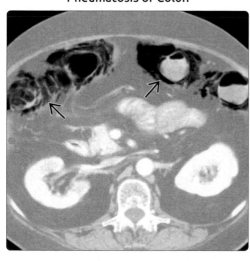

Pneumatosis of Colon

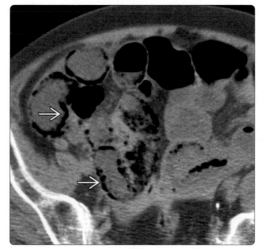

(Left) *Axial CECT shows extensive gas density in the colonic submucosa* ➡, *representing benign pneumatosis in a young woman with leukemia, presumably due to steroid and antirejection medications.* (Right) *Axial CECT shows extensive pneumatosis* ➡ *in small bowel and colon due to acute embolic infarction. The ileus helps to confirm the ischemic etiology, but correlation with clinical signs of bowel ischemia is essential.*

DIFFERENTIAL DIAGNOSIS

Common

- Ulcerative Colitis
- Cathartic Abuse
- Crohn Disease (Granulomatous Colitis)
- Senescent Change, Colon
- Toxic Megacolon

Less Common

- Ischemic Colitis
- Radiation Colitis
- Amyloidosis
- Schistosomiasis

ESSENTIAL INFORMATION

Key Differential Diagnosis Issues

- Haustra should always be present in proximal colon, but can be absent normally in distal colon
  - Haustra are sacculations of colonic lumen, separated by colonic (semilunar) folds

Helpful Clues for Common Diagnoses

- **Ulcerative Colitis**
  - Usually in chronic, burned out phase
  - Colon may appear smooth, tubular, with loss of usual transverse folds and haustra
  - Colon may be foreshortened & straightened
    - Picture frame or lead pipe appearance
  - Look for evidence of active inflammation on current or prior studies (barium enema, CT, endoscopy)
- **Cathartic Abuse**
  - Can also occur with chronic enema abuse
    - Results in neuromuscular damage
  - Look for bizarre contractions & spasm of right colon; no ulcerations
  - Colic length is usually normal, not shortened
- **Crohn Disease (Granulomatous Colitis)**
  - Chronic phase of granulomatous colitis can resemble burned out ulcerative colitis

- **Senescent Change, Colon**
  - Elderly persons often have loss of colonic folds, especially in descending colon
  - Unlike with chronic colitis, colon is not foreshortened
  - Asymptomatic and uncertain etiology
    - Some are probably due to chronic laxative & enema use
- **Toxic Megacolon**
  - Colon (especially transverse) loses normal transverse folds
  - Lumen is dilated
  - Surface irregularity = ulceration, sloughed mucosa, inflammatory pseudopolyps
  - Wall may be thin or thickened, more apparent on CT
  - Medical/surgical emergency; may perforate

Helpful Clues for Less Common Diagnoses

- **Ischemic Colitis**
  - Usually in healing or healed phase
  - Segmental loss of folds and haustra
  - Often affects splenic flexure and sigmoid colon
- **Radiation Colitis**
  - Usually takes weeks or months to develop
  - Sigmoid colon most affected, following radiation therapy for pelvic malignancies

(Left) Supine radiograph shows a shortened transverse & descending colon ➡, in a patient with chronic ulcerative colitis (UC), but no current evidence of severe exacerbation. **(Right)** Supine radiograph shows a shortened, ahaustral sigmoid colon ➡ in a patient with chronic UC.

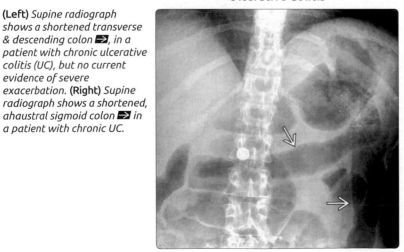

Ulcerative Colitis

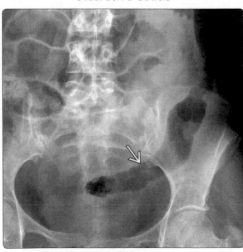

Ulcerative Colitis

Ulcerative Colitis

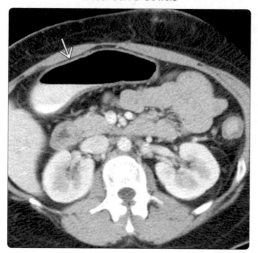

Cathartic Abuse

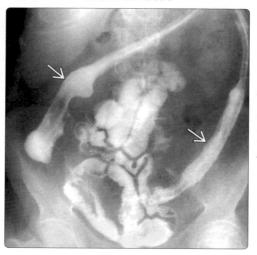

(Left) *Axial CECT shows a dilated, featureless transverse colon* ➡ *in a patient with chronic UC.* (Right) *In this elderly woman with chronic laxative use, a supine film from a contrast enema shows an ahaustral colon* ➡ *but no significant shortening. Intermittent segmental contractions were observed at fluoroscopy.*

Senescent Change, Colon

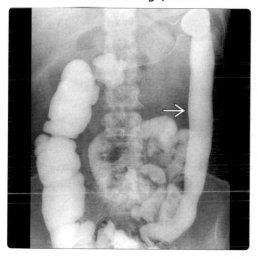

Toxic Megacolon

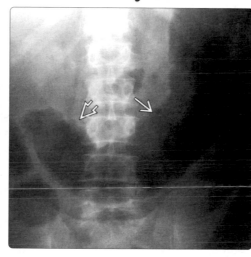

(Left) *A supine film from a contrast enema shows an ahaustral distal transverse and descending colon* ➡ *in an elderly patient with no history or clinical symptoms of colitis.* (Right) *A supine radiograph shows a dilated ahaustral transverse colon* ➡ *with a suggestion of mucosal irregularity* ➡. *Only correlation with clinical input (severe abdominal pain and guarding) distinguishes this as toxic megacolon, rather than ileus.*

Toxic Megacolon

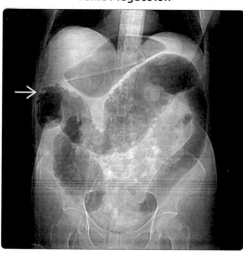

Radiation Colitis

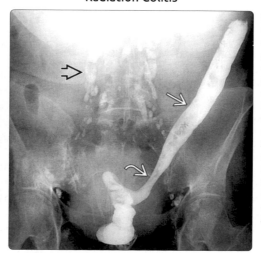

(Left) *A supine radiograph shows a shortened, ahaustral colon due to chronic granulomatous colitis (Crohn disease). Note the pseudopolyps* ➡ *and gross dilation of the transverse colon, which along with severe acute symptoms, indicated toxic megacolon.* (Right) *A supine film from a contrast enema shows a shortened, ahaustral left side of colon* ➡, *with a short stricture* ➡. *Note lymphangiographic opacification of retroperitoneal nodes* ➡.

DIFFERENTIAL DIAGNOSIS

Common

- Appendicitis
- Crohn Disease
- Pelvic Inflammatory Disease
- Pyelonephritis
- Urolithiasis (Renal Calculi)
- Mesenteric Enteritis/Adenitis

Less Common

- Infectious Colitis
- Diverticulitis
- Omental Infarct
- Epiploic Appendagitis
- Cholecystitis
- Gynecologic and Obstetric Causes
  - Ruptured Corpus Luteum
  - Uterine Fibroids
  - Hemorrhagic Ovarian Cyst
  - Ovarian Torsion
  - Endometriosis
  - Ruptured Ectopic Pregnancy
- Ischemic Enteritis
- Ischemic Colitis
- Colon Carcinoma
- Appendiceal Carcinoma
- Pancreatitis, Acute
- Foreign Body Perforation
- Abdominal Wall Trauma

Rare but Important

- Intussusception
- Meckel Diverticulitis
- Typhlitis (Neutropenic Colitis)
- Mucocele of Appendix

ESSENTIAL INFORMATION

Key Differential Diagnosis Issues

- Young men: Appendicitis, mesenteric enteritis/adenitis, epiploic appendagitis, omental infarction, acute pancreatitis, Crohn disease
- Young women: Also consider obstetric and gynecologic etiologies, cholecystitis, pyelonephritis
- Older adults: Cancer and bowel ischemia become more common considerations

Helpful Clues for Common Diagnoses

- **Appendicitis**
  - Dilated, thick-walled, blind-ending tube arising from cecal tip
  - Appendicolith in 1/3 to 1/2 of patients
  - Periappendiceal inflammation
- **Crohn Disease**
  - Thick wall, narrow lumen of distal ileum
  - Fibrofatty proliferation of mesentery
  - Cluster of right lower quadrant (RLQ) mesenteric nodes
  - Mesenteric hyperemia; engorged vessels; comb sign
- **Pelvic Inflammatory Disease**
  - Second most common etiology in young women
    - Loss of fat planes in pelvis
    - Inflamed, pus-distended fallopian tubes
    - Possible tuboovarian abscess
- **Pyelonephritis**
  - More common in girls, young women
  - Wedge-shaped or striated nephrogram; urothelial enhancement
- **Urolithiasis (Renal Calculi)**
  - Stones in renal pelvis or ureter
  - Dilated collecting system/ureter
  - Perirenal infiltration, renal swelling
- **Mesenteric Enteritis/Adenitis**
  - Distal small bowel (SB) may be inflamed in infectious ileitis (*Yersinia*, viral, *Campylobacter*)
    - Affected SB wall thickening
    - Mucosal hyperenhancement with submucosal edema
  - Cluster of mildly enlarged (~ 5 mm) nodes in RLQ
    - Without inflammation of appendix
  - Common in children & adolescents

Helpful Clues for Less Common Diagnoses

- **Infectious Colitis**
  - *Clostridium difficile* (pseudomembranous) colitis is endemic in health care facilities
  - Many other potential causes (*Campylobacter*, *Escherichia coli*, amebic, etc.)
  - Segmental or diffuse distribution
  - Mucosal hyperenhancement, submucosal edema
- **Diverticulitis**
  - May arise from cecum or ascending colon, or elongated sigmoid colon
  - Can usually identify diverticula and adjacent inflammation
    - Inflammation is **pericolonic**
    - No mucosal hyperemia or submucosal edema (unlike colitis)
- **Omental Infarct**
  - > 95% of primary type occur near ascending colon
  - 3- to 8-cm rounded mass of heterogeneous fat density with enhancing "capsule" and adjacent inflammation
    - May see whorled vessels within lesion
    - Little or no inflammation of colon or small bowel
- **Epiploic Appendagitis**
  - Small (2-4 cm) oval of fat density with capsule and inflammation near colon
    - Central dot = occluded venule
  - More common in sigmoid and descending colon
- **Cholecystitis**
  - Inflamed, distended GB may project into RLQ
    - Perforated cholecystitis may extend inflammation to adjacent organs, including ascending colon
- **Gynecologic and Obstetric Causes**
  - **Uterine fibroids**
    - May infarct, twist or bleed, leading to acute pain
  - **Hemorrhagic ovarian cyst or ovarian torsion**
    - High attenuation (CT) or echogenic material within spherical adnexal mass; young women
  - **Endometriosis**
    - Often multifocal affecting pelvic bowel segments

- Soft tissue density mass, often with inflammatory and obstructive signs
- Chronic or episodic pain with menses in young woman
  o **Ruptured ectopic pregnancy**
    - Life threatening
    - Always consider in woman of reproductive age
    - Check β-hCG pregnancy test
    - 1st imaging evaluation of pregnant patient should be by US
- **Ischemic Enteritis**
  o Embolic or thrombotic occlusion of ileocolic artery
  o Thrombosis of ileocolic or superior mesenteric vein
    - Venous thrombosis is usually in patient with prothrombotic condition
- **Ischemic Colitis**
  o Right colon involved with superior mesenteric artery (SMA) thromboembolic disease
    - More common hypoperfusion ischemic colitis affects left colon preferentially
  o Mucosal hypoenhancement, ± pneumatosis
- **Infectious Colitis**
  o Multiple possible pathogens, especially in immunocompromised patients
  o Focal, segmental, or pancolitis with wall edema, pericolonic inflammation
- **Colon or Appendiceal Carcinoma**
  o Cecal carcinoma may obstruct appendix, mimic appendicitis
    - May also perforate, with extraluminal gas and fluid
  o Look for mass in cecal or appendiceal lumen
    - Omental or mesenteric nodular mass indicates malignancy
- **Pancreatitis, Acute**
  o Inflammation may spread to ascending colon, simulating colitis
  o Characteristic inflammation of peripancreatic tissue and lab findings are key
- **Foreign Body Perforation**
  o Ingested foreign body (e.g., toothpick or animal bone)

- o Terminal ileum is most common site of obstruction or perforation of ingested foreign body
- o Look for radiopaque thin structure (bone), though others are lucent
- o Perforation results in inflammatory infiltration of bowel and mesentery
    - ± extraluminal gas and fluid
- **Abdominal Wall Trauma**
  o Hematoma or rectus muscle strain may mimic intraabdominal source of RLQ pain

Helpful Clues for Rare Diagnoses

- **Intussusception**
  o Ileocecal is most common site
  o Long segment, obstructing intussusception in adult usually has lead mass
  o Target-shaped, bowel-within-bowel appearance
- **Meckel Diverticulitis**
  o Blind-ending pouch containing particulate debris, often enteroliths
  o Located ~ 100 cm from ileocecal valve, pointed toward midline
- **Typhlitis (Neutropenic Colitis)**
  o Neutropenic colitis, in severely immunocompromised patients
  o Massive wall thickening, submucosal edema of cecum and ascending colon
- **Mucocele of Appendix**
  o Oval cystic lesion arising from tip of cecum
    - May have eggshell calcification

Appendicitis

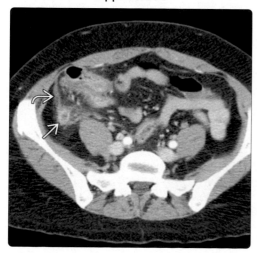

Appendicitis

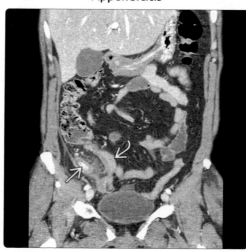

(Left) *Axial CECT shows a dilated, thick-walled appendix ➡ with inflammation of the surrounding fat planes ➡.* **(Right)** *Coronal CECT shows an appendicolith ➡ within the dilated, inflamed appendix. Note surrounding inflammatory changes, including extrinsic inflammation of terminal ileum ➡.*

Crohn Disease

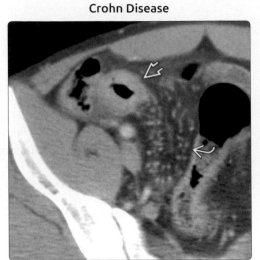

Crohn Disease

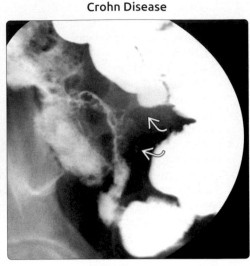

(Left) *Axial CECT shows a thick-walled terminal ileum ⇶ with increased enhancement of thickened mucosa. Also note engorged mesenteric blood vessels ➔ to the affected portion of the bowel.* (Right) *Frontal small bowel follow-through shows wall thickening and luminal narrowing of terminal ileum and cecum, and mass effect separating diseased bowel from other bowel in the right lower quadrant (RLQ). Cobblestoned mucosa (ulcerations) and sinus tracts ⇶ are noted.*

Pelvic Inflammatory Disease

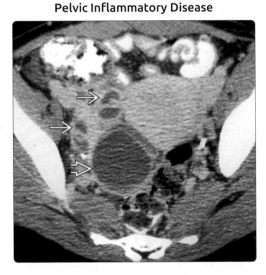

Pyelonephritis

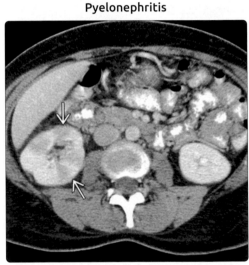

(Left) *Axial CECT shows a convoluted, dilated right pyosalpinx ➔ and a tuboovarian abscess ⇶.* (Right) *Axial CECT shows wedge-shaped and striated zones ⇶ of decreased enhancement of the right kidney, along with infiltration of the perirenal space.*

Urolithiasis (Renal Calculi)

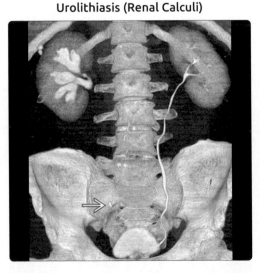

Mesenteric Enteritis/Adenitis

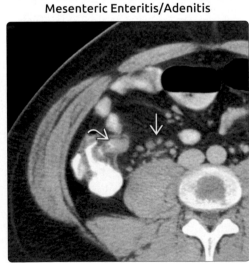

(Left) *Coronal CECT shows dilation of the right renal collecting system and delayed opacification of the right ureter, due to an obstructing ureteral calculus ⇶. Both were evident on NECT as well.* (Right) *Axial CECT shows mild thickening of the wall of the terminal ileum ➔ and a cluster of minimally enlarged mesenteric nodes ⇶; resolved spontaneously in this 24-year-old woman.*

Diverticulitis

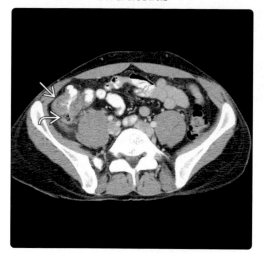

Diverticulitis

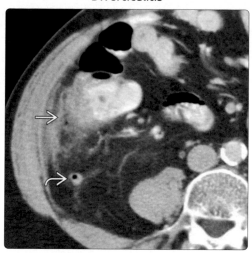

(Left) *Axial CECT shows wall thickening of the cecum* → *and diverticula* ⇉, *with adjacent inflammation.* (Right) *Axial CECT shows cecal wall thickening and infiltration of adjacent fat* →. *Note normal appendix* →. *Cecal diverticula were seen on adjacent sections.*

Omental Infarct

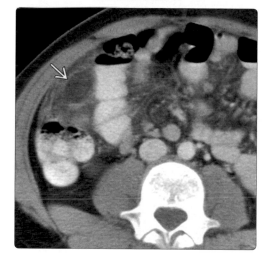

Epiploic Appendagitis

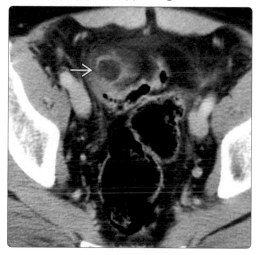

(Left) *Axial CECT shows a large oval fat density lesion* → *adjacent to the ascending colon with inflammation of the surrounding fat.* (Right) *Axial CECT shows a small, oval, fat density lesion* → *adjacent to the colon in the RLQ, with inflammation of adjacent fat.*

Cholecystitis

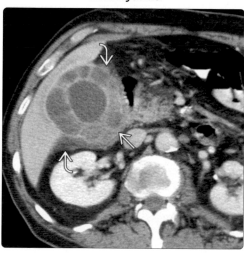

Ruptured Corpus Luteum

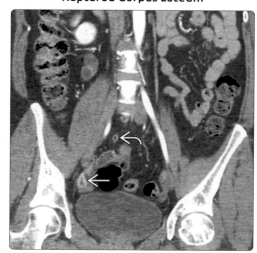

(Left) *In this patient with acute cholecystitis with perforation, axial CECT shows a thick-walled gallbladder* → *with adjacent inflammation and septate fluid collections* →. (Right) *In this young woman with acute RLQ pain, CT shows a spherical lesion with a brightly enhancing wall* → *and a small amount of adjacent, higher-than-water density fluid. The appendix* → *is normal.*

Uterine Fibroids

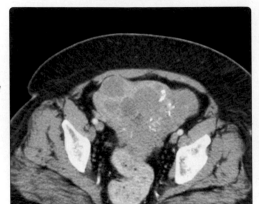

Hemorrhagic Ovarian Cyst

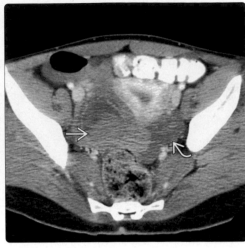

(Left) *Axial CECT shows multiple subserosal fibroids (leiomyomas) with cystic and calcified degeneration in a 51-year-old woman presenting with acute RLQ pain.* (Right) *Axial CECT shows clot within a right adnexal cyst ➡ and adjacent sentinel clot, plus hemoperitoneum ➡.*

Endometriosis

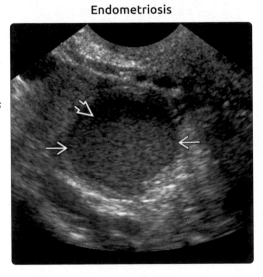

Ischemic Enteritis

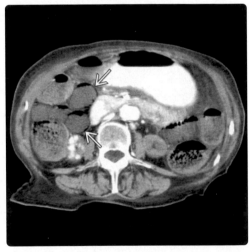

(Left) *In this young woman, sonography shows homogeneous low level echoes ➡ and a fluid level ➡ within a right lower quadrant/pelvic mass. Subsequent MR confirmed this as an endometrioma, with high signal on both T1WI and T2WI.* (Right) *Axial CECT shows diffuse ileus and gas within the wall of the distal small bowel ➡. Infarcted bowel was found at surgery.*

Ischemic Colitis

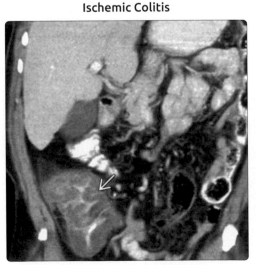

Colon Carcinoma

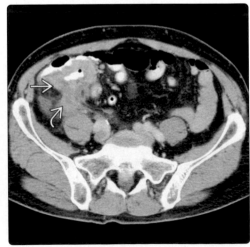

(Left) *Coronal CECT shows marked cecal mural thickening with submucosal edema ➡ and luminal narrowing. This would be difficult to distinguish from infectious colitis by CT alone.* (Right) *Axial CECT shows circumferential thickening of the wall of the cecum ➡ with a distended appendix ➡. Omental metastases were noted on adjacent sections.*

Appendiceal Carcinoma

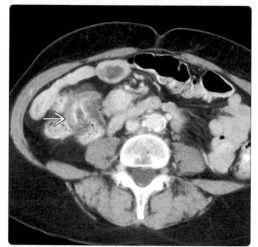

Intussusception

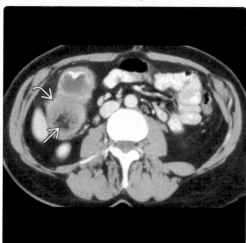

(Left) *Axial CECT shows a dilated, thick-walled appendix ➡ with infiltration of surrounding fat. Liver metastases were also seen on this CT scan.* (Right) *Axial CECT shows an ileocolic intussusception ➡ due to an appendiceal mucocele. Note the small bowel mesenteric fat ➡ within the lumen of the ascending colon.*

Meckel Diverticulitis

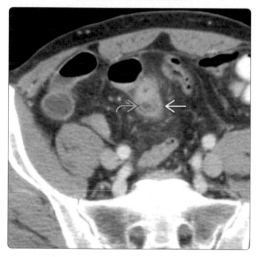

Typhlitis (Neutropenic Colitis)

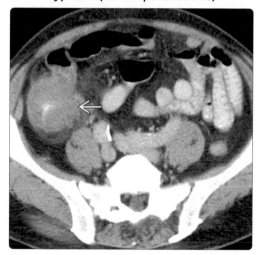

(Left) *In this patient with a perforated Meckel diverticulum, axial CECT shows a blind-ending pouch ➡ arising from the distal small bowel, containing a laminated stone ➡, with inflammation of the surrounding fat.* (Right) *Axial CECT shows marked mural thickening of the ascending colon ➡ in an elderly man receiving chemotherapy for acute myelogenous leukemia.*

Mucocele of Appendix

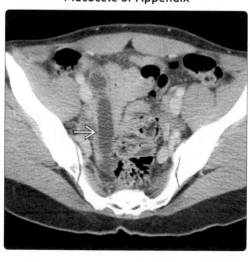

Mucocele of Appendix

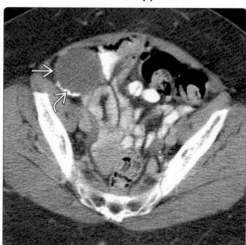

(Left) *Axial CECT shows a very distended, elongated appendix ➡ in a 46-year-old woman with only vague RLQ pain; identified as mucocele of appendix at surgical pathology.* (Right) *Axial CECT shows a pericecal mass ➡ with eggshell, though incomplete, calcification ➡.*

DIFFERENTIAL DIAGNOSIS

Common

- Diverticulitis
- Colon Carcinoma
- Epiploic Appendagitis
- Acute Colitis
  - Infectious Colitis
  - Ischemic Colitis
  - Ulcerative or Crohn Colitis
  - Fecal Impaction/Stercoral Colitis
- Gynecologic Causes
  - Adnexal Torsion
  - Endometriosis
  - Salpingitis
  - Tuboovarian Abscess
  - Uterine Fibroids
- Urolithiasis
- Sigmoid Volvulus

Less Common

- Sclerosing Mesenteritis
- Abdominal Abscess
- Peritonitis
- Renal Pathology
  - Acute Pyelonephritis
  - Renal Infarction
  - Renal Cell Carcinoma
- Coagulopathic ("Retroperitoneal") Hemorrhage
- External Hernias
  - Ventral Hernia
  - Spigelian Hernia
  - Inguinal Hernia
- Appendicitis
- Omental Infarct

ESSENTIAL INFORMATION

Key Differential Diagnosis Issues

- Most etiologies are of bowel origin, but consider genitourinary
- Don't forget to check mesentery, omentum, and abdominal wall
- CECT is imaging modality of choice, after pregnancy is taken into account

Helpful Clues for Common Diagnoses

- **Diverticulitis**
  - Most common cause in middle-aged and elderly
    - Can affect patients as young as 25
  - Usually long (10-15 cm) segment of wall thickening, luminal narrowing, pericolonic infiltration
  - Extraluminal collections of gas or fluid help confirm diagnosis
    - Look for complications (abscesses, fistulas, obstruction)
- **Colon Carcinoma**
  - Usually short segment without much pericolonic infiltration
  - Regional lymphadenopathy has strong association with carcinoma, rarely seen in diverticulitis

  - Acute symptoms may be due to colonic obstruction ± colitis proximal to obstructing mass
- **Epiploic Appendagitis**
  - Small, oval, fatty lesion (2-4 cm) with infiltration of omental fat
  - Lies immediately adjacent to colonic surface
  - Important to distinguish from diverticulitis and colitis
    - Epiploic appendagitis resolves without specific treatment
- **Acute Colitis**
  - **Infectious colitis**
    - Usually diffuse, pancolonic with impressive submucosal edema (accordion sign)
    - Hyperenhancing mucosa and engorged mesenteric vessels
    - May be segmental, including distal colon
    - Very common, especially in hospitalized patients, and those in nursing homes
  - **Ischemic colitis**
    - Hypoperfusion is most common etiology
    - Wall thickening and luminal narrowing
    - Splenic flexure, descending and sigmoid colon are affected
    - Rectum is spared (unlike ulcerative and infectious colitis)
    - Ask about prior hypotensive episode or cardiac disease
  - **Ulcerative or Crohn colitis**
    - Favors rectum and distal colon
    - Colonic wall is usually not very thickened with ulcerative colitis
    - Look for loss of haustral pattern, infiltration of pericolonic fat
    - Ask about history of prior episodes
  - **Fecal impaction/stercoral colitis**
    - Impacted stool can lead to stercoral ulceration with erosion through colonic wall
    - Look for wall perforation, perirectal infiltration, free air
- **Gynecologic Causes**
  - Many, including adnexal infection and masses, torsed ovary, endometriosis, etc.
  - Look for evidence of mass &/or inflammation centered on adnexa, rather than bowel
  - **Uterine fibroids**
    - May torse, undergo degeneration or infarction, lead to acute pain
    - Heterogeneous soft tissue masses within enlarged uterus, ± focal calcifications within masses
- **Urolithiasis**
  - Distal left ureteral stone may cause left lower quadrant (LLQ) pain
  - Diagnosis usually evident on CT
    - Ureteral calculus, hydronephrosis, perinephric stranding
- **Sigmoid Volvulus**
  - Very elongated and dilated sigmoid colon, folded back on itself (coffee bean or football sign)
  - Colon proximal to sigmoid will be dilated, but not as much as sigmoid

- o CT will show twisting of vessels in base of sigmoid mesocolon

Helpful Clues for Less Common Diagnoses

- **Sclerosing Mesenteritis**
  - o Being diagnosed much more commonly as cause of recurrent abdominal pain, usually poorly localized
  - o "Misty mesentery" with cluster of jejunal mesenteric nodes, with surrounding thin capsule
  - o Often with history of prior similar episodes
  - o May respond to steroid therapy or resolve on its own
- **Abdominal Abscess**
  - o Usually in postoperative patient, or following appendicitis, diverticulitis
  - o Loculated, rim-enhancing collection of fluid ± gas
- **Peritonitis**
  - o Often result of infected ascites or bowel perforation
    - − Perforated appendicitis, diverticulitis are most common
- **Renal Pathology**
  - o **Acute pyelonephritis**
    - − Swollen kidney with striated or wedge-shaped foci of heterogeneous enhancement
    - − Infiltrated perirenal fat; thickened, enhancing urothelium
  - o **Renal infarction**
    - − Wedge-shaped or global parenchymal nonenhancement
    - − Cortical rim sign in subacute infarct (enhanced renal capsule)
  - o **Renal cell carcinoma**
    - − Or other large neoplasm (e.g., angiomyolipoma)
    - − Spontaneous hemorrhage may cause abdominal or flank pain
- **Coagulopathic ("Retroperitoneal") Hemorrhage**
  - o Most common sites: Iliopsoas and rectus muscle compartments
    - − Often extends into adjacent retroperitoneal spaces
  - o Look for hematocrit sign, multiple sites of bleeding, active extravasation

- **External Hernias**
  - o **Ventral hernia**
    - − At site of prior laparotomy or laparoscopic incision or port
    - − Herniation of omental fat or bowel may cause focal LLQ pain
  - o **Spigelian hernia**
    - − Through defect in aponeuroses of internal oblique and transverse abdominal muscles
    - − Just lateral to rectus sheath and caudal to umbilicus
    - − External oblique muscle and aponeurosis cover herniated fat ± bowel
  - o **Inguinal hernia**
    - − Herniation and obstruction of descending colon is especially likely to be perceived as LLQ pain
- **Appendicitis**
  - o Appendix may be very long or may arise from malrotated colon, leads to left-sided symptoms
- **Omental Infarct**
  - o Primary omental infarction occurs near **ascending colon**
  - o Secondary form may occur anywhere near site of surgery, infection, radiation, etc.
  - o Heterogeneous fatty mass, larger than epiploic appendagitis
    - − Usually farther removed from surface of colon than for epiploic appendagitis
  - o Usually resolves without specific treatment

SELECTED REFERENCES

1. Singh AK et al: Acute epiploic appendagitis and its mimics. Radiographics. 25(6):1521-34, 2005
2. Horton KM et al: CT findings in sclerosing mesenteritis (panniculitis): spectrum of disease. Radiographics. 23(6):1561-7, 2003
3. Horton KM et al: CT evaluation of the colon: inflammatory disease. Radiographics. 20(2):399-418, 2000

Diverticulitis

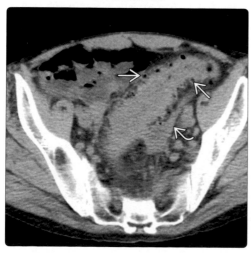

Diverticulitis

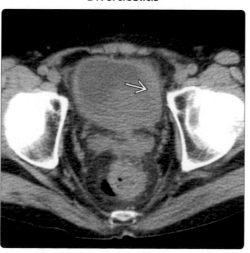

(Left) In this 40-year-old man with left lower quadrant (LLQ) pain, CT shows extensive wall thickening and diverticulosis of the sigmoid colon ➡, and surrounding inflammation, including thickening at the root of the sigmoid mesocolon ➡, indicating diverticulitis. (Right) In this 40-year-old man with diverticulitis, inflammatory thickening of the adjacent wall of the bladder ➡ raises concern for development of a colovesical fistula.

Colon Carcinoma

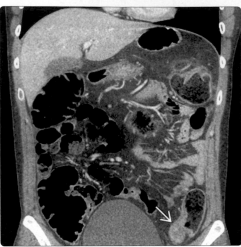

Epiploic Appendagitis

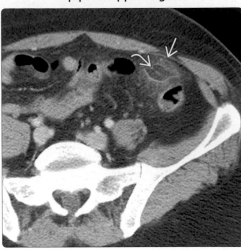

(Left) *Coronal CT shows a grossly dilated colon ending abruptly at an apple core lesion ➡ at the junction of the descending and sigmoid colon.* (Right) *CT shows a small, oval, fat-density lesion ➡ adjacent to the surface of the descending colon. The lesion has a thin, enhanced capsule, and there is a thin linear density in its center ➡ that probably represents the thrombosed vein at the center of an infarcted epiploic appendage.*

Infectious Colitis

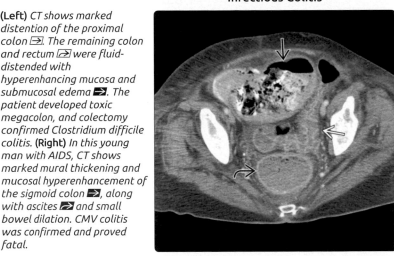

Infectious Colitis

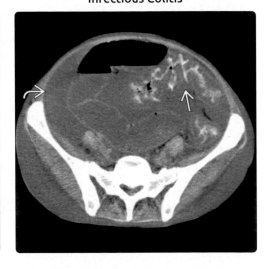

(Left) *CT shows marked distention of the proximal colon ➡. The remaining colon and rectum ➡ were fluid-distended with hyperenhancing mucosa and submucosal edema ➡. The patient developed toxic megacolon, and colectomy confirmed Clostridium difficile colitis.* (Right) *In this young man with AIDS, CT shows marked mural thickening and mucosal hyperenhancement of the sigmoid colon ➡, along with ascites ➡ and small bowel dilation. CMV colitis was confirmed and proved fatal.*

Ischemic Colitis

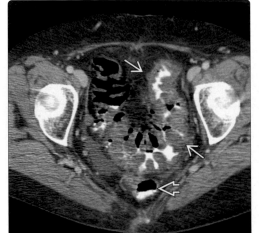

Ulcerative or Crohn Colitis

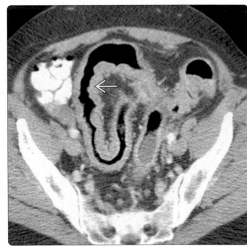

(Left) *This elderly woman with cardiac disease developed acute pain and hematochezia. CT shows marked mural thickening of the sigmoid and descending colon ➡ with sparing of the rectum ➡, typical features of ischemic colitis.* (Right) *Axial CECT shows mural thickening of the sigmoid colon ➡ and loss of normal haustration. This was an acute flare of chronic ulcerative colitis.*

Fecal Impaction/Stercoral Colitis

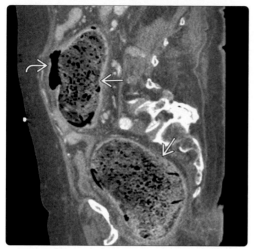

Adnexal Torsion

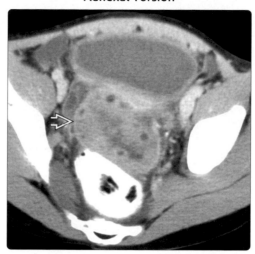

(Left) *This elderly woman with chronic constipation developed acute abdominal pain. Sagittal CT shows massive distention of the rectosigmoid colon with impacted feces ➡. Stercoral ulceration ➡ resulted in perforation of the colon and death.* **(Right)** *Axial CECT shows an enlarged ovary ➡, identified by the presence of normal follicles. The ovary is swollen and poorly enhancing due to torsion and ischemia.*

Endometriosis

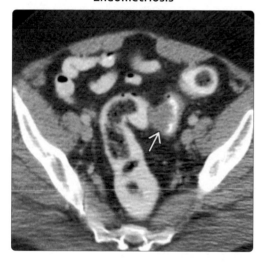

Tuboovarian Abscess

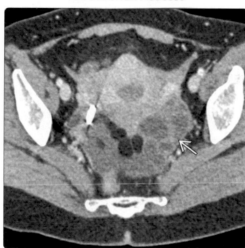

(Left) *Axial CECT shows focal eccentric narrowing and mass effect in the sigmoid colon ➡ simulating colon cancer, later proven to be endometriosis.* **(Right)** *Axial CECT shows a multiloculated tuboovarian abscess ➡ in the left adnexal region in a woman presenting with acute LLQ pain.*

Sigmoid Volvulus

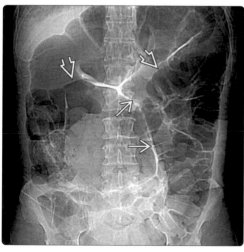

Sigmoid Volvulus

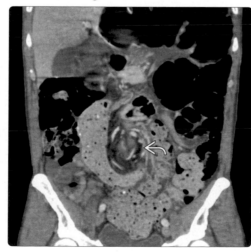

(Left) *In this 59-year-old man, a supine film of the abdomen shows marked dilation of the sigmoid colon, which is folded back upon itself. The apposed walls of the redundant sigmoid colon ➡ form the "seam" of the football (or coffee bean) shape. The sigmoid extends into the upper abdomen above the transverse colon ➡.* **(Right)** *In this 59-year-old man, coronal CT shows dramatic twisting and displacement of the base of the sigmoid colon and its mesentery ➡.*

Sclerosing Mesenteritis

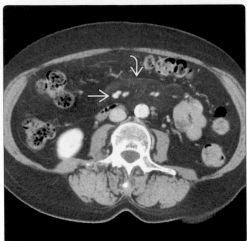

Sclerosing Mesenteritis

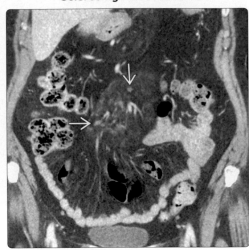

(Left) *In this 69-year-old woman with LLQ pain, CT shows infiltration of the jejunal mesentery, with a spared halo around some vessels and enlarged nodes* ➡. *A thin capsule* ➡ *marks the ventral extent of the jejunal mesenteritis.* (Right) *In this 69-year-old woman, coronal CT shows the infiltrated jejunal mesentery, along with a cluster of enlarged nodes* ➡.

Abdominal Abscess

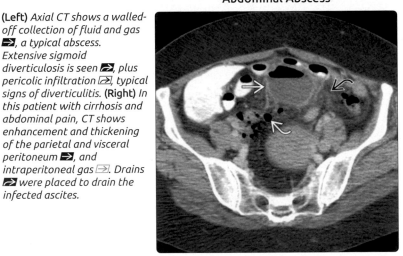

Peritonitis

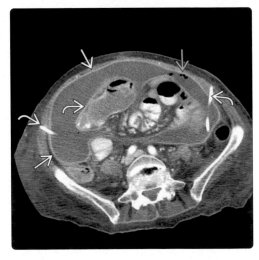

(Left) *Axial CT shows a walled-off collection of fluid and gas* ➡, *a typical abscess. Extensive sigmoid diverticulosis is seen* ➡, *plus pericolic infiltration* ➡, *typical signs of diverticulitis.* (Right) *In this patient with cirrhosis and abdominal pain, CT shows enhancement and thickening of the parietal and visceral peritoneum* ➡, *and intraperitoneal gas* ➡. *Drains* ➡ *were placed to drain the infected ascites.*

Renal Infarction

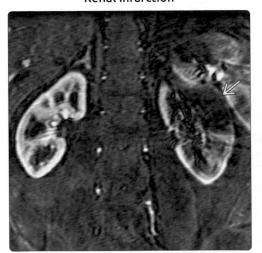

Renal Cell Carcinoma

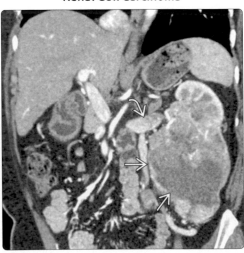

(Left) *In this man with sudden onset of LLQ and flank pain, coronal arterial-phase C+ MR shows no perfusion of the cortex or medulla of most of the upper pole of the left kidney* ➡, *due to spontaneous renal artery dissection.* (Right) *Coronal CECT shows a huge mass* ➡ *arising from and infiltrating the left kidney, with tumor thrombus in the left renal vein* ➡.

Coagulopathic ("Retroperitoneal") Hemorrhage

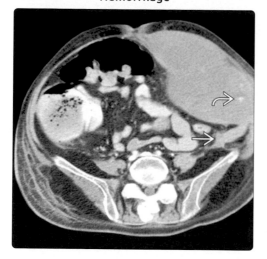

Spigelian Hernia

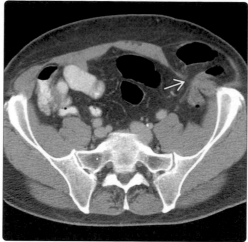

(Left) *Axial CECT shows a massive rectus sheath hematoma with foci of active bleeding* ⮑*, and some extension into the retroperitoneal spaces* ➡*.* (Right) *CT shows herniation of the descending colon through a defect* ➡ *in the aponeurosis of the transverse abdominal and internal oblique muscles, lateral to the rectus sheath.*

Inguinal Hernia

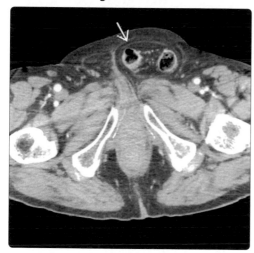

Inguinal Hernia

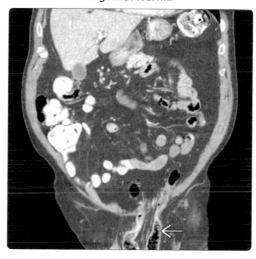

(Left) *Axial CECT shows colon and fat within a large left inguinal hernia* ➡ *that extends into the scrotum.* (Right) *Coronal CECT shows colon* ➡ *and fat within a large left inguinal hernia, extending into the scrotum.*

Ventral Hernia

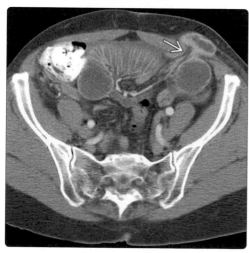

Omental Infarct

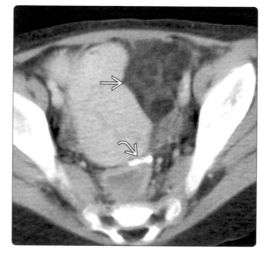

(Left) *This patient developed acute LLQ pain 2 weeks after an uneventful laparoscopic appendectomy. CT shows herniation of a segment of small bowel through one of the laparoscopy ports* ➡*, resulting in small bowel obstruction.* (Right) *Axial CECT shows a mottled fat density mass* ➡ *in the LLQ in an adolescent who had a recent colectomy; note the anastomotic staple line* ➡*. This omental infarct caused local pain, tenderness, and mass effect.*

SECTION 8
Spleen

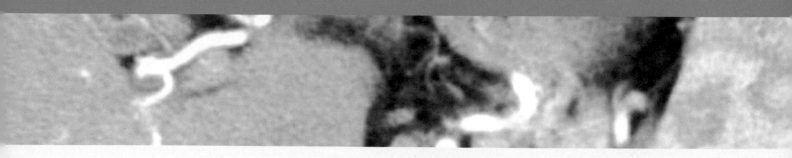

Generic Imaging Patterns

Modality-Specific Imaging Findings

COMPUTED TOMOGRAPHY

Splenomegaly

DIFFERENTIAL DIAGNOSIS

Common

- Cirrhosis With Portal Hypertension
- Congestive Heart Failure
- Hematologic Disorders
  - Hemoglobinopathies
  - Leukemia
  - Myeloproliferative Disorders
  - Myelofibrosis
- Mononucleosis
- AIDS
- Splenic Lymphoma
- Sarcoidosis
- Splenic Trauma
- Systemic Infection and Abscesses
  - Intravenous Drug Abuse

Less Common

- Primary Splenic Tumors and Metastases
- Splenic Vein Occlusion
- Splenic Infarction
- Malaria
- Collagen Vascular Diseases
- Storage Diseases
  - Amyloidosis
  - Glycogen Storage Disease

ESSENTIAL INFORMATION

Key Differential Diagnosis Issues

- Splenomegaly can usually be attributed to 1 of 5 general etiologies
  - Congestion
    - Right heart failure
    - Cirrhosis with portal hypertension
    - Portal or splenic vein thrombosis
  - Hematologic disorders
    - Polycythemia vera
    - Leukemia
    - Myelofibrosis
    - Hemoglobinopathies
    - Acute infarction
  - Inflammatory/infectious
    - Mononucleosis
    - Hepatitis
    - AIDS
    - IV drug abuse
    - Sarcoidosis
    - Collagen vascular disease
    - Malaria
  - Space-occupying masses
    - Cyst
    - Lymphoma and metastases
    - Benign tumors
  - Infiltrative diseases
    - Gaucher disease
    - Diabetes
    - Amyloidosis
    - Glycogen storage disease
    - Hemosiderosis

Helpful Clues for Common Diagnoses

- **Cirrhosis With Portal Hypertension**
  - One of the most common causes of splenomegaly in daily practice
  - Cirrhotic liver morphology (e.g., capsular nodularity, widened fissures, caudate hypertrophy) with stigmata of portal hypertension (e.g., varices, ascites, mesenteric edema, etc.)
  - Punctate foci of low T1 and T2 signal may be present in spleen due to siderotic nodules (Gamna-Gandy bodies)
- **Congestive Heart Failure**
  - Very common cause of splenomegaly in daily practice, usually on basis of right heart failure
  - Associated with imaging features of right-sided cardiac dysfunction (e.g., cardiomegaly, dilated IVC, hepatic veins, reflux of contrast into IVC on arterial phase, etc.)
- **Hematologic Disorders**
  - Wide variety of hematologic disorders can result in splenomegaly, including hemoglobinopathies (e.g., sickle cell disease, thalassemia, spherocytosis), myelofibrosis, polycythemia vera, or leukemia
  - Sickle cell disease is most common and can result in enlarged spleen in acute setting, which gradually shrinks and calcifies due to autoinfarction
  - Look for other imaging findings of hematologic disorders, such as abnormal bones, extramedullary hematopoiesis, etc.
  - Asymptomatic splenomegaly may be only sign of chronic myelogenous leukemia (CML)
  - Myelofibrosis and CML, in particular, are known for producing massive splenomegaly
- **Mononucleosis**
  - Acute infection with Ebstein-Barr virus very common cause of splenomegaly in young adolescents
  - May be associated with lymphadenopathy, including in upper abdomen, as well as mild symptomatology (sore throat, fever)
  - Can rarely result in splenic rupture (either spontaneous or after minimal trauma)
- **AIDS**
  - Spleen commonly enlarged due to chronic viremia or opportunistic infection
  - Close attention must be paid to concurrent lymphadenopathy, as splenomegaly may also result from lymphoma (common in AIDS patients)
  - Splenomegaly alone cannot predict whether HIV(+) patient has AIDS
- **Splenic Lymphoma**
  - Lymphoma (non-Hodgkin or Hodgkin) is common cause of splenomegaly and may or may not be associated with discrete lesions
    - Most common pattern is splenomegaly with diffuse infiltration and no focal mass
    - Splenomegaly can also be associated with innumerable tiny miliary lesions or discrete hypodense masses
    - Spleen may harbor lymphoma (or leukemia) without splenomegaly, and splenomegaly in lymphoma patient does not necessarily always suggest lymphomatous involvement

- **Sarcoidosis**
  - Splenic involvement generally manifests as mild splenomegaly, sometimes with innumerable small hypodense nodules (on CT, US, or MR)
  - Other ancillary imaging features include hepatomegaly, similar small hypodense hepatic lesions, upper abdominal lymphadenopathy (especially periportal nodes), and thoracic involvement (mediastinal and hilar lymphadenopathy, lung involvement)
  - Think of this diagnosis in completely asymptomatic patient with mildly enlarged spleen and multiple small splenic/liver nodules
- **Splenic Trauma**
  - Typically not diagnostic dilemma on CT, but splenic trauma with perisplenic hematoma may be misinterpreted as splenomegaly on plain radiography or ultrasound
- **Systemic Infection and Abscesses**
  - Spleen is often enlarged in patients with persistent bacteremia or viremia (e.g., IV drug users, patients with hepatitis, sepsis)
  - IV drug abusers commonly have mild splenomegaly, probably on basis of chronic, low-level sepsis from injections

Helpful Clues for Less Common Diagnoses

- **Primary Splenic Tumors and Metastases**
  - Primary splenic tumors encompass broad range of benign (hemangioma, lymphangioma, hamartoma, etc.) and malignant (e.g., angiosarcoma) lesions, which are often not easily distinguishable based on imaging
  - Splenic metastases relatively uncommon, especially in absence of metastatic disease elsewhere
  - Space-occupying masses in spleen (primary tumors or metastases) very uncommonly produce splenomegaly, instead usually replacing splenic parenchyma.
- **Splenic Vein Occlusion**
  - Splenomegaly probably occurs on basis of splenic congestion secondary to impaired outflow via splenic vein

- Spleen often will demonstrate heterogeneous enhancement and sometimes may develop frank splenic infarct
- Most common causes are chronic pancreatitis and pancreatic adenocarcinoma in tail
- **Splenic Infarction**
  - Acute infarction can result in splenic enlargement, although conversely, splenomegaly from any etiology does predispose to splenic infarction
  - Chronic focal or global splenic infarction leads to volume loss and scarring in spleen
- **Malaria**
  - Splenomegaly is often impressive feature of malarial infection
  - Repetitive bouts of malaria can result in massive splenomegaly due to abnormal immune response (hyperreactive malarial splenomegaly)
  - Very common cause of splenomegaly worldwide but uncommon in western world
- **Collagen Vascular Diseases**
  - Variety of collagen vascular diseases (e.g., rheumatoid arthritis, scleroderma, dermatomyositis, polyarteritis) can result in splenomegaly
  - Felty syndrome: Rheumatoid arthritis, splenomegaly, and granulocytopenia
    - Splenectomy may be required to treat hypersplenism that causes low white blood cell or platelet count
- **Storage Diseases**
  - **Amyloidosis**
    - Metabolic disease associated with deposition of abnormal proteins in 1 or more organs
    - May be primary or associated with other diseases (multiple myeloma, lymphoma, osteomyelitis, rheumatoid arthritis)
    - Often causes hepatosplenomegaly
  - **Glycogen storage disease**
    - Many related metabolic diseases, all caused by enzymatic defect that alters metabolism of glycogen, resulting in its storage in various tissues

Cirrhosis With Portal Hypertension

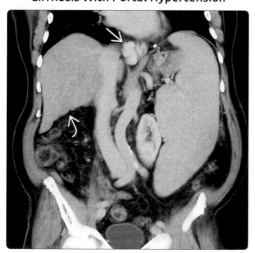

Cirrhosis With Portal Hypertension

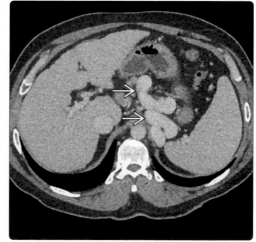

(**Left**) *Coronal volume-rendered CECT demonstrates a mildly cirrhotic liver with nodularity ⬈ along its undersurface. Notice the enlarged spleen, as well as paraesophageal varices ➡, features of portal hypertension.* (**Right**) *Axial CECT demonstrates a cirrhotic liver with capsular nodularity and widened fissures, as well as mild splenomegaly and upper abdominal varices ➡ due to portal hypertension. Portal hypertension is one of the most common causes of splenomegaly in daily practice.*

Cirrhosis With Portal Hypertension

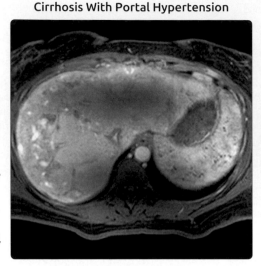

Hematologic Disorders

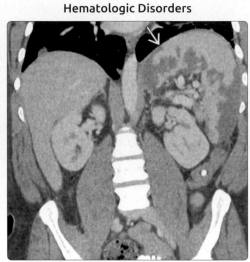

(Left) *Axial T2 FS MR demonstrates an unusual-appearing liver with differential signal between the periphery and center secondary to chronic Budd-Chiari syndrome. The spleen is mildly enlarged with small T2 hypointense foci, representing Gamna-Gandy bodies due to portal hypertension.* (Right) *Coronal CECT in a young patient with sickle cell disease demonstrates a mildly enlarged spleen ➡ with multiple splenic infarcts. Over time, sickle cell patients can demonstrate a small, calcified, autoinfarcted spleen.*

Hematologic Disorders

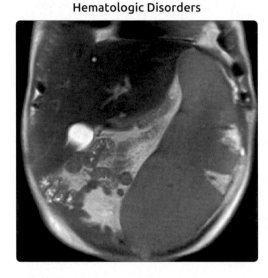

Hematologic Disorders

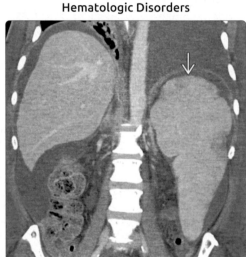

(Left) *Coronal T2 MR demonstrates a massively enlarged spleen in a patient with myelodysplastic syndrome.* (Right) *Coronal CECT demonstrates an enlarged, heterogeneous spleen ➡ in a patient with myelofibrosis.*

Mononucleosis

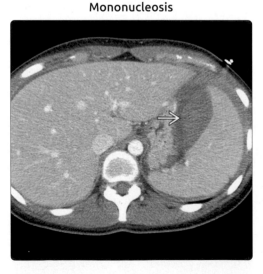

Splenic Lymphoma

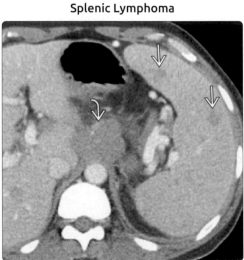

(Left) *Axial CECT demonstrates an enlarged spleen with no apparent parenchymal lesion but with surrounding high-density hematoma ➡. These findings reflect spontaneous splenic rupture due to mononucleosis infection.* (Right) *Axial CECT demonstrates splenomegaly with subtle, low-density lesions ➡ throughout the spleen, as well as gastrohepatic ligament bulky lymphadenopathy ➡, all of which is secondary to diffuse large B-cell lymphoma.*

Splenic Lymphoma

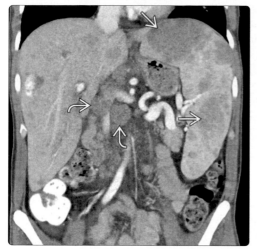

Splenic Lymphoma

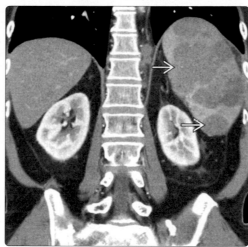

(Left) *Coronal CECT demonstrates splenomegaly with multiple hypodense, discrete splenic masses* ➡, *as well as extensive abdominal lymphadenopathy* ➡. *These findings were found to be secondary to Hodgkin lymphoma.* **(Right)** *Coronal CECT demonstrates mild splenic enlargement with multiple hypodense splenic masses* ➡ *in a patient with diffuse large B-cell lymphoma.*

Sarcoidosis

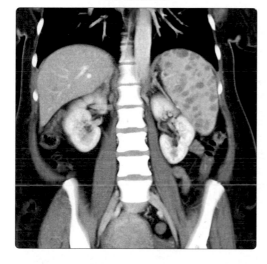

Splenic Vein Occlusion

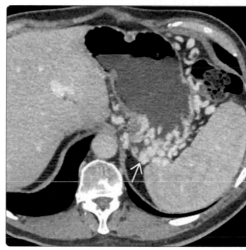

(Left) *Coronal volume-rendered CECT demonstrates mild splenomegaly with multiple low-density lesions in the spleen. The patient was asymptomatic, and this was found to be a manifestation of sarcoidosis.* **(Right)** *Axial CECT demonstrates mild splenomegaly with extensive isolated perigastric and intragastric varices* ➡. *These findings were found to be secondary to splenic vein occlusion due to a pancreatic tail ductal adenocarcinoma (not shown).*

Splenic Infarction

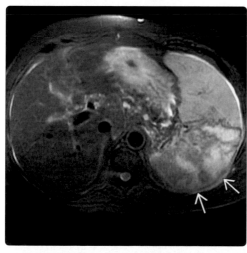

Splenic Infarction

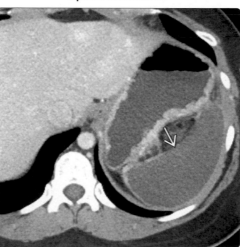

(Left) *Axial T2 FS MR demonstrates splenomegaly with a large T2 hyperintense splenic infarct* ➡. **(Right)** *Axial CECT demonstrates a diffusely low-density spleen* ➡ *secondary to global infarction.*

DIFFERENTIAL DIAGNOSIS

Common

- Healed Granulomatous Infection
- Sarcoidosis
- Vascular Abnormalities
- *Pneumocystis carinii*
- Splenic Infarction
- Splenic Cyst

Less Common

- Echinococcal (Hydatid) Cyst
- Healed Splenic Abscess
- Splenic Hematoma
- Primary Splenic Neoplasms
- Systemic Lupus Erythematosus

ESSENTIAL INFORMATION

Key Differential Diagnosis Issues

- Punctate splenic calcifications usually attributable to healed granulomatous disease (histoplasmosis, TB, etc.)

Helpful Clues for Common Diagnoses

- **Healed Granulomatous Infection**
  - Most common cause of punctate splenic calcifications is healed granulomatous infection (histoplasmosis, TB, brucellosis, toxoplasmosis, candidiasis, fungal infections)
  - **Histoplasmosis** is probably most common cause (in USA) for multiple (> 6), small, rounded calcifications
    - Calcifications with histoplasmosis tend to be larger and more numerous compared to other granulomatous infections
    - Similar calcifications in liver, lung, and thoracic lymph nodes may be present
  - **Tuberculosis** usually does not produce as many calcified granulomas as with histoplasmosis
    - May be associated with calcifications of liver, adrenal glands, and mesenteric nodes
  - **Brucellosis** may produce very large focal calcifications (> 1 cm) or rim-calcified lesions with lucent center

- **Sarcoidosis**
  - Small discrete hypodense nodules may be seen in spleen (&/or liver) in earlier stages of disease, which evolve chronically into punctate calcifications
- **Vascular Abnormalities (Mimic)**
  - Atherosclerosis may cause parallel (tram-track) splenic artery calcification, which simulate splenic calcifications
  - Splenic artery aneurysm may produce rounded eggshell calcifications near splenic hilum
- *Pneumocystis carinii*
  - *P. carinii* pneumonia infection can result in multiple tiny calcifications throughout spleen &/or liver
- **Splenic Infarction**
  - Splenic infarcts can result in splenic parenchymal scarring with peripheral subcapsular calcification or triangular calcification with apex pointed toward center of spleen
  - Sickle cell disease results in autoinfarcted spleen, which is small and diffusely calcified after multiple infarctions
- **Splenic Cyst**
  - Can demonstrate thin, peripheral eggshell calcification or thick, irregular peripheral calcification, both of which are more common with acquired cysts

Helpful Clues for Less Common Diagnoses

- **Echinococcal (Hydatid) Cyst**
  - Hydatid cysts are less frequent in spleen compared to liver or peritoneal cavity but may demonstrate either peripheral calcification or wavy, serpiginous internal calcification in chronic setting
- **Healed Splenic Abscess**
  - Any form of splenic infection may heal with calcified scar
- **Splenic Hematoma**
  - Old, resolved sites of intrasplenic hematoma may result in parenchymal calcification
- **Primary Splenic Neoplasms**
  - Lymphangiomas and hemangiomas may demonstrate calcification and may be multiple
- **Systemic Lupus Erythematosus**
  - May rarely be associated with multiple discrete splenic calcifications (which can be quite extensive)

Healed Granulomatous Infection

Healed Granulomatous Infection

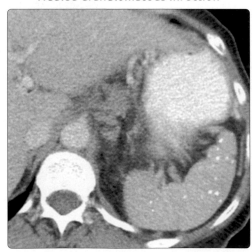

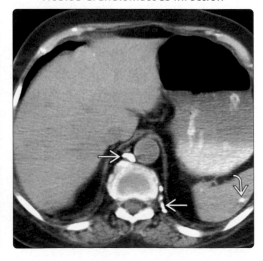

(Left) *Axial CECT demonstrates multiple punctate calcifications in the spleen, almost certainly on the basis of a healed granulomatous infection. The most common cause of such calcifications in the USA is histoplasmosis.* **(Right)** *Axial NECT shows several punctate splenic calcified granulomas* ➡ *in an elderly woman who also had calcified abdominal nodes* ➡ *and renal and adrenal lesions (not shown) from TB.*

Sarcoidosis

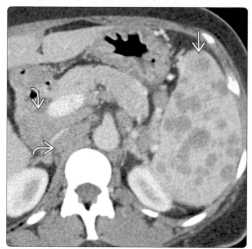

Vascular Abnormalities

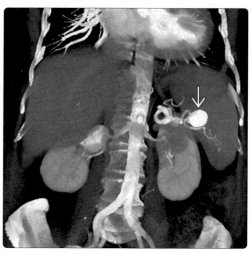

(Left) *Axial CECT in a patient with sarcoidosis demonstrates multiple small hypodense nodules* ➡ *in the spleen, as well as enlarged portacaval lymph nodes* ➡. *Multiple splenic calcifications may be seen in the more chronic setting of sarcoidosis.* **(Right)** *Coronal volume-rendered CECT demonstrates a splenic artery aneurysm* ➡ *projecting over the spleen in the left upper quadrant. While the diagnosis is obvious on CT, this could conceivably be mistaken for a splenic calcification on plain radiographs.*

Vascular Abnormalities

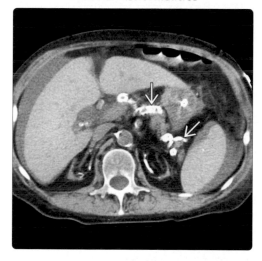

Splenic Infarction

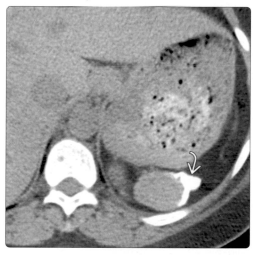

(Left) *Axial NECT shows extensive arterial atherosclerotic calcifications, including the splenic artery* ➡, *in an elderly male patient with type 1 diabetes mellitus. Note the characteristic tram-track linear configuration of these arterial calcifications.* **(Right)** *Axial CECT in a patient with sickle cell disease demonstrates a small atrophic spleen with thick subcapsular calcification* ➡ *as a result of multiple prior episodes of splenic infarction.*

Splenic Cyst

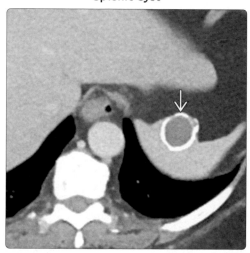

Echinococcal (Hydatid) Cyst

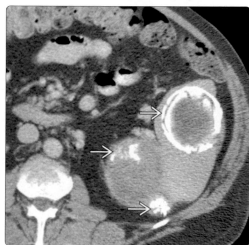

(Left) *Axial CECT demonstrates a splenic cyst* ➡ *with thick peripheral calcification. Calcification is more common in acquired splenic cysts (compared to congenital splenic cysts).* **(Right)** *Axial CECT shows multiple low-density lesions* ➡ *in the spleen, some of which have calcified walls, representing hydatid cysts in an elderly man who had similar lesions in his liver and peritoneal cavity.*

DIFFERENTIAL DIAGNOSIS

Common

- Splenic Metastases and Lymphoma
- Splenic Trauma (Mimic)
- Splenic Infarction (Mimic)
- Perfusion Artifact (Mimic)

Less Common

- Sarcoidosis
- Splenic Infection and Abscess
- Primary Splenic Tumors
- Splenic Peliosis

ESSENTIAL INFORMATION

Key Differential Diagnosis Issues

- Most solid splenic masses are benign, incidental findings that require no further evaluation or follow-up
- Given nonspecific features of most masses, suspicious lesions (based on imaging or clinical features) may require biopsy or splenectomy for diagnosis

Helpful Clues for Common Diagnoses

- **Splenic Metastases and Lymphoma**
  - Splenic metastases are almost always present in setting of widespread metastatic disease; isolated splenic metastases are exceedingly uncommon
    - Most common primary tumors are breast, lung, ovary, stomach, and melanoma
  - Lymphoma most common splenic malignancy: Usually secondary (with disease elsewhere) rather than primary
    - Imaging patterns include dominant solitary mass, multiple discrete lesions, innumerable tiny nodules, or splenomegaly without discrete lesions
    - Lesions usually solid, hypoenhancing, and homogeneous without necrosis or calcification
- **Splenic Trauma (Mimic)**
  - Intrasplenic hematoma could mimic hyperdense mass
  - Clinical history, presence of splenic laceration, and perisplenic hematoma should suggest correct diagnosis

- **Splenic Infarction (Mimic)**
  - Splenic infarct typically appears as wedge-shaped area of hypoperfusion extending to capsule but rarely appears rounded or mass-like mimicking hypodense mass
- **Perfusion Artifact (Mimic)**
  - Heterogeneous splenic enhancement (moire pattern) on arterial-phase images can mimic mass but should disappear on venous/delayed images

Helpful Clues for Less Common Diagnoses

- **Sarcoidosis**
  - Hepatosplenomegaly with multiple small hypoenhancing nodules in liver and spleen
  - Often associated with upper abdominal and thoracic lymphadenopathy ± sarcoid-related lung findings
- **Splenic Infection and Abscess**
  - Fungal microabscesses (usually in immunocompromised or HIV/AIDS patients) appear as multiple small hypodense nodules (usually just a few mm)
- **Primary Splenic Tumors**
  - Most primary splenic tumors are incidental findings, and specific diagnosis may not be possible based on imaging
  - Most common benign splenic masses include hemangioma, lymphangioma, and hamartoma
    - Hemangioma demonstrates prominent peripheral vascularity with delayed enhancement, lymphangioma appears primarily cystic, and hamartoma is nonspecific solid isoattenuating mass
  - Most common primary malignancies of spleen are lymphoma and angiosarcoma
    - Angiosarcoma is aggressive malignancy with propensity for bleeding
      - Lesions may superficially resemble hemangiomas with frequent necrotic degeneration ± calcification
- **Splenic Peliosis**
  - Very rare entity (more often reported in liver) characterized by multiple blood-filled spaces in spleen
    - Usually associated with anabolic steroids, hematologic disorders, and chronic diseases (e.g., TB, AIDS)
  - Usually appears as multiple small hypoattenuating lesions on CT/MR ± internal hematocrit levels

(Left) Axial CECT demonstrates extensive hypodense masses replacing nearly the entire spleen, representing metastatic melanoma in this patient with extensive metastatic disease elsewhere. (Right) Axial CECT demonstrates multiple homogeneous, hypodense, solid masses throughout the spleen, as well as more subtle hypodense lesions in the liver ⮡, found to represent lymphoma. Note the presence of associated gastrohepatic ligament lymphadenopathy ➡.

Splenic Metastases and Lymphoma

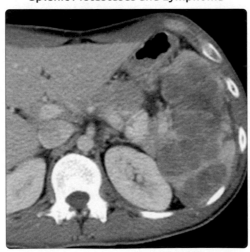

Splenic Metastases and Lymphoma

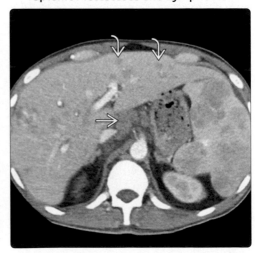

Solid Splenic Mass or Masses

Splenic Trauma (Mimic)

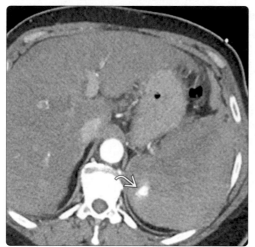

Splenic Infarction (Mimic)

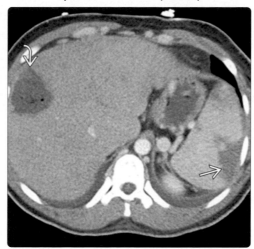

(Left) *Axial CECT in a trauma patient demonstrates a large hyperdense splenic hematoma replacing nearly the entire spleen with a focus of active extravasation ➰. **(Right)** Axial CECT in a patient after Whipple procedure demonstrates wedge-shaped infarcts ➔ in the spleen, as well as an infarct in the liver ➔, thought to be on the basis of septic emboli.*

Perfusion Artifact (Mimic)

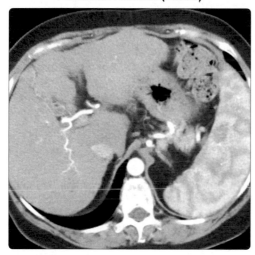

Sarcoidosis

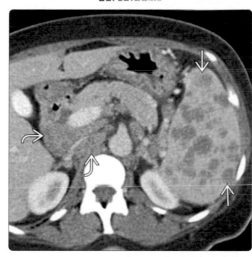

(Left) *Axial CECT shows heterogeneous enhancement of the spleen, a common normal variant on arterial-phase CECT, especially in patients such as this who have cirrhosis and portal hypertension. The spleen appeared normal on portal venous-phase CECT. **(Right)** Axial CECT in an asymptomatic patient being imaged for unrelated reasons demonstrates multiple small hypodense solid nodules ➔ in the spleen, as well as extensive upper abdominal lymphadenopathy ➔, found to represent sarcoidosis.*

Splenic Infection and Abscess

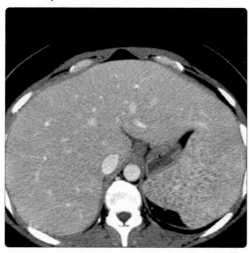

Primary Splenic Tumors

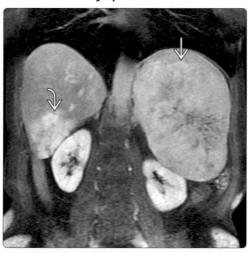

(Left) *Axial CECT shows innumerable small hypodense foci in the spleen and, more subtly, in the liver. Both the liver and spleen are enlarged. These finding were found to reflect mycobacterial infection. **(Right)** Coronal T1 C+ MR demonstrates a large, heterogeneous, enhancing splenic mass ➔ found to represent a primary splenic angiosarcoma. Note the presence of an enhancing metastasis ➔ in the liver, the most common location for metastatic disease in this aggressive malignancy.*

DIFFERENTIAL DIAGNOSIS

Common

- Splenic Cyst
- Splenic Trauma
- Splenic Infarction

Less Common

- Splenic Metastases and Lymphoma
- Splenic Infection and Abscess
- Splenic Tumors
- Pancreatic Pseudocyst

ESSENTIAL INFORMATION

Key Differential Diagnosis Issues

- While most cystic lesions of spleen are benign, metastases and lymphoma can appear low density/cystic

Helpful Clues for Common Diagnoses

- **Splenic Cyst**
  - Can be congenital (i.e., true epidermoid cyst) or acquired (e.g., trauma, infection, infarction, hematoma, etc.)
  - Usually incidental finding but can rarely be symptomatic due to size and mass effect
  - Can be entirely simple in appearance or demonstrate internal septations, necrotic debris, or peripheral calcification (either thin/eggshell or thick/irregular)
    - Should not have solid or enhancing components
  - Congenital and acquired cysts may be indistinguishable, but calcification is more common in acquired cysts
- **Splenic Trauma**
  - Acute intrasplenic hematoma is typically hyperdense on CT and may be associated with splenic laceration
  - Chronic hematoma may appear low density/cystic, while associated laceration may no longer be apparent
- **Splenic Infarction**
  - Typical appearance is wedge-shaped area of hypoperfusion at periphery of spleen but can rarely appear rounded or mass-like (and mimic cyst)

- Can evolve over time into cystic lesion, usually with immediately adjacent parenchymal scarring

Helpful Clues for Less Common Diagnoses

- **Splenic Metastases and Lymphoma**
  - Splenic metastases are rare and almost always associated with metastatic disease elsewhere
    - Isolated metastases to spleen extremely uncommon
    - Some malignancies may produce low density or cystic metastases, including melanoma, breast cancer, ovarian cancer, and endometrial cancer
  - Splenic lymphoma usually secondary (with additional disease elsewhere) rather than primary
    - Can appear as solitary dominant mass, multiple discrete lesions, innumerable tiny nodules, or splenomegaly without discrete lesions
    - Lesions typically homogeneously hypovascular on CT and can be confused for cysts
- **Splenic Infection and Abscess**
  - Pyogenic abscesses may occur due to bacteremia, septic emboli, or infection of hematoma/infarct
    - Cystic mass with thick wall ± air-fluid levels or gas
    - Less often multiloculated compared to liver abscesses
  - Echinococcal cysts are very rare in USA but appear as complex cystic masses with internal daughter cysts or internal serpiginous linear densities (water-lily sign)
  - Fungal microabscesses usually in immunocompromised patients and appear as multiple small hypodense lesions (few mm in size)
- **Splenic Tumors**
  - Primary splenic tumors are uncommon, with lymphangiomas and hemangiomas most common
    - Appearance of these lesions extremely variable, and specific diagnosis often not possible based on imaging
  - Lymphangiomas appear as thin-walled, simple-appearing cysts, although other lesions (including hemangiomas) can demonstrate cystic or necrotic components
- **Pancreatic Pseudocyst**
  - Pseudocysts can arise in pancreatic tail and spread into splenic hilum via splenorenal ligament
    - Over time, pseudocyst may invaginate into spleen

(Left) Axial CECT demonstrates a large simple-appearing splenic cyst ➡. In many cases, it is not possible on imaging to differentiate congenital and acquired splenic cysts. (Right) Coronal NECT demonstrates a splenic cyst ➡ with thick peripheral calcification. Splenic calcifications are more common in acquired splenic cysts but may be seen in congenital cysts as well.

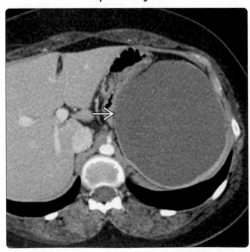

Splenic Cyst

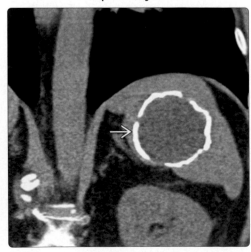

Splenic Cyst

Splenic Infarction

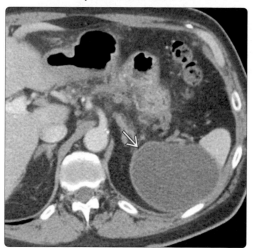

Splenic Metastases and Lymphoma

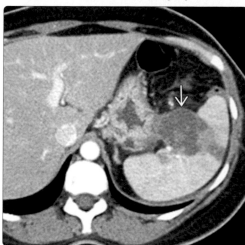

(Left) Axial CECT demonstrates a well-defined cyst ➡ in the spleen resulting from a splenic infarct a few weeks earlier. (Right) Axial CECT demonstrates a low-density mass ➡ involving the spleen and splenic hilum, representing a metastasis in this patient with metastatic ovarian cancer. Ovarian cancer is one of several malignancies (such as breast cancer, endometrial cancer, and melanoma) whose metastases can appear low density or even cystic.

Splenic Metastases and Lymphoma

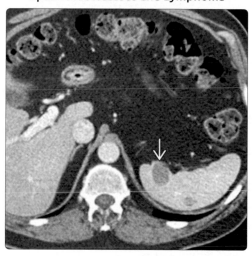

Splenic Infection and Abscess

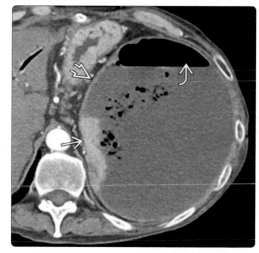

(Left) Axial CECT demonstrates a low-density lesion ➡ in the spleen, which could superficially be mistaken for a cyst. However, the lesion was new in a patient with lymphoma and represented splenic lymphoma. (Right) Axial CECT performed after splenic embolization demonstrates only a small amount of residual enhancing splenic parenchyma ➡, with the rest of the spleen replaced by a large thick-walled fluid collection ➡ containing a large amount of gas ➡ (and air-fluid level), compatible with a splenic abscess.

Splenic Tumors

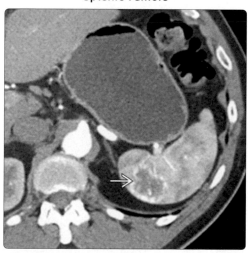

Pancreatic Pseudocyst

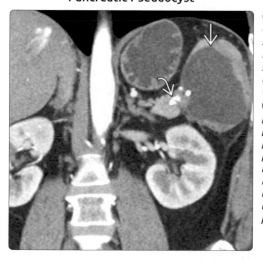

(Left) Axial CECT in the arterial phase demonstrates a splenic mass ➡ with a hypodense center and significant peripheral enhancement, compatible with a splenic hemangioma. (Right) Coronal CECT in a patient with prior history of pancreatitis demonstrates a pseudocyst ➡ in the pancreatic tail directly invaginating into the spleen. Note the calcifications ➡ in the pancreatic tail, revealing the patient's history of chronic pancreatitis.

DIFFERENTIAL DIAGNOSIS

Common

- Secondary Hemochromatosis
- Splenic Infarction
  - Sickle Cell Anemia

Less Common

- Opportunistic Infection
- Thorotrast
- Systemic Lupus Erythematosus

ESSENTIAL INFORMATION

Key Differential Diagnosis Issues

- Spleen is often used as reference standard on CT and MR by which to recognize liver pathology
  - Splenic attenuation not typically altered by metabolic processes (other than calcification and iron deposition)
- MDCT
  - Normal attenuation of spleen on NECT is roughly 10 HU lower than liver
- MR
  - Normal spleen typically demonstrates signal lower than liver and slightly greater than muscle on T1WI
  - Normal spleen typically demonstrates higher signal than liver on T2WI

Helpful Clues for Common Diagnoses

- **Secondary Hemochromatosis**
  - Primary hemochromatosis is inherited autosomal recessive disorder resulting in increased absorption of dietary iron
    - Involved organs include heart, liver, and pancreas
    - Primary hemochromatosis **does not** result in abnormal spleen MR signal or density
  - Secondary hemochromatosis (i.e., hemosiderosis) results from frequent blood transfusions, hemoglobinopathies, portacaval shunt, etc.

- Results in deposition of iron in reticuloendothelial system, including spleen, liver, and bone marrow without associated end-organ damage
- CT shows increased attenuation of liver and spleen, although CT is much less sensitive for mild degrees of iron deposition compared to MR
- MR shows decreased signal intensity in liver (± spleen) relative to muscle on both T1WI and T2WI, as well as signal loss of affected organs on in-phase GRE images (compared to out-of-phase)
  - □ Superparamagnetic effects of iron lead to shortening of T1, T2, and T2*, resulting in signal loss directly proportional to degree of iron deposition

- **Splenic Infarction**
  - Hemoglobinopathies and other causes of splenic infarction can result in segmental or subcapsular infarction, which may calcify
  - Sickle cell anemia results in repeated episodes of splenic infarctions, which by adulthood can result in small, diffusely calcified spleen (autosplenectomy)

Helpful Clues for Less Common Diagnoses

- **Opportunistic Infection**
  - Healed phase of many splenic infections results in multifocal calcifications (histoplasmosis, mycobacterial diseases, CMV, herpes), which can rarely lead to diffuse calcification of spleen
  - Diffuse calcification most likely to result from *Pneumocystis carinii* infection
  - Look for similar involvement of liver, lymph nodes, and adrenal glands
- **Thorotrast**
  - Intravascular angiographic contrast agent last used in 1950s because of its strongly carcinogenic properties (especially angiosarcoma)
  - Taken up by spleen (and to lesser extent liver) resulting in diffuse hyperdensity of affected organs, as well as parenchymal atrophy and scarring
- **Systemic Lupus Erythematosus**
  - Can result in unique pattern of diffuse splenic calcification (without atrophy)

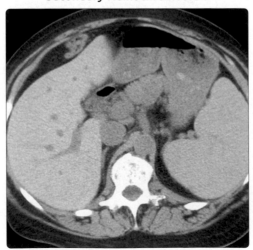

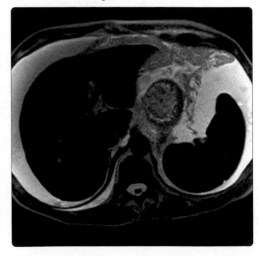

Secondary Hemochromatosis   **Secondary Hemochromatosis**

(Left) Axial NECT shows subtly increased attenuation of both the liver and spleen in this patient who had received multiple transfusions because of multiple myeloma. (Right) Axial T2 MR demonstrates diffuse low signal throughout the liver and spleen, both of which demonstrate lower signal than the paraspinal musculature. These findings reflect hemosiderosis on the basis of multiple transfusions. Note the presence of large T2 hyperintense ascites.

Secondary Hemochromatosis

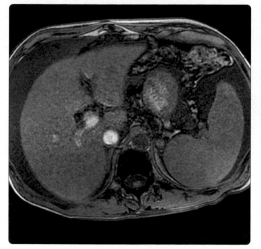

Secondary Hemochromatosis

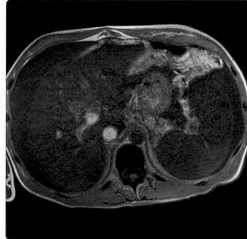

(Left) *Axial out-of-phase GRE in the same patient demonstrates fairly normal signal intensity in both the liver and spleen.* (Right) *Axial in-phase GRE in the same patient demonstrates diffuse loss of signal in both the liver and spleen, another finding consistent with iron deposition in these organs. Note that the pattern of signal loss on these dual-echo images is the opposite of fatty deposition. Unlike steatosis, which results in signal loss on the out-of-phase images, iron results in signal loss on the in-phase images.*

Sickle Cell Anemia

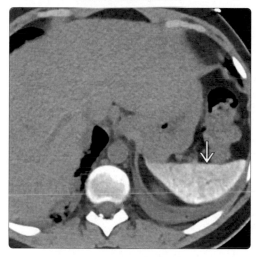

Opportunistic Infection

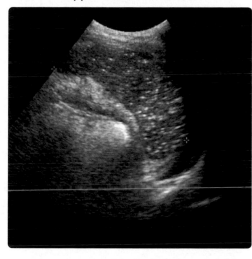

(Left) *Axial NECT in a patient with sickle cell disease demonstrates an atrophic spleen* ➡ *with diffuse calcification, compatible with splenic autoinfarction. This is a relatively common finding in sickle cell patients by adulthood.* (Right) *Transverse ultrasound of the spleen in an HIV/AIDS patient demonstrates extensive echogenic calcifications throughout the spleen, compatible with the patient's history of Pneumocystis carinii pneumonia infection.*

Opportunistic Infection

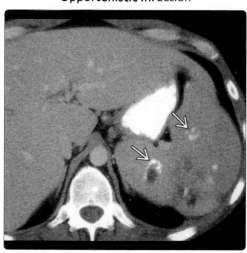

Opportunistic Infection

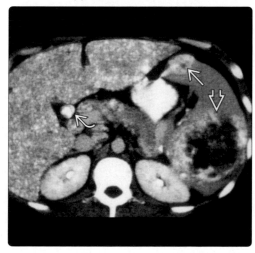

(Left) *Axial CECT in an HIV(+) patient with Pneumocystis pneumonia shows multiple calcifications* ➡ *within the spleen, some of which surround low-density abscesses.* (Right) *Axial CECT shows a more dramatic case of opportunistic infection. There are calcifications* ➡ *and an abscess* ➡ *within the spleen, as well as diffuse punctate calcifications within the liver & lymph nodes* ➡. *The spleen was removed and multiple organisms were cultured, including Pneumocystis.*

SECTION 9
Liver

Generic Imaging Patterns

Modality-Specific Imaging Findings

MAGNETIC RESONANCE IMAGING

COMPUTED TOMOGRAPHY

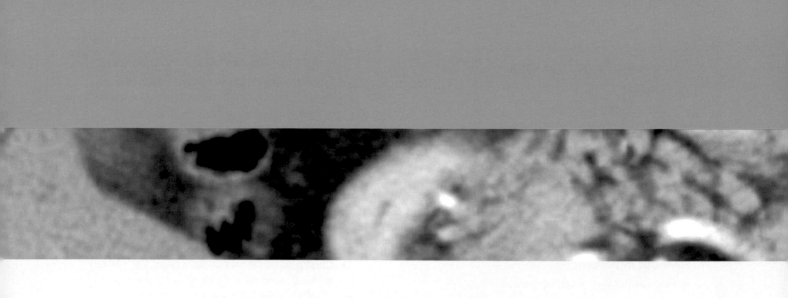

ULTRASOUND

DIFFERENTIAL DIAGNOSIS

Common

- Focal Nodular Hyperplasia
- Hepatic Cavernous Hemangioma

Less Common

- Fibrolamellar (Hepatocellular) Carcinoma
- Hepatocellular Carcinoma
- Cholangiocarcinoma (Intrahepatic, Peripheral)
- Hepatic Adenoma
- Hepatic Metastases
- Epithelioid Hemangioendothelioma

Rare but Important

- Nodular Regenerative Hyperplasia

ESSENTIAL INFORMATION

Key Differential Diagnosis Issues

- Characterize size of scar, pattern of mass enhancement, associated findings
  - Also consider whether this is solitary mass or one of many: Fibrolamellar carcinoma is almost always solitary; cholangiocarcinoma & focal nodular hyperplasia (FNH) are usually solitary; others are commonly multiple

Helpful Clues for Common Diagnoses

- **Focal Nodular Hyperplasia**
  - Larger FNH lesions (> 3 cm) usually have small central scar ± thin radiating septa
  - Homogeneous enhancement of **mass** on arterial phase
    - Isodense (isointense) to liver on all other phases
  - Central **scar** bright on T2WI; shows delayed persistent enhancement on MR and CT
    - Scar will not enhance on delayed gadoxetate (Eovist/Primovist)-enhanced scans
- **Hepatic Cavernous Hemangioma**
  - Large hemangiomas (> 5 cm) commonly have fibrotic scar that may calcify; nonscarred portions of hemangioma have typical nodular enhancement

Helpful Clues for Less Common Diagnoses

- **Fibrolamellar (Hepatocellular) Carcinoma**
  - Large, heterogeneous mass on all phases of imaging
    - Scar is large and often (> 60%) calcified
  - Aggressive signs noted at presentation in > 60%
    - Local invasion (vessels, bile ducts); metastases
- **Hepatocellular Carcinoma**
  - Large tumors, especially in noncirrhotic liver, may resemble fibrolamellar carcinoma
    - Heterogeneous hypervascular mass with washout
    - Central necrosis or scar (scar is rarely calcified in hepatocellular carcinoma)
  - Vascular invasion and metastases are common
- **Cholangiocarcinoma (Intrahepatic, Peripheral)**
  - Focal necrosis or fibrosis may resemble scar
  - Often has extensive fibrous stroma
    - With typical delayed persistent enhancement
  - Overlying capsular retraction, hepatic volume loss
  - Biliary & portal venous obstruction indicate invasive nature of lesion
- **Hepatic Adenoma**
  - Low-density foci due to fat, necrosis, old hemorrhage; not scar
  - Calcification of scar is uncommon
  - Distinction from FNH best made by Eovist-enhanced MR
- **Hepatic Metastases**
  - Target appearance; necrosis, not scar
  - Calcification of necrotic area is rare
    - Calcification can be seen with mucinous carcinoma metastases (e.g., colon, ovarian)
- **Epithelioid Hemangioendothelioma**
  - Multiple, coalescent, peripheral nodules
  - Target appearance; capsular retraction over lesions
- **Nodular Regenerative Hyperplasia**
  - Multiacinar form of nodular regenerative hyperplasia (large regenerative nodules) may have central scar
  - Usually multiple, < 4 cm in diameter
  - Usually in patients with Budd-Chiari syndrome

(Left) Axial CECT shows a homogeneously and brightly enhancing mass ➡ with a central scar ↱ on this arterial-phase image. The mass became isodense with liver on portal venous-phase CT. (Right) A 20-minute delayed, gadoxetate (Eovist)-enhanced MR section shows a large mass ➡ that retains contrast more than underlying liver. The central scar ➡ does not take up nor retain gadoxetate.

Focal Nodular Hyperplasia

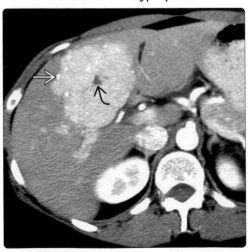

Focal Nodular Hyperplasia

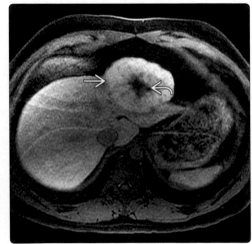

Hepatic Cavernous Hemangioma

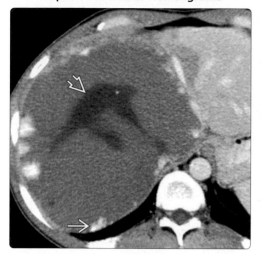

Hepatic Cavernous Hemangioma

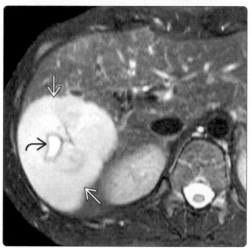

(Left) *Axial CECT shows a large mass with peripheral nodular enhancement ➡ isodense to vessels. A central scar ➡, with a small focus of calcification, did not fill in on delayed imaging. These are typical features of giant hemangiomas.* **(Right)** *Axial T2WI MR demonstrates a large mass ➡ that is very bright and well-defined on T2WI. A central scar ➡ is even more intense, typical of a large cavernous hemangioma.*

Fibrolamellar (Hepatocellular) Carcinoma

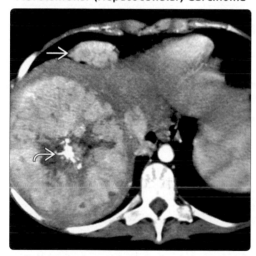

Fibrolamellar (Hepatocellular) Carcinoma

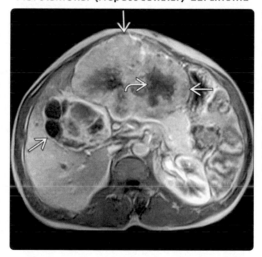

(Left) *Axial CECT shows a heterogeneous hypervascular mass with a large calcified central scar ➡ in a 22-year-old man. Note the similar enhancement of tumor in a cardiophrenic node ➡.* **(Right)** *In this 20-year-old man, MR shows a large, lobulated, encapsulated mass ➡ with a prominent central scar ➡. CT had shown focal calcifications less evident on MR.*

Hepatocellular Carcinoma

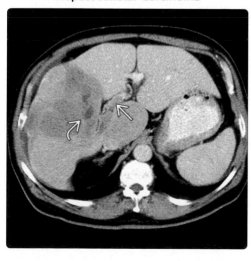

Hepatocellular Carcinoma

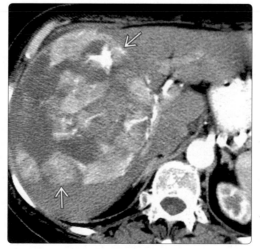

(Left) *Axial CECT shows a large mass with an eccentric scar ➡ or necrotic area. Tumor invasion of portal vein ➡ helps to identify this as hepatocellular carcinoma.* **(Right)** *In this elderly woman, arterial phase CT shows a large, heterogeneous, hypervascular mass ➡ with foci of necrosis, giving it a mottled or mosaic appearance. The age of the patient and absence of calcification favored conventional, as opposed to fibrolamellar HCC, confirmed on biopsy.*

Cholangiocarcinoma (Intrahepatic, Peripheral)

Cholangiocarcinoma (Intrahepatic, Peripheral)

(Left) *Axial CECT shows a large hepatic mass with foci of scar or necrosis ➡. Capsular retraction and occlusion of the portal vein ➡ and bile duct ➡ help confirm cholangiocarcinoma.* (Right) *CT shows a large mass ➡ in the liver with heterogeneous enhancement. The intrahepatic bile ducts are dilated ➡ and there is marked retraction of the liver capsule ➡. Delayed phase (not shown) showed persistent hyperdense enhancement of most of the tumor.*

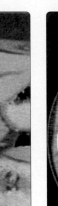
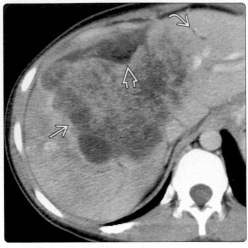

Hepatic Adenoma

Hepatic Adenoma

(Left) *Axial NECT shows a heterogeneous mass in the left lobe. At resection, the focus of high attenuation ➡ was hemorrhage and the lower density foci ➡ were necrosis and fibrosis.* (Right) *In this young woman, an encapsulated mass ➡ was hypervascular and had lipid content demonstrated on opposed-phase GRE images (not shown). The lesion remains diminished in signal intensity and does not retain contrast 20 minutes after the administration of gadoxetate (Eovist), while the normal liver has enhanced markedly.*

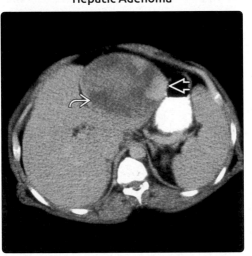
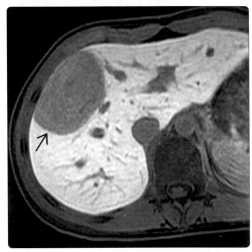

Hepatic Metastases

Hepatic Metastases

(Left) *In this elderly patient with colon cancer, precontrast CT shows multiple lesions with faint central calcification ➡.* (Right) *In this elderly patient with colon cancer, portal venous phase shows multiple metastases ➡ with central, low-density necrosis or fibrosis. The faint calcification is more difficult to recognize on contrast-enhanced imaging.*

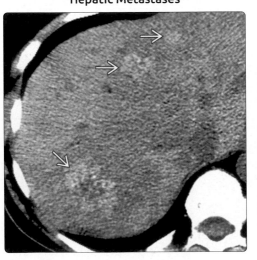
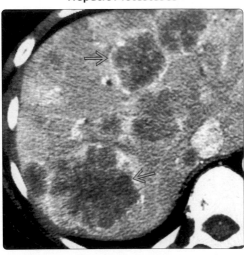

Epithelioid Hemangioendothelioma

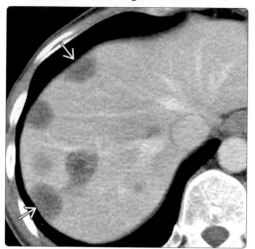

Epithelioid Hemangioendothelioma

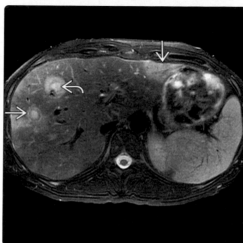

(Left) In this young woman, CECT shows multiple, peripheral hypovascular lesions with a target appearance. The subcapsular lesions are associated with retraction of the overlying liver capsule ➡. (Right) In this young woman, MR showed multiple peripheral & confluent masses ➡, many of which have central necrosis or scar ➡ that is hyperintense on T2WI. These are typical features of hepatic epithelial hemangioendothelioma.

Nodular Regenerative Hyperplasia

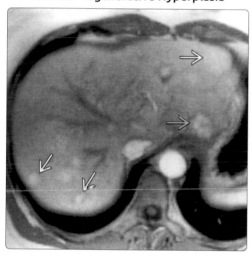

Nodular Regenerative Hyperplasia

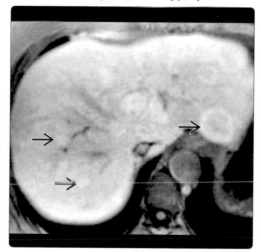

(Left) In this hypercoagulable patient, arterial phase contrast-enhanced MR shows multiple hypervascular foci ➡. Some of the lesions seem to have a hypointense rim while others have a hypointense central scar ➡. (Right) In this hypercoagulable patient, MR imaging 2 hours after IV administration of gadobenate dimeglumine shows persistent uptake and retention of the agent within the nodules ➡, indicating functional hepatocytes and deficient biliary ducts within the lesions.

Nodular Regenerative Hyperplasia

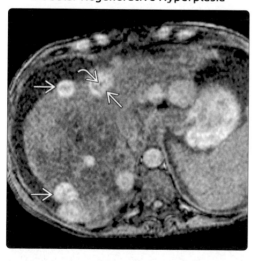

Nodular Regenerative Hyperplasia

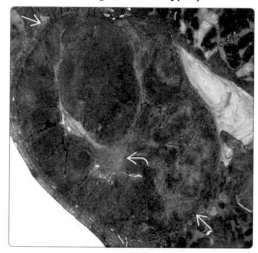

(Left) In this patient with Budd-Chiari syndrome, contrast-enhanced T1W MR shows multiple hypervascular nodules ➡, some of which have a central scar ➡. These multiple, large, regenerative nodules (NRH) confirmed transplantation. (Right) In this patient with Budd-Chiari syndrome and multiple hypervascular nodules, a trichrome stain of a specimen shows green staining of the central scar ➡ & the capsule ➡ of the nodule, typical features of the macroscopic form of NRH or large regenerative nodules.

DIFFERENTIAL DIAGNOSIS

Common

- Hepatic Trauma
- Hepatic Adenoma
- Hepatocellular Carcinoma
- Hepatic Cyst
- Autosomal Dominant Polycystic Disease, Liver

Less Common

- Coagulopathic Hemorrhage, Liver
- Hepatic Metastases
- HELLP Syndrome

ESSENTIAL INFORMATION

Key Differential Diagnosis Issues

- Hemorrhage may be detected as heterogeneous high attenuation (> 60 HU on NECT), or high-intensity foci on T1WI or spin density images, and on T2WI
- Bleeding may include subcapsular & intraperitoneal extension

Helpful Clues for Common Diagnoses

- **Hepatic Trauma**
  - Blunt or penetrating (including biopsies, TIPS, etc.)
  - Hepatic lacerations usually have linear or stellate configuration
- **Hepatic Adenoma**
  - Foci of hemorrhage within tumor is common feature on MR, less common on CT
  - Spontaneous bleeding within or around hepatic mass in young female without cirrhosis is almost diagnostic of adenoma
  - Other signs of adenoma
    - Lipid or fat content
    - Multiplicity
    - Encapsulation
- **Hepatocellular Carcinoma**
  - Spontaneous hemorrhage within tumor is uncommon
  - Spontaneous rupture through capsule is relatively common for large hepatocellular carcinoma (HCC)
  - Other signs of HCC
    - Occurrence within cirrhotic liver
    - Hypervascularity with washout
    - Encapsulation
- **Hepatic Cyst**
  - Isolated or part of autosomal dominant polycystic disease
  - Clotted blood in cyst may be mistaken for tumor but will not show enhancement

Helpful Clues for Less Common Diagnoses

- **Coagulopathic Hemorrhage, Liver**
  - Spontaneous intrahepatic or perihepatic hemorrhage is rare manifestation of coagulopathy or anticoagulant therapy
  - Spherical hematoma within liver may simulate tumor
  - Others signs of coagulopathic hemorrhage
    - Hematocrit sign (fluid level) within hematoma
    - Multiple sites of bleeding
    - Favored sites: Iliopsoas and rectus muscles
- **Hepatic Metastases**
  - Hemorrhage is uncommon, usually associated with hypervascular metastases
  - May occur following chemotherapy or transhepatic ablation of metastatic lesions
- **HELLP Syndrome**
  - Hemolysis, elevated liver enzymes, low platelets
  - Severe variation of toxemia of pregnancy
  - Foci of infarction and bleeding within liver

Hepatic Trauma   **Hepatic Trauma**

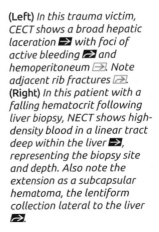
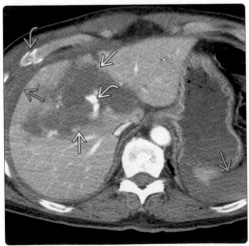
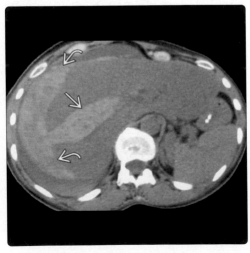

(Left) In this trauma victim, CECT shows a broad hepatic laceration ➡ with foci of active bleeding ➡ and hemoperitoneum ➡. Note adjacent rib fractures ➡. (Right) In this patient with a falling hematocrit following liver biopsy, NECT shows high-density blood in a linear tract deep within the liver ➡, representing the biopsy site and depth. Also note the extension as a subcapsular hematoma, the lentiform collection lateral to the liver ➡.

Hepatic Adenoma

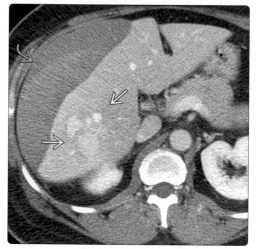

Hepatic Adenoma

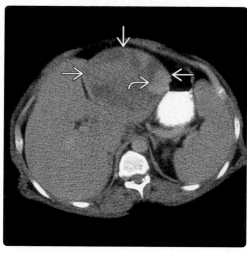

(Left) CECT in a young woman shows a hypervascular mass ➡ in the right lobe with a large, spontaneous subcapsular hematoma ➱. (Right) In this young woman with acute pain, axial NECT shows a mass ➡ in the lateral segment with high-attenuation material ➡ centrally due to an acute hematoma.

Hepatic Adenoma

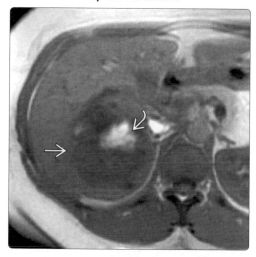

Hepatic Adenoma

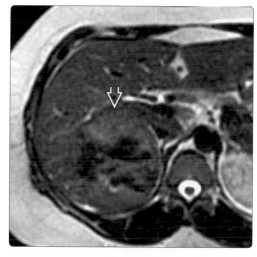

(Left) In this young woman, axial T1W MR shows a hepatic mass ➡ containing several hyperintense foci ➡ that represent hemorrhage. The foci were hyperintense on T2WI as well, distinguishing hemorrhage from fat as the etiology. (Right) In this young woman, other foci are slightly hyperintense on T2WI ➡ but these represent foci with lipid content. The latter foci showed contrast-enhancement on portal venous-phase MR. The presence of hemorrhage & lipid is typical of hepatic adenomas.

Hepatocellular Carcinoma

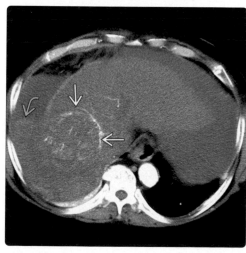

Hepatocellular Carcinoma

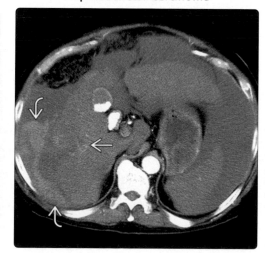

(Left) In this man with cirrhosis & sudden RUQ pain, arterial phase CT shows tumor vessels within a poorly defined, hypervascular mass ➡. Ascites and a sentinel clot ➱ overlying the hepatic mass are seen. Spontaneous rupture of an HCC was the etiology. (Right) In this man with cirrhosis & sudden RUQ pain, arterial phase CECT shows part of the hypervascular mass ➡, as well as the ascites and sentinel clot ➡ overlying the site of the capsular rupture. A catheter angiogram confirmed a bleeding HCC and it was treated with coil embolization.

Hepatocellular Carcinoma

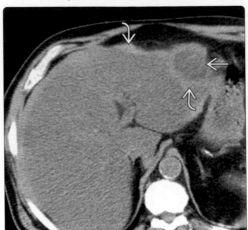

Hepatocellular Carcinoma

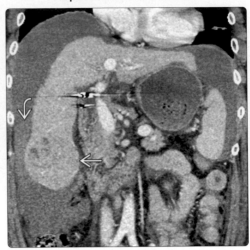

(Left) *In this 60-year-old man with alcoholic liver disease & sudden RUQ pain, NECT shows a hyperdense, sentinel clot* ➡ *within and around the liver, as well as a spherical hepatic mass* ➡. *(Right) In this woman with cirrhosis & sudden RUQ pain, coronal CT shows a heterogeneous, encapsulated mass* ➡ *that was hyperdense on arterial phase. There is generalized ascites, but also a sentinel clot* ➡ *over the mass, indicating the source of bleeding.*

Hepatic Cyst

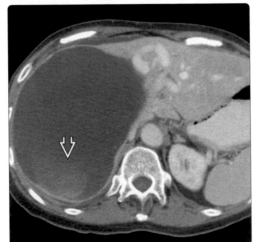

Hepatic Cyst

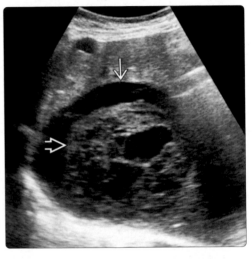

(Left) *CT shows a large mass with a thin wall, characteristic of a simple cyst. Within the cyst is a heterogeneous focus of higher attenuation* ➡, *suggestive of acute hemorrhage. Other sections showed hemorrhagic ascites. (Right) Grayscale sonography shows a hepatic cyst* ➡ *containing a heterogeneous organizing hematoma with fibrin strands* ➡.

Hepatic Cyst

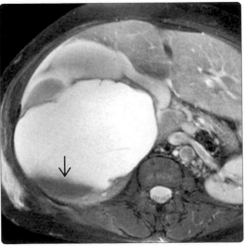

Autosomal Dominant Polycystic Disease, Liver

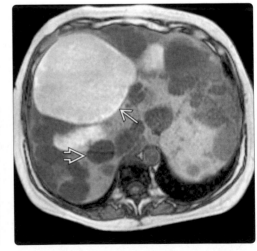

(Left) *Axial fat-suppressed T2WI MR shows a large complex cystic mass with dependent settling of material* ➡ *that is hypointense on T2WI, indicating subacute hemorrhage. (Right) Axial T1WI GRE opposed-phase MR shows many cysts within an enlarged liver. Many of the cysts are of water intensity* ➡ *(dark on this T1WI), while others* ➡ *are bright, due to hemorrhage.*

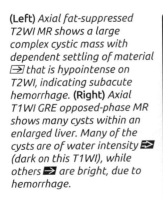

Coagulopathic Hemorrhage, Liver

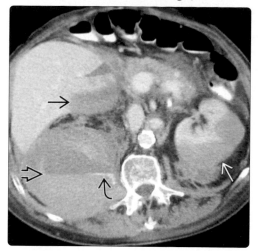

Coagulopathic Hemorrhage, Liver

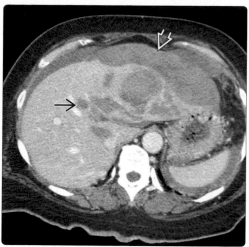

(Left) CT shows signs of coagulopathic hemorrhage, including the hematocrit sign ➾, active bleeding ➔, and multiple sites of bleeding, including hepatic ➾ and renal ➾. (Right) In this patient who was taking anticoagulant medication, CT shows hepatic defects that resemble fracture planes ➾, but there was no history of trauma. A subcapsular hematoma ➾ and hemoperitoneum are also shown. All findings resolved with withdrawal of the medication. No underlying hepatic mass or other pathology was found.

Hepatic Metastases

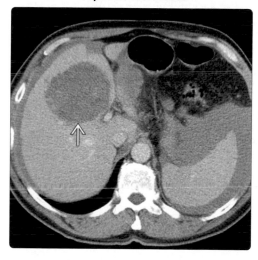

Hepatic Metastases

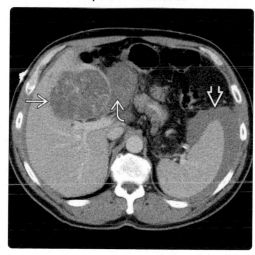

(Left) In this 55-year-old man with melanoma, CT shows metastasis to the liver ➾ that is peculiarly heterogeneous and high density, perhaps indicating bleeding within the metastasis. (Right) In this patient with metastatic melanoma & acute RUQ pain, CT shows an hepatic mass ➔. Immediately adjacent to this metastasis is a heterogeneous sentinel clot ➔ strongly suggesting bleeding from the met. Also noted is an extensive hemoperitoneum ➾ with an attenuation of 35 HU.

HELLP Syndrome

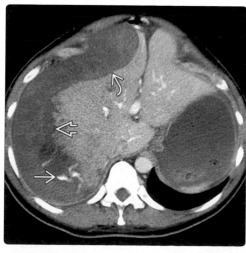

HELLP Syndrome

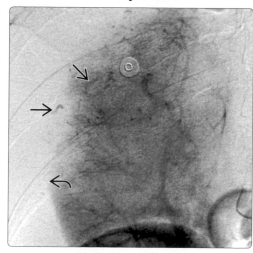

(Left) In this young woman with toxemia & sudden RUQ pain, CT shows a massive subcapsular & perihepatic hematoma ➔, along with active bleeding ➾ & heterogeneous enhancement of the hepatic parenchyma ➾. (Right) In this woman with HELLP & spontaneous bleeding, a selective hepatic arteriogram indirectly shows the subcapsular hematoma ➾ as the liver is displaced medially. It also shows multiple foci of active hemorrhage ➾, which were treated with coil embolization.

DIFFERENTIAL DIAGNOSIS

Common

- Focal Confluent Fibrosis
- Cholangiocarcinoma (Peripheral, Intrahepatic)
- Metastases and Lymphoma, Hepatic
- Hepatocellular Carcinoma
- Peritoneal Metastases (Mimic)

Less Common

- Epithelioid Hemangioendothelioma
- Hepatic Cavernous Hemangioma
- Primary Sclerosing Cholangitis
- Inflammatory Pseudotumor, Liver

ESSENTIAL INFORMATION

Key Differential Diagnosis Issues

- Capsular retraction: Focal hepatic volume loss, usually associated with fibrotic scarring
  - Any hepatic tumor that has undergone necrosis or fibrosis is likely to demonstrate this finding
  - Any process that obstructs intrahepatic bile ducts or portal veins may cause this
    - e.g., cholangiocarcinoma; any form of chronic cholangitis
  - Benign and malignant processes may have similar imaging features

Helpful Clues for Common Diagnoses

- **Focal Confluent Fibrosis**
  - Common finding in advanced cirrhosis
  - Usually affects anterior and medial segments
  - Shows delayed, persistent enhancement like all fibrotic lesions
- **Cholangiocarcinoma (Peripheral, Intrahepatic)**
  - Marked volume loss of liver distal to tumor
  - Often obstructs bile ducts and vessels
  - Delayed, persistent enhancement
  - Look for satellite tumors & peritoneal metastases
- **Metastases and Lymphoma, Hepatic**

- Untreated mets rarely causes hepatic volume loss or capsular retraction
- Effective treatment of peripheral hepatic metastases or lymphoma results in volume loss and capsular retraction
- Breast mets: May result in liver scarring and volume loss (pseudocirrhosis)
- **Hepatocellular Carcinoma**
  - Hepatocellular carcinoma following treatment (ablation, transarterial chemoembolization) often results in capsular retraction
- **Peritoneal Metastases (Mimic)**
  - Metastases to peritoneum or hepatic capsule
    - May indent liver surface and simulate capsular retraction

Helpful Clues for Less Common Diagnoses

- **Epithelioid Hemangioendothelioma**
  - Rare tumor but classically causes multiple, peripheral, confluent hepatic masses with overlying capsular retraction
- **Hepatic Cavernous Hemangioma**
  - Common tumor that rarely causes capsular retraction
  - Capsular retraction may result from fibrosis (hyalinization) of hemangioma
    - Especially within cirrhotic liver
- **Primary Sclerosing Cholangitis**
  - Peripheral hepatic fibrosis and volume loss with rounded contours of liver
  - Focal areas of hepatic injury may be mistaken for or mask cholangiocarcinoma
- **Inflammatory Pseudotumor, Liver**
  - May be indistinguishable from peripheral or hilar cholangiocarcinoma
  - Peripheral lesions result in capsular retraction; show delayed enhancement

Focal Confluent Fibrosis

Cholangiocarcinoma (Peripheral, Intrahepatic)

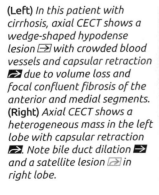

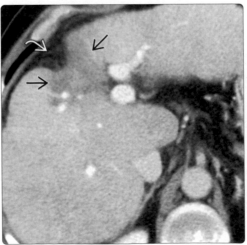

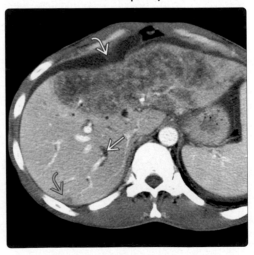

(Left) In this patient with cirrhosis, axial CECT shows a wedge-shaped hypodense lesion ➡ with crowded blood vessels and capsular retraction ➡ due to volume loss and focal confluent fibrosis of the anterior and medial segments. (Right) Axial CECT shows a heterogeneous mass in the left lobe with capsular retraction ➡. Note bile duct dilation ➡ and a satellite lesion ➡ in right lobe.

Metastases and Lymphoma, Hepatic

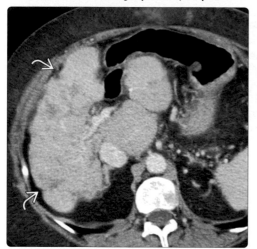

Hepatocellular Carcinoma

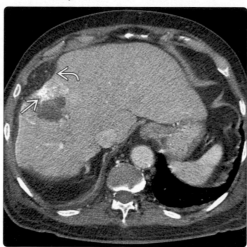

(Left) *Axial CECT shows a pseudocirrhotic-appearing liver in a woman whose hepatic metastases from breast cancer have responded to treatment, with fibrosis and volume loss and with capsular retraction* ➡. **(Right)** *In this patient who had hepatocellular carcinoma treated with chemoembolization, CT shows a necrotic mass with retained lipiodol* ➡. *Retraction of the liver capsule* ➡ *indicates volume loss of the tumor and adjacent liver.*

Peritoneal Metastases (Mimic)

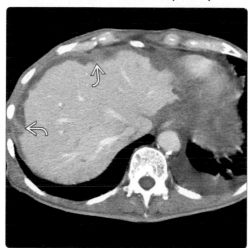

Epithelioid Hemangioendothelioma

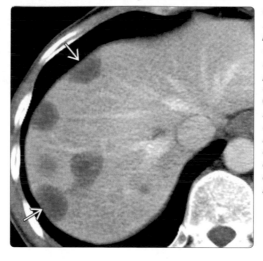

(Left) *Axial CECT shows a scalloped surface of the liver* ➡ *due to extrinsic compression by peritoneal metastases (pseudomyxoma peritonei), in this patient with appendiceal carcinoma.* **(Right)** *Axial CECT shows multiple peripheral target-type lesions with flattening or retraction of the hepatic capsule* ➡, *findings characteristic of hepatic epithelioid hemangioendothelioma.*

Primary Sclerosing Cholangitis

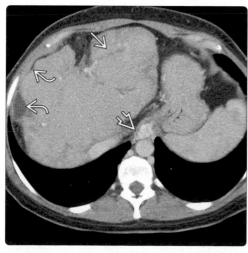

Inflammatory Pseudotumor, Liver

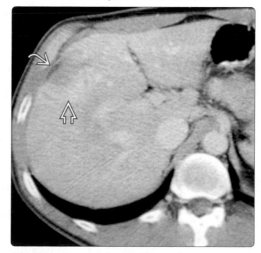

(Left) *Axial CECT shows a small liver with concave margins* ➡ *due to cirrhosis resulting from chronic primary sclerosing cholangitis. Note irregularly dilated intrahepatic bile ducts* ➡ *and esophageal varices* ➡. **(Right)** *Delayed-phase CECT shows a hepatic mass with delayed, persistent enhancement* ➡ *and retraction of the overlying capsule* ➡. *While the CT findings suggest a peripheral (intrahepatic) cholangiocarcinoma, the resected lesion proved to be an inflammatory pseudotumor.*

DIFFERENTIAL DIAGNOSIS

Common

- Steatosis (Fatty Liver) (Mimic)
- Pericaval Fat Deposition

Less Common

- Hepatocellular Carcinoma
- Hepatic Adenoma
- Hepatic Metastases
- Hepatic Angiomyolipoma
- Alcohol-Ablated Liver Tumors (Mimic)
- Fat Within Hepatic Surgical Defect (Mimic)

Rare but Important

- Teratoma or Liposarcoma
- Focal Nodular Hyperplasia
- Xanthomatous Lesions in Langerhans Cell Histiocytosis

ESSENTIAL INFORMATION

Key Differential Diagnosis Issues

- Compare attenuation (CT), intensity (MR), echogenicity (US) of lesion to internal standards
  - e.g., sites of fat and fluid
    - Many lesions simulate fat on 1 modality or sequence, but not others

Helpful Clues for Common Diagnoses

- **Steatosis (Fatty Liver) (Mimic)**
  - Focal steatosis is usually closer to water attenuation, not fat on CT
  - Vessels traverse lesion undisturbed
  - Along fissures and ligaments within liver
- **Pericaval Fat Deposition**
  - Normal variant
  - May simulate fatty mass in liver or inferior vena cava

Helpful Clues for Less Common Diagnoses

- **Hepatocellular Carcinoma**
  - Usually small foci of fat

- **Hepatic Adenoma**
  - MR shows evidence of fat (lipid) in 35-75% of adenomas; CT < 20%
- **Hepatic Metastases**
  - From liposarcoma, malignant teratoma
- **Hepatic Angiomyolipoma**
  - In 6% of patients with tuberous sclerosis
  - Look for fat-containing angiomyolipomas and cysts in kidneys
- **Alcohol-Ablated Liver Tumors (Mimic)**
  - Alcohol has fat attenuation on CT
- **Fat Within Hepatic Surgical Defect (Mimic)**
  - Omental fat may herniate or be placed into site of resection, ablation

Helpful Clues for Rare Diagnoses

- **Teratoma or Liposarcoma**
  - Primary teratoma of liver extremely rare
  - Retroperitoneal teratoma (or liposarcoma) may indent or invade liver
  - Look for fat, fluid, calcification, soft tissue
- **Focal Nodular Hyperplasia**
  - Fat within focal nodular hyperplasia is vary rare
  - May accompany diffuse steatosis
- **Xanthomatous Lesions in Langerhans Cell Histiocytosis**
  - Langerhans cell histiocytosis is malabsorption disorder of variable severity
  - Hepatic lesions usually periportal location

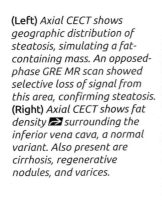

(Left) Axial CECT shows geographic distribution of steatosis, simulating a fat-containing mass. An opposed-phase GRE MR scan showed selective loss of signal from this area, confirming steatosis. (Right) Axial CECT shows fat density ⤢ surrounding the inferior vena cava, a normal variant. Also present are cirrhosis, regenerative nodules, and varices.

Steatosis (Fatty Liver) (Mimic)

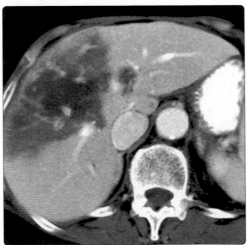

Pericaval Fat Deposition

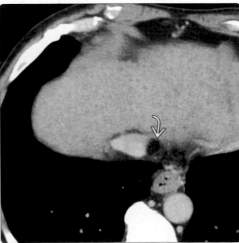

Hepatocellular Carcinoma

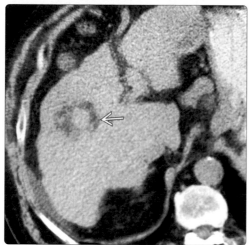

Hepatocellular Carcinoma

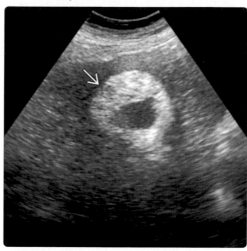

(Left) *Axial NECT shows a cirrhotic liver with a focal mass* ➡ *that has some foci of very low attenuation, indicating fatty metamorphosis. Other portions of the mass showed bright enhancement, washout, and encapsulation, typical features of a hepatocellular carcinoma.* (Right) *Sagittal ultrasound shows a very echogenic mass* ➡ *with decreased through transmission, representing hepatocellular carcinoma with fatty metamorphosis.*

Hepatic Adenoma

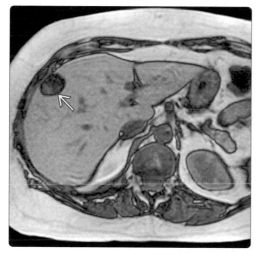

Hepatic Metastases

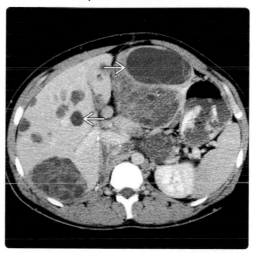

(Left) *Axial T1WI MR shows a focal mass* ➡ *that was almost isointense to liver on the in-phase T1WI, with marked signal loss on this opposed-phase image, indicating lipid content. The lesion was hypervascular & encapsulated, typical features of adenoma in a young woman without cirrhosis.* (Right) *Axial CECT shows multiple metastases from testicular malignant teratoma, some with fat attenuation* ➡.

Hepatic Angiomyolipoma

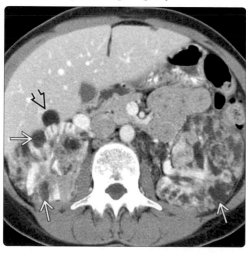

Teratoma or Liposarcoma

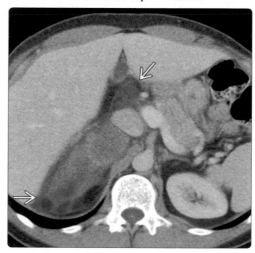

(Left) *Axial CECT shows one* ➡ *of several fatty hepatic masses in addition to innumerable angiomyolipomas in the kidneys* ➡ *in this patient with tuberous sclerosis.* (Right) *Axial CECT shows a large abdominal mass* ➡ *of mixed soft tissue and fat density, a liposarcoma, that indents the liver.*

DIFFERENTIAL DIAGNOSIS

Common

- Hepatic Cyst
- Autosomal Dominant Polycystic Disease, Liver
- Hepatic Pyogenic Abscess
- Biliary Hamartomas
- Metastases and Lymphoma, Hepatic
- Hepatic Amebic Abscess
- Biloma/Seroma
- Steatosis (Fatty Liver) (Mimic)

Less Common

- Hepatic Candidiasis
- Hepatic Hydatid Cyst
- Biliary Cystadenocarcinoma
- Biliary Intraductal Papillary Mucinous Neoplasm
- Hepatocellular Carcinoma
- Caroli Disease
- Hepatic Sarcoma (Primary)
- Intrahepatic Pseudocyst
- Hepatic Inflammatory Pseudotumor
- Ciliated Hepatic Foregut Cyst

ESSENTIAL INFORMATION

Key Differential Diagnosis Issues

- Any mural nodularity or debris level within cyst should raise concern for tumor, abscess, or hematoma
- Essential to compare current study with prior studies to observe for interval change
  - Simple cysts change size only slowly
  - Abscesses change quickly
  - Treated tumors may simulate cysts [especially gastrointestinal stromal tumor (GIST)]
- View images in multiple planes
  - Coronal & sagittal imaging often help to show true morphology, number & etiology of cystic mass

Helpful Clues for Common Diagnoses

- **Hepatic Cyst**
  - Water attenuation, no visible wall
    - No enhancement of cyst contents
    - MR: Very bright on T2WI, dark on T1WI; no enhancement or mural nodularity
    - US: Sonolucent with acoustic enhancement; no visible wall or nodularity
    - Hemorrhage within simple cyst can be difficult to distinguish from cystic neoplasm
  - 1 or 2 thin septa may be seen
  - Often multiple, of varying sizes
- **Autosomal Dominant Polycystic Disease, Liver**
  - Many cysts of varying sizes
  - Intracyst bleeding results in high-attenuation fluid and calcified cyst walls
  - May be associated with cysts in other organs
- **Hepatic Pyogenic Abscess**
  - Multiloculated, multiseptate cluster of complex cysts
  - Wall and septa may show contrast enhancement
  - Associated atelectasis and pleural effusion when abscess occurs in peripheral liver adjacent to diaphragm

- **Biliary Hamartomas**
  - These mimic cysts on CT & MR
  - Multiple small (1-1.5 cm) low-attenuation lesions ± echogenic nodules in walls
  - Lack of larger cystic lesions & cysts in other organs distinguishes this from AD polycystic disease
- **Metastases and Lymphoma, Hepatic**
  - Most common etiologies
    - From primary cystic tumor (e.g., ovarian)
    - Sarcomas, GIST, others, especially after treatment
      □ GIST metastasis treated with Gleevec may mimic simple cyst (check history and prior studies)
    - Squamous cell metastases & mucinous adenocarcinoma mets may appear cystic
  - Most have mural nodularity (CT, US, MR)
  - Lymphoma: Homogeneous masses simulate cysts on CT and ultrasound
- **Hepatic Amebic Abscess**
  - Usually solitary or few with shaggy wall
  - Uncommonly septate, unlike pyogenic abscesses
  - Imaging appearance, clinical presentation, & serology are diagnostic
- **Biloma/Seroma**
  - Following trauma, partial liver resection, radiofrequency ablation
  - In setting of liver transplantation, may result from hepatic artery thrombosis with biliary necrosis
    - Biloma in hepatic allograft is ominous finding
- **Steatosis (Fatty Liver) (Mimic)**
  - Focal deposits may be near water density on NECT (but echogenic, not cystic, on US)
  - MR also definitive, showing selective signal dropout from focal steatotic areas on opposed-phase GRE images

Helpful Clues for Less Common Diagnoses

- **Hepatic Candidiasis**
  - Innumerable microabscesses (< 1 cm) with target or wheel appearance
  - Occur in immune-compromised patients
  - Other hepatic opportunistic organisms may cause similar appearance
    - Especially fungal and mycobacterial
- **Hepatic Hydatid Cyst**
  - Solitary or multiple
  - Discrete peripheral wall ± calcification with daughter cysts
  - Daughter cysts may be smaller spheres within larger cyst, or appear as thick septations
    - Often in spoke-wheel pattern
- **Biliary Cystadenocarcinoma**
  - Asymptomatic until large
  - Solitary, multiseptate mass with discrete enhancing wall and septa
    - Rarely have no visible septa
  - Complete resection of all parts of tumor essential to prevent recurrence
  - Typically occur in middle-aged women
- **Biliary Intraductal Papillary Mucinous Neoplasm**
  - Intraductal papillary mucinous neoplasm
    - Analogous to pancreatic intraductal papillary mucinous neoplasm

- o Tumor within bile duct may rarely produce mucin that distends ducts and may simulate cystic mass
- o May see nodular, enhancing component (worrisome for cholangiocarcinoma)
- **Hepatocellular Carcinoma**
  - o Spontaneous necrosis (or following treatment) may simulate cystic mass
  - o Usually have solid component with arterial hyperenhancement & delayed washout
- **Caroli Disease**
  - o Cystic dilation of intrahepatic bile ducts
  - o Communication with bile ducts is key feature, distinguishing it from other cystic masses
    - – Recommend MRCP or ERCP
  - o Central dot sign: Dilated ducts surrounding portal vein radicle
- **Hepatic Sarcoma**
  - o Undifferentiated sarcoma, primary to liver
  - o Typical appearance is large, solitary, encapsulated mass
  - o Peripheral hypervascular solid component
  - o Central necrosis; may mimic multiseptate mass

- o Rare tumor with very aggressive clinical course
- **Intrahepatic Pseudocyst**
  - o May dissect into liver along portal triads
  - o Intrahepatic pseudocyst usually has adjacent cyst in pancreatic head
  - o Check for imaging and clinical evidence of pancreatitis
- **Hepatic Inflammatory Pseudotumor**
  - o Also called inflammatory myofibroblastic tumor
  - o Relatively rare with variable appearance
    - – Usually resemble cholangiocarcinoma with delayed, persistent enhancement
    - – Rarely has multiseptate, cystic appearance
- **Ciliated Hepatic Foregut Cyst**
  - o Rare congenital anomaly
  - o Typically small (< 3 cm) cystic mass in segment IV of liver
  - o May appear complex or solid on sonography

Hepatic Cyst

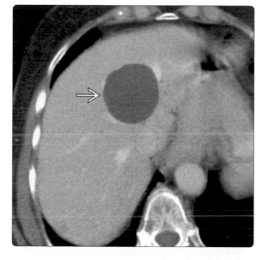

Autosomal Dominant Polycystic Disease, Liver

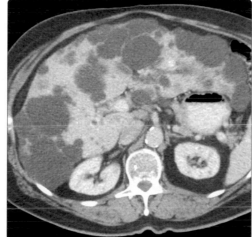

(Left) Axial CECT in this 79-year-old woman shows a spherical liver mass ➡ with water density, homogeneous contents. No internal debris or wall irregularities are present. (Right) Axial CECT shows innumerable hepatic cysts of water attenuation and varying size, causing hepatomegaly. Only a few small renal cysts are present and renal function is normal.

Biliary Hamartomas

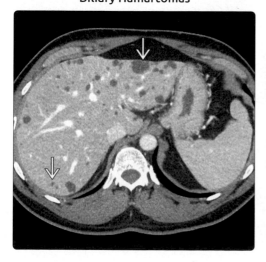

Biliary Hamartomas

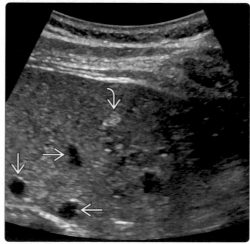

(Left) In this 53-year-old man, axial CT shows innumerable small cystic lesions ➡ throughout the liver, ranging in size from 2-15 mm. The lesions are often not perfectly spherical, and many have visible nodular enhancement within their walls. (Right) In this 53-year-old man, sonography on the same day showed only the lesions > 10 mm as cystic structures ➡ while the smaller lesions were actually hyperechoic ➡ to background liver. All are typical features of biliary hamartomas.

(Left) *CECT shows a liver mass with innumerable septa and slightly higher than water density contents. Needle aspiration yielded a small quantity of pus, and a catheter was inserted for drainage. The etiology was subacute diverticulitis.* **(Right)** *CT shows a shaggy, encapsulated, solitary cystic mass ➡ with nonenhancing contents, representing a typical amebic abscess. The imaging appearance, clinical presentation, & serology usually suffice for diagnosis.*

Hepatic Pyogenic Abscess

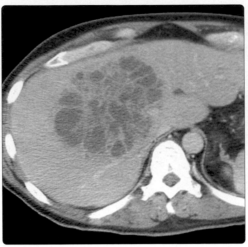

Hepatic Amebic Abscess

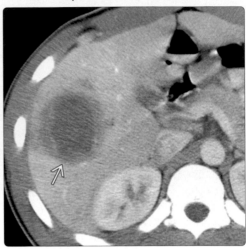

(Left) *In this immigrant from the Middle East, coronal CT shows 2 large, multiseptate, cystic masses ➡. Within the outer pericyst are the multiple daughter cysts or scolices. This imaging appearance, coupled with serology, is usually sufficient for diagnosis.* **(Right)** *In this febrile, immune-suppressed patient, axial CECT shows innumerable small hypodense lesions throughout the liver. The larger lesions have visible irregularity of their walls. Other opportunistic hepatic infections may have a similar appearance.*

Hepatic Hydatid Cyst

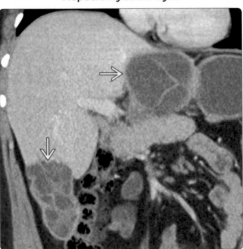

Hepatic Candidiasis

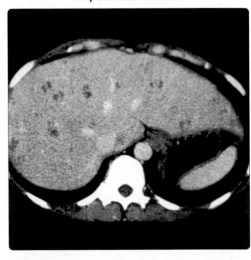

(Left) *CECT performed 3 weeks after a blunt traumatic liver laceration shows a lobulated cystic hepatic lesion ➡ that represents a combination of walled-off bile and blood, also known, respectively, as a biloma and seroma. Clinical history & comparison with prior CT scans provides confident diagnosis.* **(Right)** *Axial CECT shows a large lesion of near water attenuation that represents focal severe fatty infiltration. The presence of blood vessels coursing through this area is characteristic.*

Biloma/Seroma

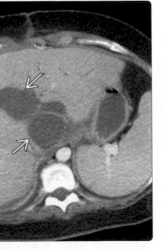

Steatosis (Fatty Liver) (Mimic)

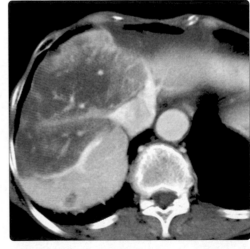

Cystic Hepatic Mass

Metastases and Lymphoma, Hepatic

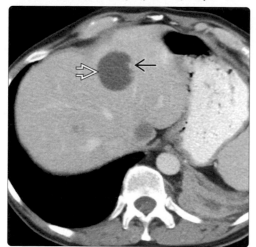

Biliary Cystadenocarcinoma

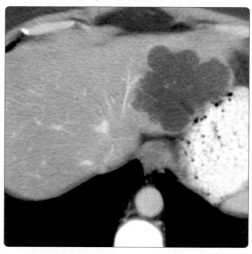

(Left) Axial CECT shows several hypodense hepatic masses, including 1 cystic lesion ⇨. The subtle mural nodule ⇨ is the clue that this is a neoplasm (metastatic thyroid cancer). (Right) In this 57-year-old asymptomatic woman, CT shows a large, solitary, water density, well-encapsulated hepatic mass with multiple thin septa. No mural nodularity is noted. Clinical & imaging features are typical of biliary cystadenoma/carcinoma.

Caroli Disease

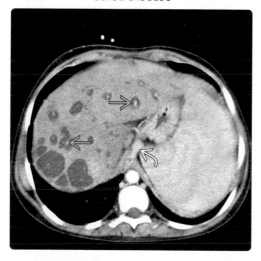

Hepatic Sarcoma (Primary)

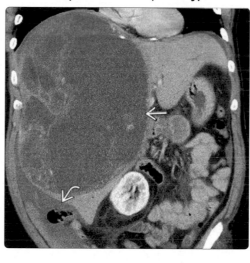

(Left) In this young woman with portal hypertension due to congenital hepatic fibrosis & Caroli disease, CT shows splenomegaly, varices ⇨, & multiple hepatic cysts. These represent dilated intrahepatic bile ducts, draped around the central dot of accompanying portal veins ⇨. (Right) In this man with RUQ pain, coronal CECT shows a huge, multiseptate, cystic mass ⇨ with enhancing peripheral components. Intraperitoneal blood ⇨ was due to capsular rupture of this undifferentiated primary hepatic sarcoma.

Biliary Intraductal Papillary Mucinous Neoplasm

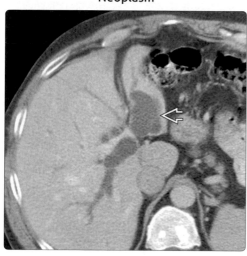

Ciliated Hepatic Foregut Cyst

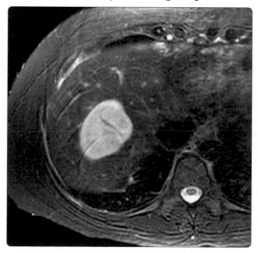

(Left) In this case of biliary IPMN with cholangiocarcinoma, axial CECT shows dilated intrahepatic bile ducts and a cystic mass ⇨. ERCP showed opacification of the cyst with contrast and the presence of surface nodularity within the bile ducts. (Right) This 29-year-old woman had a solid-appearing mass seen on US. Axial T2W MR shows a complex cystic-appearing mass in segment 4 that had no enhancement on other sequences. Resection proved this to be a ciliated hepatic foregut cyst.

DIFFERENTIAL DIAGNOSIS

Common

- Hepatic Cavernous Hemangioma
- Focal Nodular Hyperplasia
- Arterioportal Shunt
- Transient Hepatic Attenuation Difference
- Hepatocellular Carcinoma
- Hepatic Metastases
- Hepatic Adenoma

Less Common

- Hereditary Hemorrhagic Telangiectasia
- Nodular Regenerative Hyperplasia
- Fibrolamellar Hepatocellular Carcinoma
- Cholangiocarcinoma (Peripheral)
- Hepatic Angiomyolipoma
- Angiosarcoma, Liver
- Superior Vena Cava Obstruction, Abdominal Manifestations
- Peliosis Hepatis

ESSENTIAL INFORMATION

Key Differential Diagnosis Issues

- Critical to characterize morphology and hemodynamics of hepatic lesions to derive specific diagnosis; examples
  - Cavernous hemangioma, arterioportal shunt, arteriovenous malformation (AVM): Isodense to blood vessels on all phases of imaging
  - Focal nodular hyperplasia (FNH): Nearly isodense (isointense) to liver on nonenhanced, portal venous and delayed phases; homogeneously hyperdense on arterial phase
  - Hepatocellular carcinoma (HCC): Hypodense to liver on NECT, portal venous and delayed-phase imaging; heterogeneously hyperdense on arterial phase
  - Cholangiocarcinoma: Hypodense on NECT, hypo-, iso-, or hyperdense on arterial phase, hyperdense on delayed-phase imaging

Helpful Clues for Common Diagnoses

- **Hepatic Cavernous Hemangioma**
  - Small ("capillary") hemangiomas may enhance quickly and homogeneously
  - Enhanced portions of all hemangiomas remain nearly isodense to blood vessels on all phases of imaging (CT and MR)
  - Nodular, discontinuous peripheral enhancement with progressive centripetal fill in for larger hemangiomas
- **Focal Nodular Hyperplasia**
  - Common (~ 2-5%) among young women
  - Homogeneous bright enhancement on arterial phase of enhancement
  - Central scar seen in 2/3 of FNH > 3 cm
  - Nearly isodense (and isointense) to normal liver or nonenhanced, portal venous, delayed images
- **Arterioportal Shunt**
  - Common cause of small, usually peripheral, hypervascular foci within cirrhotic liver
  - Isodense (and isointense) to liver on nonenhanced portal venous and delayed imaging

- May result from percutaneous biopsy, percutaneous catheter placement, or other trauma
- Look for early filling of portal vein branch
- **Transient Hepatic Attenuation Difference**
  - Peripheral wedge-shaped hypervascular lesion seen only on arterial-phase imaging (CT or MR)
  - Usually due to obstruction of portal vein branch with compensatory increased arterial flow to involved liver
  - Can usually ignore small subcapsular lesion
    - Larger or segmental transient hepatic attenuation difference lesion usually due to mass causing occlusion or compression of portal vein branch (examples: Metastases, HCC, large benign mass, abscess)
- **Hepatocellular Carcinoma**
  - Usually heterogeneously hyperdense on arterial phase with washout to hypoattenuating on portal venous and delayed imaging
  - Look for signs of cirrhosis and invasion of veins and bile ducts
- **Hepatic Metastases**
  - Usually from endocrine primary, melanoma, or renal cell carcinoma
  - Multiplicity, heterogeneity, ring enhancement favor malignancy
- **Hepatic Adenoma**
  - In young women on oral contraceptives or individuals on anabolic steroids
  - Usually heterogeneously hypervascular
  - Often with foci of fat, necrosis, hemorrhage (more evident on MR than on CT)

Helpful Clues for Less Common Diagnoses

- **Hereditary Hemorrhagic Telangiectasia**
  - Part of multiorgan fibrovascular dysplasia (Osler-Weber-Rendu)
    - Telangiectasias and AVMs in liver and other organs (lungs, GI tract, brain, etc.)
    - Patients present with nosebleeds, GI bleeding, hemoptysis
    - Liver: Large hepatic arteries and draining veins with "vascular masses"
    - Heterogeneous enhancement of liver during arterial phase
- **Nodular Regenerative Hyperplasia**
  - In Budd-Chiari, congenital heart disease (after Fontan procedure)
  - "Large regenerative nodules" (multiacinar form of nodular regenerative hyperplasia) are common
  - Usually multiple, 1-3 cm; resemble FNH on imaging and pathology
  - Patients with Budd-Chiari also have hepatic and perihepatic venous collaterals that may appear as hypervascular lesions
- **Fibrolamellar Hepatocellular Carcinoma**
  - Large heterogeneous tumor with calcification within large scar
  - 2/3 have metastases at time of diagnosis (nodal, lung)
  - Usually diagnosed in young adults or children
- **Cholangiocarcinoma (Peripheral)**
  - Occasionally hypervascular

- o Look for delayed, persistent enhancement and capsular retraction (not seen in HCC)
- **Hepatic Angiomyolipoma**
  - o Nonfatty portions of mass are hypervascular
  - o Only 50% of hepatic angiomyolipomas (AMLs) have macroscopic fat evident on CT
    - These are difficult to distinguish from other tumors
  - o May be associated with renal AMLs, ± tuberous sclerosis complex (10%)
- **Angiosarcoma, Liver**
  - o Associated with industrial toxins
  - o Bizarre enhancement patterns; may resemble hemangioma
  - o Multiple lesions in liver and spleen
- **Superior Vena Cava Obstruction, Abdominal Manifestations**
  - o Collateral veins running along diaphragm may pass through liver to inferior vena cava
  - o Broad area of hypervascularity in left lobe on arterial phase; no mass effect
- **Peliosis Hepatis**

- o Associated with chronic wasting diseases and certain medications; also *Bartonella* infection
- o Variable appearance; sometimes resembles hemangioma

SELECTED REFERENCES

1. Colagrande S et al: Transient hepatic intensity differences: part 1. Those associated with focal lesions. AJR Am J Roentgenol. 188(1):154-9, 2007
2. Colagrande S et al: Transient hepatic intensity differences: part 2. Those not associated with focal lesions. AJR Am J Roentgenol. 188(1):160-6, 2007
3. Kamel IR et al: Incidental nonneoplastic hypervascular lesions in the noncirrhotic liver: diagnosis with 16-MDCT and 3D CT angiography. AJR Am J Roentgenol. 187(3):682-7, 2006
4. Coakley FV et al: Imaging of hepatocellular carcinoma: a practical approach. Semin Oncol. 28(5):460-73, 2001
5. Kim T et al: Discrimination of small hepatic hemangiomas from hypervascular malignant tumors smaller than 3 cm with three-phase helical CT. Radiology. 219(3):699-706, 2001

Hepatic Cavernous Hemangioma

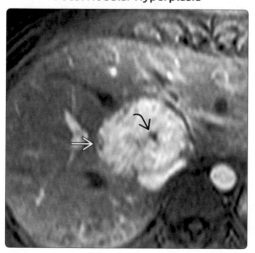

Focal Nodular Hyperplasia

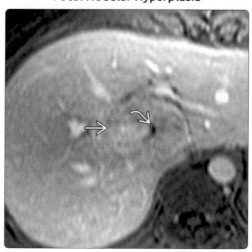

(Left) *Axial CECT shows a small hypervascular mass ⇒ that was isodense to blood pool on NECT, arterial phase, and this portal venous-phase CECT.* **(Right)** *Axial CECT shows a homogeneously hypervascular mass on arterial-phase CECT that was isodense with liver on other phases. The central scar ⇒ and early draining veins ⇒ are typical features of focal nodular hyperplasia (FNH).*

Focal Nodular Hyperplasia

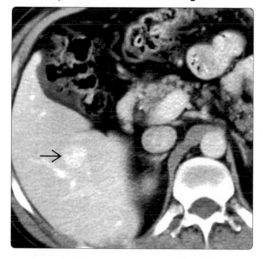

Focal Nodular Hyperplasia

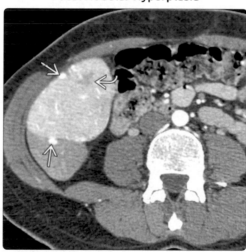

(Left) *This arterial-phase axial T1 C+ FS MR shows homogeneous bright enhancement of a hepatic mass ⇒ in this young woman. Note the central scar ⇒.* **(Right)** *This portal venous-phase axial T1 C+ FS MR shows the FNH ⇒ is nearly isointense with normal liver. The central small scar ⇒ is still well seen.*

Arterioportal Shunt

Arterioportal Shunt

(Left) *In this cirrhotic patient, arterial-phase axial CECT shows hyperdensity ➡ within the left lobe, which became isodense on portal venous phase. Early filling of the left portal vein ➡ is due to an arterioportal fistula from biopsy.* (Right) *In this patient with cirrhosis, arterial-phase CECT shows 1 of several peripheral, capsular-based, wedge-shaped hypervascular lesions ➡, all of which were invisible on venous and delayed-phase CECT. These are characteristic of arterioportal shunts within the cirrhotic liver.*

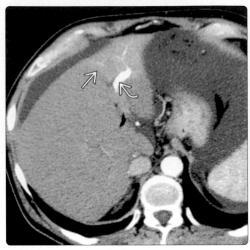

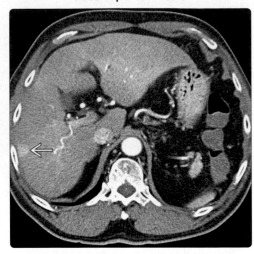

Transient Hepatic Attenuation Difference

Transient Hepatic Attenuation Difference

(Left) *In this man with hepatic metastases from pancreatic cancer, arterial-phase CECT shows peripheral, wedge-shaped zones of hepatic hyperperfusion ➡ that became isodense to liver on the portal venous phase; typical transient hepatic attenuation differences (THADs).* (Right) *In the same patient, this portal venous-phase CT shows the multiple hypodense, spherical metastases ➡ that caused the THADs seen on arterial-phase CECT. THAD lesions often result from occlusion of portal vein branches by tumor.*

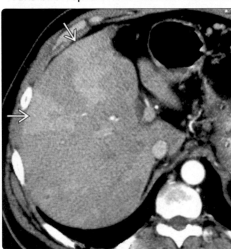

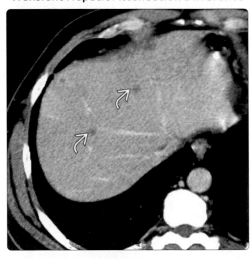

Hepatocellular Carcinoma

Hepatocellular Carcinoma

(Left) *In this man with cirrhosis, axial arterial-phase CECT shows a heterogeneously hypervascular mass ➡, that "washed out" to become hypodense on portal venous phase, characteristic findings of hepatocellular carcinoma (HCC).* (Right) *In this man with cirrhosis, this portal venous-phase CECT shows a mass ➡ that has "washed out" to become slightly hypodense to underlying liver and characteristic of HCC.*

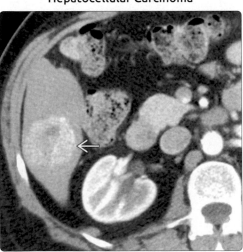

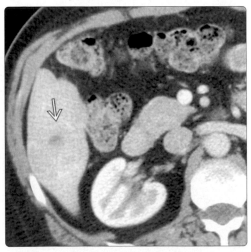

Hepatic Metastases

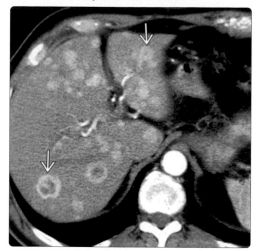

Hepatic Metastases

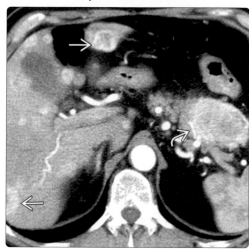

(Left) *In this man with a pancreatic endocrine tumor, arterial-phase CECT shows innumerable hypervascular metastases* ➡, *some of which are ring enhancing.* **(Right)** *In this patient with hypervascular hepatic metastases* ➡, *the primary endocrine tumor of the pancreas (malignant glucagonoma) is also evident as a hypervascular mass* ➡.

Hepatic Adenoma

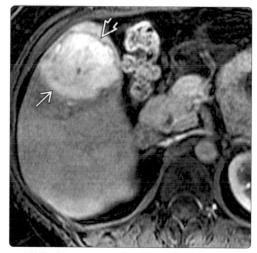

Hepatic Adenoma

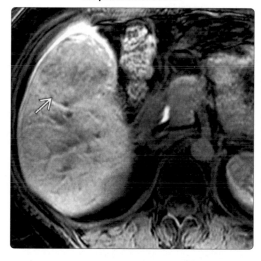

(Left) *In this young woman, axial T1 C+ MR section in the arterial phase following bolus injection of gadoxetate (Eovist) shows a hypervascular mass* ➡ *that has a capsule* ➡. **(Right)** *In this young woman, axial delayed-phase image of the Eovist-enhanced MR study shows the mass* ➡ *as heterogeneously hypointense to the normal liver. The final diagnosis was hepatic adenoma of the inflammatory subtype.*

Hereditary Hemorrhagic Telangiectasia

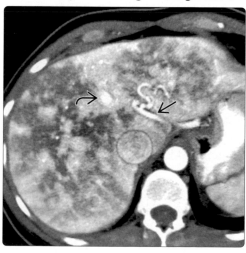

Hereditary Hemorrhagic Telangiectasia

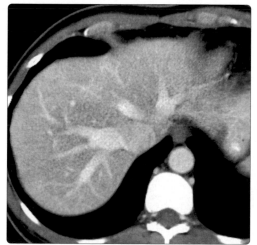

(Left) *In this middle-aged man with a family history of hereditary hemorrhagic telangiectasia (HHT), arterial-phase CT shows heterogeneous enhancement of the hepatic parenchyma, enlarged, tortuous hepatic arteries* ➡, *and early opacification of enlarged hepatic veins* ➡ *and the inferior vena cava (IVC).* **(Right)** *In this middle-aged man with HHT, portal venous-phase CECT shows homogeneous enhancement of the liver with dilated hepatic veins and IVC.*

Nodular Regenerative Hyperplasia

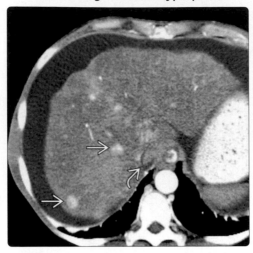

Nodular Regenerative Hyperplasia

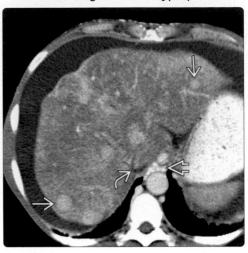

(Left) *In this patient with Budd-Chiari syndrome, arterial-phase CECT shows many small hypervascular masses ➡️ (large regenerative nodules). Note the occluded IVC ➡️, ascites, and a dysmorphic liver.* (Right) *In this patient with Budd-Chiari syndrome, portal venous CECT shows persistent hypervascularity of the large regenerative nodules ➡️ (nodular regenerative hyperplasia). Note the occluded IVC ➡️ and collateral veins ➡️.*

Fibrolamellar Hepatocellular Carcinoma

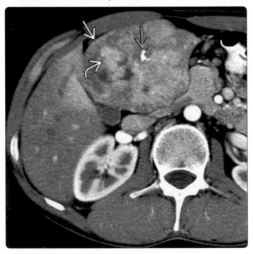

Fibrolamellar Hepatocellular Carcinoma

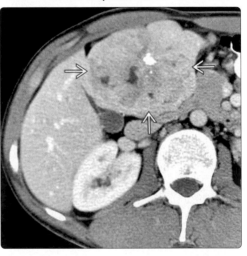

(Left) *In this 22-year-old man, arterial-phase CECT shows a mass ➡️ that is lobulated and encapsulated, with a large, calcified central scar ➡️. The mass is heterogeneously hypervascular ➡️.* (Right) *In this 22-year-old man, the hepatic mass ➡️ remains heterogeneous on portal venous-phase imaging. The liver does not appear to be cirrhotic. Porta hepatis lymphadenopathy was noted on other images.*

Cholangiocarcinoma (Peripheral)

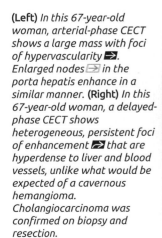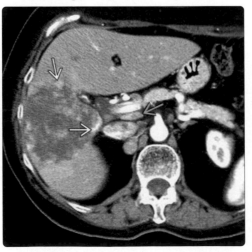

Cholangiocarcinoma (Peripheral)

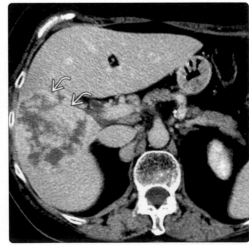

(Left) *In this 67-year-old woman, arterial-phase CECT shows a large mass with foci of hypervascularity ➡️. Enlarged nodes ➡️ in the porta hepatis enhance in a similar manner.* (Right) *In this 67-year-old woman, a delayed-phase CECT shows heterogeneous, persistent foci of enhancement ➡️ that are hyperdense to liver and blood vessels, unlike what would be expected of a cavernous hemangioma. Cholangiocarcinoma was confirmed on biopsy and resection.*

Hepatic Angiomyolipoma

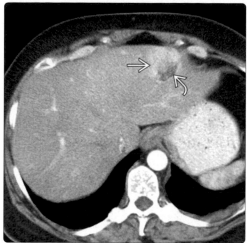
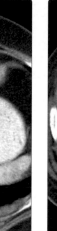

Angiosarcoma, Liver

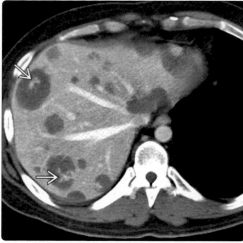

(Left) *Arterial-phase CECT shows a hypervascular mass* ➡️ *that also has foci of fat attenuation* ➡️. *Similar angiomyolipomas were present in the kidneys. While these were unsuspected findings, this patient may have a forme fruste of tuberous sclerosis complex.* (Right) *Axial CECT shows multiple tumor masses throughout the liver with peculiar eccentric enhancement and hypervascular foci* ➡️. *Similar lesions were present in the spleen and grew rapidly with a fatal outcome within several months.*

Superior Vena Cava Obstruction, Abdominal Manifestations

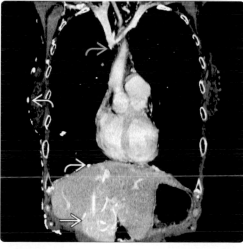

Superior Vena Cava Obstruction, Abdominal Manifestations

(Left) *In this 60-year-old woman with superior vena cava (SVC) occlusion, arterial-phase CECT shows bright enhancement of portions of the left hepatic lobe* ➡️ *along with collateral veins* ➡️ *in the chest wall and capsular surface of the liver. The liver was homogeneous on venous-phase CECT.* (Right) *In this 60-year-old woman, coronal arterial-phase CECT shows the occluded SVC* ➡️, *collateral veins* ➡️, *and the resulting early enhancement of the medial segment of liver* ➡️.

Peliosis Hepatis

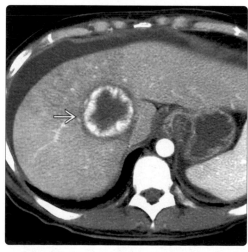

Peliosis Hepatis

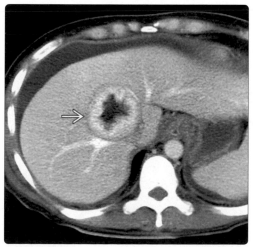

(Left) *Axial CECT shows continuous ring enhancement* ➡️ *on this arterial-phase image. Also note ascites.* (Right) *Axial CECT shows progressive fill-in* ➡️ *of the peliosis lesion, in a pattern that is similar to that of cavernous hemangioma, although hemangiomas usually have nodular enhancement.*

DIFFERENTIAL DIAGNOSIS

Common

- Passive Hepatic Congestion
- Steatosis (Fatty Liver)
- Cirrhosis
- Hepatitis

Less Common

- Budd-Chiari Syndrome
- Hereditary Hemorrhagic Telangiectasia
- Congenital Hepatic Fibrosis
- Hepatic Sarcoidosis
- Congenital Heart Disease
- Hepatic Lymphoma
- Hepatic Metastases
- Systemic Hypervolemia

ESSENTIAL INFORMATION

Key Differential Diagnosis Issues

- Mosaic liver: Enhances heterogeneously without discrete masses

Helpful Clues for Common Diagnoses

- **Passive Hepatic Congestion**
  - Most common cause; congestive heart failure, tricuspid insufficiency, constrictive pericarditis
  - Hepatic veins and inferior vena cava are engorged
  - Periportal edema is often evident
- **Steatosis (Fatty Infiltration)**
  - May cause diffuse or multifocal hypodensity within liver
  - Favors areas around hepatic veins, fissures, and ligaments
  - Hepatic vessels pass through low-density foci without being displaced or compressed
  - Selective signal dropout on opposed-phase GRE is diagnostic of steatosis
- **Cirrhosis**
  - Fibrosis, regenerating nodules, steatosis all contribute to heterogeneity of liver

- Hepatic veins normal; portal flow may be hepatofugal (reversed)
  - Widened fissures, surface nodularity
  - Signs of portal hypertension (varices, ascites, splenomegaly)
- **Hepatitis**
  - Acute viral, alcoholic, or toxic injury
  - Enlarged liver with periportal lymphedema
    - Gallbladder wall edema is also common
  - Hepatic and portal veins: Normal caliber and flow
  - Alcoholic hepatitis often has steatosis contributing to patchy hepatogram

Helpful Clues for Less Common Diagnoses

- **Budd-Chiari Syndrome**
  - Obstruction of hepatic veins &/or IVC
  - Small veins (rather than dilated as in passive hepatic congestion)
  - Intrahepatic and perihepatic venous collaterals
- **Hereditary Hemorrhagic Telangiectasia**
  - Osler-Weber-Rendu
  - Numerous arteriovenous malformations and telangiectasias connect arteries and veins
  - Large hepatic arteries and veins
- **Congenital Hepatic Fibrosis**
  - Dysmorphic liver, big arteries, portal hypertension
  - May coexist with Caroli disease, choledochal cysts, renal fibrocystic disease
- **Hepatic Sarcoidosis**
  - May simulate or cause cirrhosis
  - Hypodense granulomas and lymphadenopathy
- **Hepatic Lymphoma & Metastases**
  - Homogeneous enlargement of liver ± subtle focal masses
  - Especially common with lymphoma, metastatic breast, and melanoma
- **Systemic Hypervolemia**
  - Excessive IV hydration: Periportal lymphedema and, less often, heterogeneous hepatogram

(Left) In this 57-year-old man who had a recent myocardial infarction, CECT shows reflux of contrast material down into the dilated hepatic veins ➡. (Right) In this 57-year-old man with a recent myocardial infarction, CT shows hepatomegaly & heterogeneous parenchymal enhancement due to diminished cardiac output and delayed opacification of the dilated hepatic vein branches.

Passive Hepatic Congestion

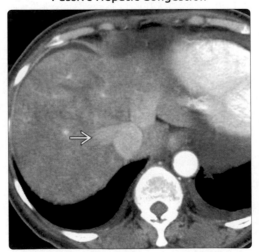

Passive Hepatic Congestion

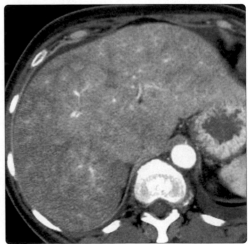

Steatosis (Fatty Liver)

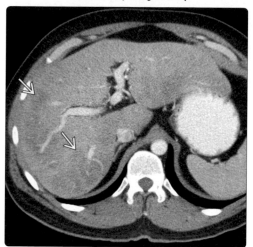

Steatosis (Fatty Liver)

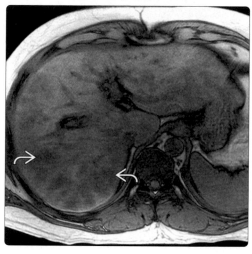

(Left) *Axial CECT shows multifocal hypodense lesions that predominantly lie in a perivascular distribution, surrounding hepatic vessels ➡. Note that the vessels are not narrowed or displaced by the hypodense lesions. MR confirmed multifocal steatosis.* (Right) *In this patient with multifocal steatosis, in-phase T1WI GRE (not illustrated) showed no apparent lesions, while the opposed-phase images clearly show signal dropout from each of the perivascular foci of steatosis ➡.*

Steatosis (Fatty Liver)

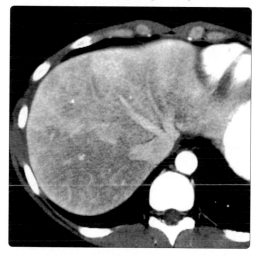

Hepatitis

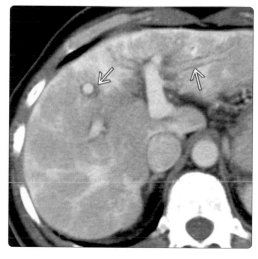

(Left) *Axial CECT shows a patchy appearance of liver, but blood vessels traverse the hypodense areas without deviation or compression, characteristic features of steatosis.* (Right) *Axial CECT shows heterogeneous enhancement of the liver and periportal lymphedema ➡. Biopsy showed severe acute and chronic viral hepatitis.*

Cirrhosis

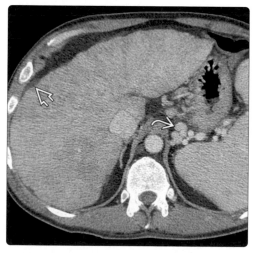

Cirrhosis

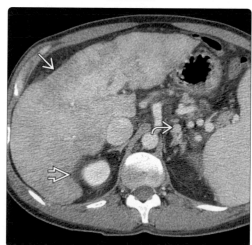

(Left) *In this 40-year-old man with alcoholic cirrhosis, the liver parenchyma is heterogeneous, likely due to steatosis and fibrosis. Note the nodular surface, varices ➡, and ascites ➡.* (Right) *In this 47-year-old man with alcoholic cirrhosis, CT shows a heterogeneous liver with ascites ➡, varices ➡, and capsular retraction ➡ overlying a focus of focal confluent fibrosis.*

(Left) *In this elderly man who is hypercoagulable due to lung cancer, massive ascites, heterogeneous mosaic enhancement of the liver parenchyma, and marked narrowing of the IVC ⮕ are shown. No patent hepatic veins are identified.* **(Right)** *In this elderly man with lung cancer and acute Budd-Chiari syndrome, the IVC is narrowed ⮕ & the hepatic veins were thrombosed, accounting for the heterogeneous hepatic enhancement and ascites.*

Budd-Chiari Syndrome

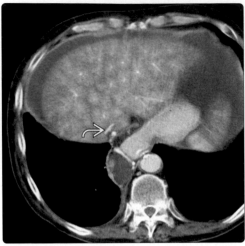

Budd-Chiari Syndrome

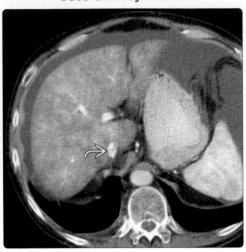

(Left) *In this 45-year-old woman with factor V Leiden deficiency, the liver enhances heterogeneously with the central right lobe & caudate enhancing normally, while the peripheral right and left lobes are poorly enhanced. Ascites and collateral veins ⮕ are noted. The IVC is thrombosed ⮕.* **(Right)** *In this 45-year-old woman with subacute BCS, CECT shows an occluded IVC ⮕ & ascites ⮕. The liver is dysmorphic with a normal density but hypertrophied caudate lobe and a shrunken peripheral liver of lower density.*

Budd-Chiari Syndrome

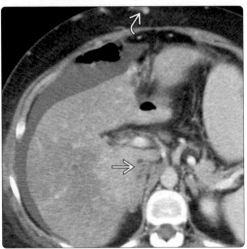

Budd-Chiari Syndrome

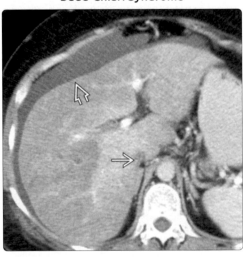

(Left) *In this middle-aged man with hereditary hemorrhagic telangiectasia, arterial-phase CT shows heterogeneous enhancement of the hepatic parenchyma due to telangiectasias & arteriovenous malformations ⮕, causing early filling of enlarged hepatic veins ⮕.* **(Right)** *In this middle-aged man with HHT, the portal venous (parenchymal)-phase CT shows a more homogeneous parenchymal enhancement and dilated IVC and hepatic veins ⮕.*

Hereditary Hemorrhagic Telangiectasia

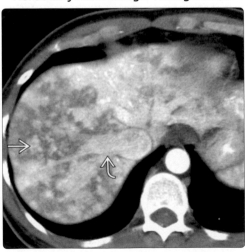

Hereditary Hemorrhagic Telangiectasia

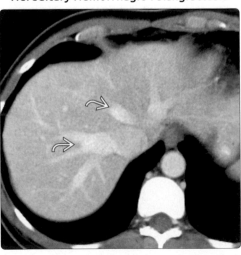

Congenital Hepatic Fibrosis

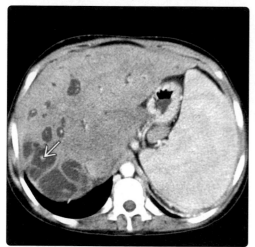

Congenital Hepatic Fibrosis

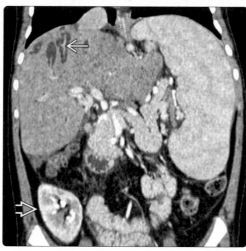

(Left) *This 40-year-old woman has congenital hepatic fibrosis and Caroli disease, accounting for her portal hypertension. Note the dysmorphic liver and the central dot sign ➡ representing the portal vein surrounded by the dilated intrahepatic ducts.* (Right) *This 40-year-old woman with biopsy-proven congenital hepatic fibrosis has dilated, deformed intrahepatic bile ducts ➡, characteristic of Caroli disease. Note the renal allograft ➡, necessitated by congenital renal fibrocystic disease.*

Hepatic Sarcoidosis

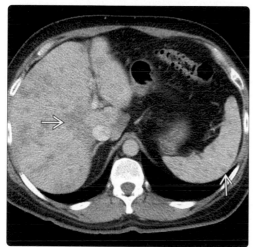

Hepatic Sarcoidosis

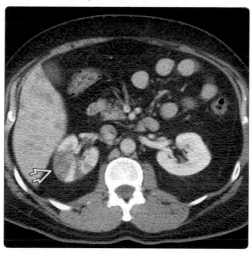

(Left) *This 45-year-old man has sarcoidosis, accounting for the low-density lesions ➡ in the liver and spleen seen on CECT. CT through the thorax showed extensive mediastinal and hilar lymphadenopathy.* (Right) *In this 45-year-old man with proven sarcoidosis in his thorax, liver, and spleen, the kidneys also showed multifocal involvement ➡.*

Hepatic Metastases

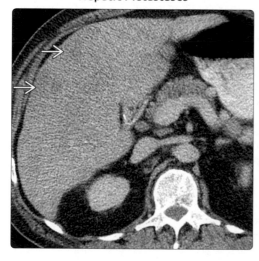

Systemic Hypervolemia

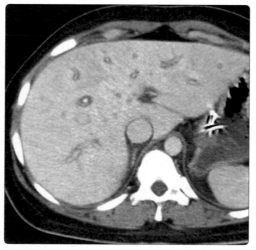

(Left) *In this man with melanoma and hepatic dysfunction, axial CECT shows diffuse low attenuation throughout the liver, suggestive of steatosis. In addition, there are several poorly defined hypodense lesions ➡. Sonography the next day confirmed innumerable focal hypoechoic metastases & no evidence of steatosis.* (Right) *Axial CECT shows an enlarged, heterogeneous liver with marked perivascular edema, all due to systemic hypervolemia (overhydration with IV fluids).*

DIFFERENTIAL DIAGNOSIS

Common

- Calcified Granuloma, Liver
- Hepatic Metastases
- Hepatic Arterial Calcification
- Ethiodol-Treated Tumor, Liver

Less Common

- Hepatic Cavernous Hemangioma
- Hepatic Hydatid Cyst
- Fibrolamellar Hepatocellular Carcinoma
- Cholangiocarcinoma (Peripheral, Intrahepatic)
- Hepatocellular Carcinoma
- Hepatic Adenoma
- Hepatic Opportunistic Infection
- Portal Vein Calcification
- Intrahepatic Biliary Calculi
- Pancreato-Biliary Parasites
- Extrahepatic Calcifications (Mimic)

Rare but Important

- Focal Nodular Hyperplasia
- Epithelioid Hemangioendothelioma
- Schistosomiasis, Hepatic

ESSENTIAL INFORMATION

Key Differential Diagnosis Issues

- Many more calcified hepatic lesions are evident on CT than on plain radiography
  - Due to greater sensitivity of CT for contrast differentiation
- MR is relatively insensitive to diagnosis of calcification
  - Visible only as focus of signal void due to immobile protons within calcified lesion
- Ultrasound detects calcifications as brightly echogenic foci with acoustic shadow
- Characterize pattern of calcification
  - Examples: Punctate, amorphous, eggshell, tram track

Helpful Clues for Common Diagnoses

- **Calcified Granuloma, Liver**
  - Most common cause of hepatic calcifications
  - Histoplasmosis > tuberculosis > coccidioidomycosis, brucellosis
  - Multiple (few to dozens), small (few millimeters) punctate calcifications
  - Often present in spleen as well
  - Usually entire lesion is densely calcified
- **Hepatic Metastases**
  - Usually have faint and amorphous, rather than dense, calcification
  - Any metastases may calcify, especially at border of viable and necrotic tumor
  - Mucinous carcinomas of colon, breast, ovary, or stomach
  - Mixture of fat and calcification seen in metastatic malignant teratoma (uncommon tumor)
  - Tumors that become necrotic in response to chemotherapy are more likely to calcify
- **Hepatic Arterial Calcification**

- Aneurysmal, eggshell, rounded, or tram-track calcification
- Diabetic arteriopathy; long segmental calcifications of medium-sized arteries, including hepatic
- **Ethiodol-Treated Tumor, Liver**
  - Iodized poppy seed oil (Lipiodol) administered intraarterially, localizes in hepatocellular carcinoma and other tumors
  - Used as adjunct to diagnosis and therapy
  - Spherical collection within tumor
  - Usually even more dense than calcified hepatic lesions
    - Check for history of angiographic treatment; check prior scans

Helpful Clues for Less Common Diagnoses

- **Hepatic Cavernous Hemangioma**
  - Large hemangiomas often have central scar that may calcify
  - Remainder of mass will show characteristic features of hemangioma
    - Peripheral nodular enhancement, progressive fill-in, isodense to blood vessels
- **Hepatic Hydatid Cyst**
  - Wall and contents may calcify
  - May get calcified hydatid sand in dependent portion of cyst
  - Complete wall calcification is usually sign of inactive hydatid infection
- **Fibrolamellar Hepatocellular Carcinoma**
  - Typically affects young adults
  - Uncommon tumor, but usually (over 60%) has large central scar with calcification
  - Tumor is large at presentation (> 10 cm) with heterogeneous enhancement
  - Most have lymphatic &/or other metastases (lung, bone) at time of presentation
- **Cholangiocarcinoma (Peripheral, Intrahepatic)**
  - Fibrotic mass arising from intrahepatic bile ducts
  - Causes volume loss of affected part of liver with capsular retraction
  - Calcification is uncommon feature
- **Hepatocellular Carcinoma**
  - Much more common than fibrolamellar HCC, but uncommonly has calcification
  - May have punctate or irregular scar calcification
- **Hepatic Adenoma**
  - Punctate or capsular calcification seen in minority of cases
  - Other features include foci of hemorrhage and fat (more evident on MR than on CT)
- **Hepatic Opportunistic Infection**
  - Cytomegalovirus, toxoplasma, pneumocystic, etc.
  - Few to innumerable punctate calcifications
  - Seen in patients with AIDS, bone marrow or organ transplantation
- **Portal Vein Calcification**
  - Calcification of wall due to portal hypertension
  - Portal vein thrombus may calcify
  - May result from bland thrombus; may follow septic thrombophlebitis
- **Intrahepatic Calculi & Biliary Parasites**

- ○ Often coexist; more common in Asian populations
- ○ Clonorchis (liver fluke) is common
- ○ Calcium bilirubinate stones in recurrent pyogenic cholangitis are often calcified
- **Extrahepatic Calcifications (Mimic)**
  - ○ Calcification in pleura, peritoneum, gallbladder, kidney, etc.
  - ○ May overlap liver and mimic hepatic calcification

Helpful Clues for Rare Diagnoses

- **Focal Nodular Hyperplasia**
  - ○ Calcification in central scar is rare and small relative to size of entire lesion
- **Epithelioid Hemangioendothelioma**
  - ○ Rare malignant tumor of lower aggressiveness
  - ○ Typically causes multiple confluent peripheral hepatic masses
    - − Characteristic retraction of overlying hepatic capsule
- **Schistosomiasis, Hepatic**
  - ○ *Schistosoma japonicum* is endemic in parts of Asia
  - ○ Causes dystrophic calcification and fibrosis in liver

SELECTED REFERENCES

1. Hale HL et al: CT of calcified liver metastases in colorectal carcinoma. Clin Radiol. 53(10):735-41, 1998
2. Stoupis C et al: The Rocky liver: radiologic-pathologic correlation of calcified hepatic masses. Radiographics. 18(3):675-85; quiz 726, 1998
3. Jacoby JH et al: Calcified liver lesions. N J Med. 87(8):651-2, 1990

Calcified Granuloma, Liver

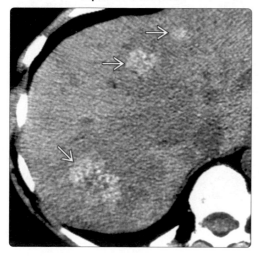

Hepatic Metastases

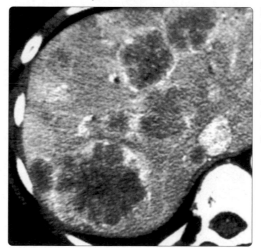

(Left) *Axial NECT shows multiple small focal calcifications ➔ in the liver and spleen, which are typically healed granulomas, usually from histoplasmosis or tuberculosis.* **(Right)** *Axial NECT shows several calcified metastases ➔ from mucinous adenocarcinoma of the colon.*

Hepatic Metastases

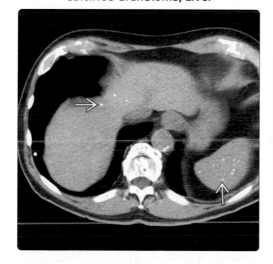

Hepatic Metastases

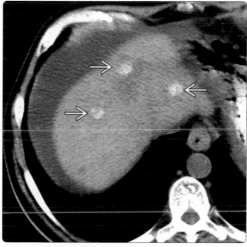

(Left) *In this man with primary colon cancer, axial NECT shows faint calcification ➔ within several metastatic foci.* **(Right)** *In the same man with primary colon cancer, axial CECT shows rim enhancement of the metastases. Note that the calcification is much less evident after contrast administration.*

(Left) Axial NECT shows calcification of medium-sized arteries, including the splenic ⮕ and left hepatic ➡ in a pattern characteristic of diabetic vasculopathy. Also note end-stage kidneys ➡. (Right) Axial CECT shows hypervascular foci of viable hepatocellular carcinoma (HCC) ➡ on this arterial-phase CECT. The very dense focus ➡ is residual Lipiodol that had been given as part of intraarterial chemotherapy.

Hepatic Arterial Calcification

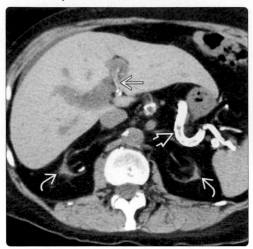

Ethiodol-Treated Tumor, Liver

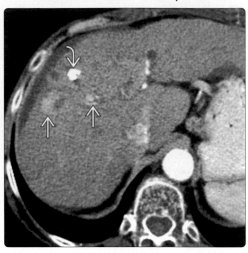

(Left) Axial CECT shows a huge hepatic cavernous hemangioma with typical peripheral nodular enhancement ➡. Note the calcification ➡ within the large central scar. (Right) In this immigrant from a sheep-raising country, coronal CT shows a large, cystic hepatic mass ➡ that has extensive peripheral (pericyst) calcification ⮕ as well as internal (daughter cyst) calcifications ➡.

Hepatic Cavernous Hemangioma

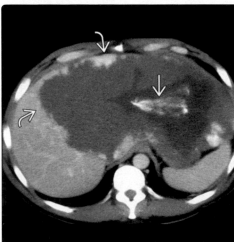

Hepatic Hydatid Cyst

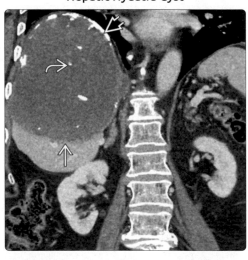

(Left) Axial CECT shows a large mass in the right lobe in this adolescent boy. Note the calcification ➡ within the large, poorly enhancing scar, and cardiophrenic lymphadenopathy ➡. Also present are lung metastases ➡. (Right) Axial CECT shows a heterogeneous left lobe mass that contains foci of fat density ➡, as well as focal calcifications ➡. While uncommon, these features are suggestive of HCC when seen in a mass within a cirrhotic liver.

Fibrolamellar Hepatocellular Carcinoma

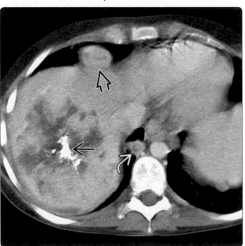

Hepatocellular Carcinoma

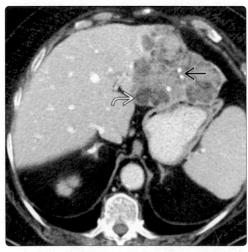

Hepatic Adenoma

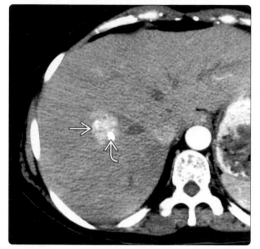

Hepatic Adenoma

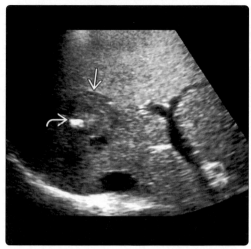

(Left) *In this young woman with a hepatic adenoma, arterial-phase CECT shows a hypervascular mass* ➡ *with eccentric calcification* ➡. **(Right)** *In this young woman with a hepatic adenoma, sagittal ultrasound shows an encapsulated mass* ➡ *with a heterogeneous echo pattern and a focus of bright signal* ➡ *with acoustic shadowing.*

Portal Vein Calcification

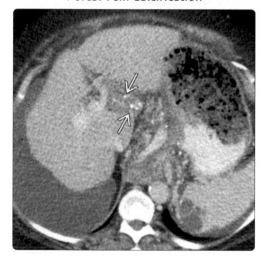

Portal Vein Calcification

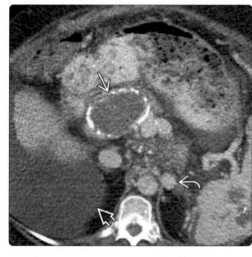

(Left) *In this 61-year-old woman with cirrhosis, axial CT shows calcification in the porta hepatis within the walls of the portal vein* ➡. **(Right)** *In this 61-year-old woman with severe cirrhosis and portal hypertension, axial CT shows an eggshell calcification* ➡ *that represents an aneurysmally dilated and thrombosed portal vein and varix. Note the other varices* ➡, *a small cirrhotic liver, and ascites* ➡.

Intrahepatic Biliary Calculi

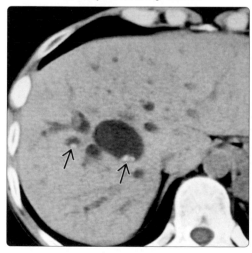

Focal Nodular Hyperplasia

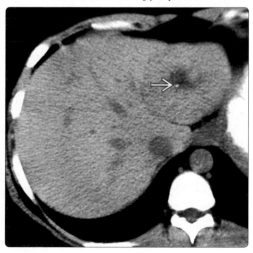

(Left) *Axial CECT shows calculi* ➡ *within massively dilated cystic dilations of the intrahepatic ducts in a patient with Caroli disease.* **(Right)** *Axial NECT shows a tiny focus of calcification* ➡ *in the central scar of an otherwise typical focal nodular hyperplasia (FNH). The mass showed bright homogeneous enhancement on arterial-phase CECT, and the calcification became less apparent. Calcification in an FNH is quite rare.*

DIFFERENTIAL DIAGNOSIS

Common

- Hepatic Pyogenic Abscess
- Hepatic Infarction
- Hepatic Tumor Following Treatment
  o Hepatocellular Carcinoma
  o Metastases and Lymphoma, Hepatic
  o Hepatic Adenoma
- Gas in Bile Ducts or Gallbladder
- Portal Venous Gas
- Hepatic Venous Gas

Less Common

- Retained Foreign Body
- Hepatic Transplantation
- Biloma
- Hepatic Amebic Abscess
- Hepatic Hydatid Cyst
- Hepatic Trauma

ESSENTIAL INFORMATION

Key Differential Diagnosis Issues

- 5 pathways to developing gas
  o Infection by gas-forming organism
  o Infarction of liver or lesion
  o Open wound or surgical drain
  o Reflux of gas into lesion from biliary tree
  o Gas within portal veins

Helpful Clues for Common Diagnoses

- **Hepatic Pyogenic Abscess**
  o 4 major routes for bacteria to liver
    – Portal vein thrombophlebitis
      □ Most often due to subacute diverticulitis or (less commonly) appendicitis
    – Ascending cholangitis
      □ Usually associated with choledocholithiasis, ± incompetence of sphincter of Oddi
      □ Surgical biliary-enteric anastomosis also predisposes to ascending cholangitis
    – Direct extension
      □ e.g., perforated ulcer or diverticulitis of colonic hepatic flexure
    – Traumatic
      □ Usually penetrating or iatrogenic (hepatic or biliary surgery)
  o Multiseptate, or cluster of grapes appearance of abscess
  o Gas is present in ~ 20% of pyogenic abscesses
    – Gas-producing organisms (*Escherichia coli* & *Klebsiella pneumoniae* most common)
  o Present in small foci or as gas-fluid level
- **Hepatic Infarction**
  o Uncommon due to dual blood supply
    – Usually requires interruption of both portal venous and hepatic arterial supply
  o Etiologies
    – Iatrogenic (cholecystectomy, hepatobiliary surgery, TIPS)
    – Liver transplantation (hepatic artery stenosis or thrombosis)
    – Blunt trauma
    – Hypercoagulable states and vasculitis
- **Hepatic Tumor Following Treatment**
  o Any treatment that results in sudden death of substantial amount of tissue (benign or malignant)
    – Chemoembolization
    – Radiofrequency or cryoablation
    – Chemotherapy, especially transarterial chemoembolization
    – Surgical ligation of hepatic arterial branch
  o Imaging, symptoms, and laboratory signs closely mimic hepatic abscess
    – Fever, leukocytosis, and pain are common
  o Presence of hepatic gas immediately following surgery does not necessarily imply infection
  o Injection of ethanol for ablation may mimic or cause intrahepatic gas
    – Ethanol is of near-gas attenuation
- **Gas in Bile Ducts or Gallbladder**
  o Many potential causes
  o Pneumobilia, incompetent sphincter of Oddi, emphysematous cholecystitis, etc.
  o Gas collects in central bile ducts near porta hepatis
- **Portal Venous Gas**
  o Mesenteric ischemia, bowel necrosis, and other causes
  o Branching pattern favoring periphery of liver
  o Look for bowel wall pneumatosis, mesenteric vascular thrombosis, and related findings

Helpful Clues for Less Common Diagnoses

- **Retained Foreign Body**
  o Retained surgical sponge: Will have opaque stripe
    – Retained sponge (gossypiboma) often leads to abscess
    – Sponge is often surrounded by larger collection of fluid with enhancing rim
  o **Oxidized surgical gelatin (Surgicel)**: Used for intraoperative hemostasis
    – Multifocal gas without fluid component
    – May have linear or curvilinear collections of gas
    – Does not imply infection
- **Hepatic Transplantation**
  o Biliary gas may be expected following biliary-enteric anastomosis
  o Portal venous gas in early posttransplant period (< 9 days) is often insignificant
  o Hepatic artery thrombosis (HAT) or stenosis may cause biliary necrosis
    – Typical appearance is branching fluid collections paralleling portal triads
    – Usually no gas within these collections unless there is biliary gas (as with biliary-enteric anastomosis)
      □ Bacterial superinfection of infarcted tissue may release gas
  o Less commonly, allograft parenchymal infarction may result from HAT
    – Gas may be found within hepatic allograft itself
- **Biloma**

- Communication with bile ducts may allow gas to enter biloma
- Infection of biloma by gas-forming organisms may release gas
- **Hepatic Amebic Abscess**
  - Usually solitary
  - Often has capsule
  - Uncommonly septate
  - Gas is rare unless abscess becomes superinfected with bacteria or ruptures into GI tract
- **Hepatic Hydatid Cyst**
  - Usually large
  - Multiseptate
  - Often has calcified wall
  - Rarely has gas unless superinfected or communicating with gut
- **Hepatic Trauma**
  - Gas may be found in hepatic or portal veins, or liver parenchyma
  - Often transient & of little significance
  - Larger areas of parenchymal gas may follow traumatic hepatic infarction
    - Due to devascularization of affected segment
- **Hepatic Venous Gas**
  - Usually iatrogenic, introduced through air in intravenous infusion lines
    - More common with femoral vein catheterization
    - More common with aggressive, rapid IV infusions

Hepatic Pyogenic Abscess

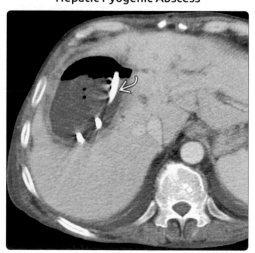

Hepatic Pyogenic Abscess

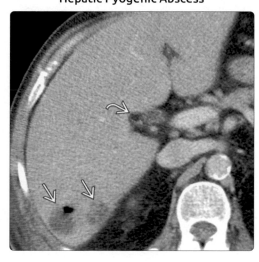

(Left) Axial CECT shows a liver abscess with fluid and gas. Also note a percutaneously placed drainage catheter ➔. (Right) Axial CECT shows 2 abscesses ➔, 1 of which contains gas. Patient has ascending cholangitis, and gas may enter the abscesses from gas-containing ducts ➔ or result from infection itself.

Liver Lesion Containing Gas

(Left) *Axial CECT shows 2 large hepatic masses* ➡️ *(metastatic breast cancer). The larger lesion has gas due to tumor infarction as a result of chemotherapy; there was no infection.* (Right) *In this man who has colon cancer, CT shows numerous metastases* ➡️*, some of which have been treated with RF ablation. One of these has gas within it* ➡️ *as well as surgical clips, the latter the result of bleeding after ablation that required intervention. The gas bubbles are not the result of infection but rather infarction of hepatic tissue (or tumor).*

Hepatic Tumor Following Treatment

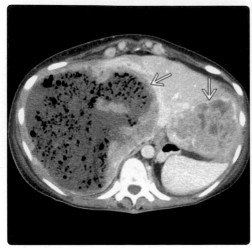

Hepatic Tumor Following Treatment

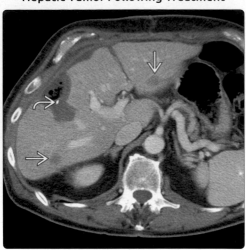

(Left) *Axial CECT shows nonenhancement of the left lobe* ➡️ *with portal venous gas* ➡️*; infarction followed attempted resection of peripheral cholangiocarcinoma.* (Right) *In this patient with acute hepatic dysfunction following cholecystectomy, CT shows marked volume loss and diffuse hypodensity of the right lobe of liver, with parenchymal gas* ➡️*. Note the surgical clip* ➡️ *that had occluded an aberrant right hepatic artery.*

Hepatic Infarction

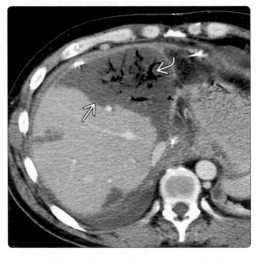

Hepatic Infarction

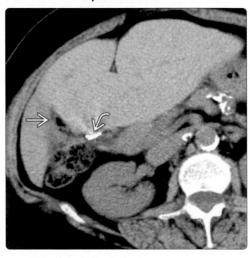

(Left) *In this woman with cirrhosis and acute abdominal pain following a hypotensive episode, US shows bubbles of gas* ➡️ *within the portal veins.* (Right) *In this woman with cirrhosis, US showed bubbles of gas within the portal veins. NECT shows pneumatosis within bowel walls* ➡️ *and luminal distention with fluid, due to bowel infarction.*

Portal Venous Gas

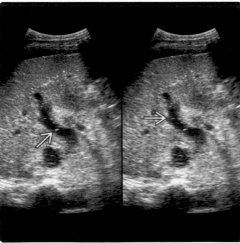
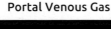

Portal Venous Gas

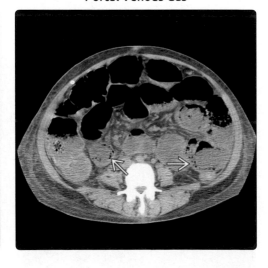

Retained Foreign Body

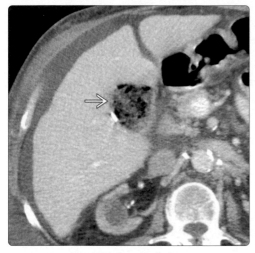

Retained Foreign Body

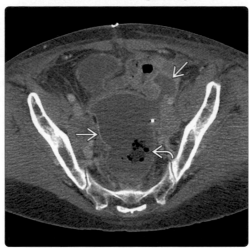

(Left) *CT shows a surgical clip & collection of gas ➡ in or adjacent to the liver. This is oxidized surgical gelatin (Surgicel) that was used as a hemostatic device & left in place. Note the relative absence of fluid within the collection.* **(Right)** *Axial CECT shows a large postoperative abscess ➡. Within the abscess, there is a tightly packed collection of gas bubbles ➡ that represents oxidized surgical cellulose (Surgicel) that had been placed to control bleeding at surgery.*

Hepatic Transplantation

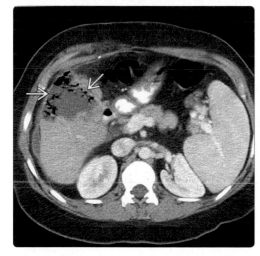

Hepatic Transplantation

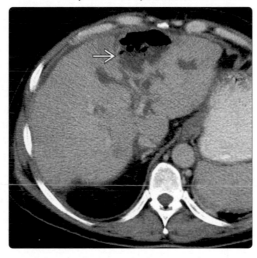

(Left) *In this patient with hepatic allograft malfunction, CT shows a wedge-shaped collection of fluid and gas ➡, representing an infected biloma due to hepatic artery thrombosis.* **(Right)** *In this patient with acute dysfunction of a hepatic allograft, CECT shows a collection of gas and fluid ➡ in the left hepatic lobe, strongly suggestive of an infected biloma due to hepatic artery stenosis or thrombosis. Arterial thrombosis was subsequently confirmed.*

Biloma

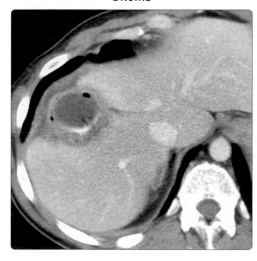

Hepatic Infarction

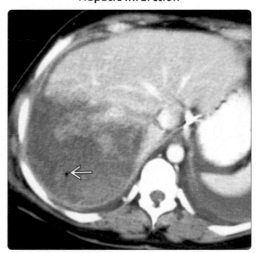

(Left) *Axial CECT shows a focal collection of fluid and gas that was the result of a deep liver laceration several days prior.* **(Right)** *Axial CECT shows devascularization of the right lobe from blunt trauma. The hepatic artery and veins to the right lobe were avulsed. The gas bubble ➡ is due to infarction, not infection.*

DIFFERENTIAL DIAGNOSIS

Common

- Ischemic Enteritis
- Ischemic Colitis
- Pneumatosis of Intestine
- Postoperative Bowel
- Pneumobilia (Mimic)

Less Common

- Diverticulitis
- Appendicitis
- Small Bowel Obstruction
- Pancreatitis, Acute
- Abdominal Abscess
- Hepatic Infarction
- Ulcerative Colitis
- Infectious Colitis
- Caustic Gastritis

ESSENTIAL INFORMATION

Key Differential Diagnosis Issues

- Almost any cause of infection, inflammation, trauma, or ischemia of any part of GI tract, including pancreas, may result in portal venous gas
- Any cause of pneumatosis may result in portal venous gas (or free intraperitoneal gas)
  - Causes include medications (especially immunosuppressive), endoscopy, bowel anastomoses
- CT and US detect portal venous gas more commonly than radiography
  - Portal venous gas detected by CT or US has better patient prognosis (75% survival); by radiography (75% mortality)

Helpful Clues for Common Diagnoses

- **Ischemic Enteritis**
  - Small bowel ischemia is more likely to progress to infarction than colonic ischemia

- Intramural pneumatosis usually accompanies portal venous gas, but these are late and ominous signs of infarction
- **Ischemic Colitis**
  - May progress to infarction with portal venous gas, but more likely to resolve spontaneously or evolve into stricture
- **Pneumatosis of Intestine**
  - Any cause of pneumatosis may lead to portal venous gas, including medications, bowel obstruction or anastomosis
  - Even benign pneumatosis cystoides of colon can cause portal venous gas
- **Pneumobilia (Mimic)**
  - Gas within bile ducts may be mistaken for portal venous gas on radiography, CT, US
  - **Gas within bile ducts tends to collect more centrally within liver**
    - **Portal venous gas flows toward periphery of liver**

Helpful Clues for Less Common Diagnoses

- **Diverticulitis and Appendicitis**
  - Chronic untreated inflammation of colon, appendix, or small bowel may result in mesenteric and portal vein thrombophlebitis
  - Veins may have thickened walls, luminal gas, progress to thrombosis
  - Look for associated pyogenic liver abscess
- **Pancreatitis, Acute**
  - Especially severe or necrotizing pancreatitis, ± infection
- **Hepatic Infarction**
  - Especially if iatrogenic (e.g., hepatic artery embolization)
  - Acute death of hepatic tissue may release gas into portal veins
- **Ulcerative or Infectious Colitis**
  - Mucosal ulceration may allow intraluminal gas to enter colonic wall and mesenteric/portal veins
  - Toxic megacolon resulting from ulcerative or infectious colitis may also lead to portal venous gas

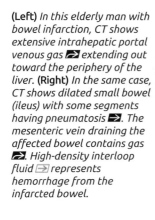

(Left) In this elderly man with bowel infarction, CT shows extensive intrahepatic portal venous gas ⬈ extending out toward the periphery of the liver. (Right) In the same case, CT shows dilated small bowel (ileus) with some segments having pneumatosis ➡. The mesenteric vein draining the affected bowel contains gas ⬈. High-density interloop fluid ➡ represents hemorrhage from the infarcted bowel.

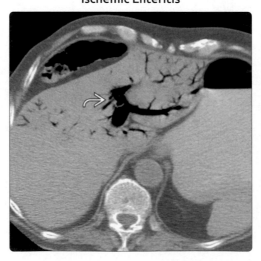

Ischemic Enteritis

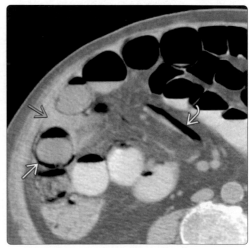

Ischemic Enteritis

Ischemic Colitis

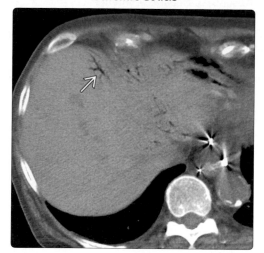

Ischemic Colitis

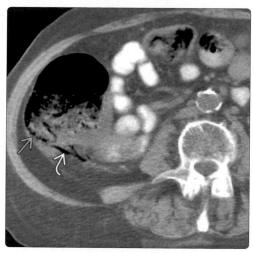

(Left) *This elderly man had acute onset of abdominal pain and hypotension. Nonenhanced CT shows gas within peripheral branches of the portal vein* ➡. **(Right)** *CT in the same case shows gas within the wall of the cecum* ⇨ *and the ileocolic vein* ➡. *The infarcted colon was resected, but the patient did not survive.*

Diverticulitis

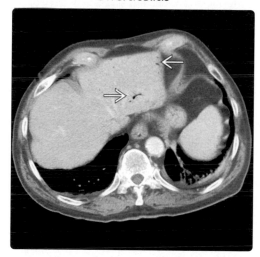

Diverticulitis

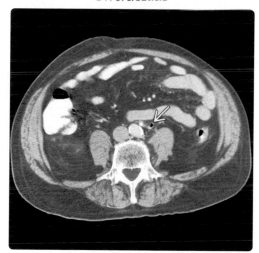

(Left) *Axial CECT shows portal venous gas* ➡ *due to diverticulitis with portal vein thrombophlebitis, which resolved with antibiotics alone.* **(Right)** *Axial CECT in the same case shows gas in the inferior mesenteric vein* ➡ *in this patient with sigmoid diverticulitis (who also had portal venous gas). This also resolved with antibiotics alone.*

Pneumatosis of Intestine

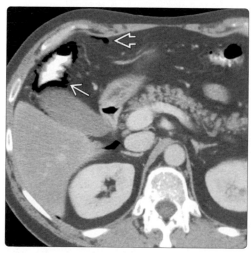

Hepatic Infarction

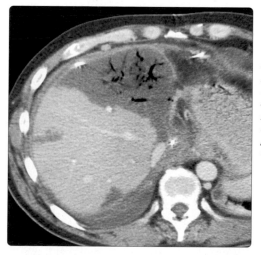

(Left) *Axial CECT shows free intraperitoneal* ⇥ *and intramural gas* ➡ *in an asymptomatic patient on steroid medication. Benign portal venous gas can also result in this setting.* **(Right)** *Axial CECT shows extensive gas in the left portal veins and infarction of the left lobe, following an aborted attempt to resect a left lobe tumor.*

DIFFERENTIAL DIAGNOSIS

Common

- Cirrhosis
- Focal Confluent Fibrosis
- Senescent Change
- Postsurgical (Mimic)

Less Common

- Congenital Absence of Hepatic Segments
- Liver Metastases
- Primary Sclerosing Cholangitis
- Congenital Hepatic Fibrosis
- Schistosomiasis

ESSENTIAL INFORMATION

Key Differential Diagnosis Issues

- Widened fissures: Congenital, acquired, or iatrogenic loss of hepatic parenchyma

Helpful Clues for Common Diagnoses

- **Cirrhosis**
  - Widening of fissures indicates fibrosis and volume loss; sensitive sign of cirrhosis
  - Look for enlarged caudate and signs of portal hypertension (varices, ascites)
- **Focal Confluent Fibrosis**
  - Common in advanced cirrhosis
  - Favors anterior and medial segments with volume loss and capsular retraction
- **Senescent Change**
  - Elderly (> 70 yr) often have asymptomatic volume loss of liver and widened fissures
  - Do not label older patient as cirrhotic without clinical correlation
- **Postsurgical (Mimic)**
  - Liver segments may be resected or tumors may have been ablated

Helpful Clues for Less Common Diagnoses

- **Congenital Absence of Hepatic Segments**
  - Most commonly affects anterior and medial segments
  - Look for deep gallbladder fossa, absence of signs of portal hypertension
- **Liver Metastases**
  - Some cancers (e.g., breast) induce fibrosis and volume loss de novo
  - Tumor volume loss and hepatic fibrosis may result from IV or arterial chemoembolization
- **Primary Sclerosing Cholangitis**
  - Results in liver volume loss even before true cirrhosis has developed
  - Liver has rounded contours due to atrophy of peripheral segments of liver and hypertrophy of deep right and caudate lobes
  - Look for irregular dilation and strictures of bile ducts
  - Check for history of inflammatory bowel disease
- **Congenital Hepatic Fibrosis**
  - Associated with autosomal recessive polycystic disease
  - Leads to portal hypertension; may simulate or develop into cirrhosis
  - Look for associated biliary or renal abnormalities
    - Caroli disease; recessive or dominant polycystic disease
  - Hepatic arteries are enlarged and tortuous
- **Schistosomiasis**
  - *Saccharina japonica* causes extensive fibrosis of liver
  - Look for periportal and pericapsular septal calcifications
  - Tortoise shell appearance

(Left) CECT shows a dysmorphic liver with signs of cirrhosis (wide fissures, caudate hypertrophy, nodular surface) and portal hypertension (splenomegaly, varices). (Right) CECT shows a hypodense mass within the anterior and medial hepatic segments ➡ with retraction of the overlying hepatic capsule ⬈, typical features of confluent hepatic fibrosis in a cirrhotic liver.

Cirrhosis

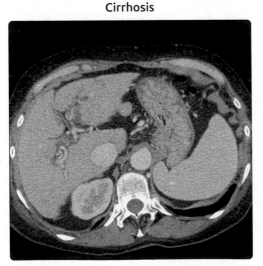

Focal Confluent Fibrosis

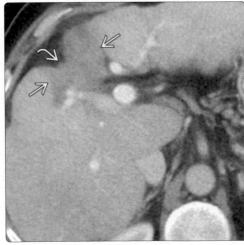

Senescent Change

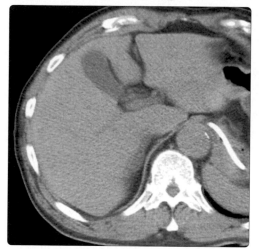

Congenital Absence of Hepatic Segments

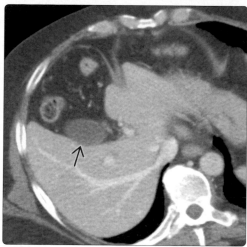

(Left) *CT shows a small medial segment with the gallbladder lying deep within the liver, and a relatively wide fissure for the falciform ligament. These findings would be suggestive of cirrhosis in a younger individual but may be normal, especially in the elderly. This man had no clinical evidence of liver disease.* (Right) *Axial CECT shows absence of the medial segment, with omental fat and colon herniating into the space between the right lobe and lateral segment. The gallbladder ⊡ marks the interlobar plane.*

Liver Metastases

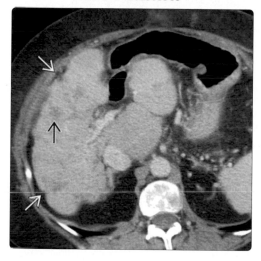

Primary Sclerosing Cholangitis

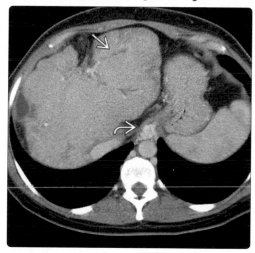

(Left) *In this woman with known hepatic metastases from breast cancer, CECT shows a dysmorphic liver with widened fissures, a lobulated and nodular contour ➡ that closely simulates cirrhosis. Subtle hypodense lesions ➡ indicate widespread metastases.* (Right) *CECT shows a cirrhotic liver with the typical beaded intrahepatic biliary ductal dilatation ➡ of PSC. The liver is small, with varices ➡, widened fissures, and rounded contours due to peripheral hepatic scarring and hypertrophy of the more central segments.*

Congenital Hepatic Fibrosis

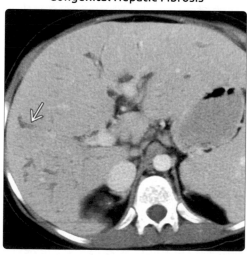

Schistosomiasis

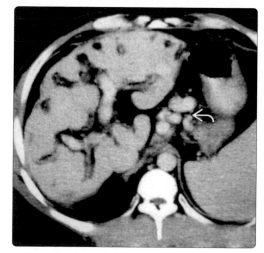

(Left) *Axial CECT shows a dysmorphic liver with widened fissures and dilated, ectatic bile ducts ➡ due to Caroli disease and congenital hepatic fibrosis.* (Right) *CECT shows signs of cirrhosis and portal hypertension, including large varices ➡. Note the extraordinarily widened hepatic fissures deeply dividing the segments of the liver along the portal vein branches. This is a characteristic feature of hepatic schistosomiasis.*

DIFFERENTIAL DIAGNOSIS

Common

- Primary Sclerosing Cholangitis
- Cirrhosis (Mimic)
  - Hepatitis
  - Peribiliary Cysts
- Portal Vein Thrombophlebitis (Mimic)
  - Diverticulitis
  - Hepatic Pyogenic Abscess
- Cholangiocarcinoma, Intrahepatic or Hilar

Less Common

- Budd-Chiari Syndrome (Mimic)
- Chemotherapy Cholangitis
- Ascending Cholangitis
- AIDS Cholangiopathy
- Fibropolycystic Liver Diseases
  - Congenital Hepatic Fibrosis
  - Caroli Disease
  - Choledochal Cyst
  - Biliary Hamartomas
  - Autosomal Dominant Polycystic Disease, Liver
- Recurrent Pyogenic Cholangitis
- Hepatic Hydatid Disease

ESSENTIAL INFORMATION

Key Differential Diagnosis Issues

- Dysmorphic liver refers to distortion and scarring of parenchyma
  - May result from inflammation, infection, ischemia, tumor
    - Or effects of treatment for these conditions
- Distinguish among dilated ducts, periportal edema, and thrombosed portal or hepatic veins
  - Appearance will vary by modality
    - US: Dilated hepatic artery in cirrhosis may simulate dilated ducts
      - Color Doppler can resolve this issue
    - CT or MR: Periportal edema may simulate dilated ducts
      - Edema usually found surrounding vessels; bile duct lie on only one side
    - CECT: Unopacified veins may simulate ducts
      - Though vessels > water attenuation
    - Cholangiography: Intrahepatic ducts may be distorted by masses or regenerating nodules, simulating cholangitis

Helpful Clues for Common Diagnoses

- **Primary Sclerosing Cholangitis**
  - Often results in chronic liver damage
    - Lobular contour of liver with preferential scarring of periphery
      - Sparing and hypertrophy of caudate and deep right lobe
      - Sometimes to degree simulating central neoplastic mass
  - Intrahepatic bile ducts show varying degrees of stricture and dilation with abnormal arborization (branching pattern)

- **Cirrhosis (Mimic)**
  - Rarely causes ductal dilation
    - But may cause pathologic processes that simulate dilated ducts
    - Regenerating nodules may compress and distort intrahepatic ducts
  - **Peribiliary cysts** are dilated peribiliary glands; may simulate dilated ducts ± small cystic masses in portal triads
  - Periportal edema may simulate ducts
  - Thrombosed portal vein branches may simulate dilated ducts on CECT or MR
    - Primary thrombosis of portal vein (hypercoagulable states)
      - Produces characteristic distortion of liver that simulates cirrhosis
- **Portal Vein Thrombophlebitis (Mimic)**
  - May be primary process in hypercoagulable states
  - May result from subacute diverticulitis or appendicitis
  - Thrombosed portal veins may simulate dilated ducts
  - Liver may be damaged by infection or ischemia
    - Pyogenic abscesses, liver infarction, volume loss, etc.
- **Cholangiocarcinoma, Intrahepatic or Hilar**
  - Arising from confluence (Klatskin) or branch ducts (intrahepatic)
  - Ducts are dilated upstream from tumor
  - Liver parenchyma shows volume loss ± visualization of tumor

Helpful Clues for Less Common Diagnoses

- **Budd-Chiari Syndrome (Mimic)**
  - Thrombosed hepatic veins may simulate dilated ducts
  - Liver is distorted with peripheral > central volume loss, scarring, hepatocellular necrosis and steatosis
- **Chemotherapy Cholangitis**
  - Intraarterial chemotherapy used for primary hepatocellular carcinoma or metastases
  - Liver distortion due to tumors and parenchymal scarring
  - Ducts are damaged and strictured with appearance like primary sclerosing cholangitis
- **Ascending Cholangitis**
  - May lead to duct strictures; rarely to chronic liver injury
  - More common are hepatic abscesses
- **AIDS Cholangiopathy**
  - Liver may be distorted by infection &/or tumor
  - Intra- and extrahepatic ducts may be strictured by infection
- **Fibropolycystic Liver Diseases**
  - Encompasses spectrum of related lesions of liver and biliary tract caused by abnormal embryologic development of ductal plates
  - Lesions may occur in isolation or in any combination; may be clinically silent
    - Or, may cause cholangitis, portal hypertension, GI bleeding, infection, etc.
  - Liver may be distorted by congenital fibrosis (simulates cirrhosis) or by scarring (especially with Caroli disease)
    - Bile ducts may be primary site of pathology (e.g., Caroli disease), coexist with primary parenchymal disease (e.g., fibrosis), or be distorted by extrinsic mass effect

Dysmorphic Liver With Abnormal Bile Ducts

- ○ **Congenital hepatic fibrosis**
  - – Dysmorphic liver, portal hypertension
  - – Enlarged and possibly supernumerary hepatic arteries
- ○ **Caroli disease**
  - – Cystic or fusiform dilation of intrahepatic ducts
  - – Liver often progressively damaged by cholangitis, obstruction
- ○ **Choledochal cyst**
  - – Fusiform or cystic dilation of intrahepatic ± extrahepatic bile duct
- ○ **Biliary hamartomas**
  - – Multiple "cysts" of nearly uniform size, up to 15 mm; no biliary connection
    - □ Mimic cysts on CT and MR but are often echogenic on sonography
  - – Liver and bile ducts are normal, unless coexisting disease, such as Caroli or congenital fibrosis
- ○ **Autosomal dominant polycystic disease, liver**
  - – Distorts liver with innumerable cysts
  - – Bile ducts intrinsically normal but may have extrinsic compression by cysts

- • **Recurrent Pyogenic Cholangitis**
  - ○ Usually in Asian, poorly nourished populations
  - ○ Liver distorted by chronic infection and biliary obstruction (abscesses, cirrhosis)
  - ○ Bile ducts enormously dilated by pus and stones
- • **Hepatic Hydatid Disease**
  - ○ Cysts may distort liver
  - ○ Cysts may communicate with ducts, leading to cholangitis

Primary Sclerosing Cholangitis

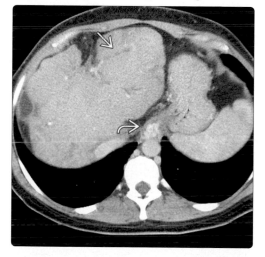

Primary Sclerosing Cholangitis

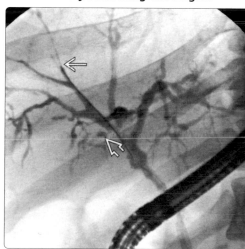

(Left) Axial CECT shows a small liver with deep scars and lobular contour, typical of cirrhosis due to primary sclerosing cholangitis. Note the irregular dilation of intrahepatic ducts ➡ and esophageal varices ➡. (Right) Anteroposterior ERCP shows segmental strictures ➡ and "diverticula" ➡ involving the intra- and extrahepatic bile ducts, resulting in a beaded appearance of the ducts.

Hepatitis

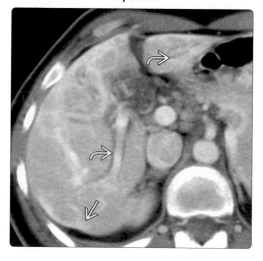

Hepatitis

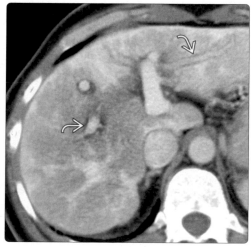

(Left) In this 47-year-old woman with liver dysfunction, CT shows a heterogeneous liver parenchyma with evidence of periportal edema ➡, a nonspecific sign often seen in acute hepatitis, among other causes. The liver contour is distorted ➡, likely due to fibrosis. Autoimmune hepatitis was the etiology. (Right) In this 47-year-old woman with autoimmune hepatitis, CT shows evidence of periportal edema ➡ that might be mistaken for dilated bile ducts, except that the lucent band extends completely around the portal vein branches.

Peribiliary Cysts

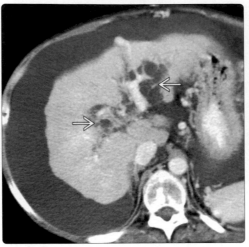

Peribiliary Cysts

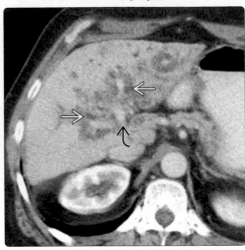

(Left) *Axial CECT shows saccular and spherical cystic lesions ➡ (peribiliary cysts) paralleling the portal triads in a patient with advanced cirrhosis and ascites.* **(Right)** *CT shows cirrhotic morphology of the liver, with reduced size of the liver, wide fissures, and ascites noted. The portal vein branches ➡ are surrounded by a collar of low density, some of which probably represents periportal edema. However, there are also discrete low-density focal lesions ➡ that represent periportal cysts within the bile duct walls.*

Portal Vein Thrombophlebitis (Mimic)

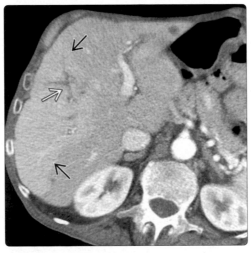

Portal Vein Thrombophlebitis (Mimic)

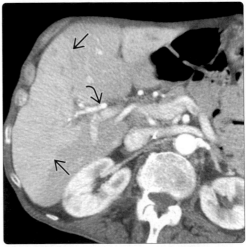

(Left) *Late arterial-phase CECT shows hyperperfusion of the anterior right lobe of the liver ➡ due to thrombosis of the anterior branch of the right portal vein. The thrombosed intrahepatic branches ➡ might be mistaken for dilated bile ducts.* **(Right)** *In this patient with THAD ➡ due to thrombosis of the anterior right portal vein, note the increased size of the right hepatic artery ➡ that is compensating for the decreased flow through the portal vein.*

Cholangiocarcinoma, Intrahepatic or Hilar

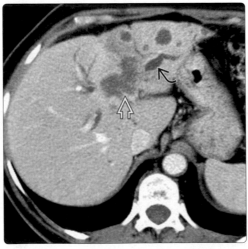

Budd-Chiari Syndrome (Mimic)

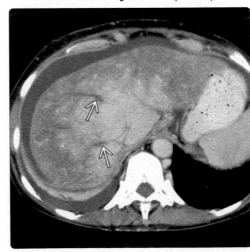

(Left) *Axial CECT shows a heterogeneous left lobe mass ➡ that obstructs intrahepatic ducts ➡ and causes volume loss of the left lobe. This was a multifocal cholangiocarcinoma.* **(Right)** *Axial CECT shows thrombosed hepatic veins ➡ that simulate dilated ducts on CECT. Ascites, peripheral hepatic damage, and central hypertrophy are typical findings of Budd-Chiari.*

Chemotherapy Cholangitis

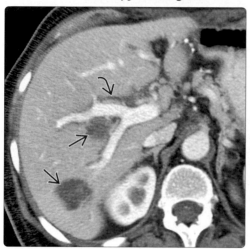

Fibropolycystic Liver Diseases

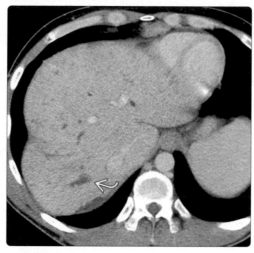

(Left) *Axial CECT shows 2 necrotic metastases ⇥ (from colon cancer) and mild dilation of the bile ducts ⇥, a result of intraarterial chemotherapy.* (Right) *Axial CECT shows a dysmorphic liver with irregular dilation of intrahepatic ducts ⇥. On lower sections, hepatic arteries were enlarged and small cystic kidneys were noted. All findings were related to fibropolycystic disease of the liver and kidneys, including congenital hepatic fibrosis.*

Caroli Disease

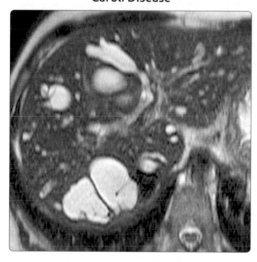

Autosomal Dominant Polycystic Disease, Liver

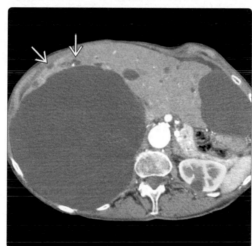

(Left) *Axial T2WI MR shows cystic and irregular cylindrical dilation of intrahepatic bile ducts, characteristic of Caroli disease. Progressive liver failure resulted in transplantation.* (Right) *Axial CECT shows 2 dominant cysts, among many smaller ones lower in the liver. Intrahepatic ducts are dilated ⇥ due to extrinsic compression.*

Recurrent Pyogenic Cholangitis

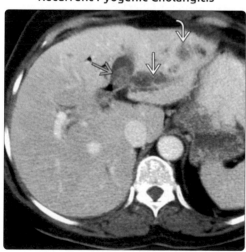

Hepatic Hydatid Disease

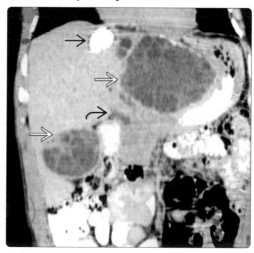

(Left) *Axial CECT shows dilated ducts ⇥ with a large pigment calculus ⇥ and a small liver abscess ⇥.* (Right) *Coronal CECT shows 2 large cystic masses ⇥ with daughter cysts and a densely calcified cyst ⇥. Bile ducts ⇥ are dilated due to communication of one of the cysts with the ducts.*

DIFFERENTIAL DIAGNOSIS

Common

- Transient Hepatic Attenuation Difference
- Cholecystitis
- Liver Metastases
- Hepatocellular Carcinoma
- Liver Biopsy or Trauma
- Arterioportal Shunt, Cirrhosis
- Anomalous Blood Supply

Less Common

- Hepatic Pyogenic Abscess
- Hepatic Cavernous Hemangioma
- Focal Nodular Hyperplasia
- Hepatic Arteriovenous Malformation
- Superior Vena Cava Obstruction, Abdominal Manifestations
- Portal Vein Occlusion
- Extrinsic Compression of Liver
- Hereditary Hemorrhagic Telangiectasia (Osler-Weber-Rendu)

ESSENTIAL INFORMATION

Key Differential Diagnosis Issues

- Transient hepatic attenuation or intensity differences (THAD or THID, respectively)
  - Focal areas of hepatic parenchymal enhancement visible only on arterial phase of contrast-enhanced imaging
    - Unique to liver, due to its dual blood supply
  - 3 major etiologies
    - Portal vein branch compression or occlusion
      - □ Metastases
      - □ Hepatocellular carcinoma (HCC)
      - □ Benign masses
      - □ Portal vein thrombosis
    - Arterioportal shunt or anomalous blood supply; diversion and mixing of blood (and contrast medium) from high-pressure arteries to low-pressure portal vein distribution
      - □ Congenital arteriovenous fistula
      - □ Post liver biopsy
      - □ Hepatocellular carcinoma
    - Siphoning or sump effect: Hypervascular mass or inflammatory process draws more arterial flow into segment of liver
      - □ Pyogenic liver abscess
      - □ Amebic abscess
      - □ Focal nodular hyperplasia (FNH)
      - □ HCC
      - □ Hypervascular metastases
- Most THAD lesions are not visible on nonenhanced CT or MR
  - Exceptions
    - Slight increased signal on T2WI may result from excess free water within zone of THID
      - □ Longstanding alterations of arterioportal supply may result in altered metabolism (e.g., focal fatty infiltration or focal sparing)

Helpful Clues for Common Diagnoses

- **Transient Hepatic Attenuation Difference**
  - Small, wedge-shaped, subsegmental, abut liver capsule
  - Presumably due to occlusion of small portal venous branch
  - "Lesion" visible only on arterial phase
- **Cholecystitis**
  - Severe acute cholecystitis may cause inflammation and hyperemia of adjacent liver
  - Origin of hot spot or rim sign surrounding gallbladder fossa on Tc-HIDA scan
- **Liver Metastases**
  - Usually from GI tract or pancreas
  - Cause occlusion of portal vein branch, eliciting compensatory increased hepatic arterial flow to segment
  - Look for spherical mass (metastasis) at apex of triangular defect (THAD or THID)
  - Hypervascular metastases may cause THAD by occlusion of portal vein &/or by drawing more arterial flow into involved segment (sump effect)
- **Hepatocellular Carcinoma**
  - 3 mechanisms cause THAD
    - Portal vein occlusion (tumor invasion)
    - Arteriovenous shunting through tumor
    - Siphon or sump effect of hypervascular tumor
  - HCC usually heterogeneously hypervascular with washout and capsule
  - Look for cirrhotic liver
- **Liver Biopsy or Trauma**
  - Arteriovenous or arterioportal shunt is common, usually transient, result
  - Early filling of veins that drain involved segment
  - Can follow any hepatic trauma or intervention
    - Liver biopsy
    - Percutaneous transhepatic biliary drain
    - Radiofrequency ablation
- **Arterioportal Shunt, Cirrhosis**
  - Often idiopathic, very common in cirrhosis
  - Usually small, peripheral, wedge-shaped
  - Larger, spherical, more central lesions are difficult to distinguish from HCC and other hypervascular tumors
  - Recommendation: Just follow small lesions on sequential scans
    - Often resolve spontaneously
- **Anomalous Blood Supply**
  - Anomalous hepatic venous drainage; common along falciform ligament, surrounding gallbladder fossa, and in segment IV
  - Common areas of THAD and also of focal fat &/or focal sparing

Helpful Clues for Less Common Diagnoses

- **Hepatic Pyogenic Abscess**
  - May compress portal vein and draw increased arterial flow into involved segment of liver
  - Usually multiseptate or cluster of grapes appearance
- **Hepatic Cavernous Hemangioma**
  - Any hepatic mass may compress portal vein branch, leading to THAD

- ○ Hemangiomas (even small) may have arterioportal shunts within mass
- **Focal Nodular Hyperplasia**
  - ○ Uncommonly causes THAD, due to mass effect on portal vein or hypervascularity of FNH lesion (sump effect)
  - ○ Uniformly & markedly hypervascular on arterial phase; isodense/intense on nonenhanced, venous and delayed phases
- **Hepatic Arteriovenous Malformation**
  - ○ May be isolated anomaly or part of systemic disorder
  - ○ Osler-Weber-Rendu or hereditary hemorrhagic telangiectasia
  - ○ Multisystemic inherited disorder with arteriovenous malformations in nose, lungs, GI tract, liver, brain
  - ○ Large hepatic arteries and hepatic veins with premature opacification of veins
  - ○ Vascular masses and telangiectasias within liver
- **Superior Vena Cava Obstruction, Abdominal Manifestations**
  - ○ Peridiaphragmatic collateral veins traverse left lobe of liver to return blood to inferior vena cava

- ○ Large zone of hypervascularity without mass effect
- ○ Collateral veins will be evident
- **Portal Vein Occlusion**
  - ○ e.g., hypercoagulable state; portal vein thrombophlebitis
    - − Thrombophlebitis often due to undiagnosed diverticulitis or appendicitis
- **Extrinsic Compression of Liver**
  - ○ e.g., subcapsular hematoma; may decrease portal perfusion, increase arterial flow
    - − Tends to affect periphery of liver in lentiform, rather than wedge-shaped, pattern

SELECTED REFERENCES

1. Colagrande S et al: Transient hepatic intensity differences: part 1, Those associated with focal lesions. AJR Am J Roentgenol. 188(1):154-9, 2007
2. Colagrande S et al: Transient hepatic intensity differences: part 2, Those not associated with focal lesions. AJR Am J Roentgenol. 188(1):160-6, 2007

Transient Hepatic Attenuation Difference

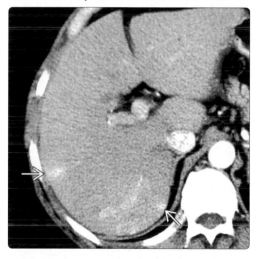

Transient Hepatic Attenuation Difference

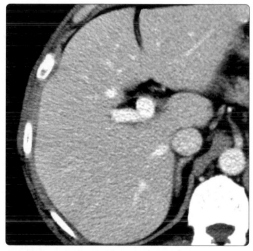

(Left) *Axial CECT shows several small, triangular, capsular-based foci of hyperattenuation* ➡, *seen only on this arterial-phase CECT. These are typical idiopathic, benign THADs.* **(Right)** *Axial CECT shows disappearance of the peripheral hyperdensities on portal venous phase, identifying them as foci of transient hepatic attenuation difference.*

Cholecystitis

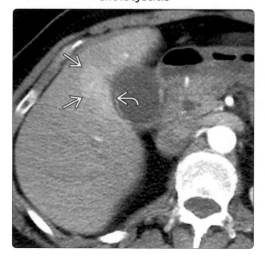

Cholecystitis

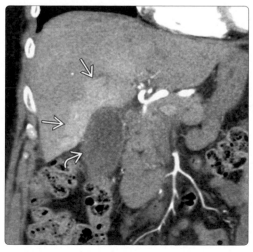

(Left) *In this 54-year-old woman with severe, acute cholecystitis, arterial-phase CECT shows a distended gallbladder that has a thickened, ill-defined wall* ➡. *The portion of the liver in apposition to the gallbladder shows abnormal bright enhancement* ➡, *indicating increased perfusion and indirectly suggesting inflammation.* **(Right)** *In this 54-year-old woman, coronal CECT shows the shaggy, thick-walled gallbladder* ➡ *and abnormally bright enhancement of the adjacent liver* ➡.

Liver Metastases

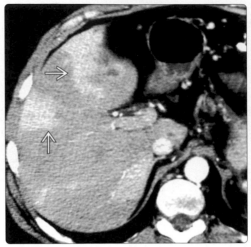

Liver Metastases

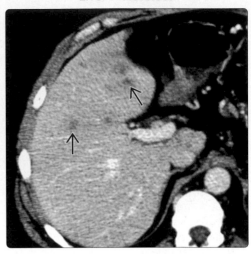

(Left) *In this patient with metastatic pancreatic carcinoma, axial CECT shows several wedge-shaped foci of hyperdensity ➡ on arterial phase. The metastatic foci that are blocking the portal venous tributaries are less clearly seen.* (Right) *In this patient with pancreatic carcinoma, portal venous-phase CECT shows disappearance of the wedge-shaped THADs but better definition of the metastases ➡ that caused them.*

Hepatocellular Carcinoma

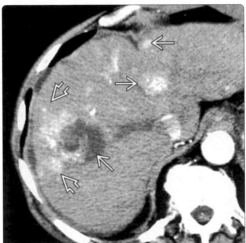

Hepatocellular Carcinoma

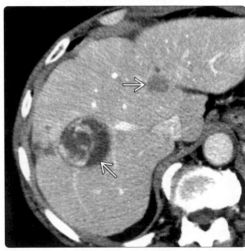

(Left) *In this 60-year-old man with cirrhosis, arterial-phase CECT shows several foci of tumor (HCC) ➡, one with a wedge-shaped zone of hypervascularity ➡ distal to the mass that is due to portal vein branch occlusion by the tumor.* (Right) *In this 60-year-old man, portal venous-phase CECT shows the HCC nodules ➡ washing out to become hypodense to the liver. Much of the THAD zone of hyperdensity is now isodense to liver.*

Liver Biopsy or Trauma

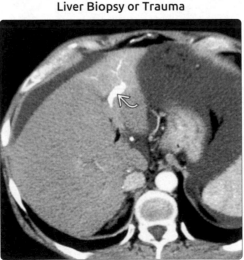

Liver Biopsy or Trauma

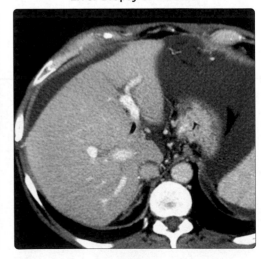

(Left) *In this 46-year-old man with cirrhosis, arterial-phase CECT shows hyperenhancement of the lateral segment and early opacification of the left portal vein ➡, the result of a percutaneous liver biopsy causing an arterial-portal shunt.* (Right) *In this 46-year-old man with cirrhosis, portal venous-phase CECT shows homogeneous enhancement of the left lobe with resolution of the THAD. This iatrogenic AP shunt resolved spontaneously.*

Arterioportal Shunt, Cirrhosis

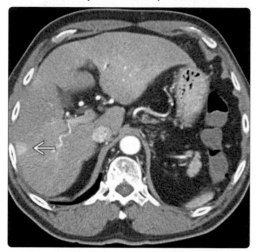

Arterioportal Shunt, Cirrhosis

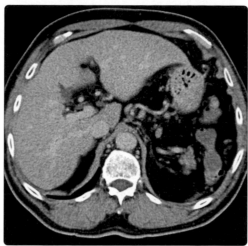

(Left) *In this 60-year-old man with cirrhosis, arterial-phase CECT shows 1* ➡ *of 9 small, wedge-shaped, capsular-based hypervascular foci (having the same features). The liver has a cirrhotic morphology with widened fissures.* (Right) *In this 60-year-old man, portal venous-phase CT shows resolution of the THAD and all of the other similar lesions. No washout or capsule is seen. On subsequent imaging studies, the AP shunts disappeared.*

Hepatic Pyogenic Abscess

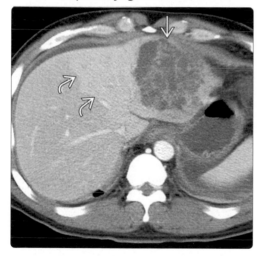

Hepatic Pyogenic Abscess

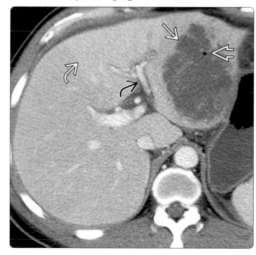

(Left) *This 41-year-old woman has a pyogenic abscess* ➡ *in the left lobe with a typical multiseptate appearance. On this early venous phase CECT, the entire left lobe of the liver is hyperenhanced with a straight line demarcation* ➡. (Right) *In this 41-year-old woman, gas is seen* ➡ *within the pyogenic abscess* ➡. *The hyperperfused left lobe* ➡ *is presumably due to the sump effect of the abscess, rather than portal vein occlusion, because the left portal vein is patent* ➡.

Hepatic Cavernous Hemangioma

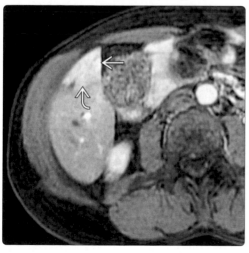

Hepatic Cavernous Hemangioma

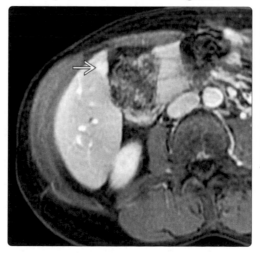

(Left) *In this 56-year-old woman, arterial-phase axial T1 C+ MR shows a brightly enhancing lesion* ➡ *and a surrounding region of transient hepatic hyperperfusion* ➡, *a THID. The enhancing lesion was a capillary hemangioma.* (Right) *In this 56-year-old woman, portal venous-phase CECT shows the small hemangioma* ➡, *but the THID has resolved.*

Focal Nodular Hyperplasia

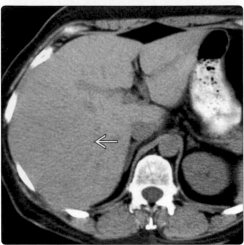

Focal Nodular Hyperplasia

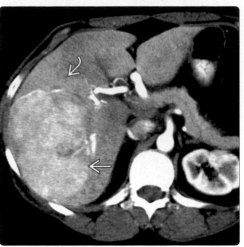

(Left) *In this 48-year-old woman, axial NECT shows a subtle mass ➡ that is almost isodense to the liver.* (Right) *In this 48-year-old woman, arterial-phase CECT shows a large, brightly enhanced mass, a focal nodular hyperplasia (FNH) ➡ with increased density of the surrounding right lobe ➡ due to sump effect. The FNH and background liver were almost isodense on venous and delayed imaging.*

Hepatic Arteriovenous Malformation

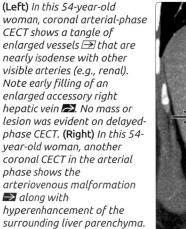
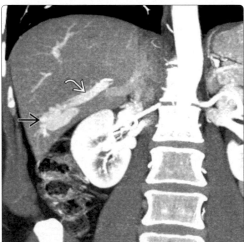

Hepatic Arteriovenous Malformation

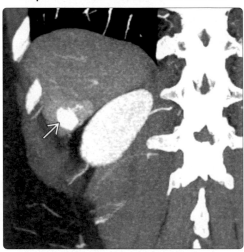

(Left) *In this 54-year-old woman, coronal arterial-phase CECT shows a tangle of enlarged vessels ➡ that are nearly isodense with other visible arteries (e.g., renal). Note early filling of an enlarged accessory right hepatic vein ➡. No mass or lesion was evident on delayed-phase CECT.* (Right) *In this 54-year-old woman, another coronal CECT in the arterial phase shows the arteriovenous malformation ➡ along with hyperenhancement of the surrounding liver parenchyma.*

Superior Vena Cava Obstruction, Abdominal Manifestations

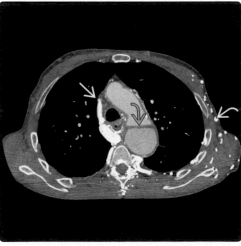

Superior Vena Cava Obstruction, Abdominal Manifestations

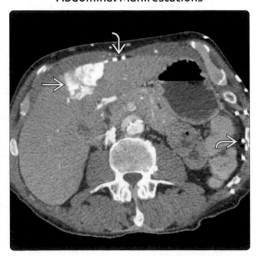

(Left) *In this 33-year-old woman with a chronic aortic dissection, arterial-phase CECT shows the aortic intimal flap ➡, along with an occluded superior vena cava (SVC) ➡ and numerous venous collaterals ➡ in the chest wall.* (Right) *In this 33-year-old woman with a chronic aortic dissection and SVC occlusion, arterial-phase CECT shows marked enhancement of the medial ("quadrate") segment ➡ due to collateral vessels ➡ traversing the liver.*

Portal Vein Occlusion

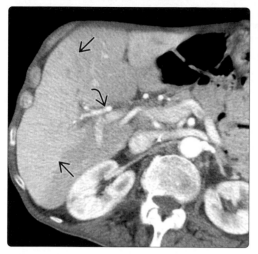

Portal Vein Occlusion

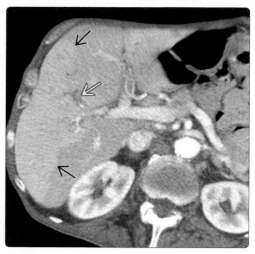

(Left) *In this 71-year-old man with liver dysfunction, early venous phase CT shows hyperperfusion of the anterior segments of the right lobe with a straight line demarcation* ➡. *The anterior branch of the right portal vein is occluded and the accompanying hepatic arterial branch* ➡ *is enlarged.* (Right) *In this 71-year-old man, early venous CECT shows hyperenhancement of the anterior hepatic segments* ➡ *and thrombosis of the anterior right portal vein* ➡.

Portal Vein Occlusion

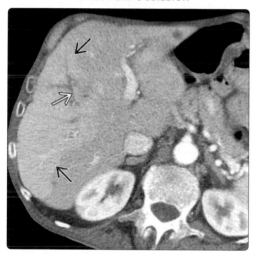

Portal Vein Occlusion

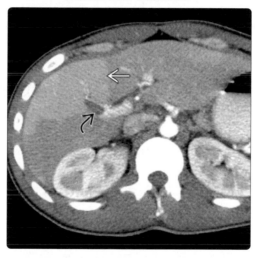

(Left) *In this 71-year-old man, the thrombosed branches of the anterior right portal vein* ➡ *might be mistaken for dilated bile ducts on early venous-phase CECT. The hyperenhanced right lobe* ➡ *is due to increased arterial flow delivered contrast opacified blood, while the remainder of the liver is perfused more by less opacified portal vein flow.* (Right) *This arterial-phase axial CECT shows a THAD* ➡ *limited to the anterior segments of the right lobe due to thrombosis of the segmental portal vein* ➡.

Hereditary Hemorrhagic Telangiectasia (Osler-Weber-Rendu)

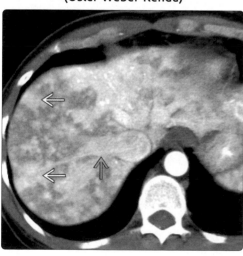

Hereditary Hemorrhagic Telangiectasia (Osler-Weber-Rendu)

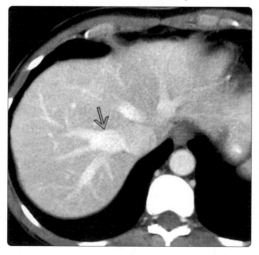

(Left) *In this middle-aged man with nosebleeds and hemoptysis, arterial-phase CECT shows multiple foci of increased hepatic enhancement* ➡ *and early filling of enlarged hepatic veins* ➡, *characteristic features of hereditary hemorrhagic telangiectasia (HHT) (Osler-Weber-Rendu syndrome).* (Right) *In this middle-aged man with HHT, the portal venous-phase CECT shows a homogeneous liver with only the enlarged hepatic veins* ➡ *as a sign of the underlying HHT.*

DIFFERENTIAL DIAGNOSIS

Common

- Metastases and Lymphoma, Hepatic
- Simple Hepatic Cysts
- Biliary Hamartoma
- Hepatic Cavernous Hemangioma
- Autosomal Dominant Polycystic Disease, Liver
- Multifocal Fatty Infiltration
- Hepatic Pyogenic Abscess
- Hepatocellular Carcinoma
- Hepatic Sarcoidosis

Less Common

- Opportunistic Infection, Hepatic
- Hepatic Adenoma
- Hepatic Amebic Abscesses
- Hepatic Hydatid Cysts
- Nodular Regenerative Hyperplasia

Rare but Important

- Hepatic Angiomyolipoma
- Epithelioid Hemangioendothelioma
- Caroli Disease

ESSENTIAL INFORMATION

Key Differential Diagnosis Issues

- On portal venous and delayed-phase CECT, almost all detectable hepatic lesions are hypodense (hypoattenuating)
- In order to narrow DDx, need to characterize contents and margins of lesions
  - e.g., water density = cysts, cystic metastases, polycystic liver, biliary hamartoma
  - Neoplasms and abscesses have less distinct walls than cysts
- Very helpful to compare with NECT and arterial-phase CECT, if available
  - e.g., contents of cysts and abscesses do not enhance; all (nonnecrotic) tumors do
  - Lesion that is hyperdense on hepatic arterial phase (HAP) but becomes hypodense on portal venous phase is definitely neoplastic

Helpful Clues for Common Diagnoses

- **Metastases and Lymphoma, Hepatic**
  - Most common cause for multiple solid hypodense lesions in adult
  - Most common primary sites: Colorectal, pancreas, breast, lung, stomach, eye
  - Most common histology: Adenocarcinoma, squamous cell, neuroendocrine, lymphoma, sarcoma
  - Almost all are hypo- or isodense to liver on portal venous phase and delayed imaging
    - Many will have hypervascular rim on HAP (not considered hypervascular)
  - Even hypervascular metastases washout to become hypodense on venous and delayed-phase imaging
- **Simple Hepatic Cysts**
  - Commonly are multiple **and of variable size**

- Larger ones will measure water density and have sharply defined walls, no or few septa
  - Small lesions: Indistinct walls and uncertain density due to volume averaging
  - Thin CT section minimizes this problem
- **Biliary Hamartoma**
  - Usually multiple to innumerable, rarely > 15-mm diameter
  - Fibrotic tissue in walls may cause nodular periphery on CECT or CEMR and echogenicity on US
  - **Biliary hamartomas are common cause of multiple "too small to characterize" lesions**
- **Hepatic Cavernous Hemangioma**
  - Multiple lesions are not rare
    - May be innumerable and in other organs and body wall (Kasabach-Merritt syndrome)
  - CT criteria: Blood pool density on NECT; nodular peripheral enhancement, isodense to blood pool on CECT
- **Autosomal Dominant Polycystic Disease, Liver**
  - Innumerable cysts, many with calcified walls and higher density (blood)
  - Cysts vary in size and often distort and enlarge liver
  - Associated cysts in kidneys and other organs; family history
- **Multifocal Fatty Infiltration**
  - May closely simulate metastases
  - Often has **perivascular distribution or follows fissures**
    - Blood vessels traverse lesion without mass effect
  - Definitive diagnosis by in- and opposed-phase GRE MR
- **Hepatic Pyogenic Abscesses**
  - Pyogenic are more common and multiple than with amebic or hydatid
  - Associated pleural effusion, atelectasis, portal vein thrombophlebitis
  - Usually multiseptate or cluster of grapes appearance
- **Hepatocellular Carcinoma**
  - Usually in cirrhotic liver or one damaged by chronic hepatitis
  - Associated signs of portal hypertension, venous invasion
  - Most lesions are heterogeneously hypervascular on arterial-phase CECT
    - Washout to hypodensity on venous and delayed-phase imaging

Helpful Clues for Less Common Diagnoses

- **Opportunistic Infection, Hepatic**
  - Innumerable "microabscesses" in immunocompromised patient
  - *Candida* is most common organism
    - Other fungi, tuberculosis, and other organisms are less common
  - Usually multiple to innumerable
  - Irregular margins; size from few mm to ~ 15 mm
- **Hepatic Adenoma**
  - Uncommon disease, but lesions are often multiple, may be innumerable (adenomatosis)
  - Larger lesions usually heterogeneous due to presence of fat, hemorrhage, or necrosis
  - Associated history of oral contraceptives, anabolic steroids, glycogen storage disease

— Obesity and steatosis predispose to multiplicity and rapid growth of adenomas
- MR evidence of capsule, intralesional lipid, and hemorrhage favor Dx of adenoma

- **Hepatic Amebic Abscesses**
  - Usually isolated or no more than a few
  - Complex fluid contents with distinct capsule
  - Imaging and demographics suggest Dx
    — Easily confirmed by serology
- **Nodular Regenerative Hyperplasia**
  - Usually occurs in Budd-Chiari syndrome
  - "Large regenerative nodules"
    — Benign hyperplastic nodules that resemble focal nodular hyperplasia (FNH) on imaging and histology
  - Usually multiple, 1-4 cm diameter
  - May have hypodense halo or rim, central scar

Helpful Clues for Rare Diagnoses

- **Hepatic Angiomyolipoma**
  - Multiple lesions are seen almost exclusively in tuberous sclerosis syndrome
  - Hepatic angiomyolipomas in kidney, cystic lesions in lungs
- **Epithelioid Hemangioendothelioma**
  - Multiple, peripheral, confluent hepatic masses
  - **Often with target appearance and overlying hepatic capsular retraction**
- **Caroli Disease**
  - Multiple cyst-like spaces within liver that communicate with biliary tree
  - Central dot sign = portal venous radicle wrapped by ectatic ducts

Other Essential Information

- In nononcology patient, appearance of benign lesions on CECT is often sufficiently characteristic to obviate additional evaluation
  - Oncology patient: Most metastases have characteristic appearance and biological behavior (e.g., interval growth or regression on therapy) to not require additional imaging evaluation

- Cysts, hemangiomas, and multifocal steatosis have characteristic appearance on MR, allowing confident diagnosis
- Biliary hamartomas are markedly underdiagnosed by radiologists
  - Comprise many "too small to characterize" lesions seen on CT

Alternative Differential Approaches

- Lesions that may be hyperdense on arterial phase but hypo- or isodense on portal venous and delayed phase
  - Benign
    — Adenomas, FNH, nodular regenerative hyperplasia
      - Note: Different types of benign lesions may coexist (cysts, hemangiomas, FNH, adenomas)
  - Malignant
    — Hepatocellular carcinoma and metastases
      - Especially from endocrine, renal, sarcoma primaries, and occasionally from primary tumors in ovary, choriocarcinoma, breast, melanoma

Metastases and Lymphoma, Hepatic

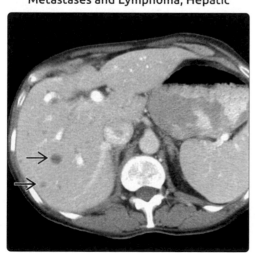

Metastases and Lymphoma, Hepatic

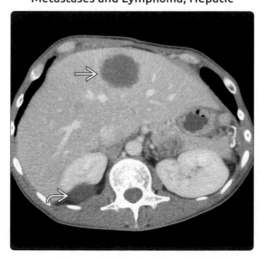

(Left) *In this woman with metastatic ovarian carcinoma, axial CECT shows multiple hypodense liver metastases ➡. The lesions are almost cystic in appearance, reflecting the cystic nature of the primary tumor.* **(Right)** *In this patient with metastatic squamous cell carcinoma, axial CECT shows 1 of several near-water density hepatic lesions ➡ that may be compared with the appearance of a simple renal cyst ➡. Indications that the hepatic lesions are not simple cysts include the subtle wall thickening and irregularity.*

(Left) *In this patient with metastatic pancreatic carcinoma, axial CECT shows multiple hypodense liver metastases* ➡️ *with poorly defined margins. Also note bilateral adrenal metastases* ⬈. **(Right)** *In this patient with AIDS and hepatic lymphoma, axial CECT shows multiple hypodense hepatic masses.*

Metastases and Lymphoma, Hepatic

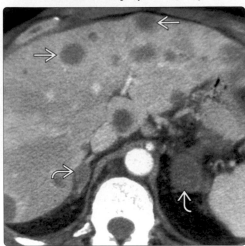

Metastases and Lymphoma, Hepatic

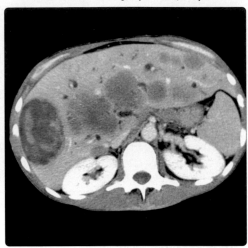

(Left) *Axial CECT shows multiple water density hepatic lesions with no discernible walls. One of the larger cysts has a thin septum* ➡️*, but there is no nodularity of the wall.* **(Right)** *Axial CECT shows 2 hepatic masses* ➡️*, each with characteristic peripheral nodular enhancement isodense with blood vessels.*

Simple Hepatic Cysts

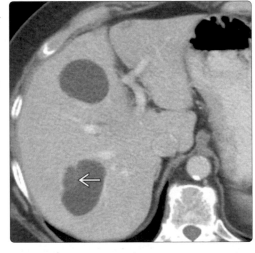

Hepatic Cavernous Hemangioma

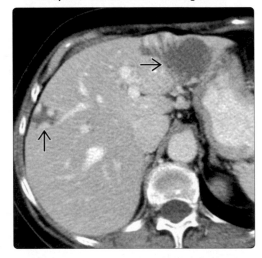

(Left) *In this asymptomatic 57-year-old man, axial CECT shows innumerable small "cystic lesions"* ➡️ *throughout the liver, ranging in size from 2-15 mm. The lesions are often not perfectly spherical, and many have visible nodular enhancement within their walls.* **(Right)** *In this 57-year-old man, sonography on the same day showed only the lesions > 10 mm as cystic structures* ➡️*, whereas the smaller lesions were actually hyperechoic* ➡️*. These are typical CT and sonographic features of biliary hamartomas.*

Biliary Hamartoma

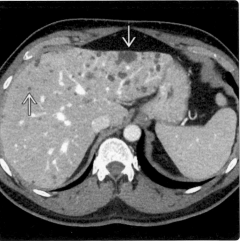

Biliary Hamartoma

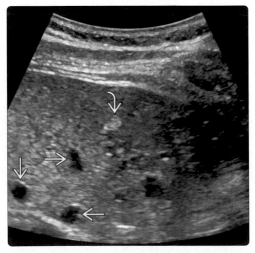

Autosomal Dominant Polycystic Disease, Liver

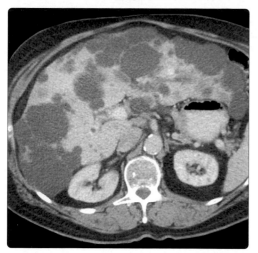

Hepatic Pyogenic Abscess

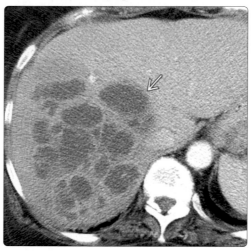

(Left) *Axial CECT shows innumerable hepatic cysts of varying size, with only small cysts noted in normally functioning kidneys.* (Right) *In this elderly woman with ascending cholangitis, CT shows a large multiseptate mass →, typical for pyogenic abscess. This was confirmed and treated with percutaneous catheter placement.*

Multifocal Fatty Infiltration

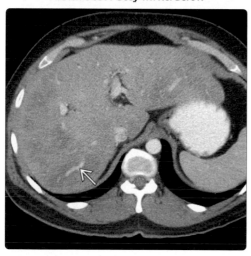

Multifocal Fatty Infiltration

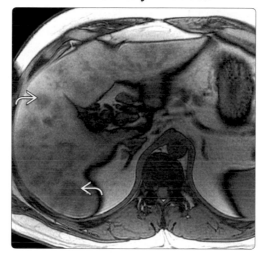

(Left) *In this 36 year-old man, axial CECT shows multifocal hypodense lesions that predominantly lie in a perivascular distribution, surrounding hepatic vessels →. Note that the vessels are not narrowed or displaced by the hypodense lesions.* (Right) *In this 36-year-old man, axial in-phase T1WI GRE showed no apparent lesions, whereas the opposed-phase images clearly show signal dropout from each of the perivascular foci of steatosis →, meaning this diagnosis was made with confidence.*

Hepatocellular Carcinoma

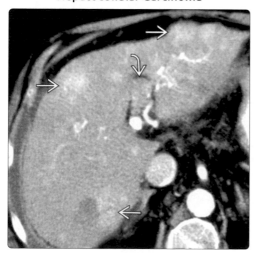

Hepatocellular Carcinoma

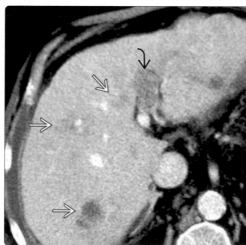

(Left) *In this 55-year-old man, arterial-phase CECT shows multiple hypervascular masses →. Also note enhancing tumor within the left portal vein →.* (Right) *In this 55-year-old man, venous-phase CECT shows multiple lesions → that are hypodense to the background liver, indicating tumor washout. Also note hypodense tumor → within the dilated left portal vein.*

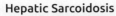

Hepatic Sarcoidosis

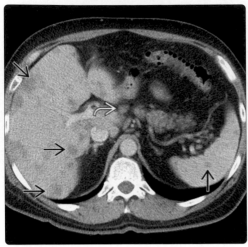

Opportunistic Infection, Hepatic

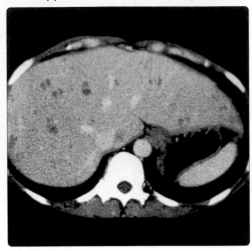

(Left) *Axial CECT shows numerous hypodense nodules or small masses in the liver and spleen ➡. On this and other sections, CT also showed upper abdominal and thoracic lymphadenopathy ➡. Biopsy confirmed sarcoidosis.* (Right) *Axial CECT shows innumerable small (< 2 cm) irregular hypodense lesions in this febrile, immunocompromised patient. Biopsy confirmed Candida microabscesses.*

Opportunistic Infection, Hepatic

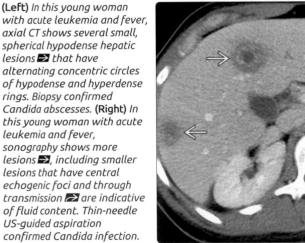

Opportunistic Infection, Hepatic

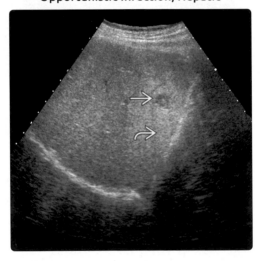

(Left) *In this young woman with acute leukemia and fever, axial CT shows several small, spherical hypodense hepatic lesions ➡ that have alternating concentric circles of hypodense and hyperdense rings. Biopsy confirmed Candida abscesses.* (Right) *In this young woman with acute leukemia and fever, sonography shows more lesions ➡, including smaller lesions that have central echogenic foci and through transmission ➡ are indicative of fluid content. Thin-needle US-guided aspiration confirmed Candida infection.*

Hepatic Amebic Abscesses

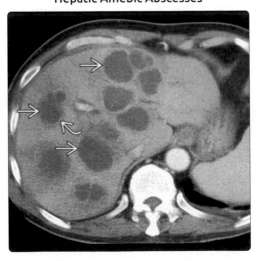

Hepatic Hydatid Cysts

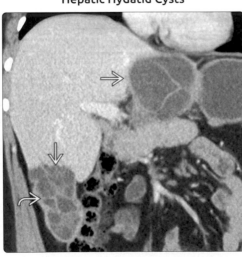

(Left) *CT shows multiple hypodense, encapsulated ➡, hepatic masses ➡. In this febrile, Hispanic immigrant, amebic abscess was considered and confirmed by serology. Amebic abscesses are rarely so numerous as in this case.* (Right) *In this young Jordanian immigrant with fever, coronal CECT shows 2 large, multiseptate hepatic masses ➡. Note the characteristic daughter cysts ➡ within one of the lesions.*

Hepatic Adenoma

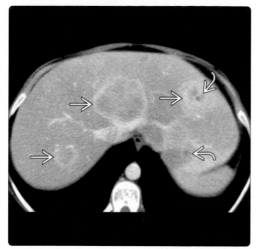

Nodular Regenerative Hyperplasia

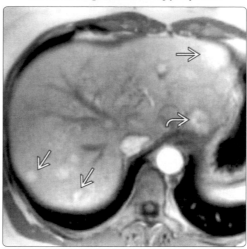

(Left) *Axial CECT shows multiple hypodense but enhancing masses with encapsulation ➡. Very low-density foci ➡ suggest fat content, which was confirmed by MR within these multiple hepatic adenomas.* (Right) *Axial T1 C+ MR shows multiple, enhancing, large regenerative nodules in this patient with Budd-Chiari syndrome. Some have a hypointense halo ➡ and others have a central scar ➡.*

Hepatic Angiomyolipoma

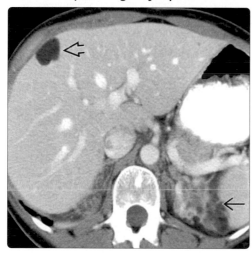

Hepatic Angiomyolipoma

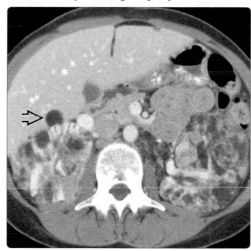

(Left) *Axial CECT shows fat density masses in the liver ➡ and kidneys ➡ in this patient with tuberous sclerosis.* (Right) *Axial CECT shows fat density masses within the liver ➡ and kidneys in this patient with tuberous sclerosis and angiomyolipomas.*

Epithelioid Hemangioendothelioma

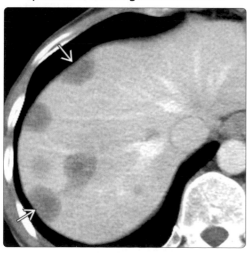

Caroli Disease

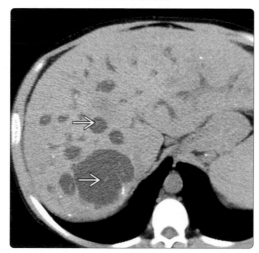

(Left) *Axial CECT shows multiple peripheral lesions with a target appearance and retraction of the overlying hepatic capsule ➡ and characteristic appearance of epithelioid hemangioendothelioma.* (Right) *Axial CECT shows multiple cystic lesions in the liver. Note the central dot sign ➡ representing the hepatic artery enveloped by the cystic bile duct dilations.*

DIFFERENTIAL DIAGNOSIS

Common

- Regenerating (Cirrhotic) Nodules
- Calcified Granulomas
- Pneumobilia

Less Common

- Hepatic Metastases
- Hepatocellular Carcinoma
- Dysplastic Nodules (Cirrhosis)
- Hepatic Adenoma
- Cholangiocarcinoma (Peripheral)
- Fibrolamellar Hepatocellular Carcinoma
- Nodular Regenerative Hyperplasia
- Hepatic Sarcoidosis
- Hepatic Hematoma
- Hereditary Hemorrhagic Telangiectasia
- Portal Vein Gas
- Hepatic Portal or Venous Collaterals

Rare but Important

- Peliosis Hepatis
- Hepatic Angiomyolipoma

ESSENTIAL INFORMATION

Key Differential Diagnosis Issues

- Most hepatic lesions are hyperintense on T2WI due to excess water content
  - Includes most inflammatory and neoplastic lesions
- Sources for hypointense appearance
  - Blood degradation products
    - Almost any liver lesion that undergoes necrosis or hemorrhage may show foci of hypointensity on T2WI
  - Macromolecules
    - Smooth muscle, fibrosis, mucin, fibrinogen, keratin
  - Necrosis
    - Especially coagulative necrosis
  - Melanin
  - Calcium
  - Flowing blood
- Relative hypointensity on T2WI
  - Lesions with fatty component
  - Depends on MR sequence used to achieve fat suppression
    - May cause signal loss from lesions that contain lipid or macroscopic fat
    - Examples
      - □ Some hepatocellular carcinoma (HCC)
      - □ Adenomas
      - □ Angiomyolipomas
      - □ Teratomas

Helpful Clues for Common Diagnoses

- **Regenerating (Cirrhotic) Nodules**
  - Usually not apparent on T1WI
  - Hypointense on T2WI, especially GRE
    - Due to presence of iron within these siderotic nodules
    - Lesions may bloom (appear larger) on GRE images
      - □ Due to increased susceptibility effects of iron

  - Usually < 1-cm diameter, hypovascular, numerous (hundreds)
- **Calcified Granulomas**
  - Common in histoplasmosis, healed TB
  - Similar lesions in spleen
  - Remainder of liver is normal
  - No mobile protons = signal void on T2WI
- **Pneumobilia**
  - Gas in bile ducts
  - More linear distribution when seen in longitudinal section
  - Signal void in air-containing structures

Helpful Clues for Less Common Diagnoses

- **Hepatic Metastases**
  - Especially likely following therapy
  - Foci of old hemorrhage or necrosis may appear hypointense on T2WI
    - Coagulative necrosis = hypointense
      - □ e.g., following ethanol or radiofrequency (RF) ablation
    - Liquefactive necrosis = hyperintense on T2WI
  - Tumors with large mucin content may appear hypointense
    - Colorectal, gastric, pancreatic, ovarian
  - Metastatic melanoma
    - Melanin within mets may cause hypointensity on T2WI, hyperintensity on T1WI (opposite of usual pattern)
- **Hepatocellular Carcinoma**
  - Usually hyperintense on T2WI
  - Potential causes for hypointense foci
    - Necrosis, old hemorrhage, iron deposits
    - Lesions treated with TACE (transarterial chemoembolization) or RF ablation
- **Dysplastic Nodules (Cirrhosis)**
  - Premalignant lesions in cirrhotic liver
  - Hyperintense on T1WI, hypointense on T2WI (opposite of HCC)
    - Hypointensity due to iron or sinusoidal blood flow within lesions
  - Usually 1-4 cm diameter, hypovascular
  - Hypovascular
  - Usually take up and retain gadoxetate (Eovist/Primovist)
- **Hepatic Adenoma**
  - Usually nearly isointense or slightly hyperintense on T2WI
    - May have foci of hypointensity due to old hemorrhage &/or necrosis
  - Fat-suppressed T2WI sequences may cause signal loss in adenomas with large amounts of lipid
- **Cholangiocarcinoma (Peripheral)**
  - Extensive fibrosis in tumor may account for hypointense foci
  - Associated with focal hepatic volume loss; delayed persistent enhancement
- **Fibrolamellar Hepatocellular Carcinoma**
  - Large mass with eccentric bands of scar tissue (fibrosis) and calcification that are hypointense on T2WI
  - Affects adolescents and young adults disproportionately
- **Nodular Regenerative Hyperplasia**

- Large regenerating nodules are macroscopic or multiacinar form of nodular regenerative hyperplasia
- Common in Budd-Chiari syndrome, congenital heart disease
- Hypervascular nodules, 1-4 cm diameter; ± halo of enhancement
- Usually more numerous and greater conspicuity on contrast-enhanced T1WI
  - Few that are detectable on T2WI are typically hypointense
- **Hepatic Sarcoidosis**
  - Liver often diffusely abnormal with innumerable ≤ 1-cm nodules
  - May be indistinguishable from cirrhosis with regenerating nodules
  - Look for lymphadenopathy, lung disease
- **Hepatic Hematoma**
  - Old hemorrhage may appear dark on T2WI
- **Hereditary Hemorrhagic Telangiectasia**
  - Osler-Weber-Rendu syndrome
  - Large feeding hepatic arteries and draining veins with telangiectasias and arteriovenous malformations
    - Flowing blood accounts for hypointense foci
  - Check for history of epistaxis, family history
- **Portal Vein Gas**
  - Signal void in vessel due to gas
  - Usually due to bowel ischemia or infection
    - e.g., diverticulitis
- **Hepatic Portal or Venous Collaterals**
  - Portal vein thrombosis with cavernous transformation
  - Also increased hepatic arterial supply to compensate for decreased portal flow
    - Flowing blood accounts for foci of hypointensity
  - Hepatic vein occlusion, with intra- or perihepatic collaterals (Budd-Chiari syndrome)

Helpful Clues for Rare Diagnoses

- **Peliosis Hepatis**
  - Rare, associated with drugs, chronic illness

- Presence of sinusoidal blood pools may account for hypointensity on T2WI
- **Hepatic Angiomyolipoma**
  - Presence of smooth muscle (macromolecules) and fat may account for foci of hypointensity

---

Regenerating (Cirrhotic) Nodules

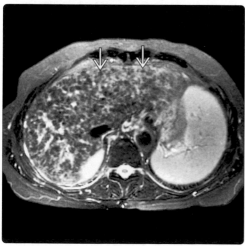

Calcified Granulomas

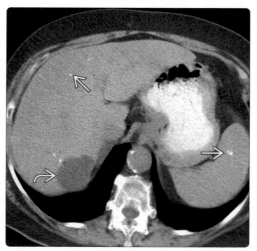

(Left) Axial T2WI MR shows innumerable tiny hypointense regenerative nodules ➡ within a cirrhotic liver. These are usually not visible on T1WI. (Right) NECT shows multiple small calcifications ➡ in the liver & spleen, typical of healed granulomas, usually histoplasmosis. A hepatic cyst ➡ is another incidental finding. The calcified granulomas were hypointense on T2W MR (not shown).

Pneumobilia

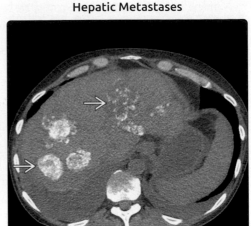

Hepatic Metastases

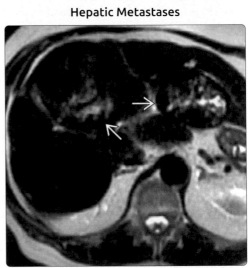

(Left) *Axial T2WI FS MR shows a gas fluid level within the common duct* ➡, *with the gas floating above the bile as a signal void.* (Right) *In this patient with colon cancer, NECT shows multiple liver metastases, some of which have scattered or heavy calcification* ➡. *These lesions were hypointense on T2W MR (not shown).*

Hepatic Metastases

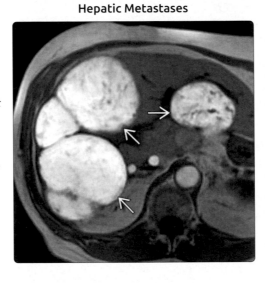

Hepatic Metastases

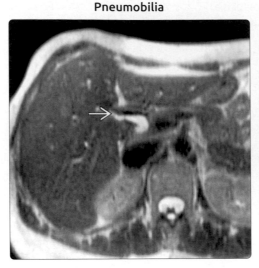

(Left) *In this patient with hepatic metastases due to melanoma, the lesions* ➡ *have the peculiar feature of being hyperintense on T1WI, which is attributed to the melanin in these lesions. Most metastases are hypo- or isointense to liver on T1WI.* (Right) *In this patient with hepatic metastases from melanoma, the lesions* ➡ *are poorly seen, but largely hypointense on T2WI due to their melanin content.*

Hepatocellular Carcinoma

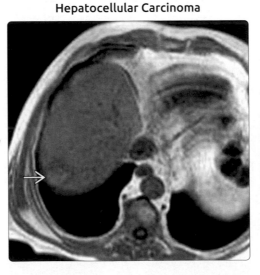

Hepatocellular Carcinoma

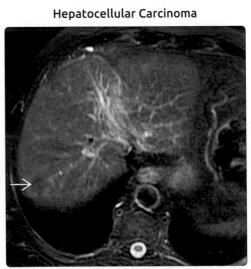

(Left) *In this man whose HCC has been treated by TACE, the mass* ➡ *is hyperintense on T1WI MR due to coagulative necrosis. The lesion was avascular on contrast-enhanced MR sequences.* (Right) *In this man whose HCC had been treated with TACE, the lesion* ➡ *is hypointense on T2W MR due to coagulative necrosis. Untreated, viable HCC is usually hyperintense on T2WI.*

Dysplastic Nodules (Cirrhosis)

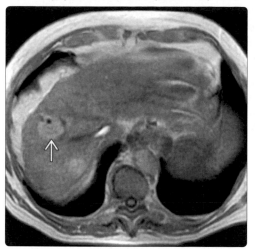

Dysplastic Nodules (Cirrhosis)

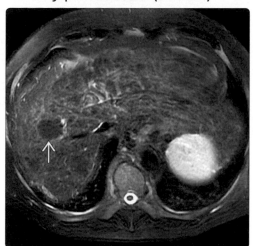

(Left) *In this man with alcoholic cirrhosis, an axial T1W MR shows a hyperintense lesion* ➜ *that was not hypervascular on contrast-enhanced sequences (not shown).* (Right) *In this man with alcoholic cirrhosis, axial T2W MR shows a hypointense lesion* ➜ *that was biopsied and proved to be a dysplastic nodule. Viable hepatocellular carcinoma (HCC) is usually hyperintense on T2WI, variable intensity on T1WI, and hypervascular.*

Nodular Regenerative Hyperplasia

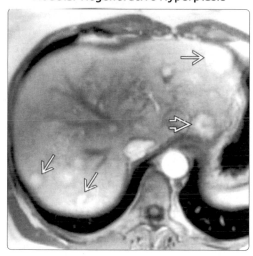

Nodular Regenerative Hyperplasia

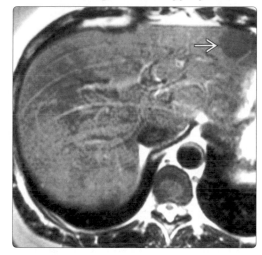

(Left) *Axial T1 C+ MR shows many hypervascular lesions* ➜ *within the liver of a patient with Budd-Chiari syndrome. At least one of the lesions* ➔ *has a central scar & a hypointense halo, a characteristic feature of multiacinar NRH (large regenerative nodule).* (Right) *Axial T2WI MR shows one* ➜ *of many focal liver lesions in a patient with Budd-Chiari syndrome that proved to be multiacinar NRH (large regenerative nodules). The lesion is hypointense on T2WI, but many more lesions were apparent on Gd-enhanced T1WI.*

Hepatic Sarcoidosis

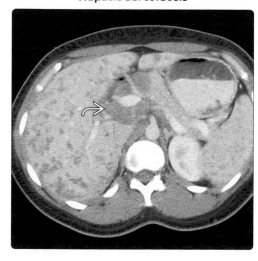

Hereditary Hemorrhagic Telangiectasia

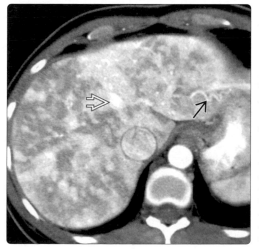

(Left) *CT shows innumerable sarcoid granulomas in the liver & spleen, along with abdominal adenopathy* ➔. *The hepatic lesions were hypointense on T2W MR.* (Right) *Arterial-phase CT shows heterogeneous enhancement of hepatic parenchyma, early filling of enlarged hepatic veins* ➔, *and enlarged, tortuous hepatic arteries* ➔. *Venous phase images showed a more homogeneous parenchymal enhancement and T2W MR showed multifocal hypointense nodules, all typical features of HHT.*

DIFFERENTIAL DIAGNOSIS

Common

- Steatosis (Fatty Liver)
- Hepatic Adenoma
- Hepatocellular Carcinoma
- Hemorrhagic Hepatic Cyst
- Dysplastic Nodules
- Liver Hematoma
- Hepatic Metastases

Less Common

- Hepatic Pyogenic Abscess
- Postoperative Packing Material
- HELLP Syndrome
- Focal Nodular Hyperplasia
- Nodular Regenerative Hyperplasia
- Hepatic Angiomyolipoma
- Peliosis Hepatis

Rare but Important

- Lipoma, Liver
- Liposarcoma, Liver
- Xanthoma, Liver
- Hepatic Adrenal Rest Tumor
- Hepatic Pseudolipoma
- Teratoma, Liver

ESSENTIAL INFORMATION

Key Differential Diagnosis Issues

- Only 4% of liver lesions are hyperintense on T1WI
- **Any lesion containing fat, hemorrhage, high protein content, or sinusoidal dilation** may appear hyperintense on T1WI
- Focal signal dropout on opposed-phase T1WI indicates intra- or intercellular lipid
- Focal signal dropout on fat-suppressed images indicates macroscopic fat
- High signal on T1WI without signal dropout on these techniques indicates presence of blood, protein, or sinusoidal dilation

Helpful Clues for Common Diagnoses

- **Steatosis (Fatty Liver)**
  - Focal fatty infiltration, can simulate mass(es)
  - Bright signal on in-phase GRE, with focal signal dropout on opposed-phase T1WI GRE is key finding
  - Presence of normal vessels coursing through "lesion" excludes neoplasm
- **Hepatic Adenoma**
  - Heterogeneous mass with ↑ signal intensity on T1WI due to fat &/or recent hemorrhage
  - 35-75% have evidence of fat on opposed-phase or fat-suppressed sequences
  - Lesion with these characteristics in young female without cirrhosis is almost diagnostic of adenoma
- **Hepatocellular Carcinoma**
  - Only about 5-10% of hepatocelluar carcinomas (HCC) have MR evidence of fat content

- Small (< 1.5 cm) well-differentiated HCCs are more often associated with diffuse-type fatty change (signal suppression on opposed phase)
- Larger tumors may have macroscopic fat (lose signal on fat-suppressed sequence)
- Heterogeneous, hypervascular mass in cirrhotic liver with these features is diagnostic of HCC
- **Treated HCCs are often hyperintense on T1WI**
  - In response to embolization or ablation
  - May represent hemorrhage &/or denatured proteins
  - Effectively treated lesions will show no enhancement
- **Hemorrhagic Hepatic Cyst**
  - Will be variably bright on both T1WI and T2WI
    - Due to blood breakdown products
  - No enhancement of contents or mural nodularity
- **Dysplastic Nodules**
  - In cirrhotic liver, dysplastic nodules are considered premalignant lesions
  - Typically appear bright on T1WI, dark on T2WI
    - Opposite findings of typical HCC
    - Also are hypovascular and dark on DWI MR
  - Most cirrhotic regenerating nodules are invisible on T1WI
    - Some are hyperintense on T1WI due to excess iron (siderotic nodules)
- **Liver Hematoma**
  - Due to trauma; much less frequently coagulopathy or hemolysis, elevated liver enzymes, low platelets (HELLP) syndrome
  - Subacute hemorrhage appears hyperintense on T1WI
    - Does not lose signal with opposed-phase or fat-suppressed sequences
- **Hepatic Metastases**
  - Rarely are bright on T1WI, except for melanoma metastases (due to melanin protein)
  - Metastases may contain fat (liposarcoma) or hemorrhage (hypervascular metastases, especially after chemotherapy)

Helpful Clues for Less Common Diagnoses

- **Hepatic Pyogenic Abscess**
  - May have bleeding within abscess to account for hyperintense portions
  - Proteinaceous debris can also be hyperintense on T1WI
- **Postoperative Packing Material**
  - Omental fat is used as packing material in hepatobiliary surgeries (e.g., focal resection or radiofrequency ablation)
  - Will be bright on T1WI but lose signal on fat-suppressed imaging sequences
- **HELLP Syndrome**
  - Complication of toxemia of pregnancy, with spontaneous hepatic infarction and hemorrhage
  - Diagnosis is usually evident clinically
- **Focal Nodular Hyperplasia**
  - Presence of fat in focal nodular hyperplasia (FNH) is rare, usually patchy distribution
    - Most FNH lesions are nearly isointense to normal liver on T1WI and T2WI
  - May occur in diffusely steatotic liver
  - May also have bright signal on T1WI due to sinusoidal dilation within lesion

- **Nodular Regenerative Hyperplasia**
  - Also known as large (multiacinar) regenerative nodules
  - Usually encountered as multiple small masses in liver damaged by Budd-Chiari syndrome
  - 75% of lesions are bright on T1WI, iso- or hypointense on T2WI
    - ± halo of low signal on T1WI
  - Show hypervascularity persisting through arterial and venous phases
  - Lesions resemble FNH on imaging and histology
- **Hepatic Angiomyolipoma**
  - Benign mesenchymal tumor composed of variable amounts of smooth muscle, fat, and proliferating blood vessels
  - Fatty component of tumor results in hyperintense foci on T1WI
  - Signal dropout on fat-suppressed sequence but not on opposed-phase images
  - More common in patients with tuberous sclerosis complex
    - Look for angiomyolipomas (AML) and cysts in kidneys
- **Peliosis Hepatis**
  - Uncommon to rare benign disorder causing sinusoidal dilation and presence of multiple blood-filled lacunar spaces
  - Associated with immunocompromised states, chronic illness, medications

Helpful Clues for Rare Diagnoses

- **Lipoma, Liver**
  - Rare; may have similar appearance as hepatic AML
- **Liposarcoma, Liver**
  - Rare, as primary hepatic tumor or metastasis or local invasion from retroperitoneal tumor
- **Xanthoma, Liver**
  - In Langerhans cell histiocytosis
  - Multisystem disorder with rare hepatic involvement
  - Uniformly hyperechoic on US, low attenuation on CT
- **Hepatic Adrenal Rest Tumor**
  - Ectopic collection of adrenocortical cells

- May be functional or nonfunctional
- **Hepatic Pseudolipoma**
  - Pseudolipoma of Glisson capsule; detached colonic epiploic appendix
  - Contains degenerated fat enveloped by liver capsule
- **Teratoma, Liver**
  - Hepatic lesion is usually invasion or metastasis from malignant tumor outside liver

Steatosis (Fatty Liver)

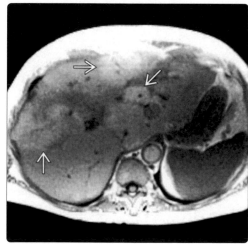

Steatosis (Fatty Liver)

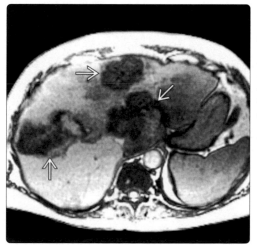

(Left) Axial T1WI MR shows a heterogeneous liver with geographic foci of high intensity ➡ on non-fat-suppressed T1WI, representing multifocal steatosis. (Right) Axial T1WI MR shows selective signal dropout from the foci of focal fatty infiltration ➡ on this opposed-phase T1 GRE image.

Hepatic Adenoma

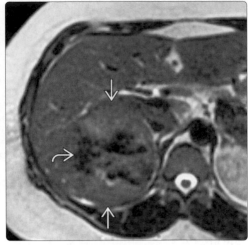

Hepatic Adenoma

(Left) *Axial T1WI MR shows a hepatic mass that has central low intensity ⬇ and peripheral high intensity ➡, the latter due to hemorrhage within the tumor.* **(Right)** *Axial T2WI MR shows a hepatic mass that has central low-intensity contents ➡ and peripheral high-intensity contents ➡, the latter due to hemorrhage within this tumor.*

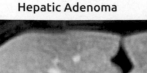
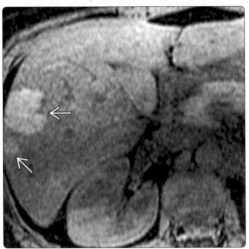

Hepatic Adenoma

Hepatic Adenoma

(Left) *In this young woman who is taking oral contraceptives, a nonenhanced, T1WI MR shows 2 spherical, hyperintense lesions ➡. These were encapsulated and heterogeneously hypervascular on other phases of imaging.* **(Right)** *Axial T1WI MR shows an exophytic hepatic mass ➡ that is hyperintense to liver on T1WI, reflecting the presence of fat within the lesion. Note also the capsule ➡.*

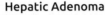
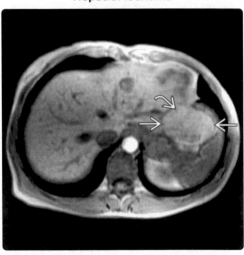

Hepatocellular Carcinoma

Hepatocellular Carcinoma

(Left) *In this 60-year-old man with cirrhosis, an axial in-phase T1WI MR shows a mass ➡ that is slightly hyperintense to background liver. On opposed-phase T1WI MR, there are multiple foci of signal dropout within the mass ➡, indicative of lipid content.* **(Right)** *In this 60-year-old man, arterial-phase T1WI C+ MR shows a heterogeneously hypervascular mass ➡ within a cirrhotic liver. On delayed-phase T1WI C+ MR, the mass ➡ shows washout and a capsule, typical of hepatocellular carcinoma (HCC).*

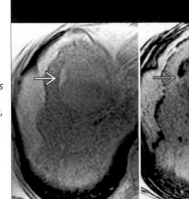
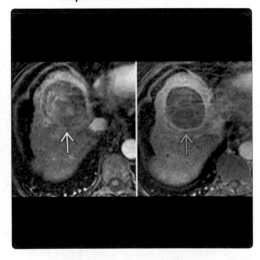

Hepatocellular Carcinoma

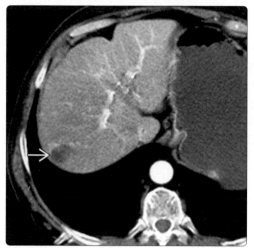

Hepatocellular Carcinoma

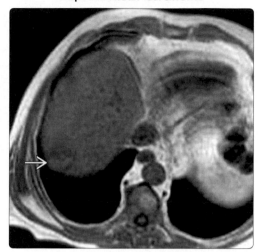

(Left) *In this 70-year-old man who had successful transarterial chemoembolization of an HCC, arterial-phase CECT shows no enhancement of the mass* ➡️*.* (Right) *In this 70-year-old patient who had successful transarterial chemoembolization of an HCC, the tumor* ➡️ *is hyperintense on unenhanced T1WI MR, indicative of denatured protein or hemorrhage*

Dysplastic Nodules

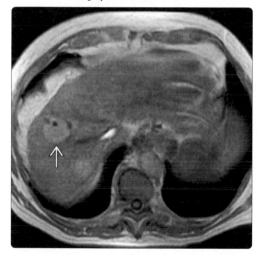

Dysplastic Nodules

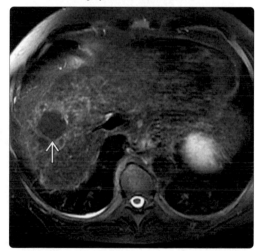

(Left) *In this 50-year-old man with cirrhosis, an unenhanced, T1WI MR shows a focal mass* ➡️ *that is hyperintense relative to the cirrhotic liver.* (Right) *In this 50-year-old man, axial T2 FS MR shows a mass* ➡️ *that is hypointense relative to the cirrhotic liver. The mass showed minimal vascularity or enhancement and was not bright on DWI, all typical features of a dysplastic nodule.*

Hemorrhagic Hepatic Cyst

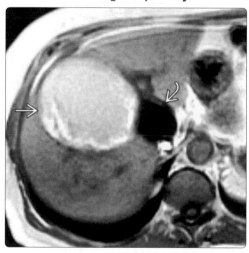

Liver Hematoma

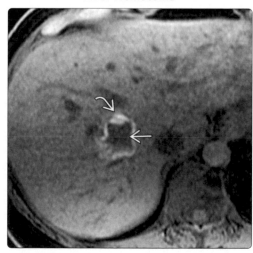

(Left) *Axial T1WI MR shows a large, somewhat complex, hyperintense cystic lesion that is a hemorrhagic cyst* ➡️*. The smaller lesion is a typical simple cyst* ➡️*, hypointense on this sequence.* (Right) *In this patient, percutaneous biopsy confirmed that a focal mass* ➡️ *represented metastasis. On this subsequent T1WI MR, the bright rim* ➡️ *surrounding the metastasis likely represents blood from the biopsy.*

Hepatic Metastases

Hepatic Metastases

(Left) *Axial T1WI MR shows multiple hyperintense masses ➡, typical of melanoma, which is due to the melanin content of the metastases. Most common hepatic metastases are hypointense on T1WI.* (Right) *In this patient with colon cancer, axial T1 FS MR shows a focal heterogeneously hyperintense mass ➡, representing metastasis.*

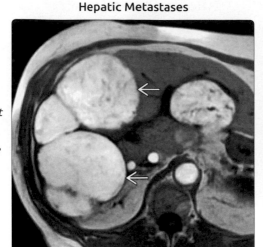

Hepatic Pyogenic Abscess

Hepatic Pyogenic Abscess

(Left) *Axial MR shows a focal, septate, hepatic mass ➡ that is hyperintense to normal liver on both T1WI and T2WI, which was aspirated and proven to be a pyogenic abscess.* (Right) *Axial T1WI MR shows a cluster of lesions in the right hepatic lobe that are mostly isointense with liver parenchyma but contain hyperintense foci ➡, representing hemorrhage (confirmed on needle aspiration of the abscesses).*

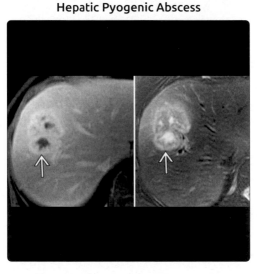

HELLP Syndrome

Focal Nodular Hyperplasia

(Left) *In this woman with toxemia of pregnancy, T1 FS MR shows a large subcapsular hematoma ➡, part of which is hyperintense ➡.* (Right) *Axial T1 FS MR shows 2 subtle hepatic masses ➡ that are almost isointense to background liver although both have some foci of hyperintensity. Both lesions showed homogeneous arterial-phase hyperenhancement and prolonged retention of gadoxetate (Eovist), diagnostic of focal nodular hyperplasia (FNH).*

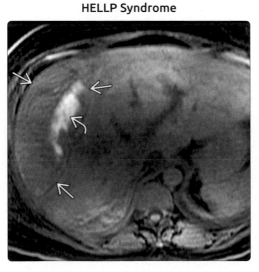

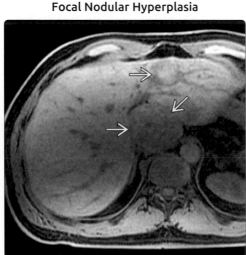

Nodular Regenerative Hyperplasia

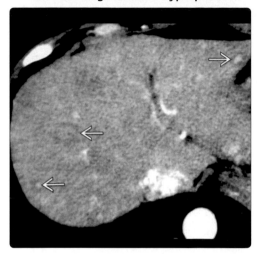

Nodular Regenerative Hyperplasia

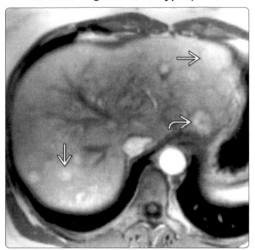

(Left) *In this woman with a hypercoagulable condition, arterial-phase CECT shows multiple, subtle, hypervascular foci ➡. (Right) In this woman with a hypercoagulable condition, axial T1 C+ MR shows multiple lesions ➡ on arterial-phase contrast-enhanced MR that were also slightly hyperintense on precontrast MR. One lesion ➡ has a capsule and central scar, simulating FNH.*

Hepatic Angiomyolipoma

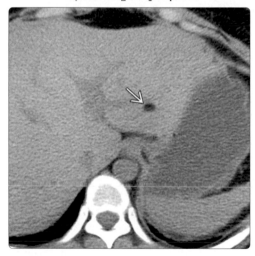

Hepatic Angiomyolipoma

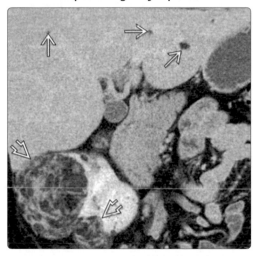

(Left) *In this 48-year-old man who has tuberous sclerosis, NECT shows a fat-density mass ➡ in the liver. (Right) In this 48-year-old man with tuberous sclerosis, coronal CECT shows multiple fat-density nodules within the liver ➡, as well as larger masses ➡ within the kidneys, all representing angiomyolipomas.*

Peliosis Hepatis

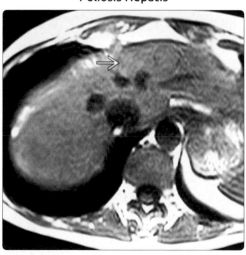

Peliosis Hepatis

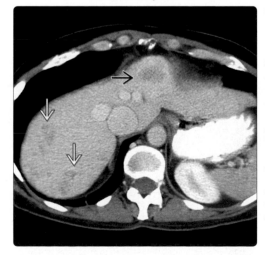

(Left) *In this 42-year-old woman with a long history of oral contraceptive use, axial T1WI MR shows a subtle mass ➡ that is just slightly hyperintense to liver. CT and contrast-enhanced MR showed multiple hypervascular foci that simulated metastases but proved to be peliosis hepatis. (Right) In this 42-year-old woman, axial CECT shows peripheral nodular enhancement of 1 ➡ of several poorly defined hepatic masses ➡. Lesions resolved following cessation of oral contraceptive use.*

DIFFERENTIAL DIAGNOSIS

Common

- Hepatic Metastases
- Hepatic Pyogenic Abscess
- Hepatocellular Carcinoma
- Hepatic Hematoma

Less Common

- Hepatic Adenoma
- Hepatic Amebic Abscess
- Hepatic Hydatid Cyst
- Focal Nodular Hyperplasia
- Nodular Regenerative Hyperplasia

ESSENTIAL INFORMATION

Key Differential Diagnosis Issues

- Most benign hepatic masses do **not** have capsule or circumferential rim evident on MR or CT
  - Most cysts, cavernous hemangiomas, focal nodular hyperplasia
- Halo = edema or compressed liver

Helpful Clues for Common Diagnoses

- **Hepatic Metastases**
  - Most common etiology for lesions with circumferential rim on MR or CT
    - Often have peritumoral halo with double ring pattern
  - Metastases are usually heterogeneously hyperintense on T2WI
- **Hepatic Pyogenic Abscess**
  - Usually multiloculated or cluster-of-grapes appearance
  - Abscess contents are hyperintense, with thick perilesional edema, also bright on T2WI
- **Hepatocellular Carcinoma**
  - In patient with cirrhosis of chronic liver injury
    - Presence of capsule in hypervascular mass with washout is diagnostic of hepatocellular carcinoma in this setting
    - Look for signs of cirrhosis, ascites, portal vein invasion

- **Hepatic Hematoma**
  - Following blunt or penetrating trauma, including iatrogenic injuries
  - Chronic hematoma may have hemosiderin in rim that is hypointense on T1WI, often hyperintense on T2WI

Helpful Clues for Less Common Diagnoses

- **Hepatic Adenoma**
  - May have thin, usually incomplete capsule that is hypointense on T2WI
  - Look for evidence of hemorrhage, fat, necrosis within mass
    - Much more evident on MR than on CT
    - e.g., MR may show lipid content by signal loss on fat-suppressed or opposed-phase GRE sequences
- **Hepatic Amebic Abscess**
  - Usually 1 or few lesions
  - Contents bright on T2WI; hypointense rim but perilesional edema bright on T2WI
  - Rarely have multiseptate appearance of pyogenic abscesses
- **Hepatic Hydatid Cyst**
  - Rim (pericyst) is hypointense on T2WI
  - Contents (daughter cysts) are very bright on T2WI
- **Focal Nodular Hyperplasia**
  - May have pseudocapsule of prominent draining veins
  - No surrounding edema or invasive features
- **Nodular Regenerative Hyperplasia**
  - In Budd-Chiari: Hypervascular nodules ± hypointense halo
  - Large regenerative nodules = macroscopic, multiacinar form of nodular regenerative hyperplasia

Hepatic Metastases

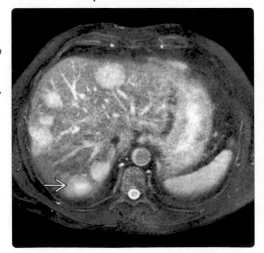

Hepatic Metastases

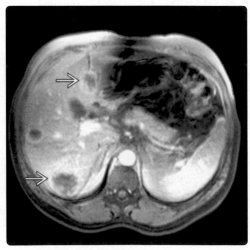

(Left) Axial T2WI MR shows multiple hepatic metastases from colon cancer, some of which have a peritumoral halo ➡. (Right) Axial T1 C+ MR shows multiple hepatic metastases from colon cancer, with a peritumoral capsule or halo ➡.

Hepatic Pyogenic Abscess

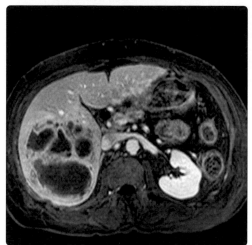

Hepatic Pyogenic Abscess

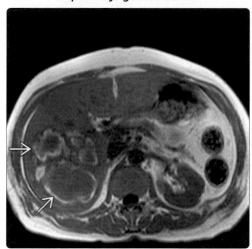

(Left) *MR shows a multiseptate mass (or cluster of adjacent masses) with contrast enhancement of its septa and the surrounding (inflamed) liver.* **(Right)** *Nonenhanced T1W MR shows an encapsulated, multiloculated abscess with heterogeneous fluid content that was hyperintense on T2WI (not shown) and components that are hyperintense on T1WI as well ➡, an unusual feature usually indicating proteinaceous or hemorrhagic fluid.*

Hepatocellular Carcinoma

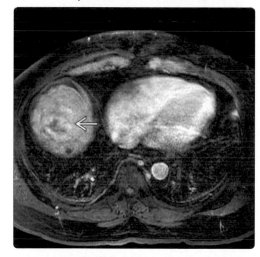

Hepatocellular Carcinoma

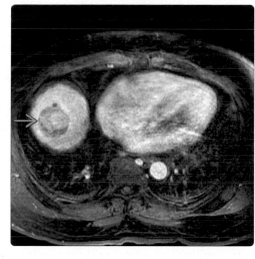

(Left) *This 56-year-old man has a mass ➡ with heterogeneous hypervascularity on arterial-phase imaging. It was also bright on T2WI and DWI (not shown).* **(Right)** *This 56-year-old man has a mass that was hypervascular, but this delayed-phase C+ image shows washout and a capsule ➡, the 2 most characteristic features of hepatocellular carcinoma (HCC).*

Hepatocellular Carcinoma

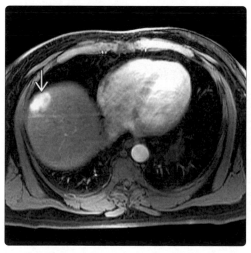

Hepatocellular Carcinoma

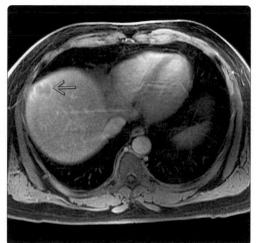

(Left) *This 54-year-old man has a hepatic mass ➡ that is heterogeneously hypervascular on arterial phase C+ T1WI MR.* **(Right)** *The hepatic mass in this 54-year-old man shows washout and a capsule ➡ on delayed-phase C+ T1WI MR, findings diagnostic of HCC in the setting of chronic liver disease.*

Hepatic Hematoma

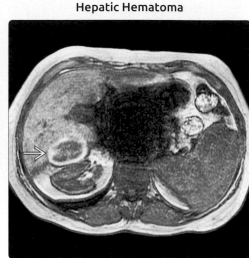

Hepatic Hematoma

(Left) *This young woman had recent liver transplantation and has an encapsulated hepatic lesion ➡ that is bright on T2WI, typical of a subacute hematoma. The midline signal void ➡ is an artifact due to metallic clips and coils.* **(Right)** *In this young woman with a perihepatic hematoma following liver transplantation, an axial T1WI FSE MR shows a lesion with a bright rim or capsule ➡.*

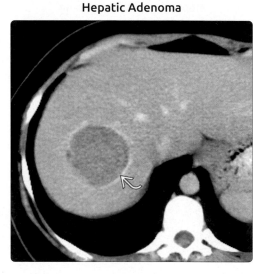

Hepatic Adenoma

Hepatic Adenoma

(Left) *This 25-year-old woman has a mass that was substantially hypodense to the liver (not shown, likely on the basis of lipid content). Arterial-phase CECT shows heterogeneous hypervascularity of the mass ➡.* **(Right)** *In this 25-year-old woman, the hepatic mass is encapsulated ➡. The hypodensity of the mass is indicative of lipid content, another typical feature of hepatic adenoma.*

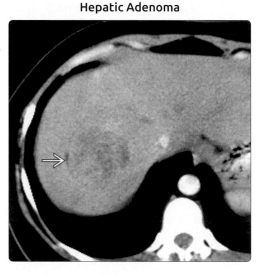

Hepatic Adenoma

Hepatic Adenoma

(Left) *This young woman has a hepatic mass ➡ that is encapsulated and slightly hyperintense to background liver on this in-phase GRE MR.* **(Right)** *This young woman has a hepatic mass that shows selective signal loss on this opposed-phase GRE T1W MR, indicative of lipid content and characteristic of hepatic adenoma.*

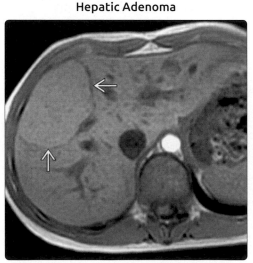

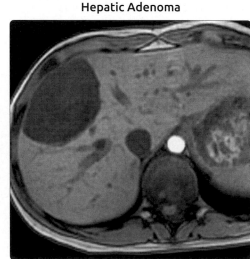

Hepatic Amebic Abscess

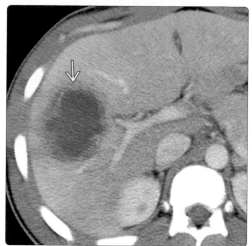

Hepatic Hydatid Cyst

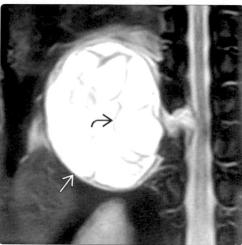

(Left) This young man has a solitary mass ➡️ with a shaggy wall or capsule. Note the hyperemia of the anterior segments of the right hepatic lobe, due in part to occlusion of the anterior branch of the right portal vein. (Right) Coronal T2WI MR shows an encapsulated, large, cystic mass ➡️. Note the presence of numerous septa ➡️ within the mass, representing scolices, or daughter cysts within the larger endocyst.

Focal Nodular Hyperplasia

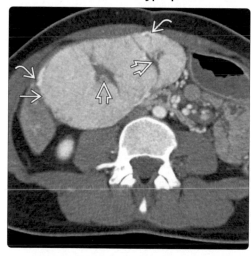

Focal Nodular Hyperplasia

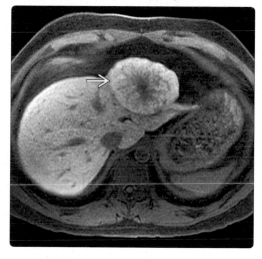

(Left) This 18-year-old woman had a palpable abdominal wall mass. Venous-phase CECT shows a hypervascular mass ➡️ with central and eccentric scar ➡️. Dilated veins ➡️ on the surface of the mass simulate a capsule. (Right) In this young man, delayed-phase Eovist-enhanced MR section shows an exophytic mass ➡️ that retains more contrast (is brighter) than background liver. Also note the central scar and a pseudocapsule, composed mostly of dilated, draining veins.

Nodular Regenerative Hyperplasia

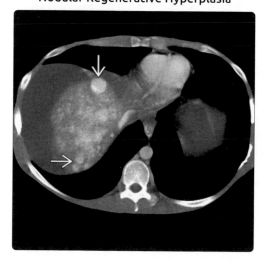

Nodular Regenerative Hyperplasia

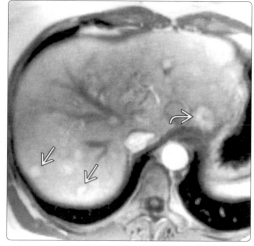

(Left) In this young man with Budd-Chiari syndrome, venous-phase CECT shows multiple hypervascular nodules ➡️ and ascites. Some of the nodules were encapsulated, and others had central scars. In this clinical setting, the findings are characteristic of the macroscopic form of nodular regenerative hyperplasia (NRH). (Right) Axial T1 C+ MR shows hypervascular masses in a patient with Budd-Chiari. Some of the lesions show a hypointense halo ➡️ and a central scar ➡️, findings typical of multiacinar NRH, or large regenerative nodules.

DIFFERENTIAL DIAGNOSIS

Common

- Cirrhotic Regenerating Nodule
- Dysplastic (Hepatic) Nodule
- Any Mass in Fatty Liver (Mimic)
- Focal Sparing in Fatty Liver
- Hepatic Metastases
- Hepatic Hematoma

Less Common

- Hemorrhage Within Hepatic Tumor
  - Hepatic Adenoma
  - Hepatocellular Carcinoma
- Calcification Within Primary Hepatic Tumor
  - Hepatic Cavernous Hemangioma
  - Fibrolamellar Carcinoma
- Hepatic Pseudotumor
  - Budd-Chiari Syndrome
  - Primary Sclerosing Cholangitis
- HELLP Syndrome

ESSENTIAL INFORMATION

Key Differential Diagnosis Issues

- Consider whether mass is abnormally dense (hyperattenuating), or whether surrounding liver is abnormally low in attenuation (e.g., steatosis)
  - Compare with spleen
  - Liver should be slightly hyperdense to spleen on NECT
- Abnormally increased attenuation due to variety of causes
  - Excessive iron
    - Siderotic regenerating nodules
  - Blood
    - Spontaneous hemorrhage in hepatic tumor
    - Trauma
    - Coagulopathic hemorrhage
    - HELLP syndrome
  - Calcification
    - Punctate or more amorphous calcification in hepatic tumors
    - Common in fibrolamellar carcinoma and mucinous adenocarcinoma metastases
- Mass may represent relatively normal liver, surrounded by liver of abnormally low attenuation
  - Focal area of sparing in diffusely steatotic liver
    - Anatomic distribution helpful in making diagnosis
  - Hepatic pseudotumor within liver with extensive damage
    - Spared area may hypertrophy and simulate mass

Helpful Clues for Common Diagnoses

- **Cirrhotic Regenerating Nodule**
  - May be hyperattenuating, due to excess iron and copper
  - Essential to recognize on NECT
    - Avoid characterizing as hypervascular because these may remain hyperattenuating on CECT
    - Regenerating nodules usually become isodense to cirrhotic liver on portal venous and delayed CECT
  - MR is good problem solver

- Regenerating nodules appear as hypointense (black) lesions on T2WI and, especially, on GRE
- **Dysplastic (Hepatic) Nodule**
  - Considered precursor to hepatocellular carcinoma (HCC)
  - Usually > 2 cm diameter; hypovascular
  - Bright on T1WI, dark on T2WI; no restricted diffusion
- **Any Mass in Fatty Liver (Mimic)**
  - Mass of soft tissue attenuation may be hyperdense within fatty liver
  - Even water attenuation cyst may appear hyperdense within severely steatotic liver
- **Focal Sparing in Fatty Liver**
  - Regions of liver surrounding gallbladder fossa and medial segment (#4) are often spared from diffuse steatosis
  - Appears hyperdense on NECT
  - Hypoechoic on US, compared to hyperechoic fatty liver
  - Spared area has normal intensity on MR sequences
    - Rest of fatty liver will show signal dropout on opposed-phase GRE
- **Hepatic Metastases**
  - Mucinous adenocarcinoma mets (calcification)
    - Colon carcinoma most common
    - Others include ovarian cystadenocarcinoma, malignant teratoma, and osteogenic carcinoma
  - Malignant melanoma
    - Melanin within metastatic foci may appear hyperdense on NECT
    - Metastases also may appear hyperintense on T1WI
      - □ Unlike most metastases that are hypo- to isointense on T1WI
- **Hepatic Hematoma**
  - Clotted blood may be hyperdense to normal liver
  - Result of blunt or penetrating trauma, including liver biopsy or other interventions
  - Rarely, spontaneous hepatic bleeding due to anticoagulation

Helpful Clues for Less Common Diagnoses

- **Hemorrhage Within Hepatic Tumor**
  - Hepatic adenoma and HCC are 2 neoplasms most likely to exhibit spontaneous hemorrhage
  - Rarely seen with hypervascular metastases, primary angiosarcoma, and others
- **Calcification Within Primary Hepatic Tumor**
  - Conventional HCC
    - Calcification is rare, usually punctate
  - Fibrolamellar carcinoma
    - 2/3 have calcification in large, irregular, stellate scar
    - Lymph node and lung metastases may be present
    - Young adult
  - Adenoma
    - Calcification in only about 5-10%, punctate
    - Most common in young women on oral contraceptives
    - MR often shows encapsulation, lipid content, focal hemorrhage
  - Hemangioma
    - Calcification rare
    - When present, usually within central scar in large (> 10 cm) hemangioma with other typical features

- **Hepatic Pseudotumor**
  - In Budd-Chiari and primary sclerosing cholangitis
  - Caudate and deep right lobe are usually spared
    - These areas may hypertrophy, but normal attenuation is maintained
  - Central spared areas appear relatively dense compared with peripheral portions of liver that are abnormally low in density
    - Peripheral low density from necrosis, fat, and fibrosis
- **HELLP Syndrome**
  - Complication of pregnancy with toxemia and disseminated intravascular coagulation
  - Hemolysis, elevated liver enzymes, low platelets (HELLP)
  - Foci of infarction ± hemorrhage within liver
    - Hematoma may be intrahepatic or subcapsular
    - May bleed into peritoneal cavity

Cirrhotic Regenerating Nodule

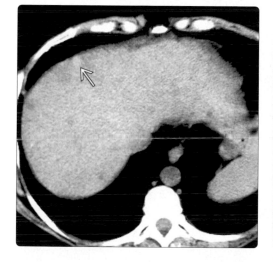

Dysplastic (Hepatic) Nodule

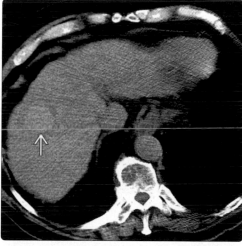

(Left) Axial NECT shows a heterogeneous cirrhotic liver with both hypo- and hyperdense nodules. The hyperdense nodule ➡ was not visible on CECT and is a benign, siderotic, regenerative nodule. (Right) In this 50-year-old man with cirrhosis, nonenhanced CT shows a spherical, hyperdense nodule ➡ that showed minimal enhancement on arterial- or venous-phase CECT. The lesion was hyperintense on T1WI, hypointense on T2WI, and retained Eovist (gadoxetate) on delayed-phase imaging (not shown).

Any Mass in Fatty Liver (Mimic)

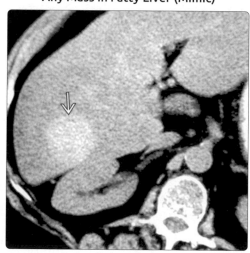

Any Mass in Fatty Liver (Mimic)

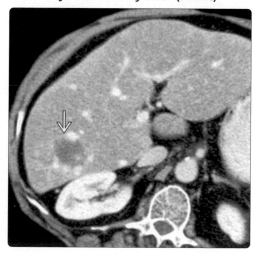

(Left) In this middle-aged woman, axial NECT shows a mass ➡ that is hyperdense to the steatotic liver and isodense to the blood pool, a proven cavernous hemangioma. (Right) In this middle-aged woman, axial CECT shows a mass ➡ with nodular peripheral enhancement that is isodense to the blood pool, typical of cavernous hemangioma.

Focal Sparing in Fatty Liver

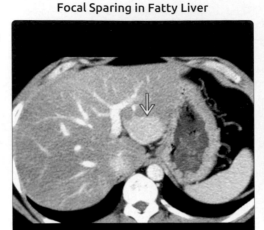

Hepatic Metastases

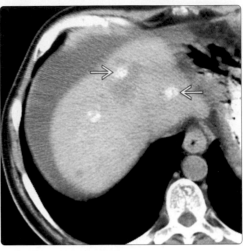

(Left) *Axial CECT shows a diffusely steatotic liver with a mass* ➡ *that represents an area of focal sparing (normal liver).* **(Right)** *Axial NECT shows several lesions* ➡ *that are hyperdense (partially calcified) representing metastases from mucinous adenocarcinoma of the colon.*

Hepatic Hematoma

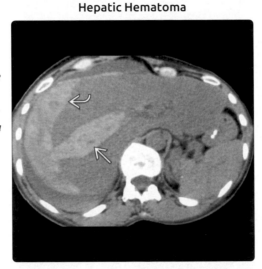

Hepatic Hematoma

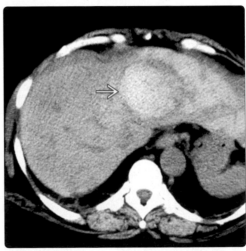

(Left) *Axial NECT shows high-density clotted blood in a crescentic collection* ➡ *around the liver and in a deep linear collection* ➡ *within the liver, due to liver biopsy.* **(Right)** *Axial NECT shows a large heterogeneous mass* ➡ *in the left lobe, representing a spontaneous hemorrhage in an anticoagulated patient. There was no underlying tumor.*

Hepatic Adenoma

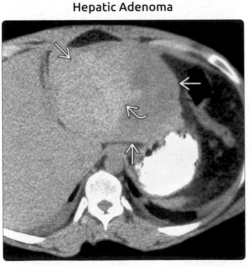

Hepatic Adenoma

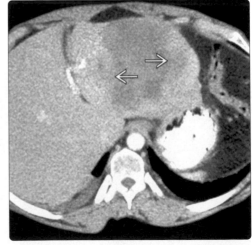

(Left) *In this young woman, axial NECT shows a mass* ➡ *in the left lobe with hyperdense foci* ➡ *representing areas of hemorrhage within a hepatic adenoma.* **(Right)** *In this young woman, axial CECT shows enhancement* ➡ *of the nonnecrotic and nonhemorrhagic portions of this hepatic adenoma.*

Hepatocellular Carcinoma

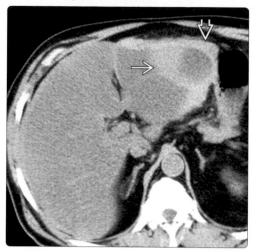

Hepatic Cavernous Hemangioma

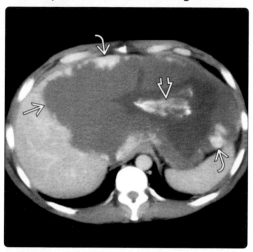

(Left) *Axial NECT shows a heterogeneous mass in the left lobe with hyperdense foci within the mass* ➡ *and around the liver* ⇒, *representing hemorrhage. CECT showed an enhancing mass, identified as hepatocellular carcinoma.* (Right) *Axial CECT shows a huge mass* ➡ *with peripheral nodular enhancement* ➚, *typical of cavernous hemangioma. A central scar* ⇒ *is partially calcified.*

Fibrolamellar Carcinoma

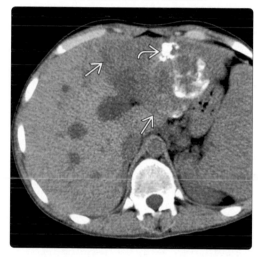

Fibrolamellar Carcinoma

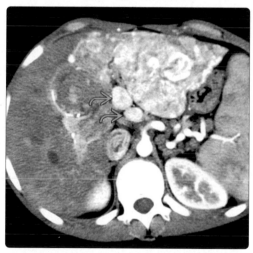

(Left) *In this 17-year-old boy, axial NECT shows a large mass* ➡ *in the left lobe. Note large foci of calcification* ➚. (Right) *In this 17-year-old boy, axial arterial-phase CECT shows heterogeneous hypervascularity within this left lobe mass. Also note hypervascular-enhancing porta hepatis lymph node metastases* ➘.

Budd-Chiari Syndrome

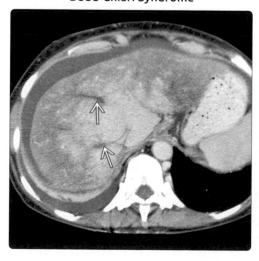

Primary Sclerosing Cholangitis

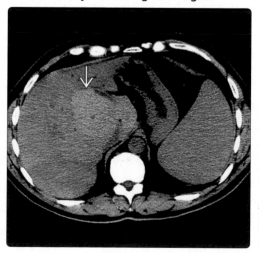

(Left) *Axial CECT shows enlargement of caudate lobe, which is hyperdense to the rest of liver, due to sparing of the caudate and peripheral atrophy and fibrosis, the characteristic pseudotumor appearance in Budd-Chiari syndrome. Thrombosed hepatic veins* ➡ *& ascites are noted.* (Right) *NECT shows massive hypertrophy and increased density of the caudate lobe* ➡, *compared with the atrophic & hypodense peripheral portions of the liver. CECT and MR showed irregular dilation of bile ducts, characteristic of PSC.*

DIFFERENTIAL DIAGNOSIS

Common

- Dilated Bile Ducts (Mimic)
- Systemic Hypervolemia
- Passive Hepatic Congestion
- Hepatitis (Acute)
  - Hepatitis, Alcoholic
  - Hepatitis, Viral
  - Hepatic Injury From Toxins
- Cholangitis
  - Ascending Cholangitis
  - Primary Sclerosing Cholangitis
  - Recurrent Pyogenic Cholangitis
  - AIDS-Related Cholangitis
  - Chemotherapy-Induced Cholangitis
- Posttransplant Liver
  - Biliary Necrosis, Posttransplantation
  - Lymphedema, Posttransplantation
- Hepatic Trauma

Less Common

- Porta Hepatis Lymphadenopathy
- Cirrhosis
  - Peribiliary Cysts
- Portal Vein Thrombosis
- Steatosis (Fatty Liver)
- Hepatocellular Carcinoma
- Cholangiocarcinoma
- Hepatic Metastases and Lymphoma

ESSENTIAL INFORMATION

Key Differential Diagnosis Issues

- Any process that increases production of hepatic extracellular fluid, or impairs capacity for lymphatics to carry this away, will result in periportal lymphedema
  - Loose areolar tissue in portal triads is easily distended by fluid
  - Common pathway for spread of fluid
    - Fluid may be lymph, bile, or blood
- Common pitfalls
  - Mistaking periportal fluid for dilated bile ducts
  - Mistaking clotted portal vein branches for dilated ducts
- MRCP or ERCP best tool for distinguishing among etiologies for branching, nonenhancing structures

Helpful Clues for Common Diagnoses

- **Dilated Bile Ducts (Mimic)**
  - Lie on only one side of portal triad
  - Periportal lucency, by definition, surrounds portal triad on all sides
  - Biliary obstruction may also cause periportal edema
  - Intrahepatic bile ducts should be less than half diameter of adjacent portal vein branch
- **Systemic Hypervolemia**
  - Overhydration, as in rapid fluid resuscitation of trauma patients
  - Liver produces lymph faster than lymphatics can carry it away
  - Look for distention of inferior vena cava (IVC)

- **Passive Hepatic Congestion**
  - e.g., congestive heart failure, constrictive pericarditis, tricuspid valve incompetence
  - Results in periportal lymphedema
  - Look for distension and reflux of vascular contrast medium into hepatic veins and IVC on arterial-phase CECT
- **Hepatitis (Acute)**
  - Any cause (alcohol, viral, toxic)
  - Often results in striking periportal edema &/or gallbladder wall edema
    - Any or all of these may cause or simulate periportal edema
- **Cholangitis**
  - Any form (ascending, primary sclerosing, recurrent pyogenic, AIDS, chemotherapy)
  - Bile duct wall thickening, periductal edema, and possibly ductal obstruction
  - **Ascending cholangitis**
    - Caused by passage of common duct stone
    - Or other etiology for incompetence of sphincter of Oddi
    - Allows reflux of duodenal contents into common bile duct
  - **Primary sclerosing cholangitis**
    - Causes irregular strictures and upstream dilation of intra- and extrahepatic ducts
    - Biliary dilation may simulate or cause periportal edema
    - Bile duct wall thickening and periportal edema are often striking on ultrasound
    - Usually associated with ulcerative colitis
  - **Recurrent pyogenic cholangitis**
    - Typically encountered in malnourished patients from Asia
    - Intra- and extrahepatic bile ducts grossly distended with pus and calculi
    - Periportal edema may coexist with biliary ductal dilation
  - **AIDS-related cholangitis**
    - Caused by opportunistic infection of bile ducts
    - Imaging findings may simulate primary sclerosis cholangitis
    - Or may be limited to stricture of common duct
  - **Chemotherapy-induced cholangitis**
    - Usually limited to patients receiving chemotherapy through direct hepatic artery catheterization and infusion
- **Posttransplant Liver**
  - Lymphatics are severed during transplantation
    - Lymphatics reform connections, but this takes some time
    - Periportal lymphedema is common and may persist for weeks; not sign of rejection
  - Biliary necrosis may occur as complication of transplantation
    - Bile ducts receive only arterial supply; hepatic arterial stenosis or thrombosis causes biliary necrosis before hepatic infarction
    - Often takes form of intrahepatic fluid collections paralleling bile ducts; may be branching or spherical

- **Hepatic Trauma**
  - Blood may spread along portal tracts in branching pattern
    - May be mistaken for dilated bile ducts or deep parenchymal laceration
    - Periportal blood is almost never only sign of hepatic trauma; usually limited to lobe of liver with intrahepatic hematoma or laceration

Helpful Clues for Less Common Diagnoses

- **Porta Hepatis Lymphadenopathy**
  - May result in lymphedema
- **Cirrhosis**
  - May cause periportal edema &/or simulate periportal edema
    - May cause peribiliary cysts (dilated peribiliary glands)
  - May cause portal vein obstruction
    - Look for nonenhancing branching structures in expected path of portal vein branches
    - Cavernous transformation of portal vein (collaterals) may also be mistaken for edema on NECT (but enhance like other vessels on CECT)
- **Portal Vein Thrombosis**
  - Portal vein branches that do not enhance on CECT are likely to be misinterpreted as dilated bile ducts or periportal edema
  - Thrombosis may result from cirrhosis (portal hypertension), hypercoagulable condition, or portal vein thrombophlebitis (e.g., from diverticulitis)
- **Steatosis (Fatty Liver)**
  - May have perivascular distribution, simulate edema
    - More likely to be mistaken on CT; steatosis should not be mistaken for fluid on US or MR
  - Often appears spherical when sectioned in short axis in dome of liver
- **Hepatocellular Carcinoma**
  - May result in nonspecific lymphedema &/or invade or obstruct bile ducts or portal vein
  - Hepatocellular carcinoma is prone to invade portal vein

- Look for distention of portal vein, enhancing tumor thrombus, contiguity with parenchymal tumor
- **Cholangiocarcinoma**
  - Peripheral or hilar
  - Possible etiologies of branching, nonenhancing structures
    - Dilated bile ducts
    - Periportal edema
    - Thickened bile duct walls
- **Hepatic Metastases and Lymphoma**
  - Any hepatic malignancy may result in excess lymphatic output, periportal edema
  - Tumors may also obstruct intrahepatic bile ducts, which may be difficult to distinguish from periportal edema in some cases

Dilated Bile Ducts (Mimic)

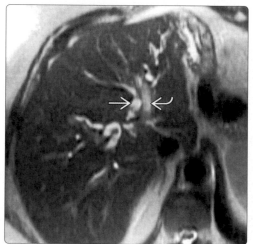

Dilated Bile Ducts (Mimic)

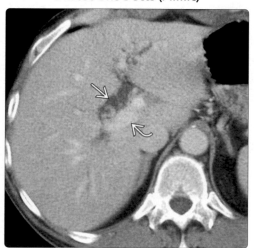

(Left) *Axial T2WI FS MR shows dilated intrahepatic bile ducts* ➡ *running parallel to, and on one side only, of the portal venous branches* ➡ *in a patient with an obstructing ductal stone.* (Right) *Axial CECT shows dilated intrahepatic bile ducts* ➡ *(due to carcinoma of the pancreatic head). The ducts lie on only one side (usually anteromedial) of the portal vein* ➡ *branches.*

Liver

Systemic Hypervolemia

Passive Hepatic Congestion

(Left) *Axial CECT shows a collar of low-density edema ⇨ surrounding portal venous branches, caused by overhydration in a healthy 22-year-old woman following a motor vehicle crash. Note distended inferior vena cava (IVC), also due to hypervolemia.* **(Right)** *Axial CECT shows periportal edema ⇨ and a distended IVC ⇨ in a 78-year-old woman with congestive heart failure.*

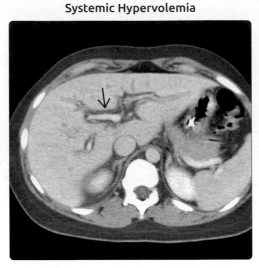

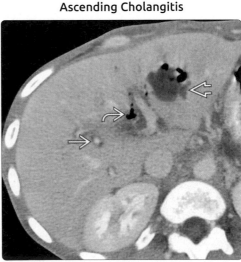

Hepatitis (Acute)

Hepatitis (Acute)

(Left) *Axial CECT shows a collar of periportal lymphedema ⇨ and porta hepatic lymphadenopathy ⇨ due to acute viral hepatitis in a 35-year-old man.* **(Right)** *Axial CECT shows marked gallbladder wall edema ⇨ and a small amount of ascites due to acute viral hepatitis in a 35-year-old man.*

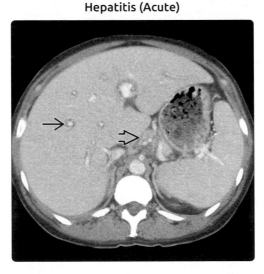

Ascending Cholangitis

Ascending Cholangitis

(Left) *Axial CECT shows periportal edema ⇨, mild dilation of ducts ⇨, and a pyogenic abscess ⇨, all due to ascending cholangitis following Whipple resection for pancreatic carcinoma.* **(Right)** *Axial CECT shows periportal lymphedema ⇨ and gas within mildly dilated ducts ⇨, plus a liver abscess ⇨, all due to ascending cholangitis following Whipple resection for pancreatic carcinoma.*

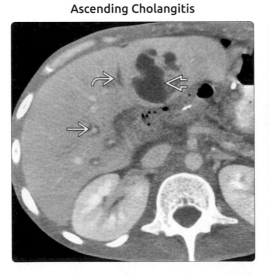

Primary Sclerosing Cholangitis

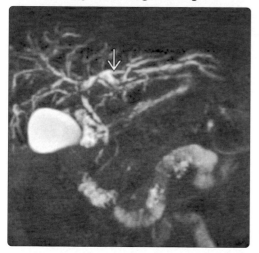

Primary Sclerosing Cholangitis

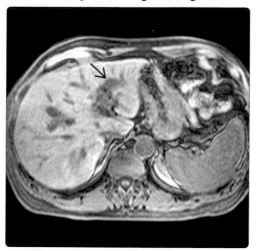

(Left) *Coronal MRCP shows irregular arborization of the intrahepatic ducts with a beaded appearance of some segments. In this 60-year-old man with ulcerative colitis and primary sclerosing cholangitis, portions of the left hepatic ducts ➡ are more dilated than the common duct.* (Right) *Axial T1WI FS MR shows low-intensity fibrosis ➡ paralleling the portal veins and mimicking dilated bile ducts in the same patient.*

Recurrent Pyogenic Cholangitis

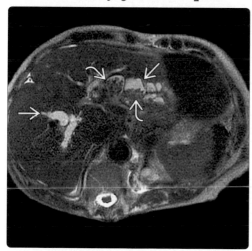

Recurrent Pyogenic Cholangitis

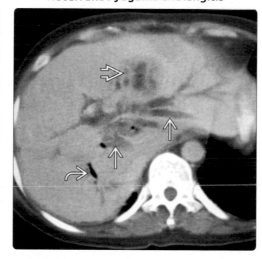

(Left) *In this elderly Asian woman, MR shows dilated intrahepatic bile ducts ➡ containing innumerable calculi ➡. Recurrent pyogenic cholangitis can cause periportal edema in addition to massively dilated bile ducts.* (Right) *Axial CECT shows grossly dilated bile ducts ➡, some of which contain gas ➡, plus a hepatic abscess ➡ in this 45-year-old Asian woman with recurrent bouts of cholangitis and sepsis.*

AIDS-Related Cholangitis

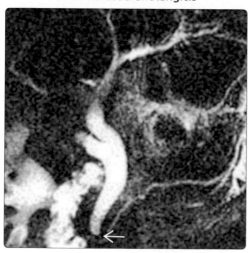

Chemotherapy-Induced Cholangitis

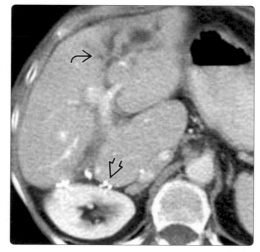

(Left) *Coronal oblique MRCP shows dilation and irregular arborization of the bile ducts and a stricture ➡ of the distal common bile duct due to AIDS-related cholangiopathy. Similar findings could be seen with primary sclerosing cholangitis.* (Right) *Axial CECT shows surgical clips ➡ from right hepatic lobectomy (for metastases). Irregular dilation of intrahepatic ducts ➡ is result of hepatic intraarterial chemotherapy.*

Biliary Necrosis, Posttransplantation

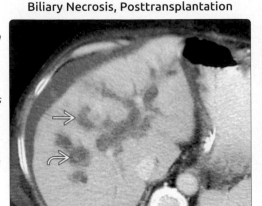

Lymphedema, Posttransplantation

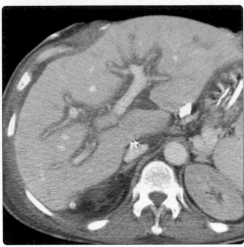

(Left) *Axial CECT shows dilated intrahepatic ducts with indistinct walls ➡ due to biliary necrosis. Intrahepatic bilomas ➡ and ascites are also noted. These are classic signs of hepatic artery stenosis or thrombosis following liver transplantation.* (Right) *Axial CECT shows classic periportal edema that surrounds the portal venous branches. This is a common finding in recent liver transplant recipients and does not imply injury to the allograft.*

Peribiliary Cysts

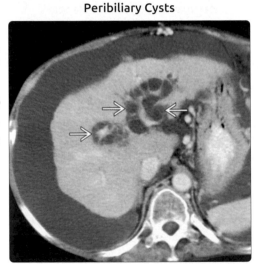

Peribiliary Cysts

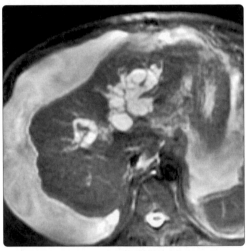

(Left) *Axial CECT shows cystic and tubular water density structures ➡ that parallel the portal veins in this 45-year-old woman with advanced cirrhosis. These are biliary cysts, not dilated ducts.* (Right) *Axial T2WI FS MR shows another view of the cystic and tubular water intensity lesions that parallel the portal veins and mimic dilated ducts in the same patient.*

Hepatic Trauma

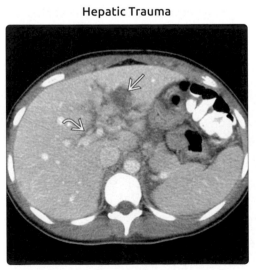

Hepatic Trauma

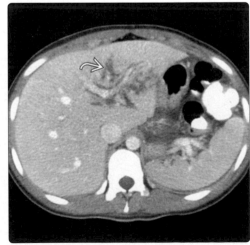

(Left) *Axial CECT shows a left lobe hepatic hematoma ➡ in a 20-year-old woman injured in a motor vehicle crash. Some of the blood tracks along the portal veins ➡ are seen.* (Right) *Axial CECT shows the left lobe irregular laceration/hematoma, with some blood ➡ tracking along portal vein branches in the same patient.*

Portal Vein Thrombosis

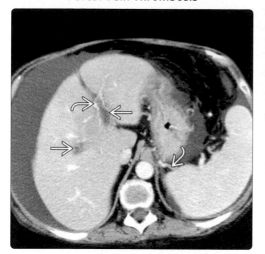

Portal Vein Thrombosis

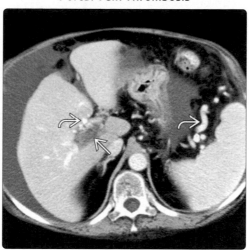

(Left) *Axial CECT shows low-density, branching structures* ➡ *that mimic dilated bile ducts but represent occluded portal vein branches. Note collateral veins* ➡ *in this 58-year-old woman who had an autologous bone marrow transplantation prior to becoming hypercoagulable.* (Right) *Axial CECT shows a thrombosed right portal vein* ➡ *that might be mistaken for a dilated duct in the same patient. Again, note collateral veins* ➡.

Steatosis (Fatty Liver)

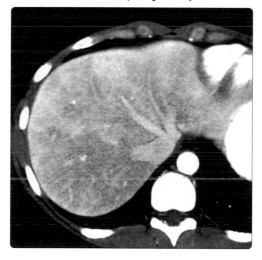

Hepatocellular Carcinoma

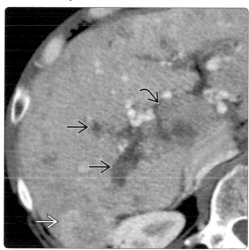

(Left) *Axial CECT shows mottled lucency in the liver, mostly in a perivascular distribution due to steatosis (fatty liver). Steatosis often favors the perivascular planes and "spares" the liver adjacent to the gallbladder fossa.* (Right) *Axial CECT shows enhancing tumor thrombus* ➡ *distending the main portal vein. Note thrombosed right portal vein* ➡ *simulating dilated ducts and the enhancing hepatocellular carcinoma* ➡ *on this arterial phase image.*

Cholangiocarcinoma

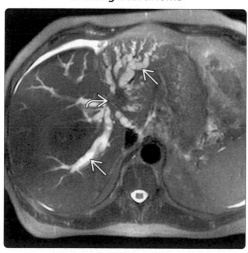

Hepatic Metastases and Lymphoma

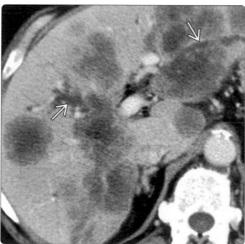

(Left) *Axial MRCP shows dilation of intrahepatic ducts* ➡ *with obstruction near the confluence of the right and left main ducts due to cholangiocarcinoma* ➡. *Malignant biliary obstruction may mimic or cause periportal edema.* (Right) *Axial CECT shows multiple hepatic metastases from colon carcinoma, with obstruction of intrahepatic bile ducts* ➡. *Metastases may also cause periportal lymphedema that may be mistaken for dilated, obstructed ducts.*

DIFFERENTIAL DIAGNOSIS

Common

- Steatosis (Fatty Liver)

Less Common

- Hepatitis
- Toxic Hepatic Injury
- Hepatic Infarction
- Hepatic Metastases and Lymphoma
- Hepatic Sarcoidosis
- Opportunistic Infections, Hepatic
- Hepatocellular Carcinoma
- Wilson Disease
- Radiation Hepatitis
- Budd-Chiari Syndrome
- Glycogen Storage Disease

ESSENTIAL INFORMATION

Key Differential Diagnosis Issues

- Look for mass effect, usually absent in steatosis, present in neoplastic etiologies

Helpful Clues for Common Diagnoses

- **Steatosis (Fatty Liver)**
  - Diffuse, geographic, or multifocal low attenuation
  - Localizes around fissures and hepatic veins
  - Blood vessels traverse low-density focus without mass effect
  - Loss of signal intensity on opposed-phase GRE MR is best sign

Helpful Clues for Less Common Diagnoses

- **Hepatitis**
  - Viral and autoimmune hepatitis usually does not alter attenuation of liver unless there is sudden, massive hepatic necrosis
    - Associated findings: Periportal edema, gallbladder wall edema
    - Necrosis accompanied by ascites is bad prognostic sign
- **Toxic Hepatic Injury**
  - Ingestion of poisonous mushrooms, carbon tetrachloride, or excess of certain medications (e.g., acetaminophen)
  - Can cause steatosis &/or necrosis
- **Hepatic Metastases and Lymphoma**
  - Lymphoma commonly causes diffuse hepatic infiltration
    - Other findings: Splenomegaly; subtle focal masses in liver & spleen; lymphadenopathy
  - Breast, lung, and melanoma are particularly likely to cause diffuse metastases
- **Hepatic Sarcoidosis**
  - Low-density, enlarged liver or innumerable small hypodense granulomas
    - Hepatic and splenic granulomas (focal hypodense lesions)
  - Look for thoracic & abdominal lymphadenopathy
- **Opportunistic Infections, Hepatic**
  - Viral, mycobacterial, etc., in AIDS patients or transplant recipients
- **Hepatocellular Carcinoma**
  - May simulate steatosis on NECT
  - Heterogeneity, hypervascular foci, and mass effect usually evident on CECT
- **Wilson Disease**
  - Causes low, not high, attenuation
- **Radiation Hepatitis**
  - Corresponding to field of external beam or distribution of radioactive embolic beads
- **Budd-Chiari Syndrome**
  - Areas of hepatocellular necrosis, usually in periphery
  - Other findings: Occlusion of inferior vena cava &/or hepatic veins; caudate hypertrophy; collateral vessels

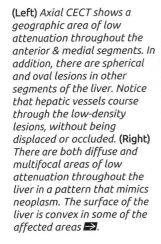

(Left) Axial CECT shows a geographic area of low attenuation throughout the anterior & medial segments. In addition, there are spherical and oval lesions in other segments of the liver. Notice that hepatic vessels course through the low-density lesions, without being displaced or occluded. (Right) There are both diffuse and multifocal areas of low attenuation throughout the liver in a pattern that mimics neoplasm. The surface of the liver is convex in some of the affected areas ➡.

Steatosis (Fatty Liver)

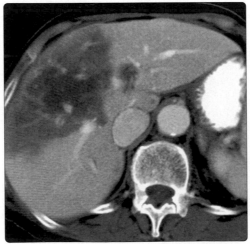

Steatosis (Fatty Liver)

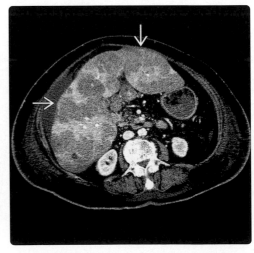

Steatosis (Fatty Liver)

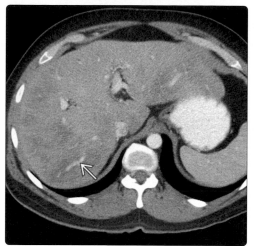

Steatosis (Fatty Liver)

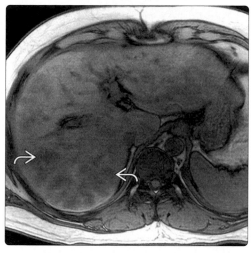

(Left) *Axial CECT shows multifocal hypodense lesions that predominantly lie in a perivascular distribution, surrounding hepatic vessels* ➡. *The vessels are not narrowed or displaced by the hypodense lesions.* (Right) *In the same case, in-phase TW GRE images were normal, while opposed-phase images show signal dropout from each of the perivascular foci of steatosis* ➡, *making this diagnosis one with confidence.*

Hepatitis

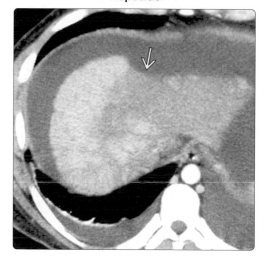

Toxic Hepatic Injury

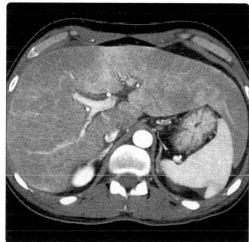

(Left) *Axial CECT shows low attenuation and volume loss of the left lobe in this patient with acute fulminant hepatitis. Note capsular retraction* ➡ *and ascites, both poor prognostic signs.* (Right) *In this young man who died due to acute alcohol & acetaminophen toxicity, CECT shows diffuse hepatomegaly with heterogeneous low attenuation throughout. Periportal edema & ascites were also noted.*

Hepatic Infarction

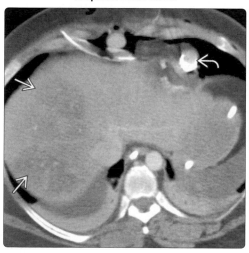

Hepatic Infarction

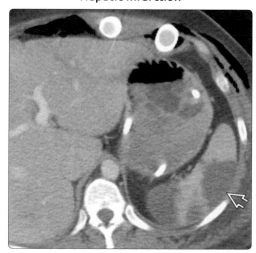

(Left) *CECT in a woman with a ventricular assist device* ➡ *& acute hepatic injury shows widespread regions of hypodensity in the liver* ➡. (Right) *CT in the same case shows peripheral, wedge-shaped defects in the spleen* ➡ *& kidneys (not shown), characteristic of acute infarction. Hepatic infarction was also biopsy proven.*

Hepatic Metastases and Lymphoma

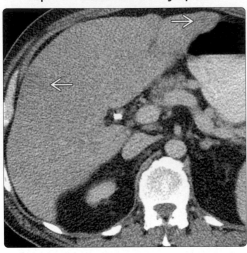

Hepatic Metastases and Lymphoma

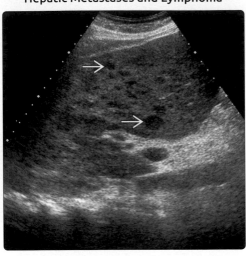

(Left) In this patient with melanoma & abnormal LFTs, axial CECT shows diffuse low attenuation throughout the liver, suggestive of steatosis. In addition, there are several poorly defined hypodense lesions ➡. (Right) In the same case, sonography the next day confirmed innumerable focal hypoechoic metastases ➡ with no evidence of the diffuse increased echogenicity that would be expected for steatosis. This represents diffuse hepatic melanoma metastases.

Hepatic Metastases and Lymphoma

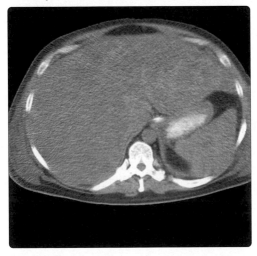

Hepatic Metastases and Lymphoma

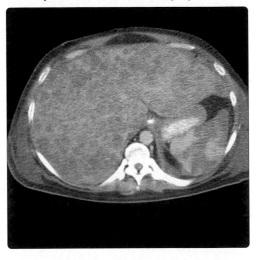

(Left) NECT shows a large and diffusely low-attenuation liver that might be misinterpreted as being due to steatosis. (Right) CECT in the same case demonstrates innumerable focal lesions in the liver and spleen. Liver biopsy confirmed non-Hodgkin lymphoma.

Hepatic Sarcoidosis

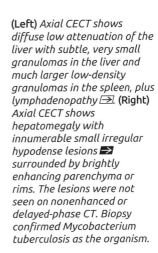

Opportunistic Infections, Hepatic

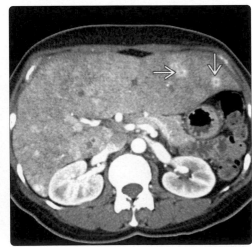

(Left) Axial CECT shows diffuse low attenuation of the liver with subtle, very small granulomas in the liver and much larger low-density granulomas in the spleen, plus lymphadenopathy ➡. (Right) Axial CECT shows hepatomegaly with innumerable small irregular hypodense lesions ➡ surrounded by brightly enhancing parenchyma or rims. The lesions were not seen on nonenhanced or delayed-phase CT. Biopsy confirmed Mycobacterium tuberculosis as the organism.

Hepatocellular Carcinoma

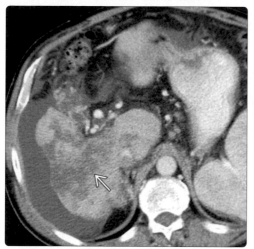

Wilson Disease

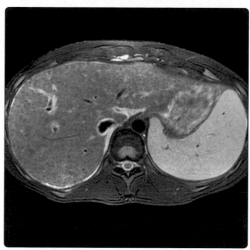

(Left) *Venous-phase CECT shows a large liver mass ➡ & obvious signs of portal hypertension, including splenomegaly & ascites. Biopsy of the mass proved hepatocellular carcinoma.* (Right) *On axial CT (not shown) and T2WI fat-suppressed MR section, the liver is less intense than the spleen. In- and opposed-phase GRE demonstrated characteristic features of steatosis and no imaging effects of the excess hepatic copper.*

Radiation Hepatitis

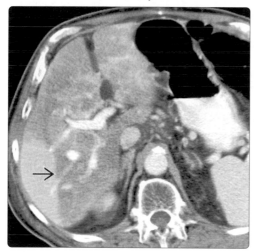

Glycogen Storage Disease

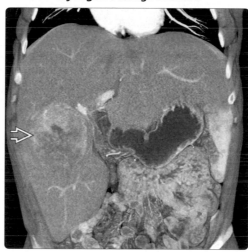

(Left) *Axial CECT shows a broad zone of low attenuation through the center of the liver, sparing the peripheral right lobe, with straight line demarcation ➡, following radiation therapy for cholangiocarcinoma.* (Right) *In this 28-year-old man with type IV glycogen storage disease, the liver is enlarged and diffusely low in attenuation. In addition, a hepatic adenoma ➡ is seen.*

Budd-Chiari Syndrome

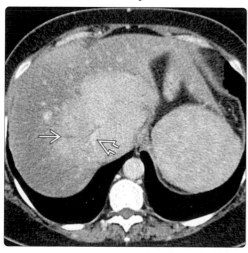

Budd-Chiari Syndrome

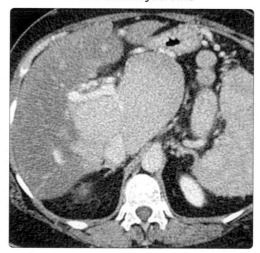

(Left) *Venous-phase CECT shows hypertrophy of the caudate and deep right lobe segments of liver, which are normal in attenuation (as compared with the spleen). The peripheral portions of the liver are decreased in volume and attenuation due to a combination of steatosis and hepatocellular necrosis. The major hepatic veins are thrombosed ➡ and the inferior vena cava is narrowed ➡.* (Right) *CT section in the same case shows the massive hypertrophy of the caudate lobe with hepatic injury in the peripheral segments.*

DIFFERENTIAL DIAGNOSIS

Common

- Focal Steatosis
- Calcified Granuloma, Liver
- Hepatic Cavernous Hemangioma
- Hepatic Metastases
- Pneumobilia
- Intrahepatic Biliary Calculi
- Pyogenic Hepatic Abscess
- Surgical Devices
- Portal Vein Gas
- Biliary Hamartomas
- Normal Anatomic Pitfalls
  - Hepatic Ligaments and Fissures
  - Diaphragmatic Leaflets
  - Refractile Artifact

Less Common

- Hepatocellular Carcinoma
- Fibrolamellar Carcinoma
- Cholangiocarcinoma
- Hepatic Adenoma
- Amebic Hepatic Abscess
- Hepatic Hydatid Cyst
- Hepatic Infarction
- Hemangioendothelioma
- Hepatic Angiomyolipoma
- Postoperative State
- Hepatic Trauma

ESSENTIAL INFORMATION

Key Differential Diagnosis Issues

- Key question
  - Is echogenic lesion a "mass" (usually spherical)?
  - Or is it linear focus [such as transjugular intrahepatic portosystemic shunt (TIPS) or gas in bile ducts]?
- There is significant overlap in US appearance of many of these entities
  - CT and MR should be considered for further evaluation of echogenic masses

Helpful Clues for Common Diagnoses

- **Focal Steatosis**
  - Typically right lobe, caudate lobe, perihilar region
    - Tends to occur along hepatic vessels
    - No mass effect, with vessels running undisplaced through lesion
  - Varied appearances
    - Hyperechoic nodule, multiple confluent hyperechoic lesions
      - □ May closely simulate metastases
      - □ Or multifocal hepatocellular carcinoma (HCC)
    - Fan-shaped lobar or segmental distribution
  - CT and MR are good problem-solving tools
    - In- and opposed-phase (OOP) GRE MR is most specific
    - Signal dropout on OOP images is essentially diagnostic of lipid content
- **Calcified Granuloma, Liver**
  - Histoplasmosis, TB, etc.

- Usually small (few mm) and multiple
  - Spleen is also usually involved
- **Hepatic Cavernous Hemangioma**
  - Hyperechoic mass in > 2/3 of cases
    - Hemangiomas may be hypoechoic relative to steatotic liver
    - Large lesions are more heterogeneous
    - Some have hyperechoic ring, rather than uniform hyperechoic appearance
  - May have posterior acoustic enhancement (due to fluid content)
- **Hepatic Metastases**
  - Hyperechoic metastases most commonly from GI tract (especially colon)
    - Others include vascular metastases from neuroendocrine tumors, melanoma, choriocarcinoma, renal cell carcinoma
  - Target metastases or bull's-eye patterns are seen in aggressive primary tumors
    - Bronchogenic carcinoma is classic example
- **Pneumobilia**
  - Echogenic shadowing foci in center of liver
    - Biliary gas flows towards porta hepatis
- **Intrahepatic Biliary Calculi**
  - Majority appear as highly echogenic foci with posterior acoustic shadowing
  - May have associated dilated ducts
  - More common in recurrent pyogenic cholangitis
- **Pyogenic Hepatic Abscess**
  - Gas within abscess may be echogenic
  - Most pyogenic abscesses are hypoechoic
- **Surgical Devices**
  - Clips, drains, shunts, catheters
  - Turn transducer to appreciate linear shape of device
- **Portal Vein Gas**
  - Echogenic, mobile, shadowing foci in periphery of liver
  - Gas in portal vein flows away from porta hepatis
    - Very obvious on real-time imaging
- **Biliary Hamartomas**
  - Common cause for lesions "too small to characterize"
  - Mimic cysts on CT and MR (near water density/intensity)
  - But may appear cystic or hyperechoic on sonography
    - Due to fibrotic foci in wall
    - Small (< 15 mm), multiple, slightly irregular in contour
- **Normal Anatomic Pitfalls**
  - Hepatic ligaments, fissures, diaphragm slips
    - Infolding of fat along these normal structures creates echogenic focus near surface of liver
    - In short-axis section, "lesions" can appear spherical and resemble masses
    - Turn US beam perpendicular to show linear shape of "lesion"
  - Refractile artifact
    - At junction of vessels, gallbladder neck

Helpful Clues for Less Common Diagnoses

- **Hepatocellular Carcinoma**
  - Small lesion more likely to be hyperechoic
  - May simulate hemangioma or focal steatosis
    - Look for background of abnormal (cirrhotic) liver

- – Generally irregular hypervascularity with Doppler
  - o Usually seen with HCCs containing micro- and macroscopic fat
- **Fibrolamellar Carcinoma**
  - o Large, heterogeneous mass in adolescent or young adult
  - o Look for central scar (may be hypo- or hyperechoic)
  - o CT or MR will show hypervascularity, nodal and other metastases in most
- **Cholangiocarcinoma**
  - o Mass with ill-defined margin
    - – Mostly hyperechoic (75%) and heterogeneous
  - o Intrahepatic (peripheral) cholangiocarcinoma usually shows dilation of intrahepatic bile ducts "upstream" from tumor
  - o CT or MR will show delayed enhancement and capsular retraction with intrahepatic cholangiocarcinoma
- **Hepatic Adenoma**
  - o Hypervascular mass ± hemorrhage in young woman on birth control pills
  - o MR will show fat content and capsule in most adenomas
    - – Fat &/or hemorrhage accounts for echogenic portions of adenomas
- **Amebic Hepatic Abscess**
  - o Usually homogeneous, hypoechoic, encapsulated, solitary
  - o Hyperechoic if complicated by bacterial superinfection or fistula to bowel
- **Hepatic Hydatid Cyst**
  - o Often cystic appearing, but one may see hyperechoic foci
    - – Hydatid sand, parenchymal invasion, calcified rim
- **Hemangioendothelioma**
  - o Infantile type: Well-defined, large hypervascular mass
  - o Epithelioid (adult) type: Multiple peripheral confluent masses
    - – CT or MR will show multifocal masses with capsular retraction
- **Hepatic Angiomyolipoma**
  - o Variable echogenicity
  - o CT/MR better for showing fat, hypervascularity
- **Postoperative State**

- o Any procedure that introduces fat or gas into liver can create echogenic, shadowing lesion
  - – Examples: Subsegmental resection of hepatic tumors
    - □ Surgeons often place omental fat or oxidized gelatin hemostatic agents within hepatic defect
    - □ Ablation (cryo- or radiofrequency) may result in gas release within necrotic tissue
- **Hepatic Trauma**
  - o Intrahepatic hematoma may be hyperechoic

Alternative Differential Approaches

- Vascular masses
  - o Cavernous hemangioma, HCC, hemangioendothelioma, some metastases
- Fat-containing masses
  - o Focal fatty infiltration, hepatic adenoma, HCC, lipid-containing metastases, angiomyolipoma, liposarcoma, teratoma (primary or metastatic to liver)
- Gas-containing masses
  - o Abscess, infarction, treated hepatic tumors with resulting sudden necrosis
- Solid masses
  - o Primary liver tumors, metastases, cholangiocarcinoma
- Masses with calcified rim
  - o Cystic masses (e.g., hydatid cyst)
  - o Some cavernous hemangiomas
- Masses with calcified scar
  - o Fibrolamellar carcinoma, cavernous hemangioma (large ones)

Focal Steatosis

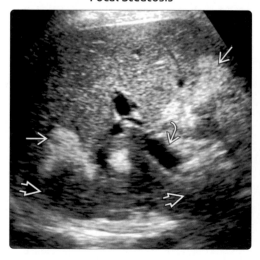

Calcified Granuloma, Liver

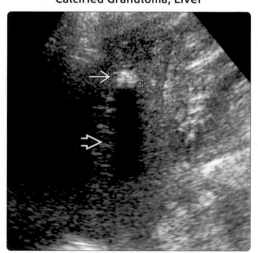

(Left) Transverse transabdominal ultrasound shows multiple hyperechoic areas ➡ with posterior acoustic shadowing ➡. Note lack of mass effect on hepatic vessels ➡. (Right) Axial ultrasound shows a coarsely calcified liver granuloma ➡ with posterior acoustic shadowing ➡. Note the amorphous appearance of the calcification.

Liver

Hepatic Cavernous Hemangioma

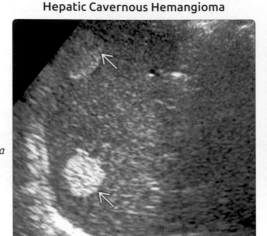

Hepatic Cavernous Hemangioma

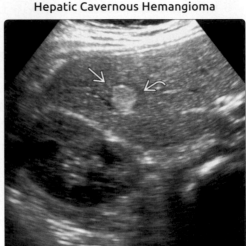

(Left) *Oblique ultrasound shows 2 hemangiomas ➡ presenting as well-defined, homogeneous, hyperechoic, rounded lesions. The appearance is typical (seen in 2/3 of hemangiomas) but is nonspecific; follow-up is usually required.* (Right) *Grayscale transabdominal ultrasound of the liver shows a hyperechoic hemangioma ➡ with small peripheral vessels forming an incomplete halo ➡ around the hemangioma, an unusual feature. Hemangiomas may have a hyperechoic rim.*

Hepatic Metastases

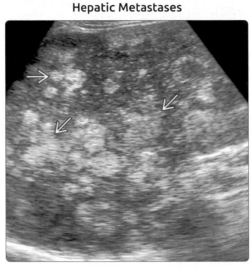

Hepatic Metastases

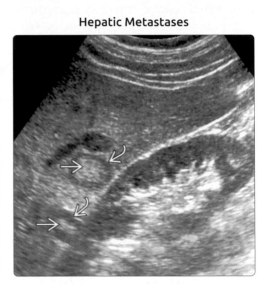

(Left) *Oblique transabdominal ultrasound shows multiple echogenic metastases ➡ from a colonic primary. Other hyperechoic metastases include neuroendocrine tumor, choriocarcinoma, and melanoma.* (Right) *Longitudinal transabdominal ultrasound shows target lesions in the liver representing metastases from lung carcinoma. The center ➡ is hyperechoic with a thick, hypoechoic rim ➡.*

Pneumobilia

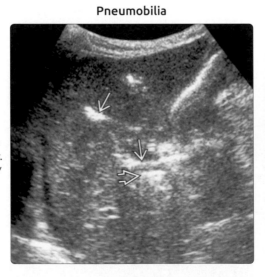

Intrahepatic Biliary Calculi

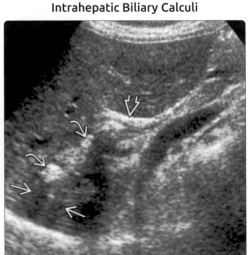

(Left) *Longitudinal transabdominal ultrasound shows linear hyperechoic structures ➡, indicating pneumobilia in intrahepatic ducts. Note reverberation artifact ➡.* (Right) *Oblique transabdominal ultrasound shows multiple intrahepatic biliary calculi in a patient with recurrent pyogenic cholangitis. The echogenic stones ➡ show acoustic shadowing ➡. Note also pneumobilia within an intrahepatic duct ➡.*

Pyogenic Hepatic Abscess

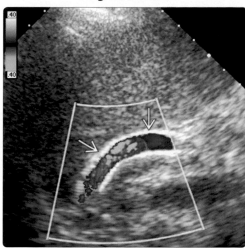

Surgical Devices

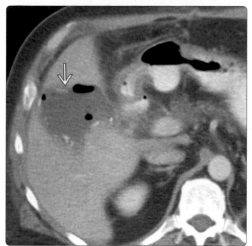

(Left) *In this woman who had a recent cholecystectomy, CT shows a collection of gas and fluid* ➔ *in the liver and gallbladder bed. Pyogenic abscesses are typically sonolucent, but gas-containing abscesses have echogenic foci.* **(Right)** *Longitudinal color Doppler ultrasound shows color flow within a transjugular intrahepatic portosystemic shunt indicating patency. The echogenic stent* ➔ *does not obstruct ultrasound interrogation and has no acoustic shadow.*

Portal Vein Gas

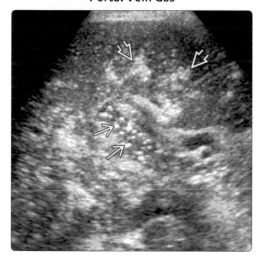

Biliary Hamartomas

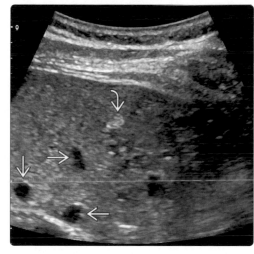

(Left) *Oblique transabdominal ultrasound shows tiny echogenic bubbles of gas* ➔ *within the portal vein. There are also echogenic patches of parenchymal gas* ➔. **(Right)** *In this patient, CT had shown innumerable small "cystic lesions" throughout the liver, ranging in size from 2-15 mm. Sonography showed some of the lesions appearing cystic* ➔, *while most were hyperechoic* ➔, *typical features of biliary hamartomas.*

Hepatic Ligaments and Fissures

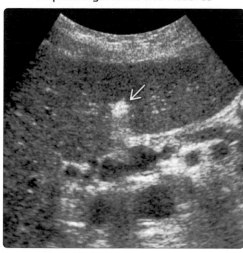

Hepatic Ligaments and Fissures

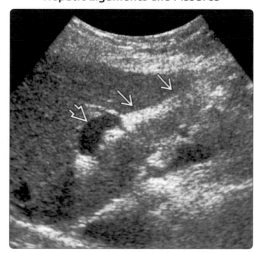

(Left) *Transverse transabdominal ultrasound shows cross section of ligamentum teres* ➔, *which appears as a round, echogenic focus in the left lobe of the liver. Its echogenicity increases with its age. It may mimic focal echogenic hepatic tumor.* **(Right)** *Sagittal ultrasound in the same patient shows the ligamentum teres* ➔ *in a longitudinal view, confirming it is not a mass. It runs from left portal vein* ➔ *to inferior tip of the left lobe.*

Diaphragmatic Leaflets

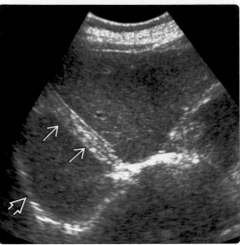

Hepatocellular Carcinoma

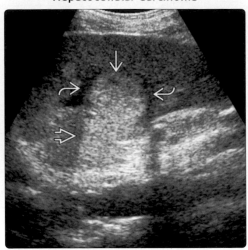

(Left) *Oblique transabdominal ultrasound shows a tubular echogenic diaphragmatic leaflet ➡ near the dome of diaphragm ➡, seen in some patients when the transducer is tilted up to the most cephalad portion of the right dome of the diaphragm.* (Right) *Oblique US shows a small, hyperechoic HCC ➡, which may be homogeneous in echotexture. Posterior acoustic enhancement ➡ makes differentiation from hemangioma difficult. Note the thin, hypoechoic halo ➡, which is generally not seen in hemangiomas.*

Hepatocellular Carcinoma

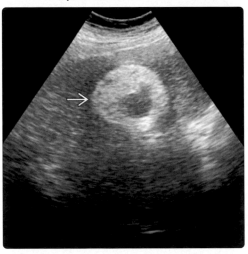

Hepatocellular Carcinoma

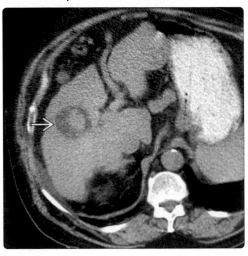

(Left) *In this 64-year-old man with cirrhosis, ultrasound shows an unusually echogenic mass ➡ that was further evaluated by CT.* (Right) *In this 64-year-old man with cirrhosis, NECT shows a mass ➡ that has portions that are unusually hypodense due to the presence of fat within the tumor. While macroscopic fat was an unusual feature, the mass was also hypervascular with washout and a capsule, characteristic features of an hepatocellular carcinoma.*

Fibrolamellar Carcinoma

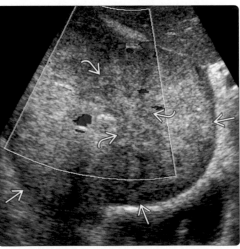

Cholangiocarcinoma

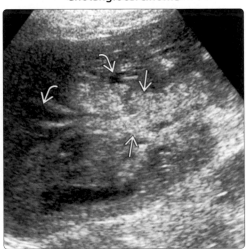

(Left) *Oblique color Doppler ultrasound shows a large, echogenic mass ➡ representing a fibrolamellar hepatocellular carcinoma. Note the central hypoechoic scar ➡, which is typically seen in fibrolamellar HCC but is not specific.* (Right) *Oblique transabdominal ultrasound shows a hilar (Klatskin) tumor ➡ causing intrahepatic biliary ductal obstruction in both lobes of liver. Note enlarged intrahepatic ducts ➡.*

Amebic Hepatic Abscess

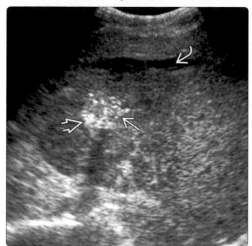

Hepatic Hydatid Cyst

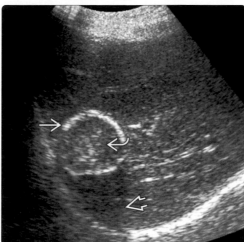

(Left) *Oblique transabdominal ultrasound shows a ruptured amebic abscess ➡, which has fistulized to the colon. Note hyperechoic gas locules ➡ within the abscess and a small amount of ascites ➡.* (Right) *Oblique transabdominal ultrasound shows the echogenic calcified wall ➡ of a hepatic hydatid cyst with posterior acoustic shadowing ➡. Note the echogenic content ➡, representing hydatid sand.*

Hepatic Hydatid Cyst

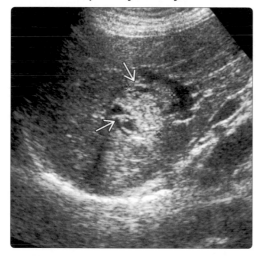

Hepatic Infarction

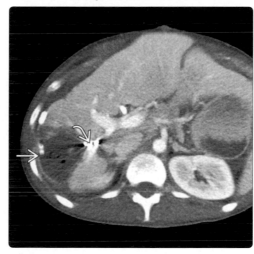

(Left) *Oblique transabdominal ultrasound shows a hepatic echinococcus cyst with echogenic hydatid sand ➡ but no apparent calcification of the cyst wall.* (Right) *This young man had a hepatic laceration with active bleeding, treated with coil embolization. A subsequent CT shows the metallic coil ➡ in the artery with a wedge-shaped collection ➡ of gas and fluid "downstream." Needle aspiration of this collection showed an infected hepatic infarction. The infarcted tissue was hyperechoic on sonography.*

Postoperative State

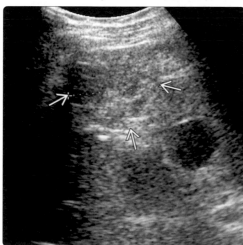

Hepatic Trauma

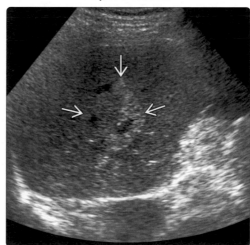

(Left) *Oblique transabdominal ultrasound shows the postsurgical appearance of the liver after subsegmental resection for hepatocellular carcinoma. The resected area is packed with fat, giving it a heterogeneous appearance ➡.* (Right) *Oblique transabdominal ultrasound shows a hyperechoic area of hemorrhage ➡ after hepatic trauma.*

DIFFERENTIAL DIAGNOSIS

Common

- Steatosis (Fatty Liver)
- Cirrhosis
- Hepatitis
- Metastases and Lymphoma, Hepatic
- Technical Artifact (Mimic)

Less Common

- Hepatocellular Carcinoma
- AIDS, Hepatic Involvement
- Hepatic Sarcoidosis
- Miliary Tuberculosis
- Schistosomiasis, Hepatic
- Biliary Hamartomas
- Mononucleosis
- Glycogen Storage Disease
- Wilson Disease

ESSENTIAL INFORMATION

Key Differential Diagnosis Issues

- Steatosis and cirrhosis account for most cases
- Distinguish between diffuse (widespread without discreet lesions) and multifocal (identifiable, individual, multiple lesions throughout liver)
  - Biliary hamartomas, granulomatous disease, and metastases are usually multifocal, rather than diffuse

Helpful Clues for Common Diagnoses

- **Steatosis (Fatty Liver)**
  - Diffuse increased echogenicity with acoustic shadowing
  - Liver often large with smooth contour
  - With increasing infiltration, vessels are pushed apart and hepatic veins take more curved course
  - Deeper portions of liver, vessels and bile ducts are often poorly depicted
- **Cirrhosis**
  - Increased, irregular echogenicity plus altered flow dynamics in hepatic and portal veins

- Nodular hepatic contour
- Signs of portal hypertension
  - Splenomegaly, ascites, varices
- **Hepatitis**
  - Chronic viral or acute alcoholic hepatitis causes increased echogenicity
  - Acute viral hepatitis usually causes decreased echogenicity
- **Metastases and Lymphoma, Hepatic**
  - Most are hypoechoic
  - Mucinous and vascular metastases may be hyperechoic
  - Breast & melanoma metastases may be diffuse & echogenic
- **Technical Artifact (Mimic)**
  - Improper transducer or gain setting

Helpful Clues for Less Common Diagnoses

- **Hepatocellular Carcinoma**
  - May be multifocal or diffuse
  - Usually in cirrhotic liver
- **AIDS, Hepatic Involvement**
  - Opportunistic hepatic infections (CMV, mycobacterial, etc.)
- **Hepatic Sarcoidosis**
  - Diffuse heterogeneous echo pattern
  - Granulomas may be hypoechoic nodules
  - Porta hepatis & upper abdominal lymphadenopathy usually present
- **Miliary Tuberculosis**
  - Innumerable small echogenic granulomas
- **Schistosomiasis, Hepatic**
  - Diffuse involvement of periportal septal thickening causes increased echogenicity
- **Biliary Hamartomas**
  - When multiple or widespread
  - Multifocal, rather than diffuse
  - Tiny (< 1.5 cm) echogenic nodules (due to fibrous tissue in walls)
  - Some lesions may appear more cystic
    - When fluid content exceeds nodularity

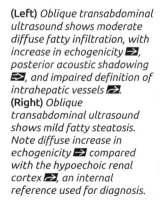

(Left) Oblique transabdominal ultrasound shows moderate diffuse fatty infiltration, with increase in echogenicity ➡, posterior acoustic shadowing ➡, and impaired definition of intrahepatic vessels ➡.
(Right) Oblique transabdominal ultrasound shows mild fatty steatosis. Note diffuse increase in echogenicity ➡ compared with the hypoechoic renal cortex ➡, an internal reference used for diagnosis.

Steatosis (Fatty Liver)

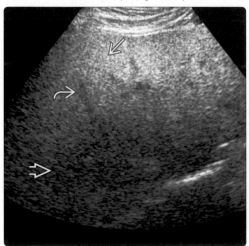

Steatosis (Fatty Liver)

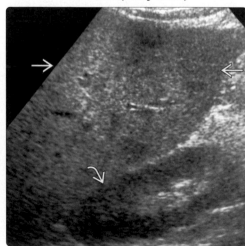

Cirrhosis

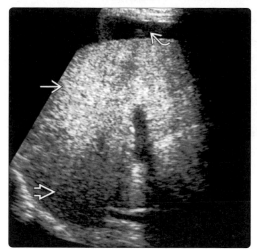

Hepatitis

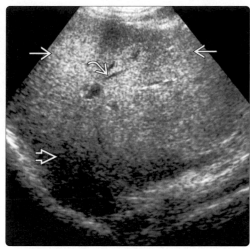

(Left) *Oblique ultrasound of a cirrhotic liver shows a small right lobe with increased echogenicity ➡, coarsened architecture, and posterior acoustic shadowing ⮕. Note ascites ⮕.* **(Right)** *Oblique transabdominal ultrasound in a case of acute alcoholic hepatitis shows increased echogenicity ➡ and posterior shadowing ⮕. The hepatic veins ➡ have a curved course.*

Metastases and Lymphoma, Hepatic

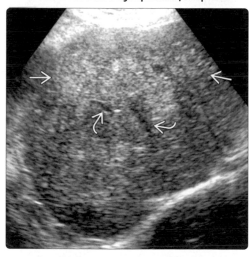

Technical Artifact (Mimic)

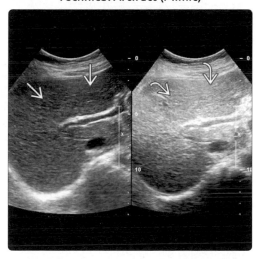

(Left) *Oblique transabdominal ultrasound of diffuse infiltrative metastases shows heterogeneous increased echogenicity ➡ and distortion of the vascular architecture ➡.* **(Right)** *Axial oblique ultrasound shows normal echogenicity of liver parenchyma ➡ on the left. Improper gain settings can cause an artifactually increased echogenicity ➡, as shown on the right.*

Hepatocellular Carcinoma

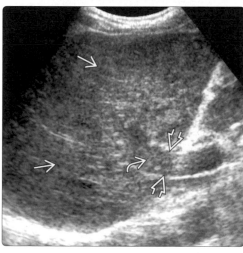

Schistosomiasis, Hepatic

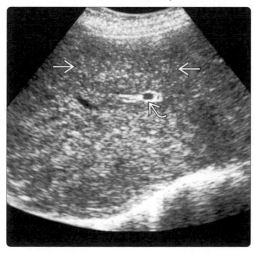

(Left) *Oblique transabdominal ultrasound shows diffuse hepatocellular carcinoma, resulting in increased echogenicity ➡ and echogenic thrombus ➡ in the portal vein ⮕. Doppler is helpful for identifying tumor thrombus.* **(Right)** *Oblique transabdominal ultrasound shows diffuse schistosomiasis involvement of liver, resulting in periportal septal fibrosis, giving an echogenic, mottled appearance ➡. Note thickened and hyperechoic portal vein walls ➡.*

DIFFERENTIAL DIAGNOSIS

Common

- Congested Liver
  - Congestive Heart Failure
  - Budd-Chiari Syndrome
- Acute Hepatitis
- Fatty Liver
- Steatohepatitis
- Fatty Cirrhosis
- Venoocclusive Disease
- Diffuse Neoplastic Infiltration
  - Infiltrative Hepatocellular Carcinoma
  - Lymphoma
  - Leukemia
  - Metastases

Less Common

- Sarcoidosis
- Glycogen Storage Disease

ESSENTIAL INFORMATION

Key Differential Diagnosis Issues

- Hepatomegaly
  - Commonly accepted to be > 15-16 cm long in mid clavicular line
    - Size varies depending on gender and body size
  - Volumetric measurements are time consuming and may not be suitable for everyday practice
- Ancillary signs used to identify hepatomegaly
  - Enlargement of caudate lobe
    - Differential diagnosis of cirrhosis
  - Extension of right lobe below right kidney
    - Differential diagnosis of Riedel lobe
  - Biconvex/rounded hepatic surface contour
  - Blunted, obtuse angle; rounded, inferior tip of right lobe
- Enlargement of left lobe (normally smaller than right)
  - Considered when left lobe is present between spleen and diaphragm

Helpful Clues for Common Diagnoses

- **Congested Liver**
  - **Congestive heart failure**
    - Dilated hepatic veins and inferior vena cava (IVC)
    - Venous "star" appearance at IVC-hepatic vein junction (instead of "rabbit ears")
    - Dilated hepatic veins may extend to periphery of liver
    - Hepatic venous flow: Turbulent appearance and pulsatile waveform on Doppler ultrasound
    - Marked pulsatility of portal vein
    - Hypoechoic parenchyma, increased posterior enhancement, soft consistency (dynamic indentation by cardiac motion)
    - Ancillary findings: Ascites, pleural effusion, thickened visceral walls (gallbladder, bowel, stomach), splenomegaly
    - Cardiomegaly
  - **Budd-Chiari syndrome**
    - Acute phase

    - Hepatomegaly and parenchymal heterogeneous echogenicity due to congestion
    - Hepatic veins/IVC: Normal or distended caliber, partially/completely filled with hypoechoic material
    - Absent or restricted flow in hepatic veins/IVC
    - Aliasing or reversed flow in patent portions of IVC due to stenosis
    - Development of small intrahepatic venous collaterals
    - Chronic phase
      - Stenotic or occluded hepatic veins/IVC
      - Compensatory hypertrophy of caudate lobe, atrophy of involved segments
      - Large regenerative nodules
- **Acute Hepatitis**
  - Diffuse decrease in echogenicity
  - Echogenicity similar to renal cortex and spleen
  - Starry sky appearance
    - Increased echogenicity of portal triad walls against background hypoechoic liver
    - Variably seen
  - Periportal hypo-/anechoic areas due to edema
  - Marked circumferential gallbladder wall edema/thickening
    - Associated with hepatitis A virus
  - Elevated hepatic artery peak velocity on Doppler US
- **Fatty Liver**
  - Increase in size of liver and change in shape as volume of infiltration increases
    - Inferior margin of right lobe has rounded contours
    - Left lobe becomes biconvex
  - Increased echogenicity
    - Liver significantly more echogenic than kidney
    - Echogenicity may vary between segments (areas of focal fatty sparing)
  - Preservation of hepatic architecture
  - Blurred margins of hepatic veins due to increased refraction and scattering of sound
  - Vessels course through liver without distortion
    - May be spread apart secondary to expansion of liver parenchyma
  - Posterior segments of liver not clearly seen due to acoustic attenuation
  - Focal fatty sparing may simulate hypoechoic lesion
  - Soft consistency: Dynamic indentation by cardiac motion
- **Steatohepatitis**
  - Characterized by inflammation accompanying fat accumulation
    - Definitive diagnosis made by liver biopsy
  - May occur in alcoholic hepatitis and nonalcoholic steatohepatitis (NASH)
  - Etiology of NASH unknown but frequently seen in following conditions
    - Obesity
    - Diabetes
    - Hyperlipidemia
    - Drugs and toxins
  - Ultrasound findings
    - Signs of fatty liver

- Firm consistency (due to inflammation) on dynamic scanning during cardiac cycle
- Irregular borders of hepatic veins due to hepatic inflammation
- Intermittent loss of visualization of hepatic veins

- **Fatty Cirrhosis**
  - Enlarged left and caudate lobes and atrophic right lobe
  - Hyperechoic but heterogeneous liver echo pattern
  - Irregular hepatic veins
  - Portal venous collaterals
  - Stiff consistency
  - Ancillary signs of portal hypertension
    - Ascites, varices, hepatofugal flow, splenomegaly

- **Venoocclusive Disease**
  - Hepatosplenomegaly and ascites
  - Periportal and gallbladder wall edema
  - Narrowing and monophasic waveform of hepatic veins due to hepatic edema
  - Slow or reversed flow in portal vein
  - Prominent hepatic arteries and elevated arterial peak systolic velocity
  - Abnormal hepatic arterial resistive index
    - < 0.55 or > 0.75 (variably seen)

- **Diffuse Neoplastic Infiltration**
  - **Infiltrative Hepatocellular Carcinoma**
    - Ill-defined area of markedly heterogeneous echotexture
      - ☐ Often indistinguishable from underlying cirrhosis
    - Color Doppler: Malignant portal vein thrombosis
      - ☐ Absence of normal blood flow and presence of hypoechoic thrombus extending into portal vein
      - ☐ Presence of arterialized flow in portal vein thrombus: High PPV but moderate sensitivity
  - **Lymphoma**
    - Diffuse/infiltrative form presents as innumerable subcentimeter hypoechoic foci
    - Miliary pattern
    - Periportal location
    - Infiltrative pattern may be indistinguishable from normal liver

- Also look for lymphadenopathy, splenomegaly or splenic lesions, bowel wall thickening, ascites
  - **Metastases**
    - Discrete nodules and masses or infiltrative pattern
    - Lung or breast cancer: Common primary showing infiltrative pattern hepatic metastases
    - Infiltrative pattern shows heterogeneous echotexture and simulates cirrhosis

Helpful Clues for Less Common Diagnoses

- **Sarcoidosis**
  - Hepatosplenic involvement
    - Most common finding: Nonspecific hepatosplenomegaly
    - Diffuse parenchymal heterogeneous echotexture
    - Numerous small nodular pattern
    - Advanced disease may cause or simulate cirrhosis
  - Can affect almost every organ
    - Most common site: Lung
  - Upper abdominal lymphadenopathy often present

- **Glycogen Storage Disease**
  - Hepatomegaly and multiple hepatic adenomas in chronically ill young patients
  - Liver may appear diffusely echogenic
    - Indistinguishable from fatty liver
  - Requires biopsy for diagnosis

SELECTED REFERENCES

1. Faraoun SA et al: Budd-Chiari syndrome: a prospective analysis of hepatic vein obstruction on ultrasonography, multidetector-row computed tomography and MR imaging. Abdom Imaging. ePub, 2015
2. Reynolds AR et al: Infiltrative hepatocellular carcinoma: what radiologists need to know. Radiographics. 35(2):371-86, 2015
3. Heller MT et al: The role of ultrasonography in the evaluation of diffuse liver disease. Radiol Clin North Am. 52(6).1163-75, 2014
4. Kratzer W et al: Factors affecting liver size: a sonographic survey of 2080 subjects. J Ultrasound Med. 22(11):1155-61, 2003

Congested Liver

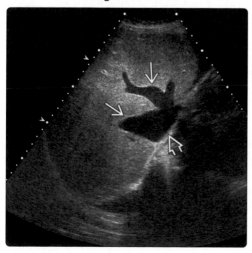

Budd-Chiari Syndrome

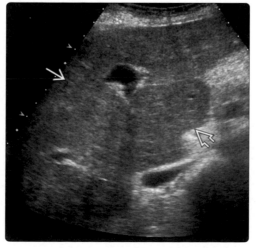

(Left) Oblique ultrasound of the liver at the level of the hepatic venous confluence shows an enlarged liver with marked dilatation of hepatic veins ➡ and inferior vena cava (IVC) ➡ indicating hepatic congestion in a patient with right heart failure. (Right) Transverse abdominal ultrasound in a patient with Budd-Chiari syndrome shows heterogeneous hepatic parenchymal echogenicity ➡ and hypertrophied caudate lobe ➡. The caudate is often hypertrophied in the setting of Budd-Chiari due to its separate venous drainage into the IVC.

(Left) *Longitudinal abdominal ultrasound in a patient with severe hepatic steatosis shows an enlarged liver measuring 21 cm in length, diffusely echogenic liver ➡ compared to the right kidney ➡, and marked attenuation of the US beam, which results in poor visualization of the diaphragm ➡. **(Right)** Longitudinal abdominal ultrasound in a patient who presented with acute liver failure from acute alcoholic hepatitis shows a markedly enlarged liver ➡ extending well below the inferior renal margin.*

Fatty Liver

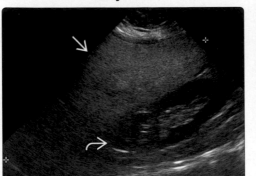

Steatohepatitis

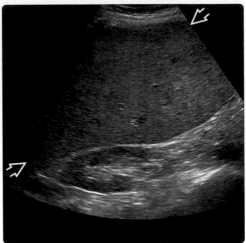

(Left) *Transverse abdominal ultrasound in a patient with venoocclusive disease shows a markedly enlarged and edematous liver resulting in narrowed hepatic veins ➡ and small-caliber inferior vena cava ➡. A small right pleural effusion is also evident ➡. **(Right)** Longitudinal abdominal ultrasound in a patient with venoocclusive disease shows marked hepatomegaly with craniocaudal length of the liver measuring 22.6 cm ➡. Liver extension well beyond the edge of the kidney is indicative of hepatomegaly.*

Venoocclusive Disease

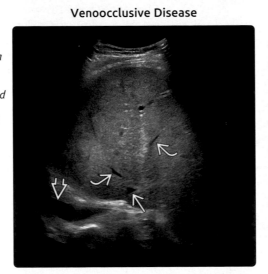

Venoocclusive Disease

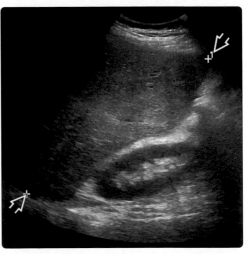

(Left) *Transverse grayscale ultrasound of the liver shows a markedly heterogeneous and enlarged liver with multiple refractive shadows ➡ caused by diffuse, infiltrative HCC. Focal echogenic lesion ➡ was shown to be a fat-containing focus of hepatocellular carcinoma (HCC). **(Right)** Transverse abdominal color Doppler ultrasound shows the right portal vein filled with echogenic material ➡, consistent with portal vein tumor thrombosis. Underlying liver is markedly heterogeneous because of diffuse HCC.*

Infiltrative Hepatocellular Carcinoma

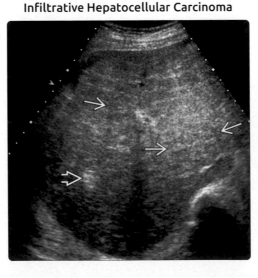

Infiltrative Hepatocellular Carcinoma

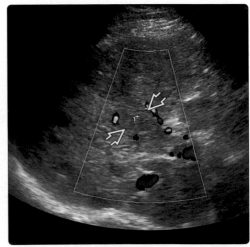

Lymphoma

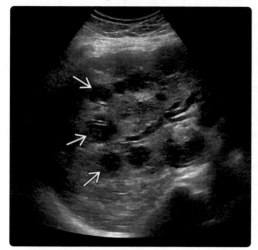

Lymphoma

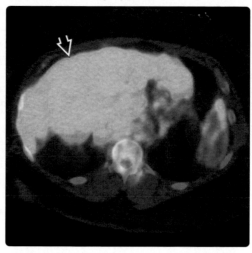

(Left) *Transverse abdominal ultrasound in a patient with lymphoma shows multiple markedly hypoechoic masses* ➡ *throughout the right lobe of the liver.* (Right) *FDG PET in the same patient with lymphoma shows the liver is enlarged and diffusely hypermetabolic throughout the entire liver parenchyma* ➡.

Metastases

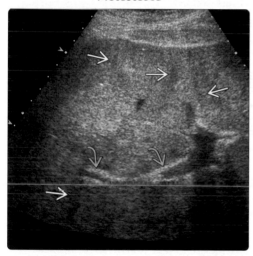

Metastases

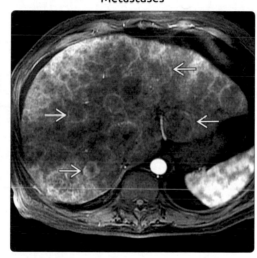

(Left) *Transverse abdominal ultrasound in a patient with hepatic metastasis from neuroendocrine tumor demonstrates enlarged and markedly heterogeneous appearance of the liver with numerous refractive shadows* ➡ *caused by underlying isoechoic metastasis. The portal veins are distorted* ➲ *by mass effect.* (Right) *T1WI C+ FS MR in the same patient demonstrates that the heterogeneous liver appearance on ultrasound is due to numerous masses* ➡, *which virtually replace the entire liver parenchyma.*

Metastases

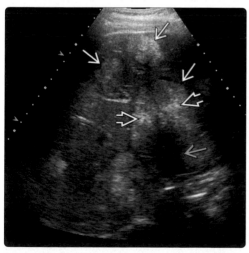

Sarcoidosis

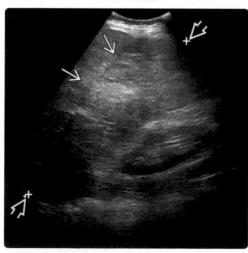

(Left) *Transverse abdominal ultrasound in a patient with colon cancer metastases in the liver shows multiple hyperechoic masses* ➡, *which enlarge the liver. Posterior acoustic shadowing* ➲ *associated with the largest mass is caused by calcifications* ➡ *in the liver metastasis.* (Right) *Transverse abdominal ultrasound in a patient with sarcoidosis shows hepatomegaly (26 cm in length)* ➡ *and heterogeneous hepatic parenchyma* ➡ *due to hepatic involvement by sarcoidosis.*

DIFFERENTIAL DIAGNOSIS

Common

- Steatosis (Fatty Liver)
- Cirrhosis
- Acute/Chronic Hepatitis
- Hepatocellular Carcinoma (Diffuse/Infiltrative)
- Infiltrative Metastasis
- Hepatic Lymphoma (Diffuse/Infiltrative)
- Biliary Hamartomas
- Technical Artifact (Mimic)

Less Common

- AIDS
- Hepatic Sarcoidosis
- Amyloidosis
- Schistosomiasis
- Glycogen Storage Disease
- Wilson Disease
- Venoocclusive Disease

ESSENTIAL INFORMATION

Key Differential Diagnosis Issues

- Diffusely increased echogenicity: Steatosis and cirrhosis account for most cases

Helpful Clues for Common Diagnoses

- **Steatosis (Fatty Liver)**
  - Diffuse increased echogenicity with acoustic attenuation
  - Liver often large with smooth contour
  - With increasing infiltration, vessels are pushed apart and hepatic veins take more curved course
- **Cirrhosis**
  - Heterogeneous parenchymal echogenicity
  - Liver surface nodularity, volume shrinkage
  - Altered flow dynamics in hepatic vasculature
- **Acute Hepatitis**
  - Decreased parenchymal echogenicity due to edema
    - Acute alcoholic hepatitis: Increased echogenicity

  - Hepatomegaly, periportal/gallbladder edema, ascites
- **Chronic Hepatitis**
  - Increased and heterogeneous parenchymal echogenicity
- **Hepatocellular Carcinoma (Diffuse/Infiltrative)**
  - Heterogeneous liver echotexture with refractive shadows
  - May accompany portal vein tumor thrombosis
- **Infiltrative Metastasis**
  - Lung or breast primary
  - May simulate cirrhosis
- **Hepatic Lymphoma (Diffuse/Infiltrative)**
  - Hepatomegaly
  - Numerous small hypoechoic foci, miliary in pattern and periportal in location
  - May be indistinguishable from normal liver
- **Biliary Hamartomas**
  - Tiny (< 1.5 cm) echogenic nodules with comet-tail artifacts
  - Numerous tiny lesions lead to inhomogeneous and coarse liver echotexture
- **Technical Artifact (Mimic)**
  - Improper transducer or gain setting

Helpful Clues for Less Common Diagnoses

- **AIDS**
  - Microabscesses from opportunistic infection (cytomegalovirus, mycobacterium, etc.)
- **Hepatic Sarcoidosis**
  - Diffuse heterogeneous echo pattern
  - Granulomas seen as hypoechoic nodules
- **Schistosomiasis**
  - Increased echogenicity caused by diffuse periportal septal thickening
- **Amyloidosis**
  - Hepatomegaly
  - Heterogeneous parenchymal echogenicity

SELECTED REFERENCES

1. Heller MT et al: The role of ultrasonography in the evaluation of diffuse liver disease. Radiol Clin North Am. 52(6):1163-75, 2014

Steatosis (Fatty Liver)

Cirrhosis

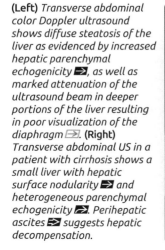
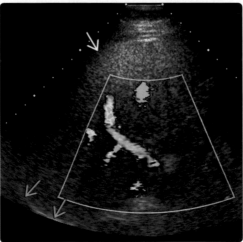
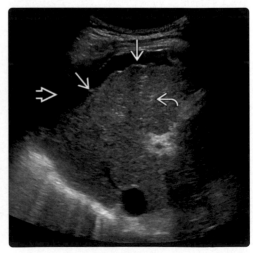

(Left) Transverse abdominal color Doppler ultrasound shows diffuse steatosis of the liver as evidenced by increased hepatic parenchymal echogenicity ➡, as well as marked attenuation of the ultrasound beam in deeper portions of the liver resulting in poor visualization of the diaphragm ⊡. (Right) Transverse abdominal US in a patient with cirrhosis shows a small liver with hepatic surface nodularity ➡ and heterogeneous parenchymal echogenicity ⬈. Perihepatic ascites ➡ suggests hepatic decompensation.

Acute/Chronic Hepatitis

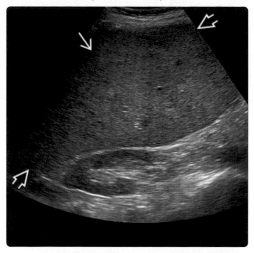

Hepatocellular Carcinoma (Diffuse/Infiltrative)

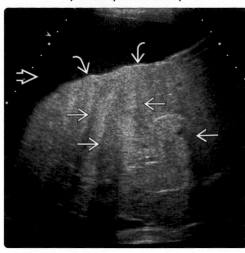

(Left) *Longitudinal abdominal ultrasound in a patient who presented with acute liver failure from acute alcoholic hepatitis shows marked hepatomegaly* ➡ *and slightly echogenic liver parenchyma* ➡. **(Right)** *Transverse abdominal ultrasound shows diffusely increased hepatic parenchymal echogenicity with multiple refractive shadows* ➡ *caused by diffuse, infiltrative hepatocellular carcinoma (HCC). Hepatic surface nodularity* ➡ *and ascites* ➡ *indicate underlying cirrhosis.*

Infiltrative Metastasis

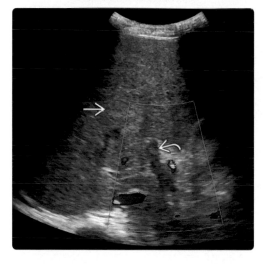

Biliary Hamartomas

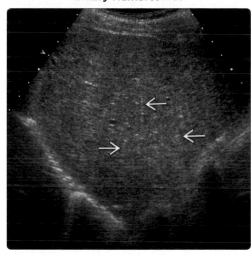

(Left) *Abdominal color Doppler ultrasound in a patient with renal cell carcinoma shows diffusely heterogeneous liver echogenicity caused by diffuse hepatic metastases* ➡. *Main portal vein is filled with hypoechoic material and shows no blood flow, suggesting thrombosis* ➡. **(Right)** *Oblique abdominal ultrasound shows diffuse and coarse liver parenchymal echotexture with multiple echogenic foci, some with associated comet-tail artifacts* ➡ *in a patient with numerous biliary hamartomas.*

Hepatic Sarcoidosis

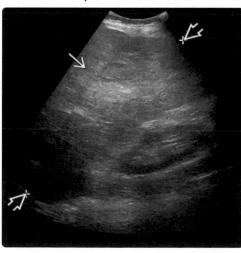

Hepatic Sarcoidosis

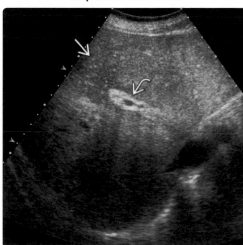

(Left) *Longitudinal abdominal ultrasound in a patient with sarcoidosis shows hepatomegaly (26 cm length)* ➡ *and heterogeneous liver parenchymal echogenicity* ➡ *due to hepatic involvement of sarcoidosis.* **(Right)** *Transverse abdominal ultrasound in a patient with amyloidosis shows heterogeneous and coarse liver echotexture* ➡ *and periportal edema* ➡ *due to hepatic involvement of amyloidosis.*

DIFFERENTIAL DIAGNOSIS

Common

- Hepatic Cyst
- Polycystic Liver Disease
- Pyogenic Hepatic Abscess
- Recent Hepatic Hemorrhage
- Biloma
- Vessels
- Biliary Cystadenoma/Cystadenocarcinoma
- Hepatic Echinococcal Cyst
- Peribiliary Cyst
- Biliary Hamartoma
- Amebic Abscess
- Dilated Bile Ducts

Less Common

- Hepatic Lymphoma
- Hepatic Metastases
- Ciliated Hepatic Foregut Cyst

Rare but Important

- Caroli Disease

ESSENTIAL INFORMATION

Key Differential Diagnosis Issues

- Lesions have few to no echoes within them
- Termed "simple"
  - When unilocular with no internal septa and not lobulated or irregular in contour
- Anechoic lesions tend to be round or oval-shaped with smooth contour on all surfaces
- Degree of posterior acoustic enhancement or shadowing and thickness of wall help limit differential diagnoses

Helpful Clues for Common Diagnoses

- **Hepatic Cyst**
  - Anechoic
  - Smooth borders but occasionally lobulated
  - Thin or imperceptible wall with no mural nodule
  - Well-defined back wall
  - Posterior acoustic enhancement
  - Often subcapsular and may bulge liver contour
  - Do not cross liver segments
  - Do not communicate with each other or bile ducts
  - No internal or mural vascularity but may distort adjacent vessels
  - May have internal echoes or septations after hemorrhage or infection
- **Polycystic Liver Disease**
  - May have concomitant autosomal dominant polycystic kidney disease
    - May make diagnosis of polycystic liver disease easier
    - Less likely to have pancreatic cysts as well
  - Individual cysts look identical to simple hepatic cysts
  - Number of cysts increases with age
  - When numerous and sizable, liver architecture is distorted, making diagnosis easier
  - Some cysts may be complicated by hemorrhage
    - Become hyperechoic or contain debris or septa

- **Pyogenic Hepatic Abscess**
  - Anechoic (50%), hyperechoic (25%), hypoechoic (25%)
  - Small or microabscesses closely simulate small cysts
    - May have internal echogenic debris when large
  - Variable in shape with thin or thick walls
  - Borders range from well defined to irregular
  - Tendency to cluster
    - Group of small pyogenic abscesses coalesce into single large cavity
  - May have adjacent hepatic parenchymal edema
    - Appears hypoechoic with coarse echo pattern ± vascularity
    - Vascularity may be seen in thick-walled portion
  - Diagnosis based on combination of clinical and sonographic features
- **Recent Hepatic Hemorrhage**
  - May be due to direct trauma, coagulopathy, surgery/biopsy
  - Initially traumatic hematoma is usually echogenic
    - Becomes anechoic after a few days
    - May have pseudowall of compressed liver parenchyma
  - Contour may be smooth or irregular
  - May be secondary hemorrhage into preexisting mass
    - Adenoma, hepatocellular carcinoma, metastasis, etc.
    - Usually not completely anechoic
- **Biloma**
  - Almost always secondary to trauma
    - Difficult to differentiate from traumatic hematoma
      - □ Hematomas show debris, septations over time
      - □ Bilomas remain anechoic
  - Round or oval in shape
  - Fluid content may be anechoic with posterior acoustic enhancement
    - Suggests fresh biloma
  - Thin capsule wall usually not discernible
  - Larger lesions may compress adjacent liver surface/architecture
  - Communicates with biliary tree
  - No vascularity within lesion
- **Vessels**
  - Portal veins: Venectasia, varicosities, collaterals from portal hypertension
  - Hepatic veins: Venectasia, Budd-Chiari, etc.
  - Hepatic arteries: Aneurysms, shunts, vascular malformation
  - Use of color Doppler
    - Confirm vascular nature and vessel type
- **Biliary Cystadenoma/Cystadenocarcinoma**
  - Well-defined, multiloculated, anechoic or hypoechoic mass
  - Highly echogenic septa
  - May see internal echoes with complex fluid, calcifications, mural/septal nodules, or papillary projections
    - More commonly associated with biliary cystadenocarcinoma
  - Color Doppler: Septal vascularity
  - Most commonly seen in middle-aged women
- **Hepatic Echinococcal Cyst**

- May be solitary or multiple
- Large, well-defined, cystic liver mass with numerous peripheral daughter cysts
- Cyst-within-cyst appearance
- Floating membrane within cyst
- Layered cyst wall is diagnostic
  - Thickness reduces posterior acoustic enhancement
- **Peribiliary Cyst**
  - Well-defined cystic lesions of round/oval/tubular shape along portal triads
  - Usually multiple; discrete or confluent configuration
  - Smooth and thin walls without internal echoes
  - Variable size from 2 mm to 2 cm
  - No communication with biliary tree
- **Biliary Hamartoma**
  - Numerous small hypoechoic/hyperechoic foci uniformly distributed throughout liver
    - Leads to inhomogeneous and coarse appearance of liver echotexture
  - Multiple echogenic foci often associated with comet-tail artifacts
  - Typically smaller lesions appear as echogenic foci while larger lesions appear cystic
    - Extent of echogenic foci on US is greater than anticipated
    - Small lesions are too small to resolve sonographically
  - Color Doppler US: Twinkling artifact may be associated with echogenic foci
- **Amebic Abscess**
  - Sharply demarcated, round or ovoid mass
  - Hypoechoic with low-level internal echoes
  - May see internal septa or wall nodularity
  - May see posterior acoustic enhancement
- **Dilated Bile Ducts**
  - Ducts may simulate anechoic nodules when viewed on cross section
  - Ducts follow periportal distribution
    - Long axis orientation with hepatic artery/portal vein provide clues to its nature

Helpful Clues for Less Common Diagnoses

- **Hepatic Lymphoma**
  - May be irregular or round/oval in shape
  - ± posterior acoustic enhancement, pseudocystic appearance
  - Extrahepatic signs such as lymphadenopathy, splenomegaly (± splenic infiltration)
- **Hepatic Metastases**
  - Anechoic hepatic metastasis
    - Suggests low degree of differentiation and high-grade malignancy
  - Usually no posterior acoustic enhancement
  - May have debris, mural nodularity, &/or thick septations
  - May have irregular margins and contour
  - Wall vascularity
- **Ciliated Hepatic Foregut Cyst**
  - Unilocular subcapsular solitary cyst located in segment 4a

Helpful Clues for Rare Diagnoses

- **Caroli Disease**
  - Central dot sign: Portal radicles within dilated intrahepatic bile ducts on color Doppler ultrasound

Technical Issues

- Important to make sure that gain settings are correct
- Gallbladder or inferior vena cava can be used as internal references for gain settings
  - These anatomic structures should normally look anechoic

SELECTED REFERENCES

1. Corvino A et al: Contrast-Enhanced Ultrasound in the Characterization of Complex Cystic Focal Liver Lesions. Ultrasound Med Biol. ePub, 2015
2. Borhani AA et al: Cystic hepatic lesions: a review and an algorithmic approach. AJR Am J Roentgenol. 203(6):1192-204, 2014
3. Lantinga MA et al: Evaluation of hepatic cystic lesions. World J Gastroenterol. 19(23):3543-54, 2013
4. Vachha B et al: Cystic lesions of the liver. AJR Am J Roentgenol. 196(4):W355-66, 2011

Hepatic Cyst

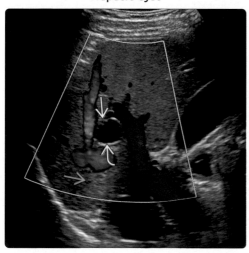

Polycystic Liver Disease

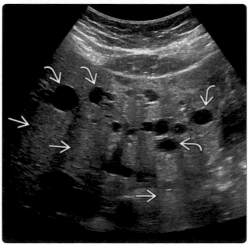

(Left) Transverse color Doppler US shows a well-defined round hepatic cyst with no internal vascularity ➡, well-defined back wall ➡, and posterior acoustic enhancement ➡ confirming the cystic nature of the lesion. (Right) Transverse grayscale US of the liver shows numerous cysts ➡ throughout the liver in a patient with polycystic liver disease. Posterior acoustic enhancement ➡ is associated with each of the cysts, confirming cystic nature of lesions.

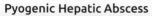

Pyogenic Hepatic Abscess

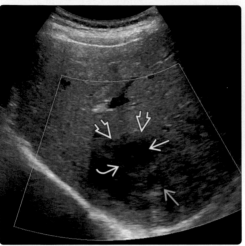

Biloma

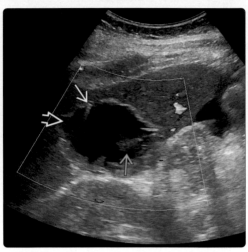

(Left) *Oblique transabdominal color Doppler ultrasound shows a centrally cystic hepatic abscess* ⇨ *with surrounding hypoechoic hepatic parenchyma* ⇉ *in the right lobe of liver. Central internal septations* ⇘ *and echogenic debris* ⇨ *are seen within the hepatic abscess.* (Right) *Transverse color Doppler US of the liver shows a biloma* ⇨ *in a resection cavity with peripheral echogenic foci* ⇨ *and ring-down artifact related to surgical clips. A small amount of internal debris is seen in the periphery of the biloma* ⇨.

Vessels

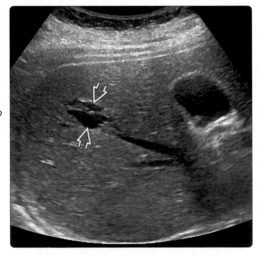

Vessels

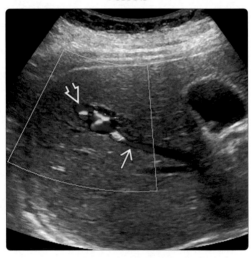

(Left) *Transverse grayscale US of the liver shows 2 adjacent well-defined tubular shaped anechoic lesions* ⇨ *in the right lobe of the liver.* (Right) *On color Doppler US in the same patient the lesion is found to represent a vascular structure* ⇨, *which drains into the middle hepatic vein* ⇨. *Color Doppler US should always be used to evaluate anechoic appearing lesions as they may in fact be vascular, as in this case of a spontaneous intrahepatic portosystemic shunt.*

Biliary Cystadenoma/Cystadenocarcinoma

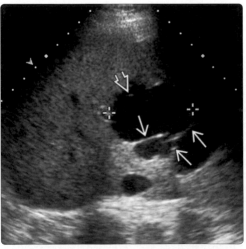

Hepatic Echinococcal Cyst

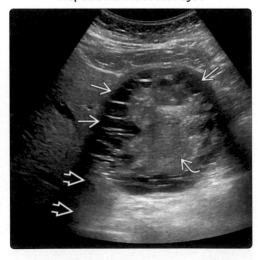

(Left) *Transverse grayscale US of the liver shows a biliary cystadenoma with sonographic imaging appearance of a complex cyst* ⇨ *with multiple septations* ⇨. *Most biliary cystadenomas are seen in middle-aged females.* (Right) *Transverse abdominal US shows an echinococcal cyst containing multiple peripheral daughter cysts* ⇨ *and central heterogeneous content* ⇉ *in the left lobe of the liver. Associated posterior acoustic enhancement* ⇨ *is seen.*

Peribiliary Cyst

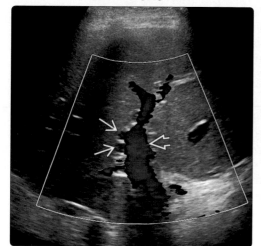

Biliary Hamartoma

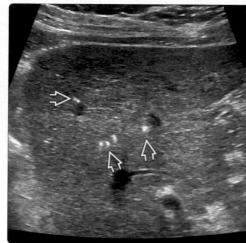

(Left) Color Doppler US shows peribiliary cysts ➡ located adjacent to the portal vein ➡. Peribiliary cysts should not be confused with biliary ductal dilatation, which would have a more tubular and continuous appearance adjacent to the portal vein. (Right) Grayscale ultrasound of the liver shows multiple tiny, echogenic foci ➡ with comet-tail artifacts generated from biliary hamartomas.

Amebic Abscess

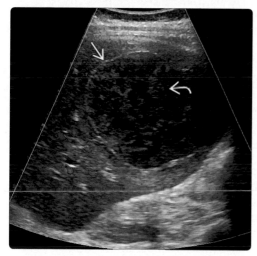

Hepatic Lymphoma

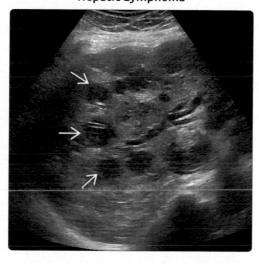

(Left) Sagittal grayscale ultrasound of the liver shows a large, well-demarcated and encapsulated hypoechoic amebic abscess ➡. The contents are heterogeneous due to floating debris ➡. No vascularity is seen within the abscess. (Right) Transverse abdominal ultrasound in a patient with lymphoma shows multiple markedly hypoechoic nodules ➡ throughout the right lobe of the liver, which have a pseudocystic appearance.

Hepatic Metastases

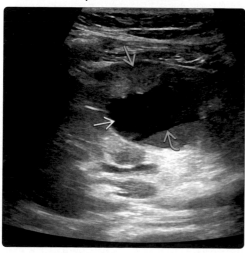

Ciliated Hepatic Foregut Cyst

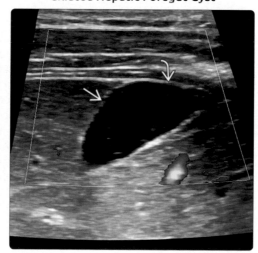

(Left) Cystic liver metastasis in a patient with metastatic cervical cancer displays a central cystic area ➡ as well as an echogenic soft tissue rim ➡ and layering debris ➡ within the dependent portion of the mass. (Right) Oblique abdominal color Doppler US in a patient with a ciliated hepatic foregut cyst shows a well-defined, ovoid, subcapsular cystic mass ➡ in segment IV of the liver ➡. Internal content of the cystic lesion is relatively homogeneous, and no vascularity is seen.

DIFFERENTIAL DIAGNOSIS

Common

- Complicated Benign Hepatic Cyst
- Hepatic Metastases
- Infection
  - Pyogenic Hepatic Abscess
  - Amebic Hepatic Abscess
  - Fungal Hepatic Abscess
- Focal Fatty Sparing
- Hepatocellular Carcinoma
- Infected Biloma

Less Common

- Hepatic Lymphoma
- Hepatic Adenoma
- Focal Nodular Hyperplasia
- Atypical Hemangioma
- Hepatic Hematoma
- Abnormal Bile Ducts
- Abnormal Vessels

ESSENTIAL INFORMATION

Key Differential Diagnosis Issues

- Lesions of lower echogenicity than liver parenchyma (compared to purely anechoic lesions)
  - With some low-level internal echogenicity
  - Solid lesion vs. complex cystic lesion

Helpful Clues for Common Diagnoses

- **Complicated Benign Hepatic Cyst**
  - Superimposed hemorrhage or infection in hepatic cyst
  - Septation/thickened wall ± mural calcification
  - Posterior acoustic enhancement
  - Solid appearance
    - If internal debris (clots or fibrin strands) dispersed within cyst
  - Fluid-debris level
    - If debris settles under influence of gravity
  - No mural nodule
  - Color Doppler
    - Absence of internal or mural vascularity
    - Adjacent vessels distorted by large cyst
- **Hepatic Metastases**
  - Hypoechoic metastases tend to be numerous and small
    - Larger lesions tend to have heterogeneous echogenicity
  - May have irregular or ill-defined borders
  - Hypoechogenicity
    - May reflect poor cellular differentiation and active growth
  - Suggest hypovascular and hypercellular tumor origin
    - Lung, breast, lymphoma
  - No posterior acoustic enhancement
  - Causes architectural distortion
    - If large or numerous
  - Color Doppler may show no vascularity
    - Most are hypovascular
  - Difficult to differentiate from lymphoma without history of known primary lesion

- **Pyogenic Hepatic Abscess**
  - Cystic mass with irregular border and debris
  - Posterior acoustic enhancement
  - Multiple thick or thin septations
  - Mural nodularity & vascularity
  - Adjacent parenchyma may be coarse & hypoechoic due to inflammation
  - "Cluster" sign: Coalescence of group of abscesses
  - May contain gas within abscess
    - Reverberation artifact or air-fluid level
  - Changes to anechoic when center becomes necrotic as center enlarges
  - Periportal distribution suggests dissemination along biliary tree
  - Random distribution suggests hematogenous spread
- **Amebic Hepatic Abscess**
  - Abuts liver capsule, under diaphragm
  - More likely to be round or oval-shaped than pyogenic abscess
  - Hypoechoic with fine internal echoes
    - More common in amebic than pyogenic abscess
  - Internal septa may be present
  - Posterior acoustic enhancement
  - No vascularity seen in wall or septa of abscess
  - Subdiaphragmatic rupture in presence of adjacent hepatic abscess
    - Suggests amebic nature of abscess
- **Focal Fatty Sparing**
  - Geographic hypoechoic area within echogenic liver
  - Due to direct drainage of hepatic flow into systemic circulation
  - Typical locations
    - Gallbladder fossa
      - Drained by cystic vein
    - Inferior aspect of segment 4b
      - Drained by aberrant gastric vein
    - Anterior to bifurcation of portal vein
      - Drained by aberrant gastric vein
    - Around hepatic veins
  - No architectural distortion
    - Vessels course through mass undistorted
    - No mass effect
  - Does not cross segments
- **Hepatocellular Carcinoma**
  - Hypoechoic: Most common US appearance of hepatocellular carcinoma
    - Solid tumor
    - May be surrounded by thin, hypoechoic halo (capsule)
  - Background cirrhotic liver
  - Associated signs of portal hypertension
    - Ascites, splenomegaly, portosystemic collaterals
  - Color Doppler
    - Irregular hypervascularity
    - Portal vein thrombus with arterial neovascularity
- **Infected Biloma**
  - Fluid collection within liver, close to biliary tree, or in gallbladder fossa
  - Debris or septa suggest infected biloma
  - Color Doppler
    - No vascularity within lesion

- Adjacent hepatic parenchyma may demonstrate reactive hypervascularity

Helpful Clues for Less Common Diagnoses

- **Hepatic Lymphoma**
  - Hypoechoic mass with irregular margins
  - Marked hypoechogenicity
    - Probably due to high cellular density and lack of background stroma
  - Large/conglomerate masses may appear to contain septa and mimic abscesses
    - May have a pseudocystic appearance
  - Other sites of involvement commonly seen
    - Lymphadenopathy, splenomegaly ± focal splenic lesions provide clues to diagnosis
- **Hepatic Adenoma**
  - Only slightly hypoechoic compared to normal liver parenchyma
    - May be isoechoic
  - May have hypoechoic rim
  - Complications: Hemorrhage, central necrosis, and rupture may be present
  - Color Doppler shows distinct venous vascularity at borders
- **Focal Nodular Hyperplasia**
  - Usually homogeneous and isoechoic to liver
    - Occasionally hypoechoic or hyperechoic
  - Central hypoechoic stellate scar with radiating fibrous septa
  - Mass effect
    - Displacement of normal hepatic vessels and ducts
  - Color Doppler: Hypervascularity
    - Spoke-wheel pattern
      - Large central feeding artery with multiple small vessels radiating peripherally
    - Large draining veins at tumor margin
    - Hemorrhage is rare
- **Atypical Hemangioma**
  - < 10% of hemangiomas are hypoechoic to liver parenchyma

- Usually with hyperechoic rim
- Typical atypical appearance
- May appear hypoechoic in fatty liver
  - Due to background hyperechoic liver
- Hypoechoic areas within large lesions
  - May represent necrosis, hemorrhage, scar, or vessels
- Smooth, well-defined borders
- May see posterior acoustic enhancement
- No visible color Doppler flow
  - Flow too slow to be detected
  - May be detected with power Doppler
- **Hepatic Hematoma**
  - Echogenicity evolves over time
    - Initially: Echogenic
    - After 4-5 days: Hypoechoic
    - After 1-4 weeks: Internal echoes and septations
- **Abnormal Bile Ducts**
  - Dilated duct with sludge or tumor
  - Interrogate in perpendicular plane to show its tubular nature
- **Abnormal Vessels**
  - Dilated portal or hepatic vein with hypoechoic thrombus
  - Interrogate in perpendicular plane to show its tubular nature

SELECTED REFERENCES

1. Corvino A et al: Contrast-Enhanced Ultrasound in the Characterization of Complex Cystic Focal Liver Lesions. Ultrasound Med Biol. ePub, 2015
2. Kunze G et al: Contrast-enhanced ultrasound in different stages of pyogenic liver abscess. Ultrasound Med Biol. 41(4):952-9, 2015
3. Klotz T et al: Hepatic haemangioma: common and uncommon imaging features. Diagn Interv Imaging. 94(9):849-59, 2013
4. Bhatnagar G et al: The varied sonographic appearances of focal fatty liver disease: review and diagnostic algorithm. Clin Radiol. 67(4):372-9, 2012
5. Bartolotta TV et al: Focal liver lesions: contrast-enhanced ultrasound. Abdom Imaging. 34(2):193-209, 2009
6. Wang ZL et al: Undetermined focal liver lesions on gray-scale ultrasound in patients with fatty liver: characterization with contrast-enhanced ultrasound. J Gastroenterol Hepatol. 23(10):1511-9, 2008
7. D'Onofrio M et al: Hypoechoic focal liver lesions: characterization with contrast enhanced ultrasonography. J Clin Ultrasound. 33(4):164-72, 2005

Complicated Benign Hepatic Cyst

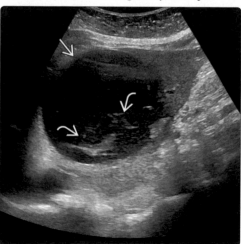

Hepatic Metastases

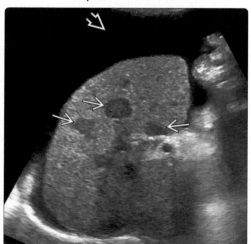

(Left) *Longitudinal oblique US of the liver shows a complicated liver cyst ➡ with internal layering debris ➡ from hemorrhage. Depending on age and amount internal hemorrhage, degree of echogenicity in a complicated cyst may vary.* **(Right)** *Grayscale abdominal US in a patient with breast cancer shows multiple well-defined hypoechoic metastatic lesions ➡ in the liver. Large amount of ascites is seen ➡.*

Hepatic Metastases

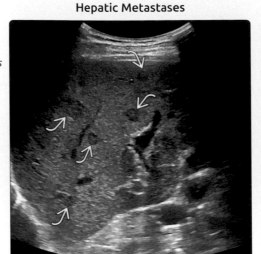

Pyogenic Hepatic Abscess

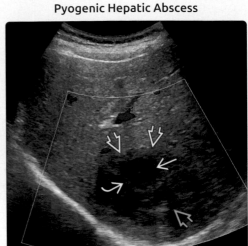

(Left) *Transverse abdominal US in a patient with colon cancer shows multiple small hypoechoic metastatic nodules in the right lobe of the liver ➟. (Right) Oblique abdominal color Doppler US shows a centrally cystic hepatic pyogenic abscess ➟ with surrounding hypoechoic hepatic parenchyma ➟ in the right lobe of the liver. Internal septations ➟ and echogenic debris ➟ are seen within the abscess.*

Amebic Hepatic Abscess

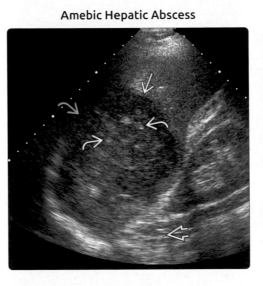

Fungal Hepatic Abscess

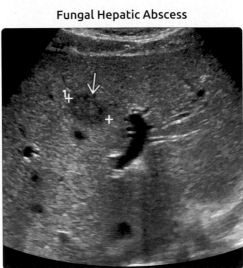

(Left) *Longitudinal abdominal US shows a large, round, hypoechoic amebic abscess in the right lobe of the liver ➟ abutting the liver capsule ➟. Internal contents are hypoechoic with heterogeneously echogenic scattered foci ➟. Mild posterior acoustic enhancement is seen ➟.* **(Right)** *Transverse abdominal US shows a hypoechoic fungal abscess in segment 4 of the liver ➟.*

Focal Fatty Sparing

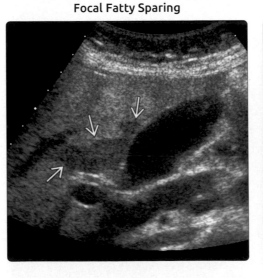

Hepatocellular Carcinoma

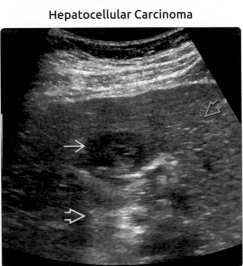

(Left) *Longitudinal abdominal US shows focal fatty sparing adjacent to the gallbladder fossa as a geographic area of decreased echogenicity ➟ in an otherwise echogenic liver due to diffuse steatosis. Liver adjacent to the gallbladder fossa is a typical location for fatty sparing.* **(Right)** *Transverse abdominal US shows a hypoechoic hepatocellular carcinoma ➟. Posterior acoustic enhancement is seen ➟. Underlying liver shows heterogeneous echotexture ➟ indicating background cirrhosis.*

Infected Biloma

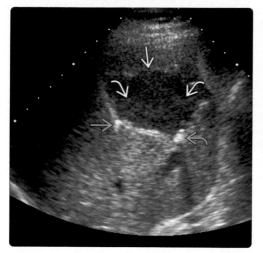

Hepatic Lymphoma

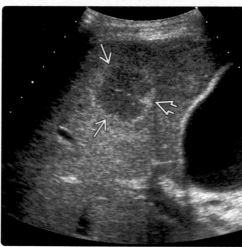

(Left) *Grayscale US shows a biloma ➡ after surgical removal of a liver mass. Low-level internal echoes ➡ suggest infected bile. Peripheral surgical suture with ring-down artifact ➡ and clip with posterior shadowing ➡ are seen along the cut liver edge.* **(Right)** *Transverse abdominal US in a patient with hepatic lymphoma shows a well-defined hypoechoic mass ➡ with thin hyperechoic rim ➡ in segment 5 of the liver.*

Hepatic Lymphoma

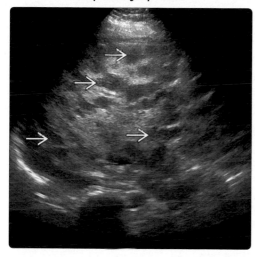

Hepatic Adenoma

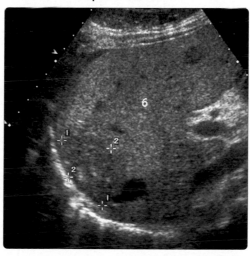

(Left) *Transverse abdominal US in a patient with hepatic lymphoma shows multiple hypoechoic nodules ➡ throughout the liver, consistent with diffuse hepatic involvement of lymphoma.* **(Right)** *Longitudinal abdominal US of the liver shows a heterogeneous slightly hypoechoic hepatic adenoma (demarcated by calipers) abutting the dome of the liver.*

Focal Nodular Hyperplasia

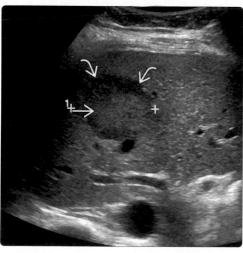

Atypical Hemangioma

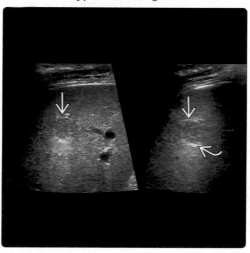

(Left) *Transverse abdominal US shows a predominantly hypoechoic focal nodular hyperplasia (FNH) ➡ with isoechoic center ➡ in the right lobe of the liver. In contrast to this case, most FNHs are isoechoic to background liver, making sonographic identification often challenging and earning the moniker "stealth lesion."* **(Right)** *Transverse abdominal US shows a hypoechoic hemangioma ➡ with thin hyperechoic rim ➡ in the right lobe of the liver, which is a "typical atypical" US finding of hepatic hemangioma.*

DIFFERENTIAL DIAGNOSIS

Common

- Focal Steatosis
- Hepatic Cavernous Hemangioma
- Hepatic Metastases
- Pyogenic Hepatic Abscess
- Normal Anatomic Pitfalls
  - Hepatic Ligaments and Fissures
  - Diaphragmatic Leaflets
  - Refractile Artifact
- Hepatocellular Carcinoma

Less Common

- Cholangiocarcinoma (Intrahepatic)
- Hepatic Adenoma
- Fibrolamellar Carcinoma
- Amebic Hepatic Abscess
- Hepatic Angiomyolipoma
- Biliary Hamartoma
- Hepatic Hydatid/Echinococcus Cyst
- Hepatic Epithelioid Hemangioendothelioma
- Hepatic Lipoma

ESSENTIAL INFORMATION

Key Differential Diagnosis Issues

- Is echogenic lesion mass or echogenic focus?
  - Mass: Usually spherical
  - Echogenic focus: Often linear, such as surgical device, pneumobilia, portal vein gas, etc.
- Significant overlap in appearance of many echogenic masses
  - Contrast-enhanced triphasic CT or MR may be needed for further characterization

Helpful Clues for Common Diagnoses

- **Focal Steatosis**
  - No mass effect, with vessels running undisplaced through lesion
  - Varied appearances
    - Hyperechoic nodule/confluent hyperechoic lesions
      - May simulate metastases
    - Fan-shaped lobar/segmental distribution
  - CT or MR are good problem-solving tools
- **Hepatic Cavernous Hemangioma**
  - Typically homogeneously hyperechoic
    - Probably due to slow blood flow rather than multiple interfaces
    - Smooth or lobulated, well-defined borders
    - May have acoustic enhancement
  - Echogenicity may vary
    - Echogenicity may change over time during imaging
    - Direction and angle of insonation may alter echogenic appearance
    - May appear hypoechoic in underlying fatty liver
    - Large lesions more heterogeneous
- **Hepatic Metastases**
  - Hyperechoic metastases: Most commonly from GI tract
  - Vascular metastases

- Neuroendocrine tumors, melanoma, choriocarcinoma, renal cell carcinoma
  - Target or bull's-eye appearance
    - Iso- or hyperechoic metastatic nodule with hypoechoic rim or halo
    - Usually from aggressive primary tumors
    - Bronchogenic carcinoma: Classic example
  - Calcified metastasis
    - Markedly echogenic interface with acoustic shadowing or diffuse small echogenic foci
    - Mucinous primary: Colon, ovary, breast
    - Calcific/ossific primary: Osteosarcoma, chondrosarcoma, neuroblastoma, malignant teratoma
    - Treated metastasis
- **Pyogenic Hepatic Abscess**
  - Echogenicity of abscess
    - Anechoic (50%), hyperechoic (25%), hypoechoic (25%)
    - Early lesions tend to be echogenic and poorly demarcated
    - May evolve into well-defined, nearly anechoic lesions
  - Cluster sign
    - Cluster of small pyogenic abscesses coalesce into single large cavity
  - Fluid level or debris, internal septa
  - Abscess wall: Hypoechoic or mildly echogenic
  - Gas within abscess: Bright echogenic foci with posterior reverberation artifact
- **Normal Anatomic Pitfalls**
  - **Hepatic ligaments and fissures, diaphragmatic leaflets**
    - Infolding of fat along these normal structures creates echogenic focus near surface of liver
    - In short axis section, "lesions" can appear spherical and resemble masses
    - Turn US beam perpendicular to show linear shape of "lesion"
  - **Refractile artifact**
    - Lateral edge shadows at junction of vessels or gallbladder neck
- **Hepatocellular Carcinoma**
  - Hyperechoic appearance indicates fatty metamorphosis/hypervascularity
    - Simulates hemangioma or focal steatosis
      - Look for background cirrhotic liver, portal vein thrombosis, risk factors (hepatitis B, C, alcohol)
      - Generally irregular intratumoral vascularity
  - Small lesions more likely to be hyperechoic

Helpful Clues for Less Common Diagnoses

- **Cholangiocarcinoma (Intrahepatic)**
  - Heterogeneous mass with ill-defined margin and satellite nodules
    - Mostly hyperechoic (75%); iso-/hypoechoic (14%)
  - Isolated intrahepatic ductal dilatation upstream to mass without extrahepatic duct dilatation
- **Hepatic Adenoma**
  - Young woman with oral contraceptive use
  - Heterogeneous and hypervascular mass with hemorrhage
  - Complex hyper-/hypoechoic mass with anechoic areas
    - Due to fat, hemorrhage, necrosis, or calcification
  - Well-defined border, round or lobulated

- **Fibrolamellar Carcinoma**
  - Large heterogeneous mass in adolescent or young adult
  - Well-defined and partially or completely encapsulated mass
  - Prominent central fibrous scar (hypo- or hyperechoic)
    - Calcification within scar common
  - Intratumoral necrosis/hemorrhage
  - Background cirrhosis or hepatitis in < 5% of patients
- **Amebic Hepatic Abscess**
  - Usually homogeneous and hypoechoic
    - Hyperechoic if complicated by bacterial superinfection or bowel fistula
  - Low-level internal echoes due to debris
  - Peripheral location: Abuts liver capsule, under diaphragm
- **Hepatic Angiomyolipoma**
  - Homogeneous/heterogeneous echogenic mass
    - Hyperechoic due to fat
  - May be hypoechoic if muscle, vascular elements, or hemorrhage predominate
- **Biliary Hamartoma**
  - Numerous small hypo /hyperechoic foci uniformly distributed throughout liver
    - When small, appear hyperechoic due to inability to resolve tiny cysts
    - Leads to inhomogeneous and coarse appearance of liver echotexture
  - Multiple echogenic foci
    - Often with associated comet-tail artifacts
  - Typically smaller lesions appear as echogenic foci, whereas larger lesions appear cystic
    - Extent of echogenic foci on US is greater than anticipated, based on comparison CT or MR
- **Hepatic Hydatid/Echinococcus Cyst**
  - Membranes ⊥ daughter cysts in complex heterogeneous mass
  - Anechoic cyst with internal debris, hydatid sand
  - *Echinococcus multilocularis*
    - Single or multiple echogenic lesions
    - Irregular necrotic areas and microcalcifications
    - Infiltrative solid masses

- Invasion of IVC and diaphragm
- **Hepatic Epithelioid Hemangioendothelioma**
  - Variable echogenicity pattern
    - Predominantly hypoechoic
    - Hyper-/isoechoic lesions; may have peripheral hypoechoic rim
  - Often associated with adjacent retracted capsule
- **Hepatic Lipoma**
  - Extremely uncommon lesion
  - Contain mature adipose tissue

Alternative Differential Approaches

- Vascular masses
  - Cavernous hemangioma, hepatocellular carcinoma (HCC), hemangioendothelioma, angiosarcoma
- Fat-containing masses
  - Focal fatty infiltration, hepatic adenoma, HCC, lipid-containing metastases, angiomyolipoma, lipoma, liposarcoma, teratoma (primary or metastatic to liver)
- Gas-containing masses
  - Abscess, infarction, treated hepatic tumors with resulting sudden necrosis
- Solid masses
  - Primary liver tumors, metastases, cholangiocarcinoma
- Masses with calcified rim
  - Chronic cystic masses
- Masses with calcified scar
  - Fibrolamellar, HCC, cavernous hemangioma (large ones)

SELECTED REFERENCES

1. Bhatnagar G et al: The varied sonographic appearances of focal fatty liver disease: review and diagnostic algorithm. Clin Radiol. 67(4):372-9, 2012
2. Kamaya A et al: Hypervascular liver lesions. Semin Ultrasound CT MR. 30(5):387-407, 2009
3. Basaran C et al: Fat-containing lesions of the liver: cross-sectional imaging findings with emphasis on MRI. AJR Am J Roentgenol. 184(4):1103-10, 2005
4. Prasad SR et al: Fat-containing lesions of the liver: Radiologic-pathologic correlation. Radiographics 25:321-331; 2005

Focal Steatosis

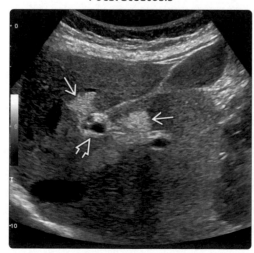

Hepatic Cavernous Hemangioma

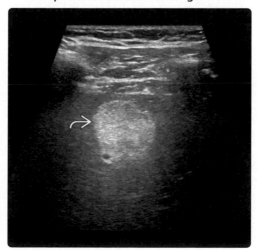

(Left) *Abdominal grayscale ultrasound shows focal fat deposition as geographic areas of increased echogenicity ⮕ around portal vein ⮕. The lesion shows no mass effect and vessels run through the lesion, features that are helpful in the diagnosis of focal steatosis.* **(Right)** *Transverse high-frequency ultrasound of the liver shows a well-defined, homogeneously echogenic cavernous hemangioma ⮕.*

(Left) *Transverse ultrasound of the right lobe of the liver shows a typical hemangioma ➦, which is homogeneously echogenic with well-defined margins.* **(Right)** *Transverse ultrasound in a patient with mucinous colon cancer demonstrates multiple large, hyperechoic metastases ➦ in the liver, containing diffuse echogenic foci ➦ related to subtle calcifications that exhibit posterior acoustic shadowing ➥. Masses distort and compress the right portal vein ➦.*

Hepatic Cavernous Hemangioma

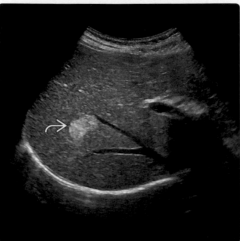

Hepatic Metastases

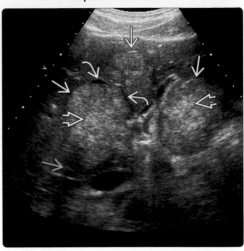

(Left) *Transverse abdominal grayscale ultrasound in a patient with carcinoid tumor shows a round, homogeneously hyperechoic metastasis in the right lobe of the liver ➦.* **(Right)** *Oblique abdominal ultrasound in a patient with melanoma shows a large, heterogeneously hyperechoic metastasis ➦ in the liver abutting the hepatic capsule. Thin, hypoechoic peritumoral halo is present ➦, a finding often seen with hepatic metastases.*

Hepatic Metastases

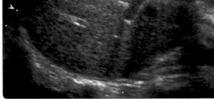
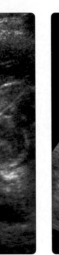

Hepatic Metastases

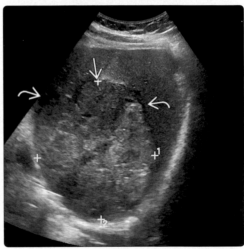

(Left) *Oblique abdominal grayscale ultrasound in a patient with liposarcoma shows a round, homogeneously hyperechoic metastasis along the margin of the right lobe of the liver ➦.* **(Right)** *Longitudinal abdominal ultrasound in a patient with bladder cancer shows multiple ill-defined, hyperechoic metastasis in the liver ➦.*

Hepatic Metastases

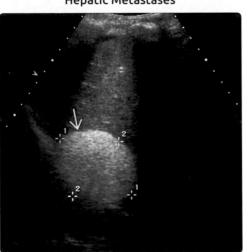

Hepatic Metastases

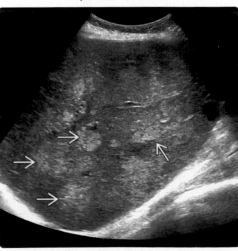

Hepatic Ligaments and Fissures

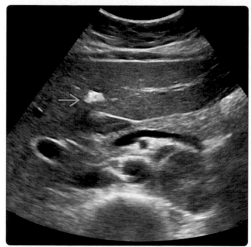

Hepatocellular Carcinoma

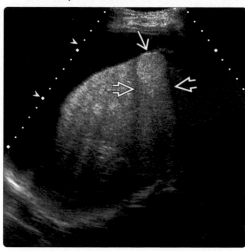

(Left) *Transverse grayscale ultrasound of the left lobe of the liver shows an echogenic falciform ligament* ➡. *The falciform ligament attaches the liver to the anterior body wall and often contains fat, which appears echogenic.* (Right) *Grayscale abdominal ultrasound shows a hyperechoic HCC in the subcapsular portion of the liver* ➡. *Lateral edge shadowing and posterior acoustic enhancement* ➡ *are seen associated with the hepatocellular carcinoma (HCC).*

Hepatic Adenoma

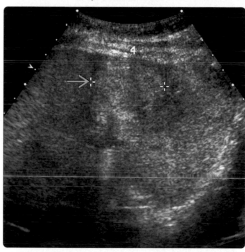

Hepatic Angiomyolipoma

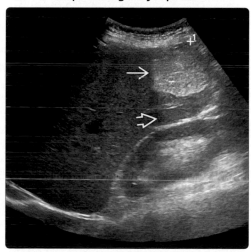

(Left) *Transverse grayscale ultrasound of the left lobe of the liver in a 22-year-old woman shows an echogenic solid mass* ➡, *which was proven to represent a hepatic adenoma.* (Right) *Longitudinal abdominal ultrasound shows a well-defined, homogeneously hyperechoic angiomyolipoma in the liver* ➡. *Slight posterior acoustic enhancement* ➡ *is seen associated with the angiomyolipoma (AML).*

Hepatic Angiomyolipoma

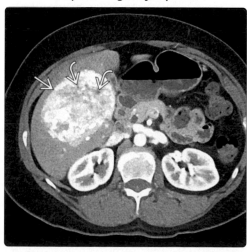

Hepatic Lipoma

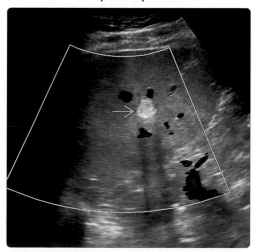

(Left) *Axial arterial phase of abdominal CECT in the same patient shows the large hypervascular AML in the right lobe of liver* ➡. *The mass contains tiny hypodense foci* ➡ *indicating fatty components.* (Right) *Color Doppler ultrasound shows a well-defined, uniformly echogenic avascular mass* ➡ *in the liver shown to represent an intrahepatic lipoma.*

DIFFERENTIAL DIAGNOSIS

Common

- Hepatic Metastases
- Hepatocellular Carcinoma
- Hepatic Lymphoma
- Hepatic Adenoma
- Fungal Hepatic Abscess
- Amebic Hepatic Abscess
- Pyogenic Hepatic Abscess

Less Common

- Hepatic Atypical Hemangioma
- Hepatic Hematoma

Rare but Important

- Sarcoidosis
- Kaposi Sarcoma

ESSENTIAL INFORMATION

Key Differential Diagnosis Issues

- Target sign: Echogenic center surrounded by hypoechoic rim
  - a.k.a. bull's-eye lesions
  - Malignancy far outnumbers other causes
- Reverse target: Hypoechoic core with hyperechoic rim

Helpful Clues for Common Diagnoses

- **Hepatic Metastases**
  - Solid central tumor with hypoechoic halo
    - Halo most likely related to compressed hepatic tissue along with zone of cancer cell proliferation
  - Alternating layers of hyper- and hypoechoic tissue
  - Usually from aggressive primary tumors
    - Classic example: Bronchogenic carcinoma
- **Hepatocellular Carcinoma**
  - Background of cirrhosis, portal hypertension, ascites
  - Rare for cirrhotic livers to develop metastases from nonhepatic primary

- Any mass in cirrhotic liver is more likely hepatocellular carcinoma than metastasis
- **Hepatic Lymphoma**
  - Vast majority are uniformly hypoechoic
  - Splenomegaly or splenic lesions, lymphadenopathy, thickened bowel wall provide clues toward diagnosis
- **Hepatic Adenoma**
  - Usually isoechoic or slightly hypoechoic
  - Complications such as hemorrhage, central necrosis make center echogenic
  - Occasional hypoechoic rim forms target-like appearance
- **Fungal Hepatic Abscess**
  - Often multiple lesions
  - Typically in immunocompromised patient
- **Amebic Hepatic Abscess**
  - Iso- to mildly hyperechoic center with hypoechoic halo
  - Abuts liver capsule
- **Pyogenic Hepatic Abscess**
  - Central hyperechoic inflammatory nodule surrounded by hypoechoic halo of fibrosis
  - Cluster sign: Cluster of small pyogenic abscesses that coalesce into single large cavity
  - Lobulated or irregular contour

Helpful Clues for Less Common Diagnoses

- **Hepatic Atypical Hemangioma**
  - Hypoechoic center with thick or thin hyperechoic rim
    - "Typical atypical" appearance (up to 40%)
    - Hypoechogenicity seem to be related to predominant fibrous stroma
- **Hepatic Hematoma**
  - May have laceration tract leading to hepatic surface
  - Multiple organs involved if traumatic cause

SELECTED REFERENCES

1. Virmani J et al: Characterization of primary and secondary malignant liver lesions from B-mode ultrasound. J Digit Imaging. 26(6):1058-70, 2013
2. Kraus GJ et al: The reverse target sign in liver disease: a potential ultrasound feature in cirrhotic liver nodules characterization. Br J Radiol. 78(928):355-7, 2005

Hepatic Metastases

Hepatic Metastases

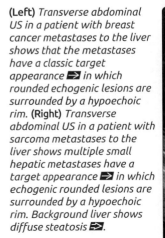
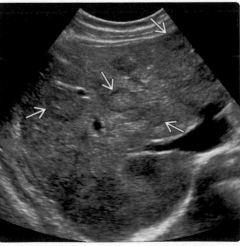
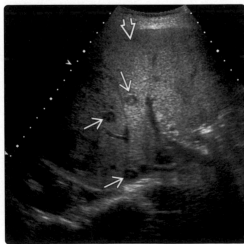

(Left) Transverse abdominal US in a patient with breast cancer metastases to the liver shows that the metastases have a classic target appearance ➡ in which rounded echogenic lesions are surrounded by a hypoechoic rim. (Right) Transverse abdominal US in a patient with sarcoma metastases to the liver shows multiple small hepatic metastases have a target appearance ➡ in which echogenic rounded lesions are surrounded by a hypoechoic rim. Background liver shows diffuse steatosis ➡.

Hepatic Metastases

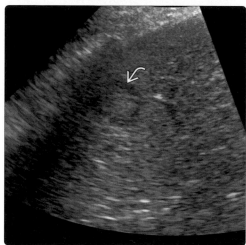

Hepatocellular Carcinoma

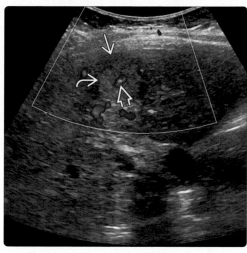

(Left) *Transverse abdominal US in a patient with lung cancer metastases to the liver shows a hepatic metastasis with a target appearance in which an isoechoic lesion is surrounded by a hypoechoic rim ➡. (Right) Transverse color Doppler US of the liver shows a hyperechoic hepatocellular carcinoma ➡ with a hypoechoic halo ➡, which creates a target appearance. Detectable internal vascularity ➡ within the tumor is seen.*

Hepatic Lymphoma

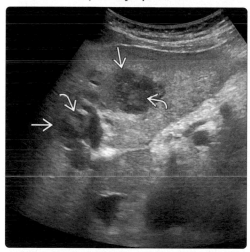

Fungal Hepatic Abscess

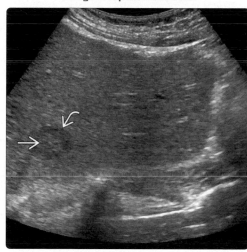

(Left) *Transverse abdominal grayscale US in a patient with lymphoma shows several hypoechoic masses with central echogenic cores ➡ surrounded by a hypoechoic rim ➡. (Right) Longitudinal grayscale US of the liver shows a fungal abscess that has an echogenic center ➡ surrounded by a hypoechoic rim ➡, which creates a target appearance.*

Pyogenic Hepatic Abscess

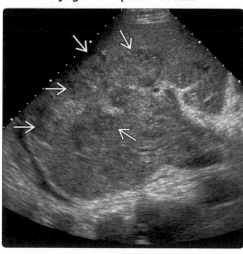

Hepatic Atypical Hemangioma

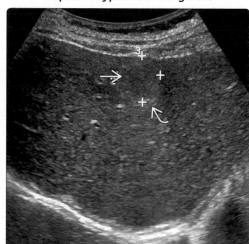

(Left) *Transverse abdominal US shows multiple hepatic abscesses ➡ that appear as isoechoic masses surrounded by thin hypoechoic rims. (Right) Longitudinal grayscale US of the liver shows an atypical hemangioma with reverse-target appearance, which is a hypoechoic mass ➡ surrounded by hyperechoic rim ➡.*

DIFFERENTIAL DIAGNOSIS

Common

- Hepatic Cysts
- Hepatic Metastases
- Hepatic Steatosis (Multifocal)
- Hepatic Hemangioma
- Hepatic Lymphoma (Discrete Form)
- Cirrhosis With Regenerative/Dysplastic Nodules
- Hepatocellular Carcinoma
- Pyogenic Hepatic Abscess
- Hepatic Microabscesses
- Cholangitis
- Vessels

Less Common

- Hepatic Echinococcus Cyst
- Hepatic Hematoma
- Biliary Hamartoma (von Meyenburg Complexes)

Rare but Important

- Caroli Disease

ESSENTIAL INFORMATION

Helpful Clues for Common Diagnoses

- **Hepatic Cysts**
  - Uncomplicated simple cyst
    - Anechoic rounded
    - Smooth or lobulated borders
    - Posterior acoustic enhancement
    - Thin or nondetectable wall
    - No septation/mural nodule/wall calcification
  - Hemorrhagic or infected cyst
    - Internal debris (clots or fibrin strands)
    - Septations/thickened wall, ± calcification
  - Autosomal dominant polycystic liver disease
    - Numerous cysts
    - Anechoic or with debris due to hemorrhage or infection
    - Calcification of some cyst walls
    - May have barely perceptible septations
    - No mural nodularity
    - Liver often distorted by innumerable cysts
    - Look for presence of renal cysts (adult polycystic kidney disease)
  - Do not demonstrate saccular configuration
    - vs. Caroli disease
  - Not associated with biliary duct dilatation
    - vs. hydatid cysts or Caroli disease
- **Hepatic Metastases**
  - Hypoechoic necrotic metastases
    - Usually from hypovascular tumors
    - Simulate cysts or abscesses
    - Abnormal intratumoral vascularity contains debris, mural nodules, or septa
  - Hyperechoic metastases
    - Simulate hemangioma or focal steatosis
    - Distort vessels and bile ducts
    - Vascular metastasis; from neuroendocrine tumors, choriocarcinoma, renal cell carcinoma, melanoma

- Target metastatic lesions
    - Solid echogenic mass with hypoechoic rim or halo
    - Usually from aggressive primary tumors
  - Cystic metastasis
    - May demonstrate posterior acoustic enhancement
    - Mural nodules, thick walls, fluid-fluid levels, internal septa, or debris
  - Calcified metastasis
    - Markedly echogenic interface with acoustic shadowing or diffuse small echogenic foci
    - Treated metastasis
- **Hepatic Steatosis (Multifocal)**
  - Focal fatty infiltration
    - Location: Right lobe, caudate lobe, perihilar
    - Hyperechoic area
  - Focal fatty sparing
    - Location: Gallbladder bed, segment IV anterior to portal bifurcation
    - Hypoechoic areas within echogenic liver
  - Geographic or fan-shaped
  - In some cases may appear as multiple echogenic nodules throughout liver
  - No mass effect
  - Vessels run undisplaced through lesion
- **Hepatic Hemangioma**
  - Well-defined margins
  - Hyperechoic mass, typically homogeneous
  - Posterior acoustic enhancement
  - Atypical features
    - Hypoechoic ± hyperechoic rim
    - Heterogeneous, calcification, irregular borders
- **Hepatic Lymphoma (Discrete Form)**
  - Well-defined nodules or masses
  - Hypoechoic or anechoic
    - Low echogenicity due to high cellular density
  - Large/conglomerate masses may appear to contain septa
    - Mimic abscesses
  - Background vascular architecture ± distortion
  - More common in immunocompromised patients
    - e.g., AIDS patients and organ transplant recipients
- **Cirrhosis With Regenerative/Dysplastic Nodules**
  - Coarse echo pattern, increased parenchymal echogenicity, other signs of cirrhosis
  - Regenerating nodules (siderotic)
    - Iso-/hypoechoic nodules (regenerating nodules)
    - Hyperechoic rim (surrounding fibrosis)
  - Dysplastic nodules
    - Hypoechoic nodule > 1 cm diameter
    - Smooth or irregular borders
    - Difficult to differentiate from small hepatocellular carcinoma
      - □ Should be further investigated with CECT or MR
- **Hepatocellular Carcinoma**
  - Most commonly hypoechoic
    - Less commonly hyperechoic or isoechoic to liver
  - Irregular hypervascularity within mass
  - Cirrhotic background liver
  - May see portal vein invasion or tumor thrombosis
- **Pyogenic Hepatic Abscess**

- o Cluster sign
  - − Cluster of small abscesses coalesce into single septated cavity
- o Complex cyst with septa and debris
- o ± ill-defined borders
- o Mural nodularity and vascularity
- o May contain gas within abscess
  - − Seen as echogenic foci of air or air-fluid level
- o Adjacent parenchyma may be coarse and hypoechoic
- o Color Doppler may show hypervascularity in inflamed surrounding liver parenchyma
- **Hepatic Microabscesses**
  - o Multiple, small, hypo-/iso-/hyperechoic lesions
  - o Central hypoechoic area of necrosis within hyperechoic lesion
  - o Target sign
    - − Central hyperechoic inflammation surrounded by hypoechoic "halo" of fibrosis
  - o Similar lesions may be found in spleen
- **Cholangitis**
  - o Circumferential bile duct wall thickening
  - o Dilatation of intra- and extrahepatic ducts
  - o Periportal hypo-/hyperechogenicity
    - − Due to periductal edema/inflammation
  - o Ascending cholangitis
    - − Obstructing calculus in extrahepatic duct
  - o Recurrent pyogenic cholangitis
    - − Biliary calculi: Cast-like and often fill duct lumen
    - − Atrophy of affected lobe/segment
- **Vessels**
  - o Portal veins: Venectasia, varicosities, collaterals from portal hypertension
  - o Hepatic veins: Venectasia, Budd-Chiari syndrome
  - o Hepatic arteries: Aneurysms, shunts, vascular malformation
  - o Use color Doppler to confirm vascular nature

Helpful Clues for Less Common Diagnoses

- **Hepatic Echinococcus Cyst**
  - o Large, well-defined hypoechoic masses

- o Numerous peripheral daughter cysts
- o Intrahepatic duct dilatation may be seen
- o May show curvilinear or ring-like pericyst calcification
- **Hepatic Hematoma**
  - o Lesions commonly in segments VI, VII, VIII
  - o Round, hyper-/hypoechoic foci
  - o Echogenicity evolves over time
    - − Echogenic initially
    - − Hypoechoic after 4-5 days
    - − Internal echoes and septations after 1-4 weeks
  - o Ancillary signs: Subcapsular hematoma, hemoperitoneum, renal or splenic laceration
- **Biliary Hamartoma (von Meyenburg Complexes)**
  - o Numerous small, hypo-/hyperechoic foci uniformly distributed throughout liver
    - − Leads to inhomogeneous and coarse appearance of liver echotexture
  - o Multiple echogenic foci
    - − Often with associated comet-tail artifacts
  - o Typically smaller lesions appear as echogenic foci, whereas larger lesions appear cystic
    - − Often extent of echogenic foci on US is greater than anticipated, based on comparison CT or MR

Helpful Clues for Rare Diagnoses

- **Caroli Disease**
  - o Hypoechoic masses
  - o Saccular or fusiform shape
  - o Central dot sign
    - − Small portal venous branches partially or completely surrounded by dilated ducts
  - o May contain calculi, which do not form casts of ducts

SELECTED REFERENCES

1. Forner A et al: Lack of arterial hypervascularity at contrast-enhanced ultrasound should not define the priority for diagnostic work-up of nodules < 2 cm. J Hepatol. 62(1):150-5, 2015
2. Kim TK et al: Contrast-enhanced ultrasound in the diagnosis of nodules in liver cirrhosis. World J Gastroenterol. 20(13):3590-6, 2014
3. Friedrich-Rust M et al: Contrast-Enhanced Ultrasound for the differentiation of benign and malignant focal liver lesions: a meta-analysis. Liver Int. 33(5):739-55, 2013

Hepatic Cysts

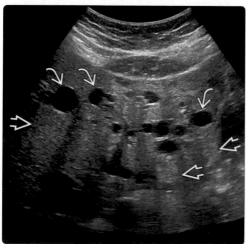

Hepatic Metastases

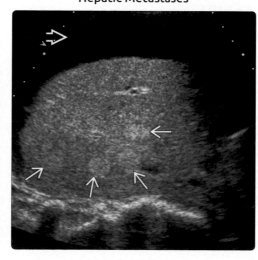

(Left) Transverse grayscale US of the liver shows innumerable cysts ➔ throughout the liver in a patient with polycystic liver disease. Posterior acoustic enhancement ➡ is seen associated with each cyst. (Right) Transverse abdominal US in a patient with carcinoid metastases to the liver shows multiple round and homogeneous hyperechoic metastatic nodules in the liver ➔. Large amount of perihepatic ascites ➡ is seen.

(Left) Transverse US in a patient with mucinous colon cancer demonstrates multiple large, hyperechoic metastases ➡ containing diffuse echogenic foci ➡ related to subtle calcifications. Note posterior acoustic shadowing caused by the calcifications ⇨. (Right) Transverse abdominal US in a patient with pancreatic cancer shows numerous small, hypoechoic metastases ➡ throughout the liver. The background liver is echogenic from hepatic steatosis, a common finding in the setting of chemotherapy.

Hepatic Metastases

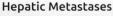

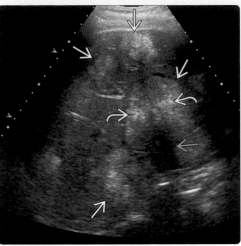

Hepatic Metastases

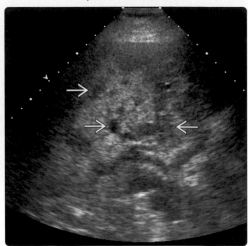

(Left) Abdominal grayscale US shows multifocal fat deposition, which appears as geographic areas of increased echogenicity ➡ around the portal vein ⇨. The lesion shows no mass effect, and vessels run through the lesion, characteristic features of fatty infiltration. (Right) Transverse abdominal US shows 2 well-defined, homogeneously hyperechoic hemangiomas in the right lobe of liver ➡.

Hepatic Steatosis (Multifocal)

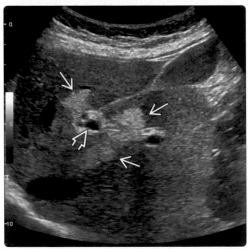

Hepatic Hemangioma

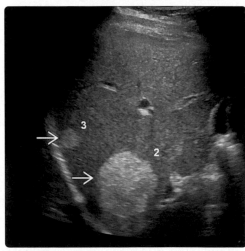

(Left) Transverse abdominal US shows 2 well-defined and homogeneously hyperechoic hemangiomas in the liver ➡. Hemangiomas in the liver are often multiple. (Right) Transverse abdominal US in a patient with lymphoma shows multiple hypoechoic masses ➡ throughout the liver. Lesions are markedly hypoechoic, resulting in a pseudocystic appearance characteristic of lymphoma.

Hepatic Hemangioma

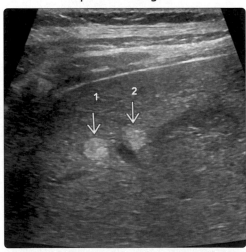

Hepatic Lymphoma (Discrete Form)

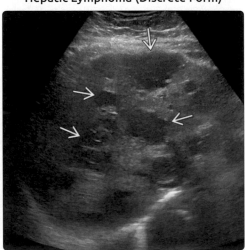

Cirrhosis With Regenerative/Dysplastic Nodules

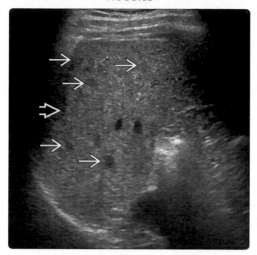

Hepatocellular Carcinoma

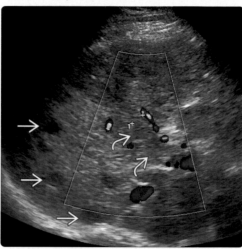

(Left) *Abdominal US in a patient with hepatitis B shows numerous small hypoechoic nodules in the liver ➡, indicating regenerative or dysplastic nodules. Coarse and heterogeneous echogenicity of liver parenchyma is consistent with underlying cirrhosis ➡.* **(Right)** *Abdominal US shows multifocal hypoechoic hepatocellular carcinomas ➡ throughout the liver. The right portal vein is thrombosed and filled with echogenic material that was found to represent tumor thrombus ➡.*

Pyogenic Hepatic Abscess

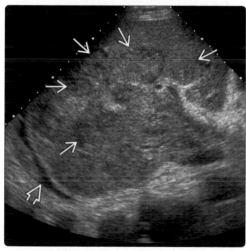

Hepatic Microabscesses

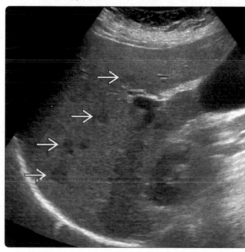

(Left) *Transverse abdominal grayscale US shows multiple hepatic abscesses ➡ in the liver, seen as ill-defined isoechoic masses surrounded by thin hypoechoic rims. A small amount of perihepatic ascites ➡ is present as well.* **(Right)** *Longitudinal abdominal grayscale US shows multiple small hypoechoic fungal microabscesses ➡ in the right lobe of liver.*

Hepatic Echinococcus Cyst

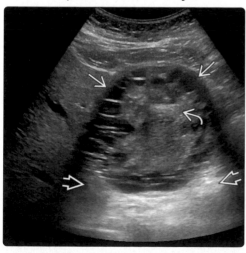

Caroli Disease

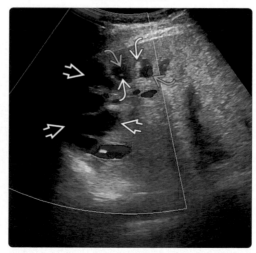

(Left) *Transverse abdominal US shows an echinococcal cyst containing multiple peripheral daughter cysts ➡ and heterogeneous material centrally ➡. Note the associated posterior acoustic enhancement ➡.* **(Right)** *Oblique abdominal US in a young patient with Caroli disease shows multiple dilated intrahepatic ducts ➡. Echogenic portal radicles ➡ are surrounded by dilated ducts. Some of the portal radicles within dilated ducts show color flow ➡, which creates the central dot sign appearance.*

Liver

DIFFERENTIAL DIAGNOSIS

Common

- Focal Nodular Hyperplasia
- Fibrolamellar Carcinoma
- Hepatocellular Carcinoma
- Hepatic Adenoma
- Hepatic Metastases

Less Common

- Atypical Hemangioma
- Hepatic Echinococcus Cyst

ESSENTIAL INFORMATION

Helpful Clues for Common Diagnoses

- **Focal Nodular Hyperplasia**
  - Mass: Typically homogeneous and isoechoic to liver
    - Occasionally hypoechoic or hyperechoic
  - Central scar: Typically hypoechoic (18% hyperechoic)
    - Contains central feeding artery
  - Color Doppler: Spoke-wheel pattern
    - Prominent central feeding artery with multiple small vessels radiating peripherally
    - Large draining veins at tumor margins
- **Fibrolamellar Carcinoma**
  - Presents in otherwise healthy young adults
    - Background cirrhosis or hepatitis in < 5% of patients
  - Well-defined, partially/completely encapsulated large mass
  - Prominent central fibrous scar
  - Calcification within scar common
  - Intralesional necrosis/hemorrhage
  - Vascular, biliary, and nodal invasion may be present
- **Hepatocellular Carcinoma**
  - Background cirrhosis ± signs of portal hypertension
  - Central tumor necrosis/fibrosis produces apparent central scar
  - Color Doppler may show irregular tumor hypervascularity or tumor thrombus in portal vein

- **Hepatic Adenoma**
  - Well-defined round or mildly lobulated contour
  - Hypo-/iso-/hyperechoic mass
  - Central fat, hemorrhage, necrosis, and calcification
    - May simulate central scar
  - Color Doppler shows hypervascular tumor supplied by hepatic artery
- **Hepatic Metastases**
  - Necrotic or treated metastases with necrotic center may simulate central scar
  - Necrotic center may be lined with irregular walls and contain debris
  - Color Doppler may not show vascularity as many metastases are hypovascular

Helpful Clues for Less Common Diagnoses

- **Atypical Hemangioma**
  - Hypoechoic center with hyperechoic rim may simulate central scar
    - "Typical atypical" hemangioma (up to 40%)
  - Posterior acoustic enhancement
  - No visible color Doppler flow in center of lesion
    - Flow too slow to be sonographically detected
- **Hepatic Echinococcus Cyst**
  - Honeycombed cyst
    - Multiple septations between daughter cysts in mother cyst
  - Spoke-wheel appearance of septa simulating central scar

SELECTED REFERENCES

1. Kong WT et al: Contrast-enhanced ultrasound in combination with color doppler ultrasound can improve the diagnostic performance of focal nodular hyperplasia and hepatocellular adenoma. Ultrasound Med Biol. 41(4):944-51, 2015
2. Kim T et al: Liver masses with central or eccentric scar. Semin Ultrasound CT MR. 30(5):418-25, 2009

(Left) *Intraoperative abdominal US using a high-frequency transducer shows a hypoechoic focal nodular hyperplasia (FNH) in the liver ➡ with a hyperechoic central scar ➡. (Right) Transverse abdominal ultrasound shows a pedunculated FNH ➡ with a slightly hyperechoic central scar ➡ arising from the lateral segment of the left lobe of the liver.*

Focal Nodular Hyperplasia

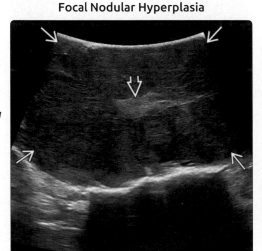

Focal Nodular Hyperplasia

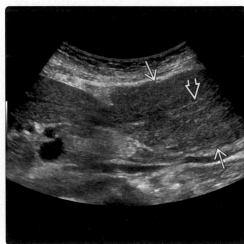

Focal Nodular Hyperplasia

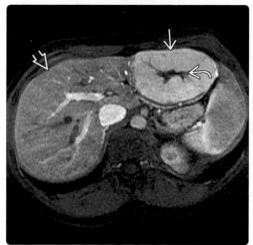

Focal Nodular Hyperplasia

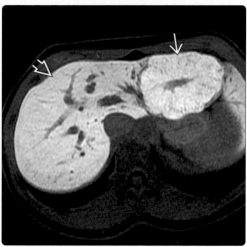

(Left) *Axial arterial phase T1 contrast-enhanced MR shows a hyperenhancing FNH* ➡, *which is hyperintense compared to adjacent liver parenchyma* ➡. *Hypointense stellate central scar* ➡ *is characteristic of FNH.* (Right) *Axial hepatobiliary phase MR obtained 20 minutes after gadoxetate injection in the same patient shows the FNH retains contrast to slightly greater degree* ➡ *than the background liver* ➡, *confirming the presence of hepatocytes in the FNH.*

Fibrolamellar Carcinoma

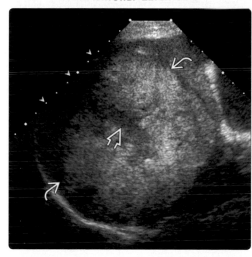

Hepatocellular Carcinoma

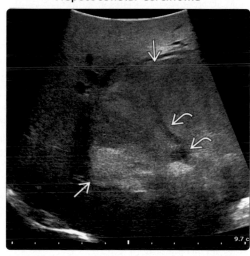

(Left) *Transverse grayscale US of the liver shows a large, predominantly echogenic mass* ➡ *with a thick, hypoechoic central scar* ➡. *The mass was proven to be a fibrolamellar carcinoma.* (Right) *Intraoperative grayscale ultrasound of the liver shows a large, heterogeneous, isoechoic hepatocellular carcinoma* ➡ *with hypoechoic central scar* ➡.

Hepatic Metastases

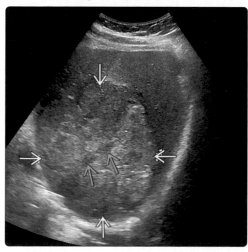

Atypical Hemangioma

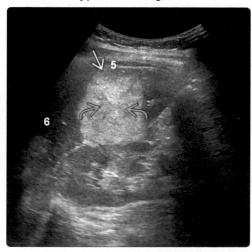

(Left) *Oblique abdominal grayscale US in a patient with melanoma shows a large, heterogeneous, hyperechoic metastasis* ➡ *in the right lobe of the liver. Central hypoechoic areas simulate a central scar* ➡. (Right) *Longitudinal grayscale abdominal US shows a hyperechoic hemangioma in the liver* ➡. *The ill-defined hypoechoic area in the center* ➡ *simulates a central scar.*

DIFFERENTIAL DIAGNOSIS

Common

- Ascending Cholangitis
- Cavernous Transformation of Portal Vein
- Portosystemic Collaterals
- Hepatic Trauma
- Acute Viral Hepatitis
- Fatty Sparing, Liver
- Diffuse/Infiltrative Hepatic Lymphoma
- Pneumobilia
- Choledocholithiasis
- Metastases

Less Common

- Peribiliary Cyst
- Hepatic Schistosomiasis
- Recurrent Pyogenic Cholangitis
- Iatrogenic Material
- Caroli Disease
- Hepatic Artery Calcification
- Cystic Duct Remnant

ESSENTIAL INFORMATION

Helpful Clues for Common Diagnoses

- **Ascending Cholangitis**
  - Periportal hypo- or hyperechogenicity adjacent to dilated intrahepatic ducts
    - Due to periductal edema/inflammation
  - Dilatation of intrahepatic bile ducts
  - Purulent bile/sludge as intraluminal echogenic material in dilated ducts
  - Circumferential thickening of bile duct wall
  - Obstructing stone in common bile duct
- **Cavernous Transformation of Portal Vein**
  - Collateralization due to portal vein occlusion
  - Usually in subacute or chronic portal vein obstruction
  - Serpiginous tubular channels along expected course of portal vein
  - Color Doppler shows hepatopetal flow
  - Signs of portal vein occlusion
    - Acute: Enlarged portal vein
    - Chronic: Small/imperceptible portal vein
    - Color Doppler: Lack of flow in portal vein
- **Portosystemic Collaterals**
  - Serpiginous hypoechoic channels in or around portal triad
  - Location
    - Intrahepatic: Portal to portal veins, portal to hepatic veins, portal to systemic veins
    - Paraumbilical vein (recanalization)
    - Gastroesophageal: Coronary and right gastric, left gastric and splenogastric
    - Lienorenal/mesenteric/retroperitoneal
  - Color Doppler
    - Shows hepatofugal flow in vessels (opposite to cavernous transformation)
    - Extent of collaterals
  - Background changes of cirrhosis/portal hypertension/portal vein thrombosis

- **Hepatic Trauma**
  - Lesions are commonly located in segments VI, VII, VIII
  - Echogenicity evolves over time
    - Initially echogenic
    - Becomes hypoechoic after 4-5 days
    - Internal echoes with septa may develop after 1-4 weeks
  - Hematoma tracking along portal triad
    - Linear, focal, or diffuse periportal lesion
  - Ancillary signs of trauma
    - Subcapsular hematoma; hemoperitoneum, renal, or splenic laceration/hematoma
  - Better evaluated by MDCT
- **Acute Viral Hepatitis**
  - Increased echogenicity of fat in periportal tissues, ligamentum venosum, and falciform ligament
  - Hepatomegaly with diffuse decrease in echogenicity
  - Starry sky appearance
    - Increased echogenicity of portal triad walls against background of hypoechoic liver
  - Periportal hypo-/anechoic area
    - Due to hydropic swelling of hepatocytes
- **Fatty Sparing, Liver**
  - Focal hypoechoic area within otherwise echogenic liver
  - No mass effect: Vessels run undisplaced through lesion
  - Due to direct drainage of hepatic blood into systemic circulation
  - Typical location
    - Next to gallbladder: Drained by cystic vein
    - Segment IV/anterior to portal bifurcation: Drained by aberrant gastric vein
- **Diffuse/Infiltrative Hepatic Lymphoma**
  - Subcentimeter periportal hypoechoic foci, miliary in pattern
  - Other evidence of lymphoma
    - Lymphadenopathy, splenomegaly/splenic lesions, bowel wall thickening, ascites
- **Pneumobilia**
  - Highly echogenic linear foci in portal triad
  - Rises to nondependent portion of liver (left lobe if patient lying supine)
  - Change in position of gas with change in patient position
  - Posterior acoustic shadowing
  - Reverberation artifact deep to lesion
  - Causes
    - Recent passage of stone from or instrumentation of biliary tree
    - Choledochoenteric fistula
    - Biliary infection by gas-forming organism
- **Choledocholithiasis**
  - Multiple echogenic foci along portal triad
  - Posterior acoustic shadowing
    - Small (< 5 mm) or soft pigmented stones may not produce posterior shadowing
  - Large stones may cause biliary obstruction, resulting in focal bile duct dilatation
- **Metastases**
  - May be located anywhere in liver
  - Usually multiple

Helpful Clues for Less Common Diagnoses

- **Peribiliary Cyst**
  - Well-defined small cystic structures adjacent to portal triads
  - More common in cirrhotic patients
  - Usually multiple
  - No communication with biliary tree
- **Hepatic Schistosomiasis**
  - Periportal fibrosis
    - Most severe at porta hepatis
    - Widened portal tracts
    - Clay-pipestem fibrosis
      - □ Hyperechoic and thickened walls of portal venules
    - Bull's-eye lesion
      - □ Anechoic portal vein surrounded by echogenic mantle of fibrous tissue
  - Mosaic pattern
    - Network of echogenic septa outlining polygonal areas of normal-appearing liver
    - Represents complete septal fibrosis
      - □ Inflammation & fibrosis in reaction to embolized eggs
    - May be discontinuous and appear mottled, nodular, or sieve-like
      - □ Partial septal fibrosis or calcification
- **Recurrent Pyogenic Cholangitis**
  - Lateral segment of left lobe and posterior segment of right lobe more commonly involved
  - Early disease with active biliary sepsis
    - Periportal hypo- or hyperechogenicity due to periductal edema/inflammation
    - Biliary duct wall thickening due to edema
    - Floating echoes within dilated ducts due to inflammatory debris
  - Late-stage disease
    - Severe atrophy of affected segment/lobe, biliary cirrhosis
    - Crowded stone-filled ducts
      - □ May appear as single heterogeneous mass

- Stones may form casts of duct
- **Iatrogenic Material**
  - Shunt, stent, embolization material, drainage tube, staples, etc.
  - Echogenic material with strong reflective surface or smooth outline
- **Caroli Disease**
  - Anechoic masses: Saccular or fusiform shape
  - Central dot sign
    - Small portal venous branches partially/completely surrounded by dilated ducts
- **Hepatic Artery Calcification**
  - Branching linear echogenic structures along portal triads
  - Often marked calcifications of splenic artery and other smaller arteries
  - Risk factors
    - Longstanding diabetes
    - Chronic renal failure
    - Conditions that predispose to heavy vascular calcifications
- **Cystic Duct Remnant**
  - History of prior cholecystectomy
  - Remnant cystic duct may be dilated

SELECTED REFERENCES

1. Shin SW et al: Usefulness of B-mode and doppler sonography for the diagnosis of severe acute viral hepatitis A. J Clin Ultrasound. 43(6):384-92, 2015
2. Spârchez Z et al: Role of contrast enhanced ultrasound in the assessment of biliary duct disease. Med Ultrason. 16(1):41-7, 2014
3. Trenker C et al: Contrast-enhanced ultrasound (CEUS) in hepatic lymphoma: retrospective evaluation in 38 cases. Ultraschall Med. 35(2):142-8, 2014
4. Wu S et al: Characteristics suggestive of focal Fatty sparing from liver malignancy on ultrasound in liver screening. Ultrasound Q. 30(4):276-81, 2014
5. Kobayashi S et al: Intrahepatic periportal high intensity on hepatobiliary phase images of Gd-EOB-DTPA-enhanced MRI: imaging findings and prevalence in various hepatobiliary diseases. Jpn J Radiol. 31(1):9-15, 2013
6. Meacock LM et al: Evaluation of gallbladder and biliary duct disease using microbubble contrast-enhanced ultrasound. Br J Radiol. 83(991):615-27, 2010
7. Passos MC et al: Ultrasound and CT findings in hepatic and pancreatic parenchyma in acute schistosomiasis. Br J Radiol. 82(979):e145-7, 2009

Ascending Cholangitis

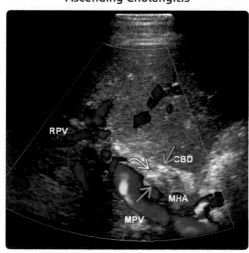

Cavernous Transformation of Portal Vein

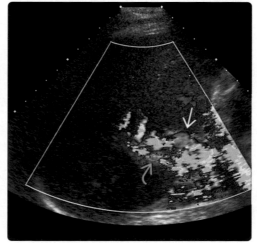

(Left) Transverse color Doppler US in a patient with ascending cholangitis shows circumferential wall thickening of the common bile duct ➡ as well as echogenic debris ➡ within the lumen. (Right) Color Doppler US shows collateralized flow ➡ in the porta hepatis in a patient with chronic portal vein thrombosis ➡. Color Doppler signal is heterogeneous because portal vein collaterals are tortuous, resulting in vessels directed toward as well as away from the transducer.

Portosystemic Collaterals

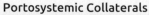

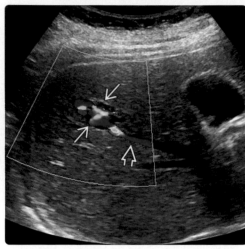

(Left) *Transverse abdominal US shows an intrahepatic portosystemic shunt between the right portal vein and right hepatic vein ➡, which appears as an entangled vascular structure that drains into the right hepatic vein ➡.*
(Right) *Transverse abdominal color Doppler US in a patient with hepatic cirrhosis shows a recanalized paraumbilical vein ➡ arising from the left portal vein ➡ and traveling anteriorly along the falciform ligament toward the inferior epigastric vein.*

Portosystemic Collaterals

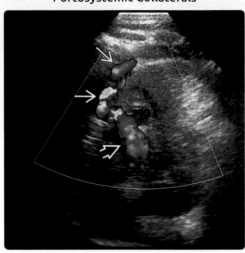

Diffuse/Infiltrative Hepatic Lymphoma

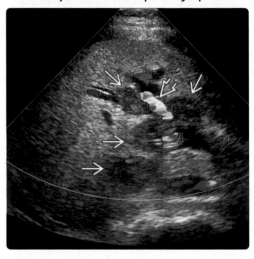

(Left) *Transverse color Doppler US in a patient with lymphoma involving the liver shows multiple markedly hypoechoic masses ➡ in a periportal distribution (right anterior portal vein ➡) in the liver. Lesions are predominantly hypovascular, a characteristic imaging appearance of lymphoma.*
(Right) *Transverse abdominal US shows linear bright hyperechoic foci ➡ caused by pneumobilia along the expected course of the biliary tree.*

Pneumobilia

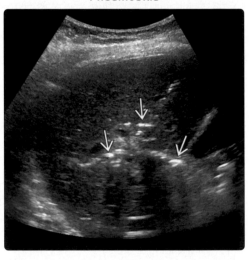

Choledocholithiasis

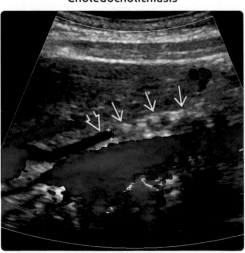

(Left) *Longitudinal color Doppler US shows multiple echogenic stones ➡ within the common bile duct, causing upstream biliary ductal dilation ➡. Color Doppler is helpful to distinguish avascular ducts from adjacent vasculature.* (Right) *Transverse abdominal color Doppler US in a patient with ovarian cancer shows an ill-defined, hypoechoic metastasis ➡ that infiltrates the left periportal region, occluding the left portal vein, which should normally be present in this region.*

Metastases

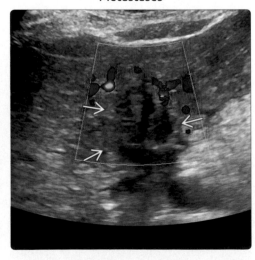

Peribiliary Cyst

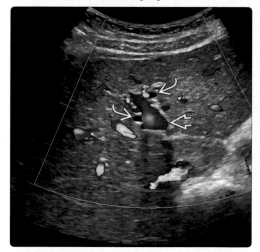

Hepatic Schistosomiasis

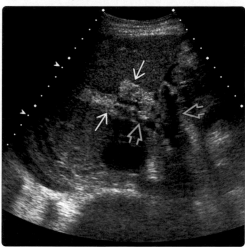

(Left) *Transverse abdominal color Doppler US shows several well-defined small peribiliary cysts* ➡ *along the left portal vein* ➡. **(Right)** *Transverse abdominal US in a patient with hepatic schistosomiasis shows thick echogenic mantle of fibrotic tissue* ➡ *in the periportal area, encasing the portal veins* ➡. *(Courtesy W. Chong, MD.)*

Recurrent Pyogenic Cholangitis

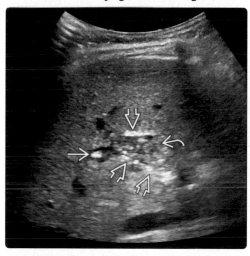

Recurrent Pyogenic Cholangitis

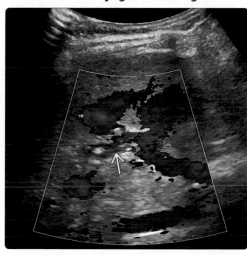

(Left) *Transverse abdominal US in a patient with recurrent pyogenic cholangitis shows echogenic intrahepatic stones* ➡ *and sludge* ➡ *within moderately dilated intrahepatic biliary ducts. Note the periductal hyperechogenicity* ➡, *related to periductal inflammation.* **(Right)** *Color Doppler US in the same patient demonstrates no flow within the dilated intrahepatic duct* ➡, *confirming the findings are indeed in the biliary tree rather than the portal or hepatic arterial system.*

Hepatic Artery Calcification

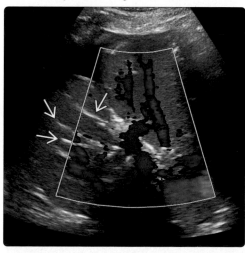

Cystic Duct Remnant

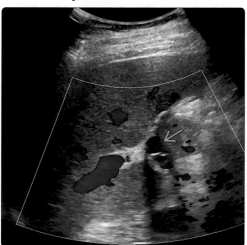

(Left) *Transverse abdominal color Doppler US shows multifocal linear branching echogenic structures* ➡ *that are hepatic artery calcifications related to end-stage renal disease.* **(Right)** *Longitudinal color Doppler US in a patient who underwent cholecystectomy shows a cystic duct remnant* ➡ *that appears as a round cystic lesion in the region of the porta hepatis.*

DIFFERENTIAL DIAGNOSIS

Common

- Cirrhosis
- Subcapsular Hepatic Neoplasm
- Hepatic Metastasis
- Infiltrative Hepatocellular Carcinoma
- Postsurgical Hepatic Resection

Less Common

- Hepatic Rupture
- Schistosomiasis

ESSENTIAL INFORMATION

Helpful Clues for Common Diagnoses

- **Cirrhosis**
  - Nodular surface contour
    - Micronodular (< 1 cm in diameter): Due to alcoholism
    - Macronodular: Due to viral hepatitis
  - Hypertrophy of caudate lobe and lateral segment of left lobe
  - Atrophy of right lobe and medial segment of left lobe
  - Widening of fissures
  - Coarse/nodular/heterogeneous parenchymal echotexture
- **Subcapsular Hepatic Neoplasm**
  - Primary or secondary subcapsular neoplasm may distort surface contour when large or numerous
  - Lesions cause architectural distortion of liver parenchyma
- **Hepatic Metastasis**
  - Commonly due to gastric, ovarian, breast, or pancreatic primary
  - Treated metastases (e.g., from breast) may shrink and fibrose, simulating nodular contour of cirrhotic liver
- **Infiltrative Hepatocellular Carcinoma**
  - Margins of tumor often indistinct
  - May see refractive shadows emanating from hepatic parenchyma
  - Portal triads may be effaced or invaded
  - Often associated with tumor thrombus in the portal vein or hepatic vein (less common)
- **Postsurgical Hepatic Resection**
  - Combination of surgical defect and surrounding scarring causes irregularity of contour
  - Surgical material ± fat in surgical defect causes further heterogeneity of surgical site

Helpful Clues for Less Common Diagnoses

- **Hepatic Rupture**
  - Echogenic blood clot on surface of liver
  - May see breach of hepatic capsule or irregularity of capsular surface if underlying lesion is hepatocellular carcinoma
  - Hemoperitoneum may be present
    - More echogenic than ascites
  - Underlying cause
    - Large or exophytic hepatocellular carcinoma or other tumor
    - Spontaneous hepatic rupture associated with HELLP (hemolysis, elevated liver enzymes, and low platelets) syndrome
      - Thought to be secondary to endothelial dysfunction and thrombotic microangiopathy
- **Schistosomiasis**
  - Irregular/notched, liver surface
  - Echogenic periportal fibrotic bands (most severe at porta hepatis)
  - Mosaic pattern: Network of echogenic septa outlining polygonal areas of normal-appearing liver
    - Represents complete septal fibrosis (inflammation and fibrosis as reaction to embolized eggs)

SELECTED REFERENCES

1. Goel A et al: Pregnancy-related liver disorders. J Clin Exp Hepatol. 4(2):151-62, 2014
2. Irshad A et al: Current role of ultrasound in chronic liver disease: surveillance, diagnosis and management of hepatic neoplasms. Curr Probl Diagn Radiol. 41(2):43-51, 2012
3. Tchelepi H et al: Sonography of diffuse liver disease. J Ultrasound Med. 21(9):1023-32; quiz 1033-4, 2002

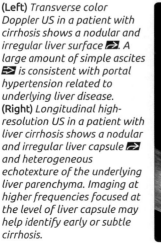

(Left) Transverse color Doppler US in a patient with cirrhosis shows a nodular and irregular liver surface ➡. A large amount of simple ascites ⧀ is consistent with portal hypertension related to underlying liver disease. (Right) Longitudinal high-resolution US in a patient with liver cirrhosis shows a nodular and irregular liver capsule ➡ and heterogeneous echotexture of the underlying liver parenchyma. Imaging at higher frequencies focused at the level of liver capsule may help identify early or subtle cirrhosis.

Cirrhosis

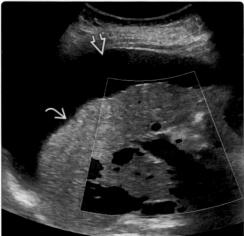

Cirrhosis

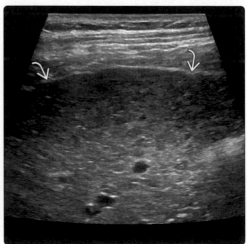

Subcapsular Hepatic Neoplasm

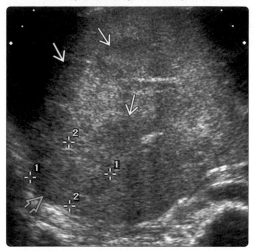

Subcapsular Hepatic Neoplasm

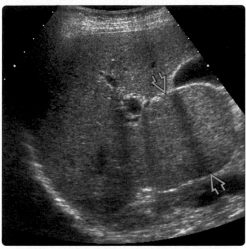

(Left) *Transverse grayscale US of the liver shows an isoechoic liver metastasis ⇰ from breast cancer that bulges and slightly distorts the liver surface. Multiple other subtle hypoechoic breast cancer metastases are seen throughout the rest of the liver ➡.* (Right) *Transverse grayscale US of the liver shows a large isoechoic mass in the caudate lobe of the liver which creates a rounded bulge upon the hepatic surface in this area. This mass was a focal nodular hyperplasia ⇰.*

Hepatic Metastasis

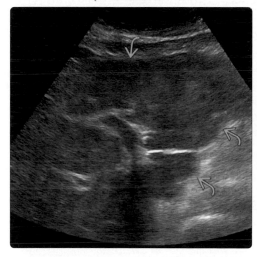

Infiltrative Hepatocellular Carcinoma

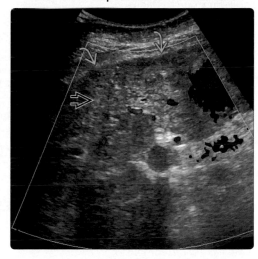

(Left) *Transverse grayscale US of the left lobe of the liver in a patient with breast cancer shows markedly irregular and nodular liver surface due to diffuse hepatic involvement with metastases ⇗.* (Right) *Transverse color Doppler US in a patient with infiltrative hepatocellular carcinoma throughout the liver shows the infiltrative tumor causes both markedly heterogeneous echotexture ⇰ as well as irregular hepatic surface ⇗.*

Hepatic Rupture

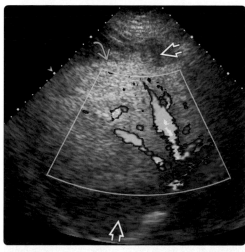

Schistosomiasis

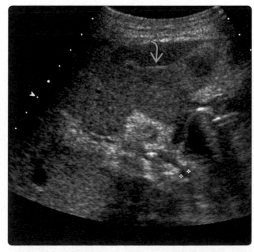

(Left) *Transverse color Doppler image in a patient with liver rupture from HELLP syndrome shows a large amount of perihepatic and subcapsular blood ➡ which causes the liver margin ⇗ to appear irregular. Acute blood can be so echogenic that the liver margin can be obscured by the blood.* (Right) *Transverse grayscale US of a patient with schistosomiasis and periportal fibrosis as well as hepatic capsular irregularity ⇗ is shown. (Courtesy W. Chong, MD.)*

DIFFERENTIAL DIAGNOSIS

Common

- Portal Hypertension
- Portosystemic Collaterals
- Bland Portal Vein Thrombosis
- Portal Vein Tumor Thrombus
- Pulsatile Portal Vein

Less Common

- Portal Vein Gas

ESSENTIAL INFORMATION

Helpful Clues for Common Diagnoses

- **Portal Hypertension**
  - Decreased portal vein mean velocity (< 16 cm/s)
  - Portal venous pressure ≥ 10 mm Hg more than inferior vena cava pressure
  - Hepatofugal portal vein flow in severe portal hypertension
  - Absent (aphasic) portal venous flow due to stagnation
    - Lack of respiratory phasicity
    - Severe portal hypertension
  - Development of portosystemic shunts
  - Background cirrhosis, splenomegaly, ascites, thickened bowel wall
- **Portosystemic Collaterals**
  - Common locations
    - Inferior hepatic margin via gastroepiploic vein
    - Gastroesophageal junction via left gastric vein
    - Anterior abdominal wall via ligamentum teres (recanalized paraumbilical vein)
    - Lienorenal ligament via lienorenal collaterals
  - Color Doppler shows low velocity hepatofugal flow
- **Bland Portal Vein Thrombosis**
  - Echogenic material within portal vein (acute thrombosis)
  - Poor visualization of portal vein (chronic thrombosis)
  - Cavernous transformation of portal vein in chronic thrombosis

- Color Doppler: Interrupted/irregular flow in portal vein
- Signs of liver dysfunction or portal hypertension
  - Cirrhosis, ascites, splenomegaly, portosystemic collaterals
- **Portal Vein Tumor Thrombus**
  - Majority arise from hepatocellular carcinoma
  - Echogenic material within portal vein
  - Suspect tumor thrombus in case of adjacent hepatic malignancy
  - Color Doppler may show tumor neovascularity within thrombus
- **Pulsatile Portal Vein**
  - Normal portal vein waveform
    - Hepatopetal and mildly phasic (gentle undulation)
  - Increased pulsatility (pulsatile waveform)
    - When there is large difference between peak systolic velocity and end diastolic velocity
      - Tricuspid regurgitation
      - Right-sided congestive heart failure
      - Arterioportal shunting in cirrhosis
      - Arteriovenous fistula in hereditary hemorrhagic telangiectasia

Helpful Clues for Less Common Diagnoses

- **Portal Vein Gas**
  - Highly reflective foci (gas) travels within portal vein
  - Poorly defined, highly reflective parenchymal foci
  - Gas moves to periphery of liver (as opposed to biliary gas, which moves towards liver hilum)
  - High intensity transient signals (HITS) with spectral Doppler
    - Strong transient spikes superimposed on portal venous flow pattern

SELECTED REFERENCES

1. Manzano-Robleda Mdel C et al: Portal vein thrombosis: what is new? Ann Hepatol. 14(1):20-7, 2015
2. McNaughton DA et al: Doppler US of the liver made simple. Radiographics. 31(1):161-88, 2011
3. Abboud B et al: Hepatic portal venous gas: physiopathology, etiology, prognosis and treatment. World J Gastroenterol. 15(29):3585-90, 2009

(Left) Spectral Doppler US of the liver in a patient with portal hypertension shows retrograde (hepatofugal) flow in the portal vein ➡, a finding that appears blue on the color Doppler US and is displayed below the baseline on the spectral waveform ➡. (Right) Transverse abdominal color Doppler US in a patient with hepatic cirrhosis shows a recanalized paraumbilical vein ➡ arising from the left portal vein ➡ and traveling anteriorly along the falciform ligament towards the inferior epigastric vein.

Portal Hypertension

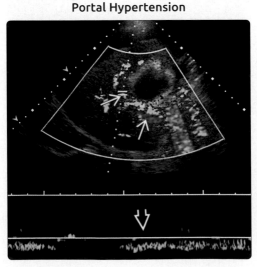

Portosystemic Collaterals

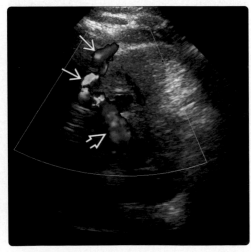

Bland Portal Vein Thrombosis

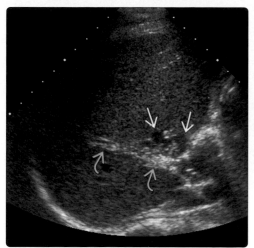

Bland Portal Vein Thrombosis

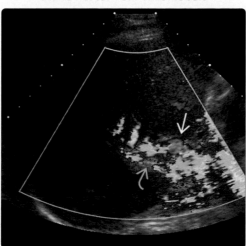

(Left) *Grayscale US shows an echogenic, chronically thrombosed main portal vein* ⟱ *and adjacent collateralized flow* ➡ *indicating cavernous transformation of the portal vein.* (Right) *Color Doppler US in the same patient shows collateralized flow* ➡ *in the porta hepatis in this patient with chronic portal vein thrombosis* ⟱. *Color Doppler signal is heterogeneous because portal vein collaterals are tortuous, resulting in vessels directed towards as well as away from the transducer.*

Portal Vein Tumor Thrombus

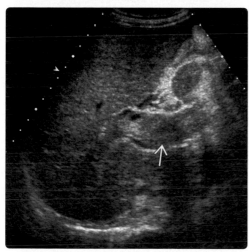

Portal Vein Tumor Thrombus

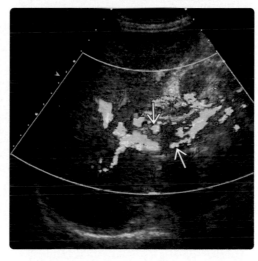

(Left) *Transverse grayscale US of the liver in a patient with hepatocellular carcinoma shows an expansile echogenic tumor thrombus in the main portal vein* ➡. (Right) *Color Doppler US in the same patient shows multiple small feeding vessels* ➡ *in the tumor thrombus with a dot-dash pattern. Tumor thrombus in the setting of hepatocellular carcinoma is almost always associated with infiltrative tumor and carries a poor prognosis.*

Pulsatile Portal Vein

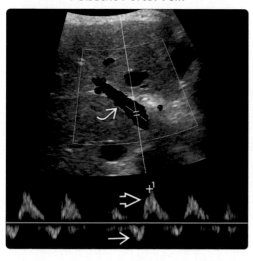

Portal Vein Gas

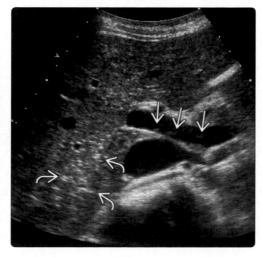

(Left) *Spectral Doppler US in a patient with right heart failure shows a pulsatile waveform with flow above* ➡ *and below* ➡ *baseline in the main portal vein* ➡. *The waveform is characterized as predominantly antegrade, pulsatile, and biphasic-bidirectional.* (Right) *Oblique US of the liver shows several echogenic foci in the main portal vein* ➡ *representing gas bubbles. Bright echogenic patches* ➡ *in the liver parenchyma more peripherally represent intraparenchymal portal venous gas.*

SECTION 10
Gallbladder

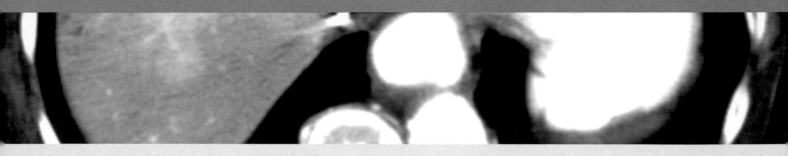

DIFFERENTIAL DIAGNOSIS

Common

- Decreased Vagal Stimulation
  - Postvagotomy State
  - Anticholinergic Medications
  - Diabetes Mellitus
- Decreased Cholecystokinin Secretion
  - Hyperalimentation
  - Prolonged Fasting
- Obstructed Flow of Bile
  - Calculous Cholecystitis
  - Choledocholithiasis
  - Pancreatic Ductal Adenocarcinoma
- Inflammation of Gallbladder by Intrinsic or Adjacent Process
- Acalculous Cholecystitis

Less Common

- Gallbladder Hydrops
- Gallbladder Empyema
- Choledochal Cyst (Mimic)

ESSENTIAL INFORMATION

Key Differential Diagnosis Issues

- No absolute size criteria, but gallbladder (GB) considered distended when > 5 cm in diameter or 10 cm in length
- GB contracts and empties in response to vagal stimulation and cholecystokinin (secreted in response to fatty foods)
  - Vagal stimulation causes GB contraction; cholecystokinin causes GB contraction and relaxation of sphincter of Oddi
- Normal emptying requires patent cystic duct and common bile duct (CBD)

Helpful Clues for Common Diagnoses

- Causes can be divided into 5 major categories
  - **Decreased Vagal Stimulation**
    - Vagotomy, anticholinergic medicines, or diabetic neuropathy can reduce vagal stimulation and result in GB distension

  - **Decreased Cholecystokinin Secretion**
    - Prolonged fasting, hyperalimentation, and low fat (and high alcohol) diet result in diminished cholecystokinin secretion & consequent GB distension
  - **Obstructed Flow of Bile**
    - Cystic/common duct calculus, tumors of GB, bile ducts, ampulla, or pancreas, or CBD strictures resulting from chronic pancreatitis can obstruct bile flow from GB, resulting in distension
    - Courvoisier law: Massive distension of GB in patient with painless jaundice raises concern for malignant obstruction
    - Calculous cholecystitis often presents with distended GB due to obstruction of cystic duct by stone
  - **Inflammation of GB by Intrinsic or Adjacent Process**
    - AIDS cholangiopathy, hepatitis, pancreatitis, or perforated duodenal ulcer may cause secondary GB inflammation and distension
  - **Acalculous Cholecystitis**
    - Most often diagnosed in critically ill or ICU patients (particularly when not eating)
    - Distended GB with wall thickening, pericholecystic fluid, and positive sonographic Murphy sign

Helpful Clues for Less Common Diagnoses

- **Gallbladder Hydrops**
  - Distended GB with simple fluid contents resulting from chronic obstruction (usually due to stones)
  - No wall thickening, pericholecystic fluid, or Murphy sign
  - May result in right upper quadrant pain without fever
- **Gallbladder Empyema**
  - Distended GB filled with infected material (pus) due to acute cholecystitis with intraluminal infection
  - Usually associated with other features of cholecystitis (wall thickening, pericholecystic fluid, etc.)
  - Fluid within GB appears complex with internal debris
- **Choledochal Cyst (Mimic)**
  - Choledochal cysts may extend into porta hepatis and mimic GB
  - Other upper abdominal cysts (hepatic, renal, pancreatic) can also theoretically mimic appearance of GB

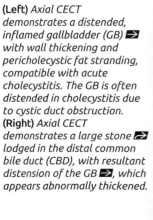

(Left) *Axial CECT demonstrates a distended, inflamed gallbladder (GB)* ➡ *with wall thickening and pericholecystic fat stranding, compatible with acute cholecystitis. The GB is often distended in cholecystitis due to cystic duct obstruction.* (Right) *Axial CECT demonstrates a large stone* ➡ *lodged in the distal common bile duct (CBD), with resultant distension of the GB* ➡*, which appears abnormally thickened.*

Calculous Cholecystitis

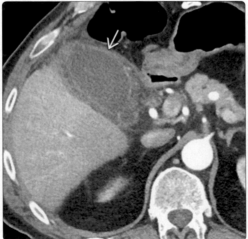

Choledocholithiasis

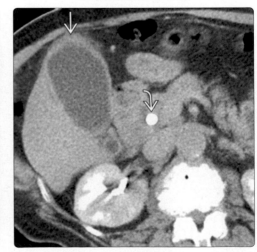

Pancreatic Ductal Adenocarcinoma

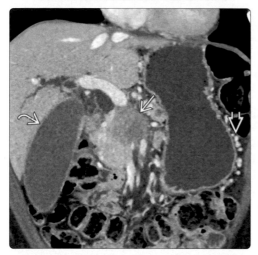

Pancreatic Ductal Adenocarcinoma

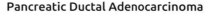
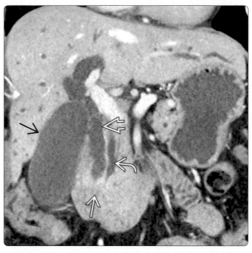

(Left) *Coronal CECT demonstrates a large hypodense mass ➡ centered in the pancreatic head, with resultant upstream biliary obstruction and distension of the GB ➡. The mass also obstructs the portal superior mesenteric vein confluence with multiple gastroepiploic varices ➡. (Right) Coronal CECT demonstrates a classic double-duct sign due to a subtle obstructing pancreatic adenocarcinoma ➡, with dilatation of the CBD ➡ and pancreatic duct ➡. Note the gallbladder distension ➡ due to biliary obstruction.*

Inflammation of Gallbladder by Intrinsic or Adjacent Process

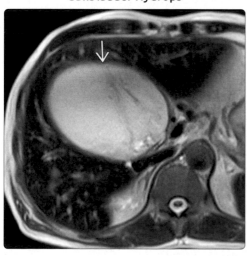

Inflammation of Gallbladder by Intrinsic or Adjacent Process

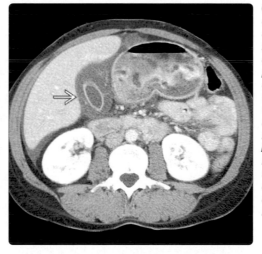

(Left) *Axial CECT demonstrates a severely atrophic pancreas with a markedly dilated pancreatic duct ➡ and parenchymal/intraductal calcifications ➡, compatible with chronic pancreatitis. The CBD was obstructed in this case (not shown), with resultant distension of the GB ➡. (Right) Axial CECT shows marked GB wall thickening ➡ that is more impressive than distention of the GB lumen in a patient with acute viral hepatitis.*

Gallbladder Hydrops

Choledochal Cyst (Mimic)

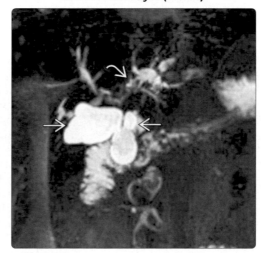

(Left) *Axial T2 MR demonstrates a massively distended GB ➡ with some internal debris and sludge. The patient had no clinical signs of infection, suggesting GB hydrops. (Right) Coronal MRCP shows a complex cystic structure ➡ in the porta hepatis that might be mistaken for a dilated GB. This is a choledochal cyst that had been partially removed, along with the GB at surgery. Note the dilation & strictures ➡ of the intrahepatic ducts.*

DIFFERENTIAL DIAGNOSIS

Common

- Biliary Sphincterotomy
  - Biliary Stent Placement
- Choledocholithiasis
- Patulous Sphincter of Oddi
- Surgical Biliary-Enteric Anastomosis
- Portal Vein Gas (Mimic)
- Hepatic Artery Calcification (Mimic)

Less Common

- Emphysematous Cholecystitis
- Gas Within Gallstones
- Duodenal Diverticulum
- Gallstone Ileus
- Duodenal Ulcer
- Inflammation Near Ampulla
- Cholangitis, Chemotherapy Induced
- Biliary Infection
  - Recurrent Pyogenic Cholangitis
- Ampullary and Periampullary Tumors

Rare but Important

- Bile Sump Syndrome
- Bronchobiliary Fistula
- Trauma
- Transarterial Hepatic Chemoembolization

ESSENTIAL INFORMATION

Key Differential Diagnosis Issues

- Gas in biliary system (pneumobilia or aerobilia) is sequelae of abnormal sphincter of Oddi function or communication between biliary tree and bowel
  - In most (but not all) cases, pneumobilia is incidental imaging finding of little significance, most often attributable to prior surgery or biliary intervention
  - Pneumobilia should be carefully distinguished from portal venous gas, since although most causes of pneumobilia are benign, portal venous gas almost always heralds presence of critical illness/ischemia
  - Large amounts of pneumobilia can reflux into gallbladder lumen itself, and should not be confused with emphysematous cholecystitis
- Gas in biliary system is usually much more evident on CT than on other imaging modalities
  - Pneumobilia not uncommonly visualized on US as brightly echogenic branching reflector (± dirty posterior acoustic shadowing)
  - Pneumobilia typically low signal on MR and can sometimes be confused for low-signal gallstones

Helpful Clues for Common Diagnoses

- **Biliary Sphincterotomy**
  - Entails cutting muscles of sphincter of Oddi (usually during ERCP) for variety of indications, including stone removal, treating strictures, placing biliary stents, treating duct leaks, etc.
  - Allows reflux of gas from duodenal lumen into bile ducts and is very common cause of pneumobilia

- Concurrent placement of biliary stent results in greater degrees of pneumobilia
- **Choledocholithiasis**
  - Passage of stones may lead to scarring and distortion of sphincter of Oddi, which leads to incompetence, allowing reflux of duodenal gas into bile duct
- **Patulous Sphincter of Oddi**
  - May occur spontaneously, especially in elderly, but resulting pneumobilia is usually quite minimal
- **Surgical Biliary-Enteric Anastomosis**
  - Bile duct is anastomosed to a loop of bowel (usually Roux-en-Y loop of jejunum), allowing direct reflux of bowel gas into biliary tree
  - May be seen in setting of liver transplantation, Whipple procedure, and many other hepatobiliary surgeries
- **Portal Vein Gas (Mimic)**
  - May be mistaken for biliary gas
  - Pneumobilia collects near porta hepatis **centrally**, while portal venous gas flows toward and collects in **periphery** of liver
  - Portal venous gas appears mobile with small bubbles on US, while biliary gas is less mobile with larger collections of gas
- **Hepatic Artery Calcification (Mimic)**
  - Relatively uncommon, except with chronic renal failure, but might be mistaken for biliary or portal venous gas on US

Helpful Clues for Less Common Diagnoses

- **Emphysematous Cholecystitis**
  - Rare complication due to gallbladder infection with gas-forming organism (usually *Clostridium perfringens*)
    - Gas in gallbladder wall or lumen may reflux into biliary tree, although this is relatively uncommon
  - Most commonly occurs in elderly or diabetic patients
  - US demonstrates echogenic reflectors in gallbladder (i.e., gas) wall or lumen with dirty posterior acoustic shadowing
- **Gas Within Gallstones**
  - Gas-fissuring within gallstones is incidental finding and does not imply infection or complication
  - Often has Mercedes Benz appearance with branching or chevron pattern of gas within stone
- **Duodenal Diverticulum**
  - Periampullary diverticulum may lead to sphincter of Oddi dysfunction, allowing reflux of gas
- **Gallstone Ileus**
  - Small bowel obstruction caused by impaction of gallstone within bowel (usually terminal ileum)
    - Occurs when large gallstone erodes through adherent walls of inflamed gallbladder and duodenum (usually cholecystoduodenal fistula)
    - Results in Rigler triad of findings, including pneumobilia, small bowel obstruction, and gallstone
- **Duodenal Ulcer**
  - Ulcer may erode into bile duct or gallbladder resulting in choledochoduodenal or cholecystoduodenal fistula
- **Inflammation Near Ampulla**
  - Any periampullary inflammation may result in incompetence of sphincter of Oddi, with reflux of gas

○ Can be complication of any surrounding inflammatory process, including ulcer, pancreatitis, duodenitis, Crohn disease, etc.

- **Biliary Infection**
  ○ May result in pneumobilia due to gas-forming infection or by resulting in incompetent sphincter of Oddi
    - Gas-containing liver abscess may communicate with biliary tree and lead to pneumobilia
  ○ Recurrent pyogenic cholangitis
    - Results in massive dilation of bile ducts (especially extrahepatic duct and central intrahepatic ducts), which are filled with pus and stones
    - Chronic pyogenic infection of biliary tree
    - Almost always occurs in patients either living in or originally from southeast Asia
- **Ampullary and Periampullary Tumors**
  ○ Any benign or malignant tumor arising in the ampullary or periampullary region may lead to sphincter incompetence with gas reflux
  ○ Malignant tumors may also result in spontaneous biliary-enteric fistula

Helpful Clues for Rare Diagnoses

- **Bile Sump Syndrome**
  ○ After side-to-side choledochoduodenostomy (performed to improve bile drainage), sphincter of Oddi dysfunction may lead to distal CBD serving as reservoir for static bile and stones
  ○ Bile sump syndrome occurs when distal CBD accumulates stones, bile, and debris, and becomes nidus for cholangitis
  ○ Associated with pneumobilia
- **Bronchobiliary Fistula**
  ○ Extremely rare condition which is most often caused by hepatic/subphrenic abscesses or sequelae of hepatic intervention (liver resection, ablation, TACE)
  ○ Patients present with chronic cough and biliptysis
  ○ Imaging may show communication between biliary tree and bronchial tree with frequent large-volume pneumobilia
- **Trauma and Transarterial Hepatic Chemoembolization**
  ○ Rare causes of spontaneous biliary-enteric fistulas (usually cholecystoduodenal fistula)

Biliary Sphincterotomy

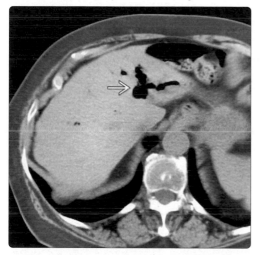

Biliary Sphincterotomy

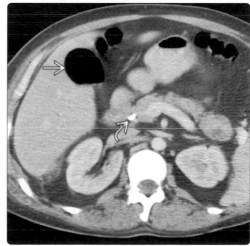

(Left) *Axial NECT shows pneumobilia, predominantly located in the central, larger bile ducts ➡ within the nondependent portions of the liver.* (Right) *Axial CECT performed shortly after the placement of a biliary stent ➡ shows extensive gaseous distention of the gallbladder lumen ➡. Placement of a biliary stent can lead to greater degrees of pneumobilia compared to sphincterotomy alone.*

Biliary Sphincterotomy

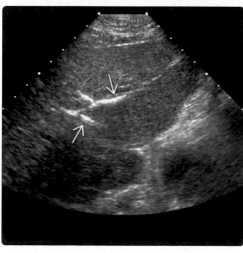

Biliary Sphincterotomy

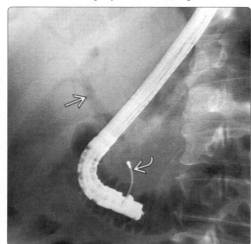

(Left) *Transverse ultrasound in a patient with history of sphincterotomy demonstrates the classic ultrasound appearance of pneumobilia, with branching echogenic reflectors ➡ following the expected course of the bile ducts, predominantly in the central aspect of the liver.* (Right) *Oblique ERCP shows gas in the bile ducts ➡ and the endoscope with a sphincterotomy device ➡ in place.*

(Left) *Axial CECT shows gas in the bile ducts ➡, clearly separate from the contrast-opacified portal veins ➯. Stones were found within the common bile duct on MRCP.* **(Right)** *Frontal radiograph demonstrates the classic radiographic appearance of pneumobilia with a branching gas pattern ➡ limited to the porta hepatis. The patient had undergone prior small bowel and liver transplantation with biliary-enteric anastomosis.*

Choledocholithiasis

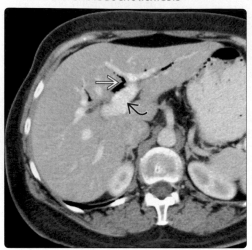

Surgical Biliary-Enteric Anastomosis

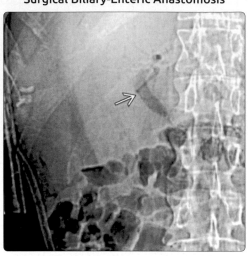

(Left) *Coronal CECT in a patient status-post Whipple procedure nicely demonstrates the hepaticojejunostomy, with gas tracking from the right upper quadrant small bowel loop ➡ into the biliary tree ➡. The hepaticojejunal anastomosis is often best appreciated in the coronal plane.* **(Right)** *Coronal CECT demonstrates gas ➡ outlining the central bile ducts in a patient status post hepaticojejunostomy as part of a Whipple procedure.*

Surgical Biliary-Enteric Anastomosis

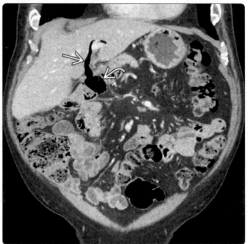

Surgical Biliary-Enteric Anastomosis

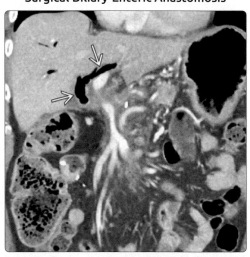

(Left) *Axial NECT demonstrates extensive portal venous gas ➡ at the periphery of the liver in a patient with mesenteric ischemia. Unlike most cases of pneumobilia, portal venous gas is a critical imaging finding which should raise concern for ischemia.* **(Right)** *Transverse ultrasound image in a patient with bowel ischemia demonstrates the characteristic appearance of portal venous gas, with ill-defined, mobile, small echogenic reflectors ➡ primarily located at the periphery of the liver.*

Portal Vein Gas (Mimic)

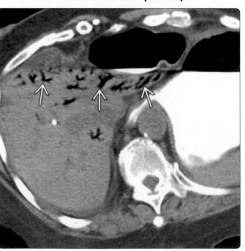

Portal Vein Gas (Mimic)

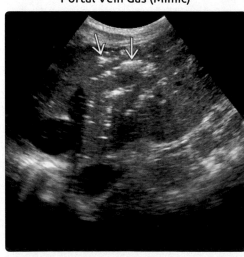

Hepatic Artery Calcification (Mimic)

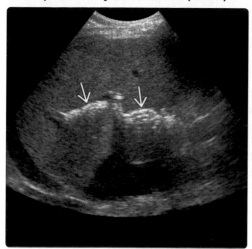

Emphysematous Cholecystitis

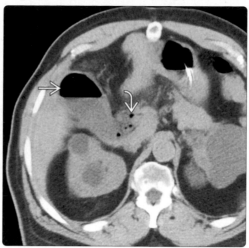

(Left) *Sagittal ultrasound image in a patient with renal failure demonstrates extensive linear echogenic reflectors* ➡ *with posterior acoustic shadowing branching in the central liver. Correlation with CT (not shown) demonstrated that these represented extensive hepatic artery calcifications.* (Right) *Axial NECT shows gas within the gallbladder lumen* ➡ *and pneumobilia* ➡ *due to emphysematous cholecystitis in an elderly diabetic man.*

Gas Within Gallstones

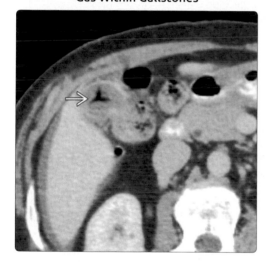

Gallstone Ileus

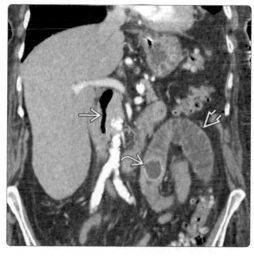

(Left) *Axial CECT shows a classic Mercedes Benz-shaped gas fissure* ➡ *within a gallstone. This is an incidental finding which should not be confused with emphysematous cholecystitis.* (Right) *Coronal CECT demonstrates the classic features of a gallstone ileus, including a large gallstone* ➡ *impacted in the small bowel, obstruction and dilatation of the more proximal small bowel* ➡, *and biliary gas nicely filling the common bile duct* ➡.

Gallstone Ileus

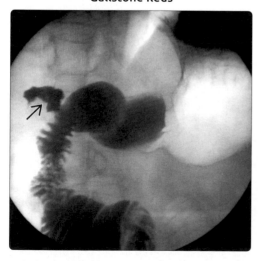

Recurrent Pyogenic Cholangitis

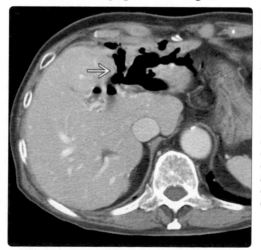

(Left) *Upper GI fluoroscopic image in a patient with gallstone ileus nicely demonstrates filling of the gallbladder* ➡ *via a cholecystoduodenal fistula.* (Right) *Axial CECT shows gross dilation and distortion of the bile ducts* ➡ *which are filled with gas and pus. The left lobe is affected more than the right and shows parenchymal atrophy as a result of chronic infection. These findings are classic for recurrent pyogenic cholangitis.*

DIFFERENTIAL DIAGNOSIS

Common

- Hyperplastic Cholecystoses
- Gallbladder Carcinoma

Less Common

- Xanthogranulomatous Cholecystitis
- Porcelain Gallbladder
- Gallbladder Metastases and Lymphoma
- Gallbladder Wall Polyps
- Intramural Hematoma, Gallbladder

ESSENTIAL INFORMATION

Key Differential Diagnosis Issues

- Normal gallbladder (GB) wall measures ≤ 3 mm and appears as thin echogenic line on US and is barely perceptible on CT
- Significant overlap in imaging appearance of GB carcinoma, xanthogranulomatous cholecystitis, and large polyps, but cholecystectomy should be recommended in suspicious cases to exclude malignancy

Helpful Clues for Common Diagnoses

- **Hyperplastic Cholecystoses**
  - Adenomyomatosis results in GB wall thickening due to formation of intramural diverticula (Rokitansky-Aschoff sinuses) with smooth muscle and epithelial proliferation
  - Can demonstrate focal or segmental forms
    - Focal form most common at fundus and may appear mass-like with internal cystic spaces, intramural echogenic foci, and comet-tail/twinkling artifacts
    - Segmental form may cause annular thickening or strictures of GB resulting in hourglass appearance
  - Diagnosis easily made on MR, which demonstrates T2 bright cystic spaces (string-of-beads appearance)
- **Gallbladder Carcinoma**
  - May present with discrete polyploid mass, focal or diffuse wall thickening, or mass replacing GB

- Wall thickening tends to be irregular and nodular, often with other suspicious features (e.g., invasion of adjacent liver, bulky local lymphadenopathy, metastases)
    - Usually associated with color flow vascularity on US and heterogeneous enhancement on CT/MR
  - Eccentric and substantial GB wall thickening distinguishes GB carcinoma from simple cholecystitis

Helpful Clues for Less Common Diagnoses

- **Xanthogranulomatous Cholecystitis**
  - Focal or diffuse wall thickening with low-attenuation intramural bands/nodules and pericholecystic fluid
  - Low-attenuation bands/nodules (representing foamy cell infiltrate) may show signal loss on out-of-phase MR
  - Imaging features often indistinguishable from GB carcinoma, and definitive diagnosis only after resection
- **Porcelain Gallbladder**
  - Calcifications in GB wall can be diffuse or segmental, as well as either thin or thick/irregular
  - Debatable association with GB carcinoma, although focal calcification possibly associated with higher risk than diffuse calcification
  - Presence of discrete soft tissue adjacent to calcification should raise concern for carcinoma
- **Gallbladder Metastases and Lymphoma**
  - Metastases to GB uncommon, but melanoma is most common primary tumor (enhancing nodule/mass)
    - Usually in setting of widespread metastatic disease
  - Lymphoma of GB almost always secondary involvement (primary GB lymphoma incredibly rare)
    - Higher-grade lymphomas present as larger masses
- **Gallbladder Wall Polyps**
  - Inflammatory or neoplastic polyps may arise in GB wall
  - Size is biggest predictor of malignancy, as 100% of polyps ≥ 2 cm are malignant
  - Polyps ≥ 10 mm generally treated with cholecystectomy, while serial follow-up utilized for smaller polyps
- **Intramural Hematoma, Gallbladder**
  - Uncommon result of trauma with GB injury
  - Usually associated with blood in GB lumen/hemobilia

Hyperplastic Cholecystoses

Hyperplastic Cholecystoses

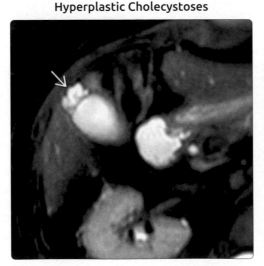
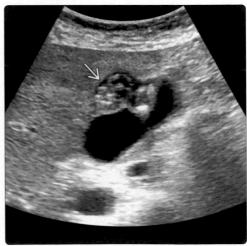

(Left) *Axial T2 FS MR demonstrates multiple T2 hyperintense cystic spaces ➡ at the gallbladder fundus, characteristic of focal adenomyomatosis.* **(Right)** *Ultrasound shows a focal heterogeneously echogenic mass ➡ in the gallbladder that proved to be focal adenomyomatosis. Note the multiple internal echogenic foci within the mass, some of which are associated with comet-tail artifact.*

Gallbladder Carcinoma

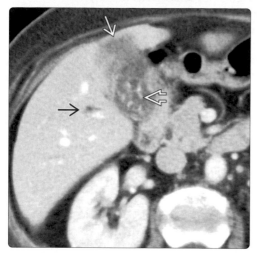

Gallbladder Carcinoma

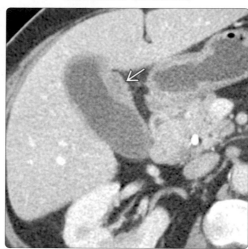

(Left) *Axial CECT shows an eccentric soft tissue density mass* ➡ *arising from the gallbladder with direct invasion of the liver. Note the presence of gallstones* ➡ *and dilated intrahepatic ducts* ➡. (Right) *Axial CECT demonstrates focal thickening* ➡ *of the medial gallbladder wall, found to represent gallbladder carcinoma at surgical resection. Focal, nodular, or irregular gallbladder thickening should raise suspicion for malignancy.*

Xanthogranulomatous Cholecystitis

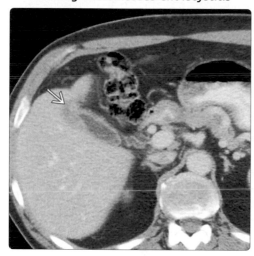

Porcelain Gallbladder

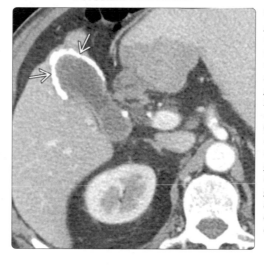

(Left) *Axial CECT shows a focally thickened wall* ➡ *of the gallbladder fundus. There is an indistinct border with the liver, initially thought to be suspicious for carcinoma, but found to represent xanthogranulomatous cholecystitis at resection.* (Right) *Axial CECT demonstrates focal thick calcification* ➡ *of the gallbladder fundus, compatible with a porcelain gallbladder. The association between porcelain gallbladder and gallbladder cancer is now considered debatable.*

Gallbladder Metastases and Lymphoma

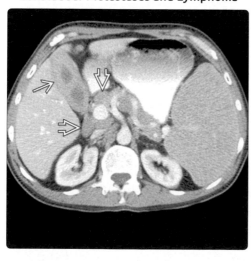

Gallbladder Wall Polyps

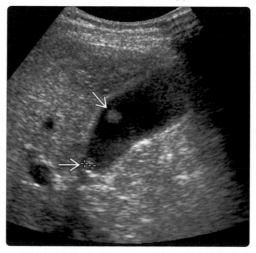

(Left) *Axial CECT demonstrates retroperitoneal lymphadenopathy* ➡ *with soft tissue thickening of the gallbladder wall* ➡. *The gallbladder in this case represents rare lymphomatous involvement.* (Right) *Ultrasound image demonstrates 2 distinct polyps* ➡ *arising from the gallbladder wall. The management of gallbladder polyps is based on size, with polyps measuring ≥ 10 mm, typically requiring cholecystectomy.*

DIFFERENTIAL DIAGNOSIS

Common

- Acute Calculous Cholecystitis
- Chronic Cholecystitis
- Hyperplastic Cholecystosis (Adenomyomatosis)
- Wall Thickening Due To Systemic Diseases
  - Congestive Heart Failure
  - Renal Failure
  - Hepatic Cirrhosis
  - Hypoalbuminemia

Less Common

- Acute Acalculous Cholecystitis
- Acute Pancreatitis
- Acute Hepatitis
- Perforated Peptic Ulcer
- Gallbladder Carcinoma
- Lymphoma
- AIDS-Related Cholangiopathy
- Gallbladder Varices

Rare but Important

- Xanthogranulomatous Cholecystitis
- Dengue Fever

ESSENTIAL INFORMATION

Key Differential Diagnosis Issues

- Clinical information is essential to derive differential diagnosis
- Presence of sepsis and right upper quadrant (RUQ) pain favor acute cholecystitis
- Presence of known systemic diseases: Congestive heart failure, renal failure, hypoalbuminemia are important considerations
- Presence of regional disease: Acute hepatitis or pancreatitis, cirrhosis affect gallbladder wall
- Known malignancy

Helpful Clues for Common Diagnoses

- **Acute Calculous Cholecystitis**
  - Clinical: RUQ pain, fever, positive Murphy sign
  - Acute gallbladder (GB) inflammation secondary to calculus obstructing cystic duct
  - Gallstones ± impaction in GB neck
  - Diffuse GB wall thickening (> 3 mm)
    - Striated appearance: Alternating bright and dark bands within thick GB wall
    - GB wall lucency halo sign: Sonolucent middle layer due to edema
  - Distended gallbladder (GB hydrops)
  - Positive sonographic Murphy sign
  - Presence of pericholecystic fluid
  - Complicated cholecystitis
    - Gangrenous cholecystitis
      - □ Asymmetric wall thickening
      - □ Marked wall irregularities
      - □ Intraluminal membranes
    - GB perforation
      - □ Defect in GB wall

- □ Pericholecystic abscess or extraluminal stones
  - Emphysematous cholecystitis
    - □ Gas in GB wall/lumen
  - Empyema of GB
    - □ Intraluminal echoes, purulent exudate/debris
- **Chronic Cholecystitis**
  - Mostly asymptomatic
  - Diffuse GB wall thickening
    - Mean thickness ~ 5 mm
    - Smooth/irregular contour
  - Contracted GB
    - GB lumen may be obliterated in severe cases
  - Presence of gallstones in nearly all cases
- **Hyperplastic Cholecystosis (Adenomyomatosis)**
  - Adenomyomatosis of GB
  - Clinically asymptomatic, usually incidental US finding
  - Focal or diffuse GB wall thickening
  - Tiny echogenic foci in GB wall producing comet-tail artifacts
  - Presence of cystic spaces within GB wall
  - Fundal adenomyomatosis: Smooth thickening or focal mass in fundal region ± ring down artifact
  - Hourglass GB: Narrowing of mid portion of GB
- **Wall Thickening Due To Systemic Diseases**
  - Clinical correlation is key to explain presence of GB wall thickening
  - Appearance of wall thickening is nonspecific
  - Other ancillary US findings
    - **Congestive heart failure**: Engorged hepatic veins and IVC, diffuse hypoechoic liver echo pattern
    - **Renal failure**: Small kidneys with increased parenchymal echogenicity
    - **Hepatic cirrhosis**: Coarse liver echo pattern, irregular/nodular liver contour, signs of portal hypertension (e.g., ascites, splenomegaly, varices)
    - **Hypoalbuminemia**: Presence of ascites, diffuse bowel wall thickening

Helpful Clues for Less Common Diagnoses

- **Acute Acalculous Cholecystitis**
  - More commonly seen in critically ill patients (e.g., post major surgery, severe trauma, sepsis, etc.)
  - US features are similar to acute calculous cholecystitis except for absence of impacted gallstone
    - GB wall thickening: Hypoechoic, layered/striated appearance
    - GB distension: Often filled with sludge
    - Positive sonographic Murphy sign
    - Pericholecystic fluid
- **Acute Pancreatitis**
  - Spread of inflammation to GB fossa
  - Nonspecific GB wall thickening
  - Diffuse/focal, swollen, hypoechoic pancreas
- **Acute Hepatitis**
  - Clinical history: General malaise, vomiting, deranged liver function test with hepatitic pattern
  - Hepatomegaly with diffuse decrease in echogenicity
  - Starry-sky appearance: Increased echogenicity of portal triad walls against hypoechoic liver parenchyma
  - Periportal hypo-/anechoic area

- o Gallbladder lumen less dilated than in acute cholecystitis
- **Perforated Peptic Ulcer**
  - o Penetrating ulcer in duodenal wall causes sympathetic GB wall thickening
  - o Presence of extraluminal fluid/gas
- **Gallbladder Carcinoma**
  - o Asymmetric or irregular GB wall thickening
  - o Mass replacing GB with locally advanced tumor
  - o Presence of gallstones
  - o Invasion of adjacent structures (e.g., liver, duodenum)
  - o Regional nodal and liver metastases
- **Lymphoma**
  - o Rare involvement of GB by secondary lymphoma
  - o Nonspecific diffuse GB wall thickening
  - o Presence of intraabdominal lymphomatous lymph nodes
- **AIDS-Related Cholangiopathy**
  - o Biliary inflammatory lesions caused by AIDS-related opportunistic infections leading to biliary stricture/obstruction or cholecystitis
  - o Diffuse GB wall thickening
  - o Bile duct wall thickening/inflammation
    - – Periductal hyper-/hypoechoic areas
  - o Focal biliary stricture and dilatation
- **Gallbladder Varices**
  - o Usually seen in portal hypertension or cavernous transformation of main portal vein
  - o Tubular structures in GB wall readily confirmed with color/power Doppler and pulsed Doppler

Helpful Clues for Rare Diagnoses

- **Xanthogranulomatous Cholecystitis**
  - o Rare form of chronic cholecystitis
  - o Diffuse irregular wall thickening, may appear infiltrative; mimics GB carcinoma
- **Dengue Fever**
  - o Rash, fever, headache and joint pains after travel to endemic area
  - o GB wall thickening from acute viral hepatic infection leading to hepatic failure

Other Essential Information

- Fever, leucocytosis, liver function tests

Alternative Differential Approaches

- Etiology of GB wall thickening
  - o Inflammatory conditions
    - – Acute calculous cholecystitis
    - – Acute acalculous cholecystitis
    - – Chronic cholecystitis
    - – AIDS-related cholangiopathy
    - – Secondary causes: Acute hepatitis, perforated peptic ulcer, pancreatitis
  - o Systemic diseases
    - – Congestive heart failure
    - – Renal failure
    - – Liver cirrhosis
    - – Hypoalbuminemia
  - o Neoplastic infiltration
    - – GB carcinoma
    - – Leukemic/lymphomatous infiltration

SELECTED REFERENCES

1. Garg PK et al: Xanthogranulomatous inflammation of gallbladder and bile duct causing obstructive jaundice masquerades gallbladder cancer: a formidable diagnostic challenge continues. J Gastrointest Cancer. Suppl 1:178-81, 2014
2. Runner GJ et al: Gallbladder wall thickening. AJR Am J Roentgenol. 202(1):W1-W12, 2014
3. Zemour J et al: Gallbladder tumor and pseudotumor: Diagnosis and management. J Visc Surg. 151(4):289-300, 2014
4. Teefey SA et al: Acute cholecystitis: do sonographic findings and WBC count predict gangrenous changes? AJR Am J Roentgenol. 200(2):363-9, 2013
5. Charalel RA et al: Complicated cholecystitis: the complementary roles of sonography and computed tomography. Ultrasound Q. 27(3):161-70, 2011
6. O'Connor OJ et al: Imaging of cholecystitis. AJR Am J Roentgenol. 196(4):W367-74, 2011
7. Ito K et al: Imaging findings of unusual intra- and extrahepatic portosystemic collaterals. Clin Radiol. 64(2):200-7, 2009
8. Furlan A et al: Gallbladder carcinoma update: multimodality imaging evaluation, staging, and treatment options. AJR Am J Roentgenol. 191(5):1440-7, 2008
9. van Breda Vriesman AC et al: Diffuse gallbladder wall thickening: differential diagnosis. AJR Am J Roentgenol. 188(2):495-501, 2007
10. Levy AD et al: Gallbladder carcinoma: radiologic-pathologic correlation. Radiographics. 21(2):295-314; questionnaire, 549-55, 2001

Acute Calculous Cholecystitis

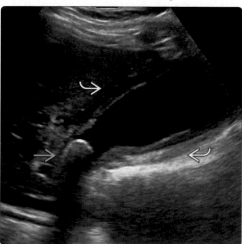

Congestive Heart Failure

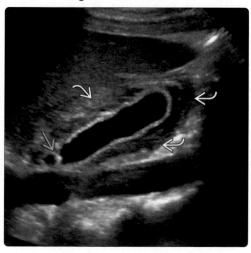

(Left) *Longitudinal oblique ultrasound of acute calculous cholecystitis shows an impacted stone ➡ in the gallbladder neck. There is diffuse edema and thickening of the gallbladder wall ➡.* **(Right)** *Longitudinal oblique ultrasound shows diffuse gallbladder wall edema secondary to heart failure. There is striated wall thickening ➡ and a fold in the gallbladder neck ➡.*

(Left) *Longitudinal oblique ultrasound in gangrenous acute calculous cholecystitis shows a markedly abnormal gallbladder with shadowing stones ⇨. There is asymmetric wall thickening with intramural fluid collections ⇨ and focal thinning of the wall at the fundus ⇨. (Right) Transverse ultrasound in a patient with acute hepatitis and fulminant liver failure shows that the gallbladder wall is circumferentially thickened ⇨ with striations. Ascites ⇨ is noted.*

Acute Calculous Cholecystitis

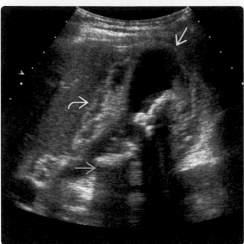

Acute Hepatitis

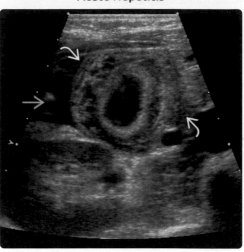

(Left) *Longitudinal ultrasound shows the gallbladder in a patient with perforated acute calculous cholecystitis. The gallbladder wall is asymmetrically thickened ⇨ and there is intraluminal debris with linear membranes ⇨. (Right) Axial CECT of the same patient shows multiple calcified gallstones ⇨ in an abscess cavity ⇨ outside the perforated gallbladder ⇨.*

Acute Calculous Cholecystitis

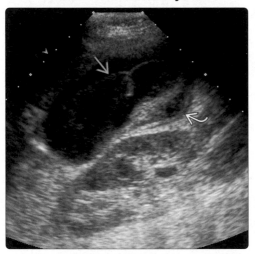

Acute Calculous Cholecystitis

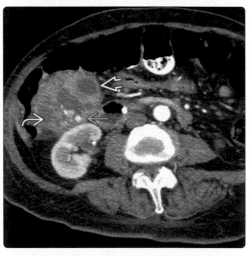

(Left) *Longitudinal ultrasound in a patient with adenomyomatosis shows diffuse thickening of the gallbladder wall ⇨ with several tiny focal polypoid lesions ⇨. (Right) Longitudinal ultrasound in a patient with segmental adenomyomatosis shows diffuse thickening of the gallbladder wall in the fundus ⇨ with multiple small, echogenic foci. There is a transition zone ⇨ (waisting) in the body with normal wall thickness in the neck ⇨.*

Hyperplastic Cholecystosis (Adenomyomatosis)

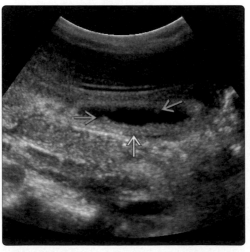

Hyperplastic Cholecystosis (Adenomyomatosis)

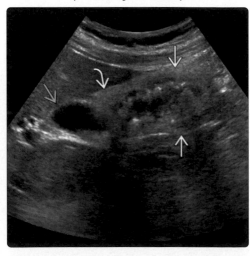

Hepatic Cirrhosis

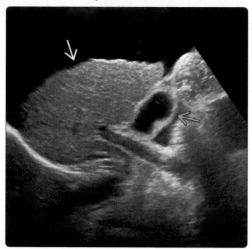

AIDS-Related Cholangiopathy

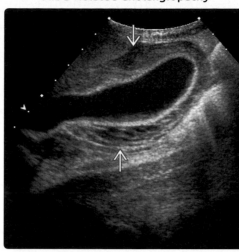

(Left) *Longitudinal oblique ultrasound through the liver and gallbladder shows a nodular cirrhotic liver ➡ surrounded by ascites. The gallbladder wall ➡ is mildly uniformly thickened. There were no stones.* **(Right)** *Longitudinal oblique ultrasound in a patient with HIV/AIDS shows a thick-walled gallbladder with no gallstones. There are linear strands in the edematous wall ➡ compatible with striated edema.*

Gallbladder Carcinoma

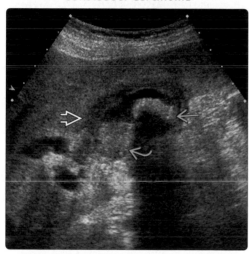

Gallbladder Carcinoma

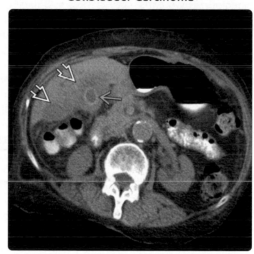

(Left) *Transverse ultrasound of gallbladder carcinoma shows a shadowing stone ➡ with sludge ➡. The gallbladder wall was thick and indistinct with loss of echogenicity ➡ at its interface with the liver.* **(Right)** *Axial NECT of the same patient shows a gallstone ➡. The gallbladder wall is thick and hypodense, with infiltration of the adjacent liver ➡.*

Gallbladder Varices

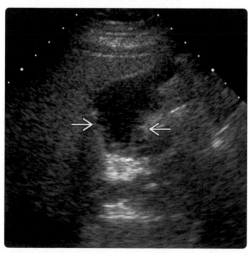

Gallbladder Varices

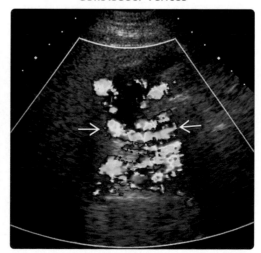

(Left) *Transverse ultrasound in a patient with cavernous transformation of the main portal vein secondary to pancreatitis shows small cystic spaces in the wall at the gallbladder neck and body ➡.* **(Right)** *Transverse color Doppler ultrasound in the same patient shows multiple collateral veins ➡ in the gallbladder wall and around the porta hepatis.*

DIFFERENTIAL DIAGNOSIS

Common

- Vicarious Excretion of Contrast
- Layering of Small Gallstones
- Intraluminal Contrast After Cholangiography
- Biliary Stent
- Gallbladder Sludge

Less Common

- Biliary or Hepatic Trauma
- Milk of Calcium Bile
- Biliary-Enteric Fistula or Anastomosis
- Porcelain Gallbladder (Mimic)
- Gallbladder Carcinoma (Mimic)
- Hemorrhagic Cholecystitis

ESSENTIAL INFORMATION

Key Differential Diagnosis Issues

- Most common causes of high-density bile are iatrogenic (e.g., vicarious excretion, cholangiography, stents)

Helpful Clues for Common Diagnoses

- **Vicarious Excretion**
  - Excretion of intravenous contrast by organs other than the kidneys, including hepatobiliary excretion
  - Given sensitivity of CT, contrast in gallbladder (GB) on day after contrast administration is normal, although visualization of contrast in GB on radiographs suggests ↓ renal function
- **Layering of Small Gallstones**
  - Using wide window level on CT may allow visualization of discrete stones, although may not always be possible to distinguish from other causes of hyperdense bile
- **Intraluminal Contrast After Cholangiography**
  - High-density contrast may be seen in GB and biliary tree after ERCP or transhepatic cholangiogram
- **Biliary Stent**
  - May allow reflux of enteric contrast material and gas into GB and biliary tree

- **Gallbladder Sludge**
  - Layering high-density material within GB lumen, which appears echogenic on US
  - May or may not have attenuation > bile on CT (depending on concentration of cholesterol crystals)
  - Associated with rapid weight loss, TPN, critical illness, and certain medications

Helpful Clues for Less Common Diagnoses

- **Biliary or Hepatic Trauma**
  - Injury to bile ducts, GB, or adjacent liver can result in hemobilia (including high-density blood in GB)
  - Hemobilia should prompt careful search for posttraumatic pseudoaneurysm, liver laceration adjacent to bile ducts, or GB injury
- **Milk of Calcium Bile**
  - High-density calcium carbonate precipitate within bile resulting from chronic cystic duct obstruction and biliary stasis (including chronic TPN)
  - High attenuation bile (> 150 HU on NECT) in GB which can extend into cystic duct or CBD
- **Biliary-Enteric Fistula or Anastomosis**
  - May allow reflux of enteric contrast and gas into GB and bile ducts
  - Spontaneous cholecystenteric fistulas are rare, but can result from gallstone ileus, trauma, tumor, or peptic ulcer disease
- **Porcelain Gallbladder (Mimic)**
  - Typically wall of GB is calcified (and hyperdense), rather than intraluminal bile itself
- **Gallbladder Carcinoma (Mimic)**
  - Usually focal hypodense wall thickening or discrete soft tissue density mass, but enhancing tumor can theoretically mimic high density intraluminal bile
  - Tumors often associated with gallstones
- **Hemorrhagic Cholecystitis**
  - Rare form of complicated cholecystitis that can be associated with blood in GB lumen or bile ducts (± active contrast extravasation)

(Left) Axial NECT demonstrates vicarious excretion of contrast into the gallbladder (GB). This can be a normal finding on CT after contrast administration, and does not necessarily imply diminished renal function. (Right) Frontal radiograph demonstrates dense persistent enhancement of the kidneys ➡ and high-density contrast within the GB ➡, following an angiogram that caused or contributed to acute renal failure.

Vicarious Excretion of Contrast

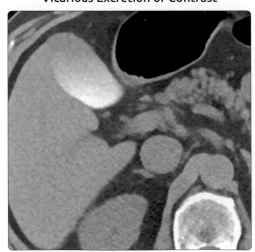

Vicarious Excretion of Contrast

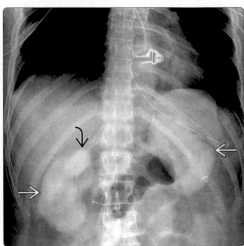

Layering of Small Gallstones

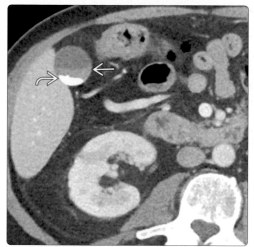

Intraluminal Contrast After Cholangiography

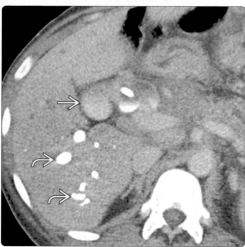

(Left) *Axial CECT demonstrates high-density stones ⊿ layering within the GB. Although subtle, sludge ➡ (which is lower in density than stones but higher in density than bile) is seen layering above the stones.* (Right) *Axial CECT in a patient after a cholangiogram demonstrates residual high-density contrast within the right hepatic lobe ducts ➡, as well as contrast within the GB ➡. Contrast can normally be seen in the biliary system if CT is performed immediately after a cholangiogram.*

Biliary or Hepatic Trauma

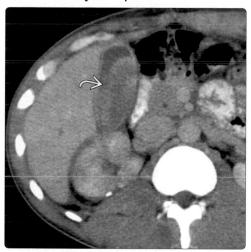

Milk of Calcium Bile

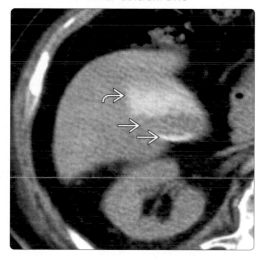

(Left) *Axial NECT in a trauma patient demonstrates high-density clotted blood ➡ within the GB lumen, either due to to direct injury to the GB or passage of blood into the GB lumen through the cystic duct.* (Right) *Axial NECT shows multiple layers within the GB, including a layer consisting of milk of calcium bile ➡ and 2 layers of small stones ➡.*

Porcelain Gallbladder (Mimic)

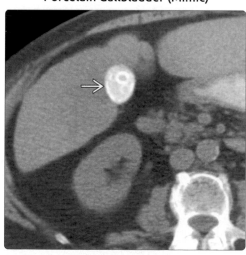

Hemorrhagic Cholecystitis

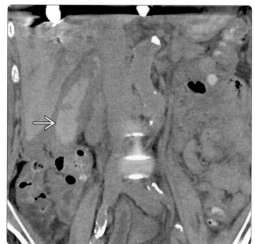

(Left) *Axial NECT shows a calcified wall of the GB ➡ (porcelain GB) as well as milk of calcium bile and gallstones.* (Right) *Coronal NECT demonstrates high-density blood products ➡ within the GB in a patient with hemorrhagic cholecystitis.*

DIFFERENTIAL DIAGNOSIS

Common

- Large Gallstone
- Porcelain Gallbladder
- Contracted Gallbladder With Gallstones
- Gas-Filled Duodenal Bulb

Less Common

- Hyperplastic Cholecystosis
- Adherent Gallstones
- Emphysematous Cholecystitis
- Gallbladder Fistula
- Iatrogenic

ESSENTIAL INFORMATION

Key Differential Diagnosis Issues

- Differentiate gas-filled duodenum from abnormal gallbladder by location and repositioning patient
- Duodenum may be mistaken for gallbladder post cholecystectomy
  - Relevant surgical history is key
  - Look for cholecystectomy scars if no history is available
  - Correlate with other imaging
- Gas in gallbladder may be surgical emergency
  - If unclear, confirm with CT

Helpful Clues for Common Diagnoses

- **Large Gallstone**
  - Strong acoustic impedance at wall-stone interface with posterior shadowing
  - Wall-echo-shadow appearance (optimize technique)
  - Mobile on changing patient's position unless stone is very large and gallbladder is contracted around it
- **Porcelain Gallbladder**
  - Diffuse gallbladder wall calcification
    - Echogenic curvilinear line in gallbladder fossa
    - Dense posterior acoustic shadowing
  - Segmental form: Interrupted echogenic line on anterior wall

  - Or multiple separate coarse echogenic foci/clumps in wall with posterior acoustic shadowing
- **Contracted Gallbladder With Gallstones**
  - Multiple, closely packed echogenic stones without bile mimic echogenic gallbladder wall
  - Thickened gallbladder wall
  - Gallstones may not move on changing patient's position if gallbladder is severely contracted
- **Gas-Filled Duodenal Bulb**
  - Observe peristalsis
  - Move patient to move gas or have patient drink water to confirm

Helpful Clues for Less Common Diagnoses

- **Hyperplastic Cholecystosis**
  - Focal, diffuse or segmental gallbladder wall thickening
  - Tiny echogenic foci in gallbladder wall with characteristic comet-tail artifacts
  - Segmental form: Transition from normal to thick wall in mid gallbladder producing "hourglass" gallbladder
- **Adherent Gallstones**
  - Not curvilinear in configuration or mobile
- **Emphysematous Cholecystitis**
  - Complicated form of acute cholecystitis
  - Clinical evidence of fulminant biliary sepsis is usually present
  - Gas in gallbladder wall/lumen
    - Echogenic crescent in gallbladder with reverberation artifacts ("dirty" shadowing)
  - More common in diabetes and immunosuppressed patients
- **Gallbladder Fistula**
  - Spontaneous fistula from erosion of gallstone into duodenum: Gallstone ileus
  - Fistula to gallbladder from adjacent bowel malignancy
- **Iatrogenic**
  - Known history of intervention such as endoscopic retrograde cholangiopancreatography or biliary stent
  - Gas in gallbladder without signs of cholecystitis

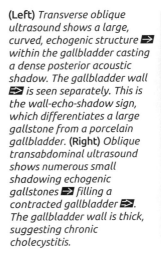
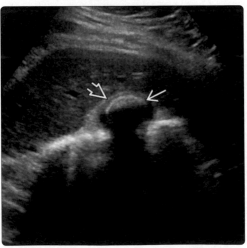

Large Gallstone

Contracted Gallbladder With Gallstones

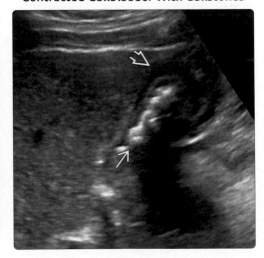

(Left) *Transverse oblique ultrasound shows a large, curved, echogenic structure ➡ within the gallbladder casting a dense posterior acoustic shadow. The gallbladder wall ➡ is seen separately. This is the wall-echo-shadow sign, which differentiates a large gallstone from a porcelain gallbladder.* (Right) *Oblique transabdominal ultrasound shows numerous small shadowing echogenic gallstones ➡ filling a contracted gallbladder ➡. The gallbladder wall is thick, suggesting chronic cholecystitis.*

Porcelain Gallbladder

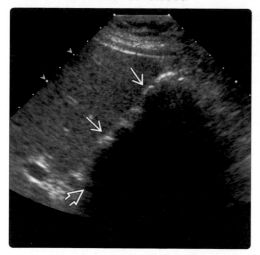

Porcelain Gallbladder

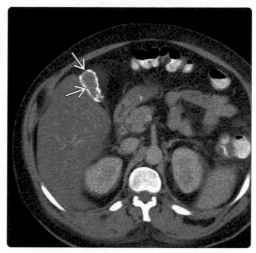

(Left) *Oblique transabdominal ultrasound shows curvilinear echogenicity* ➔ *in the gallbladder wall casting dense posterior acoustic shadowing* ⇥. *Absence of wall-echo-shadow sign suggests porcelain gallbladder.* (Right) *Axial CECT of the same patient confirms the thin diffuse gallbladder wall calcification* ➔ *in a contracted gallbladder.*

Gas-Filled Duodenal Bulb

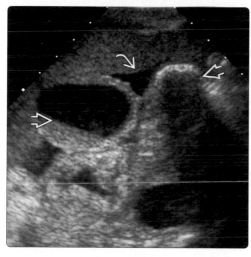

Hyperplastic Cholecystosis

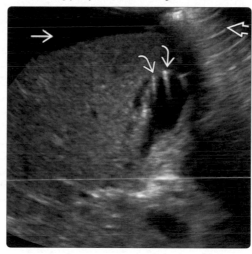

(Left) *Transverse ultrasound shows the duodenal bulb containing gas* ⇥. *The gallbladder contains sludge in this patient with ascites* ➔ *and cirrhosis. The duodenum may be mistaken for a gallbladder.* (Right) *Transverse oblique ultrasound shows multiple areas of comet-tail artifact* ➔ *emanating from the thick wall of the gallbladder. Reverberation artifact is noted from bowel* ⇥, *and there is ascites* ➔ *in this patient with chronic liver disease.*

Emphysematous Cholecystitis

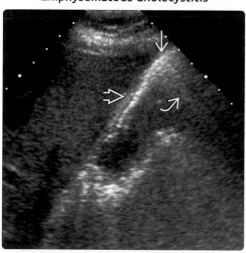

Iatrogenic

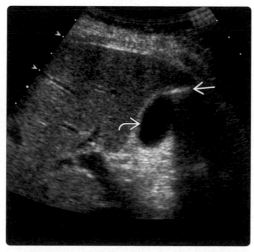

(Left) *Longitudinal ultrasound shows the gallbladder fundus in a diabetic patient with fever and right upper quadrant pain. A linear bright echo* ➔ *within a thick wall* ⇥ *produces dirty shadowing* ➔ *that is highly suggestive of gas. This was confirmed with CT. Surgery was performed for emphysematous cholecystitis.* (Right) *Transverse oblique ultrasound shows a bright linear echo with dirty shadowing* ➔ *representing gas in the gallbladder fundus post ERCP. The gallbladder* ➔ *was normal.*

DIFFERENTIAL DIAGNOSIS

Common
- Cholelithiasis
- Sludge/Sludge Ball/Echogenic Bile

Less Common
- Blood Clot
- Complicated Cholecystitis
- Gas Within Gallbladder Lumen
- Drainage Catheter
- Tumor
- Parasitic Infestation

ESSENTIAL INFORMATION

Helpful Clues for Common Diagnoses
- **Cholelithiasis**
  - Highly reflective intraluminal structure within gallbladder lumen
  - Posterior acoustic shadowing
  - Gravity-dependent and mobile
  - Variants
    - Bright echoes with acoustic shadowing in gallbladder fossa representing gallbladder packed with stones
    - Nonshadowing gallstones, usually small (< 5 mm)
    - Double-arc shadow sign or wall-echo-shadow (WES) sign
    - Immobile adherent/impacted gallstones
  - Complication: Acute calculous cholecystitis
    - Gallbladder distension and wall thickening, sonographic Murphy sign, pericholecystic fluid
- **Sludge/Sludge Ball/Echogenic Bile**
  - Amorphous, mid-/high-level echoes within gallbladder, lack of shadowing
  - Sediment in dependent portion
  - Mobile on changing patient's position without posterior acoustic shadowing
  - Sludge ball: Aggregate with well-defined, round contour, moves slowly

- Can be isoechoic to liver resulting in "hepatization" of gallbladder

Helpful Clues for Less Common Diagnoses
- **Blood Clot**
  - Echogenic/mixed echoes or blood fluid level within gallbladder
  - Occasionally retractile, conforming to gallbladder shape
  - Post trauma, post surgery, or after hepatobiliary intervention; associated with gastrointestinal bleed
- **Complicated Cholecystitis**
  - Gangrenous cholecystitis: Intraluminal echogenic debris and membranes
    - Asymmetric wall thickening, marked wall irregularities
  - Emphysematous cholecystitis: Gas in gallbladder wall and lumen
  - Gallbladder empyema
    - Distended pus filled gallbladder, echogenic contents, no shadowing
- **Gas Within Gallbladder Lumen**
  - Iatrogenic from interventional procedure or endoscopy
  - Secondary to fistula with bowel as in gallstone ileus
    - Small bowel obstruction and pneumobilia, CT more definitive
- **Drainage Catheter**
  - History of percutaneous or endoscopic drainage
  - Tubular, parallel echogenic lines, ± pig-tail loop, man-made configuration
- **Tumor**
  - Primary cancers involve wall ± endoluminal mass, stones, and extension to liver
  - Hematogenous metastases most commonly from melanoma
    - Multiple > single broad-based, hypoechoic, polypoid lesions, ± wall thickening
  - Look for color Doppler flow in mass, confirm with spectral Doppler
- **Parasitic Infestation**
  - Tubular, parallel echogenic lines

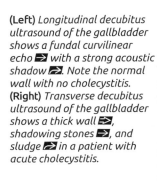

(Left) Longitudinal decubitus ultrasound of the gallbladder shows a fundal curvilinear echo ➡ with a strong acoustic shadow ➡. Note the normal wall with no cholecystitis. (Right) Transverse decubitus ultrasound of the gallbladder shows a thick wall ➡, shadowing stones ➡, and sludge ➡ in a patient with acute cholecystitis.

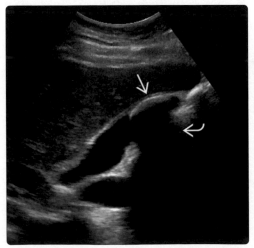

Cholelithiasis

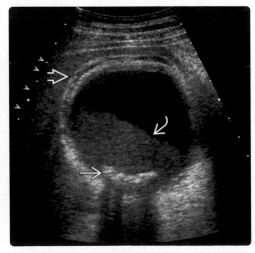

Cholelithiasis

Sludge/Sludge Ball/Echogenic Bile

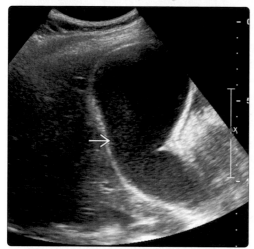

Sludge/Sludge Ball/Echogenic Bile

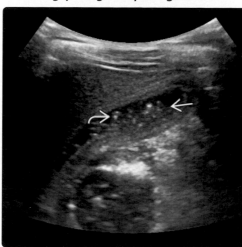

(Left) Transverse ultrasound of the right upper quadrant shows a markedly distended sludge-filled gallbladder ➜ in acalculous cholecystitis. Although the wall was not thick, the patient was treated with percutaneous drainage. (Right) Longitudinal decubitus ultrasound of a nondistended gallbladder shows intraluminal echoes from small nonshadowing sludge balls ➜. Some display the comet-tail artifact ➜.

Complicated Cholecystitis

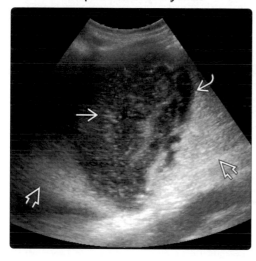

Complicated Cholecystitis

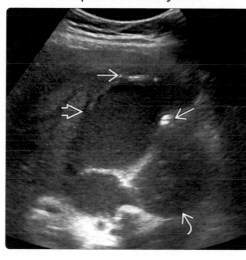

(Left) Transverse ultrasound of the gallbladder fossa shows the gallbladder lumen to be filled with membranes ➜ with no wall. There is pericholecystic fluid ➜ and echogenic fat ➜ in this diabetic patient with gangrenous cholecystitis. (Right) Transverse ultrasound shows a distended gallbladder with intraluminal sludge, discontinuous wall ➜, pericholecystic abscess ➜, and gas in the wall ➜ from emphysematous cholecystitis.

Drainage Catheter

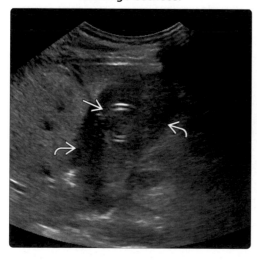

Tumor

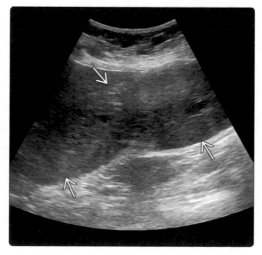

(Left) Transverse ultrasound was taken following percutaneous drainage for acalculous cholecystitis in a sick patient. The pig-tail catheter ➜ is looped in the gallbladder lumen, which contains sludge ➜. The wall is indistinct. (Right) Longitudinal ultrasound shows a markedly distended gallbladder (15 cm) with low level intraluminal echoes ➜. The lumen was filled with necrotic adenocarcinoma with muscle invasion in the neck only.

DIFFERENTIAL DIAGNOSIS

Common

- Physiologic Dilatation
- Acute Calculous Cholecystitis
- Acute Acalculous Cholecystitis

Less Common

- Mucocele/Hydrops
- Drugs
- Post Vagotomy
- Choledochal Cyst
- Gallbladder Carcinoma
- Gallbladder Hemorrhage
- Acute Hemorrhagic Cholecystitis
- Other Causes of Cholecystitis
  - Obstruction Post Biliary Stenting
  - Ischemia Post Transarterial Hepatic Chemoembolization or in Setting of Severe Hypotension or Sepsis
  - Infectious Cholecystitis

Rare but Important

- Mucin-Producing Gallbladder Carcinoma
- Gallbladder Torsion/Volvulus
- Systemic Lupus Erythematosus
- Henoch-Schönlein Purpura

ESSENTIAL INFORMATION

Key Differential Diagnosis Issues

- Determine if gallbladder is obstructed or not
  - Look for intrinsic lesion such as stone, polyp, or mass
  - Look for extrinsic mass, collection, or inflammation
- Differentiate acute surgical from nonsurgical gallbladder distension
- Look for secondary signs of inflammation
  - Wall thickness, pericholecystic fluid, or inflamed fat
- Correlate with patient history, signs, and laboratory results

Helpful Clues for Common Diagnoses

- **Physiologic Dilatation**
  - Distended > 5 x 5 x 10 cm
  - Otherwise normal-appearing gallbladder
  - Secondary to
    - Prolonged fasting
    - Postoperative state
    - Total parenteral nutrition
    - Post vagotomy
- **Acute Calculous Cholecystitis**
  - Distension with
    - Gallstones
    - Wall thickening
    - Pericholecystic fluid
  - Presence of sonographic Murphy sign is key for diagnosis of acute cholecystitis
- **Acute Acalculous Cholecystitis**
  - Distension without gallstones
  - Sludge, wall thickening of gallbladder
  - Ill patient with sepsis, postoperative or post trauma
  - Increased risk of wall necrosis and gangrene

- Difficult diagnosis as sonographic Murphy sign may not be elicited in obtunded or sedated patients
- Confirm with HIDA
- Or diagnostic/therapeutic percutaneous cholecystotomy

Helpful Clues for Less Common Diagnoses

- **Mucocele/Hydrops**
  - Distended gallbladder filled with watery mucoid material
  - Thin gallbladder wall
  - Secondary to gallbladder outlet obstruction
    - Obstructing polyp or stone
    - Obstructing masses such as pancreaticobiliary and ampullary carcinoma
    - Acute or chronic pancreatitis
  - Courvoisier sign
    - Distended nontender palpable gallbladder in setting of jaundice is rarely due to obstructing gallstones
      - Stones are associated with chronic inflammation and lack of gallbladder distensibility
      - Or they produce acute obstruction with less gallbladder distension
    - Neoplasms such as pancreatic carcinoma are more likely as they produce chronic lower grade obstruction
- **Drugs**
  - Various drugs may decrease gallbladder contraction
    - Including atropine, somatostatin, arginine, nifedipine, progesterone, trimebutine, loperamide, and ondansetron
- **Post Vagotomy**
  - Gallbladder volumes increase after vagotomy secondary to vagal denervation
  - Predisposes to gallstone formation
- **Choledochal Cyst**
  - Large cyst may compress or obstruct gallbladder or mimic distended gallbladder
  - Associated with biliary dilatation
  - Can be confirmed with MRCP or ERCP
- **Gallbladder Carcinoma**
  - Typically thick irregular wall or solid tumor in lumen
  - Extension into liver
  - Gallstones typically present
  - Mucin-producing variant may produce distended mucin filled gallbladder
    - Smaller mural/polypoid mass
- **Gallbladder Hemorrhage**
  - Mobile internal echoes
  - Increasing echogenic luminal content over time if active bleeding
  - Retracting clot
  - Post hepatobiliary intervention or biopsy
  - Post trauma or surgery
  - Secondary to neoplasms, anticoagulation or bleeding disorder
  - Post aneurysm rupture
  - Present with
    - Pain
    - Jaundice
    - Hemobilia
    - Hematemesis
    - Hematochezia

- **Acute Hemorrhagic Cholecystitis**
  - Intraluminal hemorrhage with signs of acute cholecystitis
  - Underlying
    - Atherosclerosis
    - Diabetes
    - Bleeding diathesis
    - Anticoagulation therapy
- **Other Causes of Cholecystitis**
  - Following metal bile duct stent placed for malignant biliary stricture
    - Cholecystitis from cystic duct obstruction
  - Ischemic cholecystitis
    - Following transarterial hepatic chemoembolization for liver malignancy
    - Following prolonged hypotension post trauma, hemorrhage, sepsis
  - Infectious cholecystitis
    - Ultrasound findings similar to acute acalculous cholecystitis
    - Bacteria
      - *Salmonella typhi*: Acute and chronic infection
      - *Escherichia coli, Klebsiella, Staphylococcus* species
      - Leptospirosis
    - Viral
      - Hepatitis A and B viruses, CMV, dengue virus
    - Diagnoses made by clinical picture and laboratory tests
    - Hydatid
      - In endemic regions
      - Intraluminal gallbladder membranes or cysts
      - Curvilinear calcifications
      - Typically associated with liver cysts
    - Ascariasis
      - Intraluminal living or dead worms
      - Obstructed cystic duct causing cholecystitis
    - Malaria
      - Can cause acalculous cholecystitis

Helpful Clues for Rare Diagnoses

- **Gallbladder Torsion/Volvulus**
  - Elderly thin women with wandering gallbladder
  - Features of cholecystitis, but difficult preoperative diagnosis
  - Markedly dilated gallbladder
  - May be displaced from normal location
  - Twisting of cystic duct and artery
    - Whirl sign on color Doppler
- **Systemic Lupus Erythematosus**
  - Acalculous cholecystitis due to vasculitis of gallbladder wall and bile ducts
  - Treated nonsurgically with corticosteroids
- **Henoch-Schönlein Purpura**
  - Associated with gallbladder hydrops or acalculous cholecystitis
  - Characteristic skin rash

SELECTED REFERENCES

1. Eachempati SR et al: Acute cholecystitis in the sick patient. Curr Probl Surg. 51(11):441-66, 2014
2. Revzin MV et al: The gallbladder: uncommon gallbladder conditions and unusual presentations of the common gallbladder pathological processes. Abdom Imaging. 40(2):385-99, 2015
3. Sebastian S et al: Managing incidental findings on abdominal and pelvic CT and MRI, Part 4: white paper of the ACR Incidental Findings Committee II on gallbladder and biliary findings. J Am Coll Radiol. 10(12):953-6, 2013
4. Boonstra EA et al: Torsion of the gallbladder. J Gastrointest Surg. 16(4):882-4, 2012
5. Charalel RA et al: Complicated cholecystitis: the complementary roles of sonography and computed tomography. Ultrasound Q. 27(3):161-70, 2011
6. Gore RM et al: Gallbladder imaging. Gastroenterol Clin North Am. 39(2):265-87, ix, 2010

Physiologic Dilatation

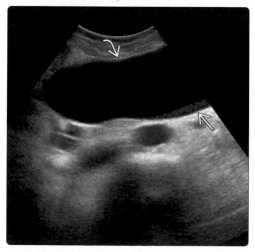

Physiologic Dilatation

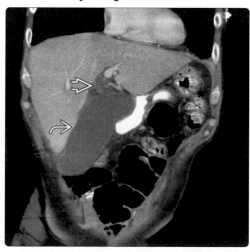

(Left) Transverse oblique ultrasound of the gallbladder in a ventilated patient on total parenteral nutrition. The gallbladder is distended ➡ with minimal sludge ➡. There is no wall thickening. (Right) CECT of the same patient shows the distended gallbladder ➡ and cystic duct ➡ without signs of inflammation or obstructing lesion.

(Left) *Longitudinal oblique ultrasound of the gallbladder shows an obstructing stone in the neck* ➡️. *The gallbladder is distended with diffuse hypoechoic wall thickening* ➡️ *in this patient with acute calculous cholecystitis.* (Right) *Longitudinal oblique ultrasound shows a distended gallbladder with fundal stones* ➡️ *and wall thickening* ➡️. *The patient had a positive Murphy sign consistent with acute calculous cholecystitis.*

Acute Calculous Cholecystitis

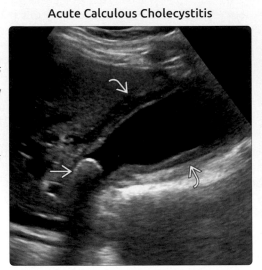

Acute Calculous Cholecystitis

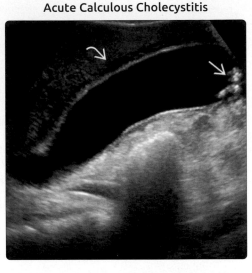

(Left) *Sagittal CECT of the same patient shows a distended gallbladder* ➡️ *with diffuse wall thickening* ➡️. *The stones were not visible on CT.* (Right) *Transverse ultrasound shows a gangrenous gallbladder with no stones. The wall is edematous* ➡️ *with a focal defect anteriorly* ➡️. *A pericholecystic abscess had developed (not shown).*

Acute Calculous Cholecystitis

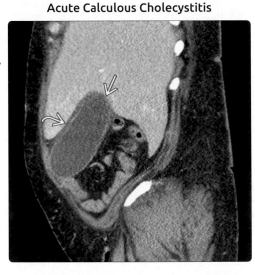

Acute Acalculous Cholecystitis

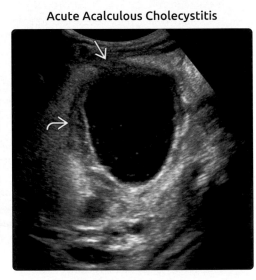

(Left) *Longitudinal oblique ultrasound of the gallbladder in a patient with obstructive jaundice from a pancreatic head carcinoma shows a distended but otherwise normal gallbladder* ➡️ *(the Courvoisier sign).* (Right) *Axial CECT of the same patient was taken after placement of a metal bile duct stent* ➡️ *to relieve biliary obstruction. There is now edema of the gallbladder wall and pericholecystic stranding* ➡️ *from acute cholecystitis, which later perforated.*

Mucocele/Hydrops

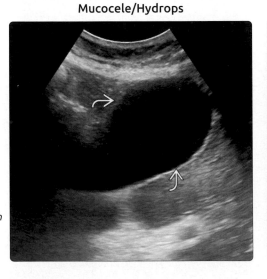

Mucocele/Hydrops

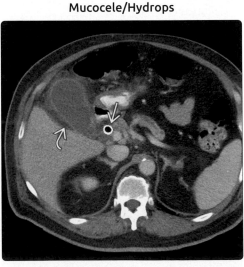

Mucocele/Hydrops

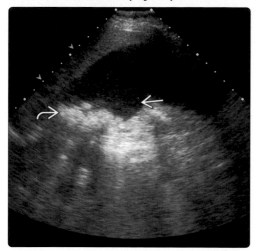

Mucocele/Hydrops

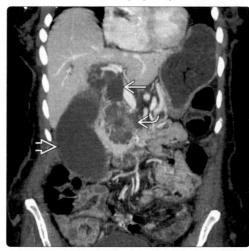

(Left) *Longitudinal oblique ultrasound of the gallbladder in an elderly patient with jaundice shows a dilated gallbladder with stones* ➡ *and sludge* ➡. *The wall was normal. The common bile duct was dilated secondary to a pancreatic lesion.* (Right) *CECT of the same patient better demonstrates the obstructing multicystic serous cystadenoma in the head of pancreas* ➡ *obstructing the bile duct* ➡ *and causing gallbladder distension* ➡.

Gallbladder Carcinoma

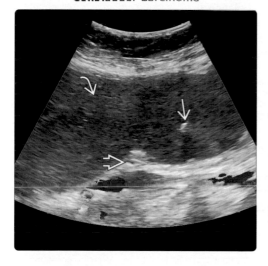

Gallbladder Carcinoma

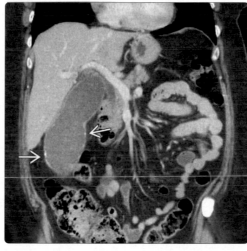

(Left) *Oblique color Doppler ultrasound shows a distended gallbladder filled with avascular low level echoes* ➡ *with one small stone* ➡. *The posterior wall is irregular* ➡. *The lumen was filled with necrotic adenocarcinoma.* (Right) *CECT shows a dilated gallbladder with low-density contents. There is subtle wall calcification* ➡ *and internal heterogeneity. This was largely necrotic adenocarcinoma with a small invasive tumor in the gallbladder neck.*

Acute Hemorrhagic Cholecystitis

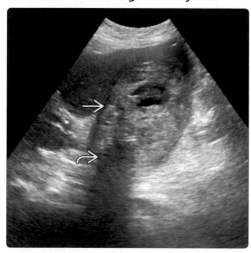

Acute Hemorrhagic Cholecystitis

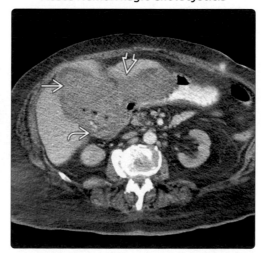

(Left) *Longitudinal oblique ultrasound shows a markedly abnormal gallbladder filled with bright echoes* ➡ *in a patient with a dropping hematocrit and signs of infection. Shadowing is noted* ➡ *but the stone is indistinct.* (Right) *Axial CECT of the same patient shows a perforated gallbladder with gallstones* ➡ *and luminal hemorrhage* ➡. *There is an adjacent hematoma* ➡. *Active bleeding was treated by embolization.*

DIFFERENTIAL DIAGNOSIS

Common

- Choledocholithiasis
- Ascending Cholangitis
- Recurrent Pyogenic Cholangitis
- Pancreatic Ductal Carcinoma
- Cholangiocarcinoma
- Choledochal Cyst

Less Common

- Sludge
- Periampullary Tumor
- Sclerosing Cholangitis
- Parasitic Infestation
- AIDS-Related Cholangiopathy
- Biliary Intraductal Papillary Mucinous Neoplasm

ESSENTIAL INFORMATION

Helpful Clues for Common Diagnoses

- **Choledocholithiasis**
  - Most common location is in common bile duct (CBD)
  - Round echogenic focus with marked posterior acoustic shadowing
- **Ascending Cholangitis**
  - Imaging may reveal biliary duct wall thickening, intraluminal debris, or obstructing biliary stone
  - Periportal inflammatory hypo-/hyperechogenicity may be seen
- **Recurrent Pyogenic Cholangitis**
  - Bacterial colonization of brown pigment stones in both intrahepatic and extrahepatic bile ducts
  - Densely packed intrahepatic stones
  - Atrophy of involved lobe/segment of liver in later stages
- **Pancreatic Ductal Carcinoma**
  - Ill-defined, solid mass in pancreatic head
  - Pancreatic duct dilatation that abruptly tapers at point of pancreatic carcinoma
  - Vascular encasement ± regional nodal/liver metastases

- **Cholangiocarcinoma**
  - Extrahepatic cholangiocarcinoma involves biliary ducts in hepatoduodenal ligament
    - Intra- and extrahepatic biliary dilatation
    - May see: Irregular soft tissue thickening of extrahepatic bile duct or polypoidal mass within CBD
    - May present as a periampullary mass in the pancreatic head
  - Intrahepatic cholangiocarcinoma: Ill-defined, infiltrative, iso-/hyperechoic mass often with capsular retraction
- **Choledochal Cyst**
  - Congenital biliary malformation characterized by fusiform duct dilatation
  - Most commonly involves CBD
  - Cystic extrahepatic mass separated from gallbladder and communicating with CHD or intrahepatic ducts
  - Fusiform dilatation of extra- ± intrahepatic bile ducts
  - Abrupt change in caliber at junction of dilated segment to normal ducts

Helpful Clues for Less Common Diagnoses

- **Sclerosing Cholangitis**
  - Autoimmune disease that causes multiple intra- and extrahepatic biliary strictures with dilatation
- **Biliary Intraductal Papillary Mucinous Neoplasm**
  - Ductal intraluminal mass with frond-like papillary projections
  - Hypersecretion of mucin as well as anatomic obstruction leads to markedly dilated intra- and extrahepatic biliary ducts

SELECTED REFERENCES

1. Plentz RR et al: Clinical presentation, risk factors and staging systems of cholangiocarcinoma. Best Pract Res Clin Gastroenterol. 29(2):245-252, 2015
2. Raman SP et al: Abnormalities of the Distal Common Bile Duct and Ampulla: Diagnostic Approach and Differential Diagnosis Using Multiplanar Reformations and 3D Imaging. AJR Am J Roentgenol. 203(1):17-28, 2014
3. Attasaranya S et al: Choledocholithiasis, ascending cholangitis, and gallstone pancreatitis. Med Clin North Am. 92(4):925-60, x, 2008
4. Lim JH et al: Biliary intraductal papillary-mucinous neoplasm manifesting only as dilatation of the hepatic lobar or segmental bile ducts: imaging features in six patients. AJR Am J Roentgenol. 191(3):778-82, 2008

Choledocholithiasis

Ascending Cholangitis

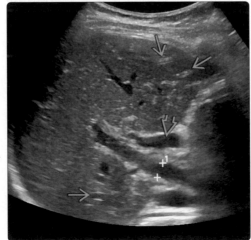
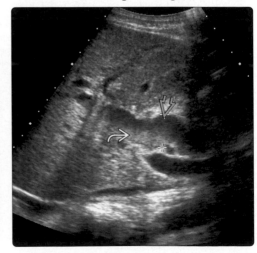

(Left) Grayscale ultrasound of the liver shows mild biliary ductal dilatation of the common bile duct ➡ as well as mildly prominent intrahepatic biliary ducts creating subtle double ducts ➡. The cause of mild biliary ductal dilatation was due to an obstructing stone in the common bile duct (not shown). (Right) Longitudinal oblique grayscale US of the liver shows a markedly dilated common duct ➡ with layering debris ➡ in a patient with ascending cholangitis.

Recurrent Pyogenic Cholangitis

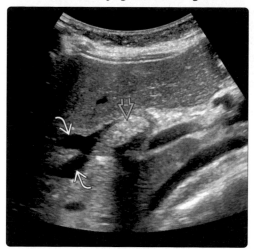

Cholangiocarcinoma

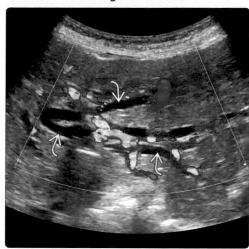

(Left) *Grayscale US of the liver shows a large intrahepatic stone ⇒ causing upstream biliary ductal dilatation ➡ in a patient with recurrent pyogenic cholangitis.* (Right) *Transverse color Doppler US of the left lobe of the liver shows moderate biliary ductal dilatation ➡ caused by an obstructing central cholangiocarcinoma.*

Cholangiocarcinoma

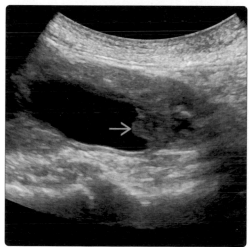

Choledochal Cyst

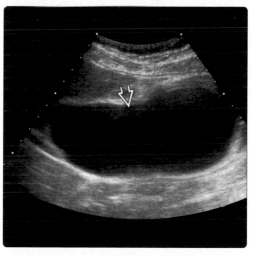

(Left) *Longitudinal oblique US of the common bile duct demonstrates an obstructing soft tissue mass ➡, which was proven to represent an intraluminal cholangiocarcinoma.* (Right) *Longitudinal oblique US of the right upper quadrant in a 14-year-old girl shows a markedly dilated tubular structure ➡, which was found to be a large type I choledochal cyst.*

Biliary Intraductal Papillary Mucinous Neoplasm

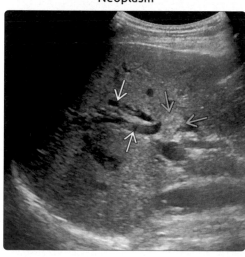

Biliary Intraductal Papillary Mucinous Neoplasm

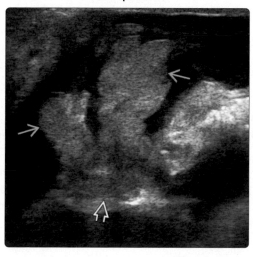

(Left) *Transverse US of the liver shows moderate intrahepatic ductal dilatation ➡, which was caused by a biliary intraductal papillary mucinous neoplasm ➡. Biliary ductal dilatation was seen both proximal as well as distal to the lesion due to copious mucin production.* (Right) *Intraoperative grayscale ultrasound in the same patient shows the biliary intraductal papillary neoplasm has frond-like projections ➡ into the biliary tree. The point where the biliary IPMN arises from the biliary duct wall ➡ is evident on this image.*

DIFFERENTIAL DIAGNOSIS

Common

- Acute Cholecystitis
- Gallstones
  - Cholelithiasis
  - Choledocholithiasis
- Acute Hepatitis
- Hepatic Steatosis (Fatty Liver)
- Ascending Cholangitis
- Acute Pancreatitis
- Duodenal Ulcer

Less Common

- Acute Colitis
- Appendicitis
- Omental Infarct
- Epiploic Appendagitis
- Hepatic Pyogenic Abscess
- Passive Hepatic Congestion
- Diverticulitis
- Pyelonephritis
- Thoracic Infection or Inflammation
- Hepatic Tumor

ESSENTIAL INFORMATION

Key Differential Diagnosis Issues

- Hepatobiliary etiologies (e.g., cholecystitis, hepatitis, cholelithiasis, choledocholithiasis) are most common causes of right upper quadrant (RUQ) pain
- In most cases, when patients present with classic signs and symptoms of gallbladder-related disease, US serves as best 1st-line screening modality
- Although CT lacks sensitivity and specificity for gallbladder-related disorders, it is superior modality for many other entities on differential diagnosis and may be required if US does not provide firm diagnosis
- MRI/MRCP is best noninvasive imaging modality for evaluation of biliary tree (particularly for biliary stones)

Helpful Clues for Common Diagnoses

- **Acute Cholecystitis**
  - 90-95% of patients with cholecystitis have gallstones, with acute calculous cholecystitis far more common than acalculous cholecystitis
  - Patients present with fever, RUQ pain, and elevated WBC
  - US remains best diagnostic modality, with imaging features including GB wall thickening, presence of gallstones, sonographic Murphy sign, pericholecystic fluid, and wall hyperemia (on color Doppler)
  - Important complications include gangrenous cholecystitis, emphysematous cholecystitis, hemorrhagic cholecystitis, and perforation
- **Gallstones (Cholelithiasis and Choledocholithiasis)**
  - Patients may present with biliary colic (dull RUQ pain with radiation to back or right shoulder)
  - US and MR have superior sensitivity for stones compared to CT (~ 80%), with CT often missing pure cholesterol stones which are isodense to bile

- US is best initial imaging modality, but given that distal CBD often obscured by bowel gas on US, MRCP much better for identifying stones in common bile duct
- **Acute Hepatitis**
  - Any cause of hepatitis (alcohol, viral, toxic) may result in liver swelling that stretches liver capsule and causes RUQ pain
  - All imaging modalities are usually normal in setting of acute hepatitis, but in severe cases, enlarged liver may appear abnormally low density on CT or hypoechoic on US with prominent portal triads (starry-sky appearance)
  - Marked reactive gallbladder wall thickening is common ancillary feature
- **Hepatic Steatosis (Fatty Liver)**
  - Usually asymptomatic, although acute fatty infiltration may stretch liver capsule and cause pain
  - Most common definitions of steatosis include liver lower in attenuation than spleen on NECT or absolute attenuation of liver on NECT of < 40 HU
  - MR with chemical shift imaging is most sensitive modality for diagnosing steatosis
- **Ascending Cholangitis**
  - Pyogenic infection of biliary tree due to biliary obstruction (most often due to distal obstructing stone)
  - Biliary dilatation with thickened, hyperenhancing bile duct walls, debris within duct lumen, and heterogeneous liver enhancement (most often on arterial-phase images)
    - Frequent association with pyogenic liver abscesses (25%)
  - Other forms of cholangitis (e.g., primary sclerosing and recurrent pyogenic cholangitis) may also cause acute RUQ pain
- **Acute Pancreatitis**
  - Enlarged, edematous pancreas (with loss of normal fatty lobulation) with peripancreatic fat stranding, free fluid, and inflammation (± parenchymal necrosis, ± peripancreatic fluid collections)
  - Vast majority of cases secondary to alcohol abuse or gallstones
  - While primarily centered in midabdomen, inflammation frequently spreads laterally toward gallbladder and right colon, explaining frequent presentation with RUQ pain
- **Duodenal Ulcer**
  - Most likely to be symptomatic when penetrating or perforated
  - Look for thickened duodenum with adjacent extraluminal gas or enteric contrast media (although < 50% of patients have ectopic gas/contrast)
  - Inflammation centered around duodenum in anterior pararenal space, but may spread laterally to involve adjacent structures (e.g., colon, gallbladder)

Helpful Clues for Less Common Diagnoses

- **Acute Colitis**
  - Any form of acute colitis (e.g., pseudomembranous, infectious, ulcerative, ischemic) that affects ascending colon can cause RUQ pain
  - Colonic wall thickening and submucosal edema with pericolonic fat stranding and inflammation
- **Appendicitis**

- While more often presenting with right lower quadrant (RLQ) pain, tip of appendix may extend upwards to RUQ and cause upper abdominal pain
- Dilated, thickened appendix with periappendiceal fat stranding and free fluid (± ectopic gas or fluid collections in cases with rupture)

- **Omental Infarct**
  - Omental fat necrosis caused by disruption of arterial blood supply
  - Most cases are located in right abdomen adjacent to ascending colon, and can present with RLQ or RUQ pain
    - Usually no evidence of other constitutional symptoms or elevated WBC
  - Ill-defined fat stranding or discrete encapsulated, fat-containing mass in omentum (± whorled pattern of vessels leading to infarct)

- **Epiploic Appendagitis**
  - Primary thrombosis or torsion of epiploic appendage
  - Can occur anywhere, but much more common in left lower quadrant adjacent to descending/sigmoid colon
  - Similar in appearance to omental infarct, with a small fat-containing mass abutting colon with adjacent fat stranding (± central dot sign)

- **Hepatic Pyogenic Abscess**
  - Can be associated with variety of causes, including recent surgery, cholangitis, septic thrombophlebitis (related to GI tract infections), etc.
  - Multiloculated cluster of thick-walled fluid collections in liver with surrounding low-density parenchymal edema (± internal gas)
  - Patients usually symptomatic with pain, fever, and elevated WBC

- **Passive Hepatic Congestion**
  - Although usually asymptomatic, enlargement and edema of liver may stretch capsule and cause RUQ pain
  - Enlarged, edematous liver may demonstrate mosaic or nutmeg pattern of heterogeneous enhancement

- Often other ancillary findings of right heart dysfunction, including cardiomegaly (with relative enlargement of right heart), dilatation of hepatic veins and IVC, and retrograde opacification of IVC/hepatic veins on arterial-phase imaging

- **Diverticulitis**
  - Right-sided diverticulitis is uncommon in western world, but much more common in certain ethnic groups (especially Asian populations)
  - Findings similar to diverticulitis elsewhere, with multiple diverticula (including at least one focally inflamed diverticulum), colonic wall thickening, and pericolonic fat stranding (± ectopic gas or fluid collections)

- **Pyelonephritis**
  - Infection of right kidney can result in RUQ pain
    - Patients typically febrile with flank tenderness and elevated WBC
  - Enlarged kidney with asymmetric perinephric stranding and striated or wedge-shaped areas of diminished enhancement on CECT (particularly in delayed nephrographic phase)

- **Thoracic Infection or Inflammation**
  - Any inflammatory process in right lower lung can cause RUQ pain, including pneumonia, pulmonary embolus, pulmonary infarct, pleural effusion, empyema, myocardial infarct, or pericarditis
  - Lung bases should be carefully evaluated in any patient presenting with RUQ pain

- **Hepatic Tumor**
  - Any tumor that is large or exophytic can stretch hepatic capsule and cause pain (even benign lesions such as giant hemangioma or large cyst)
  - Hepatocellular carcinoma and hepatic adenoma, in particular, are prone to spontaneous bleeding or rupture through liver capsule with hemoperitoneum

Acute Cholecystitis

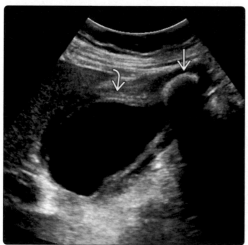

Acute Cholecystitis

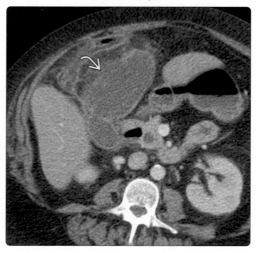

(Left) *Sagittal ultrasound image demonstrates a large gallstone* ➡ *lodged in the gallbladder (GB) neck with diffuse GB wall thickening* ➡. *Sonographic Murphy sign was positive, compatible with acute calculous cholecystitis.* (Right) *Axial CECT demonstrates a distended, thick-walled GB with extensive surrounding inflammation, compatible with acute cholecystitis. Note the irregularity and absent enhancement of the right lateral wall* ➡, *suggesting gangrenous cholecystitis.*

Gallstones

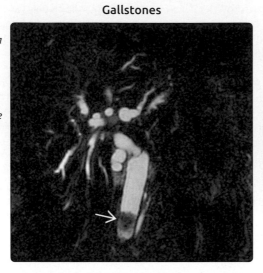

Gallstones

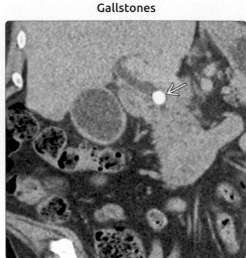

(Left) *Coronal MRCP with MIP reconstruction demonstrates a large low-signal stone ➡ in the distal common bile duct (CBD) causing proximal biliary obstruction. MR is the best noninvasive modality for the evaluation of extrahepatic bile duct stones.* **(Right)** *Coronal NECT demonstrates a high-density calcified stone ➡ in the distal CBD causing mild proximal obstruction. The sensitivity of CT for gallstones is better than commonly thought, approaching 80%.*

Acute Hepatitis

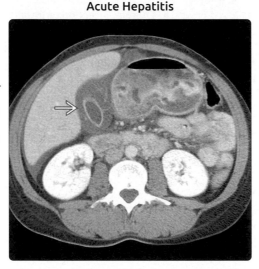

Hepatic Steatosis (Fatty Liver)

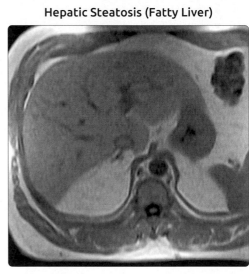

(Left) *Axial CECT shows marked thickening of the GB wall ➡ and ascites in this patient with acute viral hepatitis, who presented with symptoms of acute right upper quadrant (RUQ) pain. While the liver often appears normal on imaging in acute hepatitis, dramatic GB wall thickening is a common feature.* **(Right)** *Axial in-phase GRE image demonstrates homogenous signal throughout the liver.*

Hepatic Steatosis (Fatty Liver)

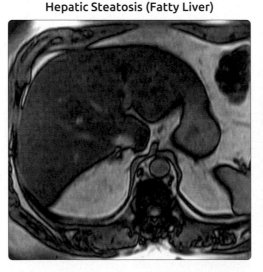

Ascending Cholangitis

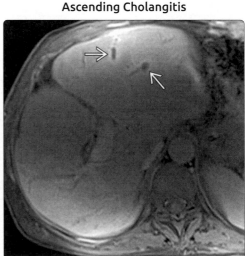

(Left) *Axial GRE opposed-phase image in the same patient demonstrates diffuse signal loss throughout the liver, compatible with diffuse hepatic steatosis. MR with chemical shift imaging is the most sensitive imaging modality for steatosis.* **(Right)** *Axial T1 C+ FS MR after liver transplant in a patient with fever demonstrates scattered dilated peripheral intrahepatic ducts ➡ with wall thickening and hyperenhancement, compatible with ascending cholangitis.*

Acute Pancreatitis

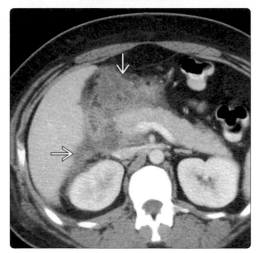

Duodenal Ulcer

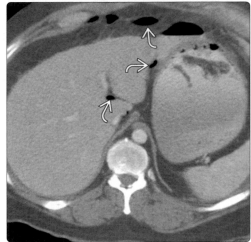

(Left) *Axial CECT demonstrates extensive infiltration of the fat planes in the RUQ* ➡ *in a patient with acute pancreatitis, with inflammation spreading to involve the ascending colon as well.* (Right) *Axial CECT shows extraluminal gas* ➡ *under the diaphragm and in the porta hepatis from a perforated duodenal ulcer.*

Duodenal Ulcer

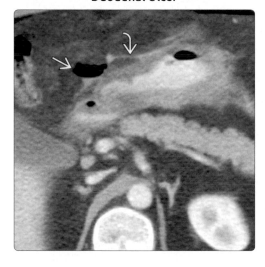

Acute Colitis

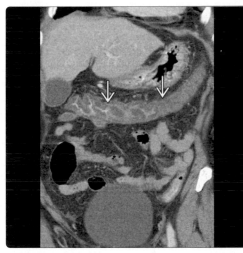

(Left) *Axial CECT shows extraluminal gas* ➡ *and enteric contrast media* ➡ *just ventral to the duodenal bulb and antrum, ultimately confirmed to represent a perforated duodenal ulcer.* (Right) *Coronal CECT shows marked thickening of the colonic wall, including the hepatic flexure and transverse colon* ➡*, representing acute infectious pseudomembranous colitis.*

Infectious Colitis

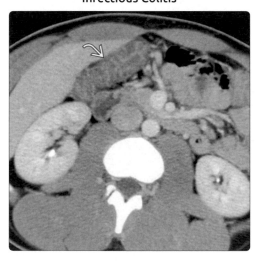

Appendicitis

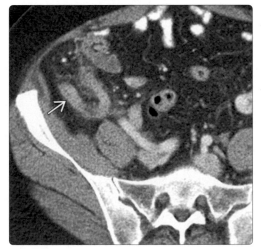

(Left) *Axial CECT shows right side colitis* ➡ *with mural edema and mucosal enhancement. This was found to represent infectious Campylobacter colitis.* (Right) *Axial CECT demonstrates a thick-walled appendix* ➡ *with adjacent fat-stranding and inflammation, compatible with acute uncomplicated appendicitis.*

Appendicitis

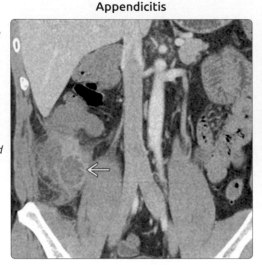

Omental Infarct

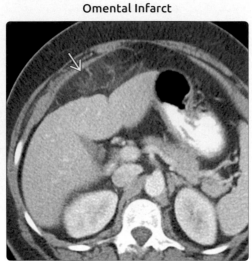

(Left) Axial CECT in a patient with right abdominal pain and fever demonstrates a large pericolonic fluid collection ➡ with extensive adjacent inflammation, found to represent the sequelae of perforated appendicitis. (Right) Axial CECT in a patient presenting with RUQ pain demonstrates an encapsulated fat-containing mass ➡ in the anterior omentum, a classic appearance for an omental infarct.

Epiploic Appendagitis

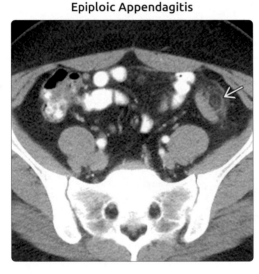

Hepatic Pyogenic Abscess

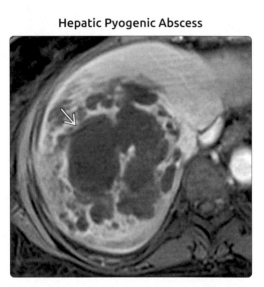

(Left) Axial CECT demonstrates a small fat-containing mass ➡ abutting the sigmoid colon with adjacent stranding and inflammation, a characteristic appearance for epiploic appendagitis. (Right) Axial T1 C+ FS MR demonstrates a large multiloculated cystic liver mass ➡ with a thick peripheral rind of enhancement, compatible with a liver abscess in this patient with abdominal pain and fever.

Hepatic Pyogenic Abscess

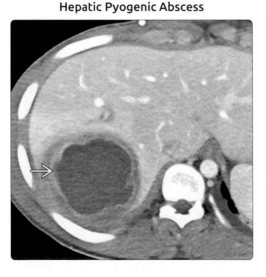

Passive Hepatic Congestion

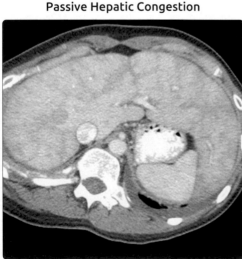

(Left) Axial CECT demonstrates a large thick-walled cystic mass ➡ in the right hepatic lobe with subtle surrounding low-density parenchymal edema, compatible with a large liver abscess. (Right) Axial CECT in a patient with cardiac dysfunction demonstrates the classic heterogeneous nutmeg enhancement of the liver suggestive of passive hepatic congestion.

Diverticulitis

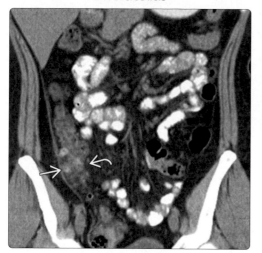

Diverticulitis

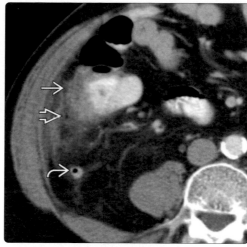

(Left) *Coronal CECT in a patient with right abdominal pain demonstrates thickening of the right colon* ⮕ *and its adjacent facia with several cecal diverticula* ⮕, *compatible with acute cecal diverticulitis.* (Right) *Axial CECT shows mural thickening and extensive adjacent inflammatory change* ⮕ *around the ascending colon, with a small bubble of ectopic gas* ⮕. *Note the normal appendix* ⮕. *These findings were secondary to cecal diverticulitis.*

Pyelonephritis

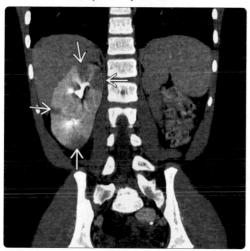

Hepatic Tumor

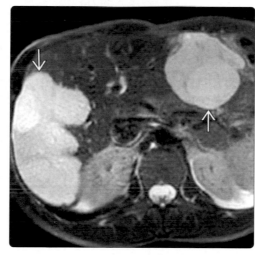

(Left) *Axial CECT demonstrates multiple wedge-shaped areas of low attenuation* ⮕ *within the right kidney, compatible with acute pyelonephritis.* (Right) *Axial T2 FS MR demonstrates multiple giant hemangiomas* ⮕ *throughout the liver, each of which demonstrates striking T2 hyperintensity. Even benign liver lesions, such as hemangiomas or cysts, can cause pain when they are very large as a result of stretching the liver capsule.*

Hepatic Tumor

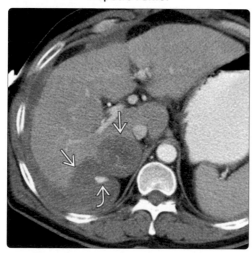

Hepatic Tumor

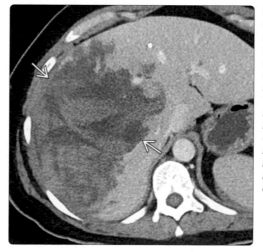

(Left) *Axial CECT demonstrates at least 2 masses* ⮕ *along the margin of the right hepatic lobe with evidence of active extravasation* ⮕ *and bleeding into the perihepatic space. This was found to represent hepatocellular carcinoma with hemorrhage.* (Right) *Axial CECT demonstrates a large hemorrhagic mass* ⮕ *in the right hepatic lobe, found to represent a bleeding hepatic adenoma.*

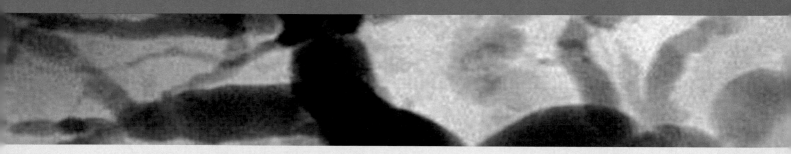

SECTION 11
Biliary Tract

Generic Imaging Patterns

Modality-Specific Imaging Findings

MAGNETIC RESONANCE IMAGING

DIFFERENTIAL DIAGNOSIS

Common

- Choledocholithiasis
- Postcholecystectomy Dilatation of Common Bile Duct
- Senescent & Postoperative Dilatation
- Pancreatic Ductal Adenocarcinoma
- Chronic Pancreatitis

Less Common

- Other Ampullary, Periampullary, & Pancreatic Neoplasms
  - Distal Common Bile Duct Cholangiocarcinoma
  - Ampullary Tumors
  - Periampullary Duodenal Adenocarcinoma
  - Mucinous Pancreatic Cystic Tumors
    - Mucinous Cystic Neoplasm
    - Intraductal Papillary Mucinous Neoplasm
- Gallbladder Carcinoma
- Primary Sclerosing Cholangitis
- Pancreatic Pseudocyst
- AIDS Cholangiopathy
- Recurrent Pyogenic Cholangitis
- Biliary Trauma
- Small Bowel Obstruction
- Choledochal Cyst

Rare but Important

- Other Pancreatic Masses
- Biliary Intraductal Papillary Mucinous Neoplasm
- Pancreatobiliary Parasites

ESSENTIAL INFORMATION

Key Differential Diagnosis Issues

- When common bile duct (CBD) is only borderline enlarged, decision to pursue further testing will depend on presence of clinical & biochemical markers of biliary obstruction
  - Presence of elevated bilirubin (direct & indirect), alkaline phosphatase, & transaminases should raise concern for CBD obstruction
  - **Painful** jaundice suggests acute or subacute obstruction, usually on basis of gallstones or cholangitis
  - **Painless** jaundice suggests chronic obstruction, & should raise concern for malignant obstruction or longstanding inflammatory obstruction [such as primary sclerosing cholangitis (PSC)]
- Size thresholds for CBD are generally controversial, but CBD size should generally be < 6 mm (+ 1 mm for each decade over 60 years)
  - Some suggest size up to 1 cm may be within normal limits after cholecystectomy, although this is controversial
- Presence of intrahepatic & extrahepatic biliary dilatation generally more concerning for distal obstruction than dilated CBD alone

Helpful Clues for Common Diagnoses

- **Choledocholithiasis**
  - CT sensitivity for stones is ~ 80%, with "pure" cholesterol stones often missed due to isodensity with bile
    - Gallstones on CT are variable in density, ranging from soft tissue density to calcified

- Stones can be very difficult to perceive in CBD on CT, particularly when CBD is not dilated
  - Stones (usually) appear as signal void on all MR pulse sequences, with T2WI most sensitive
    - Some pigment stones are rarely hyperintense on T1WI
    - MR is clearly best modality for identification of CBD stones, although impacted stones in ampulla can still be difficult to perceive in some cases
  - Gallstones appear echogenic on US, but distal CBD usually poorly evaluated due to overlying bowel gas
  - Patients with CBD stones almost always have GB stones
- **Senescent & Postoperative Dilatation**
  - It is generally accepted (although not without debate) that CBD seems to increase in diameter with advanced age & following cholecystectomy
    - CBD dilatation especially common if CBD was dilated prior to cholecystectomy
- **Pancreatic Ductal Adenocarcinoma**
  - Most common cause of painless jaundice
  - Poorly marginated hypodense mass centered in pancreatic head resulting in abrupt narrowing of distal CBD & pancreatic duct (double-duct sign) with upstream pancreatic atrophy
  - Often infiltrates posteriorly to encase mesenteric vasculature
- **Chronic Pancreatitis**
  - May produce smooth, tapered narrowing & stricture of distal CBD as it traverses pancreatic head
  - Other stigmata include dilated, beaded pancreatic duct with parenchymal/intraductal calcifications
  - Can result in focal fibroinflammatory mass in pancreatic head, which may be difficult to distinguish from pancreatic cancer

Helpful Clues for Less Common Diagnoses

- **Other Ampullary, Periampullary, & Pancreatic Neoplasms**
  - **Distal Common Bile Duct Cholangiocarcinoma**
    - Only 20% of extrahepatic bile duct cholangiocarcinomas arise in distal 1/3 of duct, but 95% of these lesions result in CBD obstruction
    - May present as ill-defined soft tissue mass or as discrete duct wall thickening with hyperenhancement
    - Does not typically obstruct pancreatic duct or cause pancreatic atrophy
  - **Ampullary Tumors**
    - Encompasses wide range of histologic tumor types, including ampullary adenoma, ampullary carcinoma, & ampullary carcinoid
    - Tumor typically small & not uncommonly difficult to definitively visualize
    - May present as discrete nodule at ampulla or subtle wall thickening of medial duodenal wall at ampulla
    - Almost always obstructs CBD, but only obstructs pancreatic duct in ~ 50% & does not usually cause pancreatic atrophy
  - **Periampullary Duodenal Adenocarcinoma**
    - Distinction between ampullary carcinoma & periampullary duodenal adenocarcinoma may not be possible on imaging
    - Frequent obstruction of distal CBD, but pancreatic atrophy or pancreatic ductal obstruction uncommon

- **Mucinous Pancreatic Cystic Tumors**
  - Majority of mucinous cystic neoplasms (MCNs) & intraductal papillary mucinous neoplasms (IPMNs) do not cause CBD obstruction
  - IAP consensus guidelines for management of IPMN/MCN suggests presence of CBD obstruction/jaundice is "high-risk" feature that should prompt concern for invasive malignancy
  - MCN usually appears as unilocular cyst (± thick wall or mural nodularity), while IPMN presents as cystic lesion that communicates with pancreatic duct
  - MCN more often located in tail segment, while IPMN most common in head
- **Gallbladder Carcinoma**
  - Frequently causes CBD obstruction as result of either direct tumor extension or metastatic lymphadenopathy
  - More typically obstructs mid- or proximal CBD (rather than distal CBD), with intrahepatic biliary dilatation predominating over CBD dilatation
- **Primary Sclerosing Cholangitis**
  - Much more likely to cause strictures of CBD & intrahepatic ducts rather than impressive dilation
  - Prominent dilation of CBD or intrahepatic ducts as result of dominant CBD stricture is unusual, & should raise concern for superimposed cholangiocarcinoma
- **Pancreatic Pseudocyst**
  - Pseudocysts arising in pancreatic head may cause CBD obstruction due to extrinsic mass effect
  - Obstruction in this setting may not be cured by draining pseudocyst, as CBD obstruction is often actually caused by coexisting fibrotic stricture of intrapancreatic CBD
- **AIDS Cholangiopathy**
  - Now uncommon diagnosis due to widespread utilization of HAART for HIV/AIDS
  - Can result in multiple intrahepatic & extrahepatic ductal strictures that are very similar to PSC
  - Classically results in papillary stenosis & CBD dilatation, with distal CBD narrowing usually smooth & tapered
- **Recurrent Pyogenic Cholangitis**
  - Almost always diagnosed in patients from Southeast Asia

- Results in biliary dilatation that disproportionately affects extrahepatic duct & central intrahepatic ducts (with frequent intraductal stones & purulent debris)
- **Biliary Trauma**
  - CBD injury can result in stricture or transection of duct with proximal biliary dilatation
  - Usually iatrogenic (especially during cholecystectomy or other biliary surgeries), rather than truly trauma-related
  - Usually abrupt narrowing of CBD ± adjacent biloma
- **Small Bowel Obstruction**
  - Obstruction of duodenum or Roux loop can result in increased intraluminal pressures that may impair biliary drainage & cause proximal biliary dilatation
- **Choledochal Cyst**
  - Type I choledochal cyst results in isolated fusiform CBD dilation, while type IV choledochal cyst results in cystic dilatation of intrahepatic & extrahepatic bile duct

Helpful Clues for Rare Diagnoses

- **Other Pancreatic Masses**
  - Range of other pancreatic tumors can theoretically cause CBD obstruction, particularly when large
  - Pancreatic neuroendocrine tumors & serous cystadenomas do not typically cause CBD or pancreatic duct obstruction, although very large tumors can obstruct CBD due to mass effect
  - Lymphoma of pancreas does not usually cause pancreatic or biliary ductal obstruction
- **Biliary Intraductal Papillary Mucinous Neoplasm**
  - Mucin-producing neoplasm arising from biliary mucosa
  - Can result in localized or diffuse massive dilatation of bile ducts as result of distension with mucin (± visible intraductal mural nodularity or soft tissue)
- **Pancreaticobiliary Parasites**
  - Uncommon in western world, but parasites can involve biliary tree, resulting in ductal dilatation & strictures
  - Ascariasis can involve any portion of biliary tree, while fascioliasis preferentially involves extrahepatic duct & large intrahepatic ducts
  - Parasite may be visible within duct as filling defect

Choledocholithiasis

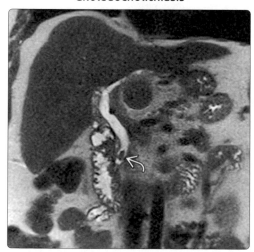

Choledocholithiasis

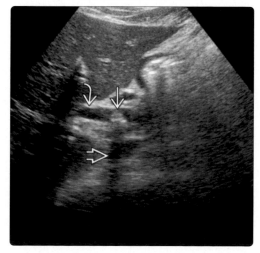

(Left) Coronal T2 HASTE MR demonstrates a low-signal stone ➡ in the distal common bile duct (CBD). Although there are some rare exceptions, gallstones typically appear low signal on all MR pulse sequences. (Right) US demonstrates a mildly dilated CBD ➡ secondary to a gallstone ➡ with posterior acoustic shadowing ➡. US is often relatively insensitive for choledocholithiasis due to overlying bowel gas.

(Left) Coronal FIESTA image demonstrates a low-signal stone ➡ impacted in the distal CBD at the level of the ampulla, resulting in significant proximal CBD and intrahepatic biliary dilatation. (Right) Axial T2 FS MR demonstrates a low-signal filling defect ➡ within the distal CBD, compatible with choledocholithiasis.

Choledocholithiasis

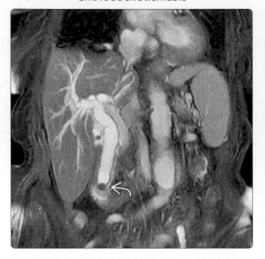

Choledocholithiasis

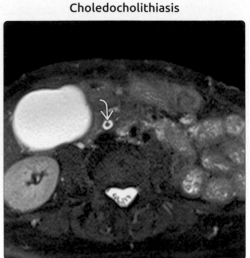

(Left) Axial CECT shows mild dilatation of the common duct ➡ in a patient status post cholecystectomy. There were no signs or symptoms of biliary obstruction, and these findings were attributed to her prior cholecystectomy. (Right) Axial CECT shows dilation of the intrahepatic bile ducts ➡ in an elderly woman with a prior cholecystectomy, but no symptoms or signs of biliary obstruction.

Postcholecystectomy Dilatation of Common Bile Duct

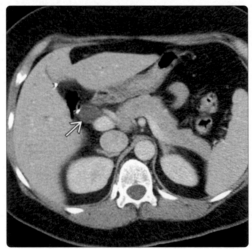

Postcholecystectomy Dilatation of Common Bile Duct

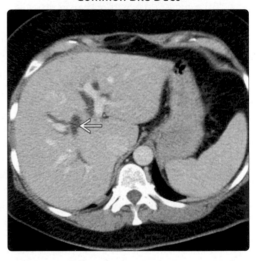

(Left) Coronal MRCP with MIP reconstruction in a patient with pancreatic adenocarcinoma demonstrates a classic double-duct sign, including a markedly dilated biliary tree with abrupt narrowing of the distal CBD ➡ due to the patient's malignancy. (Right) Coronal CECT demonstrates an ill-defined, hypodense mass ➡ in the pancreatic head, resulting in obstruction and dilatation of both the CBD ➡ and pancreatic duct ➡, compatible with pancreatic adenocarcinoma.

Pancreatic Ductal Adenocarcinoma

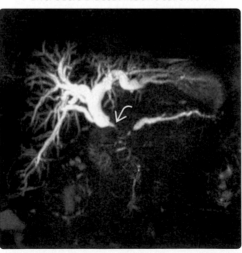

Pancreatic Ductal Adenocarcinoma

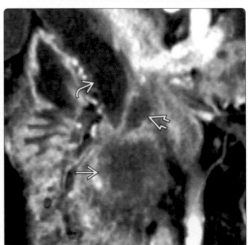

Pancreatic Ductal Adenocarcinoma

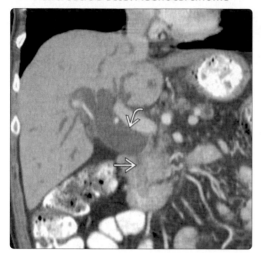

Chronic Pancreatitis

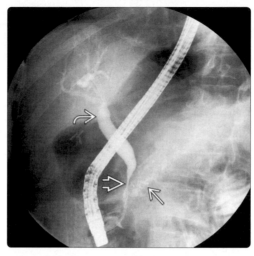

(Left) *Coronal CECT demonstrates an infiltrative mass ⟳ in the pancreatic head, representing the patient's known pancreatic adenocarcinoma, resulting in obstruction and severe dilatation of the CBD ⟹ and biliary tree.* **(Right)** *Frontal projection from an ERCP in a patient with chronic pancreatitis demonstrates long, smooth tapering of the distal CBD ⟹ as a result of a distal stricture, with mild associated proximal CBD dilatation ⟹. In addition, the pancreatic duct ⟹ appears beaded and very irregular.*

Chronic Pancreatitis

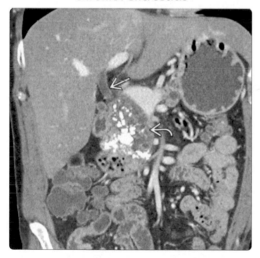

Distal Common Bile Duct Cholangiocarcinoma

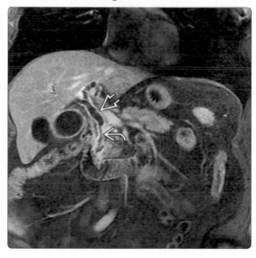

(Left) *Coronal CECT demonstrates an extensively calcified soft tissue mass in the pancreatic head, representing a focal fibroinflammatory mass ⟳ related to the patient's known chronic pancreatitis. There is mild resultant CBD dilatation ⟹.* **(Right)** *Coronal T1 C+ FS MR demonstrates mild dilatation of the proximal extrahepatic bile duct ⟹, with abrupt transition to a strictured distal CBD ⟹. This stricture was found to be malignant, representing a distal CBD cholangiocarcinoma.*

Distal Common Bile Duct Cholangiocarcinoma

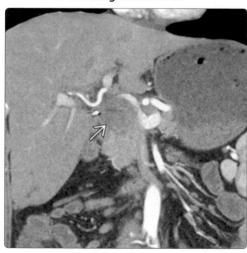

Ampullary Tumors

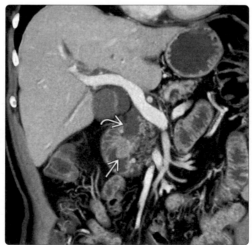

(Left) *Coronal CECT demonstrates an infiltrative hypodense mass ⟳ centered in the porta hepatis, in close proximity to the extrahepatic bile duct, found at resection to represent a distal CBD cholangiocarcinoma.* **(Right)** *Coronal CECT demonstrates a round, soft tissue nodule ⟹ at the ampulla resulting in obstruction of the CBD ⟹, found to represent an ampullary carcinoma at resection.*

Ampullary Tumors

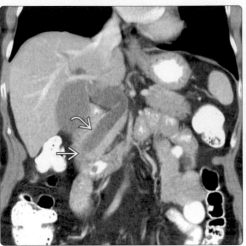

Periampullary Duodenal Adenocarcinoma

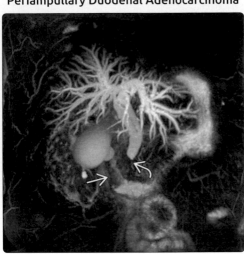

(Left) *Coronal CECT demonstrates severe CBD dilatation ⇶ with abrupt narrowing near the ampulla. Although subtle, there is minimal hypodense soft tissue ⇶ present at the ampulla, representing a small ampullary carcinoma.* **(Right)** *Coronal MRCP with MIP reconstruction demonstrates a diffusely dilated biliary tree with abrupt narrowing of the distal CBD ⇶. Although subtle on this heavily T2 weighted image, there is circumferential wall thickening ⇶ of the duodenum, representing duodenal adenocarcinoma.*

Periampullary Duodenal Adenocarcinoma

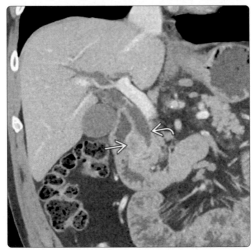

Gallbladder Carcinoma

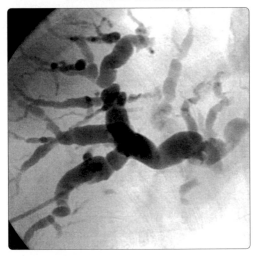

(Left) *Coronal CECT demonstrates mass-like thickening ⇶ of the medial duodenum near the ampulla, resulting in obstruction of the CBD ⇶. This was found to be a periampullary duodenal adenocarcinoma at resection.* **(Right)** *Percutaneous cholangiogram shows massive dilation of the intrahepatic ducts with abrupt obstruction near the confluence, secondary to a carcinoma of the gallbladder neck involving the common duct.*

Pancreatic Pseudocyst

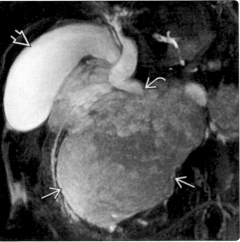

AIDS Cholangiopathy

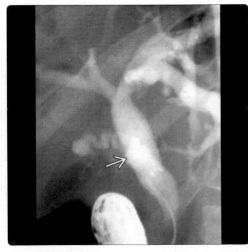

(Left) *Coronal MRCP with MIP reconstruction demonstrates obstruction of the CBD ⇶ by a large pseudocyst ⇶. Note the distension of the gallbladder ⇶ secondary to biliary obstruction. The patient underwent a successful surgical procedure with enteric cyst drainage into the duodenum.* **(Right)** *Frontal ERCP shows diffuse dilatation of the CBD ⇶ (secondary to papillary stenosis), compatible with the patient's known AIDS cholangiopathy.*

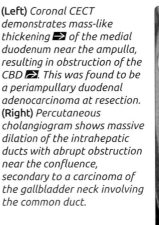
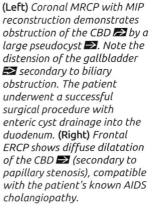

Recurrent Pyogenic Cholangitis

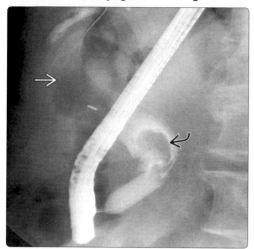

Recurrent Pyogenic Cholangitis

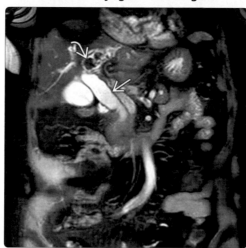

(Left) *Frontal ERCP demonstrates a massively dilated CBD with large stones within the CBD ➯, compatible with the patient's history of recurrent pyogenic cholangitis. There is also a large amount of gas ➡ within the ducts.* (Right) *Coronal FIESTA demonstrates severe dilatation of the CBD ➡, along with dilatation of the left hepatic lobe ducts, which are filled with multiple T2-hypointense stones ➚. These findings are compatible with recurrent pyogenic cholangitis.*

Choledochal Cyst

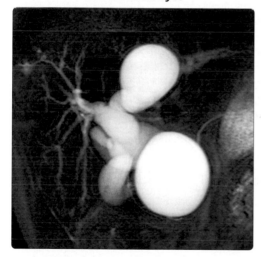

Choledochal Cyst

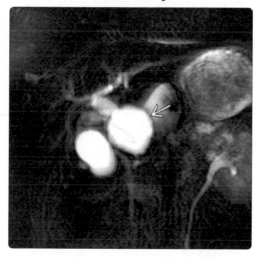

(Left) *Coronal MRCP with MIP reconstruction demonstrates extensive cystic dilatation of the intrahepatic and extrahepatic bile ducts, compatible with a type IV choledochal cyst.* (Right) *Coronal MRCP with MIP reconstruction demonstrates focal fusiform dilatation ➡ of the CBD, with the intrahepatic ducts appearing normal. This represents a type I choledochal cyst.*

Choledochal Cyst

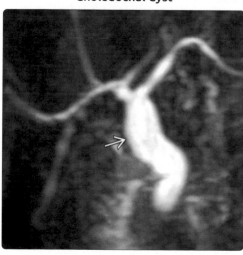

Biliary Intraductal Papillary Mucinous Neoplasm

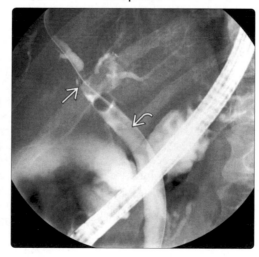

(Left) *Coronal MRCP with MIP reconstruction demonstrates diffuse, fusiform dilation of the extrahepatic common duct ➡, a type I choledochal cyst in the Todani classification.* (Right) *Frontal projection ERCP demonstrates diffuse dilatation of the CBD, with a discrete mass within the proximal CBD ➡. There is also heterogeneous filling of the CBD with contrast ➚, likely as a result of mucin. These findings were found to represent a biliary intraductal papillary mucinous neoplasm.*

DIFFERENTIAL DIAGNOSIS

Common

- Primary Sclerosing Cholangitis
- Malignant Obstruction
  - Cholangiocarcinoma
  - Gallbladder Carcinoma
  - Liver Tumors
  - Periportal Lymphadenopathy
- Ascending Cholangitis

Less Common

- AIDS Cholangiopathy
- Recurrent Pyogenic Cholangitis
- Pancreato-Biliary Parasites
- Hepatic Hydatid Cyst
- Chemotherapy Cholangitis
- Biliary Intraductal Papillary Mucinous Neoplasm
- IgG4-Related Sclerosing Cholangitis
- Ischemic Cholangitis
- Caroli Disease
- Mirizzi Syndrome

ESSENTIAL INFORMATION

Key Differential Diagnosis Issues

- Disproportionate dilatation of intrahepatic bile ducts (relative to extrahepatic bile duct) most often results from either one of several forms of cholangitis or obstructing mass
- Presence of significant isolated intrahepatic biliary dilatation (whether diffuse, lobar, or segmental) should always prompt careful evaluation for obstructing mass or malignant stricture
- Many different forms of cholangitis may appear similar radiographically, requiring correlation with clinical history or biopsy to make more specific diagnosis

Helpful Clues for Common Diagnoses

- **Primary Sclerosing Cholangitis**
  - Immune-mediated form of cholangitis resulting in fibrosis, inflammation, and strictures of bile ducts
  - Beaded strictures with intervening sites of normal or dilated ducts
    - Usually involves both intrahepatic and extrahepatic ducts, but isolated or disproportionate involvement of intrahepatic ducts can occur
      - □ Main right and left ducts are often most severely involved
    - Chronic involvement can result in unique form of cirrhosis with rounded, lobulated contour of liver with peripheral atrophy and severe hypertrophy of caudate/central liver (pseudotumoral enlargement)
  - Most often diagnosed in young male patients (30-40 yr) with strong association with ulcerative colitis and autoimmune diseases
- **Malignant Obstruction**
  - **Cholangiocarcinoma**
    - Tumors arising either at liver hilum/confluence of ducts (i.e., Klatskin tumor) or peripherally in liver itself can result in proximal intrahepatic biliary dilatation

- Tumors classically demonstrate prominent delayed enhancement on multiphase imaging (CT or MR)
  - □ Liver peripheral to tumor may demonstrate atrophy or capsular retraction
  - □ Tumor may appear as discrete mass, subtle asymmetric soft tissue along margin of duct, or focal duct wall thickening and enhancement
  - **Gallbladder Carcinoma**
    - Gallbladder cancers frequently extend to involve proximal extrahepatic duct or hepatic duct confluence, producing intrahepatic biliary dilatation
    - May be difficult on imaging to confidently differentiate primary gallbladder carcinoma from hilar cholangiocarcinoma
    - Frequently associated with liver metastases, bulky lymphadenopathy, and carcinomatosis
  - **Liver Tumors**
    - Any tumor involving liver or liver hilum (e.g., hepatocellular carcinoma, metastases, lymphoma, etc.) can theoretically invade and obstruct intrahepatic ducts
    - Even benign masses, when large, may displace and dilate ducts due to extrinsic mass effect
  - **Periportal Lymphadenopathy**
    - Periportal lymphadenopathy can obstruct proximal extrahepatic duct due to extrinsic compression and result in intrahepatic biliary dilatation
- **Ascending Cholangitis**
  - Acute pyogenic infection due to biliary obstruction, most often on basis of distal obstructing stone or reflux of bowel contents (e.g., biliary-enteric anastomosis)
  - Biliary dilatation proximal to site of obstruction with evidence of bile duct wall thickening and enhancement on CT/MR
    - Often associated with heterogeneous liver enhancement, particularly on arterial-phase images
  - Results in inflammatory bile duct strictures with abnormal biliary tree arborization and branching

Helpful Clues for Less Common Diagnoses

- **AIDS Cholangiopathy**
  - Increasingly uncommon entity (due to widespread utilization of HAART) seen in late-stage AIDS patients (usually CD4 < 100 mm³)
    - Inflammation of biliary tree caused by opportunistic infection
  - Beaded strictures of intrahepatic or extrahepatic ducts that may closely resemble primary sclerosing cholangitis (PSC)
    - Strictures may be associated with bile duct wall thickening and enhancement on CT/MR
    - Gallbladder not uncommonly involved with wall thickening and surrounding inflammation
  - Classically associated with papillary stenosis [tapered narrowing of distal common bile duct (CBD)]
- **Recurrent Pyogenic Cholangitis**
  - Disease almost always diagnosed in patients living in or immigrating from Southeast Asia, likely related to parasitic or bacterial infection of biliary tree
  - Results in significant dilatation of bile ducts which frequently demonstrate internal stones

- o Tends to involve extrahepatic and central intrahepatic ducts preferentially and may be localized to one portion of liver (especially left hepatic lobe)
  - − Involved portions of liver often demonstrate parenchymal atrophy
- **Pancreato-Biliary Parasites**
  - o Parasites (such as ascariasis, clonorchiasis, fascioliasis) can involve biliary tree and result in biliary dilatation
    - − Distribution of biliary involvement will depend on parasite type (e.g., clonorchiasis involves small peripheral intrahepatic ducts)
  - o Parasite may be seen within dilated duct as filling defect
- **Hepatic Hydatid Cyst**
  - o Endemic in sheep-raising countries (Mediterranean, Africa, South America)
  - o May cause biliary dilatation if hepatic echinococcal cyst communicates with bile duct or frank rupture of cyst into biliary tree
  - o Direct communication between hydatid cyst and bile duct may rarely be directly visualized with wall defect in cyst leading into adjacent dilated bile duct
- **Chemotherapy Cholangitis**
  - o Form of cholangitis resulting from intraarterial chemotherapy (such as transarterial chemoembolization)
  - o Imaging features similar to PSC, including multifocal biliary strictures
  - o Distribution of strictures based on hepatic arterial supply to bile ducts, with preferential involvement of proximal extrahepatic bile duct and biliary confluence
- **Biliary Intraductal Papillary Mucinous Neoplasm**
  - o Mucin-producing neoplasm arising from biliary mucosa which is analogous to pancreatic intraductal papillary mucinous neoplasm
  - o Results in severely dilated bile ducts filled with mucin ± enhancing mural nodularity or discrete intraductal soft tissue mass
  - o Can involve ducts diffusely or be localized
  - o Typically diagnosed in elderly patients from East Asia who present with jaundice and repetitive bouts of cholangitis

- **IgG4-Related Sclerosing Cholangitis**
  - o Entity characterized by lymphoplasmacytic infiltration of biliary tree
    - − Often associated with IgG4-related sclerosing disease in other organs (especially autoimmune pancreatitis)
  - o Strictures most commonly seen in distal CBD, but can be seen anywhere in biliary tree
    - − Involved bile ducts appear thickened and hyperenhancing
  - o Look for other stigmata of IgG4-related sclerosing disease, including findings of autoimmune pancreatitis (such as sausage-shaped enlargement of pancreas, low-density halo/capsule, narrowing of pancreatic duct)
- **Ischemic Cholangitis**
  - o Entity most often seen in setting of liver transplant resulting either from hepatic artery compromise (stenosis or thrombosis) or other microangiopathic/immunologic injuries
  - o Results in multiple intrahepatic and extrahepatic strictures that may not be distinguishable from PSC without clinical history (including beaded appearance of biliary tree)
    - − Tendency to involve middle 1/2 of CBD and hepatic duct confluence
    - − Often associated with hyperdense (or T1 hyperintense) cast material filling bile ducts
- **Caroli Disease**
  - o Congenital cystic dilatation of intrahepatic ducts with normal caliber extrahepatic bile duct
    - − Caroli syndrome also associated with hepatic fibrosis and portal hypertension
  - o Cystic dilatation of intrahepatic ducts can be focal, segmental, or diffuse with frequent intraductal stones
  - o Associated with central dot sign on CT/MR due to enhancing portal radicle at center or periphery of dilated duct
- **Mirizzi Syndrome**
  - o Obstruction of proximal extrahepatic bile duct due to gallstone impacted within cystic duct or gallbladder neck
  - o Results in dilatation of intrahepatic bile ducts and proximal extrahepatic duct

Primary Sclerosing Cholangitis

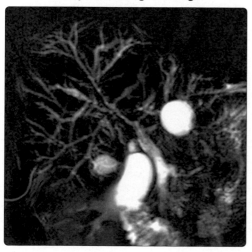

Primary Sclerosing Cholangitis

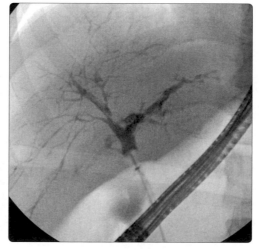

(Left) Coronal MRCP with MIP reconstruction in a patient with primary sclerosing cholangitis (PSC) demonstrates mild diffuse intrahepatic biliary ductal dilatation with the ducts showing a subtle beaded morphology. (Right) Frontal projection from an ERCP cholangiogram demonstrates the characteristic features of PSC, including mild diffuse biliary dilatation and a classic beaded appearance of the ducts (with alternating sites of dilated, narrowed, or normal ducts).

Cholangiocarcinoma

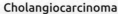
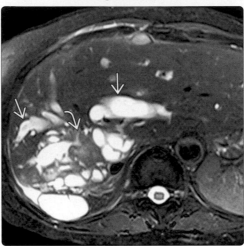

Cholangiocarcinoma

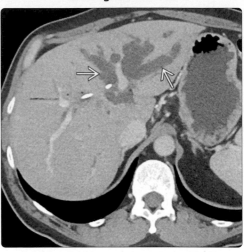

(Left) *Axial T2 FS MR demonstrates severely dilated bile ducts ⮕ throughout the right hepatic lobe with subtle T2-hyperintense infiltrating tumor ⮕ causing obstruction. This was ultimately found to represent an intrahepatic cholangiocarcinoma.* **(Right)** *Axial CECT demonstrates severe dilatation of the intrahepatic bile ducts ⮕ in the left hepatic lobe. Although a discrete obstructing mass is difficult to identify on imaging, this was ultimately found to be an obstructing cholangiocarcinoma.*

Gallbladder Carcinoma

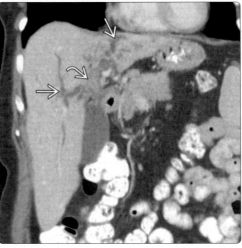
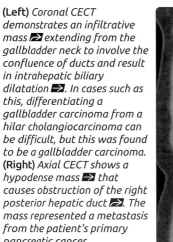

Liver Tumors

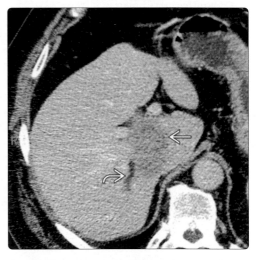

(Left) *Coronal CECT demonstrates an infiltrative mass ⮕ extending from the gallbladder neck to involve the confluence of ducts and result in intrahepatic biliary dilatation ⮕. In cases such as this, differentiating a gallbladder carcinoma from a hilar cholangiocarcinoma can be difficult, but this was found to be a gallbladder carcinoma.* **(Right)** *Axial CECT shows a hypodense mass ⮕ that causes obstruction of the right posterior hepatic duct ⮕. The mass represented a metastasis from the patient's primary pancreatic cancer.*

Ascending Cholangitis

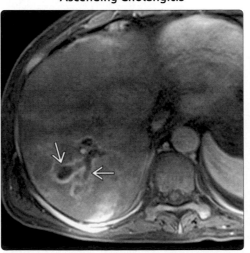

AIDS Cholangiopathy

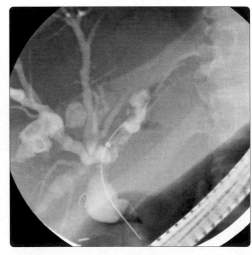

(Left) *Axial T1 C+ arterial-phase MR in a liver transplant patient with ascending cholangitis demonstrates focally dilated ducts ⮕ in the right hepatic lobe with wall thickening and hyperenhancement, as well as heterogeneous background liver enhancement.* **(Right)** *Frontal ERCP cholangiogram in an AIDS patient with low CD4 count demonstrates diffuse, irregular, beaded, biliary dilatation, found to represent AIDS cholangiopathy.*

AIDS Cholangiopathy

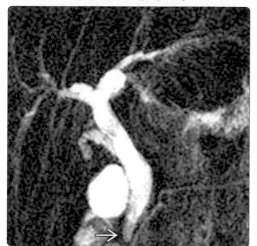

Recurrent Pyogenic Cholangitis

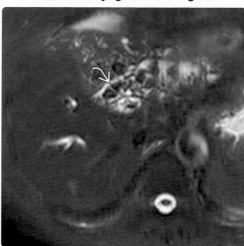

(Left) *Coronal MRCP shows irregular arborization of the intrahepatic bile ducts and a stricture of the distal common bile duct ➡, typical findings of AIDS cholangiopathy with papillary stenosis.* **(Right)** *Axial T2 FS MR in an Asian patient demonstrates severely dilated bile ducts in the left hepatic lobe filled with T2-hypointense stones ➡, a classic appearance for recurrent pyogenic cholangitis.*

IgG4-Related Sclerosing Cholangitis

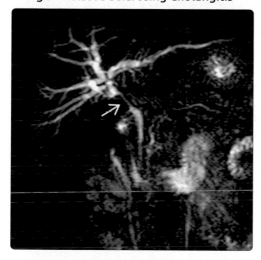

Ischemic Cholangitis

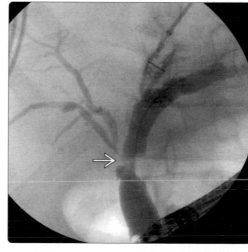

(Left) *Coronal MRCP with MIP reconstruction demonstrates a dominant stricture ➡ in the proximal extrahepatic duct, found to be a manifestation of IgG4-cholangiopathy in a patient with evidence of retroperitoneal fibrosis (also thought to be IgG4 related).* **(Right)** *Frontal ERCP cholangiogram in a liver transplant patient with known hepatic artery thrombosis demonstrates a dominant biliary stricture ➡ at the confluence of ducts with associated intrahepatic biliary dilatation, compatible with ischemic cholangiopathy.*

Biliary Intraductal Papillary Mucinous Neoplasm

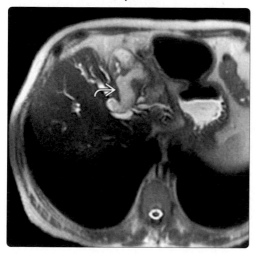

Caroli Disease

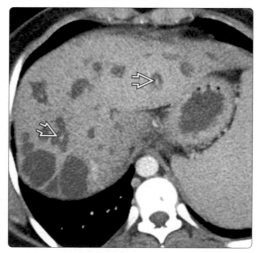

(Left) *Axial T2 MR shows massive dilation of the left intrahepatic ducts ➡ and mild dilation of the right ducts. No obstructing mass or stricture is identified downstream, and these findings were found to be secondary to a biliary IPMN.* **(Right)** *Axial CECT demonstrates extensive cystic dilatation of the intrahepatic bile ducts, with a few of the dilated ducts demonstrating a characteristic central dot sign ➡. This constellation of imaging features is classic for Caroli disease.*

DIFFERENTIAL DIAGNOSIS

Common

- Primary Sclerosing Cholangitis
- Ascending Cholangitis
- Posttransplant Liver and Ischemic Cholangiopathy
- Cirrhosis (Mimic)

Less Common

- AIDS Cholangiopathy
- Cholangiocarcinoma
- Recurrent Pyogenic Cholangitis
- Caroli Disease
- Chemotherapy Cholangitis
- Hepatic Metastases (Mimic)
- Pancreatobiliary Parasites
- Autoimmune (IgG4) Cholangitis
- Radiation Therapy
- Portal Biliopathy

ESSENTIAL INFORMATION

Key Differential Diagnosis Issues

- Sclerosing cholangitis is general term for disorders which result in fibrosis and stricturing of biliary tree
  - Most common cause is idiopathic form: Primary sclerosing cholangitis (PSC)
  - **Many** other secondary causes generally grouped together as "secondary" sclerosing cholangitis (including many rare causes)
- Most common causes of multiple biliary strictures have significant overlap in imaging appearance, making correlation with clinical history critical for diagnosis
- **Multiple** biliary strictures are typically benign, although development of new or dominant stricture can herald development of superimposed cholangiocarcinoma (particularly in PSC patients)
- MR/MRCP is best noninvasive modality for demonstrating distribution, length, and morphology of strictures

Helpful Clues for Common Diagnoses

- **Primary Sclerosing Cholangitis**
  - Immune-mediated disorder resulting in inflammation and fibrosis of intrahepatic and extrahepatic ducts, most often diagnosed in young male patients (30-40 years old)
  - Multifocal beaded strictures with intervening sites of normal or dilated ducts
    - Active inflammation associated with bile duct wall thickening and enhancement on CECT and MR
    - Chronic involvement results in pruned appearance of biliary tree
  - Chronic inflammation can result in cirrhotic liver with massive enlargement of central liver (pseudotumoral hypertrophy), atrophy of peripheral liver, and rounded/lobulated hepatic contour
    - Periphery of liver may be hypodense on CECT and mildly T2 hyperintense on MR due to fibrosis
  - Strong association with inflammatory bowel disease and other autoimmune diseases
  - Any new dominant stricture should raise concern for superimposed cholangiocarcinoma
- **Ascending Cholangitis**

- Pyogenic infection of biliary tree due to biliary obstruction [most often due to gallstones in distal common bile duct (CBD)]
- Dilated bile ducts with wall thickening, hyperenhancement of duct wall, and patchy heterogeneous hepatic enhancement (particularly on arterial phase-images)
  - May be associated with debris within bile duct, liver abscesses, or portal vein thrombosis
- Results in strictures of biliary tree, as well as abnormal arborization pattern of intrahepatic ducts
  - Biliary tree may communicate with hepatic abscesses
- **Posttransplant Liver and Ischemic Cholangiopathy**
  - Nonanastomotic strictures may develop in transplant liver due to hepatic artery thrombosis/stenosis or immunologic injury (prolonged warm/cold ischemic time, blood antigen incompatibility, etc.)
    - Beaded strictures of biliary tree (similar to PSC) with predominant involvement of middle 1/3 of CBD and hepatic duct confluence
    - Often associated with bile duct "casts" filling dilated bile ducts (hyperdense on CT, high signal on T1WI MR)
  - Biliary strictures in transplant liver may also develop at anastomotic site or due to cholangitis
- **Cirrhosis (Mimic)**
  - Regenerating nodules and hepatic fibrosis can distort, displace, and compress ducts due to mass effect, mimicking appearance of strictures

Helpful Clues for Less Common Diagnoses

- **AIDS Cholangiopathy**
  - Opportunistic infections of biliary tree in AIDS patients with very low CD4 counts (usually < 100 cells/mm³)
    - Now uncommon due to widespread HAART
  - Tapered, smooth narrowing of distal CBD (e.g., papillary stenosis) with long segment extrahepatic duct strictures and beaded strictures of intrahepatic ducts (similar to PSC)
  - May be associated with concomitant gallbladder wall thickening due to acalculous cholecystitis
- **Cholangiocarcinoma**
  - May present as discrete mass (i.e., "mass-forming" cholangiocarcinoma), subtle focal wall thickening (i.e.,"'periductal infiltrating") or as intraductal nodule/mass
  - Tumor classically characterized by increasing delayed enhancement due to fibrotic nature of tumor
  - Tumor often narrows or obstructs biliary tree with upstream biliary dilatation
    - May produce multiple strictures due to single large mass obstructing biliary tree in several locations, or due to satellite lesions/metastases
- **Recurrent Pyogenic Cholangitis**
  - Occurs almost always in patients either living in or originally from Southeast Asia, likely due to parasitic infection of biliary tree
  - Results in dilation of intrahepatic and extrahepatic ducts (especially extrahepatic and central intrahepatic ducts) with multiple intrahepatic strictures, abnormal intrahepatic duct arborization, and stones throughout biliary tree

- Can affect localized portions of liver, especially left hepatic lobe and right posterior lobe
- Chronic disease can result in atrophy of affected portions of liver
○ Duct dilation and intraductal stones tend to be more prominent than biliary strictures

- **Caroli Disease**
  ○ Congenital multifocal saccular dilatation of large intrahepatic ducts with alternating biliary strictures
    - Appears as multiple cysts throughout liver, which communicate with biliary tree
    - Characteristic central dot sign on CECT or MR with enhancing portal radicle surrounded by dilated duct
    - Hepatolithiasis and sludge may appear as filling defects within dilated ducts
  ○ Caroli syndrome also associated with hepatic fibrosis and portal hypertension
  ○ Commonly associated with polycystic hepatorenal syndrome (especially autosomal recessive), hepatic fibrosis, and medullary sponge kidney
  ○ Usually known diagnosis, as most patients present in childhood or young adulthood due to cholangitis or liver dysfunction

- **Chemotherapy Cholangitis**
  ○ Iatrogenic cholangitis related to intraarterial chemotherapy or transarterial chemoembolization for hepatic malignancies
  ○ Results in biliary strictures which tend to involve proximal extrahepatic duct and biliary confluence more commonly that peripheral intrahepatic ducts
    - Necrosis of peripheral ducts can result in biloma or abscess formation
  ○ Duct strictures and necrosis result from either direct toxic effect of drug on bile ducts, or due to occlusion of peribiliary vascular plexus with resultant ischemic cholangiopathy

- **Hepatic Metastases (Mimic)**
  ○ Masses may distort, displace, and narrow bile ducts due to mass effect, simulating appearance of strictures and resulting in upstream biliary dilatation

- **Pancreatobiliary Parasites**

○ Parasites can cause strictures &/or biliary dilation, with parasite often visible as filling defect within duct
  - Sites of involvement within biliary tree depend on individual parasite (e.g., clonarchiasis typically involves peripheral intrahepatic ducts)
○ Although uncommon in western world, many biliary parasites are endemic in developing world

- **Autoimmune (IgG4) Cholangitis**
  ○ Can result in strictures anywhere in biliary tree, but most commonly involves CBD
    - Smooth, long strictures without irregularity
    - Can rarely appear mass-like and mimic tumor (inflammatory pseudotumor)
  ○ Involved bile duct segments demonstrate wall thickening and hyperenhancement on CT/MR
  ○ May be associated with diffuse gallbladder wall thickening
  ○ Frequently associated with other manifestations of IgG4-related sclerosing disease (e.g., autoimmune pancreatitis, retroperitoneal fibrosis, etc.)

- **Radiation Therapy**
  ○ Radiation therapy (when liver is included in radiation portal) can acutely result in radiation-induced hepatitis, and chronically may produce biliary strictures
  ○ Biliary stigmata typically take many years to become apparent (often over 10 years)
  ○ Distribution in liver will depend on which portions of liver exposed to radiation

- **Portal Biliopathy**
  ○ Refers to abnormalities of bile ducts and gallbladder in patients with portal hypertension
  ○ Most commonly results in strictures of CBD, but can result in pruning and strictures of intrahepatic ducts as well
    - Filling defects within ducts may actually represent venous collaterals protruding into duct lumen
  ○ Likely related to ischemic bile duct injury, with biliary abnormalities most commonly present in patients with portal vein occlusion and cavernous transformation

Primary Sclerosing Cholangitis

Primary Sclerosing Cholangitis

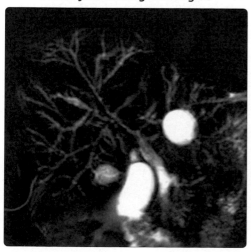

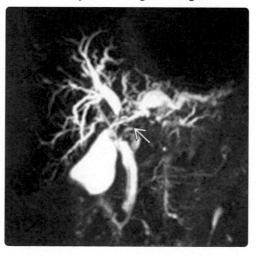

(Left) *Coronal MRCP with MIP reconstruction demonstrates the characteristic appearance of primary sclerosing cholangitis (PSC), with extensive beaded strictures throughout the intrahepatic biliary tree.* **(Right)** *Coronal MRCP with MIP reconstruction demonstrates extensive beading and irregularity of the biliary tree, compatible with the patient's PSC. Note the dominant stricture ➡ involving the proximal common duct and the central right and left hepatic ducts.*

(Left) *Axial CECT in the same patient demonstrates an infiltrating hypodense mass* ➥ *accounting for the dominant stricture, representing a cholangiocarcinoma. Cholangiocarcinoma should always be considered with dominant or new strictures in PSC patients.* **(Right)** *Axial T1 C+ MR in the arterial phase in a patient with cholangitis demonstrates diffusely heterogeneous parenchymal enhancement and dilated bile ducts in the right lobe, which communicate with small abscesses* ➥.

Primary Sclerosing Cholangitis

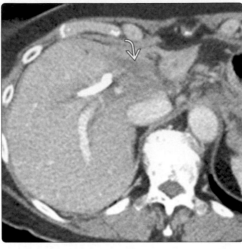

Ascending Cholangitis

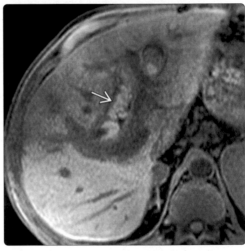

(Left) *Cholangiogram in a liver transplant patient with severe hepatic artery stenosis demonstrates extensive strictures and irregularity of the biliary tree, representing ischemic cholangitis.* **(Right)** *Axial noncontrast T1 MR in a liver transplant patient with hepatic artery thrombosis demonstrates diffuse biliary dilatation due to ischemic cholangiopathy, with T1-hyperintense cast material* ➥ *filling the central bile ducts.*

Posttransplant Liver and Ischemic Cholangiopathy

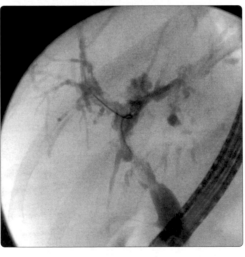

Posttransplant Liver and Ischemic Cholangiopathy

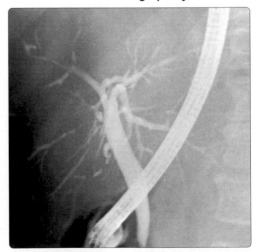

(Left) *ERCP in a patient with AIDS demonstrates extensive beading, irregularity, and strictures of the intrahepatic ducts, as well as dilatation of the common bile duct (CBD), found to represent AIDS cholangiopathy.* **(Right)** *ERCP demonstrates multiple strictures of the intrahepatic ducts, as well as dilatation of the CBD, found to represent AIDS cholangiopathy. The findings in this case are not easily distinguishable from PSC.*

AIDS Cholangiopathy

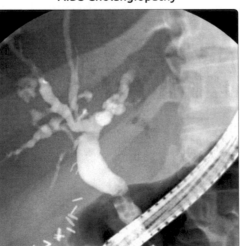

AIDS Cholangiopathy

Cholangiocarcinoma

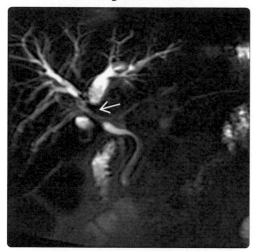

Recurrent Pyogenic Cholangitis

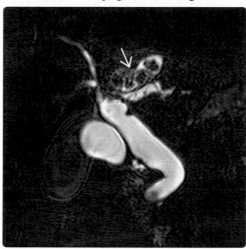

(Left) *Coronal MRCP with MIP reconstruction demonstrates a large stricture* ➡ *involving the CBD and central right/left hepatic ducts, found to be secondary to a large cholangiocarcinoma.* **(Right)** *Coronal MRCP with MIP reconstruction in an Asian patient demonstrates localized dilatation of the left hepatic lobe ducts* ➡ *with multiple low-signal stones filling the dilated ducts, compatible with recurrent pyogenic cholangitis.*

Caroli Disease

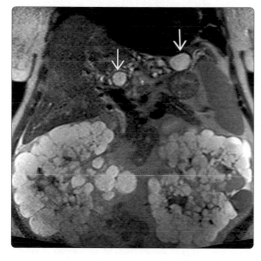

Chemotherapy Cholangitis

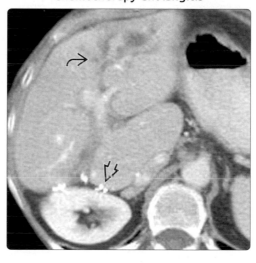

(Left) *Coronal T2 MR demonstrates extensive enlargement of both kidneys with innumerable cysts, compatible with autosomal dominant polycystic disease. There are multiple cysts* ➡ *in the left hepatic lobe communicating with dilated bile ducts, compatible with Caroli disease.* **(Right)** *Axial CECT shows surgical clips* ➦ *from right hepatic lobectomy (for metastases). Irregular dilation of the intrahepatic ducts* ➨ *in this case was the result of hepatic intraarterial chemotherapy.*

Autoimmune (IgG4) Cholangitis

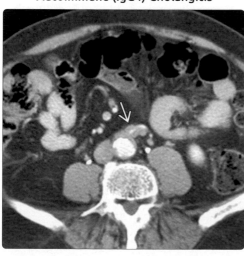

Autoimmune (IgG4) Cholangitis

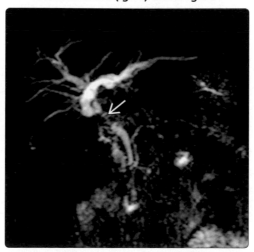

(Left) *Axial CECT demonstrates soft tissue* ➡ *infiltrating along the course of the inferior mesenteric artery, found to represent retroperitoneal fibrosis (RPF).* **(Right)** *Coronal MRCP with MIP reconstruction in the same patient demonstrates a stricture* ➡ *of the proximal common duct with mild upstream intrahepatic biliary dilatation. This was found to represent IgG4 cholangiopathy, which is often associated with other autoimmune diseases (such as RPF).*

DIFFERENTIAL DIAGNOSIS

Common

- Choledocholithiasis
- Pneumobilia
- Susceptibility Artifact (Mimic)
- Contraction of Sphincter of Oddi (Mimic)
- Respiratory Motion Artifact (Mimic)
- Hemobilia
- Portal Vein Gas (Mimic)
- Flow Artifact (Mimic)
- Pulsatile Vascular Compression (Mimic)
- Cystic Duct Insertion (Mimic)

ESSENTIAL INFORMATION

Key Differential Diagnosis Issues

- While MR is most sensitive modality for identifying stones in extrahepatic bile duct, knowledge of common artifacts and pitfalls is critical to avoid misinterpretation
- Optimally, any potential abnormality should be seen on more than 1 pulse sequence to confirm its veracity
- Always be certain to look at thin-section source 3D MRCP images; relying on MIP reconstructions alone increases risk of interpretation error

Helpful Clues for Common Diagnoses

- **Choledocholithiasis**
  - Most common cause of hypointense (signal void) intraductal filling defect on MR
  - Gallstones are typically low signal on all MR pulse sequences, although some pigments stones may rarely demonstrate high T1 signal
  - Typically multiple with stones also usually present in GB
- **Pneumobilia**
  - Gas bubbles appear low signal on all pulse sequences, but float ventrally with air-fluid levels on axial images
  - Be very cognizant of this pitfall in patients who have undergone prior biliary-enteric anastomosis, sphincterotomy, or other biliary intervention
- **Susceptibility Artifact (Mimic)**

- Any metallic foreign body (e.g., surgical clip, coil, stent) or gas-filled structure (e.g., gas in stomach/duodenum) may produce signal void, which might mimic stone
  - Signal void due to susceptibility generally increases in size on in-phase GRE images (which accentuate susceptibility artifacts) compared to opposed phase
  - New titanium surgical clips cause less artifact
- **Contraction of Sphincter of Oddi (Mimic)**
  - Contraction of sphincter with distal narrowing may mimic stone or stricture in the distal CBD
  - Pitfall can be avoided by acquiring several sequential 2D thick-slab MRCP acquisitions to visualize opening of sphincter of Oddi
- **Respiratory Motion Artifact (Mimic)**
  - Suboptimal breath holds may result in signal loss that might theoretically mimic filling defect
- **Hemobilia**
  - Can produce low-signal filling defect
  - Generally occurs due to trauma, intervention, or biliary/hepatic tumors
- **Portal Vein Gas (Mimic)**
  - Particularly on axial images, gas in portal venous system might be be mistaken for pneumobilia or stones
- **Flow Artifact (Mimic)**
  - Very common cause of pseudo filling defect, particularly on any sequence relying on single-shot fast spin echo technique (usually HASTE in abdomen)
  - Filling defect in center of duct (rather than layering dependently), and not present on other sequences
- **Pulsatile Vascular Compression (Mimic)**
  - Arteries (e.g., hepatic, cystic, and gastroduodenal arteries) can compress biliary tree during systole, simulating stricture or filling defect
  - Band of signal loss, rather than discrete filling defect
  - Most commonly seen across common hepatic duct or left hepatic duct due to right hepatic artery
- **Cystic Duct Insertion (Mimic)**
  - When cystic duct is large, redundant, or tortuous, it could mimic presence of filling defect at its site of insertion on common hepatic duct

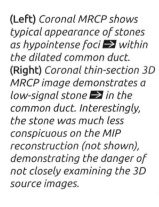

(Left) Coronal MRCP shows typical appearance of stones as hypointense foci ➡ within the dilated common duct. (Right) Coronal thin-section 3D MRCP image demonstrates a low-signal stone ➡ in the common duct. Interestingly, the stone was much less conspicuous on the MIP reconstruction (not shown), demonstrating the danger of not closely examining the 3D source images.

Choledocholithiasis

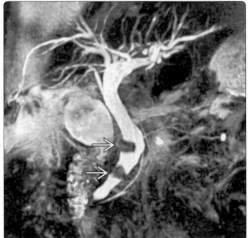

Choledocholithiasis

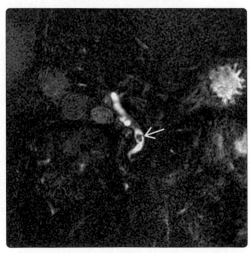

Pneumobilia

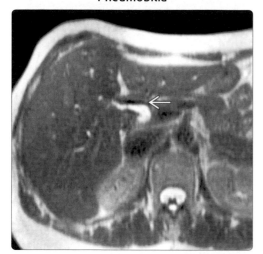

Pneumobilia

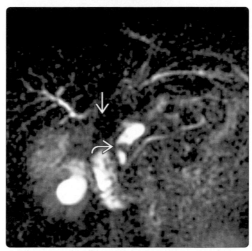

(Left) *Axial T2WI MR shows an air-fluid level within the bile ducts as a signal void* ➡ *with a linear interface with the high-signal bile in the dependent position of the bile duct.* (Right) *Coronal oblique MRCP shows a focal defect in the bile duct that represents a stone* ➡, *but also a broad signal void in the more proximal duct* ➡ *due to pneumobilia.*

Susceptibility Artifact (Mimic)

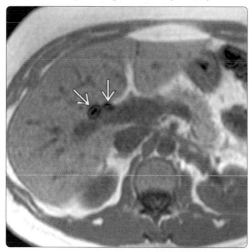

Flow Artifact (Mimic)

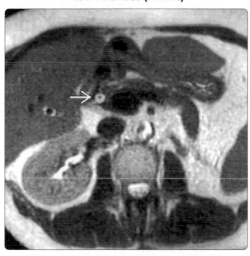

(Left) *Axial T1WI MR in-phase GRE shows 2 hypointense lesions in the porta hepatis caused by cholecystectomy clips* ➡. *These signal voids result from susceptibility artifact.* (Right) *T2 HASTE MR shows a signal void* ➡ *in the center of the bile duct that was not present on the coronal or MRCP sequences. This is a typical flow artifact. As in this case, flow artifacts are much more common with single shot fast spin-echo technique.*

Pulsatile Vascular Compression (Mimic)

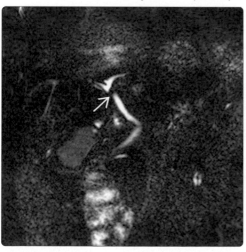

Pulsatile Vascular Compression (Mimic)

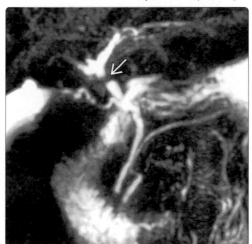

(Left) *Coronal MRCP with MIP reconstruction demonstrates a band-like signal void* ➡ *extending across the proximal common hepatic duct, a classic appearance and location for vascular pulsation artifact.* (Right) *Coronal MRCP shows a signal void* ➡ *in the common hepatic duct due to compression by the hepatic artery that crosses the duct at this level.*

SECTION 12

Pancreas

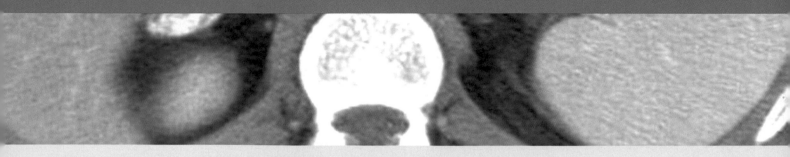

Generic Imaging Patterns

Modality-Specific Imaging Findings

ULTRASOUND

DIFFERENTIAL DIAGNOSIS

Common

- Pancreatic Ductal Adenocarcinoma
- Chronic Pancreatitis
- Normal Anatomic Variants of Pancreas (Mimic)
- Mucinous Cystic Neoplasm
- Peripancreatic Lymphadenopathy (Mimic)
- Unopacified Bowel (Mimic)
- Duodenal Diverticulum (Mimic)

Less Common

- Pancreatic Serous Cystadenoma
- Ampullary Carcinoma
- Pancreatic Metastases and Lymphoma
- Cholangiocarcinoma
- Pancreatic Neuroendocrine Tumor
- Solid Pseudopapillary Neoplasm
- Acute Pancreatitis
- Autoimmune Pancreatitis
- Groove Pancreatitis
- Agenesis of Dorsal Pancreas
- Adjacent Masses (Mimic)
  - Duodenal Carcinoma
  - Gastric Tumors
    - Gastrointestinal Stromal Tumor
  - Carcinoid Tumor
  - Desmoid Tumor
  - Retroperitoneal Sarcoma
  - Retroperitoneal Lymphoma
  - Peripancreatic Vascular Lesions
  - Adrenal Mass
    - Adrenal Carcinoma
    - Pheochromocytoma

Rare but Important

- Schwannoma
- Giant Cell Carcinoma
- Acinar Cell Carcinoma

ESSENTIAL INFORMATION

Key Differential Diagnosis Issues

- Masses that arise from structures adjacent to pancreas may simulate pancreatic mass (e.g., duodenum, adrenal, etc.)
- Pancreatitis may be very difficult to differentiate from ductal adenocarcinoma, including chronic pancreatitis (CP), focal autoimmune pancreatitis, and groove pancreatitis
- Pancreatic adenocarcinoma is most common solid hypovascular pancreatic mass
  - Pancreatic duct obstruction and parenchymal atrophy are very common with ductal adenocarcinoma but less common with other entities in differential diagnosis

Helpful Clues for Common Diagnoses

- **Pancreatic Ductal Adenocarcinoma**
  - Hypodense, poorly marginated mass with tendency to extend posteriorly and involve mesenteric vasculature
  - Usually causes pancreatic duct and biliary obstruction with upstream parenchymal atrophy

- MR: Typically T1 hypointense (compared to high T1 signal of pancreas), variable signal on T2WI, and hypoenhancing on T1 C+ (with delayed enhancement)
  - Commonly metastasizes to liver, peritoneum, and lung
- **Chronic Pancreatitis**
  - May produce fibroinflammatory mass in pancreatic head, appearing identical to ductal adenocarcinoma
    - Can result in double-duct sign similar to malignancy with pancreatic duct and biliary obstruction
    - May require biopsy or imaging surveillance to exclude malignancy
  - Other features of CP include dilated pancreatic duct and parenchymal/intraductal calcifications
  - Gland often appears diffusely atrophic (particularly body), with ↓ T1 signal and ↓ arterial enhancement on MR (with ↑ delayed enhancement)
- **Normal Anatomic Variants of Pancreas (Mimic)**
  - Pancreatic head can appear lobulated and enlarged but probably normal if enhancement is identical to rest of gland with no ductal obstruction
  - Asymmetric fatty infiltration of pancreatic head
    - Most commonly in anterior pancreatic head due to embryologic development of dorsal/ventral pancreas
    - May mimic hypodense mass on CT but sharply demarcated from normal density posterior head and not associated with mass effect or ductal obstruction
    - MR can confirm diagnosis easily with signal loss within "mass" on out-of-phase images
- **Mucinous Cystic Neoplasm**
  - Most often seen in middle-aged women and usually located in pancreatic tail
  - Typically cystic in appearance, but complex mucinous cystic neoplasm with invasive malignancy may show substantial soft tissue component and may mimic solid mass
  - No pancreatic duct communication or obstruction
- **Peripancreatic Lymphadenopathy (Mimic)**
  - Lymphadenopathy abutting pancreas may mimic pancreatic mass, especially metastatic lymphadenopathy from upper abdominal primary tumors
  - Gallbladder cancer classically results in bulky peripancreatic adenopathy and biliary obstruction, which can be mistaken for pancreatic cancer
- **Unopacified Bowel (Mimic)**
  - Collapsed duodenum/jejunum may mimic mass
- **Duodenal Diverticulum (Mimic)**
  - Diverticulum can abut pancreas and mimic hypodense mass (particularly when filled with fluid or debris)

Helpful Clues for Less Common Diagnoses

- **Pancreatic Serous Cystadenoma**
  - Lesions with preponderance of septations can appear solid without apparent microcystic component
    - Lesions can appear hypovascular or hypervascular
  - Lesions appear well circumscribed with lobulated contour and peripheral vascularity ± central calcification
- **Ampullary Carcinoma**
  - May not be easily distinguishable from pancreatic head adenocarcinoma
  - Can produce double-duct sign, although pancreatic duct only obstructed in ~ 50%

- o Usually does not cause upstream pancreatic atrophy
- **Pancreatic Metastases and Lymphoma**
  - o Melanoma, lung, and breast are most common hypovascular metastases to pancreas
    - – Lack of ductal obstruction and presence of primary tumor should suggest correct diagnosis
  - o Primary lymphoma of pancreas is very rare, but pancreas can be secondarily involved in generalized lymphoma
    - – Vessels surrounded by tumor without attenuation or narrowing (unlike ductal adenocarcinoma)
    - – Bulky lymphadenopathy almost always present
- **Cholangiocarcinoma**
  - o May not be easily distinguishable from pancreatic head adenocarcinoma or ampullary carcinoma
  - o Obstructs bile duct, but usually no pancreatic ductal obstruction or pancreatic atrophy
  - o Can present as discrete mass or as focal common bile duct (CBD) wall thickening
- **Pancreatic Neuroendocrine Tumor**
  - o Usually hypervascular but rarely hypovascular
  - o Tumors may calcify or invade mesenteric veins, features uncommon with ductal adenocarcinoma
  - o Do not typically obstruct pancreatic duct or CBD
- **Solid Pseudopapillary Neoplasm**
  - o Typically well circumscribed, solid, and hypovascular but can demonstrate cystic component ± internal hemorrhage
  - o Almost always diagnosed in young female patients
- **Acute Pancreatitis**
  - o Focal inflammation or necrosis can be mass-like and mimic tumor
  - o Tumor typically infiltrates posteriorly into retroperitoneum, whereas pancreatitis almost always infiltrates anteriorly into mesentery
  - o Presence of dilated pancreatic duct or CBD should raise concern for malignancy
  - o Pancreatic cancer can rarely (~ 5%) present with pancreatitis, so equivocal cases may require short-interval follow-up or endoscopic US
- **Autoimmune Pancreatitis**

- o Most often presents with diffuse pancreatic involvement, including sausage-like enlargement of pancreas, hypodense halo around pancreas, and lack of peripancreatic inflammation
- o Can rarely present as focal "mass"
- o Does not usually obstruct pancreatic duct or CBD, although IgG4 cholangiopathy can cause biliary dilatation
- **Groove Pancreatitis**
  - o Form of CP that results in sheet-like, curvilinear soft tissue thickening (+ cystic change) in pancreaticoduodenal groove
  - o Can result in mild pancreatic or biliary ductal dilatation
  - o Difficult to differentiate from pancreatic or duodenal malignancy, and may require surgery for diagnosis
- **Agenesis of Dorsal Pancreas**
  - o Pancreatic head may be hypertrophied (mimicking mass), while absent body/tail may be mistaken for atrophy upstream from mass
  - o May also mimic mass on ERCP, as injection of ventral duct ends abruptly at head
- **Adjacent Masses (Mimic)**
  - o **Duodenal carcinoma**
    - – Can be difficult to differentiate from pancreatic adenocarcinoma but does not usually cause pancreatic duct obstruction or parenchymal atrophy

Helpful Clues for Rare Diagnoses

- **Schwannoma**
  - o Well-circumscribed, homogeneous mass (± cystic change)
  - o Variable enhancement, but most often mildly hypervascular (mimicking neuroendocrine tumor)
- **Giant Cell Carcinoma**
  - o Large, heterogeneous, hypodense mass most often arising from pancreatic body/tail
- **Acinar Cell Carcinoma**
  - o Large, well-circumscribed mass with cystic/necrotic degeneration and frequent exophytic component
  - o Does not usually cause pancreatic duct or CBD dilatation
  - o More often confused with neuroendocrine tumors due to well-circumscribed margins and enhancement

Pancreatic Ductal Adenocarcinoma

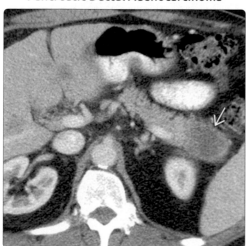

Pancreatic Ductal Adenocarcinoma

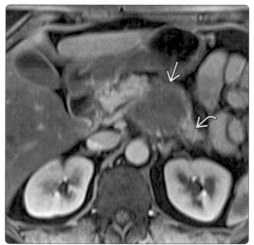

(Left) Axial CECT demonstrates a poorly marginated, hypodense mass ➡ in the pancreatic tail, characteristic of pancreatic adenocarcinoma. (Right) Axial T1 C+ MR in the arterial phase demonstrates a hypodense, poorly enhancing mass ➡ in the body/tail with associated severe upstream pancreatic atrophy ➹, compatible with pancreatic adenocarcinoma.

Chronic Pancreatitis

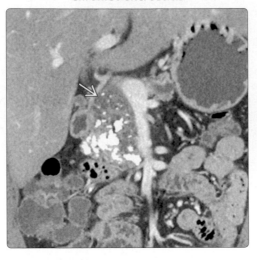

Chronic Pancreatitis

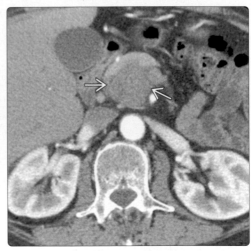

(Left) *Coronal CECT demonstrates a large, hypodense mass* ➡ *in the pancreatic head with extensive internal calcifications, compatible with a fibroinflammatory mass related to chronic pancreatitis (CP). Close surveillance or biopsy may be necessary to exclude malignancy.* (Right) *Axial CECT demonstrates a hypodense mass* ➡ *in the pancreatic head/uncinate. Although thought to be a pancreatic adenocarcinoma, this was found to be a fibroinflammatory mass related to CP at resection.*

Normal Anatomic Variants of Pancreas (Mimic)

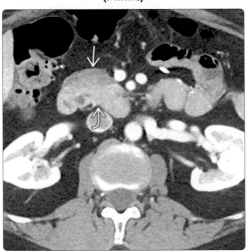

Mucinous Cystic Neoplasm

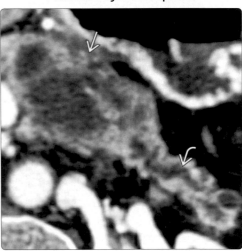

(Left) *Axial CECT demonstrates the characteristic appearance of focal fatty infiltration of the dorsal anlage. Note the low-density area in the anterior head* ➡ *(without ductal dilatation) clearly demarcated from the normal-appearing posterior head* ➡. (Right) *Axial CECT demonstrates an MCN with malignant degeneration. The mass* ➡ *itself appears predominantly cystic with clear solid components and results in upstream ductal dilatation* ➡ *and atrophy, features strongly suggestive of malignancy.*

Peripancreatic Lymphadenopathy (Mimic)

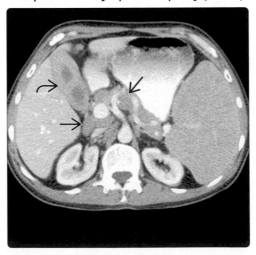

Pancreatic Serous Cystadenoma

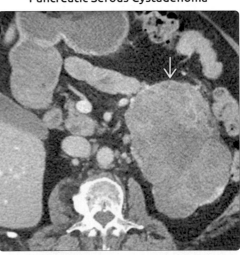

(Left) *Axial CECT shows hypodense masses* ➡ *surrounding the pancreas, gallbladder wall thickening* ➡, *and splenomegaly. This was found to be non-Hodgkin lymphoma with peripancreatic lymphadenopathy.* (Right) *Axial CECT demonstrates a lobulated, well-circumscribed mass* ➡ *arising from the pancreatic tail. The mass appears relatively solid, with some subtle internal cystic components. This represents a serous cystadenoma, which can appear solid when septations predominate over cystic components.*

Ampullary Carcinoma

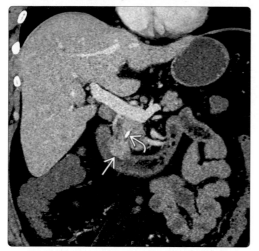

Pancreatic Metastases and Lymphoma

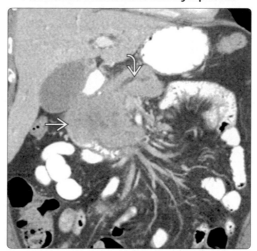

(Left) *Coronal CECT demonstrates a hypodense mass ➡ centered near the ampulla, found to be an ampullary carcinoma at resection. A biliary stent ➡ is partially visualized.* (Right) *Coronal CECT demonstrates a hypodense mass ➡ in the pancreatic head resulting in mild obstruction of the pancreatic duct ➡. This is an unusual case of pancreatic lymphoma, which does not usually obstruct the common bile duct (CBD) or pancreatic duct, and is usually associated with more significant lymphadenopathy.*

Pancreatic Metastases and Lymphoma

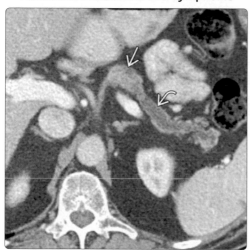

Pancreatic Metastases and Lymphoma

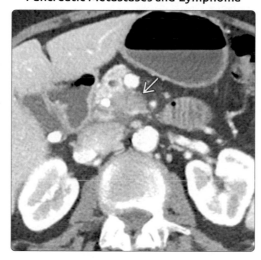

(Left) *Axial CECT demonstrates a small pancreatic mass ➡ causing pancreatic duct dilatation ➡ and atrophy. Originally thought to be adenocarcinoma, this was found to be a colon cancer metastasis. Metastases do not usually obstruct the pancreatic duct.* (Right) *Axial CECT demonstrates an infiltrative hypodense mass ➡ in the uncinate process. While pancreatic adenocarcinoma could appear virtually identical, this lesion represents a metastasis from the patient's breast cancer.*

Pancreatic Metastases and Lymphoma

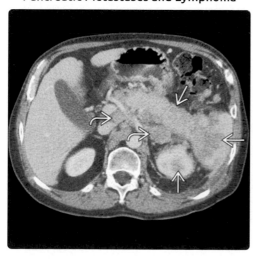

Cholangiocarcinoma

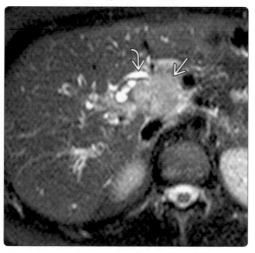

(Left) *Axial CECT shows a diffuse hypodense mass that infiltrates pancreas ➡, spleen, kidney, and left adrenal gland. Note the presence of extensive retroperitoneal lymphadenopathy ➡, which suggests the correct diagnosis of non-Hodgkin lymphoma.* (Right) *Axial T2 FS MR demonstrates T2-hyperintense mass ➡ obstructing distal CBD ➡, found to be distal cholangiocarcinoma (CCA) at resection. Distal CCA is sometimes difficult to differentiate from pancreatic head adenocarcinoma or ampullary carcinoma.*

Solid Pseudopapillary Neoplasm

Acute Pancreatitis

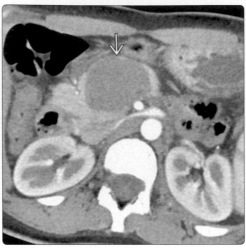

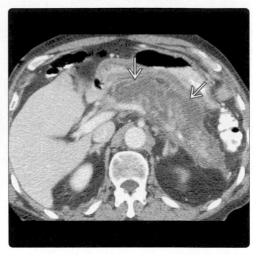

(Left) *Axial CECT in a young female patient demonstrates a well-circumscribed, hypodense mass* ➡ *in the pancreas, a typical appearance of a solid pseudopapillary tumor.* (Right) *Axial CECT shows a heterogeneous, hypodense, mass-like enlargement* ➡ *of the pancreas due to necrotizing pancreatitis. Such patients are invariably very ill with metabolic derangements that help to distinguish them from patients with an infiltrating carcinoma of the pancreas.*

Autoimmune Pancreatitis

Autoimmune Pancreatitis

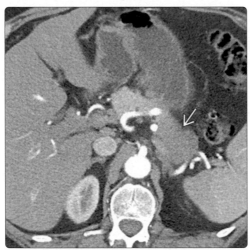

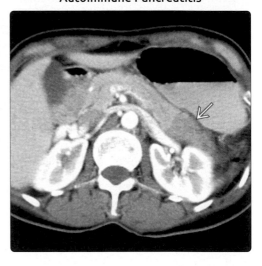

(Left) *Axial CECT demonstrates a focal hypodense mass* ➡ *in the pancreatic tail. While virtually indistinguishable from an adenocarcinoma on imaging, this was found to be focal autoimmune pancreatitis at resection.* (Right) *Axial CECT shows a hypodense "mass"* ➡ *in the pancreatic tail. The presence of an elevated serum IgG4 and resolution of all imaging findings with steroid medication confirmed the diagnosis of autoimmune pancreatitis.*

Groove Pancreatitis

Groove Pancreatitis

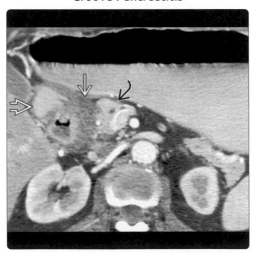

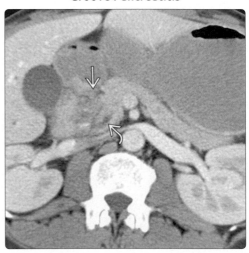

(Left) *Axial CECT demonstrates a hypodense, sheet-like mass* ➡ *in groove between the pancreatic head* ➡ *& 2nd portion of duodenum* ➡*, along with gastric outlet obstruction due to duodenal luminal stricture. These findings are classic for groove pancreatitis.* (Right) *Axial CECT demonstrates sheet-like soft tissue* ➡ *centered in the pancreaticoduodenal groove with mild dilatation of the pancreatic duct* ➡*. Virtually impossible to differentiate from malignancy, this was found to be groove pancreatitis at resection.*

Duodenal Carcinoma

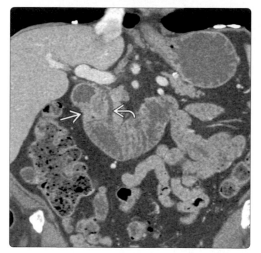

Gastrointestinal Stromal Tumor

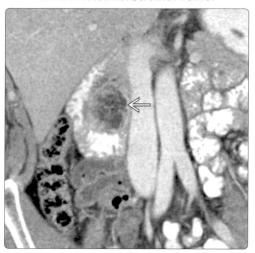

(Left) *Coronal CECT demonstrates an annular constricting mass ➡ in the duodenum resulting in mild CBD dilatation ➡, found to be a duodenal adenocarcinoma at resection.* **(Right)** *Coronal CECT demonstrates a hypodense mass ➡ centered between the duodenum and pancreatic head, mimicking a primary pancreatic mass. This was found to be a duodenal gastrointestinal stromal tumor at resection.*

Retroperitoneal Sarcoma

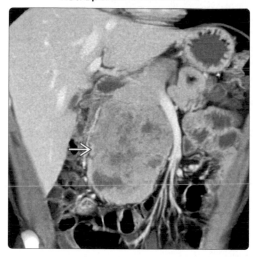

Adrenal Carcinoma

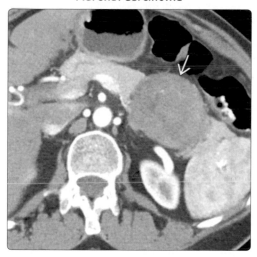

(Left) *Coronal CECT demonstrates a large, mixed solid & cystic mass ➡ in the retroperitoneum, abutting the pancreatic head but with an intervening fat plane. In cases like this with large masses, the site of origin can be difficult to determine, but this was a primary retroperitoneal sarcoma arising from the IVC.* **(Right)** *Axial CECT shows a large, hypodense mass ➡ centered near pancreatic tail. While originally thought to be a primary pancreatic mass, this was found at resection to be an adrenal carcinoma abutting the pancreas.*

Pheochromocytoma

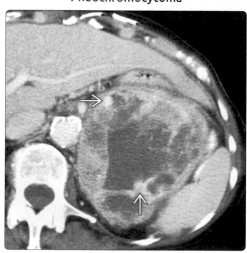

Acinar Cell Carcinoma

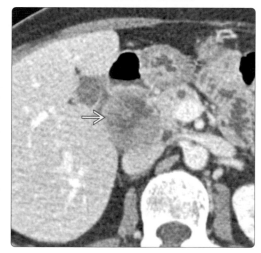

(Left) *Axial CECT shows a heterogeneous left upper quadrant mass with extensive necrosis but foci of hypervascularity ➡. This mass simulates a GIST or pancreatic mass but is a large adrenal pheochromocytoma.* **(Right)** *Axial CECT demonstrates a well-circumscribed, hypodense mass ➡ in the pancreatic head. This was found to be an acinar cell carcinoma at resection. These lesions are very difficult to prospectively differentiate from an adenocarcinoma or neuroendocrine tumor.*

DIFFERENTIAL DIAGNOSIS

Common

- Pancreatic Neuroendocrine Tumor

Less Common

- Pancreatic Metastases
- Pancreatic Serous Cystadenoma
- Accessory Spleen (Mimic)
- Peripancreatic Vascular Abnormalities
- Retroperitoneal Paraganglioma (Mimic)
- Adrenal Pheochromocytoma (Mimic)
- Renal Cell Carcinoma (Mimic)
- Gastrointestinal Stromal Tumor (Mimic)
- Carcinoid Tumor (Mimic)
- Splenic Tumors (Mimic)

Rare but Important

- Acinar Cell Carcinoma
- Pancreatic Schwannoma
- Solitary Fibrous Tumor

ESSENTIAL INFORMATION

Key Differential Diagnosis Issues

- Differentiate true pancreatic masses from lesions originating from adjacent organs (stomach, spleen, adrenal, kidney)
  - Look for plane of demarcation separating mass and pancreas
    - Multiplanar reformations and curved planar reconstructions may be helpful for identifying true origin of lesion
  - Distinction between pancreatic and peripancreatic masses not always possible with certainty, although making distinction prospectively may not alter surgical treatment
- Vast majority of hypervascular lesions truly arising from pancreas itself represent neuroendocrine tumors
  - Consider possibility of neuroendocrine tumor strongly in patients with predisposing syndromes, including multiple endocrine neoplasia type I, von Hippel-Lindau syndrome, and tuberous sclerosis
- While pancreatic neuroendocrine tumors are more common, always consider metastases in patients with history of renal cell carcinoma (RCC) or prior nephrectomy
  - RCC can metastasize to pancreas many years after initial surgical resection of renal tumor
- Always consider possibility of benign accessory spleen when confronted with hypervascular lesion near pancreatic tail, and recommend nuclear medicine study (Tc-99m heat-denatured RBC study) in equivocal cases

Helpful Clues for Common Diagnoses

- **Pancreatic Neuroendocrine Tumor**
  - Can be benign or malignant, but much better prognosis compared to pancreatic adenocarcinoma
  - Now divided into syndromic and nonsyndromic tumors depending on whether lesion produces clinical syndrome due to hormone secretion
    - Syndromic tumors (such as insulinomas, gastrinomas, glucagonomas, etc.) tend to be smaller (< 3 cm) at presentation
    - Nonsyndromic tumors are often larger and more heterogeneous/aggressive in appearance with more frequent necrosis, cystic change, and calcification
  - Well-circumscribed hypervascular mass with noninfiltrative margins and frequent internal calcifications (either central or diffuse)
    - Usually avidly vascular and typically most conspicuous on arterial phase, but can, in atypical cases, be more evident on venous phase or appear hypodense
    - Cystic and necrotic change more common with larger tumors
      □ Tumors can rarely appear primarily cystic (with peripheral mural enhancement) and mimic other cystic pancreatic neoplasms
    - Most often no biliary or pancreatic ductal obstruction unless lesion is large or in rare cases where tumors secrete hormones (such as serotonin) that result in ductal stricture
    - May invade (rather than encase) mesenteric veins
    - Metastases (most often liver and lymph nodes) have similar imaging characteristics to primary tumor
      □ Liver metastases may be very T2 hyperintense on MR (mimicking cysts or hemangiomas) and demonstrate internal fluid-fluid levels on T2WI MR

Helpful Clues for Less Common Diagnoses

- **Pancreatic Metastases**
  - RCC most common source of hypervascular metastases to pancreas
  - Patients may present with pancreatic metastases from RCC many years after nephrectomy
  - Indistinguishable from neuroendocrine tumors in absence of history
  - Does not commonly obstruct pancreatic duct
  - Isolated RCC metastasis to pancreas may be amenable to surgical resection
- **Pancreatic Serous Cystadenoma**
  - Classic microcystic or sponge lesion is mass with multiple internal enhancing septations, multiple (> 6) small internal cystic spaces, and central calcification
  - Lesions with extensive internal septations that predominate over cystic spaces may appear solid and avidly enhancing (i.e., solid serous adenoma) without appreciable cystic component
    - May have central scar with calcification (similar to classic microcystic serous cystadenoma)
    - Does not usually obstruct pancreatic duct
    - Often associated with considerable neovascularity, including hypertrophied feeding vessels draped around margins of mass
    - MR might be able to better demonstrate internal cystic component or microcystic architecture in some cases
- **Accessory Spleen (Mimic)**
  - Benign ectopic splenic tissue of congenital origin usually located near splenic hilum
  - Pancreatic tail is 2nd most common location for splenules (20% of cases)
    - Usually located < 3 cm from pancreatic tail

- Diagnosis usually easier with multiphase imaging, as splenule should follow enhancement pattern of normal spleen on all phases
  - Arterial phase often most valuable, as splenules demonstrate serpiginous differential enhancement of red and white pulp (similar to normal spleen)
  - Should follow signal of normal spleen on all MR pulse sequences
  - Can be differentiated from other masses due to their uptake of radiotracer on either Tc-99m sulfur colloid or Tc-99m heat-denatured RBC scans
- **Peripancreatic Vascular Abnormalities**
  - Splenic artery aneurysms or pseudoaneurysms may mimic vascular mass
    - Should follow blood pool on all phases
  - Large splenic or portal vein abutting pancreas or varices (in cirrhosis/portal hypertension) may superficially mimic pancreatic mass
- **Retroperitoneal Paraganglioma (Mimic)**
  - Neuroendocrine tumors arising from autonomic nervous system most often seen in young and middle-aged patients
  - Avidly enhancing retroperitoneal (extrapancreatic) mass that may abut pancreas and mimic primary pancreatic mass
- **Adrenal Pheochromocytoma (Mimic)**
  - Pheochromocytoma arising from left adrenal gland may abut pancreatic tail and mimic hypervascular pancreatic mass
  - Lesions avidly enhance and classically demonstrate Hounsfield attenuation > 100 on arterial-phase images
- **Renal Cell Carcinoma (Mimic)**
  - Masses (especially clear cell variant of RCC) arising from upper pole of kidney may simulate primary pancreatic mass
- **Gastrointestinal Stromal Tumor (Mimic)**
  - From stomach or duodenum may simulate mass in pancreatic body or head
  - Variable enhancement, but some lesions can appear markedly vascular and hyperenhancing

- **Carcinoid Tumor (Mimic)**
  - Lesion arising from duodenum or ampulla, or mesenteric metastasis abutting pancreas, may mimic pancreatic mass
  - Usually avidly vascular with arterial-phase hyperenhancement and frequent hypervascular locoregional lymphadenopathy
- **Splenic Tumors (Mimic)**
  - Hemangioma, angiosarcoma, or hypervascular metastases to splenic hilum could simulate mass in pancreatic tail

Helpful Clues for Rare Diagnoses

- **Acinar Cell Carcinoma**
  - Very rare pancreatic tumor that may be associated with hypersecretion of lipase and unique clinical syndrome (skin rashes, arthralgias, fevers, and fat necrosis)
  - Typically large (average > 6 cm) well-defined mass with enhancing capsule and tendency to exophytically extend from pancreas
    - Does not typically obstruct common bile duct or pancreatic duct
  - Variable enhancement but may be hypovascular or hypervascular
  - Commonly demonstrates internal hemorrhage, necrosis, and cystic degeneration
  - Most often confused for neuroendocrine tumors on imaging
- **Pancreatic Schwannoma**
  - Rare, typically benign mass that may be of pancreatic or peripancreatic origin
  - Well-circumscribed mass that is typically mildly hypervascular (albeit less vascular than neuroendocrine tumors)
  - May show internal cystic or necrotic change
- **Solitary Fibrous Tumor**
  - Rare, usually benign tumor that appears large, exophytic, and hypervascular
  - May demonstrate calcification, cystic change, or necrosis
  - Indistinguishable from pancreatic neuroendocrine tumor

Pancreatic Neuroendocrine Tumor

Pancreatic Neuroendocrine Tumor

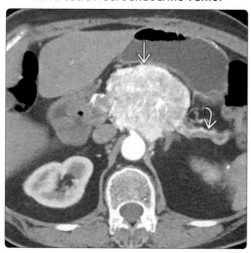

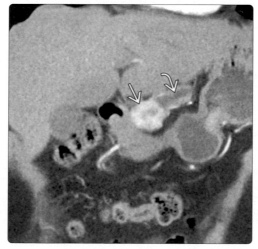

(Left) Axial CECT in the arterial phase demonstrates a markedly hypervascular mass ➡ arising from the pancreatic body, compatible with a neuroendocrine tumor. Note the upstream atrophy ⇗ of the pancreas, a relatively unusual feature for neuroendocrine tumors. (Right) Coronal CECT in the arterial phase demonstrates an avidly enhancing pancreatic neuroendocrine tumor ➡. The pancreatic duct ⇗ is obstructed by the mass, an unusual feature for neuroendocrine tumors.

Pancreatic Neuroendocrine Tumor

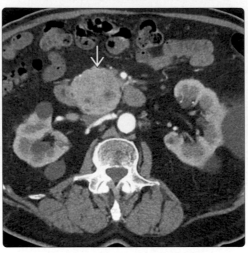

Pancreatic Neuroendocrine Tumor

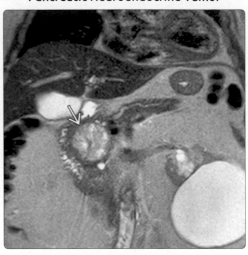

(Left) *Axial CECT demonstrates an avidly enhancing neuroendocrine tumor* ➡ *in the pancreatic head. These lesions are almost always most conspicuous in the arterial phase of enhancement.* (Right) *Coronal T2 HASTE MR in the same patient demonstrates that the mass* ➡ *is T2 hyperintense. Neuroendocrine tumors on MR imaging tend to be T1 hypointense and T2 hyperintense with similar enhancement characteristics on post gadolinium images compared to CT.*

Pancreatic Neuroendocrine Tumor

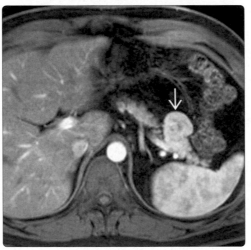

Pancreatic Neuroendocrine Tumor

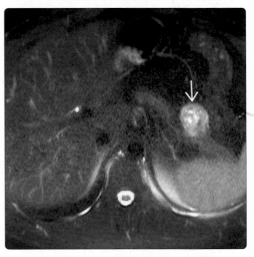

(Left) *Axial T1 C+ MR demonstrates an avidly enhancing mass* ➡ *in the pancreatic tail, found to be an insulinoma in a patient with classic symptoms of Whipple triad. As with CT, these tumors tend to be most conspicuous on the arterial phase of enhancement on MR.* (Right) *Axial T2 FS MR in the same patient demonstrates that the mass* ➡ *is moderately T2 hyperintense.*

Pancreatic Metastases

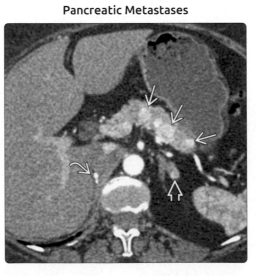

Pancreatic Metastases

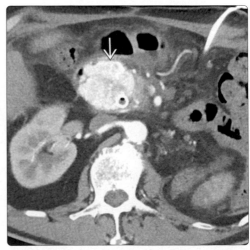

(Left) *Axial CECT in the arterial phase demonstrates multiple hypervascular lesions in the pancreas* ➡. *While these could represent multiple neuroendocrine tumors, absence of the right kidney* ➡ *suggests the correct diagnosis of metastatic renal cell carcinoma (RCC). Note additional metastasis to left adrenal gland* ➡. (Right) *Axial CECT demonstrates a large hypervascular mass* ➡ *in the pancreatic head. The clue to the diagnosis in this case is the absent left kidney, suggesting this mass represents a metastasis from RCC.*

Pancreatic Serous Cystadenoma

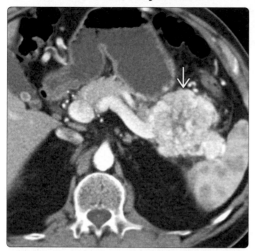

Accessory Spleen (Mimic)

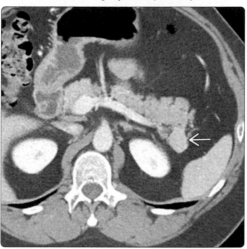

(Left) *Axial CECT demonstrates a large hypervascular mass* ➔ *arising from the pancreatic tail with a central scar. Indistinguishable from a neuroendocrine tumor, this was found to be a solid serous cystadenoma at resection.* (Right) *Axial CECT demonstrates an enhancing mass* ➔ *abutting the pancreatic tail. While a neuroendocrine tumor is a theoretical possibility, notice that the lesion demonstrates identical enhancement to the adjacent spleen, in keeping with a benign splenule.*

Retroperitoneal Paraganglioma (Mimic)

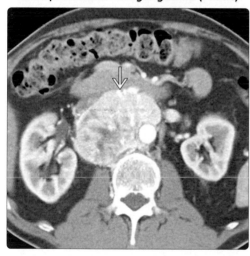

Gastrointestinal Stromal Tumor (Mimic)

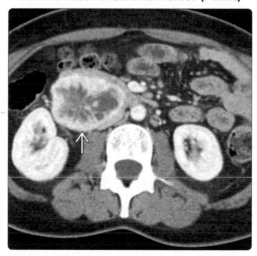

(Left) *Axial CECT demonstrates a hypervascular mass* ➔ *in the retroperitoneum. Note that the mass abuts the pancreas but does not appear to be arising from the pancreas itself. This was found to be a paraganglioma at resection.* (Right) *Axial CECT demonstrates a hypervascular mass* ➔ *near the pancreatic head. While the mass does abut the pancreas, the mass was prospectively thought to be of duodenal origin. The mass was found to be a duodenal gastrointestinal stromal tumor at resection.*

Carcinoid Tumor (Mimic)

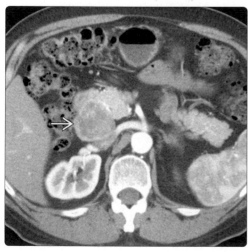

Acinar Cell Carcinoma

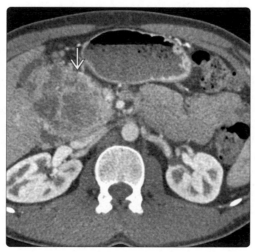

(Left) *Axial CECT demonstrates a hypervascular mass* ➔ *abutting the pancreatic head. On careful examination, the mass arises from the duodenum (not the pancreas) and was found to be a duodenal carcinoid tumor at resection.* (Right) *Axial CECT demonstrates an enhancing mass* ➔ *in the pancreatic head with internal necrosis. While a neuroendocrine tumor was prospectively thought to be most likely, this was found to represent a rare acinar cell carcinoma at resection.*

DIFFERENTIAL DIAGNOSIS

Common

- Intraductal Papillary Mucinous Neoplasm
- Pancreatic Pseudocyst
- Pancreatic Serous Cystadenoma
- Mucinous Cystic Neoplasm
- Lesser Sac Ascites (Mimic)
- Duodenal Diverticulum (Mimic)

Less Common

- Solid Pseudopapillary Neoplasm
- Pancreatic Neuroendocrine Tumor
- Pancreatic Ductal Adenocarcinoma
- Nonneoplastic Pancreatic Cysts
  - Autosomal Dominant Polycystic Disease
  - Cystic Fibrosis
  - Von Hippel-Lindau Disease
- Lymphoepithelial Cyst
- Pseudoaneurysm (Mimic)
- Portal Vein Aneurysm (Mimic)
- Metastases and Lymphoma
- Gastrointestinal Stromal Tumor (Mimic)
- Choledochal Cyst (Mimic)

Rare but Important

- Hydatid Cyst
- Retroperitoneal Teratoma
- Duodenal Duplication Cyst

ESSENTIAL INFORMATION

Key Differential Diagnosis Issues

- Pancreatic cystic lesions are increasingly being discovered incidentally due to widespread use of CT and MR
- In many (but not all) cases, making specific diagnosis based on imaging alone may not be possible
  - Clinical history, demographics, and imaging must be used in conjunction to narrow differential diagnosis
    - Age and sex (e.g., young woman: Solid pseudopapillary neoplasm)
    - History of prior pancreatitis or imaging stigmata of chronic pancreatitis (suggestive of pseudocyst)
    - Location of lesion [e.g., body/tail for mucinous cystic neoplasm (MCN)]
    - Communication with pancreatic duct [favors intraductal papillary mucinous neoplasm (IPMN)]
    - Calcification within lesion (e.g., central calcification in serous cystadenoma)
    - Mural nodularity (worrisome for invasive malignancy)
  - Endoscopic US now routinely used in lesions judged to be at high risk based on CT/MR, providing high-resolution images of internal cyst architecture, facilitating cyst aspiration
- Pseudocysts are uncommon in absence of clear history of pancreatitis, and all cystic masses should therefore be considered potential neoplasms

Helpful Clues for Common Diagnoses

- **Intraductal Papillary Mucinous Neoplasm**
  - Most common in elderly men (50-70 years)

  - Side-branch IPMN: Well-defined cystic lesion communicating with main pancreatic duct (MPD), which can be unilocular, multilocular, or tubular
    - Identifying communication of cyst with MPD is key to diagnosis and can be easier on MR
    - Mural nodularity suggests invasive malignancy; dilatation of MPD suggests main duct involvement
    - Often multiple, with presence of multiple pancreatic cysts strongly suggesting multifocal IPMN
  - Main-duct IPMN: Dilated (either segmental or diffuse), tortuous main pancreatic duct, which may demonstrate internal mural nodularity or calcification
    - ↑ risk of malignancy compared with side-branch IPMN
  - Combined-type IPMN: Cystic lesion in communication with dilated main pancreatic duct
- **Pancreatic Pseudocyst**
  - Uncommon in absence of known history of pancreatitis or imaging features of chronic pancreatitis
  - Usually well-defined cystic lesion with clearly demarcated wall (± peripheral calcification)
  - Lesions adjacent to pancreas may demonstrate residual communication with pancreatic duct
  - May have internal septations but should not demonstrate mural nodularity or soft tissue component
- **Pancreatic Serous Cystadenoma**
  - Benign pancreatic tumor, which is most common in older women and is almost always incidentally identified
    - Most common in pancreatic head
  - 3 primary morphologic patterns
    - Microcystic adenoma: Honeycomb pattern with many (> 6) small (< 2 cm) internal cysts, enhancing septations, and central scar with calcification
    - Macrocystic serous cystadenoma: Oligocystic variant with few (or none) internal septations
      □ Difficult to distinguish from MCN
    - "Solid" serous adenoma: Internal septations predominate over cystic component, producing apparently solid, hypervascular mass
  - Easier diagnosis on MR, which better delineates internal septations and microcystic morphology
- **Mucinous Cystic Neoplasm**
  - Almost always occurs in middle-aged women (99%)
  - "Macrocystic" lesion, which is either unilocular or composed of few (< 6) large (> 2 cm) locules
    - Most common in body or tail segments; may have calcification at periphery or in septations; thick wall, mural nodularity, or thick septations raise suspicion for malignancy
  - No communication with pancreatic duct (unlike IPMN)
- **Lesser Sac Ascites (Mimic)**
  - Most commonly seen in setting of acute pancreatitis, gastric ulcer, peritonitis, or peritoneal carcinomatosis; nonloculated fluid without definable wall bounded only by ligamentous margins of lesser sac
- **Duodenal Diverticulum (Mimic)**
  - Fluid-filled diverticulum arising from 2nd or 3rd portions of duodenum may simulate pancreatic head cyst, particularly when completely filled with fluid (without gas or enteric contrast)

Helpful Clues for Less Common Diagnoses

- **Solid Pseudopapillary Neoplasm**

- o Almost always in young women under 35 years of age
- o Well-defined, encapsulated mass, which is most often solid but can demonstrate variable internal cystic components and internal hemorrhage
  - Frequent peripheral or central calcification (~ 50%); internal hemorrhage very characteristic and usually easiest to appreciate on MR
- **Pancreatic Neuroendocrine Tumor**
  - o Some tumors can appear nearly completely cystic and can closely mimic other pancreatic cystic neoplasms
    - Presence of mural nodularity or peripheral rim of hypervascularity on arterial-phase images should strongly suggest this diagnosis
  - o Larger tumors more likely to demonstrate cystic or necrotic degeneration
- **Pancreatic Ductal Adenocarcinoma**
  - o Very rarely cystic, although hypovascular or necrotic tumors may simulate cystic mass; tumors arising from underlying IPMN may demonstrate associated cystic component
- **Nonneoplastic Pancreatic Cysts**
  - o Relatively rare in absence of predisposing syndrome and in such cases may not be easily distinguished from pancreatic cystic neoplasms
    - Usually simple in appearance without mural nodularity or other suspicious imaging features; do not typically communicate with pancreatic duct
  - o Most common predisposing syndromes include
    - **Autosomal dominant polycystic disease**: Multiple asymptomatic cysts in pancreas and other organs (kidneys, liver)
    - **Cystic fibrosis**: Pancreas can demonstrate 1 or multiple cysts (usually later in disease course)
    - **Von Hippel-Lindau disease**: Pancreas can demonstrate small, simple pancreatic cysts, as well as ↑ prevalence of serous cystadenoma
- **Lymphoepithelial Cyst**
  - o Rare benign cysts, which typically occur in older men
  - o Classically described as being complex in appearance with internal loculations and calcification

- May demonstrate internal macroscopic or microscopic fat (usually easier to appreciate on MR)
- o Can appear extrapancreatic (abutting pancreas) or exophytic
- **Pseudoaneurysm (Mimic)**
  - o Thrombosed pseudoaneurysm arising from splenic or gastroduodenal artery can mimic cystic pancreatic mass (particularly when no residual internal flow)
- **Portal Vein Aneurysm (Mimic)**
  - o Portal vein can be markedly dilated, usually due to portal hypertension, and thrombosis of portal vein can theoretically simulate cystic mass in pancreas
- **Metastases and Lymphoma**
  - o Lymphoma is rarely truly cystic (in absence of treatment), although hypodense lymph nodes abutting pancreas can superficially mimic cystic lesion; metastases to pancreas or adjacent lymph nodes may appear cystic depending on primary tumor type
- **Gastrointestinal Stromal Tumor (Mimic)**
  - o Lesions arising exophytically from stomach or duodenum may simulate pancreatic mass; can appear cystic, necrotic
- **Choledochal Cyst (Mimic)**
  - o Cystic dilation of common bile duct (CBD) can simulate cystic pancreatic lesion, including fusiform dilatation of CBD itself or diverticulum arising from CBD; cystic lesion should be in contiguity with CBD, often easier to appreciate on MR/MRCP, not CT

Helpful Clues for Rare Diagnoses

- **Hydatid Cyst**
  - o Very rare diagnosis, even in endemic areas, although similar imaging features to hydatid cysts elsewhere; cystic mass, which may demonstrate multiple internal cysts (daughter cysts), serpiginous internal bands (water lily sign), or peripheral/internal calcification
- **Retroperitoneal Teratoma**
  - o Mature teratomas may appear primarily cystic but often demonstrate macroscopic fat or calcification
- **Duodenal Duplication Cyst**
  - o Most often arise along medial wall of 2nd/3rd duodenum, potentially mimicking pancreatic head cyst

Intraductal Papillary Mucinous Neoplasm

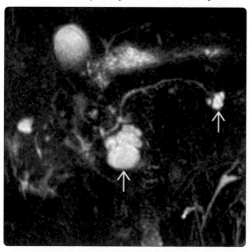

Intraductal Papillary Mucinous Neoplasm

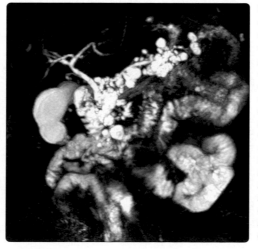

(Left) Coronal MRCP with MIP reconstruction demonstrates 2 cystic lesions ➡ directly communicating with the pancreatic duct in the head and tail, compatible with side-branch intraductal papillary mucinous neoplasms (IPMNs). MRCP is the best radiologic modality to demonstrate communication of a cyst with the pancreatic duct. (Right) Coronal MRCP with MIP reconstruction demonstrates innumerable pancreatic cysts replacing the entire pancreas, compatible with multifocal IPMNs. Multiplicity is a common feature of IPMN.

Intraductal Papillary Mucinous Neoplasm

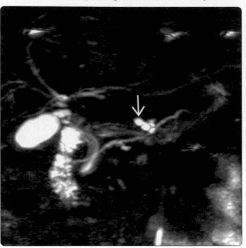

Intraductal Papillary Mucinous Neoplasm

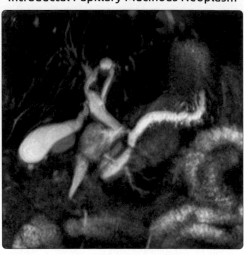

(Left) *Coronal MRCP with MIP reconstruction demonstrates a cystic lesion* ➡ *with a "cluster of grapes" morphology communicating with the pancreatic duct, suggestive of side-branch IPMN. While IPMN can be unilocular, tubular, or multicystic, IPMNs are relatively common.* (Right) *Coronal MRCP with MIP reconstruction demonstrates a diffusely dilated main pancreatic duct with ectatic side branches. Mucin was seen extruding from the ampulla at endoscopy, and this was found to be a main-duct IPMN.*

Pancreatic Pseudocyst

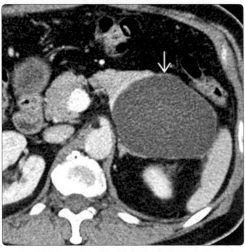

Pancreatic Pseudocyst

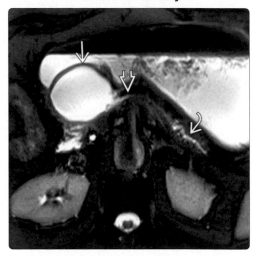

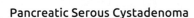

(Left) *Axial CECT in a patient with a known history of pancreatitis demonstrates a large cyst* ➡ *in the pancreatic tail. While a cystic neoplasm is certainly a possibility based on imaging alone, the patient's history allowed the correct diagnosis of a pseudocyst.* (Right) *Axial T2 FS MR in a patient with a history of recurrent pancreatitis demonstrates a pseudocyst* ➡ *in the pancreatic head with apparent communication* ➡ *with the pancreatic duct. Note the pancreatic atrophy with ductal ectasia* ➡ *secondary to chronic pancreatitis.*

Pancreatic Serous Cystadenoma

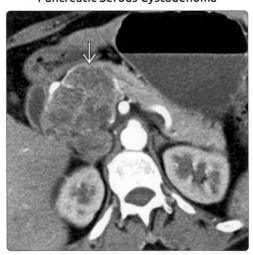

Pancreatic Serous Cystadenoma

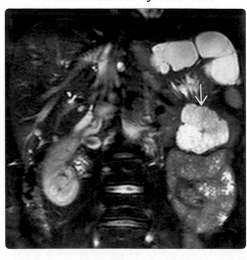

(Left) *Axial CECT demonstrates a classic microcystic serous cystadenoma* ➡ *of the pancreas with innumerable internal tiny cystic components, enhancing septations, a lobulated contour, and peripheral vascularity.* (Right) *Coronal MRCP with MIP reconstruction demonstrates a classic serous cystadenoma* ➡. *As seen in this case, the internal microcystic architecture of these lesions is almost always better assessed on MR.*

Mucinous Cystic Neoplasm

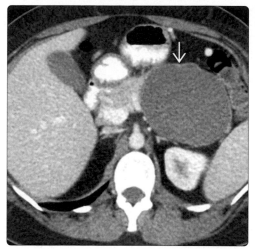

Mucinous Cystic Neoplasm

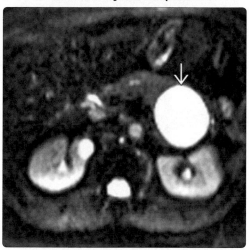

(Left) *Axial CECT in a middle-aged woman demonstrates a large simple-appearing pancreatic cyst* ➡️ *arising from the pancreatic tail. While a specific diagnosis is difficult based on imaging alone, the location of the cyst in the tail and patient demographics allow the correct diagnosis of a mucinous cystic neoplasm (MCN).* **(Right)** *Axial T2 FS MR demonstrates a large simple-appearing MCN* ➡️ *in the pancreatic tail. As seen in this case, these lesions usually arise in the pancreatic tail and typically occur in middle-aged women.*

Duodenal Diverticulum (Mimic)

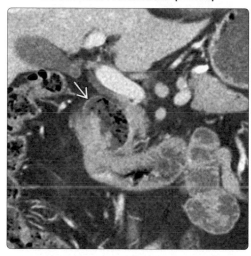

Solid Pseudopapillary Neoplasm

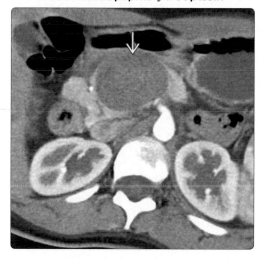

(Left) *Coronal CECT demonstrates a classic duodenal diverticulum* ➡️ *filled with fluid and gas invaginating directly into the pancreatic head. When filled with fluid, diverticula can mimic a pancreatic cystic lesion.* **(Right)** *Axial CECT in a young woman demonstrates a homogeneous cystic lesion* ➡️ *in the pancreatic head/neck, found to be a solid pseudopapillary neoplasm (SPEN) at surgical resection, always a primary consideration when confronted with a pancreatic cyst in a young woman.*

Solid Pseudopapillary Neoplasm

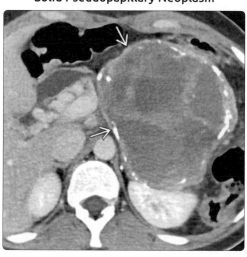

Pancreatic Neuroendocrine Tumor

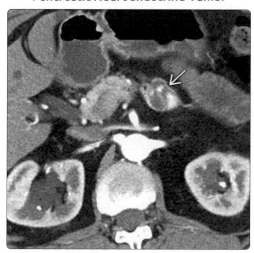

(Left) *Axial CECT demonstrates a large complex cystic mass* ➡️ *arising from the pancreatic tail in a young woman, found to be a SPEN at resection. SPENs can demonstrate either peripheral or internal calcification, internal hemorrhage, and a combination of cystic and solid components.* **(Right)** *Axial CECT in the arterial phase demonstrates a cystic lesion* ➡️ *in the pancreatic body with hypervascular mural nodularity, a feature strongly suggestive of a cystic neuroendocrine tumor.*

Pancreatic Neuroendocrine Tumor

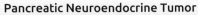
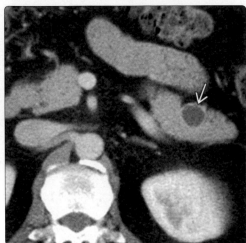

Pancreatic Ductal Adenocarcinoma

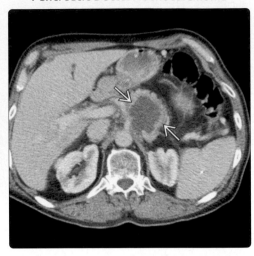

(Left) *Axial CECT demonstrates a relatively simple-appearing cystic lesion ➡ arising from the pancreatic tail. Note, however, the subtle rim of enhancement around the margins of the cyst, a feature that allows the correct diagnosis of a cystic neuroendocrine tumor.* (Right) *Axial CECT demonstrates an unusually low-density or necrotic pancreatic ductal carcinoma ➡. While pancreatic adenocarcinoma is rarely ever truly cystic, it can rarely simulate a cystic mass due to internal necrosis or low-density components.*

Autosomal Dominant Polycystic Disease

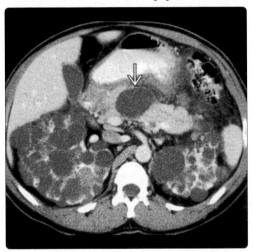

Cystic Fibrosis

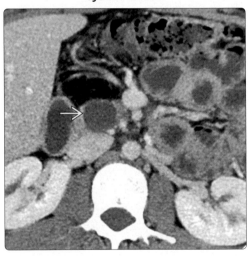

(Left) *Axial CECT in a patient with autosomal dominant polycystic kidney disease demonstrates cystic enlargement of both kidneys, as well as 1 cyst in the pancreas ➡, likely due to the patient's syndrome.* (Right) *Axial CECT demonstrates a simple cyst ➡ in the pancreatic head in a patient with cystic fibrosis (CF). Nonneoplastic simple cysts are a known feature of CF, most often in the later stages of the disorder.*

Von Hippel-Lindau Disease

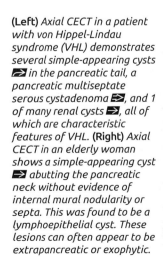
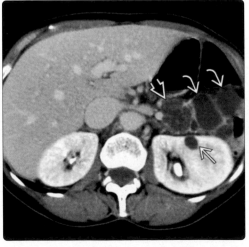

Lymphoepithelial Cyst

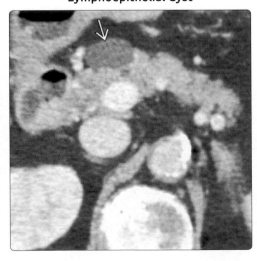

(Left) *Axial CECT in a patient with von Hippel-Lindau syndrome (VHL) demonstrates several simple-appearing cysts ➡ in the pancreatic tail, a pancreatic multiseptate serous cystadenoma ➡, and 1 of many renal cysts ➡, all of which are characteristic features of VHL.* (Right) *Axial CECT in an elderly woman shows a simple-appearing cyst ➡ abutting the pancreatic neck without evidence of internal mural nodularity or septa. This was found to be a lymphoepithelial cyst. These lesions can often appear to be extrapancreatic or exophytic.*

Lymphoepithelial Cyst

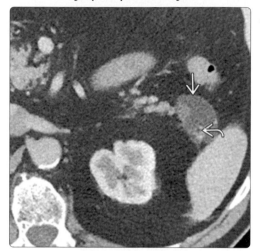

Pseudoaneurysm (Mimic)

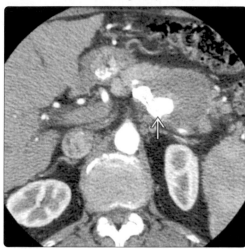

(Left) *Axial CECT demonstrates a complex cyst* ➡ *abutting the pancreatic tail with internal mural nodularity and a subtle focus of macroscopic fat* ➡. *This lesion was found to be a lymphoepithelial cyst at resection.* (Right) *Axial CECT demonstrates a splenic artery pseudoaneurysm, with enhancement* ➡ *of a portion of the pseudoaneurysm sac. The thrombosed portion of the aneurysm sac could superficially resemble a pancreatic cyst.*

Choledochal Cyst (Mimic)

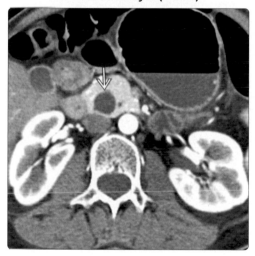

Choledochal Cyst (Mimic)

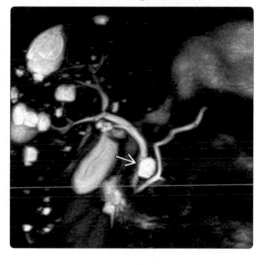

(Left) *Axial CECT demonstrates a cystic lesion* ➡ *in the pancreatic head that superficially appears to be of pancreatic origin.* (Right) *Coronal MRCP with MIP reconstruction in the same patient better demonstrates that the cystic lesion seen on CT is actually a diverticulum* ➡ *arising from the common bile duct, compatible with a choledochal cyst.*

Hydatid Cyst

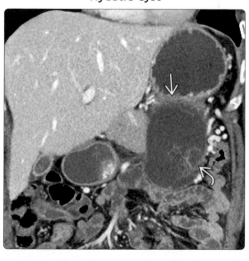

Hydatid Cyst

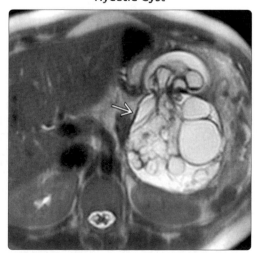

(Left) *Coronal CECT in a recent immigrant from abroad demonstrates a complex cystic lesion* ➡ *in the pancreatic tail with internal septations and subtle internal daughter cysts* ➡. *This was found to be an echinococcal cyst at resection.* (Right) *Axial T2 MR in the same patient better demonstrates the markedly complex internal architecture of this lesion* ➡ *with extensive internal septations and daughter cysts. The internal morphology of these lesions is often easier to appreciate on MR compared to CT.*

DIFFERENTIAL DIAGNOSIS

Common

- Chronic Pancreatitis
- Senescent Change
- Obesity
- Diabetes Mellitus
- Cystic Fibrosis, Pancreas
- Cushing Syndrome & Steroid Medications

Less Common

- Asymmetric Fatty Infiltration (Normal Variant)
- Lipomatous Pseudohypertrophy
- Shwachman-Diamond Syndrome
- Agenesis of Dorsal Pancreas

ESSENTIAL INFORMATION

Key Differential Diagnosis Issues

- Fatty infiltration & atrophy does not necessarily imply pathologic condition (pancreas can become fat infiltrated & less glandular in setting of advanced age, diabetes, obesity, & certain medications)
- Differentiate benign **diffuse** pancreatic atrophy from **upstream** pancreatic atrophy in setting of obstructed pancreatic duct (which raises concern for malignancy)
  - o Pancreatic adenocarcinoma often obstructs pancreatic duct & results in severe atrophy of pancreas **upstream** from site of obstruction
  - o Malignant atrophy not associated with fatty infiltration

Helpful Clues for Common Diagnoses

- **Chronic Pancreatitis**
  - o Typically associated with parenchymal atrophy that is most apparent in body/tail
  - o Other CT features include parenchymal/intraductal calcifications, dilated pancreatic duct, & pseudocysts
  - o MR findings more sensitive for early CP, including ↓ T1 parenchymal signal, ↓ arterial phase enhancement, ↑ delayed enhancement, & duct side-branch ectasia
- **Senescent Change**

- o Atrophy & fatty infiltration with mild pancreatic ductal dilation is normal finding in elderly
- o Can mimic CP, as elderly may also demonstrate small parenchymal calcifications, ↓ parenchymal T1 signal, & ↓ enhancement on MR
- **Obesity**
  - o Particularly common in patients with type II diabetes
- **Cystic Fibrosis, Pancreas**
  - o Commonly results in complete fatty replacement of pancreas (often by end of teenage years)
  - o May also be associated with small pancreatic cysts
- **Cushing Syndrome & Steroid Medications**
  - o Hypercortisolism (including cases secondary to steroid medications) can result in pancreatic fatty atrophy
  - o Steroid medications more likely to result in fatty infiltration at higher doses for prolonged time periods

Helpful Clues for Less Common Diagnoses

- **Asymmetric Fatty Infiltration (Normal Variant)**
  - o Focal accumulation of fat in anterior pancreatic head due to embryologic development of dorsal/ventral pancreas
  - o Low-density area in anterior head of pancreas sharply demarcated from normal density posterior head
  - o May simulate hypodense mass, but should not demonstrate mass effect or ductal dilatation
- **Lipomatous Pseudohypertrophy**
  - o Focal or diffuse enlargement of pancreas with fatty replacement (but preserved exocrine function)
  - o Unknown etiology, but possibly potentiated by cirrhosis, viral infection, or abnormal metabolism
- **Shwachman-Diamond Syndrome**
  - o Rare disorder characterized by pancreatic exocrine insufficiency, bone marrow dysfunction, & dwarfism
  - o Can produce fatty infiltration similar to cystic fibrosis
  - o Enlarged gland in early stages that gradually atrophies
  - o No pancreatic calcifications or cysts (unlike cystic fibrosis)
- **Agenesis of Dorsal Pancreas**
  - o Pancreatic head & uncinate are normal in appearance, while body & tail segments are either absent (complete agenesis) or truncated (partial agenesis)

Chronic Pancreatitis

Senescent Change

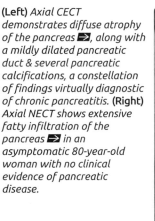

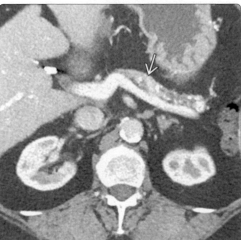

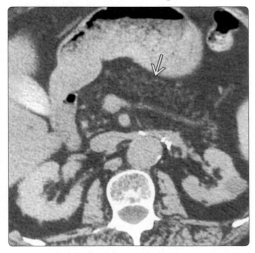

(Left) *Axial CECT demonstrates diffuse atrophy of the pancreas ➡, along with a mildly dilated pancreatic duct & several pancreatic calcifications, a constellation of findings virtually diagnostic of chronic pancreatitis.* (Right) *Axial NECT shows extensive fatty infiltration of the pancreas ➡ in an asymptomatic 80-year-old woman with no clinical evidence of pancreatic disease.*

Cystic Fibrosis, Pancreas

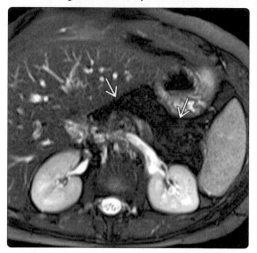

Asymmetric Fatty Infiltration (Normal Variant)

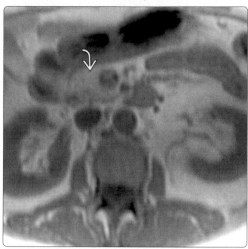

(Left) *Axial T2 FS MR in a patient with cystic fibrosis demonstrates diffuse fatty replacement ➜ of the pancreas. This finding is present in many cystic fibrosis patients by their late teenage years.* **(Right)** *Axial in-phase GRE MR demonstrates homogenous high signal in the entire pancreatic head ➜.*

Asymmetric Fatty Infiltration (Normal Variant)

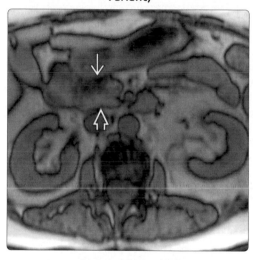

Lipomatous Pseudohypertrophy

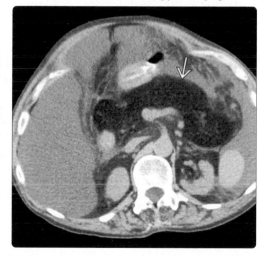

(Left) *Axial out-of-phase GRE MR in the same patient demonstrates focal signal dropout in the anterior pancreatic head ➜, characteristic of focal fatty infiltration. Note that the posterior pancreatic head ➜ does not lose signal on the out-of-phase image. MR is the best modality to confirm this diagnosis.* **(Right)** *Axial NECT shows lipomatous pseudohypertrophy of the pancreas ➜, likely attributable to chronic alcohol abuse & cirrhosis in this patient.*

Agenesis of Dorsal Pancreas

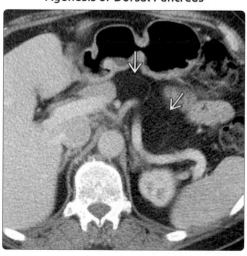

Agenesis of Dorsal Pancreas

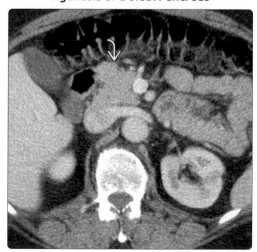

(Left) *Axial CECT incidentally demonstrates absence of the pancreatic body & tail with fat attenuation ➜ in place of the normal pancreatic parenchyma.* **(Right)** *Axial CECT in the same patient demonstrates a normal appearance of the pancreatic head ➜. This constellation of findings is compatible with agenesis of the dorsal pancreas.*

DIFFERENTIAL DIAGNOSIS

Common

- Pancreatic Ductal Adenocarcinoma
- Chronic Pancreatitis
- Senescent Change, Pancreas
- Intraductal Papillary Mucinous Neoplasm
- Pancreatic Divisum

Less Common

- Ampullary Carcinoma
- Duodenal Adenocarcinoma
- Pancreatic Neuroendocrine Tumor
- Choledocholithiasis

ESSENTIAL INFORMATION

Key Differential Diagnosis Issues

- Normal pancreatic duct measures 3 mm in head, 2 mm in body, and 1 mm in tail
  - Normal duct should taper gradually toward body and tail
- Unexplained dilatation of pancreatic duct (in absence of clear stigmata of chronic pancreatitis) should raise concern for occult obstructing mass
  - Additional imaging features, which increase suspicion for obstructing mass include
    - Abrupt or irregular narrowing of pancreatic duct
    - Pancreatic atrophy upstream from stricture
    - Double-duct sign [i.e., dilatation of both common bile duct (CBD) and pancreatic duct], which carries higher risk of malignancy compared to isolated dilatation of pancreatic duct alone
    - Locoregional lymphadenopathy or metastatic disease
  - In cases with such features, even if discrete obstructing mass is not visualized, endoscopic ultrasound may be necessary to exclude small occult lesion
- Pancreatic adenocarcinoma is, by far, most common tumor to obstruct pancreatic duct
  - Neuroendocrine tumors, lymphoma, metastases to pancreas, and focal autoimmune pancreatitis do not typically cause pancreatic ductal obstruction

Helpful Clues for Common Diagnoses

- **Pancreatic Ductal Adenocarcinoma**
  - Hypoenhancing, poorly marginated, infiltrative mass arising from pancreas
    - Tumors tend to be hypointense on T1WI MR (nicely juxtaposed against T1 hyperintense normal pancreas), variable in signal on T2WI, and hypoenhancing on T1 C+
  - Mass results in abrupt narrowing of pancreatic duct with upstream ductal dilatation and parenchymal atrophy
    - CBD typically obstructed when tumor located in pancreatic head
    - Some tumors located in uncinate may not result in pancreatic or biliary ductal obstruction
  - Tumor commonly infiltrates posteriorly into retroperitoneum with frequent vascular encasement and narrowing

- 5% of all pancreatic adenocarcinomas are isodense to normal pancreas on CT, and secondary signs (dilated ducts, parenchymal atrophy) may be only clue to presence of subtle tumor
  - Endoscopic US may be necessary to identify these isodense lesions as well as very small masses, which are not discretely seen on CT
- Bulky lymphadenopathy uncommon, but metastases most frequent to liver, peritoneum, and lungs
- **Chronic Pancreatitis**
  - Dilated, beaded pancreatic duct with multiple sites of stricture and associated diffuse pancreatic atrophy
    - Chronic pancreatitis is most common cause of benign pancreatic duct strictures, although benign strictures can also be seen in setting of prior trauma or surgery
  - Pancreatic parenchymal and intraductal calcifications virtually diagnostic of chronic pancreatitis
    - Intraductal stones/calcifications can obstruct pancreatic duct
  - Pseudocysts may be present and may demonstrate communication with pancreatic duct on MRCP
  - Focal fibroinflammatory mass (usually in pancreatic head) due to chronic pancreatitis can be very difficult (or impossible) to distinguish from malignancy
  - MR more sensitive (compared to CT) for early changes of chronic pancreatitis, including ectasia of pancreatic duct side branches, loss of normal T1WI parenchymal signal, lack of duct distension with secretin, and ↓ exocrine function with secretin
    - Parenchyma may demonstrate diminished arterial-phase enhancement with increased delayed enhancement due to fibrosis
  - Groove pancreatitis, an unusual form of chronic pancreatitis resulting in curvilinear soft tissue in pancreaticoduodenal groove, can also result in dilatation of upstream pancreatic duct and CBD
- **Senescent Change, Pancreas**
  - Mild pancreatic parenchymal atrophy and mild dilation of pancreatic duct are normal findings in elderly and should not be misinterpreted as pathologic enlargement
    - No published consensus on what duct diameter constitutes "mild" degree of dilatation
    - Even in cases of senescent dilatation pancreatic duct should still taper normally towards body and tail
    - No evidence of pancreatic duct strictures or intraductal stones
  - Elderly patients may demonstrate tiny foci of calcification, diminished parenchymal signal on T1WI MR, and parenchymal hypoenhancement on T1WI C+ MR, which can mimic chronic pancreatitis
  - Moderate or severe degrees of pancreatic ductal dilatation, particularly with evidence of abrupt ductal obstruction/cut-off, are not normal in elderly and should prompt further evaluation
- **Intraductal Papillary Mucinous Neoplasm**
  - Main duct or combined-type intraductal papillary mucinous neoplasm (IPMN) may result in diffuse or segmental dilatation of main pancreatic duct
    - Main pancreatic duct usually measures ≥ 5 mm
    - Amorphous calcifications may be seen within duct lumen

- Pancreas often atrophic overlying dilated segments of duct
- Intraductal nodularity or soft tissue suggests presence of invasive malignancy
- Presence of discrete cyst communicating with dilated pancreatic duct suggests combined-type IPMN
  - Dilated duct may result in bulging of papilla of Vater into duodenum, and mucin may be seen extruding from ampulla on endoscopy
- **Pancreatic Divisum**
  - Anatomic variant of pancreatic ductal anatomy with dominant dorsal duct entering minor papilla, short ventral duct entering major papilla, and no communication between dorsal and ventral ducts
  - Dorsal pancreatic duct is commonly mildly dilated with loss of normal tapering toward pancreatic tail, likely due to functional stenosis or poor drainage of pancreatic secretions at minor papilla
    - Dilated duct may also be attributable to chronic pancreatitis due to association between divisum and pancreatitis
  - While diagnosis can be suggested based on CT, divisum easiest to appreciate on MRCP

Helpful Clues for Less Common Diagnoses

- **Ampullary Carcinoma**
  - Tumors arising from ampulla of Vater can be indistinguishable on imaging from pancreatic head adenocarcinoma or duodenal adenocarcinoma
  - Ampullary carcinoma encompasses several different histologic tumors types, each with variable prognosis
  - Lesions almost always obstruct common bile duct, but only ~ 50% of lesions obstruct pancreatic duct
  - Even lesions that obstruct pancreatic duct do not typically cause pancreatic parenchymal atrophy (unlike pancreatic adenocarcinoma)
- **Duodenal Adenocarcinoma**

  - Paraampullary duodenal adenocarcinomas that involve ampulla of Vater may be difficult to distinguish from pancreatic head adenocarcinoma, although pancreatic atrophy and pancreatic ductal obstruction are uncommon
  - Look for tumor centered in duodenal wall or within lumen of duodenum
  - Other duodenal tumors (such as villous adenoma, carcinoid) can also theoretically result in ductal obstruction
  - Duodenal adenocarcinoma has superior prognosis compared to both ampullary carcinoma and pancreatic adenocarcinoma
- **Pancreatic Neuroendocrine Tumor**
  - Well-circumscribed hypervascular tumor, which is typically best visualized on arterial-phase images
  - Neuroendocrine tumors do not typically cause pancreatic duct obstruction
  - Large tumors can obstruct pancreatic duct due to mass effect, and some small tumors have been shown to secrete hormones (especially serotonin) that may cause ductal stricture and obstruction
- **Choledocholithiasis**
  - Stone lodged in distal common channel can obstruct both pancreatic and common bile ducts
  - Stones lodged in this location typically far easier to identify on MR compared to CT, although even MR can struggle with stones lodged in ampulla
    - Gallstones typically demonstrate low signal on all pulse sequences
  - May cause "gallstone pancreatitis" with edema and inflammation of pancreatic head
    - Correlate with history of sudden onset of pain and elevated pancreatic enzymes

SELECTED REFERENCES

1. Raman SP et al: Abnormalities of the distal common bile duct and ampulla: diagnostic approach and differential diagnosis using multiplanar reformations and 3D imaging. AJR Am J Roentgenol. 203(1):17-28, 2014
2. Kawamoto S et al: Small serotonin-producing neuroendocrine tumor of the pancreas associated with pancreatic duct obstruction. AJR Am J Roentgenol. 197(3):W482-8, 2011

Pancreatic Ductal Adenocarcinoma

Pancreatic Ductal Adenocarcinoma

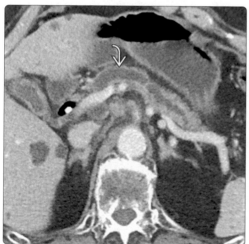

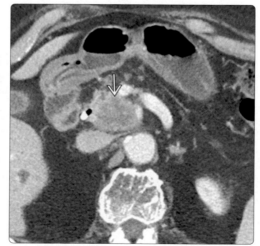

(Left) *Axial CECT demonstrates a diffusely dilated pancreatic duct ➚, an imaging feature that should prompt a careful search for an obstructing mass.* **(Right)** *Axial CECT in the same patient demonstrates a poorly margined hypodense mass ➙ in the pancreatic head/uncinate causing the pancreatic ductal obstruction, compatible with a pancreatic adenocarcinoma.*

Pancreatic Ductal Adenocarcinoma

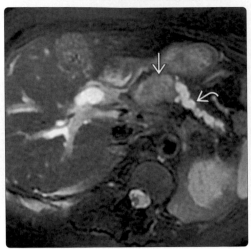

Chronic Pancreatitis

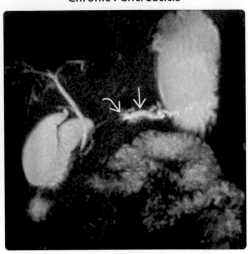

(Left) *Axial T2 FS MR demonstrates a mildly T2 hyperintense mass ➡ in the pancreatic head causing upstream parenchymal atrophy and dilatation of the pancreatic duct ➡, characteristic features of pancreatic adenocarcinoma.* **(Right)** *Coronal MRCP demonstrates dilatation ➡ of the pancreatic duct in the body/tail segment, a focal stricture ➡ of the duct in the body, and ectasia of duct side branches. These findings were found to be secondary to chronic pancreatitis.*

Chronic Pancreatitis

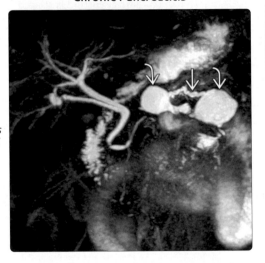

Chronic Pancreatitis

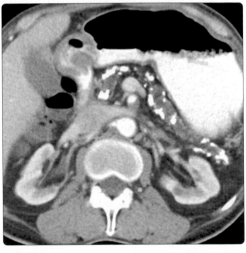

(Left) *Coronal MRCP with MIP reconstruction demonstrates dilatation and beading of the pancreatic duct ➡ in the body/tail. At least 2 fluid collections ➡ appear to communicate with the pancreatic duct. This constellation of findings represents chronic pancreatitis with pseudocysts.* **(Right)** *Axial CECT demonstrates an atrophic pancreas with a diffusely dilated pancreatic duct and multiple parenchymal/intraductal calcifications, features which are diagnostic of chronic pancreatitis.*

Intraductal Papillary Mucinous Neoplasm

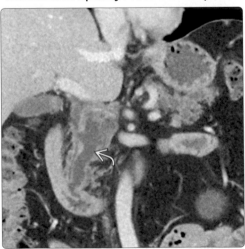

Intraductal Papillary Mucinous Neoplasm

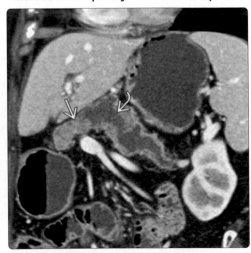

(Left) *Coronal CECT demonstrates a diffusely dilated main pancreatic duct ➡, which appears to "bulge" into the ampulla. This was found to represent a main-duct intraductal papillary mucinous neoplasm (IPMN) at endoscopy, where mucin was seen extruding from the ampulla.* **(Right)** *Curved MPR demonstrates a severely dilated main pancreatic duct ➡ with enhancing soft tissue ➡ in the downstream duct, compatible with a main-duct IPMN and likely associated invasive carcinoma.*

Pancreatic Divisum

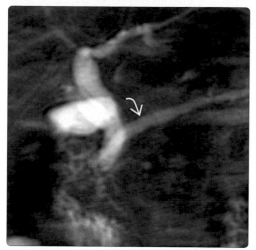

Ampullary Carcinoma

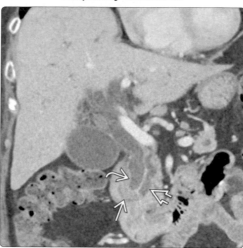

(Left) *MRCP with MIP reconstruction demonstrates the main pancreatic duct* �){ *crossing behind the common bile duct (CBD) to enter the minor papilla, compatible with pancreatic divisum. As in this case, divisum can be associated with mild pancreatic ductal dilatation.* (Right) *Coronal CECT demonstrates a mass* ➡ *centered at the ampulla obstructing both the common bile duct* ➔ *and pancreatic duct* ➡. *This was found to be an ampullary carcinoma at surgery.*

Ampullary Carcinoma

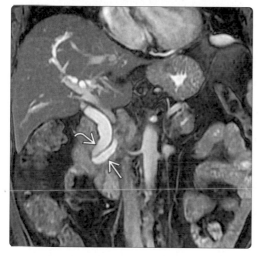

Duodenal Adenocarcinoma

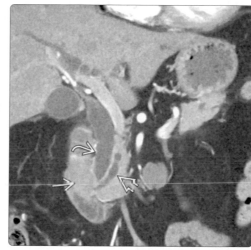

(Left) *Coronal FIESTA image demonstrates a double-duct sign, with dilatation of both the CBD* ➔ *and pancreatic duct* ➡. *No mass was visible, but a small obstructing ampullary carcinoma was discovered at endoscopic ultrasound.* (Right) *Coronal CECT demonstrates a soft tissue mass* ➡ *centered in the duodenum obstructing both the CBD* ➔ *and pancreatic duct* ➡. *This was found to be a paraampullary duodenal adenocarcinoma, which more commonly obstructs the CBD than the pancreatic duct.*

Pancreatic Neuroendocrine Tumor

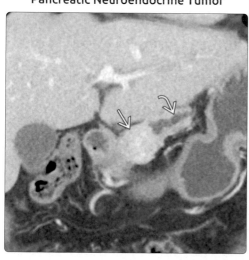

Pancreatic Neuroendocrine Tumor

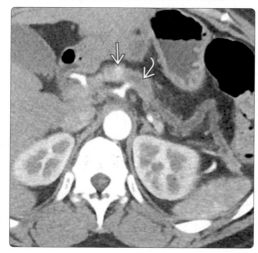

(Left) *Coronal CECT demonstrates an avidly enhancing mass* ➡ *obstructing the pancreatic duct* ➔ *and resulting in upstream atrophy. Neuroendocrine tumors only rarely cause ductal obstruction due to large size/mass effect or secretion of hormones that cause ductal stricture.* (Right) *Axial CECT demonstrates nodular enhancement* ➡ *in the pancreatic head, representing a small neuroendocrine tumor. The ductal dilatation* ➔ *and atrophy in this case are atypical features.*

DIFFERENTIAL DIAGNOSIS

Common

- Acute Pancreatitis
- Pancreatic Ductal Carcinoma
- Anasarca
- Portal Hypertension
- Traumatic Pancreatitis
- Duodenal Ulcer
- Gastric Ulcer

Less Common

- Shock Pancreas
- Sclerosing Mesenteritis
- Autoimmune Pancreatitis
- Groove Pancreatitis
- Lymphoma
- Duodenal Diverticulitis
- Diverticulitis

ESSENTIAL INFORMATION

Key Differential Diagnosis Issues

- Any inflammatory or neoplastic process originating from structures abutting pancreas may cause infiltration of peripancreatic fat planes
  - Most commonly seen due to inflammatory conditions arising in anterior pararenal space (pancreas, duodenum, ascending colon, and descending colon)
  - Utilizing multiplanar reformations can help better determine source of inflammation
- Acute pancreatitis is overwhelmingly most common cause of infiltration of peripancreatic fat planes
- Clinical history is critical in formulating diagnosis, as several entities (e.g., traumatic pancreatitis, shock pancreas) can appear virtually identical to acute pancreatitis on imaging

Helpful Clues for Common Diagnoses

- **Acute Pancreatitis**
  - Pancreas typically appears enlarged and edematous with loss of normal fatty lobulation
    - Pancreas and surrounding fat planes can appear essentially normal in mild cases
  - Inflammation (including stranding and free fluid) spreads **ventrally** into mesentery and **laterally** within anterior pararenal space
    - May result in thickening of anterior perirenal (Gerota) fascia (forms posterior border of anterior pararenal space)
    - May produce reactive wall thickening of left/right colon and duodenum
  - Look for evidence of abnormal pancreatic enhancement to suggest necrotizing pancreatitis
  - Pancreatic enzyme (e.g., lipase) levels can confirm diagnosis
- **Pancreatic Ductal Carcinoma**
  - Hypodense, poorly marginated mass that tends to infiltrate **dorsally** into retroperitoneum to involve mesenteric vasculature
  - ~ 5% of patients with pancreatic cancer may present with clinical/biochemical signs of acute pancreatitis

- Presence of dorsal infiltration, dilated pancreatic duct, common bile duct (CBD) obstruction, parenchymal atrophy, or metastatic disease should suggest presence of underlying tumor
- **Anasarca and Portal Hypertension**
  - Any entity that results in anasarca can cause generalized edema and infiltration, including edema of mesenteric and peripancreatic fat
  - Peripancreatic infiltration from anasarca or portal hypertension may be indistinguishable from that seen with acute pancreatitis, although generalized nature of edema should suggest correct diagnosis
- **Traumatic Pancreatitis**
  - Imaging features similar to acute pancreatitis, although clinical history and presence of fracture plane through pancreas, contusion, or peripancreatic hematoma suggest correct diagnosis
    - Fluid separating pancreas from splenic vein is sensitive sign of pancreatic injury
  - May not be evident immediately, can appear at 24-48 hr
  - May be associated with fluid collection/pseudocyst if trauma results in pancreatic duct disruption
- **Duodenal Ulcer**
  - Perforated duodenal ulcer may cause infiltration of right anterior pararenal space surrounding pancreatic head/neck
  - Multiplanar reformations may better demonstrate that inflammation is centered around duodenum (rather than pancreas)
    - Extraluminal gas or enteric contrast suggests correct diagnosis but may not always be present
  - Ulcer can rarely penetrate into pancreas and cause secondary pancreatitis
- **Gastric Ulcer**
  - Most commonly perforates into lesser sac (between posterior wall of stomach and pancreas)
    - Gastric wall usually thickened with adjacent inflammation
    - Extraluminal gas and enteric contrast allow confident diagnosis but may not always be present
  - Ulcer can rarely penetrate posteriorly into body of pancreas and cause secondary pancreatitis

Helpful Clues for Less Common Diagnoses

- **Shock Pancreas**
  - Part of hypoperfusion complex, which results from severe traumatic injury or hypotension
    - Most often seen after head/spine trauma or significant blood loss
    - Often victims of blunt trauma who were hypotensive on arrival to emergency department
  - Patients have usually been fluid resuscitated prior to CT scan, but mesenteric, bowel wall, and peripancreatic edema may persist (or worsen temporarily)
    - CT findings usually resolve within 24 hr
  - Pancreas appears enlarged, edematous, and hypoenhancing, mimicking both acute pancreatitis and posttraumatic pancreatitis
    - May be impossible to distinguish from traumatic injury by imaging alone, but lack of fracture plane and presence of other imaging signs of shock complex make traumatic pancreatitis less likely

- Other features of shock complex include diffuse small bowel wall thickening with mucosal enhancement, hyperenhancement of kidneys and adrenal glands, and small aorta/inferior vena cava
- **Sclerosing Mesenteritis**
  - Idiopathic inflammatory and fibrotic disorder affecting mesentery (also known as retractile mesenteritis, fibrosing mesenteritis, or panniculitis)
  - Imaging appearance variable depending on acuity
    - Acute mesenteritis: Left upper quadrant "misty mesentery" with fat stranding and induration, thin surrounding pseudocapsule, and multiple prominent mesenteric lymph nodes with halo of spared surrounding fat
      □ Infiltrated fat planes usually in jejunal mesentery (caudal to pancreas), and process is not truly peripancreatic
      □ Any other cause of "misty mesentery" can infiltrate peripancreatic fat planes as well
    - Chronic mesenteritis: Fibrotic soft tissue mass with desmoplastic reaction and calcification
- **Autoimmune Pancreatitis**
  - Can involve pancreas diffusely (most common) or focally
  - Pancreas enlarged and edematous with thin hypodense halo (which may demonstrate delayed enhancement)
  - General paucity of peripancreatic infiltration and fat stranding compared with acute edematous or necrotizing pancreatitis
  - Pancreatic duct is normal in size or narrowed (not dilated or obstructed)
  - Often associated with other autoimmune diseases, including retroperitoneal fibrosis, IgG4 cholangiopathy, and Riedel thyroiditis
    - Bile ducts may be dilated with wall thickening and hyperenhancement (especially distal CBD) as result of concomitant IgG4 cholangiopathy
- **Groove Pancreatitis**
  - Rare form of chronic pancreatitis resulting in sheet-like, curvilinear soft tissue thickening in pancreaticoduodenal groove (between 2nd portion of duodenum and pancreatic head)

- May be associated with cysts in groove and medial wall of duodenum
  - Can be very difficult to differentiate prospectively from pancreatic head adenocarcinoma or duodenal adenocarcinoma, and most patients undergo Whipple resection to exclude malignancy
- **Lymphoma**
  - Primary pancreatic lymphoma is very rare (usually in immunocompromised or elderly patients), with most cases representing secondary lymphomatous involvement of pancreas
    - Almost always significant lymphadenopathy elsewhere and other sites of lymphomatous involvement
  - Homogeneous soft tissue mass that may infiltrate pancreas and peripancreatic fat planes, potentially mimicking acute pancreatitis on imaging (but not clinically)
  - Tumor encases peripancreatic vasculature without attenuation, narrowing, or occlusion
  - No obstruction of CBD or pancreatic duct
  - No atrophy of pancreas upstream from mass
- **Duodenal Diverticulitis**
  - May perforate spontaneously or after intubation, resulting in surrounding inflammation (i.e., duodenal diverticulitis)
  - Inflammation can involve pancreatic head, simulating acute pancreatitis
  - Recognizing that inflammation is centered around diverticulum and presence of extraluminal gas or enteric contrast are keys to diagnosis
  - Duodenal diverticulum (especially when large) may be predisposing factor for acute pancreatitis
- **Diverticulitis**
  - Inflammation can extend into anterior pararenal space when diverticulitis originates from ascending/descending colon
    - May spread medially within anterior pararenal space to peripancreatic region, potentially simulating acute pancreatitis

Acute Pancreatitis

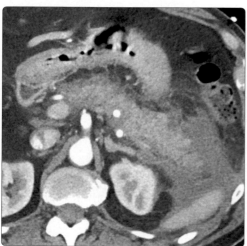

Acute Pancreatitis

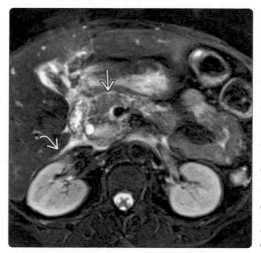

(Left) Axial CECT demonstrates pancreatic edema with loss of normal pancreatic lobulation and diffuse peripancreatic fat stranding and fluid, compatible with acute pancreatitis. (Right) Axial T2 FS MR demonstrates edema and T2 hyperintensity of the pancreatic head ➡ with T2 bright fluid tracking from the pancreas into the right anterior pararenal space ➡, compatible with acute pancreatitis. Fat-suppressed T2WIs are the most sensitive sequence for identifying pancreatitis.

(Left) *Axial T2 FS MR demonstrates extensive edema in the pancreatic bed, with a fluid collection ➡️ replacing much of the pancreatic body and tail. Only a small portion of the normal pancreas ➡️ is identified, compatible with acute necrotizing pancreatitis.* **(Right)** *Axial T2 FS MR demonstrates enlargement of the pancreas (which appears abnormally T2 hyperintense), with fluid tracking into the left anterior pararenal space ➡️, compatible with acute pancreatitis.*

Acute Pancreatitis

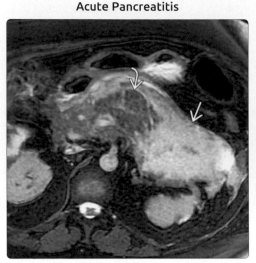

Acute Pancreatitis

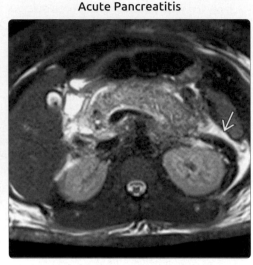

(Left) *Axial CECT demonstrates a poorly marginated, hypodense mass ➡️ arising from the pancreas, compatible with pancreatic adenocarcinoma.* **(Right)** *Axial T2 MR in the same patient demonstrates that the pancreatic mass ➡️ is relatively T2 hypointense. Pancreatic adenocarcinoma can be quite variable in signal on T2WI, making this pulse sequence generally less important for lesion identification.*

Pancreatic Ductal Carcinoma

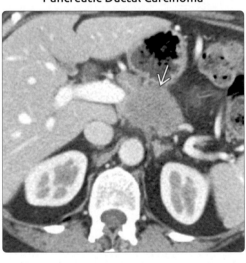

Pancreatic Ductal Carcinoma

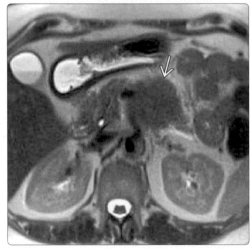

(Left) *Axial CECT demonstrates an infiltrative mass ➡️ arising from the pancreatic body with encasement of the celiac trunk ➡️, a classic appearance for pancreatic adenocarcinoma. Unlike pancreatitis, pancreatic adenocarcinoma infiltrates dorsally into the retroperitoneum.* **(Right)** *Axial CECT demonstrates diffuse tumor infiltration replacing the entire pancreas, a rare manifestation of pancreatic adenocarcinoma.*

Pancreatic Ductal Carcinoma

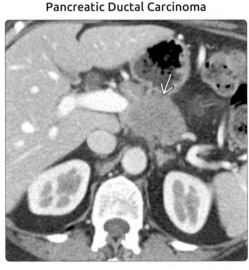

Pancreatic Ductal Carcinoma

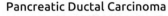

Portal Hypertension

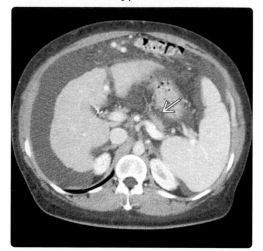

Traumatic Pancreatitis

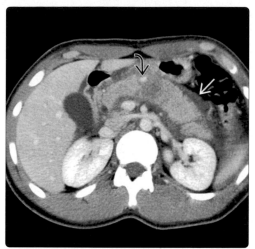

(Left) *Axial CECT shows cirrhosis with multiple stigmata of portal hypertension, including ascites, varices, and splenomegaly. In this setting, the resulting peripancreatic edema* ➡ *is impossible to distinguish from acute pancreatitis.* (Right) *Axial CECT shows a fracture plane through the pancreatic body with extensive peripancreatic edema* ➡ *and active bleeding* ➡*, compatible with acute traumatic pancreatic injury.*

Traumatic Pancreatitis

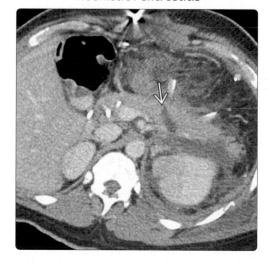

Duodenal Ulcer

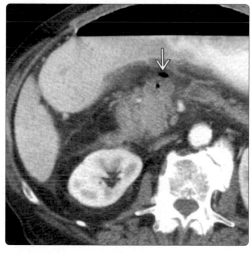

(Left) *Axial CECT after a gunshot wound to the abdomen demonstrates a fracture plane* ➡ *through the pancreatic body with extensive peripancreatic fat stranding and fluid, compatible with a posttraumatic pancreatic laceration with pancreatitis.* (Right) *Axial CECT demonstrates inflammatory changes surrounding the 2nd portion of the duodenum and head of pancreas with a tiny focus of adjacent extraluminal gas* ➡*, compatible with a perforated duodenal ulcer.*

Gastric Ulcer

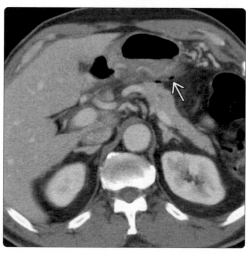

Shock Pancreas

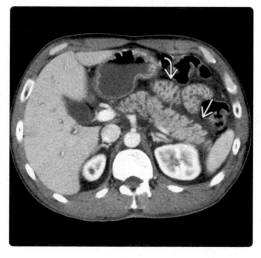

(Left) *Axial CECT demonstrates mural thickening of the stomach, adjacent infiltration of fat planes, and several bubbles of gas in the lesser sac* ➡*. A perforated gastric ulcer was confirmed at surgery.* (Right) *Axial CECT demonstrates infiltration of fat planes* ➡ *around the pancreas and in the mesentery, along with intense mucosal enhancement and submucosal edema of the entire small bowel* ➡ *(shock bowel). The pancreatic findings do not reflect direct traumatic injury, but rather, shock pancreas.*

(Left) *Axial CECT in the setting of shock physiology demonstrates marked edema/infiltration of the peripancreatic fat planes. Also note the collapsed cava sign ➡, a flattened appearance of the inferior vena cava due to hypovolemia.* **(Right)** *Axial CECT demonstrates extensive infiltration of the jejunal mesentery, caudal to the pancreas, with a thin capsule ➡ and small mesenteric nodes ➡, a classic appearance for sclerosing mesenteritis.*

Shock Pancreas

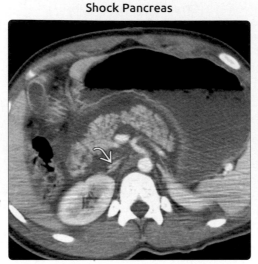

Sclerosing Mesenteritis

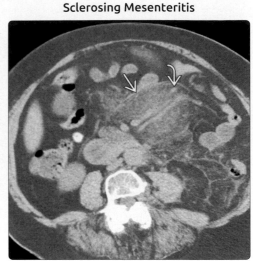

(Left) *Axial CECT demonstrates focal soft tissue ➡ surrounding the superior mesenteric artery, initially thought to represent an uncinate process pancreatic adenocarcinoma. Surprisingly, this was found to represent sclerosing mesenteritis at biopsy.* **(Right)** *Axial T2 FS MR demonstrates enlargement and T2 hyperintensity of the pancreatic body/tail ➡, with a paucity of peripancreatic fat stranding or inflammation. The patient's IgG4 was elevated, and this was found to be autoimmune pancreatitis that resolved after steroids.*

Sclerosing Mesenteritis

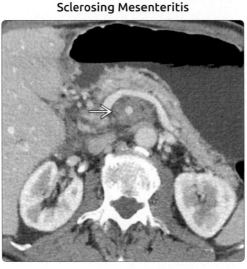

Autoimmune Pancreatitis

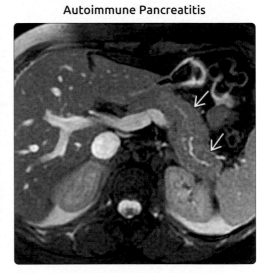

(Left) *Axial CECT demonstrates induration ➡ surrounding the pancreatic body and tail with extension along the left anterior pararenal space. This was found to represent autoimmune pancreatitis.* **(Right)** *Axial CECT shows sausage-shaped enlargement of the pancreatic body with subtle infiltration of surrounding fat, seemingly limited by a thin capsule ➡. This was found to be a manifestation of autoimmune pancreatitis.*

Autoimmune Pancreatitis

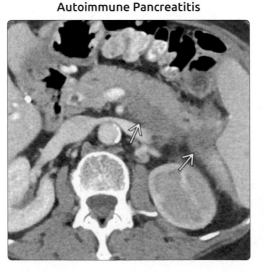

Autoimmune Pancreatitis

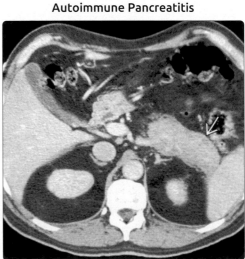

Groove Pancreatitis

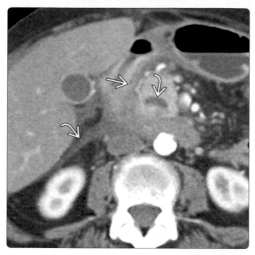

Groove Pancreatitis

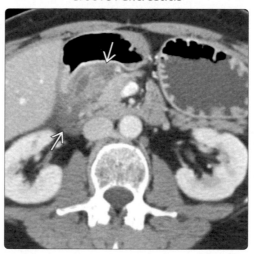

(Left) *Axial CECT demonstrates induration in the pancreaticoduodenal groove* ➡️*, a cystic focus* ➡️ *in the pancreatic head, and fluid tracking along the right anterior pararenal space. This was found to be groove pancreatitis, although peripancreatic fluid is a relatively unusual feature.* **(Right)** *Axial CECT demonstrates hypodense soft tissue thickening* ➡️ *in the pancreaticoduodenal groove. Although malignancy was suspected, this was found to be groove pancreatitis at resection.*

Lymphoma

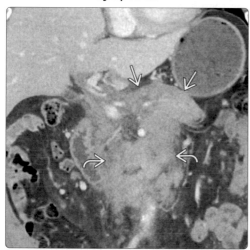

Lymphoma

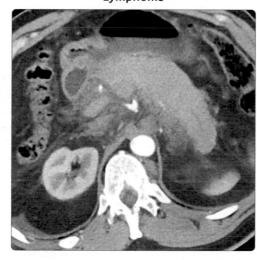

(Left) *Coronal CECT demonstrates lymphomatous infiltration of the pancreas* ➡️*, which appears abnormally hypodense and infiltrated. Note the extensive surrounding lymphadenopathy* ➡️*, which is almost always present in these cases.* **(Right)** *Axial CECT in the same patient demonstrates extensive stranding and infiltration of peripancreatic fat planes, with the pancreas itself appearing enlarged and edematous. Although representing lymphoma, this appearance could be easily confused for acute pancreatitis.*

Lymphoma

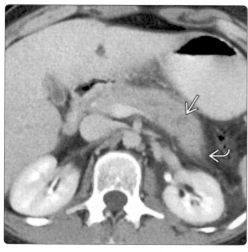

Duodenal Diverticulitis

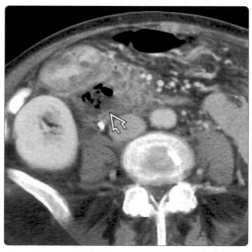

(Left) *Axial CECT shows 1 of several small hypodense pancreatic masses* ➡️*, along with infiltration of the surrounding fat* ➡️*. These findings were found to represent acute lymphoblastic lymphoma with pancreatic involvement.* **(Right)** *Axial CECT shows extraluminal gas and fluid* ➡️ *near the 2nd portion of duodenum and pancreatic head, along with extensive inflammatory infiltration, representing the sequelae of a perforated duodenal diverticulum.*

DIFFERENTIAL DIAGNOSIS

Common

- Chronic Pancreatitis
- Senescent Change, Pancreas
- Peripancreatic Vascular Lesions (Mimic)
- Choledocholithiasis (Mimic)
- Duodenal Diverticulum (Mimic)

Less Common

- Calcified Cystic or Solid Pancreatic Masses
  - Pancreatic Neuroendocrine Tumor
  - Pancreatic Serous Cystadenoma
  - Mucinous Cystic Neoplasm
  - Solid Pseudopapillary Neoplasm
  - Pancreatic Pseudocyst
  - Intraductal Papillary Mucinous Neoplasm
  - Pancreatic Metastases
- Cystic Fibrosis, Pancreas
- Hereditary Pancreatitis

Rare but Important

- Kwashiorkor
- Hyperparathyroidism

ESSENTIAL INFORMATION

Key Differential Diagnosis Issues

- While true parenchymal calcifications are most common with chronic pancreatitis, a few tiny calcifications can be seen in elderly patients with senescent change
- Splenic artery vascular calcifications much more common than pancreatic parenchymal calcifications and should not be misinterpreted to suggest chronic pancreatitis
- Calcifications can be seen with variety of cystic and solid pancreatic masses
  - Pancreatic adenocarcinoma almost **never** demonstrates calcification and presence of calcification should suggest alternative diagnosis
  - Pancreatic neuroendocrine tumor is most common pancreatic solid mass to show calcification
  - Many pancreatic cystic lesions can demonstrate calcification, and pattern of calcification may help in diagnosis
    - e.g., serous cystadenoma: Central calcification in scar; mucinous cystic neoplasm: Curvilinear peripheral calcification

Helpful Clues for Common Diagnoses

- **Chronic Pancreatitis**
  - Pancreatic parenchymal fibrosis resulting from chronic, progressive inflammation, most often on basis of alcohol abuse
  - Calcifications (usually multiple) can be either parenchymal or intraductal, ranging in size from punctate to large (~ 1 cm)
    - Calcifications most commonly occur in pancreatic head (and may be clustered in that location)
  - Other CT stigmata of chronic pancreatitis include dilated, beaded pancreatic duct (± strictures), parenchymal atrophy, and pseudocysts

- Large intraductal stones can contribute to pancreatic ductal obstruction and dilatation
  - Degree of pancreatic calcification related to severity of patient's fibrosis and disease
    - Calcifications most common with chronic pancreatitis due to alcohol (90% with calcification have history of alcohol abuse)
- **Senescent Change, Pancreas**
  - Elderly patients may demonstrate features that mimic chronic pancreatitis, including mild pancreatic ductal dilatation, parenchymal atrophy, and a few punctate parenchymal calcifications
    - Usually a few scattered punctate (1-3 mm) calcifications (parenchymal or intraductal)
  - Typically patients over age of 70 without symptoms of pancreatic endocrine or exocrine deficiency
- **Peripancreatic Vascular Lesions (Mimic)**
  - Vascular calcifications adjacent to pancreas can mimic primary pancreatic calcification
    - Tram-track atherosclerotic calcifications of splenic artery are very common (more common than true pancreatic calcifications)
    - Splenic artery aneurysms can demonstrate peripheral or eggshell calcification
    - Chronic splenic vein thrombus may demonstrate calcification or appear as mural wall thickening with calcification
- **Choledocholithiasis (Mimic)**
  - Calcified stone in distal common bile duct may be difficult to distinguish from pancreatic calcification
    - Often associated with proximal biliary dilatation
  - Use multiplanar reformations to localize stone to distal common bile duct
- **Duodenal Diverticulum (Mimic)**
  - High-density oral contrast (or medication) within diverticulum (when diverticulum abuts pancreas) may mimic parenchymal calcification

Helpful Clues for Less Common Diagnoses

- **Calcified Cystic or Solid Pancreatic Masses**
  - **Pancreatic neuroendocrine tumors**
    - Internal calcifications are common and frequently coarse and irregular (central > eccentric)
      - Most common etiology for calcified **solid** pancreatic mass
      - Small masses can rarely appear almost completely calcified
      - Nonsyndromic tumors and large masses with central necrosis more likely to develop calcification
    - Typically hypervascular tumors, which avidly enhance on arterial phase images
  - **Pancreatic serous cystadenoma**
    - Classic appearance is microcystic adenoma: Honeycomb or sponge pattern with multiple (> 6) small (< 2 cm) internal cysts, central scar, and central calcification
    - Calcifications usually appear dystrophic in center of lesion (in scar) or as thin calcification within septation
    - Usually asymptomatic lesion found in older women (grandmother tumor)
  - **Mucinous cystic neoplasm**

- Premalignant or frankly malignant cystic tumor found most often in middle-aged females
- Unilocular or multilocular cystic lesion, which may demonstrate thick wall, septations, or mural nodularity
  □ Most often found in pancreatic tail
- Curvilinear calcifications can be seen frequently (16%) in either cyst wall or septations
○ **Solid pseudopapillary neoplasm**
- Almost always seen in young (< 35 yr) female patients
- Usually solid, encapsulated mass (typically large at presentation) with enhancing capsule (± cystic components)
  □ Does not usually obstruct pancreatic or common bile ducts
  □ May demonstrate internal hemorrhage (usually easier to appreciate on MR)
- Calcifications are very common (~ 50%) and can be peripheral or central
○ **Pancreatic pseudocyst**
- Longstanding or chronic pseudocysts may demonstrate peripheral calcification
- Usually associated with clinical history or imaging stigmata of prior pancreatitis
○ **Intraductal papillary mucinous neoplasm**
- Mucin-producing tumor that arises from main pancreatic duct or side branches
- Can present as dilated pancreatic duct [main-duct intraductal papillary mucinous neoplasm (IPMN)] or cystic lesion in communication with main pancreatic duct (side-branch IPMN)
- Side-branch IPMN can demonstrate peripheral or septal calcification in 20%
- Main-duct IPMN can demonstrate amorphous calcifications within dilated main pancreatic duct
○ **Pancreatic metastases**
- Metastases to pancreas are rare, but metastases from mucinous tumors of gastrointestinal tract can be associated with calcification
- **Cystic Fibrosis, Pancreas**

○ Pancreatic findings include small parenchymal or intraductal calcifications, fatty replacement of pancreas, and small pancreatic cysts
  - Calcifications are usually tiny and punctate
○ Most common cause of pancreatic calcification in children
  - Usually not diagnostic dilemma due to characteristic lung findings and known clinical history
  - Pancreatic calcifications in cystic fibrosis (CF) usually imply advanced pancreatic fibrosis (often associated with diabetes)
    □ Pancreatic calcifications only seen in minority of patients with CF
- **Hereditary Pancreatitis**
  ○ Autosomal dominant trait associated with several gene mutations
  ○ Results in chronic pancreatitis in unusually young patients (often < 20 yr) with peak incidence at 5 yr of age
  ○ 50% develop intraductal calcifications, which are often large and round in morphology (compared to tiny punctate calcifications in CF)
  ○ Consider this diagnosis in presence of parenchymal/intraductal calcifications or other imaging features of chronic pancreatitis in young patient
  ○ Associated with high risk for pancreatic cancer

Helpful Clues for Rare Diagnoses

- **Kwashiorkor**
  ○ Clinical syndrome associated with severe malnutrition and protein deficiency
    - Virtually never diagnosed in developing world, but can be seen in developing world in areas of famine
  ○ May be associated with pancreatic calcification, as well as clinical signs of pancreatic insufficiency (diabetes and steatorrhea)
- **Hyperparathyroidism**
  ○ Can be associated with pancreatic calcifications either on basis of recurrent pancreatitis or hypercalcemia

---

Chronic Pancreatitis

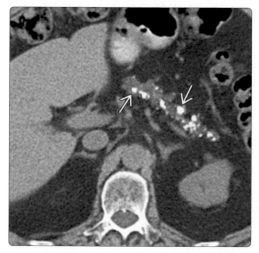

Chronic Pancreatitis

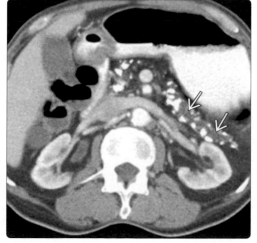

(Left) Axial NECT demonstrates diffuse pancreatic atrophy and multiple pancreatic calcifications ➡ in a patient with chronic pancreatitis. Chronic pancreatitis is, by far, the most common cause of pancreatic calcification. (Right) Axial CECT in a patient with chronic pancreatitis demonstrates characteristic imaging features, including glandular atrophy, a dilated pancreatic duct ➡, and multiple calcifications.

(Left) *Axial CECT shows a rim-calcified lesion* ➡️ *that represents a thrombosed portal vein aneurysm in a patient with cirrhosis and portal hypertension. An abnormality such as this could easily be mistaken for a calcified pancreatic cystic mass.* **(Right)** *Coronal NECT demonstrates a calcified stone* ➡️ *in the distal common bile duct (CBD). When viewed in the axial plane, a stone in this location could conceivably be confused for a pancreatic calcification.*

Peripancreatic Vascular Lesions (Mimic)

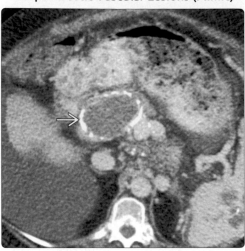

Choledocholithiasis (Mimic)

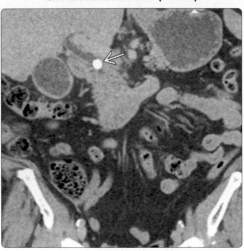

(Left) *Axial CECT demonstrates an enhancing mass* ➡️ *in the pancreatic tail with coarse, dystrophic internal calcifications* ➡️. *This was found to be a neuroendocrine tumor at resection.* **(Right)** *Axial CECT demonstrates a solid mass* ➡️ *in the pancreatic tail with significant internal calcifications, found to be a neuroendocrine tumor at resection. Neuroendocrine tumors represent the most common solid pancreatic mass to demonstrate calcification.*

Pancreatic Neuroendocrine Tumor

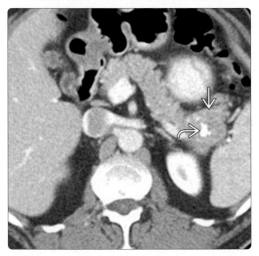

Pancreatic Neuroendocrine Tumor

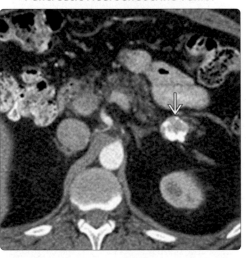

(Left) *Axial CECT demonstrates a low-density mass* ➡️ *in the pancreatic head with multiple internal speckled calcifications. Although subtle, there is the suggestion of septations within the lesion, and this was found to be a serous cystadenoma.* **(Right)** *Axial CECT demonstrates a large cystic mass with multiple internal septations and large cystic spaces, found to be an atypical oligocystic serous cystadenoma. Note the central dystrophic calcification* ➡️ *and more subtle calcifications in septations* ➡️.

Pancreatic Serous Cystadenoma

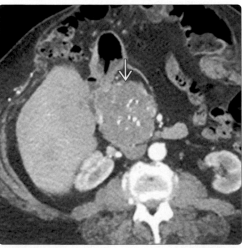

Pancreatic Serous Cystadenoma

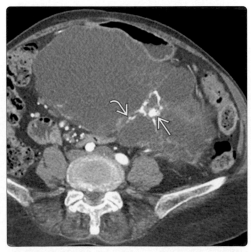

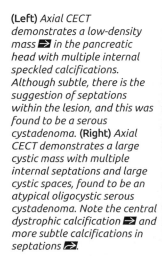

Mucinous Cystic Neoplasm

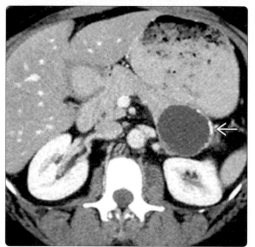

Solid Pseudopapillary Neoplasm

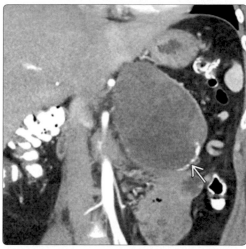

(Left) Axial CECT demonstrates a cystic mass in the pancreatic tail with thin curvilinear peripheral calcification ➡, a classic pattern for a mucinous cystic neoplasm. (Right) Coronal CECT in a young female patient demonstrates a low-density pancreatic mass with peripheral calcification ➡, confirmed to represent a solid pseudopapillary neoplasm (SPEN) at resection. Calcifications in SPEN can be central or peripheral.

Solid Pseudopapillary Neoplasm

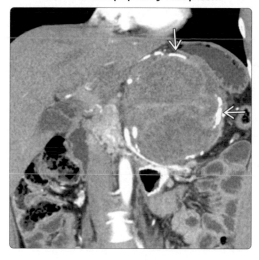

Intraductal Papillary Mucinous Neoplasm

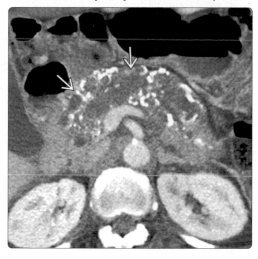

(Left) Coronal CECT in a young female patient demonstrates a heterogenous pancreatic mass with thick peripheral calcification ➡, found to be a SPEN at resection. Higher density internal components could represent solid tumor or hemorrhage. (Right) Axial CECT shows multiple amorphous calcifications within a markedly dilated pancreatic duct ➡. At surgery, the dilated duct was found to be secondary to a main-duct IPMN with associated invasive malignancy.

Pancreatic Pseudocyst

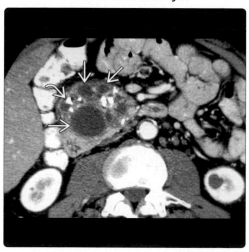

Cystic Fibrosis, Pancreas

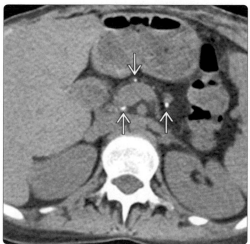

(Left) Axial CECT demonstrates multiple coarse calcifications ➡ in the pancreatic head, as well as multiple round cystic lesions ➡ with thick enhancing rims, consistent with pancreatic pseudocysts in the setting of chronic pancreatitis. (Right) Axial NECT in a patient with cystic fibrosis (CF) demonstrates characteristic fatty atrophy of the pancreas with subtle punctate calcifications ➡. Calcifications are present in a minority of patients with CF and usually suggest significant pancreatic fibrosis.

DIFFERENTIAL DIAGNOSIS

Common

- Pancreatic Pseudocyst
- Serous Cystadenoma of Pancreas
- Mucinous Cystic Neoplasm
- Intraductal Papillary Mucinous Neoplasm

Less Common

- Necrotic Pancreatic Ductal Carcinoma
- Solid Pseudopapillary Neoplasm
- Cystic Pancreatic Neuroendocrine Tumor
- Congenital Cyst
- Lymphoepithelial Cyst
- Cystic Metastases

ESSENTIAL INFORMATION

Key Differential Diagnosis Issues

- US can characterize simple or macrocystic pancreatic lesions
  - Most represent pancreatic pseudocysts
- Remaining benign and malignant cystic pancreatic lesions may appear echogenic due to numerous microcystic interfaces, soft tissue components, or complex content
- CECT or CEMR is necessary to adequately characterize internal features that are not well assessed with transabdominal ultrasound
- Endoscopic ultrasound (EUS) also provides high-resolution imaging but is invasive and requires conscious sedation
  - Can be used for biopsy or fluid aspiration in indeterminate cases
- Key features that guide differential diagnosis
  - Location and size
  - Wall thickness
  - Loculation and number of locules
  - Internal septations and septal thickness
  - Presence of solid components and vascularity
  - Central scar
  - Calcification and location
  - Communication with pancreatic duct
  - Fluid characterization/presence of hemorrhage
  - Pancreatic and biliary diameter
  - Upstream pancreatic atrophy
  - Evidence of acute or chronic pancreatitis
  - Locoregional adenopathy and hepatic metastases
- Consider clinical context
  - Patient demographics, pancreatitis, obstructive symptomatology, familial syndromes

Helpful Clues for Common Diagnoses

- **Pancreatic Pseudocyst**
  - Common late complication of pancreatitis
    - Develops 4-6 weeks after onset of acute pancreatitis
    - Evolves over time, whereas neoplastic lesions persist without change
  - Generally well circumscribed, smooth walled, unilocular, anechoic with posterior acoustic enhancement
  - May be complicated
    - Multilocular
    - Internal echoes with fluid-debris level or septations
    - Wall calcification

- But shows no vascularized soft tissue elements
- Associated with other findings of acute or chronic pancreatitis
  - Parenchymal atrophy or calcification, fat stranding on CT, ductal strictures on MR
  - Generally not seen with mucinous cystic neoplasm (MCN), primary mimic of pseudocyst

- **Serous Cystadenoma of Pancreas**
  - Benign pancreatic tumor
  - Commonly in pancreatic body and tail; 30% occur in pancreatic head
  - Typically composed of small cystic areas separated by internal septations
  - Septa coalesce to form central echogenic scar with "sunburst" calcification
  - Can mimic nonspecific solid and cystic tumor
    - Heterogeneous echogenic appearance due to numerous interfaces
    - Intralesional color Doppler flow in fibrovascular septa
  - Characteristic honeycomb appearance on CT, MR, and endoscopic ultrasound
  - Less commonly, may see oligocystic variant that may be indistinguishable from MCN by imaging
    - EUS-guided cyst aspiration may be helpful in making diagnosis
  - Usually seen in older women (mean age: 61 years)

- **Mucinous Cystic Neoplasm**
  - Tumors range in grade from benign with malignant potential to invasive carcinoma
  - More common location: Pancreatic body and tail
  - Anechoic or hypoechoic, thick-walled, cystic mass ± mildly thickened septa
  - Can demonstrate peripheral calcification
  - May be indistinguishable from pseudocyst
  - Lacks additional findings/history of pancreatitis
  - EUS-guided biopsy may be helpful in making diagnosis
  - Solid components or marked septal thickening suggests carcinoma
  - Seen almost exclusively in middle-aged women (mean age: 50 years)

- **Intraductal Papillary Mucinous Neoplasm**
  - Tumor with varying malignant potential: Branch type generally benign with low malignant potential; main duct intraductal papillary mucinous neoplasm thought to be precursor to invasive pancreatic ductal adenocarcinoma
  - Typically in head of pancreas/uncinate process
  - Main duct type: Marked pancreatic ductal dilatation
    - When diffuse, may simulate chronic pancreatitis
      - However, calcification and parenchymal atrophy are not typically seen
    - If segmental, can mimic fluid collection or mucinous cystic tumor
  - Side branch type: Collections of dilated side branches
    - Anechoic or hypoechoic cyst or collection of small anechoic cysts
    - Look for communication with pancreatic duct, which is distinguishing feature compared to other cystic neoplasms
    - May be multifocal, whereas serous cystadenoma and MCN are typically solitary
  - Occur most frequently in older men (mean age: 65 years)

Helpful Clues for Less Common Diagnoses

- **Necrotic Pancreatic Ductal Carcinoma**
  - Most common pancreatic neoplasm
  - Malignant lesion
  - Commonly in head of pancreas
  - Typically appears as ill-defined, solid, hypoechoic mass with ductal obstruction
  - May show complex cystic areas due to tumor necrosis, side branch obstruction or adjacent pseudocyst
    - Uncommon form of common neoplasm
  - Infiltrative appearance ± vascular invasion distinguishes this entity from other solid malignancies that may show cystic change
  - Obstructive symptomatology
- **Solid Pseudopapillary Neoplasm**
  - Tumor with low-grade malignant potential
  - Commonly in pancreatic tail
  - Well-defined, large heterogeneous echogenic solid and cystic mass
  - Cystic areas are secondary to tumor degeneration and vary in size and morphology
  - Prominent vascular soft tissue components
  - Often shows intratumoral hemorrhage
  - Typically seen in young women (< 35 years)
- **Cystic Pancreatic Neuroendocrine Tumor**
  - All tumors > 5 mm considered malignant
  - Typically round, solid, hypoechoic mass with internal color Doppler flow
  - Central cyst formation may occur due to tumor degeneration
    - Uncommon form of uncommon neoplasm
  - Identification of hypervascular rim can be challenging
  - Familial syndromes: Multiple endocrine neoplasia type I; von Hippel-Lindau; neurofibromatosis type I; tuberous sclerosis
    - May have multiple lesions
    - Occurs in younger patients (< 40 years)
- **Congenital Cyst**
  - True epithelial lining with serous fluid
    - Consider in patients with autosomal dominant polycystic kidney disease, von Hippel-Lindau and cystic fibrosis
      - Usually multiple; can replace entire pancreas (e.g., in cystic fibrosis)
- **Lymphoepithelial Cyst**
  - Rare, benign, lesion usually in tail of pancreas
  - Nonneoplastic, no malignant behavior
  - Macrocystic morphology, multilocular or unilocular cysts
  - May see characteristic T1 hyperintensity and low T2 signal due to keratin content
  - Almost exclusively in middle-aged to elderly men
- **Cystic Metastases**
  - Pancreatic metastases are uncommon
  - Can occur with renal cell carcinoma, melanoma, breast cancer, lung cancer, gastric cancer, colorectal carcinoma

SELECTED REFERENCES

1. Kim YS et al: Rare nonneoplastic cysts of pancreas. Clin Endosc. 48(1):31-8, 2015
2. Goh BK et al: Are the Sendai and Fukuoka consensus guidelines for cystic mucinous neoplasms of the pancreas useful in the initial triage of all suspected pancreatic cystic neoplasms? A single-institution experience with 317 surgically-treated patients. Ann Surg Oncol. 21(6):1919-26, 2014
3. Sahani DV et al: Diagnosis and management of cystic pancreatic lesions. AJR Am J Roentgenol. 200(2):343-54, 2013
4. Megibow AJ et al: The incidental pancreatic cyst. Radiol Clin North Am. 49(2):349-59, 2011
5. Hutchins G et al: Diagnostic evaluation of pancreatic cystic malignancies. Surg Clin North Am. 90(2):399-410, 2010
6. Kalb B et al: MR imaging of cystic lesions of the pancreas. Radiographics. 29(6):1749-65, 2009

Pancreatic Pseudocyst

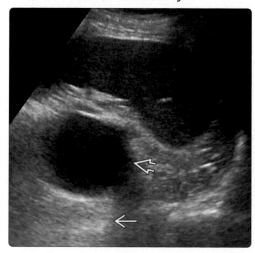

Pancreatic Pseudocyst

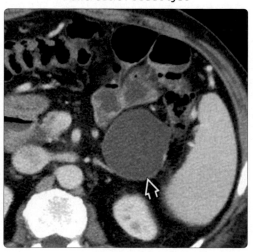

(Left) *Transverse transabdominal ultrasound shows a well-demarcated, anechoic lesion* ➡ *with through transmission* ➡ *in the tail of the pancreas, compatible with a pseudocyst.* (Right) *Axial CECT in the same patient demonstrates a well-demarcated, low-density cystic lesion* ➡ *with a thin wall in the tail of the pancreas. Note the lack of enhancing components and marked pancreatic atrophy.*

(Left) *Transverse transabdominal ultrasound in the region of the pancreas shows a well-circumscribed, unilocular cystic lesion ⇨ with through transmission. Note the echogenic internal contents and layering debris ⇨ compatible with a complex pseudocyst.* **(Right)** *Transverse transabdominal ultrasound shows pancreatic ductal dilation ⇨ and 2 well-circumscribed, elongated fluid collections ⇨ with internal echoes in the neck and body of the pancreas, compatible with complex pseudocysts from severe pancreatitis.*

Pancreatic Pseudocyst

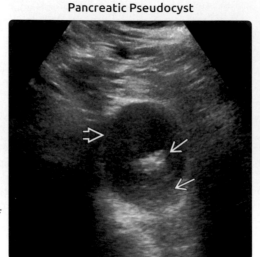

Pancreatic Pseudocyst

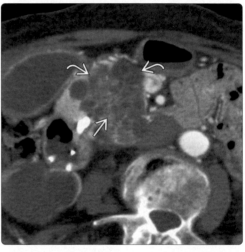

(Left) *Transverse transabdominal ultrasound shows a hyperechoic, solid-appearing mass in the head of the pancreas with small cystic components ⇨ and more echogenic center ⇨.* **(Right)** *Corresponding axial CECT better characterizes numerous small cysts ⇨ within the lesion, separated by thin septa, which appear more coalescent centrally ⇨.*

Serous Cystadenoma of Pancreas

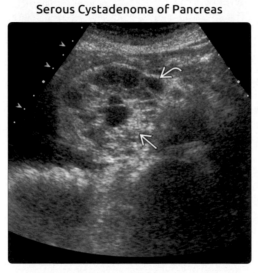

Serous Cystadenoma of Pancreas

(Left) *Transverse transabdominal ultrasound shows a heterogeneous lesion ⇨ in the tail of the pancreas composed of innumerable tiny cysts separated by linear septations, which result in a hyperechoic appearance due to the highly reflective interfaces.* **(Right)** *Axial CECT shows the classic honeycomb appearance of a serous cystadenoma ⇨: A microcystic lesion with thin enhancing septa delineating small cysts. Note the scattered central calcifications and lack of wall thickening, which are also typical features.*

Serous Cystadenoma of Pancreas

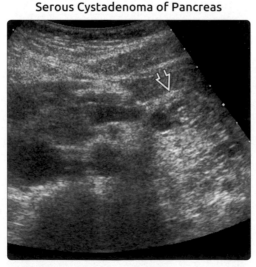

Serous Cystadenoma of Pancreas

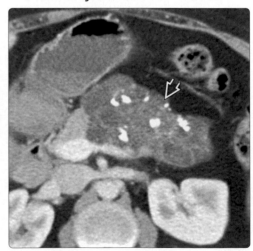

Mucinous Cystic Neoplasm

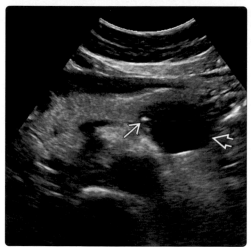

Mucinous Cystic Neoplasm

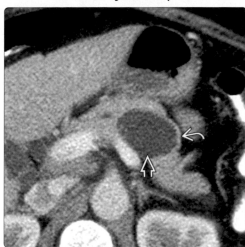

(Left) *Transverse transabdominal ultrasound shows a well-defined, anechoic cystic lesion* ⇒ *in the body of the pancreas with a few hyperechoic peripheral foci* ⇒*.* **(Right)** *Corresponding axial CECT shows an encapsulated oval, hypodense mass* ⇒ *in the body of the pancreas with a thickened enhancing cyst wall* ⇒*. The lesion contained internal septations, not seen on CT.*

Intraductal Papillary Mucinous Neoplasm

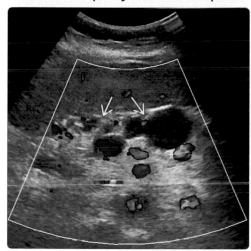

Intraductal Papillary Mucinous Neoplasm

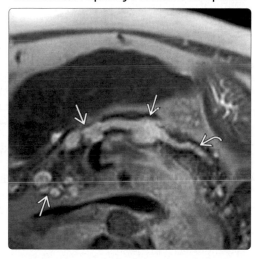

(Left) *Transverse transabdominal color Doppler ultrasound shows a collection of multiple small, round and oval cysts* ⇒ *within the body of the pancreas.* **(Right)** *Axial T2 HASTE MR in the same patient better demonstrates multifocal involvement of the pancreas. Numerous T2-bright cysts* ⇒ *are seen throughout the pancreas, several of which appear contiguous with a dilated pancreatic duct* ⇒*, compatible with a mixed, branch, and main duct intraductal papillary mucinous neoplasm.*

Cystic Pancreatic Neuroendocrine Tumor

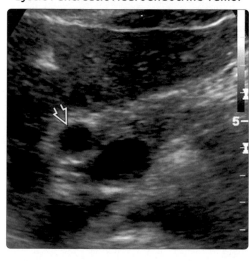

Cystic Pancreatic Neuroendocrine Tumor

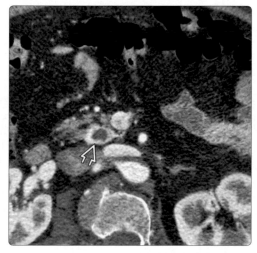

(Left) *Transverse transabdominal ultrasound of the pancreas shows a round, well-circumscribed, cystic lesion* ⇒ *extending exophytically from the neck of the pancreas. This was amenable to endoscopic US-guided biopsy, which showed a cystic neuroendocrine tumor.* **(Right)** *Axial CECT in a different patient shows a round cystic lesion* ⇒ *in the uncinate process with a peripheral rim of hypervascular enhancement, a typical appearance for a small cystic neuroendocrine tumor.*

DIFFERENTIAL DIAGNOSIS

Common

- Pancreatic Ductal Carcinoma
- Focal Acute Pancreatitis
- Chronic Pancreatitis
- Pancreatic Neuroendocrine Tumor
- Serous Cystadenoma of Pancreas
- Mucinous Cystic Neoplasm of Pancreas

Less Common

- Metastasis
- Lymphoma
- Solid Pseudopapillary Neoplasm
- Intrapancreatic Splenule

ESSENTIAL INFORMATION

Key Differential Diagnosis Issues

- Correlate with clinical information (e.g., history of pancreatitis, obstructive symptomatology)
- Pancreatic duct dilatation favors diagnosis of pancreatic ductal carcinoma
  - Biliary dilatation present as well in pancreatic head ductal carcinoma
- Other ancillary findings to look for include
  - Cystic component
  - Internal septation
  - Presence of intralesional calcification
  - Vascular encasement
  - Regional lymph node and liver metastases
- Clues to detection of small tumor
  - Focal contour irregularity
  - Subtle pancreatic duct/bile duct dilatation
- CECT or CEMR improves ability to detect and characterize solid pancreatic lesions
  - Can evaluate for vascular encasement
- Endoscopic ultrasound is invasive; however, increases sensitivity for lesion detection and can be used to guide biopsy for diagnosis

Helpful Clues for Common Diagnoses

- **Pancreatic Ductal Carcinoma**
  - Arises from ductal epithelium of exocrine pancreas
  - Location: Head of pancreas (60-70%), body (20%), diffuse (15%), tail (5%)
  - Average size: ~ 2-3 cm
  - Pathology: Scirrhous infiltrative adenocarcinoma with dense cellularity and sparse vascularity
  - Typical US findings
    - Poorly defined, homogeneous or heterogeneous, hypoechoic mass
    - Pancreatic duct dilatation upstream from tumor with abrupt tapering at site of obstruction
    - Bile duct dilatation seen in pancreatic head tumor
    - Necrosis/cystic component is rarely seen
    - Displacement/encasement of adjacent vascular structures (e.g., superior mesenteric vessels, splenic artery, hepatic artery, gastroduodenal artery)
    - Presence of liver and regional nodal metastases
    - Ascites due to peritoneal metastases

- **Focal Acute Pancreatitis**
  - Clinical information very important for correct imaging interpretation
    - Acute onset of epigastric pain, fever, and vomiting
    - Raised serum amylase and lipase
    - Presence of underlying predisposing factors: Biliary stone, alcoholism, drugs (e.g., steroid), trauma, etc.
  - Focal, ill-defined, hypoechoic enlargement of pancreatic parenchyma
    - Heterogeneous appearance in cases with intrapancreatic necrosis/hemorrhage
  - Blurred pancreatic outline/margin
  - Presence of peripancreatic fluid collection
  - Lack of pancreatic duct dilatation
  - No parenchymal calcification

- **Chronic Pancreatitis**
  - Longstanding clinical symptoms, recurrent attacks of epigastric pain, typically radiates to back
  - Most common US features
    - Diffuse atrophy
    - Main pancreatic duct beading and side branch dilatation
    - Parenchymal and ductal calcifications
  - Can have focal involvement with mass-like appearance
  - Look for smoothly stenotic or normal main duct penetrating abnormal region on MRCP

- **Pancreatic Neuroendocrine Tumor**
  - Functioning and nonfunctioning subtypes have distinct appearances
    - Functioning tumor usually small, solid, well-circumscribed, hypo-/isoechoic mass
    - Nonfunctioning tumors tend to be larger with more heterogeneous echo pattern due to necrosis, calcification, and cystic change
    - Solid components are typically hypervascular on power Doppler US and hyperenhancing on CT and MR
  - Detection may be difficult with small functioning tumors
  - Endoscopic US detects tumors in pancreatic head and body
  - Intraoperative US is useful for tumor localization
  - Liver and regional lymph node metastases seen in 60-90% at clinical presentation
    - Hyperechoic liver metastases more suggestive of neuroendocrine tumors than ductal carcinoma

- **Serous Cystadenoma of Pancreas**
  - Commonly in pancreatic body and tail; 30% occur in pancreatic head
  - Composed of tiny cysts separated by internal septations
  - Septa coalesce to form central echogenic scar with "sunburst" calcification
  - US appearance depends on size of individual cysts
    - Slightly echogenic, solid-appearing mass (small cysts provide numerous acoustic interfaces)
    - Partly solid-appearing mass with anechoic cystic areas; cysts usually at periphery due to central scar
    - Multicystic mass with internal septations and solid component
  - Typically no pancreatic duct dilatation
    - However, large lesions in head of pancreas can behave more aggressively
  - Intralesional color Doppler flow in fibrovascular septa

o Usually seen in older women (6th decade)

- **Mucinous Cystic Neoplasm of Pancreas**
  o More common in pancreatic body and tail
  o Well-demarcated, anechoic or hypoechoic, thick-walled, cystic mass
    – Uni-/multilocular cysts separated by thick echogenic septations
  o Solid papillary tissue protruding into tumor suggests malignancy
  o Liver metastases appear as thick-walled cystic hepatic lesions
  o Seen almost exclusively in middle-aged women

Helpful Clues for Less Common Diagnoses

- **Metastasis**
  o Nonspecific imaging findings
  o Focal or diffuse involvement
  o Renal cell carcinoma: Most common primary; often solitary
  o Other sources: Lung, GI, breast, melanoma, ovary, liver; typically disseminated disease
- **Lymphoma**
  o Secondary lymphoma more common than primary lymphoma
    – Known clinical history of systemic lymphomatous involvement
  o Large, homogeneous, solid mass
  o Presence of peripancreatic nodal masses
  o Peripancreatic vessels displaced or stretched
- **Solid Pseudopapillary Neoplasm**
  o Most common in pancreatic tail
  o Well-demarcated, large, heterogeneous echogenic solid and cystic mass
  o Small cystic areas often present due to tumor degeneration
    – Often with intratumoral hemorrhage
  o Dystrophic calcification occasionally seen
  o No pancreatic duct dilatation or calcification
  o Prominent vascular soft tissue components
    – → hypervascular pattern with color Doppler

o Liver metastases seen in ~ 4% of patients
o Typically seen in young women (< 35 years)

- **Intrapancreatic Splenule**
  o Congenital anomaly arising from aberrant splenic embryologic fusion
  o 2nd most common location for accessory spleens is in the pancreatic tail
  o Appears as small, well-circumscribed solid mass, usually at tip and not > 3 cm from tail
  o Can easily be mistaken for primary pancreatic mass, particularly neuroendocrine tumor
  o Follows attentuation of spleen on all phases of CT imaging and intensity of spleen on all MR sequences
  o Confirm with Tc-99m labeled heat damaged red blood cells

SELECTED REFERENCES

1. Al-Hawary MM et al: Mimics of pancreatic ductal adenocarcinoma. Cancer Imaging. 13(3):342-9, 2013
2. Bhosale PR et al: Vascular pancreatic lesions: spectrum of imaging findings of malignant masses and mimics with pathologic correlation. Abdom Imaging. 38(4):802-17, 2013
3. Dimcevski G et al: Ultrasonography in diagnosing chronic pancreatitis: new aspects. World J Gastroenterol. 19(42):7247-57, 2013
4. Coakley FV et al: Pancreatic imaging mimics: part 1, imaging mimics of pancreatic adenocarcinoma. AJR Am J Roentgenol. 199(2):301-8, 2012
5. Raman SP et al: Pancreatic imaging mimics: part 2, pancreatic neuroendocrine tumors and their mimics. AJR Am J Roentgenol. 199(2):309-18, 2012

Pancreatic Ductal Carcinoma

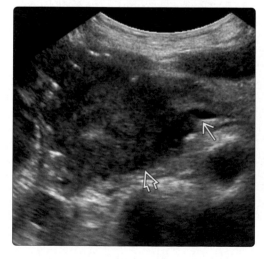

Pancreatic Ductal Carcinoma

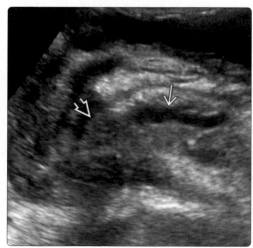

(Left) *Transverse transabdominal ultrasound shows a large infiltrative, solid, hypoechoic mass in the head of the pancreas* ➡ *abutting the superior mesenteric vein* ➡, *raising concern for vascular encasement.* (Right) *Transverse transabdominal ultrasound shows a poorly defined infiltrative hypoechoic mass* ➡ *in the head of the pancreas, obstructing the pancreatic duct, which is dilated upstream* ➡.

(Left) *Longitudinal oblique power Doppler ultrasound shows an ill-defined, solid hypoechoic mass* ⮞ *in the pancreatic head resulting in obstruction of the terminal portion of the common bile duct* ➡. **(Right)** *Transverse transabdominal ultrasound shows a poorly marginated, solid, hypoechoic mass* ⮞ *in the body of the pancreas, narrowing the splenic vein* ➡.

Pancreatic Ductal Carcinoma

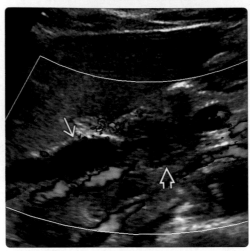

Pancreatic Ductal Carcinoma

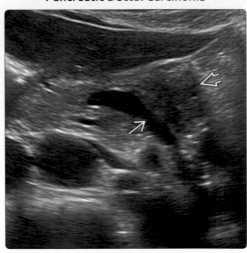

(Left) *Transverse transabdominal ultrasound shows focal enlargement* ⮞ *of the distal pancreas with a homogeneous hypoechoic appearance relative to the normal pancreas* ➡. *Note the absence of ductal dilatation.* **(Right)** *Transverse ultrasound shows parenchymal calcifications* ➡ *in the enlarged pancreatic head. Note the dilated pancreatic* ⮞ *and common bile* ➡ *ducts and the pancreatic margins are indistinct.*

Focal Acute Pancreatitis

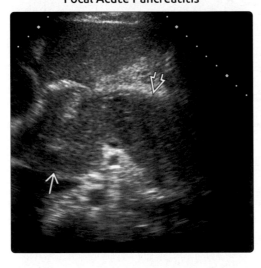

Chronic Pancreatitis

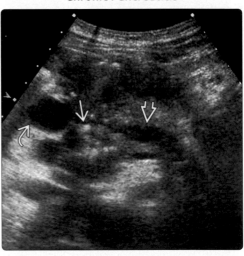

(Left) *Transverse intraoperative ultrasound shows a well-defined, hypoechoic, solid mass* ➡ *in the body of the pancreas, which was a biopsy-proven pancreatic neuroendocrine tumor.* **(Right)** *Transverse transabdominal ultrasound shows a well-circumscribed solid and cystic mass* ⮞ *with peripheral loculations* ➡. *There are also tiny cystic spaces with thin linear septations* ➡.

Pancreatic Neuroendocrine Tumor

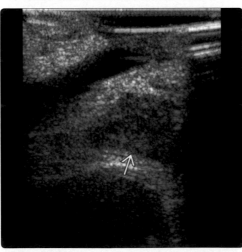

Serous Cystadenoma of Pancreas

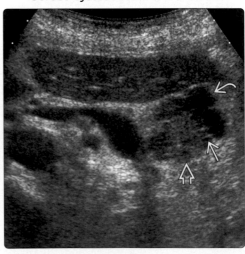

Solid Pancreatic Lesion

Serous Cystadenoma of Pancreas

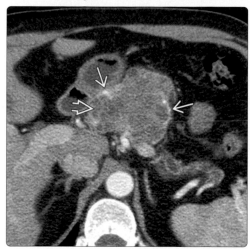

Mucinous Cystic Neoplasm of Pancreas

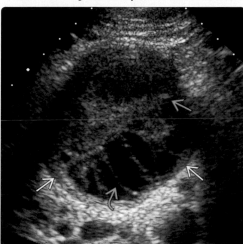

(Left) *Axial CECT demonstrates clusters of tiny cysts ⇒ separated by thin enhancing septations, in a honeycomb pattern characteristic of serous cystadenoma. Note the thin calcifications ➡.* (Right) *Transverse transabdominal ultrasound shows a well-circumscribed, heterogeneous, multilocular cystic mass in the pancreas with thick ➡ and thin ➔ internal septations and a thick wall ➡.*

Metastasis

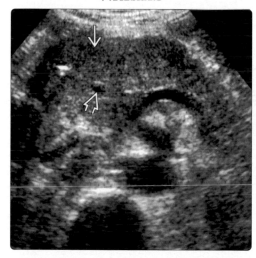

Lymphoma

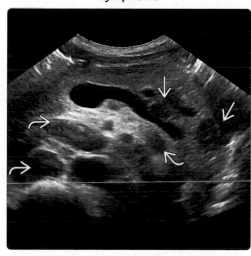

(Left) *Transverse transabdominal ultrasound shows an ill-defined, solid, hypoechoic mass ➡ involving the head and body of the pancreas. The common hepatic artery is encased ➡. Note the absence of pancreatic duct dilatation.* (Right) *Transverse ultrasound of the pancreas shows multiple round masses in the pancreatic tail ➡, compatible with lymphomatous involvement. Other abnormal nodes were present in the retroperitoneum ➡ from disseminated non-Hodgkin lymphoma.*

Solid Pseudopapillary Neoplasm

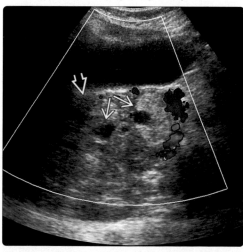

Intrapancreatic Splenule

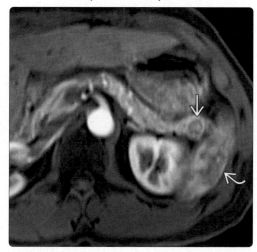

(Left) *Longitudinal ultrasound demonstrates a well-circumscribed, large, heterogeneous, echogenic solid mass ➡ in a 17-year-old girl. Note color Doppler flow in the periphery of the lesion and heterogeneous cystic areas of degeneration ➡.* (Right) *Axial postcontrast T1 FS MR in the arterial phase shows a small, round, well-circumscribed lesion in the tip of the tail of the pancreas ➡. The lesion demonstrates heterogeneous arterial phase enhancement, which matches that of the spleen ➡.*

Pancreas

DIFFERENTIAL DIAGNOSIS

Common

- Chronic Pancreatitis
- Pancreatic Ductal Carcinoma
- Periampullary Tumor

Less Common

- Obstructing Distal Common Bile Duct Stone
- Intraductal Papillary Mucinous Neoplasm

ESSENTIAL INFORMATION

Key Differential Diagnosis Issues

- Pancreatic ductal dilatation: > 3 mm possibly with tortuous configuration
  - May see abrupt tapering at site of obstruction
  - Should prompt thorough search for obstructing lesion at papilla or in pancreatic head
    - US may not provide adequate visualization due to overlying bowel gas or body habitus
    - CT, MR, &/or endoscopic US should be considered
- Isolated pancreatic duct dilatation
  - Most commonly due to chronic pancreatitis
  - High possibility of pancreatic cancer if no evidence of chronic pancreatitis
  - Mild, idiopathic dilatation without tortuosity, frequently seen in elderly patients
- When associated with biliary duct dilatation, termed "double duct" sign
  - Etiology more likely malignant disease; most commonly pancreatic ductal adenocarcinoma
  - Obstructing common bile duct stone or benign stenosis are also possibilities if patient does not have jaundice or mass

Helpful Clues for Common Diagnoses

- **Chronic Pancreatitis**
  - Clinical history of longstanding recurrent attacks of epigastric pain; typically radiates to back
  - Atrophic pancreas with irregular outline and heterogeneous, hypo-/hyperechoic echo pattern
  - Pancreatic calcification: Intraductal and parenchymal
  - May see dilated side branches when severe
  - MR may show duct dilatation with strictures → more suggestive of chronic pancreatitis than intraductal papillary mucinous neoplasm (IPMN)
- **Pancreatic Ductal Carcinoma**
  - Causes pancreatic duct obstruction as tumor arises from ductal epithelium of exocrine pancreas
  - Irregular, ill-defined, solid, hypoechoic mass
  - Pancreatic duct dilatation upstream from tumor
  - Bile duct dilatation with tumor in pancreatic head
  - Lack of pancreatic calcification or ductal calculus
  - May see liver and regional lymph node metastases

Helpful Clues for Less Common Diagnoses

- **Obstructing Distal Common Bile Duct Stone**
  - Obstructive jaundice and epigastric pain
  - Presence of bile duct dilatation
- **Intraductal Papillary Mucinous Neoplasm**
  - Main duct type shows marked diffuse pancreatic ductal dilatation ± pancreatic atrophy
    - Calcification not typically seen and is more suggestive of chronic pancreatitis
    - Mural/intraluminal nodularity or associated soft tissue mass is suggestive of malignancy
  - Side branch duct type may show mild ductal dilatation communicating with cystic pancreatic lesion
    - Grape-like cluster of cysts with IPMN vs. unilocular cyst with chronic pancreatitis

SELECTED REFERENCES

1. Cohen J et al: Double-duct sign in the era of endoscopic ultrasound: the prevalence of occult pancreaticobiliary malignancy. Dig Dis Sci. 59(9):2280-5, 2014
2. Kim JH et al: Intraductal papillary mucinous neoplasm of the pancreas: differentiate from chronic pancreatitis by MR imaging. Eur J Radiol. 81(4):671-6, 2012
3. Tanaka S et al: Slight dilatation of the main pancreatic duct and presence of pancreatic cysts as predictive signs of pancreatic cancer: a prospective study. Radiology. 254(3):965-72, 2010

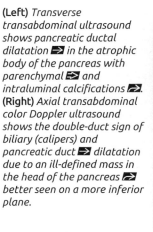

(Left) *Transverse transabdominal ultrasound shows pancreatic ductal dilatation* ➡ *in the atrophic body of the pancreas with parenchymal* ➡ *and intraluminal calcifications* ➡. (Right) *Axial transabdominal color Doppler ultrasound shows the double-duct sign of biliary (calipers) and pancreatic duct* ➡ *dilatation due to an ill-defined mass in the head of the pancreas* ➡ *better seen on a more inferior plane.*

Chronic Pancreatitis

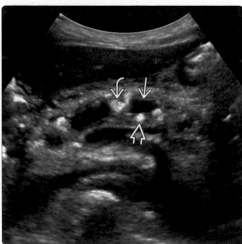

Pancreatic Ductal Carcinoma

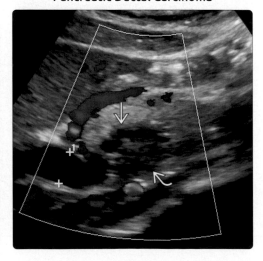

Chronic Pancreatitis

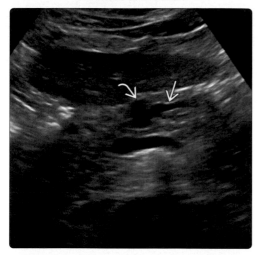

Chronic Pancreatitis

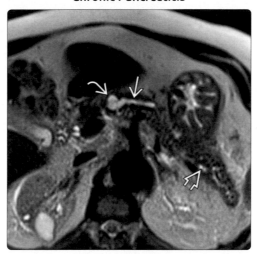

(Left) *Transverse transabdominal ultrasound shows a dilated pancreatic duct* ➡ *communicating with a small pseudocyst* ➡ *in the body of the pancreas.* (Right) *Axial T2 HASTE MR better demonstrates mild pancreatic ductal dilatation* ➡ *communicating with the small pseudocyst* ➡. *Note the tiny dilated side branches* ➡ *in the tail of the pancreas. Pancreatic duct strictures were also seen (not shown) in this patient with a history of pancreatitis.*

Pancreatic Ductal Carcinoma

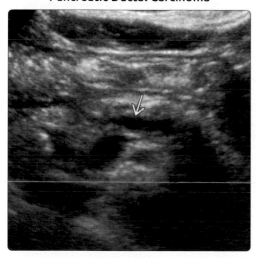

Pancreatic Ductal Carcinoma

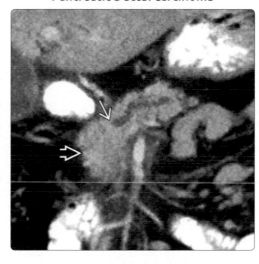

(Left) *Transverse oblique transabdominal ultrasound shows pancreatic ductal dilation in the body of the pancreas* ➡. (Right) *Coronal CECT was performed in the same patient to further characterize the cause of the pancreatic ductal dilatation. The dilated duct terminates abruptly* ➡ *at the site of a large, ill-defined mass in the pancreatic head* ➡.

Intraductal Papillary Mucinous Neoplasm

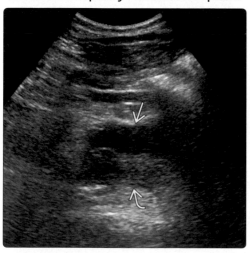

Intraductal Papillary Mucinous Neoplasm

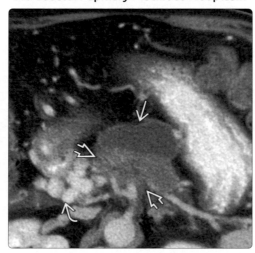

(Left) *Transverse transabdominal ultrasound shows marked pancreatic ductal dilatation* ➡ *with low-level internal echoes and an ill-defined hypoechoic mass posteriorly* ➡. (Right) *Axial CECT demonstrates marked pancreatic ductal dilatation* ➡ *with an infiltrative soft tissue mass posteriorly* ➡, *encasing the celiac axis. Note cavernous transformation of the portal vein* ➡ *due to venous occlusion from the mass which was proven by biopsy to be malignant transformation of a main duct type IPMN.*

SECTION 13
Retroperitoneum

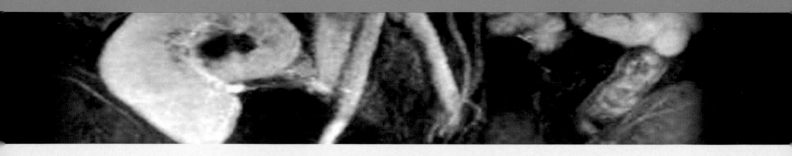

Generic Imaging Patterns

DIFFERENTIAL DIAGNOSIS

Common

- Renal Cystic Masses
  - Renal Cyst
  - Renal Cell Carcinoma (Cystic)
  - Multilocular Cystic Nephroma
- Pancreatic Cystic Masses
  - Pancreatic Pseudocyst
  - Mucinous Cystic Neoplasm
  - Serous (Microcystic) Cystadenoma
  - Islet Cell Tumor
  - Solid and Pseudopapillary Neoplasm
  - Metastases

Less Common

- Adrenal Cystic Masses
  - Adrenal Adenoma (Mimic)
  - Adrenal Cyst
  - Adrenal Seroma (Liquefied Hematoma)
- Retroperitoneal Cystic Masses
  - Retroperitoneal Seroma (Liquefied Hematoma)
  - Retroperitoneal Sarcoma (Mimic)
  - Retroperitoneal Lymphocele
  - Urinoma
  - Retroperitoneal Abscess
  - Lymphangioma

Rare but Important

- Cystic Retroperitoneal Mesothelioma
- Lymphangioleiomyomatosis, Retroperitoneum
- Tailgut Cyst
- Necrosis of Solid Neoplasm
- Pseudomyxoma Retroperitonei

ESSENTIAL INFORMATION

Key Differential Diagnosis Issues

- Most retroperitoneal cystic masses are easily recognized as arising from solid organs
  - Kidney
  - Pancreas
  - Adrenal
- "Cyst mass" may be fluid collection
  - Evolving hematoma
  - Seroma
  - Urinoma

Helpful Clues for Common Diagnoses

- Renal Cystic Masses
  - Renal cyst
    - By far, most common "retroperitoneal" cystic mass (> 50% of older adults)
  - Renal cell carcinoma (cystic)
    - Small percentage are cystic, but usually have mural nodularity to exclude simple cyst
    - Look for claw sign to determine renal origin
  - Multilocular cystic nephroma
    - Complex, multicystic mass with invagination into renal hilum
    - Indistinguishable from cystic renal cell carcinoma

- Biphasic age distribution
  - Boys between 3 months and 2 years old (90% tumors)
  - Females: < 5 years and peak in 5th and 6th decades
- Pancreatic Cystic Masses
  - Pancreatic pseudocyst
    - Most common mass, especially in symptomatic patient with history of alcohol abuse or gallstones
  - Mucinous cystic neoplasm
    - Most common cystic pancreatic tumor
    - Multiseptated mass in body/tail, with mural nodularity
    - Middle-aged or older woman
  - Serous (microcystic) cystadenoma
    - Sponge or honeycomb appearance of well-encapsulated mass
    - Much less common is macrocystic variant, with fewer and larger cystic spaces
  - Other pancreatic cystic masses
    - Islet cell tumor
    - Solid and pseudopapillary neoplasm
    - Metastases

Helpful Clues for Less Common Diagnoses

- Adrenal Cystic Masses
  - Adrenal adenoma (mimic)
    - Lipid-rich adenoma appears near water attenuation on NECT, but enhances, unlike cysts
  - Adrenal cyst
    - Water density
    - No enhancement
    - No visible wall
  - Adrenal seroma (liquefied hematoma)
    - Evolving hematoma will become more homogeneous and lower in attenuation
- Retroperitoneal Cystic Masses
  - Retroperitoneal seroma (liquefied hematoma)
    - Evolving retroperitoneal hematoma (e.g., following ruptured aortic aneurysm, or anticoagulation-induced hemorrhage)
    - May become homogeneous, near water attenuation collection
    - Compare with prior studies, history of hemorrhage
  - Retroperitoneal sarcoma (mimic)
    - Myxoid liposarcoma may have near-water attenuation on CT, but it is solid mass
    - Lower attenuation is myxoid element, or mixture of poorly differentiated fat and other tumor elements
  - Retroperitoneal lymphocele
    - Lymph "pseudocyst" resulting from surgical disruption of pelvic or retroperitoneal lymphatics
    - Renal or pancreatic transplant
    - Common after node dissection/resection for prostate or bladder cancer
  - Urinoma
    - Perirenal or general retroperitoneal collection of urine, following ureteral obstruction and disruption of renal collecting system or ureter
  - Retroperitoneal abscess
    - Complex appearing, may contain gas
    - Perirenal is most common

– Retroperitoneal perforation of appendix or diverticulitis are also well-recognized sources
– Patient is symptomatic (fever, increased white count)

○ **Lymphangioma**
– Discrete, asymmetrical water (or less than water) density mass
– Many thin septations, ± calcifications
– Very soft, easily indented by adjacent vessels

Helpful Clues for Rare Diagnoses

• **Cystic Retroperitoneal Mesothelioma**
○ Much less common than pleural or peritoneal mesothelioma
○ May be unilocular

• **Lymphangioleiomyomatosis, Retroperitoneum**
○ Proliferation of smooth muscle cells within lymphatics causes obstruction and mass

• **Tailgut Cyst**
○ Found in retrorectal (presacral) space
○ May be either unilocular or multilocular

○ Filled with mucoid material, which may be echogenic on ultrasound

• **Necrosis of Solid Neoplasm**
○ Any retroperitoneal tumor may be hypovascular or necrotic enough to simulate cystic mass

• **Pseudomyxoma Retroperitonei**
○ May occur in isolation, without intraperitoneal disease

SELECTED REFERENCES

1. Al-Hawary MM et al: Pancreatic solid and cystic neoplasms: diagnostic evaluation and intervention. Radiol Clin North Am. 53(5):1037-48, 2015
2. Loock MT et al: MR imaging features of nongynaecologic cystic lesions of the pelvis. Clin Imaging. 37(2):211-8, 2013
3. Tsai CF et al: Huge urinoma presenting as a bulging mass. Nephrology (Carlton). 18(6):477, 2013
4. Wilkinson C et al: Adult multilocular cystic nephroma: report of six cases with clinical, radio-pathologic correlation and review of literature. Urol Ann. 5(1):13-7, 2013
5. Katabathina VS et al: Cystic renal neoplasms and renal neoplasms associated with cystic renal diseases in adults: cross-sectional imaging findings. J Comput Assist Tomogr. 36(6):659-68, 2012
6. Shanbhogue AK et al: Uncommon primary pelvic retroperitoneal masses in adults: a pattern-based imaging approach. Radiographics. 32(3):795-817, 2012

Renal Cyst

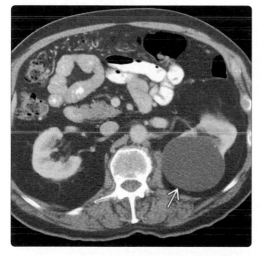

Renal Cyst

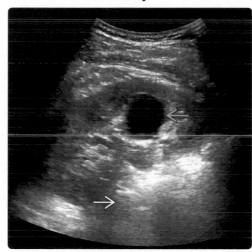

(Left) Axial CECT shows a typical simple cyst ➡, having no enhancement of the water attenuation contents, no mural nodularity or septa, and having a well-marginated exophytic component. (Right) Longitudinal ultrasound shows a simple cyst ➡ within the inferior pole of the kidney. The cyst is simple-appearing due to its imperceptible wall, anechoic contents, and posterior through transmission ➡. Application of color Doppler (not shown) revealed no flow within the cyst.

Renal Cell Carcinoma (Cystic)

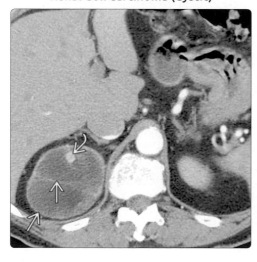

Renal Cell Carcinoma (Cystic)

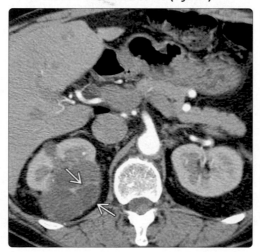

(Left) Axial CECT shows a complex mass arising from the superior pole of the right kidney. The mass shows a discernible, contrast-enhancing peripheral wall, enhancing septa ➡, and a focal, enhancing nodule ➡ along its anterior aspect. Pathology was consistent with cystic renal cell carcinoma. (Right) Axial CECT shows a lobulated, complex cystic mass with numerous, enhancing septa and a thin, barely perceptible, peripheral wall ➡.

Multilocular Cystic Nephroma

Multilocular Cystic Nephroma

(Left) *Axial CECT shows a complex cystic mass with thin enhancing septa ➡. Note invagination into the renal hilum ➡, a characteristic feature of this tumor.* **(Right)** *Transverse ultrasound of the right kidney demonstrates an encapsulated, multiloculated cystic mass ➡ that herniates into the renal sinus, characteristic of a multilocular cystic nephroma.*

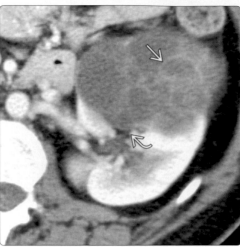

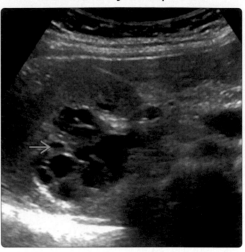

Pancreatic Pseudocyst

Mucinous Cystic Neoplasm

(Left) *Axial CECT shows 2 retroperitoneal cystic masses that are pseudocysts ➡, following an episode of necrotizing pancreatitis. The pseudocyst dorsal to the descending colon has higher density contents and an enhancing wall due to infection. The gallbladder ➡ is also seen.* **(Right)** *Axial CECT shows a complex cystic pancreatic mass ➡ with relatively few large cystic spaces separated by enhancing septa ➡. There is minimal dilation of the upstream pancreatic duct ➡ and no parenchymal atrophy.*

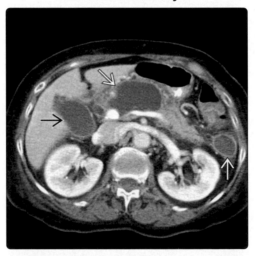

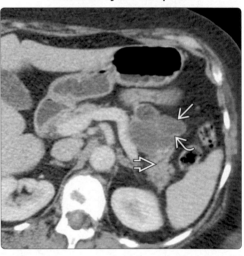

Serous (Microcystic) Cystadenoma

Adrenal Adenoma (Mimic)

(Left) *Axial CECT shows a large mass ➡ arising from the pancreatic head, with a sponge or honeycomb appearance due to innumerable tiny cystic spaces. Some of the septa have focal calcifications ➡.* **(Right)** *Axial NECT shows a water density, but solid, mass ➡ in the right adrenal, a typical appearance of a lipid-rich adenoma on NECT. The lesion enhanced to "soft tissue density" (40 HU) after contrast administration.*

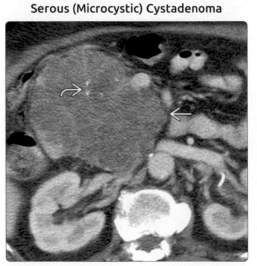

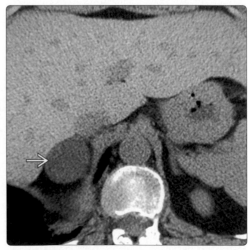

Adrenal Cyst

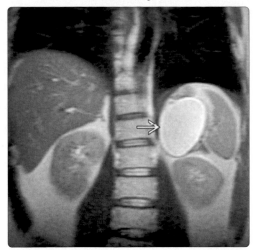

Adrenal Seroma (Liquefied Hematoma)

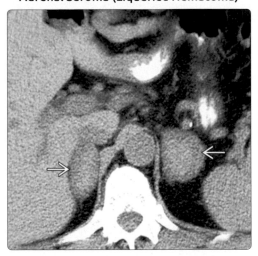

(Left) *Coronal T2WI MR shows a uniformly high-intensity mass ➡ in the left suprarenal region, a typical appearance for an adrenal cyst.* (Right) *Axial NECT shows bilateral heterogeneously high-attenuation masses ➡ in the adrenal glands due to acute hemorrhage. These evolved into water density seromas.*

Adrenal Seroma (Liquefied Hematoma)

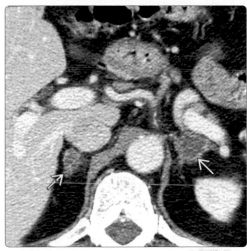

Retroperitoneal Seroma (Liquefied Hematoma)

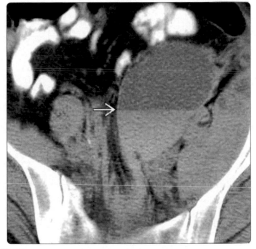

(Left) *Axial CECT shows bilateral small water density, nonenhancing masses ➡ in the adrenal glands, 12 weeks after a prior CT scan had shown larger, heterogeneously high-attenuation masses due to acute hemorrhage.* (Right) *Axial NECT shows a retroperitoneal hemorrhage centered in the iliopsoas compartment. Note the hematocrit sign ➡ with a cell-fluid level indicative of a coagulopathic hemorrhage.*

Retroperitoneal Seroma (Liquefied Hematoma)

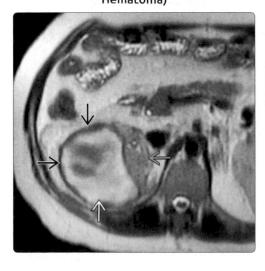

Retroperitoneal Sarcoma (Mimic)

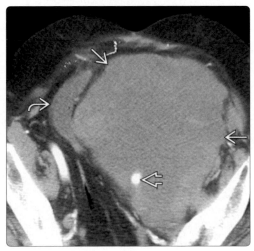

(Left) *Axial T2WI FS MR shows a heterogeneous mass in right perinephric space that compresses kidney ➡. Thin, low signal intensity outer rim ➡ surrounds high signal intensity inner rim ➡, both of which surround an intermediate signal intensity center. Findings are consistent with a subacute hematoma.* (Right) *Axial CECT shows a large retroperitoneal mass ➡ of near water attenuation due to poorly differentiated liposarcoma with myxoid elements. The mass displaces the urinary bladder ➡ and left iliac vessels ➡.*

Retroperitoneal Sarcoma (Mimic)

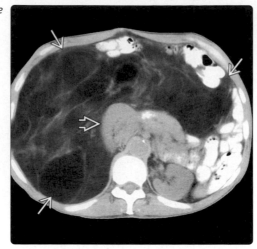

Retroperitoneal Sarcoma (Mimic)

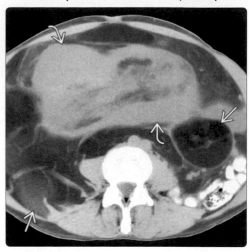

(Left) *Axial CECT shows a huge retroperitoneal mass* ➡ *that is mostly of near fat density, representing a liposarcoma. Note displacement of retroperitoneal structures, including the right kidney* ➡ *and ascending colon.* (Right) *Axial CECT shows a huge retroperitoneal mass* ➡ *that contains large foci of fat density and others of soft tissue or "water" attenuation* ➡*, the latter representing myxoid or poorly differentiated sections of the tumor.*

Retroperitoneal Lymphocele

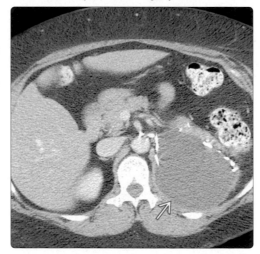

Retroperitoneal Lymphocele

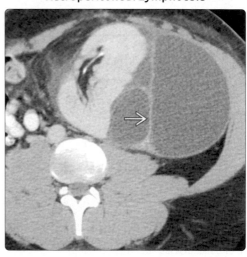

(Left) *Axial CECT shows a water density, nonenhancing mass* ➡ *in the left nephrectomy bed. The patient was asymptomatic following resection for renal cell carcinoma.* (Right) *Axial CECT shows a water density mass with several thin internal septa* ➡ *displacing a renal allograft.*

Retroperitoneal Lymphocele

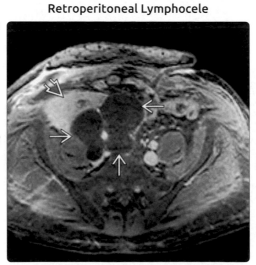

Retroperitoneal Lymphocele

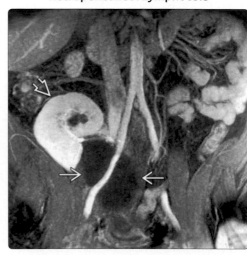

(Left) *Axial T1 C+ FS MR shows a septate cystic mass* ➡ *medial and inferior to a renal allograft* ➡*, a typical appearance of a posttransplant lymphocele.* (Right) *Coronal T1 C+ FS MR shows a septate, cystic mass* ➡*, medial and inferior to a renal allograft* ➡*, that caused partial obstruction of the ureter and transplant dysfunction.*

Urinoma

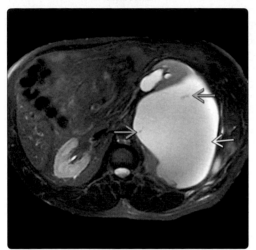

Urinoma

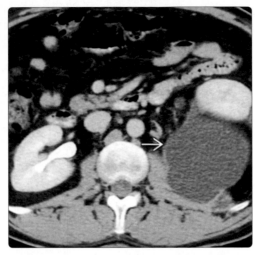

(Left) Axial T2W MR with fat saturation shows homogenous high signal intensity within a large perinephric space urinoma ➡; a few thin septa ➡ are noted. *(Right)* Axial CECT shows a water density retroperitoneal urinoma ➡ due to ureteral injury that occurred during resection of the left colon.

Retroperitoneal Abscess

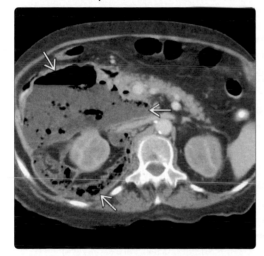

Lymphangioma

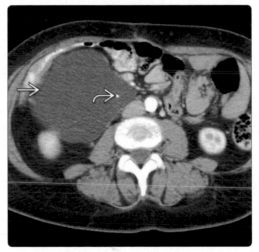

(Left) Axial CECT shows a huge collection ➡ of fluid (pus) and gas in the retroperitoneum as a result of duodenal perforation, caused by endoscopic papillotomy & biliary stone extraction. *(Right)* Axial CECT shows a large water density cyst ➡ that displaces abdominal and retroperitoneal structures. The presence of a small calcification ➡ suggests thin septa that are difficult to detect by CT.

Lymphangioleiomyomatosis, Retroperitoneum

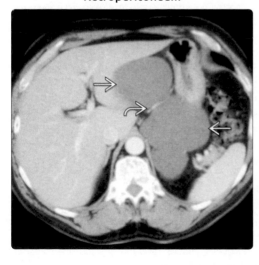

Lymphangioleiomyomatosis, Retroperitoneum

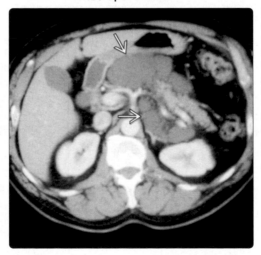

(Left) Axial CECT of a 53-year-old man shows a septate cystic retroperitoneal (or lesser sac) mass ➡. The left gastric artery ➡ indents the mass, a finding indicating the lesion's soft consistency. *(Right)* Axial CECT shows contiguous cystic, septate retroperitoneal masses ➡ that surround the pancreas and celiac axis but cause no obstructive signs or symptoms.

DIFFERENTIAL DIAGNOSIS

Common

- Lymphoma
- Metastases
- Sarcoma
- Retroperitoneal Hemorrhage
- Posttransplant Lymphoproliferative Disorder
- Infectious/Inflammatory Nodes
- Duplications and Anomalies of Inferior Vena Cava
- Collateral Vessels and Varices
- Retroperitoneal Fibrosis
- Unopacified Bowel (Mimic)

Less Common

- Nerve Sheath Tumors
  - Neurofibroma
  - Ganglioneuroma
  - Plexiform Neurofibroma
  - Malignant Peripheral Nerve Sheath Tumor
  - Neurilemoma, Retroperitoneal
  - Paraganglioma
- Leukemia, Abdominal Manifestations
- Malignant Fibrous Histiocytoma
- Hemangiopericytoma, Retroperitoneal

Rare but Important

- Extramedullary Hematopoiesis
- Lymphangioleiomyomatosis
- Primary Retroperitoneal Seminoma
- Primary Retroperitoneal Teratoma
- Chordoma

ESSENTIAL INFORMATION

Key Differential Diagnosis Issues

- Determine location and origin of mass
  - Determine if arising from retroperitoneal organ (e.g., kidney, adrenal, pancreas)
  - Look for beak sign (distortion of contour of organ by exophytic mass arising from it)
  - If it causes anterior displacement of retroperitoneal structure [e.g., ascending or descending colon, aorta, inferior vena cava (IVC)], it is retroperitoneal
    - If not arising from organ, it is considered primary retroperitoneal mass
- Most retroperitoneal masses are malignant
  - Lymphoma > metastases > primary sarcoma

Helpful Clues for Common Diagnoses

- **Lymphoma**
  - Non-Hodgkin > Hodgkin for abdominal disease, especially with mesenteric nodes
  - Discrete or confluent nodes surrounding aorta and IVC; symmetrical
- **Metastases**
  - Most common primary sites: Pelvic malignancy > melanoma, breast, lung, others; asymmetrical
- **Sarcoma**
  - Large eccentric mass that displaces abdominal viscera
  - Liposarcoma is most common type

- Often contains foci of near-fat density, but also areas of water or soft tissue attenuation [representing myxoid or poorly differentiated (high-grade) portions of tumor]
- Myxoid regions appear hyperintense on T2WI and show delayed enhancement
- However, other fibrous tumors may have similar delayed enhancement (neurogenic tumors and malignant fibrous histiocytoma)
  - Leiomyosarcoma
    - Large, encapsulated, soft tissue density mass with foci of necrosis
- **Retroperitoneal Hemorrhage**
  - Coagulopathic or ruptured aneurysm
  - Fluid of high density dissects along fascial planes
- **Infectious/Inflammatory Nodes**
  - Hepatitis, mononucleosis, tuberculosis, sarcoid
- **Duplications and Anomalies of Inferior Vena Cava**
  - Cylindrical shape, characteristic enhancement pattern
  - Left-sided IVC joins left renal vein
- **Collateral Vessels and Varices**
  - Bypassing occluded or absent IVC
  - Portal hypertension (varices often shunt to renal and gonadal veins)
- **Retroperitoneal Fibrosis**
  - Mantle of tissue encasing lower aorta, IVC, ureters
  - Often causes ureteral obstruction and medial deviation

Helpful Clues for Less Common Diagnoses

- **Neurofibroma**
  - Benign nerve sheath tumor
  - May occur as isolated finding or as part of neurofibromatosis
  - High signal on T2WI
- **Plexiform Neurofibroma**
  - Invariably associated with neurofibromatosis, type 1
    - Other findings of NF1 include acoustic nerve schwannomas, meningiomas, café au lait skin pigmentation
  - Plexiform tumors are benign, elongated, symmetrical masses that parallel psoas muscle; may extend into presacral pelvis
  - Usually hypodense to muscle on CECT; may have swirled pattern of enhancement
- **Malignant Peripheral Nerve Sheath Tumor**
  - Also part of NF1 complex
  - Suggested by asymmetrical retroperitoneal mass in patient with this syndrome
- **Neurilemoma, Retroperitoneal**
  - More often spherical (rather than elongated like other masses)
  - Well encapsulated; central necrosis
- **Paraganglioma**
  - Occur along sympathetic nerve chain
  - Often hypervascular with central necrosis
  - Very bright on T2WI
  - Same histology and biochemistry as pheochromocytoma
- **Malignant Fibrous Histiocytoma**
  - Most common soft tissue sarcoma in adults
  - But only 15% arise in retroperitoneum or abdomen

- ○ Nonspecific appearance of soft tissue density, asymmetric mass
- **Hemangiopericytoma, Retroperitoneal**
  - ○ May extend into pelvis
  - ○ Asymmetric large mass with foci of necrosis
  - ○ Most characteristic feature is hypervascularity
    - − Most other retroperitoneal tumors are hypovascular

Helpful Clues for Rare Diagnoses

- **Extramedullary Hematopoiesis**
  - ○ In patients with myelodysplastic conditions or hemoglobinopathies
  - ○ Can affect virtually any organ or site
    - − Paraspinal and perirenal masses may result
    - − Other abdominal sites include liver and spleen
- **Primary Retroperitoneal Seminoma**
  - ○ Most or all represent metastases from testicular primary germ cell malignancy
  - ○ Testicular mass is often clinically silent and may be represented only by scarred lesion

SELECTED REFERENCES

1. Barrington SF et al: Role of imaging in the staging and response assessment of lymphoma: consensus of the International Conference on Malignant Lymphomas Imaging Working Group. J Clin Oncol. 32(27):3048-58, 2014
2. Lubner MG et al: Primary malignant tumors of peritoneal and retroperitoneal origin: clinical and imaging features. Surg Oncol Clin N Am. 23(4):821-45, 2014
3. Allen-Auerbach M et al: PET/computed tomography and lymphoma. Radiol Clin North Am. 51(5):833-44, 2013
4. Caiafa RO et al: Retroperitoneal fibrosis: role of imaging in diagnosis and follow-up. Radiographics. 33(2):535-52, 2013
5. Eberhardt SC et al: Oncology imaging in the abdomen and pelvis: where cancer hides. Abdom Imaging. 38(4):647-71, 2013
6. George V et al: Chronic fibrosing conditions in abdominal imaging. Radiographics. 33(4):1053-80, 2013
7. Manzella A et al: Abdominal manifestations of lymphoma: spectrum of imaging features. ISRN Radiol. 2013:483069, 2013
8. Osman S et al: A comprehensive review of the retroperitoneal anatomy, neoplasms, and pattern of disease spread. Curr Probl Diagn Radiol. 42(5):191-208, 2013
9. Shanbhogue AK et al: Uncommon primary pelvic retroperitoneal masses in adults: a pattern-based imaging approach. Radiographics. 32(3):795-817, 2012

Lymphoma

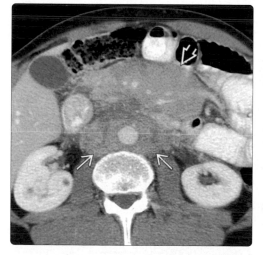

Lymphoma

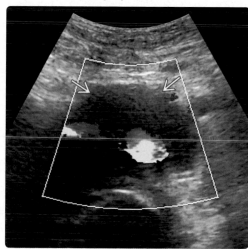

(Left) Axial CECT shows retroperitoneal lymphadenopathy ➡ that surrounds the aorta and inferior vena cava (IVC), and mesenteric adenopathy ➡ that surrounds the mesenteric vessels (sandwich sign). (Right) Transverse color Doppler US shows a soft tissue mass ➡ surrounding the aorta and IVC due to non-Hodgkin lymphoma.

Lymphoma

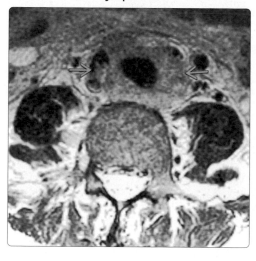

Lymphoma

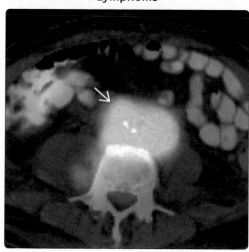

(Left) Axial T2WI MR SS FSE in the same patient shows that the periaortic mass ➡ has intermediate to high signal intensity. (Right) Axial PET/CT in the same patient demonstrates that the non-Hodgkin lymphoma adenopathy ➡ is intensely FDG-avid.

Lymphoma

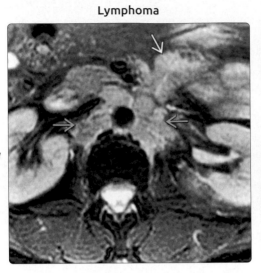

Sarcoma

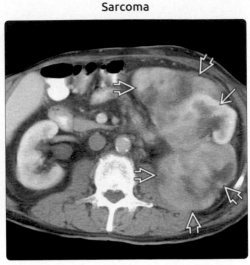

(Left) *Axial T2WI MR with fat suppression shows high signal intensity in confluent paraaortic* ➡ *and mesenteric* ➡ *adenopathy due to non-Hodgkin lymphoma.* (Right) *Axial CECT shows a huge mass* ➡ *that displaces and envelopes the kidney* ➡. *In spite of the apparent absence of fat-density tissue, this was a liposarcoma, predominantly poorly differentiated (pleomorphic; myxoid).*

Metastases

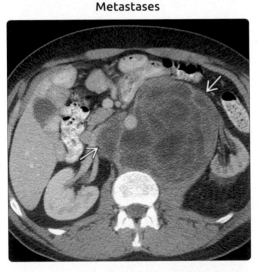

Metastases

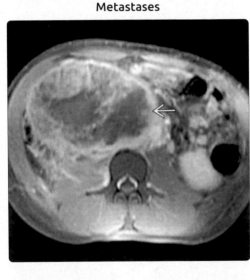

(Left) *Axial CECT shows a huge mass of retroperitoneal nodes* ➡ *from metastatic testicular carcinoma. Note the low density and asymmetric shape of the nodal mass, both common features of this disease, but unusual for lymphoma.* (Right) *Axial T1 C+ MR with fat saturation reveals a large, retroperitoneal mass* ➡ *that is partially necrotic. Its location to the right of midline reflects that the metastasis is ipsilateral to the primary tumor in the right testis (not shown).*

Retroperitoneal Hemorrhage

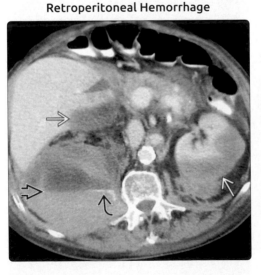

Retroperitoneal Hemorrhage

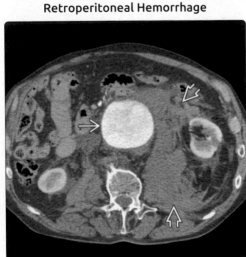

(Left) *Axial CECT shows multiple classic signs of a coagulopathic hemorrhage, including involvement of the iliopsoas compartment, the hematocrit sign* ➡, *multiple sites of hemorrhage* ➡, *and active bleeding* ➡. (Right) *Axial CECT shows a classic retroperitoneal hemorrhage due to a ruptured abdominal aortic aneurysm, including a large aneurysm* ➡, *and contiguous blood that tracks through multiple compartments of the retroperitoneum* ➡.

Posttransplant Lymphoproliferative Disorder

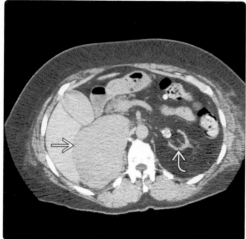

Infectious/Inflammatory Nodes

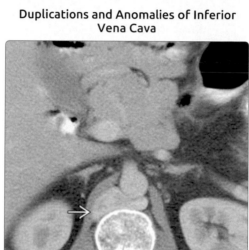

(Left) *Axial NECT shows massive right retroperitoneal adenopathy* ➡ *due to posttransplant lymphoproliferative disorder in a patient with a renal transplant. Note the end-stage left kidney* ➡. *(Right) Axial CECT shows enlarged retroperitoneal and mesenteric nodes* ➡ *in a patient with AIDS due to systemic HIV infection.*

Duplications and Anomalies of Inferior Vena Cava

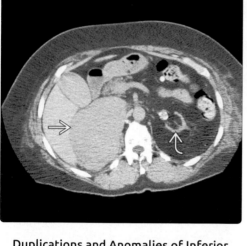

Duplications and Anomalies of Inferior Vena Cava

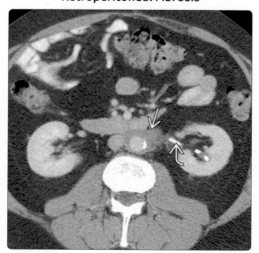

(Left) *Axial CECT shows both renal veins* ➡ *draining into the IVC, which does not continue cephalad, but extends behind the right crus as an azygous continuation* ➡. *(Right) Axial CECT shows azygous continuation of an interrupted IVC* ➡, *simulating a retrocrural mass.*

Collateral Vessels and Varices

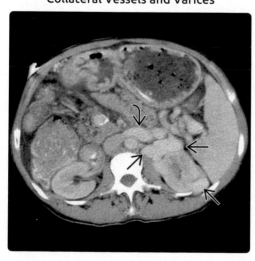

Retroperitoneal Fibrosis

(Left) *Axial CECT shows enormous varices* ➡ *that surround the left kidney and empty into the IVC through a spontaneous splenorenal shunt* ➡. *If the varices had not been opacified by an adequate IV bolus of contrast media, they might have been mistaken for a retroperitoneal mass.* **(Right)** *Axial CECT shows the classic appearance of a mantle of soft tissue* ➡ *that encases the aorta and IVC and obstructs the ureters. Note the left ureteral stent* ➡.

Retroperitoneal Fibrosis

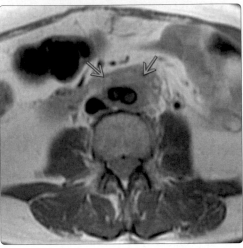

Retroperitoneal Fibrosis

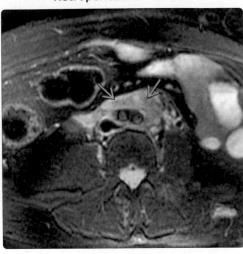

(Left) *Axial T1WI MR shows a mantle of soft tissue ➡ surrounding the anterior and lateral aspects of the iliac bifurcation. The soft tissue has low to intermediate signal intensity.* (Right) *Axial T2WI MR with fat suppression in the same patient demonstrates high signal intensity of the soft tissue mass ➡ that surrounds the iliac bifurcation, consistent with active fibrosis.*

Unopacified Bowel (Mimic)

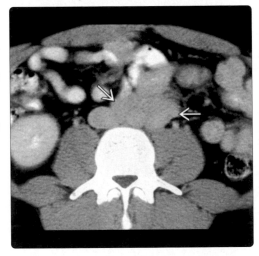

Ganglioneuroma

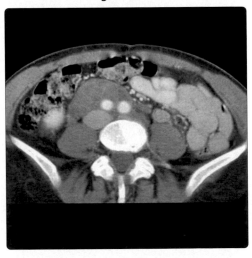

(Left) *Axial CECT shows what appears to be a soft tissue density mass ➡ around the aorta that actually represents unopacified bowel.* (Right) *Axial CECT shows an eccentric soft tissue density mass that had a cylindrical shape and paralleled the IVC and right iliac vessels but did not invade or obstruct the ureters (confirmed ganglioneuroma).*

Ganglioneuroma

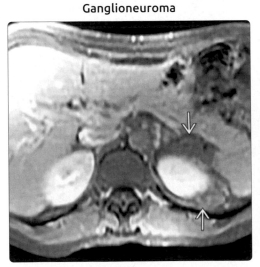

Plexiform Neurofibroma

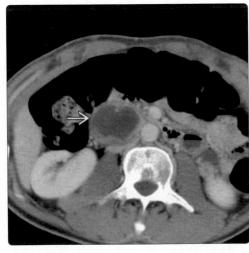

(Left) *Axial T1WI C+ MR with fat suppression shows heterogeneous enhancement of a left perirenal soft tissue mass ➡. Pathology proved ganglioneuroma.* (Right) *Axial CECT shows part of an extensive abdominal and retroperitoneal mass ➡ in a patient with neurofibromatosis type 1, representing plexiform neurofibroma.*

Neurilemoma, Retroperitoneal

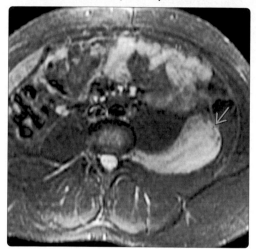

Paraganglioma

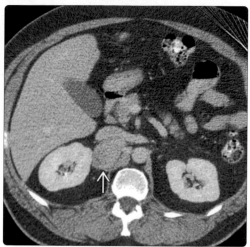

(Left) Axial T2WI MR with fat suppression reveals slightly heterogeneous, high signal intensity within the left retroperitoneal mass ➡. Surgical pathology was consistent with a benign neurilemoma. (Right) Axial CECT shows a right retroperitoneal mass ➡ that proved to be a paraganglioma on MIBG scan and resection.

Paraganglioma

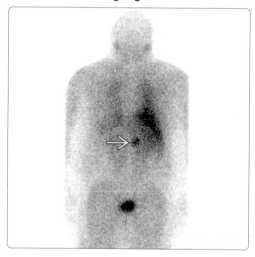

Leukemia, Abdominal Manifestations

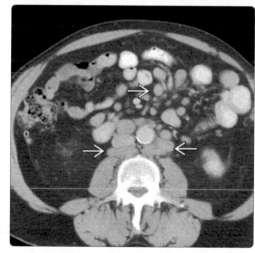

(Left) Coronal MIBG scintigraphy shows a focal uptake of MIBG ➡ in the right paraspinal region, suggesting a pheochromocytoma in the adrenal gland, or a paraganglioma in extra-adrenal tissue along the sympathetic axis. (Right) Axial CECT shows retroperitoneal and mesenteric adenopathy ➡, resembling that typical of lymphoma, but in a patient with chronic lymphocytic leukemia.

Malignant Fibrous Histiocytoma

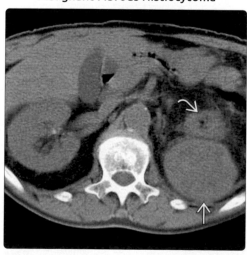

Malignant Fibrous Histiocytoma

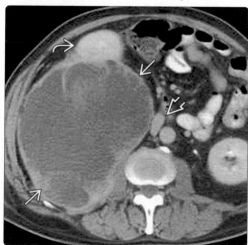

(Left) Axial NECT shows a large, soft tissue density mass ➡ that displaces the kidney ➡ forward. There is no means of distinguishing this from other retroperitoneal tumors, such as a leiomyosarcoma, on imaging alone. (Right) Axial CECT shows a large, heterogeneous retroperitoneal mass ➡ that displaces the kidney ➡ forward and the IVC to the left ➡.

DIFFERENTIAL DIAGNOSIS

Common

- Liposarcoma
- Angiomyolipoma, Renal
- Adrenal Myelolipoma

Less Common

- Metastases, Retroperitoneal
- Pyelonephritis, Xanthogranulomatous
- AIDS Lipodystrophy
- Lipoma, Retroperitoneal
- Teratoma, Retroperitoneum
- Pelvic Lipomatosis

ESSENTIAL INFORMATION

Key Differential Diagnosis Issues

- 2 key features distinguish liposarcoma from renal angiomyolipoma (AML)
  - Liposarcoma is less vascular than AML
  - AML will replace part of kidney (claw sign)

Helpful Clues for Common Diagnoses

- **Liposarcoma**
  - Usually large when discovered
  - Usually has fat and soft tissue density (myxoid) components
  - Usually compresses and displaces retroperitoneal organs; invasion is uncommon
- **Angiomyolipoma, Renal**
  - Benign hamartoma composed of blood vessels, muscle, and fat
  - Large angiomyolipoma may simulate liposarcoma (both contain fat)
  - Renal parenchymal defect and enlarged vessels favor AML
- **Adrenal Myelolipoma**
  - Fat and soft tissue components ± calcification; benign

Helpful Clues for Less Common Diagnoses

- **Metastases, Retroperitoneal**
  - Testicular or ovarian malignant teratomas
  - Growing retroperitoneal mixed fatty density mass in patient with treated nonseminomatous germ cell tumor may represent residual teratoma
- **Pyelonephritis, Xanthogranulomatous**
  - Chronic obstruction and infection
  - Closely related: Replacement lipomatosis of kidney
- **AIDS Lipodystrophy**
  - Proliferation of retroperitoneal and mesenteric fat in response to medications used to treat AIDS
  - No discrete focal mass
- **Lipoma, Retroperitoneal**
  - Less heterogeneous than liposarcoma
  - May arise from duodenum
- **Teratoma, Retroperitoneum**
  - Uncommon to rare as primary retroperitoneal tumor
- **Pelvic Lipomatosis**
  - Nonencapsulated overgrowth of benign fatty tissue in perirectal and perivesical spaces
  - Straightens and lifts rectosigmoid colon
  - Pear-shaped, nondistensible bladder compressed by extensive perivesical fat

SELECTED REFERENCES

1. Schieda N et al: Pitfalls of adrenal imaging with chemical shift MRI. Clin Radiol. Nov;69(11):1186-97, 2014
2. Hekimoglu K: Giant retroperitoneal liposarcomas: diagnostic approach with multidetector computed tomography and magnetic resonance imaging. JBR-BTR. 96(6):375-7, 2013
3. Osman S et al: A comprehensive review of the retroperitoneal anatomy, neoplasms, and pattern of disease spread. Curr Probl Diagn Radiol. 42(5):191-208, 2013
4. Goenka AH et al: Imaging of the retroperitoneum. Radiol Clin North Am. 50(2):333-55, vii, 2012
5. Kani KK et al: Extrahepatic, nonneoplastic, fat-containing lesions of the abdominopelvic cavity: spectrum of lesions, significance, and typical appearance on multidetector computed tomography. Curr Probl Diagn Radiol. 41(2):56-72, 2012

Liposarcoma

Liposarcoma

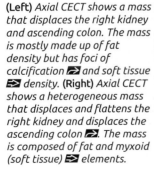

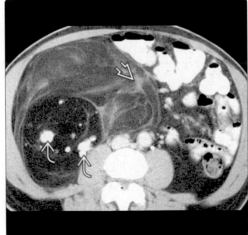

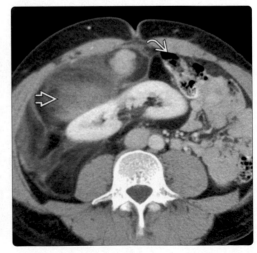

(Left) *Axial CECT shows a mass that displaces the right kidney and ascending colon. The mass is mostly made up of fat density but has foci of calcification ➡ and soft tissue ➡ density.* (Right) *Axial CECT shows a heterogeneous mass that displaces and flattens the right kidney and displaces the ascending colon ➡. The mass is composed of fat and myxoid (soft tissue) ➡ elements.*

Angiomyolipoma, Renal

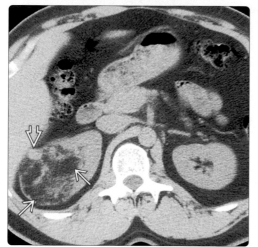

Angiomyolipoma, Renal

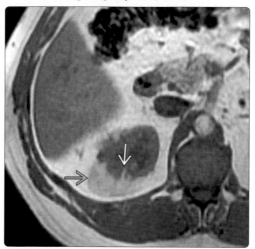

(Left) *Axial NECT shows a heterogeneous renal mass that contains fat ➡️ and soft tissue density ⬌, features of a typical angiomyolipoma.* (Right) *Axial T2 MR shows a lesion ➡️ with signal intensity similar to fat arising from the posterior renal cortex via a small defect ➡️.*

Angiomyolipoma, Renal

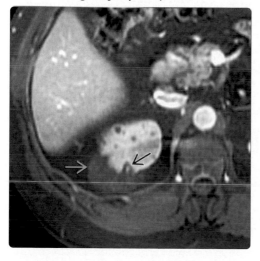

Adrenal Myelolipoma

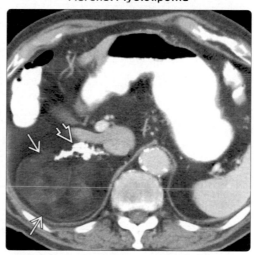

(Left) *Axial post-contrast T1 MR with fat suppression in the same patient shows that the lesion ➡️ loses signal intensity with application of fat saturation. A cortical defect (notch sign) and a feeding vessel ➡️ are shown.* (Right) *Axial CECT shows a large, suprarenal mass ➡️ made up mostly of fat and with large foci of calcification ⬌.*

AIDS Lipodystrophy

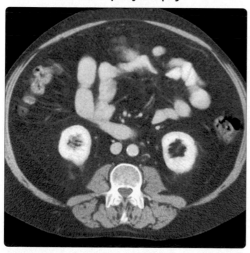

Pelvic Lipomatosis

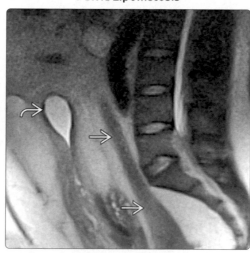

(Left) *Axial CECT shows massive, generalized proliferation of retroperitoneal and mesenteric fat, out of proportion to the subcutaneous fat, in a young man with AIDS who noted increasing abdominal girth.* (Right) *Sagittal T2 MR demonstrates the inverted pear- or teardrop-shaped bladder that is displaced superoanteriorly ➡️. The rectum ➡️ is compressed and elongated due to the lipomatosis.*

DIFFERENTIAL DIAGNOSIS

Common

- Renal Trauma
- Pelvic Trauma
- Coagulopathic (Retroperitoneal) Hemorrhage
- Ruptured Abdominal Aortic Aneurysm

Less Common

- Hepatic Trauma
- Perirenal Hemorrhage
  o Renal Cell Carcinoma
  o Angiomyolipoma, Renal
- Adrenal Hemorrhage
- Adrenal Carcinoma

ESSENTIAL INFORMATION

Key Differential Diagnosis Issues

- Key to distinguishing ruptured aneurysm [abdominal aortic aneurysm (AAA)] from coagulopathic hemorrhage
  o Coagulopathic: Hematocrit sign (cellular-fluid level); multiple sites; blood limited to iliopsoas or involving rectus muscles
  o Ruptured AAA: Aneurysm > 4-cm diameter; interrupted intimal calcification; eccentric shape of aneurysm; blood contiguous with > 3-cm length of aneurysm
- Renal tumors
  o Renal cell carcinoma
    - Most common neoplastic cause of retroperitoneal hemorrhage
    - Typically heterogeneous, hypervascular mass
  o Angiomyolipoma
    - Contains fat and soft tissue components in most cases
    - Adrenal tumors may be obscured by hemorrhage or distorted anatomy

Helpful Clues for Common Diagnoses

- **Renal Trauma**
  o Perirenal hemorrhage accompanies any significant renal injury

  o Linear wedge-shaped parenchymal defect ± active extravasation of blood or urine
- **Pelvic Trauma**
  o Extraperitoneal bleeding often extends cephalad along anterior margin of spine and psoas muscles into retroperitoneum

Helpful Clues for Less Common Diagnoses

- **Hepatic Trauma**
  o Injury to bare area of liver may result in retroperitoneal hemorrhage
- **Perirenal Hemorrhage**
  o Renal tumors may bleed spontaneously or after trauma
    - Look for spherical mass with claw sign (parenchymal defect)
  o Angiomyolipoma, Renal
    - Look for fat component of mass (may be obscured by bleeding)
- **Adrenal Hemorrhage**
  o Common in neonates
  o May result from trauma, sepsis, shock, post partum, coagulopathy, underlying tumor or cyst, surgery
  o Bilateral hemorrhage is usually not due to direct trauma, tumor, or surgery
  o Liver transplantation often results in asymptomatic right adrenal hemorrhage
- **Adrenal Carcinoma**
  o Any adrenal mass (pheochromocytoma, metastasis, cyst) may bleed

SELECTED REFERENCES

1. Kasotakis G: Retroperitoneal and rectus sheath hematomas. Surg Clin North Am. 94(1):71-6, 2014
2. Goenka AH et al: Imaging of the retroperitoneum. Radiol Clin North Am. 50(2):333-55, vii, 2012
3. Tonolini M et al: Hemorrhagic complications of anticoagulant therapy: role of multidetector computed tomography and spectrum of imaging findings from head to toe. Curr Probl Diagn Radiol. 41(6):233-47, 2012
4. Furlan A et al: Spontaneous abdominal hemorrhage: causes, CT findings, and clinical implications. AJR Am J Roentgenol. 193(4):1077-87, 2009

Renal Trauma

Coagulopathic (Retroperitoneal) Hemorrhage

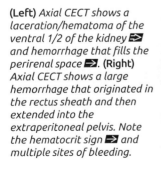

(Left) Axial CECT shows a laceration/hematoma of the ventral 1/2 of the kidney ➡ and hemorrhage that fills the perirenal space ➡. (Right) Axial CECT shows a large hemorrhage that originated in the rectus sheath and then extended into the extraperitoneal pelvis. Note the hematocrit sign ➡ and multiple sites of bleeding.

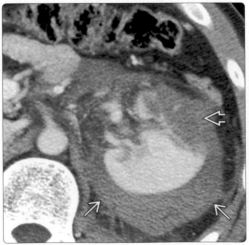

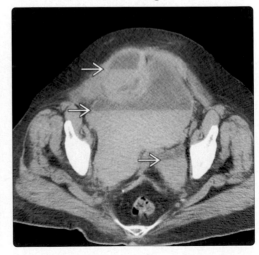

Coagulopathic (Retroperitoneal) Hemorrhage

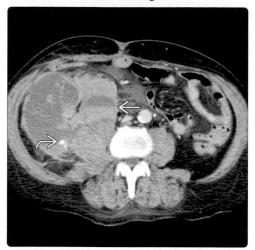

Ruptured Abdominal Aortic Aneurysm

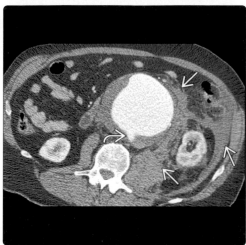

(Left) *Axial CECT shows a large hemorrhage into the posterior abdominal wall and retroperitoneum. Note the hematocrit sign ⮕ and foci of active bleeding ⮕.* (Right) *Axial CECT shows a large aneurysm with hemorrhage ⮕ into the retroperitoneum. Clot is contiguous with the aorta. Note the probable site of rupture ⮕.*

Perirenal Hemorrhage

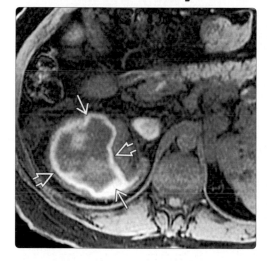

Perirenal Hemorrhage

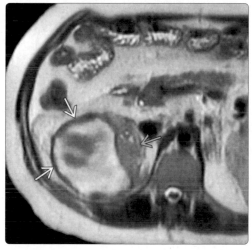

(Left) *Axial T1WI MR with fat saturation shows a heterogeneous mass in the right perinephric space. Note there is a thin, low signal intensity outer rim ⮕ surrounding a high signal intensity inner rim ⮕, both of which surround an intermediate signal intensity center. Findings are consistent with a subacute hematoma.* (Right) *Axial T2WI MR in the same patient better demonstrates a low signal intensity outer rim ⮕. Note that the right kidney ⮕ is compressed and displaced medially.*

Renal Cell Carcinoma

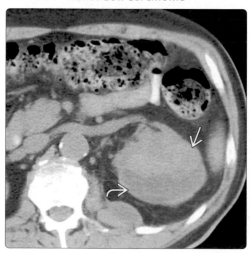

Angiomyolipoma, Renal

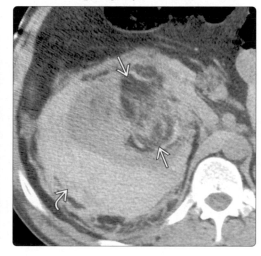

(Left) *Axial NECT shows a small end-stage left kidney surrounded by spontaneous perirenal hemorrhage ⮕. An exophytic mass ⮕ is seen. The mass proved to be renal cell carcinoma in this dialysis-dependent patient.* (Right) *Axial NECT shows extensive bleeding ⮕ into the perirenal space from an angiomyolipoma, which is the underlying, heterogeneous, fat density mass ⮕.*

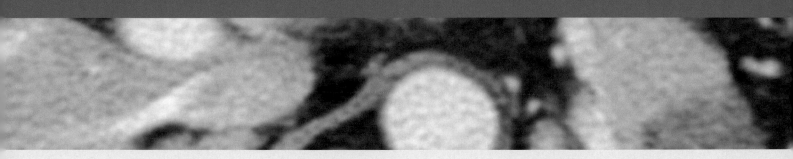

SECTION 14
Adrenal

Generic Imaging Patterns

DIFFERENTIAL DIAGNOSIS

Common

- Adrenal Adenoma
- Metastases and Lymphoma, Adrenal
- Adrenal Hemorrhage
- Pheochromocytoma
- Adrenal Cyst
- Retroperitoneal Varices or Vessels (Mimic)

Less Common

- Adrenal Myelolipoma
- Adrenal TB and Fungal Infection
- Adrenal Carcinoma
- Renal Cell Carcinoma (Mimic)
- Gastric Diverticulum (Mimic)
- Adrenal Hyperplasia
- Adrenal Ganglioneuroma

Rare but Important

- Adrenal Collision Tumor
- Adrenal Hemangioma

ESSENTIAL INFORMATION

Key Differential Diagnosis Issues

- Primary diagnostic consideration, particularly in oncologic population: Differentiate between adrenal metastasis and incidental adrenal adenoma
- Imaging intensive approach advocated by specialty societies to confirm adenomas, though vast majority of adrenal incidentalomas are statistically adenomas
- Combination of imaging (CT or MR) and clinical history usually allows confident diagnosis
  - CT and MR protocols geared towards identifying intracytoplasmic lipid in adenomas
  - Lipid-poor adenomas may be problematic, though washout kinetics, clinical history (malignancy), and extraadrenal findings (additional metastases) aid diagnosis
- Cushing syndrome: Excess cortisol; 75-80% due to pituitary adenoma secreting excess ACTH
- Conn syndrome: Excess aldosterone; 75-80% due to adrenal adenoma (small)
- Addison syndrome: Adrenal insufficiency; due to autoimmune disease (80% in Western countries), bilateral metastases, adrenal hemorrhage, or systemic infection
- Clinical history (hypertension) may suggest pheochromocytoma, but biochemical work-up (urine metanephrines) confirms diagnosis

Helpful Clues for Common Diagnoses

- **Adrenal Adenoma**
  - Well-circumscribed, round or oval, homogeneous, low-density (0-20 HU) mass on NECT
    - < 10 HU threshold: Highly specific for lipid-rich adenoma
    - Histology of lipid-rich adenomas characterized by intravoxel signal drop out at out-of-phase T1WI
  - Lipid-poor adenomas are best diagnosed on CT, with unenhanced, enhanced, and 15-minute delayed imaging to calculate washout

- Absolute washout: > 60%
- Relative washout: > 40%
  □ Rare false-positives: hepatocellular carcinoma, renal cell carcinoma metastases, pheochromocytoma
- Web-based calculators readily available

- **Metastases and Lymphoma, Adrenal**
  - Metastases: Primary sites include lung, breast, kidney, melanoma
    - Cannot always be distinguished from lipid-poor adenoma by imaging alone
    - Clinical history, comparison to prior studies, identification of additional (extraadrenal) disease aid diagnosis
    - PET/CT very useful in oncology patients; may help to identify FDG-avid adrenal metastases
  - Lymphoma: Non-Hodgkin lymphoma most common
    - Rounded or triangular shape; mild enhancement
    - FDG-avid on PET/CT

- **Adrenal Hemorrhage**
  - Acute: Homogeneous, round, nonenhancing, hyperdense mass (50-90 HU)
  - Chronic: Mass with hypoattenuating center (pseudocyst), calcification
  - Unilateral, usually due to direct trauma or iatrogenic (e.g., liver transplantation)
  - Bilateral usually in response to shock; postpartum; severe burns, sepsis

- **Pheochromocytoma**
  - Well circumscribed, round, 3- to 5-cm diameter (symptomatic lesions)
    - Pheochromocytoma that occurs as part of syndrome may be detected as smaller, asymptomatic mass
    - Syndromes associated with pheochromocytoma: Multiple endocrine neoplasia (types II and III); neurofibromatosis; von Hippel Lindau; Carney syndrome; tuberous sclerosis
  - Hyperintense on T2WI with heterogeneous bright enhancement
  - ± hemorrhage, necrosis, calcification
  - Supporting history (e.g., hypertension, palpitations, headache) and biochemical data (urine metanephrines) drive diagnosis

- **Adrenal Cyst**
  - Well-defined, nonenhancing water-density mass ± calcification (eggshell)
    - Thin wall, septa calcification favor cyst rather than lipid-rich adenoma at NECT
  - Rarely large lesion ± internal hemorrhage

- **Retroperitoneal Varices or Vessels (Mimic)**
  - Tortuous splenic artery and varices often lie in suprarenal space
  - Contrast-enhanced CT or MR or color Doppler US can usually establish diagnosis

Helpful Clues for Less Common Diagnoses

- **Adrenal Myelolipoma**
  - Uncommon, nonfunctioning benign tumor
  - Macroscopic fat intersperse with soft tissue (myeloid elements, hemorrhage) at NECT

- Coronal reconstructions may help determine organ of origin: Adrenal myelolipoma vs. exophytic renal angiomyelolipoma
  - o Hyperintense on T1WI, focal areas of signal loss on fat-suppressed techniques
    - Interface between fat and soft tissue elements will lose signal on opposed phase GRE series
  - o Echogenic mass at ultrasound: May be indistinguishable from surrounding retroperitoneal fat unless mass effect
  - o CT and MR findings are diagnostic in most cases
    - No treatment needed in most cases, though large myelolipomas may hemorrhage
    - Resection advocated for large, asymptomatic, or atypical lesions
- **Adrenal TB and Fungal Infection**
  - o Heterogeneous, poorly enhancing mass(es) during acute infection
  - o Acute: Mild to marked enlargement of adrenal glands with preserved contour
  - o Chronic: Small calcified adrenal glands
    - Adrenal TB = most common cause of Addison syndrome (adrenal insufficiency) in 3rd world countries
- **Adrenal Carcinoma**
  - o Nonfunctioning tumors typically large (> 10 cm) at presentation
  - o Functioning tumors may be smaller (< 5 cm)
  - o Early invasion of IVC accounts for poor prognosis
  - o ± necrosis, hemorrhage, calcification (30%)
- **Renal Cell Carcinoma (Mimic)**
  - o Large tumor from upper pole of kidney may simulate adrenal carcinoma
  - o Look for claw sign (defect in renal cortex at origin of mass), coronal CT reconstruction or MR helpful to determine organ of origin
- **Gastric Diverticulum (Mimic)**
  - o Rounded mass in suprarenal site
  - o May contain fluid, gas, contrast material
  - o Give extra oral contrast or gas granules; place patient prone to make diagnosis

- **Adrenal Hyperplasia**
  - o Adrenal glands may appear normal; normal shape but increased thickness (> 10 mm); or may be nodular
  - o Nodular hyperplasia can be difficult to distinguish from small adrenal adenomas or other lesions (e.g., metastases)
  - o Hyperplasia or swelling may occur in response to stress, pituitary ACTH-secreting tumor (accounts for 75-80% of Cushing syndrome cases), congenital adrenal hyperplasia, or ectopic source of ACTH

Helpful Clues for Rare Diagnoses

- **Adrenal Collision Tumor**
  - o Coexistence of 2 contiguous but histologically distinct tumors within same adrenal gland
  - o Adenoma and myelolipoma; adenoma and metastases most common combinations
- **Adrenal Hemangioma**
  - o > 10 cm, central low attenuation (necrosis or fibrosis) ± calcification

Alternative Differential Approaches

- Bilateral adrenal masses: Metastases, hyperplasia, lymphoma, hemorrhage, TB, or fungal infection, pheochromocytoma (10%), adenoma (10%), or combination of 2 types of masses (e.g., adenoma on 1 side, myelolipoma on other)

SELECTED REFERENCES

1. Allen BC et al: Adrenal imaging and intervention. Radiol Clin North Am. 53(5):1021-35, 2015
2. Siegelman ES: Adrenal MRI: techniques and clinical applications. J Magn Reson Imaging. 36(2):272-85, 2012
3. Johnson PT et al: Adrenal imaging with multidetector CT: evidence-based protocol optimization and interpretative practice. Radiographics. 29(5):1319-31, 2009 Review. Erratum in: Radiographics. Nov;29(7):2198, 2009
4. Johnson PT et al: Adrenal mass imaging with multidetector CT: pathologic conditions, pearls, and pitfalls. Radiographics. 29(5):1333-51, 2009
5. Park BK et al: Comparison of delayed enhanced CT and chemical shift MR for evaluating hyperattenuating incidental adrenal masses. Radiology. 243(3):760-5, 2007

Adrenal Adenoma

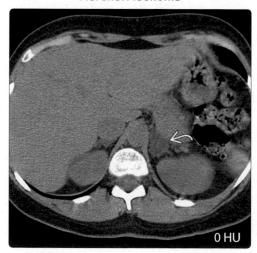

Adrenal Adenoma

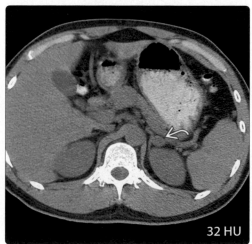

(Left) NECT of 45-year-old man shows an incidental uniform 2-cm, low-attenuation (0 HU) left adrenal lesion ➦. Its attenuation is characteristic of a lipid-rich adenoma. (Right) NECT shows an incidental, indeterminate (32 HU) left adrenal lesion ➦. Although it is still statistically a benign adenoma, a dedicated contrast-enhanced adrenal mass CT was performed. Washout > 60% confirmed a lipid-poor adenoma.

Adrenal Adenoma

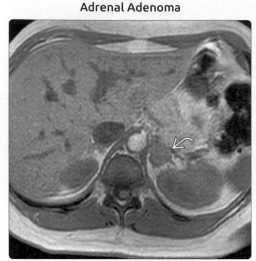

Adrenal Adenoma

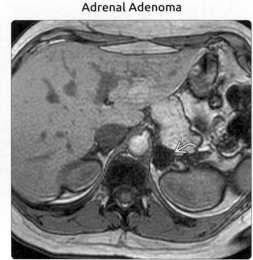

(Left) *T1 in-phase MR shows a well-circumscribed, indeterminate signal intensity left adrenal lesion ➥. (Right) The corresponding out-of-phase T1W MR shows signal suppression of the left adrenal lesion ➥. Low attenuation (< 10 HU) at NECT and signal dropout at chemical shift MR are characteristic features of lipid-rich adenomas.*

Adrenal Adenoma

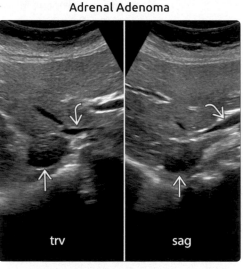

Metastases and Lymphoma, Adrenal

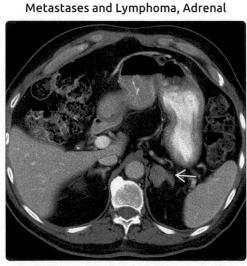

(Left) *Transverse and sagittal ultrasound images of a 70-year-old woman with ↑ liver function tests show an incidental solid right adrenal lesion ➥ posterior to the IVC ➥. The appearance at ultrasound is nonspecific; NECT confirmed a lipid-rich adenoma. (Right) Ultrasound performed on a patient with known lung carcinoma shows a solid right adrenal lesion ➥. A dedicated CECT adrenal CT showed prolonged absolute washout kinetics (< 60%). Ultrasound-guided biopsy confirmed a metastasis.*

Metastases and Lymphoma, Adrenal

Metastases and Lymphoma, Adrenal

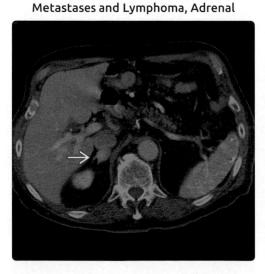

(Left) *PET/CT shows an FDG-avid adrenal metastasis ➥ in a patient with esophageal carcinoma. Identification of extraadrenal metastases typically makes characterization of adrenal masses in oncology patients unnecessary, but PET may be useful for confirming solitary adrenal metastases prior to adrenalectomy. (Right) CECT of a patient with a history of lung cancer shows a new, isolated adrenal mass ➥. Although a relative washout of 42% suggests a lipid-poor adenoma, a metastasis was confirmed at adrenalectomy.*

Metastases and Lymphoma, Adrenal

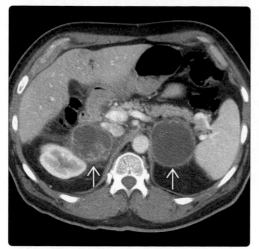

Metastases and Lymphoma, Adrenal

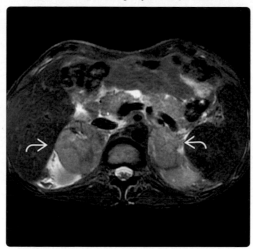

(Left) *CECT of a patient with back pain and lethargy, and a history of lung carcinoma, shows large, necrotic adrenal metastases ➡. Lab data (↓ Na, ↑ K) and an ACTH stimulation test confirmed profound adrenal insufficiency.* (Right) *T2 TSE performed on a 36-year-old man with malaise and adrenal insufficiency shows bilateral bulky T2-intense adrenal masses ➡.*

Metastases and Lymphoma, Adrenal

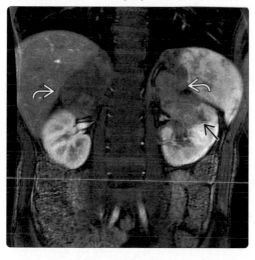

Adrenal Hemorrhage

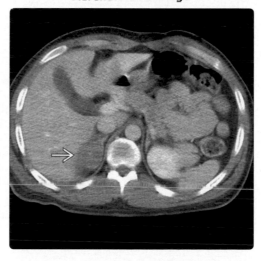

(Left) *Coronal T1 C+ MR in same patient shows mild enhancement of both masses ➡ & extension of tumor into left kidney ➡. Absence of disease elsewhere & clinical history suggested adrenal lymphoma. Biopsy confirmed diffuse B-cell lymphoma; patient was successfully treated with CHOP and Rituxan.* (Right) *CECT of a young male patient post trauma shows right adrenal hematoma ➡. Traumatic adrenal hemorrhage is typically associated with other visceral injuries & high injury severity scores.*

Adrenal Hemorrhage

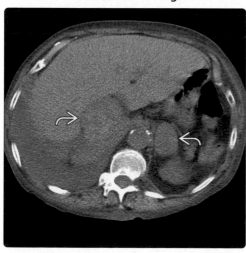

Pheochromocytoma

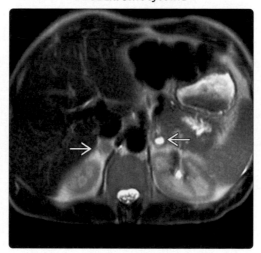

(Left) *NECT of a hypotensive patient with metastatic lung carcinoma shows bilateral adrenal hematomas ➡. Small adrenal metastases were shown on a prior staging CT.* (Right) *T2W MR of a man with MEN 2A syndrome and ↑ urinary metanephrines shows small bilateral adrenal pheos ➡. Hereditary pheos are typically small and often bilateral.*

Pheochromocytoma

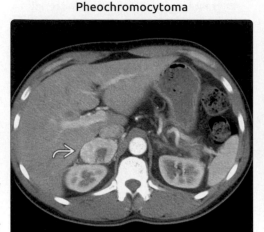

Pheochromocytoma

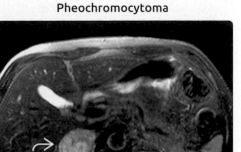

(Left) *CECT of a 26-year-old man shows marked enhancement of a 4-cm right adrenal pheochromocytoma ➡. Genetic testing, prompted by the patient's young age, confirmed an atypically large hereditary pheochromocytoma.* (Right) *T2W MR of the same patient shows a slightly T2 intense right pheochromocytoma ➡. Marked, light bulb, T2 hyperintensity was considered a characteristic feature of these lesions in the early MR literature, but this is often not the case.*

Pheochromocytoma

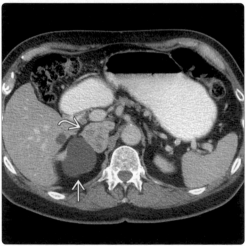

Pheochromocytoma

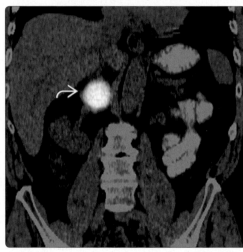

(Left) *Metanephrine evaluation was performed on this elderly patient after dedicated adrenal CT showed a vascular right adrenal mass ➡ with minimal washout. Note the adjacent renal cyst ➡.* (Right) *I-123 MIBI CT-SPECT exam on the same patient (performed to exclude metastases) confirmed a solitary 4-cm right adrenal pheochromocytoma ➡. Sporadic pheochromocytomas tend to occur in older patients and classic symptoms (headache, hypertension, palpitations, sweating) may be absent.*

Adrenal Cyst

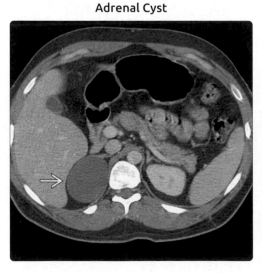

Adrenal Cyst

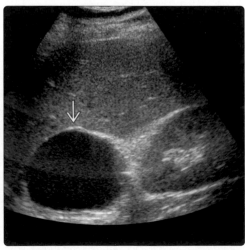

(Left) *CECT shows an incidental nonenhancing right adrenal cyst ➡. Differentiation of adrenal cysts from adenomas at NECT may be difficult, but septations and thin calcification favor cysts.* (Right) *Ultrasound performed on the same patient shows a simple suprarenal (adrenal) cyst ➡. Lack of cyst complexity might suggest an endothelial cyst, but pseudocysts are the most common type of adrenal cysts in surgical series.*

Adrenal Myelolipoma

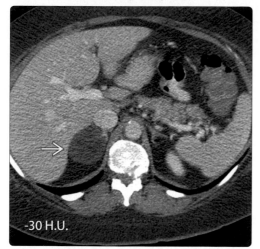

-30 H.U.

Adrenal TB and Fungal Infection

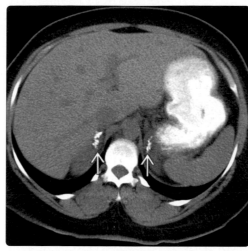

(Left) *CECT shows a fat attenuation (-30 HU) adrenal lesion* ➡️*, an appearance pathognomonic of an adrenal myelolipoma. The differential diagnosis of large myelolipomas includes retroperitoneal liposarcomas and renal angiomyolipomas.* **(Right)** *NECT shows calcified adrenals* ➡️*, likely due to prior granulomatous infection. These calcifications are typically incidental, though in undeveloped countries, they may suggest adrenal tuberculosis, a common cause of adrenal insufficiency in these populations.*

Adrenal Carcinoma

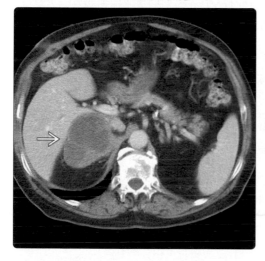

Adrenal Carcinoma

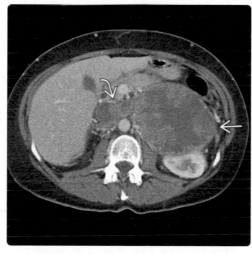

(Left) *CECT of an elderly male patient with mild flank pain shows a large, heterogeneous right adrenal mass* ➡️*. Resection performed after metanephrine screening confirmed an adrenal carcinoma. Large, solid, unilateral adrenal masses with invasive margins should raise index of suspicion for adrenal carcinoma.* **(Right)** *CECT shows a huge left adrenal carcinoma* ➡️ *& tumor thrombus within left renal vein* ➡️*. These highly malignant tumors are often large at presentation & have a predilection for venous invasion.*

Adrenal Hyperplasia

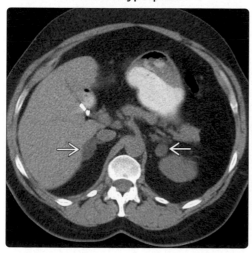

Adrenal Hyperplasia

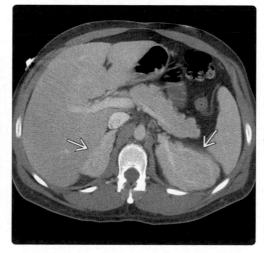

(Left) *NECT of a female patient with Cushing syndrome, a suppressed ACTH, and abnormal dexamethasone suppression shows nodular adrenal glands* ➡️*. ACTH independent macronodular hyperplasia was confirmed at resection.* **(Right)** *CECT shows massively enlarged adrenals* ➡️*, a characteristic feature of congenital adrenal hyperplasia This autosomal recessive disease is usually due to 21-hydroxylase deficiency, is typically diagnosed in the neonatal period, and is responsible for most adrenogenital syndromes.*

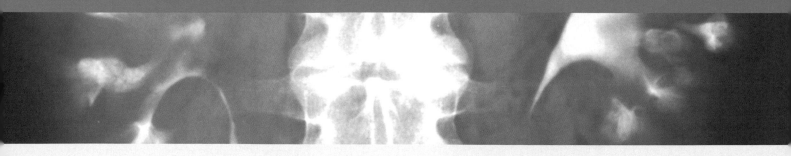

SECTION 15
Kidney

Generic Imaging Patterns

Modality-Specific Imaging Findings

ULTRASOUND

DIFFERENTIAL DIAGNOSIS

Common

- Renal Cell Carcinoma
- Wilms Tumor (Nephroblastoma)
- Column of Bertin (Mimic)
- Fetal Lobation
- Pyelonephritis

Less Common

- Hyperdense Renal Cyst (Mimic)
- Angiomyolipoma, Renal
- Renal Oncocytoma
- Metastases and Lymphoma, Renal
- Urothelial Cell Carcinoma
- Pyelonephritis, Xanthogranulomatous
- Renal Trauma
- Aneurysm, Renal Artery (Mimic)
- Arteriovenous Malformation, Renal (Mimic)

Rare but Important

- Renal Medullary Carcinoma
- Renal Tumors, Atypical and Rare
  - Mesenchymal Tumor, Renal
  - Juxtaglomerular Tumor
  - Plasmocytoma, Renal
  - Small Cell Carcinoma, Renal

ESSENTIAL INFORMATION

Key Differential Diagnosis Issues

- Solid, expansile mass in adult is usually renal cell carcinoma, unless
  - Mass contains fat (probably angiomyolipoma)
  - Patient has fever, urosepsis (consider pyelonephritis and renal abscess)
  - Patient is immunocompromised (consider lymphoma, posttransplant lymphoproliferative disorder)
  - Patient has known other primary cancer (consider metastases)
- Role of biopsy is evolving but definitely has role in diagnosing renal lymphoma and metastases
  - Useful in diagnosing oncocytoma, angiomyolipoma (AML)
  - Morphology and immunohistochemical features are key pathologic findings
  - Routinely performed prior to percutaneous ablation: ~ 20% of small (< 4 cm) enhancing renal masses are benign (i.e., non-fat-containing AML, oncocytoma)
- Morphology of lesion also aids diagnosis: "beans" vs. "balls"
  - Infiltrating tumor maintains reniform ("bean") shape: Consider urothelial carcinoma, collecting duct carcinoma, medullary carcinoma
  - Well-circumscribed ("ball") tumor: Consider renal cell carcinoma (RCC) (clear cell, papillary, chromophobe)
- Clinical history is key in diagnosing renal trauma, infection, metastases, lymphoma
  - Not usually helpful in diagnosing primary renal tumors
- CT or MR evaluation of renal mass must include nonenhanced and parenchymal phase images

- Arterial phase good for diagnosing column of Bertin; pyelographic phase essential for diagnosing transitional cell cancer

Helpful Clues for Common Diagnoses

- **Renal Cell Carcinoma**
  - Usually discovered as incidental finding
    - May have hematuria or flank pain
  - Variable appearance and histology
    - From mostly cystic, to hypovascular (papillary), to hypervascular (most RCCs)
    - Large tumors may have lipoid degeneration, invade renal sinus or perirenal fat, simulate angiomyolipoma
    - Large tumors may also have osseous metaplasia
    - Common RCC subtypes (WHO classification): Clear cell, papillary, chromophobe
    - Additional rare, aggressive renal epithelial tumors may be suggested by central infiltrative growth pattern (collecting duct, medullary carcinoma)
  - Large RCC with predilection for renal vein, inferior vena cava invasion
- **Wilms Tumor (Nephroblastoma)**
  - Most common solid renal mass in children
  - Highly variable appearance
- **Column of Bertin (Mimic)**
  - Hypertrophied column of septal cortex that protrudes into renal sinus
    - Usually between upper and middle calyces
  - Same enhancement characteristics (and echogenicity) as renal cortex
  - Utilize power (color) Doppler to confirm similar vascularity of adjacent cortex if identified at screening ultrasound
- **Fetal Lobation**
  - Persistent cortical lobulation, reflecting fetal renal development as multiple separate lobes
  - Enhances like normal cortex and medulla
- **Pyelonephritis**
  - Severe focal pyelonephritis, renal abscess, or xanthogranulomatous pyelonephritis may be indistinguishable from tumor by imaging alone
  - Consider clinical presentation; needle aspiration and drainage of abscess

Helpful Clues for Less Common Diagnoses

- **Hyperdense Renal Cyst (Mimic)**
  - High-density ("hyperdense" or "hemorrhagic") renal cyst is indistinguishable from tumor on either NECT or CECT alone
    - Cyst will not enhance, while viable tumor almost always enhances ≥ 20 HU (beware papillary RCC)
    - Sonography useful to show sonolucent contents and acoustic enhancement of hyperdense cyst
    - Large cyst with extensive hemorrhage may be impossible to distinguish from necrotic tumor
    - Attenuation > 70 HU at NECT strongly suggests high-attenuation ("hyperdense") CT rather than RCC
- **Angiomyolipoma, Renal**
  - Most common benign renal solid mass
  - 95% have identifiable fat on CT or MR
    - Use NECT or MR to identify small foci of fat

- AML without fat is difficult or impossible to distinguish from RCC by imaging (often hyperdense to kidney on NECT)
- Highly echogenic at ultrasound, though imaging overlap with small echogenic RCC
  - □ Features favoring RCC: Halo, cystic components
  - Multiple and bilateral in tuberous sclerosis
  - May result in spontaneous bleeding
- **Renal Oncocytoma**
  - Benign epithelial tumor
  - Often has central stellate scar (30-50%), though not specific finding
  - Segmental inversion pattern suggested, though specificity also disputed
    - Hypervascular component on corticomedullary phase deenhances on nephrographic phase
    - Hypovascular component on corticomedullary phase retains contrast on nephrographic phase
- **Metastases and Lymphoma, Renal**
  - Often multiple, in patient with known primary tumor
  - Usually less vascular and less exophytic than RCC
  - Multiple renal lymphoma patterns: Multifocal or infiltrating tumor, diffuse bilateral enlargement
  - Consider lymphoma if large tumor and retroperitoneal adenopathy without renal vein invasion
- **Urothelial Cell Carcinoma**
  - More infiltrative, less expansile than RCC
  - May be part of multifocal tumor
    - Bladder > kidney > ureter
  - Most low-grade, superficial papillary masses
  - 15% aggressive: Invade renal sinus and parenchyma
- **Renal Trauma**
  - Renal hematoma may be indistinguishable from tumor
    - History (including possible invasive procedure like biopsy) is key
  - Traumatic injury will evolve quickly
- **Aneurysms and Arteriovenous Malformations (Mimic)**
  - Vascular lesions can mimic tumor
  - Key is multiphasic CT or MR during rapid bolus of contrast medium or color Doppler

Helpful Clues for Rare Diagnoses

- **Renal Medullary Carcinoma**
  - Rare, highly aggressive tumor
  - Usually affects men with sickle cell trait
- **Renal Tumors, Atypical and Rare**
  - May arise from any mesenchymal component of renal capsule, cortex, or medulla
  - Generally cannot be diagnosed by imaging

Alternative Differential Approaches

- Lesions that may be hyperdense on NECT: Hyperdense cyst, RCC, oncocytoma, non-fat-containing AML, transitional cell carcinoma

SELECTED REFERENCES

1. Moch H et al: The 2016 WHO Classification of Tumours of the Urinary System and Male Genital Organs-Part A: Renal, Penile, and Testicular Tumours. Eur Urol. ePub, 2016
2. Sidhar K et al: Renal cell carcinomas: sonographic appearance depending on size and histologic type. J Ultrasound Med. 35(2):311-20, 2016
3. Schieda N et al: Diagnostic accuracy of segmental enhancement inversion for diagnosis of renal oncocytoma at biphasic contrast enhanced CT: systematic review. Eur Radiol. 24(6):1421-9, 2014
4. Woo S et al: Comparison of segmental enhancement inversion on biphasic MDCT between small renal oncocytomas and chromophobe renal cell carcinomas. AJR Am J Roentgenol. 201(3):598-604, 2013
5. Choudhary S et al: Renal cell carcinoma: recent advances in genetics and imaging. Semin Ultrasound CT MR. 30(4):315-25, 2009
6. Sahni VA et al: Biopsy of renal masses: when and why. Cancer Imaging. 9:44-55, 2009
7. Jonisch AI et al: Can high-attenuation renal cysts be differentiated from renal cell carcinoma at unenhanced CT? Radiology. 243(2):445-50, 2007
8. Silverman SG et al: Hyperattenuating renal masses: etiologies, pathogenesis, and imaging evaluation. Radiographics. 27(4):1131-43, 2007
9. Prasad SR et al: Common and uncommon histologic subtypes of renal cell carcinoma: imaging spectrum with pathologic correlation. Radiographics. 26(6):1795-806; discussion 1806-10, 2006
10. Blitman NM et al: Renal medullary carcinoma: CT and MRI features. AJR Am J Roentgenol. 185(1):268-72, 2005
11. Browne RF et al: Transitional cell carcinoma of the upper urinary tract: spectrum of imaging findings. Radiographics. 25(6):1609-27, 2005
12. Curry NS: Imaging the small solid renal mass. Abdom Imaging. 27(6):629-36, 2002

Renal Cell Carcinoma

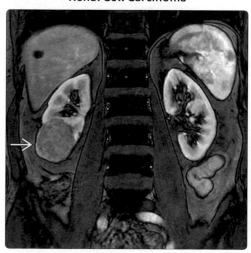

Renal Cell Carcinoma

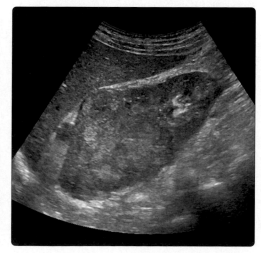

(Left) T1 C+ FS MR performed to evaluate an incidental mass identified at ultrasound shows a right lower pole tumor ➡. Enhancement is the hallmark of renal neoplasia, and most large solid lesions are renal cell carcinomas (RCCs). Clear cell carcinoma was confirmed at nephrectomy. (Right) Ultrasound performed for evaluation of hematuria shows a large, isoechoic right upper pole mass. Renal venous invasion (not shown) indicated at least Robson stage 3a RCC, which was confirmed at CT and nephrectomy.

Renal Cell Carcinoma

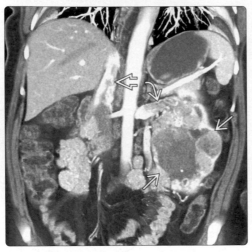

Renal Cell Carcinoma

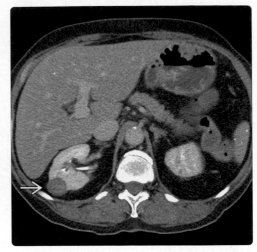

(Left) *CECT shows a large RCC ⮡ replacing lower 2/3 of kidney, with invasion of renal vein ⮡ and inferior vena cava ⮡. Coronal CT or MR are particularly helpful for assessing level of caval involvement.* **(Right)** *CECT shows an incidental, exophytic 42 HU right renal mass ⮡. Based on this single phase, it is impossible to differentiate between an RCC and a high-attenuation cyst, but slight enhancement (18HU) and a solid appearance at US indicated neoplasia. Biopsy performed prior to ablation confirmed papillary RCC.*

Wilms Tumor (Nephroblastoma)

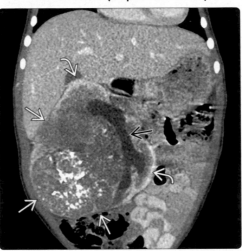

Column of Bertin (Mimic)

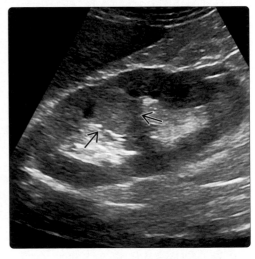

(Left) *Coronal CECT of a 2 year old with a palpable mass shows a huge enhancing, partially calcified tumor ⮡ that replaces most of the kidney ⮡ and obstructs the collecting system ⮡. Wilms tumor is the most common malignant abdominal neoplasm in children < 9 years. CT is the staging modality of choice.* **(Right)** *Sagittal ultrasound shows an isoechoic "mass" ⮡ that protrudes into the renal sinus fat. Power Doppler ultrasound and CECT confirmed a column of Bertin.*

Pyelonephritis

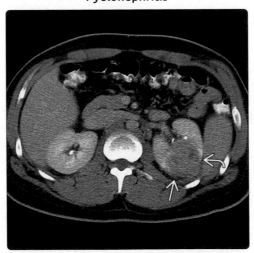

Angiomyolipoma, Renal

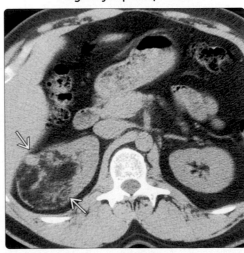

(Left) *CECT of a young male patient with fatigue shows a heterogeneous left renal lesion ⮡. Nephrectomy eventually confirmed acute and chronic MRSA pyelonephritis. Clinical history (fever, leukocytosis) more typically leads to a correct diagnosis of pyelonephritis. Subtle perinephric fat infiltration ⮡ was the only suggestive imaging sign in this case.* **(Right)** *Axial NECT shows a right renal mass ⮡ composed primarily of fat, a feature indicating a benign AML. Large (> 4 cm) AMLs are prone to hemorrhage.*

Renal Oncocytoma

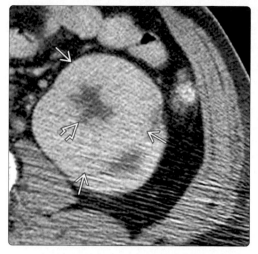

Metastases and Lymphoma, Renal

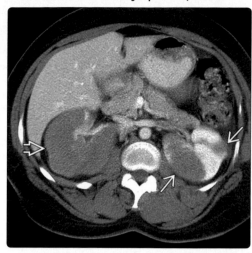

(Left) *Axial CECT shows a large, spherical mass ➡ with almost the same attenuation as the kidney. There is a central scar ⇢ within the mass, a characteristic but uncommon and nonspecific sign of oncocytoma.* (Right) *CECT of a 53-year-old woman with multiple sclerosis shows an infiltrating right renal mass ⇢ and multiple left renal masses ➡. B-cell non-Hodgkin lymphoma was confirmed at ultrasound-guided biopsy.*

Metastases and Lymphoma, Renal

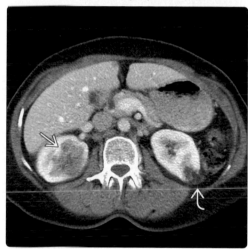

Urothelial Cell Carcinoma

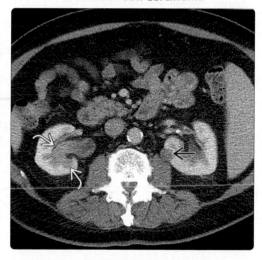

(Left) *CECT of a middle-aged man with a history of lung cancer shows an infiltrating right upper pole renal mass ➡ and a contralateral AML ➡. Ultrasound-guided biopsy confirmed a lung metastasis.* (Right) *CECT of an elderly man with hematuria and a history of noninvasive bladder carcinoma post TURBT shows an infiltrating midcalyceal urothelial carcinoma ➡ that invades the renal pelvis. Note the contralateral high-attenuation left renal cyst ➡ (confirmed at ultrasound).*

Renal Trauma

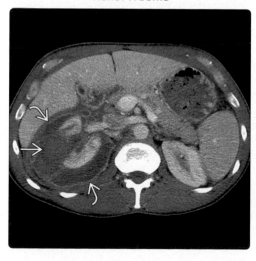

Arteriovenous Malformation, Renal (Mimic)

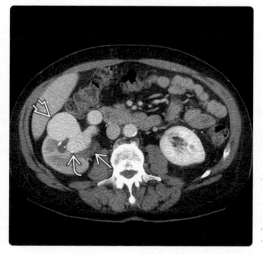

(Left) *CECT performed 10 days post trauma shows residual clot ➡ within a deep interpolar laceration and subacute perinephric hemorrhage ➡. Only a residual scar was identified on a CT performed 6 months later.* (Right) *CECT of a patient with hematuria and hypertension shows brisk enhancement of a huge right interpolar AVM ➡. Note the subtle wall calcification ➡ and a nephrogram delay, which is likely due to a combination of shunting and mass effect upon a partially obstructed renal pelvis ➡.*

DIFFERENTIAL DIAGNOSIS

Common

- Renal Cysts
- Renal Sinus Cysts
- Renal Cell Carcinoma
- Wilms Tumor
- Abscess, Renal
- Focal Hydronephrosis
- Trauma, Renal

Less Common

- Multilocular Cystic Nephroma
- Metastases and Lymphoma, Renal
- Angiomyolipoma, Renal
- Localized Cystic Renal Disease
- Segmental Multicystic Dysplastic Kidney
- Renal Tumors, Atypical and Rare

ESSENTIAL INFORMATION

Key Differential Diagnosis Issues

- Bosniak classification of renal cysts: CT triage system (ultrasound, MR as adjunct modalities)
  - I: Benign, simple cyst
    - Spherical, near water attenuation (or sonolucent), no enhancement, no visible wall
    - Sharp delineation with renal parenchyma, no calcification
    - Malignancy risk < 1% (no follow-up needed)
  - II: Minimally complicated, benign
    - High-attenuation cyst; spherical, nonenhancing, partially exophytic
    - < 1-mm septation (hairline thin): But no enhancing mural nodularity
    - Fine calcification with septa or wall
    - Malignancy risk < 3% (no follow-up needed)
  - IIF: Cystic lesion with mild abnormality
    - Subjective: Between II and III
    - Slightly thick wall, many thick, but perceptible septa
    - Slightly thick, but regular calcifications
    - Malignancy risk: 5-10% (follow-up recommended)
  - III: Complicated cyst; possibly malignant
    - Thick wall or septa; enhancement of wall or septum (includes multilocular cystic nephroma and some cystic renal cell carcinomas; often indistinguishable by imaging)
    - Thick, irregular calcifications
    - Malignancy risk: 40-60% (resection recommended)
  - IV: Cystic neoplasm; probably malignant
    - Enhancing mural nodularity (enhancing tissue is almost always neoplastic)
    - Solid enhancing elements, independent of septa
    - Malignancy risk > 80% (resection recommended)
- Sonography is complementary study when CT suggests cyst
  - Caution
    - Homogeneous tumor [like papillary renal cell carcinoma (RCC) or lymphoma] may appear anechoic on US
    - US tends to accentuate thickness of septa, may make Bosniak type II cyst look like type III

- MR also useful adjunct if CT contraindication
  - Like ultrasound, septation may be accentuated at T2
  - Qualitative assessment of wall, septal enhancement
  - Calcification not perceived

Helpful Clues for Common Diagnoses

- **Renal Cysts**
  - Extremely common, increased prevalence and size with age
  - Typical appearance
    - Ultrasonography: Sonolucent with acoustic enhancement; no mural nodularity; no or thin septa
    - CT: Near water attenuation; no enhancement; no mural nodularity; no or thin septa or calcification; pseudoenhancement of small intrarenal cysts is problem with helical CT (often see apparent increase in attenuation by up to 15 HU)
    - To make valid assessment of enhancement of mass, must use same slice thickness, same imaging factors, same scanner on same day
    - MR: Homogeneously hypointense on T1WI, very hyperintense on T2WI; no enhancement
  - Most are cortical, exophytic
  - Thin, nonenhancing septa are not worrisome, even with thin calcification
    - Usually result of prior infection or hemorrhage within cyst
  - Large cyst with extensive hemorrhage may be impossible to distinguish from necrotic tumor
- **Renal Sinus Cysts**
  - Includes peri- and parapelvic cysts and parapelvic lymphangiectasia
  - Often indistinguishable
    - Peripelvic cysts: Lymphatic origin
    - Parapelvic cysts: Extension of renal cysts into renal pelvis
    - Renal lymphangiomatosis: Developmental malformation
  - May be single cyst or multiple cysts that surround calices and renal vessels
    - Easily mistaken for hydronephrosis on US or CT, unless excretory-phase images are obtained
- **Renal Cell Carcinoma**
  - Some renal cell carcinomas (RCC) are predominantly cystic, even when small
    - Imaging will almost always show wall irregularity and enhancement with IV contrast administration
    - Many cysts and cystic renal cell carcinomas: Consider von Hippel Lindau
  - Some RCC are hypovascular (especially papillary type)
    - These are homogeneous and low density (CT); intensity (T1W MR); hypoechoic (US) and easily mistaken for cysts
    - CT will usually show slow and mild (20-30 HU) enhancement
- **Wilms Tumor**
  - Many morphological variations, including partially cystic
  - Some tumors have foci of calcification &/or fat
- **Abscess, Renal**
  - Usually has shaggy, enhancing wall and infiltration of perirenal fat

- Complex cyst containing low-level echoes at ultrasound
- Clinical history and needle aspiration are keys to diagnosis
- **Focal Hydronephrosis**
  - Obstructed calyx or infundibulum (e.g., TB, transitional cell carcinoma)
  - Duplicated collecting system with obstruction of ureter from upper pole moiety
  - May be mistaken for upper pole renal cystic mass
- **Trauma, Renal**
  - Evolving renal hematoma or urinoma may simulate cystic mass

Helpful Clues for Less Common Diagnoses

- **Multilocular Cystic Nephroma**
  - Benign mass comprises multiple noncommunicating cysts: Bosniak III or IV lesion
    - Arises from metanephric blastema
  - Wall and septa enhance and may calcify
  - Cystic mass herniates into renal hilum
  - Cannot be distinguished from RCC by imaging alone
  - Demographics: Young male patients, middle-aged women
- **Metastases and Lymphoma, Renal**
  - May be homogeneous, minimally enhancing, multiple
  - Dedicated renal mass imaging protocols (CT, MR, US) will confirm solid nature of masses
  - Typically in context of disseminated extrarenal tumor
    - Renal metastases: Common primary tumor include bronchogenic carcinoma, breast carcinoma, melanoma
    - Renal lymphoma: Typically non-Hodgkin (large cell) lymphoma
- **Angiomyolipoma, Renal**
  - Fat component may be mistaken for water density on CT, especially if small and evenly distributed
  - US: Highly echogenic, unlike cyst
- **Localized Cystic Renal Disease**
  - Old term unilateral polycystic disease

- Unilateral conglomerate mass consisting of multiple thin-walled cysts
  - May be separated by normal renal parenchyma
  - Lack of surrounding capsule helps to distinguish from multilocular cystic nephroma
- May involve entire kidney
- Not related to autosomal dominant polycystic disease
- **Segmental Multicystic Dysplastic Kidney**
  - Conglomeration of different-sized cysts with little or no renal parenchyma in affected portion of kidney
- **Renal Tumors, Atypical and Rare**
  - Other rare tumors, such as renal angiosarcoma, may appear as complex cystic mass
  - Mixed epithelial and stromal tumor has similar imaging appearance as multilocular cystic nephroma, cystic RCC
    - Benign cystic neoplasm containing stromal and epithelial elements
    - Almost exclusively found in perimenopausal women

SELECTED REFERENCES

1. Wood CG 3rd et al: CT and MR imaging for evaluation of cystic renal lesions and diseases. Radiographics. 35(1):125-41, 2015
2. Bosniak MA: The Bosniak renal cyst classification: 25 years later. Radiology. 262(3):781-5, 2012
3. Smith AD et al: Bosniak category IIF and III cystic renal lesions: outcomes and associations. Radiology. 262(1):152-60, 2012
4. Jonisch AI et al: Can high-attenuation renal cysts be differentiated from renal cell carcinoma at unenhanced CT? Radiology. 243(2):445-50, 2007
5. Israel GM et al: Evaluation of cystic renal masses: comparison of CT and MR imaging by using the Bosniak classification system. Radiology. 231(2):365-71, 2004
6. Israel GM et al: Follow-up CT of moderately complex cystic lesions of the kidney (Bosniak category IIF). AJR Am J Roentgenol. 181(3):627-33, 2003
7. Bosniak MA: Diagnosis and management of patients with complicated cystic lesions of the kidney. AJR. 169: 819, 1997
8. Bosniak MA: The current radiological approach to renal cysts. Radiology. 158(1):1-10, 1986

Renal Cysts

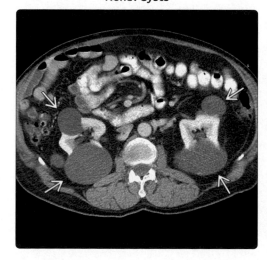

Renal Cysts

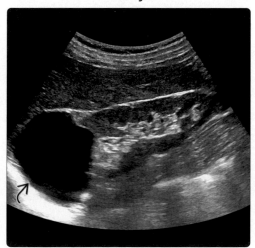

(Left) *CECT of a 62-year-old man with abdominal pain shows multiple simple, exophytic renal cortical cysts ➡. Features of these Bosniak I cysts include water attenuation, the lack of an enhancing wall, septa, or calcifications.* **(Right)** *Right upper quadrant US shows a large exophytic simple right upper pole renal cyst ➷. Ultrasound is an adjunct modality in Bosniak classification system and is a useful technique to differentiate between high-attenuation cysts and true solid renal lesions.*

Renal Cysts

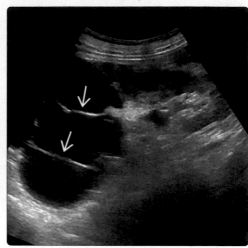

Renal Cysts

(Left) *Coronal Gd-enhanced T1W MR shows a Bosniak II cyst, i.e., minimally complicated, but benign cyst. Hairline-thin septations ➡ are perceptible. A subtype Bosniak II cyst is the high-attenuation (> 20 HU) cyst. Either CECT, MR, or US is needed to differentiate between a high-attenuation cyst and a solid renal lesion. No follow-up is needed for these cysts.* **(Right)** *US of the same patient shows thicker septations ➡. Exaggerated septal thickness prompted an inappropriate Bosniak IIF classification.*

Renal Sinus Cysts

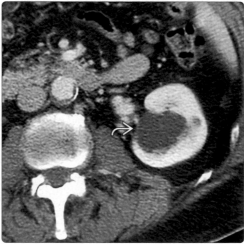

Renal Sinus Cysts

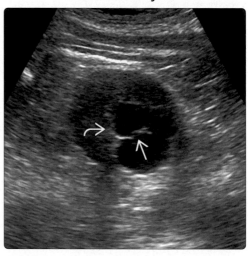

(Left) *CECT shows a Bosniak I left parapelvic cyst ➡. Such a cyst is invariably benign, and no imaging follow-up is needed. Benign renal cysts are present in 20-30% of middle-aged adults, and the incidence increases with age.* **(Right)** *US of the same patient performed to assess for potential renal calculi shows a central cyst ➡ with a septation ➡. Cyst septation is accentuated at ultrasound and often erroneously prompts Bosniak up-classification.*

Renal Sinus Cysts

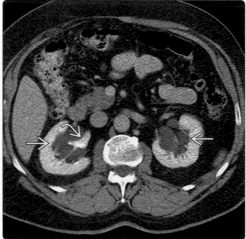

Renal Cell Carcinoma

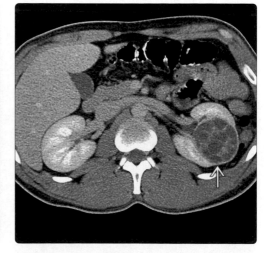

(Left) *CECT shows bilateral peripelvic cysts ➡. Note compression of opacified right renal pelvis by the cysts ➡. Care should be taken to differentiate noncommunicating peripelvic cysts from hydronephrosis at ultrasound. Excretory phase CECT may be confirmatory.* **(Right)** *CECT of a 28-year-old man with flank pain and hematuria shows a complex cystic left renal lesion ➡. Irregular, enhancing septa and nodules indicate a Bosniak IV cyst. Cystic clear cell carcinoma was shown at nephrectomy.*

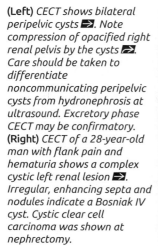

Abscess, Renal

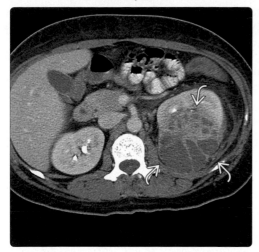

Abscess, Renal

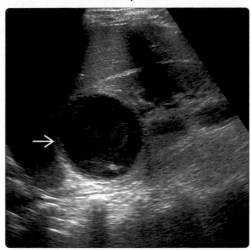

(Left) CECT of a patient with fever, leukocytosis, and flank pain shows a complex left upper pole renal-perirenal abscess ⮧. Complexity and perinephric infiltration suggest an abscess, but clinical history, urinalysis, and aspiration confirm the diagnosis. (Right) Sonography performed before catheter drainage on a different patient with fever, gram-negative bacteremia, and leukocytosis shows a complex right upper pole cyst ⮧ containing low-level echoes. Aspiration of frank pus confirmed an abscess.

Multilocular Cystic Nephroma

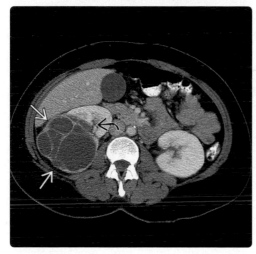

Multilocular Cystic Nephroma

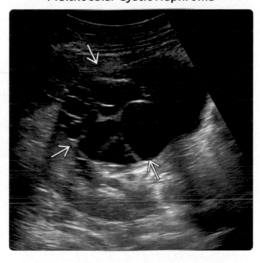

(Left) CECT of a middle-aged woman with flank pain shows a complex, encapsulated cystic lesion ⮧ that invaginates into the renal hilum ⮧. Enhancing thick septa indicate a Bosniak III cyst. A multilocular cystic nephroma was confirmed at resection. (Right) US of a 51-year-old woman with vague right flank discomfort shows a complex cystic renal lesion ⮧ with thick septations. Clear-cut septal enhancement at CECT prompted resection of this multilocular cystic nephroma.

Localized Cystic Renal Disease

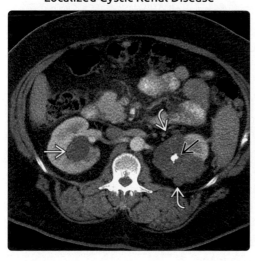

Renal Tumors, Atypical and Rare

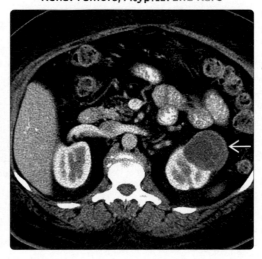

(Left) CECT shows a right parapelvic cyst ⮧ and left upper pole localized cystic renal disease ⮧ (and calculus ⮧). The characteristic imaging appearance of this acquired (not hereditary) entity is a nonencapsulated collection of cysts. (Right) CECT of a perimenopausal woman shows a complex, exophytic cystic lesion ⮧. Thick enhancing septa indicate a Bosniak III cyst. Partial nephrectomy confirmed a mixed epithelial and stromal tumor, a rare benign cystic renal neoplasm.

DIFFERENTIAL DIAGNOSIS

Common

- Simple Renal Cysts
- Uremic Cystic Disease (Acquired Cystic Kidney Disease)
- Autosomal Dominant Polycystic Disease, Kidney
- Von Hippel-Lindau Disease
- Tuberous Sclerosis

Less Common

- Lithium Nephropathy
- Medullary Cystic Disease

Rare but Important

- Glomerulocystic Disease

ESSENTIAL INFORMATION

Key Differential Diagnosis Issues

- Imaging features of renal cysts
  - Consider number, size, and location of renal cysts to narrow differential diagnosis
- Kidney size
  - May help narrow differential diagnosis
- Ancillary imaging findings
  - e.g., presence of renal tumors; presence of cysts or tumors in other organs
- Clinical factors
  - e.g., presence, degree, and type of renal dysfunction
  - Use of medications such as lithium

Helpful Clues for Common Diagnoses

- **Simple Renal Cysts**
  - Imaging features of renal cysts
    - Often multiple and of variable size
    - Usually less numerous than in congenital cystic syndromes
    - Usually of water attenuation
      - □ Hyperdense cysts are not uncommon and usually coexist with simple cysts
    - Location
      - □ Cortex
      - □ Renal sinus: Parapelvic (peripelvic) cysts
  - Kidney size
    - Normal size and function
- **Uremic Cystic Disease (Acquired Cystic Kidney Disease)**
  - ≥ 3 cysts per kidney in patients with end-stage renal disease and no history of hereditary cystic disease
  - Imaging features of renal cysts
    - Multiple, located in both cortex and medulla
    - Variable size; up to several centimeters
  - Kidney size
    - Small, atrophic
    - Cysts and kidneys may become larger
      - □ Advanced cases of acquired cystic disease may be indistinguishable from autosomal dominant polycystic disease, kidney
  - Ancillary imaging features
    - Prone to spontaneous bleeding into cysts or perirenal space
    - Increased risk of renal cell carcinoma

  - □ Enhancing mass in end-stage kidneys = renal cell carcinoma (until proven otherwise)
  - Clinical factors
    - Patients are almost always dialysis dependent
    - Cysts will persist even if patient receives renal transplantation
- **Autosomal Dominant Polycystic Disease, Kidney**
  - Imaging features of renal cysts
    - Multiple and of variable size
    - Number and size of cysts increase over time
    - Attenuation (CT) and signal intensity (MR) of renal cysts are variable
      - □ Hyperdense contents and calcified wall due to prior hemorrhage
  - Kidney size
    - Increased renal size
    - Progressive increase in volume of cysts and kidneys
  - Ancillary imaging features
    - Cysts in other organs
      - □ Liver, pancreas, seminal vesicles
      - □ Intracranial arterial aneurysm
  - Clinical factors
    - Family history
    - Progressive loss of renal function; 50% evolve to end-stage renal disease by 6th decade
    - Gene mutations: PHD1, PKD2
      - □ PKD2 gene mutation associated with milder, later presentation and fewer renal cysts
- **Von Hippel-Lindau Disease**
  - Imaging features of renal cysts
    - Multiple and of various size
    - 59-63% of patients have renal cysts
  - Ancillary imaging features
    - Renal cell carcinoma
      - □ Present in 25-45% of patients
      - □ Histology: Clear cell type; location: Bilateral in 75% of cases
    - Pancreas: Cysts, serous microcystic adenomas, neuroendocrine (islet cell) tumors
    - Adrenal: Pheochromocytoma (often recurrent, multiple)
    - CNS: Hemangioblastomas of cerebellum, brainstem, spinal cord
  - Clinical factors
    - Multisystem disorder, autosomal dominant disease
- **Tuberous Sclerosis**
  - Imaging features of renal cysts
    - Multiple and of various size
  - Ancillary imaging features
    - Kidneys: Hamartomas = angiomyolipomas (often multiple and bilateral)
    - Hamartomatous tumors in brain, lung, heart, skin
  - Clinical factors
    - Multisystem disorder, autosomal dominant disease

Helpful Clues for Less Common Diagnoses

- **Lithium Nephropathy**
  - Imaging features of renal cysts
    - Multiple, bilateral
    - Microcysts (1-2 mm)

- Location: Cortex and medulla
  o Kidney size
    - Normal to small
  o Clinical factors
    - Occurs in patients who take lithium long term (for bipolar disease or other affective disorders)
    - Causes diabetes insipidus and renal insufficiency
      □ Patients are rarely dialysis dependent, unlike patients with acquired cystic disease of uremia
- **Medullary Cystic Disease**
  o Imaging features of renal cysts
    - Small size
      □ 0.1-1.5 cm
    - Renal medulla and corticomedullary junction
  o Kidney size
    - Small to normal-sized kidneys
  o Clinical factors
    - Nephronophthisis or salt-wasting nephropathy
    - Progressive renal failure and anemia in young patient

Helpful Clues for Rare Diagnoses

- **Glomerulocystic Disease**
  o Imaging features of renal cysts
    - Small cysts in renal cortex
      □ Arise from proximal convoluted tubules and Bowman space
  o Clinical factors
    - Sporadic or familial occurrence
    - Rare condition associated with renal insufficiency but rarely end-stage renal failure
    - Affects children and young adults

Alternative Differential Approaches

- Multicystic renal diseases associated with tumors
  o Uremic cystic disease: Renal cell carcinoma, especially papillary type
  o von Hippel-Lindau disease: Renal cell carcinoma + tumors of pancreas, adrenal (pheochromocytoma) and CNS (hemangioblastomas)
  o Tuberous sclerosis: Angiomyolipomas and, rarely, renal cell carcinoma

Simple Renal Cysts

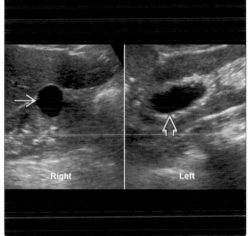

Simple Renal Cysts

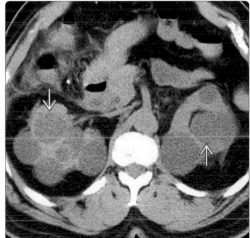

(Left) *Longitudinal renal ultrasound shows a simple anechoic ➡ cyst in the cortex of the right kidney and a large left parapelvic cyst ⇒. (Right) Axial NECT shows multiple, bilateral cysts ➡ but preservation of normal cortex (and function) in an 86-year-old man.*

Uremic Cystic Disease (Acquired Cystic Kidney Disease)

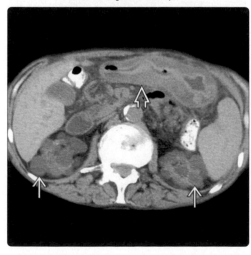

Uremic Cystic Disease (Acquired Cystic Kidney Disease)

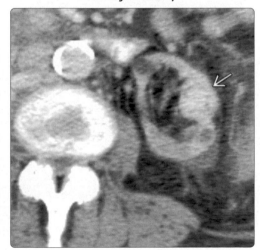

(Left) *Axial NECT shows small kidneys with innumerable cysts ➡. Gastric wall ⇒ is thickened due to gastritis induced by immunosuppressive drugs in this patient who had a renal transplant following years of dialysis therapy. (Right) Axial CECT shows a brightly enhancing solid mass ➡ (renal cell carcinoma) in a patient with dialysis-dependent renal failure. Note the small kidney with innumerable cysts.*

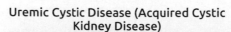

Uremic Cystic Disease (Acquired Cystic Kidney Disease)

Autosomal Dominant Polycystic Disease, Kidney

(Left) *Coronal T2WI MR in a patient with end-stage renal disease and acquired cystic renal disease shows atrophic kidneys with multiple, simple cysts* ➡. **(Right)** *Coronal T2WI MR in a 25-year-old man with autosomal dominant polycystic kidney disease (ADPKD) shows enlarged kidneys replaced by innumerable cysts* ➡ *of various size and signal intensity. Liver cysts are the most common extrarenal manifestation in patients with ADPKD.*

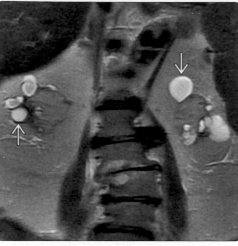
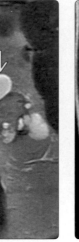

Autosomal Dominant Polycystic Disease, Kidney

Autosomal Dominant Polycystic Disease, Kidney

(Left) *Axial NECT shows massive enlargement of both kidneys with innumerable cysts of varying size and attenuation, some of which have internal hemorrhage* ➡. **(Right)** *Axial NECT shows innumerable cysts of varying size and attenuation in the kidneys* ➡ *and liver* ➡.

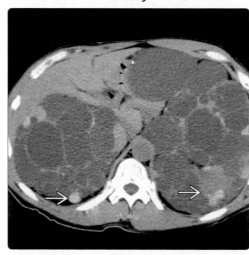
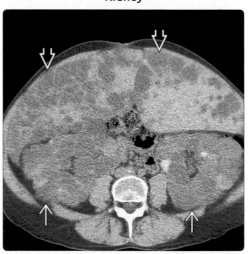

Autosomal Dominant Polycystic Disease, Kidney

Von Hippel-Lindau Disease

(Left) *Axial CECT shows innumerable small cysts* ➡, *mostly in the cortex, in this 62-year-old man with preserved renal function and presumed type 2 ADPKD.* **(Right)** *Axial CECT shows multiple renal cysts* ➡ *and a solid enhancing mass* ➡ *(renal cell carcinoma) in a patient with von Hippel-Lindau disease.*

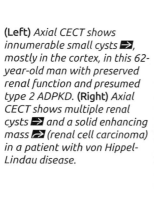
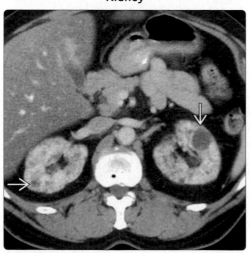
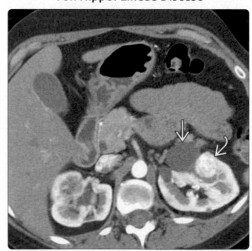

Von Hippel-Lindau Disease

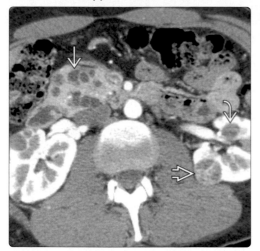

Tuberous Sclerosis

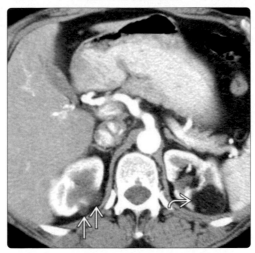

(Left) *Axial CECT shows multiple cysts in the pancreas ➡ and kidneys ➡ as well as one of several solid enhancing masses ➡ (renal cell carcinoma). These are classic features of von Hippel-Lindau syndrome.* **(Right)** *Axial CECT shows 2 of many simple renal cysts ➡ and a fat-containing mass ➡ (angiomyolipoma) in the left kidney.*

Tuberous Sclerosis

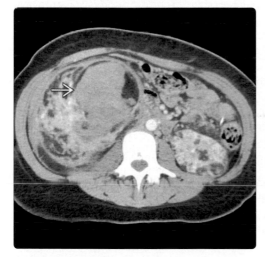

Lithium Nephropathy

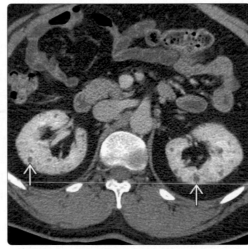

(Left) *Axial CECT shows innumerable small fat density angiomyolipomas (AMLs) in both kidneys. Spontaneous hemorrhage ➡ is associated with one of the larger AMLs. Due to partial volume averaging, it is difficult to distinguish small AMLs from simple cysts, both of which are usually present in patients with tuberous sclerosis.* **(Right)** *Axial CECT in a patient with lithium nephropathy shows innumerable, bilateral microcysts ➡ in normal-size kidneys.*

Lithium Nephropathy

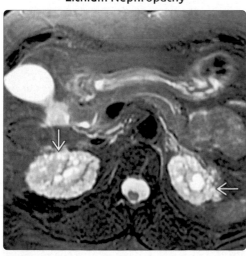

Medullary Cystic Disease

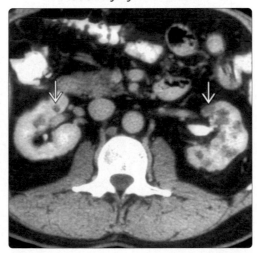

(Left) *Axial T2WI MR shows innumerable tiny cysts ➡ throughout the cortex and medulla of both kidneys in a 69-year-old woman receiving long-term lithium therapy for bipolar disorder. The kidneys are diminished in size and function.* **(Right)** *Axial CECT shows multiple medullary and cortical cysts ➡ in a patient with progressive renal failure, anemia, and salt-wasting nephropathy, all of which are typical imaging and clinical features of medullary cystic disease.*

DIFFERENTIAL DIAGNOSIS

Common

- Acute Pyelonephritis
- Renal Transitional Cell Carcinoma
- Renal Cell Carcinoma
- Renal Lymphoma

Less Common

- Xanthogranulomatous Pyelonephritis
- Renal Metastases
- HIV Nephropathy
- Renal Tuberculosis
- Renal Infarction

Rare but Important

- Renal Medullary Carcinoma
- Renal Squamous Cell Carcinoma
- Collecting Duct Carcinoma
- Renal Sarcoma
- Renal Parenchymal Malakoplakia
- IgG4-Related Sclerosing Disease

ESSENTIAL INFORMATION

Key Differential Diagnosis Issues

- Infiltrative refers to processes that replace renal parenchyma without distorting its reniform shape
  - Lack of sharp border of demarcation with normal parenchyma
- Diagnosis requires imaging characterization, plus clinical data

Helpful Clues for Common Diagnoses

- **Acute Pyelonephritis**
  - Enlarged kidney with striated or wedge-shaped foci of decreased enhancement on CECT or Gd-enhanced MR
    - Perinephric inflammatory changes (perinephric fat stranding and fluid; ± renal, perirenal abscess)
  - More common in young women; usually presenting with high fever and bacteria in urine

- **Renal Transitional Cell Carcinoma**
  - Irregular filling defect in renal pelvis with tumor infiltration of parenchyma
  - Renal mass much less common than polypoid uroepithelial tumor of urinary bladder or renal pelvis
- **Renal Cell Carcinoma**
  - Usually expansile mass, but may infiltrate diffusely simulating renal transitional cell carcinoma (TCC)
    - ± renal vein thrombosis
  - Infiltration of renal parenchyma is more common with TCC than with renal cell carcinoma (RCC), but RCC is more common tumor
- **Renal Lymphoma**
  - Most commonly it is secondary to systemic disease
  - Presenting with multiple bilateral renal masses or infiltration of renal parenchyma/sinus with maintenance of reniform shape
    - ± adenopathy, splenomegaly

Helpful Clues for Less Common Diagnoses

- **Xanthogranulomatous Pyelonephritis**
  - Chronic renal infection, destruction of renal parenchyma and replacement by lipid-laden macrophages
  - Enlarged, nonfunctioning kidney, ± large, central calculus
- **Renal Metastases**
  - More frequently presenting as multiple solid masses rather than infiltrative pattern
  - Common etiologies: Bronchogenic carcinoma; breast carcinoma; GI malignancies; melanoma
- **Renal Infarction**
  - Wedge-shaped perfusion defect
  - Clinical history (vasculitis, thromboembolic disease) key

Helpful Clues for Rare Diagnoses

- **Renal Medullary Carcinoma**
  - Young patient with sickle cell trait
- **Renal Squamous Cell Carcinoma**
  - Chronic calculus disease

Renal Transitional Cell Carcinoma

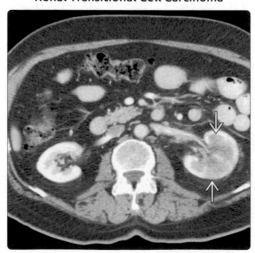

Renal Transitional Cell Carcinoma

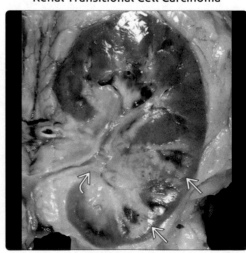

(Left) *Axial CECT shows classic infiltration and enlargement of the medullary portions of the lower pole of the left kidney* ➡ *by transitional cell carcinoma.* **(Right)** *Gross pathology of the resected left kidney in the same patient (coronal plane) shows tumor along the surface of the inferior pole of the collecting system* ➡ *with infiltration of the medullary portion of the lower pole* ➡ *with sparing of the cortex.*

Acute Pyelonephritis

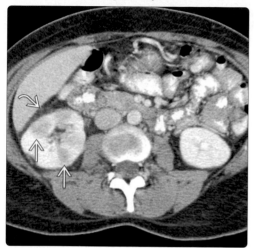

Renal Cell Carcinoma

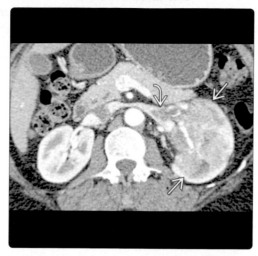

(Left) *Axial CECT shows an enlarged right kidney with striated nephrogram pattern* ➡, *characteristic, but not diagnostic, of acute pyelonephritis. Note perinephric fat infiltration* ➡. (Right) *Axial CECT shows infiltration of the left kidney by a mass. The hypervascularity of the mass* ➡ *and the invasion of the renal vein* ➡ *suggest the diagnosis of renal cell carcinoma, rather than transitional cell carcinoma.*

Renal Lymphoma

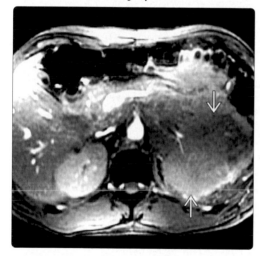

Xanthogranulomatous Pyelonephritis

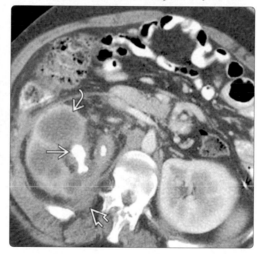

(Left) *Axial T2* GRE MR shows an infiltrating left renal mass* ➡ *extending to the perirenal space, biopsy-proven B-cell non-Hodgkin lymphoma. Systemic adenopathy was also present (not shown in this image).* (Right) *Axial CECT shows an enlarged and nonfunctioning right kidney with an obstructing calculus* ➡. *Low-density xanthomatous inflammation* ➡ *replaces the renal parenchyma and spreads to the perirenal space* ➡.

Renal Infarction

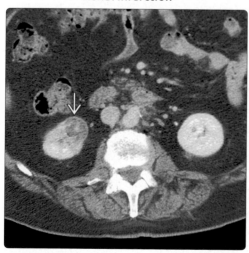

Renal Medullary Carcinoma

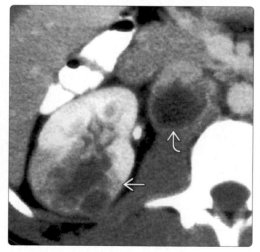

(Left) *Axial CECT shows heterogeneous decreased enhancement of the lower pole of the right kidney* ➡, *simulating an infiltrative mass, but proved to be due to acute renal infarction.* (Right) *Axial CECT shows an infiltrative mass* ➡ *in the lower pole of the right kidney with direct invasion of the inferior vena cava* ➡ *in a young man with sickle cell trait and renal medullary carcinoma.*

DIFFERENTIAL DIAGNOSIS

Common

- Perirenal & Subcapsular Hemorrhage
  - Renal Trauma
  - Coagulopathic ("Retroperitoneal") Hemorrhage
  - Hemorrhagic Neoplasms
  - Vascular: Vasculitis & Aneurysms
- Renal Metastases & Lymphoma
- Renal, Perirenal Abscess

Less Common

- Pyelonephritis, Xanthogranulomatous
- Pancreatitis, Acute
- Extramedullary Hematopoiesis
- Urinoma
- Accessory Spleen
- Retroperitoneal Fibrosis
- Nephroblastomatosis

Rare but Important

- Renal Lymphangiomatosis
- Multiple Myeloma
- Rosai-Dorfman Disease
- Erdheim-Chester Disease
- IgG4-Related Sclerosing Disease

ESSENTIAL INFORMATION

Key Differential Diagnosis Issues

- Key to differential diagnosis: Imaging plus clinical
  - Seek evidence for
    - Trauma
    - Infection
    - Tumor (primary or metastatic)

Helpful Clues for Common Diagnoses

- **Perirenal & Subcapsular Hemorrhage**
  - Trauma: Blunt, penetrating, or iatrogenic
    - Renal biopsy
    - Retrograde pyelography or ureteral catheterization
    - Percutaneous nephrostomy
    - Lithotripsy
  - Spontaneous coagulopathic
    - Hemophilia
    - Anticoagulant therapy
  - Tumor
    - Angiomyolipoma & renal cell carcinoma are most common
    - Large tumors extend into perirenal space
    - May bleed into perirenal space
    - Metastases quite uncommon
  - Vasculitis
    - Polyarteritis nodosa
    - Lupus erythematosus
    - Other small & medium vessel arteritides
  - Ruptured aneurysm or arteriovenous fistula: Aortic or renal artery
- **Renal Metastases & Lymphoma**
  - Metastases: More often discrete masses within kidney &/or perirenal space

- Melanoma is most common primary tumor
  - Lymphoma: More often confluent masses
- **Renal, Perirenal Abscess**
  - Marked infiltration of perirenal space; thickened perirenal fascia
  - Abscess contents do not enhance
    - May contain gas

Helpful Clues for Less Common Diagnoses

- **Pyelonephritis, Xanthogranulomatous**
  - Usually infiltrates & replaces kidney & perirenal space with heterogeneous, low-density mass
    - Low density is due to lipid-laden macrophages
    - Attenuation is usually lower than water but higher than "pure" fat
  - Almost always associated with large calculus obstructing renal pelvis or infundibulum
    - Affected portion (or entire) kidney is usually nonfunctional
- **Pancreatitis, Acute**
  - May spread to perirenal space, usually through renal hilum (rarely through perirenal fascia)
  - Pseudocyst may form within perirenal space
    - Density of pseudocyst may vary; often higher than water density when acute due to blood & proteinaceous contents
- **Extramedullary Hematopoiesis**
  - Associated with chronic anemia, leukemia, extensive bone tumor
  - May infiltrate kidney & perirenal space
  - May also see other sites
    - Spleen, paraspinal masses, etc.
- **Urinoma**
  - Due to obstruction of ureter & rupture of renal fornix
  - Urine collects within perirenal space, usually caudal to kidney
  - Density of "mass" depends on use of contrast media
    - On NECT will be near water density
    - On CECT, pyelographic phase, should see densely opacified urine within perirenal space
- **Accessory Spleen**
  - May "migrate" along splenorenal ligament to result in perirenal mass
  - Similar density & enhancement pattern as spleen
  - Tc sulfur colloid scan is definitive test
- **Retroperitoneal Fibrosis**
  - Causes confluent mass that encases distal aorta, inferior vena cava, & ureters
  - Fibrotic mass may extend into perirenal spaces
  - Caliectasis, hydronephrosis, & urinoma may all result from ureteral obstruction
- **Nephroblastomatosis**
  - Multiple masses in renal cortex & perirenal space, bilateral; precursor of Wilms tumor

Helpful Clues for Rare Diagnoses

- **Renal Lymphangiomatosis**
  - Rare benign malformation of perirenal lymphatics
  - Unilateral or bilateral perirenal & peripelvic septate cystic collections
    - Anechoic on US

– Innumerable cystic, water attenuation cystic spaces on CECT

- **Multiple Myeloma**
  - Perirenal spaces may be involved with masses of proliferating plasmacytes
- **Rosai-Dorfman Disease**
  - Rare disorder that results in proliferation & accumulation of histiocytes (WBC) in lymph nodes & extranodal tissues
  - Sites of extranodal disease include skin, CNS, kidney/perirenal, & gut
- **Erdheim-Chester Disease**
  - a.k.a. polyostotic sclerosing histiocytosis
  - Rare multisystem disease characterized by progressive involvement of bones, organs & tissues by xanthogranulomatous infiltration (lipid-laden histiocytes & giant cells)
  - Presents with leg pain & shows sclerosis of metaphyses of lower extremities
  - Kidneys, heart, lungs, pleura, orbits, CNS, & meninges can be involved
- **IgG4-Related Sclerosing Disease**

  - Potentially multisystem autoimmune inflammatory process (e.g., autoimmune pancreatitis, cholangitis, thyroiditis)
  - Can infiltrate kidneys & perirenal spaces

SELECTED REFERENCES

1. Glockner JF et al: Magnetic Resonance Imaging of Perirenal Pathology. Can Assoc Radiol J. ePub, 2016
2. Heller MT et al: Acute conditions affecting the perinephric space: imaging anatomy, pathways of disease spread, and differential diagnosis. Emerg Radiol. 19(3):245-54, 2012
3. Heller MT et al: Neoplastic and proliferative disorders of the perinephric space. Clin Radiol. 67(11):e31-41, 2012
4. Diaz JR et al: Spontaneous perirenal hemorrhage: what radiologists need to know. Emerg Radiol. 18(4):329-34, 2011
5. Surabhi VR et al: Neoplastic and non-neoplastic proliferative disorders of the perirenal space: cross-sectional imaging findings. Radiographics. 28(4):1005-17, 2008
6. Westphalen A et al: Differential diagnosis of perinephric masses on CT and MRI. AJR Am J Roentgenol. 183(6):1697-702, 2004

Renal Trauma

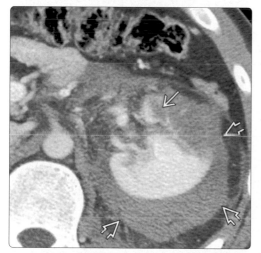

Hemorrhagic Neoplasms

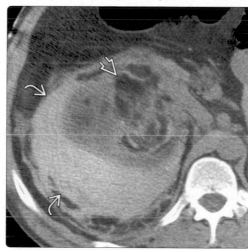

(Left) *Axial CECT shows hemorrhage ⊟ filling the perirenal space due to a parenchymal laceration ➡.* (Right) *Axial NECT shows blood ⊟ filling the perirenal space that is hyperdense to the renal parenchyma. Note the heterogeneous fat density mass ⊟, an acute myeloid leukemia, that was the source of the hemorrhage.*

Renal Metastases & Lymphoma

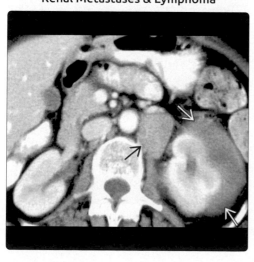

Renal Metastases & Lymphoma

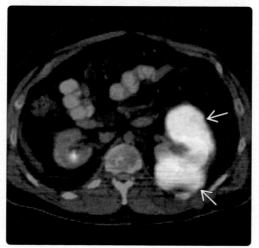

(Left) *Axial CECT shows a soft tissue density mass ⊟ filling the perirenal space, and retroperitoneal lymphadenopathy ⊟, both due to non-Hodgkin lymphoma.* (Right) *Axial PET shows intense FDG uptake ⊟ in and around the left kidney due to metastatic melanoma.*

Renal, Perirenal Abscess

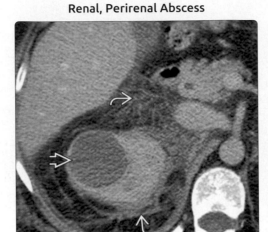

Renal, Perirenal Abscess

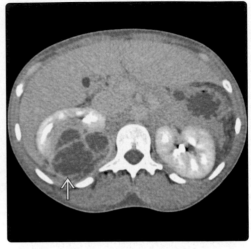

(Left) Axial CECT shows an encapsulated, spherical abscess ➡ and diffuse infiltration of the perirenal space ➡. (Right) Axial CECT shows a multiseptate renal and perirenal mass ➡, a typical appearance of an abscess.

Pyelonephritis, Xanthogranulomatous

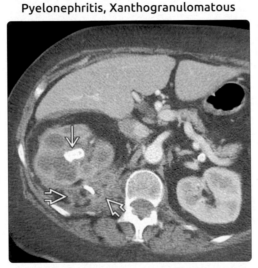

Pancreatitis, Acute

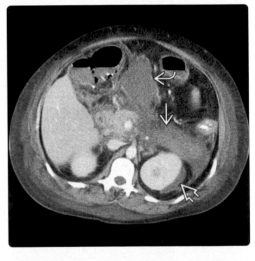

(Left) Axial CECT shows a nonfunctional right kidney with a large central calculous ➡. The proliferated, chronically inflamed fat and pus distend the perirenal space ➡. (Right) Axial CECT shows severe pancreatitis with necrosis of the body/tail segments ➡ and spread of inflammation into the mesentery ➡, retroperitoneum, and even the left perirenal space ➡.

Extramedullary Hematopoiesis

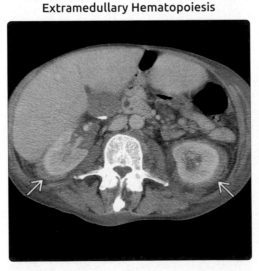

Extramedullary Hematopoiesis

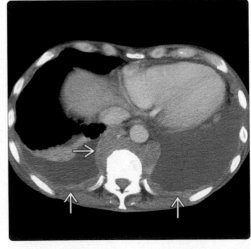

(Left) Axial CECT in a 64-year-old man with myelofibrosis shows bilateral perirenal masses ➡ due to extramedullary hematopoiesis. Similar masses were seen in the paraspinal region. (Right) Another CT in the same patient shows paraspinal and pleural masses ➡, typical features of extramedullary hematopoiesis, along with pleural effusions.

Urinoma

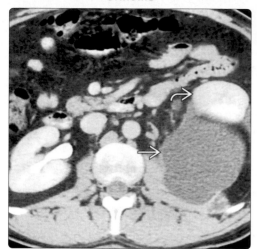

Urinoma

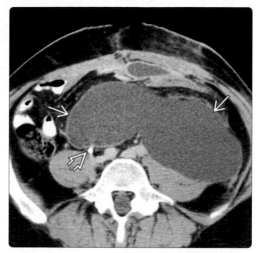

(Left) *Axial CECT shows a water density mass* ➡ *in the left perirenal space that displaces the kidney* ➡. *The left ureter had been injured during a colonic resection, causing a stricture and urinary leak.* **(Right)** *A more caudal axial CECT in the same case shows more of the large urinoma* ➡. *Note the opacified right ureter* ➡ *and the absence of an opacified left ureter.*

Retroperitoneal Fibrosis

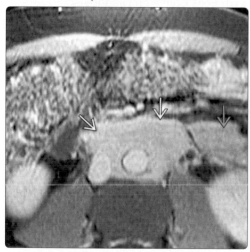

Renal Lymphangiomatosis

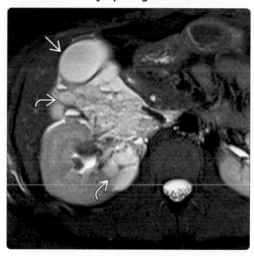

(Left) *Axial T1 C+ FS MR shows an unusually large mass of fibrotic tissue* ➡ *that encases the aorta and inferior vena cava and that extends along the renal hila* ➡ *into the perirenal spaces.* **(Right)** *Axial T2 FS MR shows a multiseptate fluid intensity mass* ➡ *that fills the perirenal space and replaces part of the kidney* ➡, *a typical appearance of a lymphangioma.*

Erdheim-Chester Disease

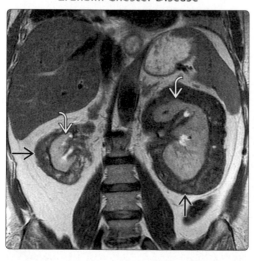

IgG4-Related Sclerosing Disease

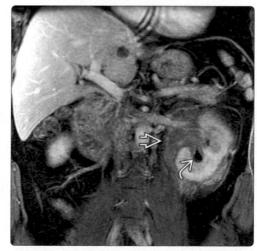

(Left) *Coronal T2 MR shows encasement of the kidneys* ➡ *by heterogeneous perinephric space tissue* ➡. *These findings plus pleural thickening and sclerosis of the metaphyseal regions of the femur are characteristic features of Erdheim-Chester disease.* **(Right)** *Coronal T1 C+ MR shows a delayed nephrogram and hydronephrosis* ➡ *along with perirenal infiltration* ➡. *Renal biopsy confirmed IgG4 sclerosing disease. The process improved with steroid therapy.*

DIFFERENTIAL DIAGNOSIS

Common

- Chronic Glomerulonephritis
- Renal Cortical Necrosis
- Renal Allograft Rejection
- Sickle Cell Anemia

Less Common

- Chronic Hypercalcemia
- Oxalosis (Primary or Secondary)
- Alport Syndrome
- Ethylene Glycol (Antifreeze) Poisoning
- Tuberculosis

ESSENTIAL INFORMATION

Key Differential Diagnosis Issues

- Nephrocalcinosis: Cortical (5%) much less common than medullary (95%)
- Most common etiologies of cortical nephrocalcinosis: Chronic glomerulonephritis > cortical necrosis > rejected renal allograft
- Focal areas of dystrophic calcification in renal masses or infection are not considered nephrocalcinosis
- Tuberculosis (mimic): Focal amorphous calcification at sites of caseating infection
  - Diffuse: Dense calcification throughout autonephrectomized kidney (putty kidney)
  - Renal scarring and volume loss
- Opportunistic infections (mimic)
  - Usually in patients with AIDS
  - Cytomegalovirus, mycobacterium avium intracellulare, pneumocystis
  - Usually multiple punctate calcifications in cortex and medulla

Helpful Clues for Common Diagnoses

- **Chronic Glomerulonephritis**
  - Punctate and curvilinear, cortical
  - Decreased renal size and function

- **Renal Cortical Necrosis**
  - Usually due to shock (e.g., placental abruption, severe hypotensive episode)
  - Also associated with nephrotoxins (e.g., amphotericin B)
  - Thin peripheral rim of calcification just beneath renal capsule; may extend into septum of Bertin
    - Tram line calcification or punctate calcifications in renal cortex
  - CECT: Hypoattenuating band between cortical calcification and opacified medulla; no or minimal concentration and excretion of contrast medium
  - US: Hyperechoic peripheral renal cortex with shadowing
- **Renal Allograft Rejection**
  - Allograft usually in iliac fossa
  - Calcification: Cortex or entire organ
  - Allograft diminished in size
- **Sickle Cell Anemia**
  - Chronic ischemia → small, peripherally calcified kidneys
  - Analogous to spleen changes in sickle cell
  - Sclerotic bones in long-standing disease

Helpful Clues for Less Common Diagnoses

- **Chronic Hypercalcemia**
  - Milk-alkali ingestion; vitamin D excess
- **Oxalosis (Primary or Secondary)**
  - Primary: Autosomal recessive disorder
  - Secondary: Over ingestion of oxalic acids or its precursors
  - Dense calcification of cortex ± medulla
  - Kidneys normal to small size; hyperdense bones
- **Alport Syndrome**
  - X-linked recessive disorder
  - Kidney involvement: Glomerulonephritis and interstitial fibrosis
  - Kidneys: Atrophic/echogenic in longstanding disease

(Left) AP radiograph shows cortical nephrocalcinosis in patient with chronic glomerulonephritis. Note the patient has not received any intravenous contrast material. The cortical calcification is dystrophic due to longstanding inflammation. Chronic glomerulonephritis is the most common cause of cortical nephrocalcinosis. (Right) Axial NECT shows coarse calcifications ➡ in renal cortical regions in patient with chronic glomerulonephritis. Exophytic cyst in the left kidney ➡ is secondary to chronic dialysis.

Chronic Glomerulonephritis

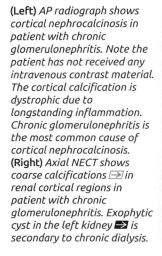
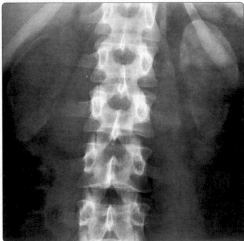

Chronic Glomerulonephritis

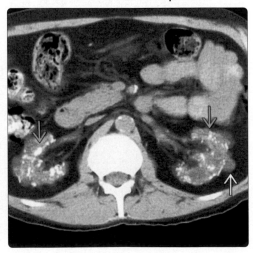

Renal Cortical Necrosis

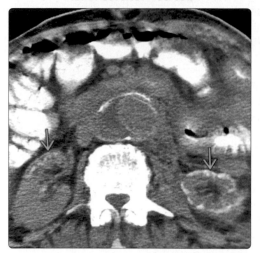

Renal Allograft Rejection

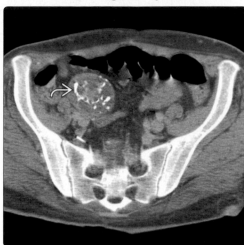

(Left) *Axial NECT shows a patient who experienced renal cortical necrosis due to an episode of hypotension during repair of an acutely ruptured abdominal aortic aneurysm. Note thin rim of cortical nephrocalcinosis* ➡ *bilaterally. Most cases of renal cortical necrosis are due to an episode of profound hypotension* **(Right)** *Axial NECT shows cortical calcifications within atrophic renal allograft* ➡ *in right iliac fossa. Cortical calcifications of renal allograft are associated with a nonfunctional, failed transplant.*

Sickle Cell Anemia

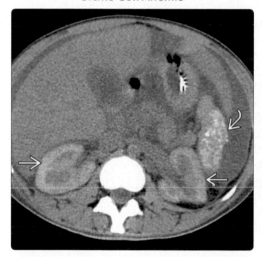

Oxalosis (Primary or Secondary)

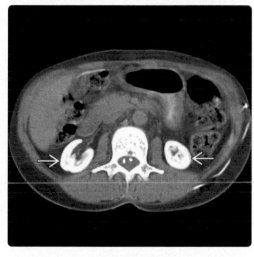

(Left) *Axial NECT shows cortical calcification of both kidneys* ➡ *and the spleen* ➡, *along with dense bones and ascites in a patient with sickle cell anemia.* **(Right)** *Axial NECT shows small, densely calcified and nonfunctional kidneys* ➡, *along with dense bones, typical findings for oxalosis. Alport syndrome can have identical imaging findings.*

Alport Syndrome

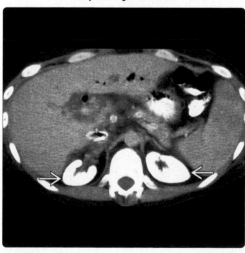

Tuberculosis

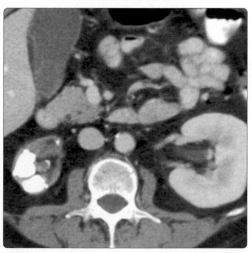

(Left) *Axial NECT shows dense diffuse calcification and small size of both kidneys* ➡ *in a patient with Alport syndrome.* **(Right)** *Axial CECT shows a small, nonfunctional right kidney with cortical and medullary calcifications.*

DIFFERENTIAL DIAGNOSIS

Common

- Hyperparathyroidism
- Renal Tubular Acidosis
- Medullary Sponge Kidney
- Hypercalcemia/Hypercalciurina

Less Common

- Oxalosis
- Papillary Necrosis
- Sarcoid
- Infections (Tuberculosis, Chronic Pyelonephritis)
- Milk-Alkali Syndrome
- Hypervitaminosis D
- Syndromic (e.g., Cushing Syndrome)
- Medications
- Multiple Myeloma

ESSENTIAL INFORMATION

Key Differential Diagnosis Issues

- Medullary nephrocalcinosis refers to deposition of calcium salts in renal medulla
  - Medulla can show focal or diffusely increased echogenicity or have ring-like appearance on US
- Medullary nephrocalcinosis is most common form of nephrocalcinosis
  - 20x more common than cortical nephrocalcinosis
- Most conditions that cause medullary nephrocalcinosis also cause nephrolithiasis
  - Calcium deposits rupture through renal papillae into collecting system
- Imaging is limited in distinguishing among numerous etiologies

Helpful Clues for Common Diagnoses

- **Hyperparathyroidism**
  - Primary form accounts for 40% of all cases of medullary nephrocalcinosis

  - Clusters of round calcifications primarily in renal pyramids; may fill ureters
  - Still visible on CT and radiographs after IV contrast administration (unlike medullary sponge kidney)
- **Renal Tubular Acidosis**
  - Imaging findings identical to hyperparathyroidism
  - Occurs in both familiar and secondary forms
- **Medullary Sponge Kidney**
  - Renal tubular ectasia; tiny calculi within diluted tubules; disappear after IV contrast administration
  - Excretory CECT and urography: Renal pyramid "brush," dilated tubules
- **Hypercalcemia/Hypercalciuria**
  - Of many potential causes
  - May cause cortical and medullary calcinosis

Helpful Clues for Less Common Diagnoses

- **Oxalosis**
  - Dense calcification of cortex ± medulla
  - Kidneys normal to small size
  - Skeletal hyperdensity
  - Alport syndrome: Similar appearance
- **Papillary Necrosis**
  - Often in setting of analgesic abuse
  - Entire papilla may be calcified
- **Sarcoid**
  - Associated with adenopathy and pulmonary fibrosis
- **Infections (Tuberculosis, Chronic Pyelonephritis)**
  - **Pyelonephritis, Chronic**
    - Punctate or focal calcifications in cortex and medulla
    - Cortical thinning over dilated calyces
    - Kidneys decreased in size and function
  - **Opportunistic Infections**
    - Usually in patients with AIDS: *Mycobacterium avium-intracellulare*, pneumocystis, CMV
  - **Tuberculosis, Renal**
    - Focal or diffuse calcification at sites of caseated infection
- **Medications**
  - Amphotericin, furosemide, acetazolamide

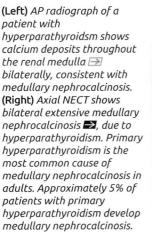

(Left) AP radiograph of a patient with hyperparathyroidsm shows calcium deposits throughout the renal medulla ➡ bilaterally, consistent with medullary nephrocalcinosis. (Right) Axial NECT shows bilateral extensive medullary nephrocalcinosis ➡, due to hyperparathyroidism. Primary hyperparathyroidism is the most common cause of medullary nephrocalcinosis in adults. Approximately 5% of patients with primary hyperparathyroidism develop medullary nephrocalcinosis.

Hyperparathyroidism

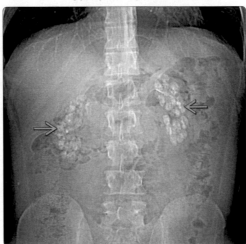

Hyperparathyroidism

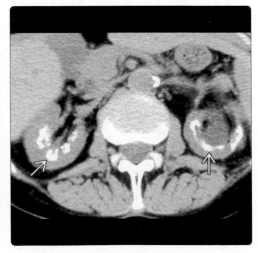

Renal Tubular Acidosis

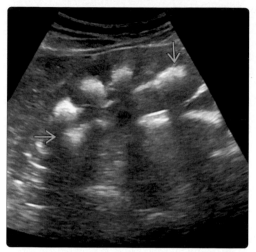

Renal Tubular Acidosis

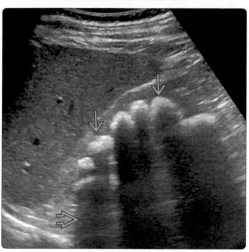

(Left) *Sagittal US of the kidney in a patient with renal tubular acidosis shows increased echogenicity ➡ of the renal medulla due to diffuse medullary nephrocalcinosis. Note the shadowing posterior to the pyramids. Medullary nephrocalcinosis can also produce ring-like echogenicity.* **(Right)** *Sagittal US demonstrates extensive medullary nephrocalcinosis ➡ in a patient with renal tubular acidosis. Note the extensive posterior shadowing ➡ that obscures the posterior aspect of the kidney.*

Renal Tubular Acidosis

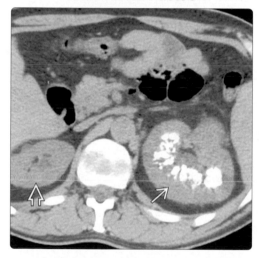

Medullary Sponge Kidney

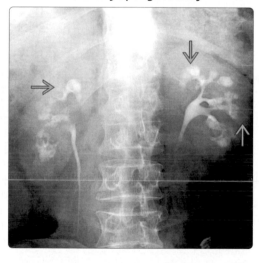

(Left) *Axial NECT shows dense medullary nephrocalcinosis in the left kidney ➡ but no involvement of the right ➡, an unusual degree of asymmetry in medullary nephrocalcinosis. Renal tubular acidosis occurs in both familial and secondary forms.* **(Right)** *Frontal excretory urography shows a classic paint brush appearance ➡ of the dilated renal tubules in the renal pyramids bilaterally. The many small calculi within the tubules are obscured by the opacified urine.*

Medullary Sponge Kidney

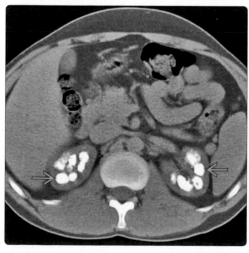

Papillary Necrosis

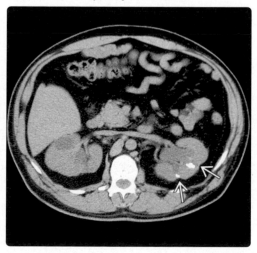

(Left) *Axial NECT in the same patient reveals the extensive, dense calcifications ➡ in the renal medulla bilaterally. Unlike medullary sponge kidney, medullary nephrocalcinosis due to hyperparathyroidism and renal tubular acidosis is usually very dense.* **(Right)** *Axial NECT shows small kidneys. Note the cortical scarring overlying the medullary calcifications ➡ and the dilated calices, all due to chronic reflux and infection.*

DIFFERENTIAL DIAGNOSIS

Common

- Renal Trauma
- Renal Angiomyolipoma
- Renal Cell Carcinoma
- Coagulopathic Hemorrhage
- Ruptured Abdominal Aortic Aneurysm
- Acquired Cystic Disease of Uremia
- Adrenal Hemorrhage
- Perirenal Abscess (Mimic)
- Renal Lymphoma (Mimic)

Less Common

- Vasculitides
- Autosomal Dominant Polycystic Kidney Disease
- Renal Artery Aneurysm/Pseudoaneurysm
- Renal Vein Thrombosis
- Renal Arteriovenous Malformation
  - Arteriovenous Fistula
- Acute Pancreatitis
- Pheochromocytoma
- Adrenocortical Carcinoma

ESSENTIAL INFORMATION

Key Differential Diagnosis Issues

- History (trauma, tumor, anticoagulation, known vasculitis) is extremely helpful
- Trauma
  - Penetrating or high-impact blunt trauma
- Tumor
  - Tumors may cause spontaneous hemorrhage or may bleed with trauma
    - Consider underlying pathology if amount of perirenal hemorrhage exceeds what would be expected based on severity of trauma
  - Look for claw sign identifying mass arising from kidney
  - Repeat imaging after resolution of hematoma may be necessary to detect underlying pathology
- Anticoagulation
  - Look for other sites of bleeding, especially into abdominal wall muscles
  - Hematocrit sign (cellular-fluid level) strongly suggests coagulopathy as cause of hemorrhage
- Acute spontaneous perirenal hemorrhage has been referred to as **Wunderlich syndrome**

Helpful Clues for Common Diagnoses

- **Renal Trauma**
  - Most common cause of perirenal hemorrhage
  - Perirenal fluid may be combination of blood and urine
    - For any renal laceration evident on CT, delayed scans should be obtained to evaluate for urinary extravasation
  - Look for extravasation of contrast indicating active bleeding
  - Consider iatrogenic causes
    - Percutaneous biopsy, nephrostomy, retrograde ureteral catheterization, lithotripsy
- **Renal Angiomyolipoma**
  - Accounts for almost 50% of all cases of spontaneous perirenal hemorrhage
    - Hemorrhage more common in tumors > 4 cm
  - Look for fat-containing mass in kidney
    - Mass may be obscured by hemorrhage
    - ~ 5% of angiomyolipomas (AMLs) contain minimal fat (lipid-poor AML) not detectable by imaging modalities
    - Calcification is extremely rare in AML; if present, suspect renal cell carcinoma (RCC)
  - 80% of patients with tuberous sclerosis have numerous bilateral AMLs: Higher risk of complications
  - AML complicated by hemorrhage is usually treated by embolization (coil, Embosphere, foam, etc.)
- **Renal Cell Carcinoma**
  - Lower chance of bleeding than AML
  - Heterogeneous enhancing mass
  - May have calcification (seen in < 10%; helpful to differentiate from AML)
  - Rarely may show macroscopic fat
  - Up to 25% of sporadic cases of RCC are multifocal
- **Coagulopathic Hemorrhage**
  - Usually in patients receiving heparin or Coumadin
  - Bleeding usually starts in iliopsoas compartment; spreads into retroperitoneum
  - Look for hematocrit sign
- **Ruptured Abdominal Aortic Aneurysm**
  - Can bleed into any or all retroperitoneal compartments
    - May follow renal vessels into perirenal space
  - Hematoma is contiguous with aneurysm sac
- **Acquired Cystic Disease of Uremia**
  - ≥ 3 cysts in kidneys in patient with history of end-stage renal disease (ESRD)
    - No correlation with underlying cause of ESRD or method of dialysis
  - Hemorrhage into cysts occurs in ~ 50% cases
  - Rarely rupture and cause perinephric hematoma
  - Look for associated RCC
    - 3-6% prevalence of RCC in patients with acquired cystic disease of uremia
- **Adrenal Hemorrhage**
  - More common in neonates but can be seen in children and adults as well
  - Seen with both traumatic and nontraumatic causes
  - Unilateral hemorrhage more common in trauma
  - Nontraumatic etiologies typically present with bilateral hemorrhage
    - Stress (including recent surgery or hypotension)
    - Hemorrhagic diathesis or coagulopathy
    - Bleeding adrenal tumor
    - Sepsis (Waterhouse-Friderichsen syndrome)
- **Perirenal Abscess (Mimic)**
  - High-attenuation pus may occasionally simulate blood
  - Present clinically with fever, flank pain, and increased white cell count
- **Renal Lymphoma (Mimic)**
  - Non-Hodgkin lymphoma may cause perirenal infiltrative mass that might mimic hemorrhage
  - Look for lymphadenopathy and other findings of lymphoma

Helpful Clues for Less Common Diagnoses

- **Vasculitides**
  - Most likely diagnosis in absence of renal trauma, mass, aneurysm, or anticoagulation
  - Most common causes
    - Polyarteritis nodosa, lupus, granulomatosis with polyangiitis (previously known as Wegener granulomatosis)
  - Segmental arterial mediolysis: Increasingly recognized noninflammatory vascular disease
    - Caused by lysis of smooth muscle, of unknown etiology
    - Affecting medium-sized arteries causing stenosis, dissection, and aneurysm
- **Autosomal Dominant Polycystic Kidney Disease**
  - Bleeding into cysts is common; cyst rupture may rarely result in perirenal hemorrhage
- **Renal Artery Aneurysm (Pseudoaneurysm)**
  - Risk factors
    - True aneurysm: Arteriosclerosis, fibromuscular dysplasia, AML, pregnancy
    - Pseudoaneurysm: Trauma, inflammation, infection, vasculitis
  - Risk of rupture is directly proportional to size of aneurysm
  - Increased risk of rupture in pregnancy
- **Renal Vein Thrombosis**
  - Rare cause of spontaneous perirenal hemorrhage
  - Vein thrombosis → congestion → venous ischemia/infarction → hemorrhage
  - Risk factors: Hypercoagulable state, nephrotic syndrome, dehydration, infection, tumor
  - Affected kidney is enlarged and edematous
- **Renal Arterlovenous Malformation**
  - Abnormal communication between artery and vein through nidus
    - Congenital; seen with Osler-Weber-Rendu syndrome
  - Seen as focus of abnormal enhancement during arterial phase with premature opacification of renal vein
  - **Arteriovenous Fistula**

- Direct communication between artery and vein, without nidus
- Mostly acquired and caused by trauma
  - Most have remote history of penetrating trauma (including iatrogenic, such as biopsy)
- Both feeding artery and draining vein are enlarged (due to decreased resistance and resultant increased flow)
- Doppler US with spectral interrogation shows high-velocity flow and pulsatile wave in draining vein
- **Acute Pancreatitis**
  - May infiltrate perirenal (and other retroperitoneal) spaces and mimic perirenal hemorrhage
  - History and findings of pancreatitis with predominantly peripancreatic location of collections are clue to diagnosis
- **Pheochromocytoma**
  - Highly vascular adrenal tumor prone to hemorrhage, necrosis
    - Hemorrhage may extend into perirenal space
  - Clinical presentation and lab data may be helpful in making diagnosis
- **Adrenocortical Carcinoma**
  - Large suprarenal mass often containing hemorrhagic, cystic, and calcific areas
  - Look for vascular invasion
    - Renal vein, inferior vena cava
- **Hemorrhagic Fever With Renal Syndrome**
  - Multisystem infectious disease caused by Hanta viruses (carried by rodents)

SELECTED REFERENCES

1. Flum AS et al: Update on the diagnosis and management of renal angiomyolipoma. J Urol. ePub, 2015
2. Diaz JR et al: Spontaneous perirenal hemorrhage: what radiologists need to know. Emerg Radiol. 18(4):329-34, 2011
3. Katabathina VS et al: Wunderlich syndrome: cross-sectional imaging review. J Comput Assist Tomogr. 35(4):425-33, 2011
4. Sheth S et al: Imaging of renal lymphoma: patterns of disease with pathologic correlation. Radiographics. 26(4):1151-68, 2006
5. Harris AC et al: CT findings in blunt renal trauma. Radiographics. 21 Spec No:S201-14, 2001

Renal Trauma

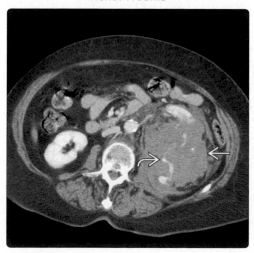

Renal Trauma

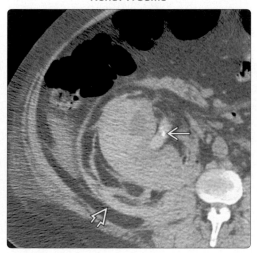

(Left) *Axial CECT shows a large perirenal hemorrhage ➡ due to a parenchymal laceration through the dorsal 1/2 of the kidney. Note extravasation of contrast-opacified blood ➡.* **(Right)** *Axial NECT shows perirenal hemorrhage ➡ and a small stone in the renal pelvis ➡ following lithotripsy and previous placement of a nephrostomy tube in an attempt to clear the renal calculi.*

(Left) *Axial NECT shows hyperdense blood throughout the perirenal space* ⇨ *due to spontaneous rupture of an angiomyolipoma, marked by its heterogeneous fat density* ⇨. **(Right)** *Axial CECT shows large perinephric hematoma* ⇨ *caused by spontaneous bleeding from the exophytic, hypervascular renal mass* ⇨ *which was proven to be clear cell-type renal cell carcinoma.*

Renal Angiomyolipoma

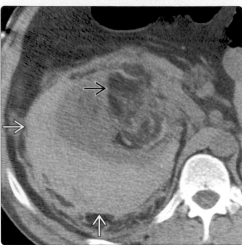

Renal Cell Carcinoma

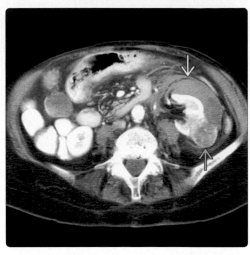

(Left) *Axial CECT shows a large perirenal hemorrhage* ⇨ *due to spontaneous bleeding in a patient receiving heparin for anticoagulation therapy.* **(Right)** *Axial CECT in this coagulopathic patient shows left perirenal hemorrhage* ⇨, *as well as bleeding into the subhepatic* ⇨ *and iliopsoas compartments. Note the hematocrit sign* ⇨ *and active extravasation* ⇨ *of blood.*

Coagulopathic Hemorrhage

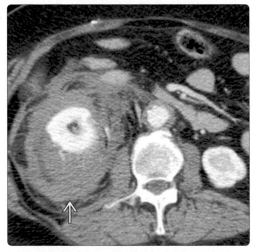

Coagulopathic Hemorrhage

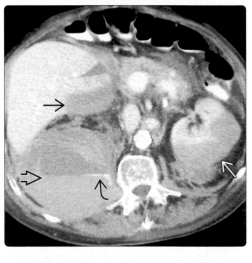

(Left) *Axial CECT shows a large abdominal aortic aneurysm (AAA)* ⇨ *with hemorrhage that dissects throughout the retroperitoneum, including the left perirenal space* ⇨. **(Right)** *Axial CECT shows the lower end of a large AAA that ruptured into the retroperitoneum with bleeding into the perirenal and other retroperitoneal spaces.*

Ruptured Abdominal Aortic Aneurysm

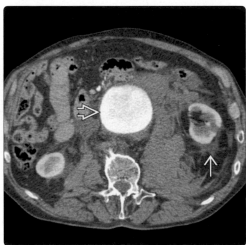

Ruptured Abdominal Aortic Aneurysm

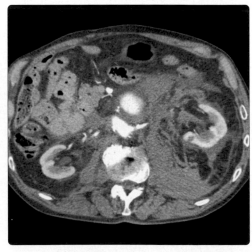

Acquired Cystic Disease of Uremia

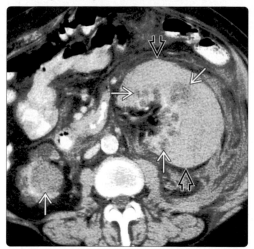

Perirenal Abscess (Mimic)

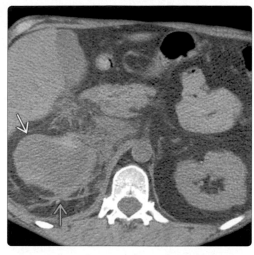

(Left) *Axial CECT in patient with history of end-stage renal disease who is on hemodialysis shows small kidneys containing innumerable cysts ➡ compatible with acquired cystic disease of uremia. Note the large left perirenal hemorrhage ⭲ due to spontaneous hemorrhage.* (Right) *Axial NECT in patient who presented with acute flank pain shows an exophytic right renal mass ➡ with extensive infiltration in the perirenal space ⭲. A repeat CECT after antibiotic therapy showed an evolving renal abscess.*

Renal Lymphoma (Mimic)

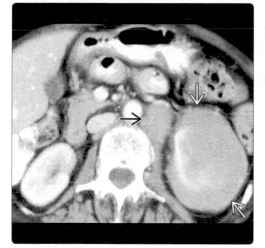

Autosomal Dominant Polycystic Kidney Disease

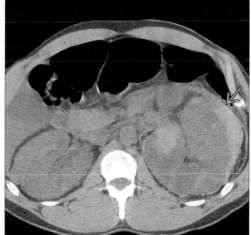

(Left) *Axial CECT shows high-density homogeneous tissue distending the perirenal space ➡ and extending into the renal sinus. The presence of similar tissue in retroperitoneal lymph nodes ⭲ helps to identify this as renal and perirenal lymphoma.* (Right) *Axial NECT in patient presenting with acute flank pain shows enlarged kidneys replaced by innumerable simple and hyperdense cysts compatible with autosomal dominant polycystic kidney disease and acute left perinephric hematoma ⭲.*

Renal Arteriovenous Malformation

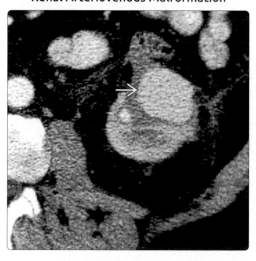

Renal Arteriovenous Malformation

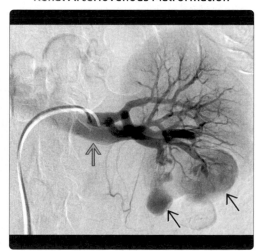

(Left) *Axial CECT shows a mass within the left kidney ➡ that is nearly isodense with blood vessels. Subsequent sonography confirmed a renal arteriovenous malformation (AVM), and this was embolized via angiographic catheterization.* (Right) *Catheter angiography shows contrast injection of the renal artery with premature opacification of the renal vein ⭲ due to large AVMs ⭲ that were subsequently embolized.*

DIFFERENTIAL DIAGNOSIS

Common

- Renal Angiomyolipoma
- Wilms Tumor

Less Common

- Fat in Renal Scar
- Renal Junction Line
- Renal Cell Carcinoma
- Retroperitoneal Liposarcoma (Mimic)
- Adrenal Myelolipoma (Mimic)
- Xanthogranulomatous Pyelonephritis (Mimic)
- Renal Lipomatosis
- Renal Oncocytoma

ESSENTIAL INFORMATION

Key Differential Diagnosis Issues

- Expansile renal mass that contains fat in adult is diagnostic of angiomyolipoma (AML), with rare exceptions
  - Suspect malignancy, not AML, when following findings are present
    - Intratumoral calcifications
    - Invasion of perirenal or sinus fat
    - Large necrotic mass with foci of fat
    - Nodal or venous invasion

Helpful Clues for Common Diagnoses

- **Renal Angiomyolipoma**
  - Most common benign renal tumor
    - Majority incidentally found
    - 90% single and unilateral; 10% bilateral and multiple, usually associated with tuberous sclerosis
  - Ultrasound
    - Well-defined hyperechoic mass
    - Up to 30% of small renal cell carcinomas (RCC) may appear hyperechoic
    - Detection of hyperechoic renal lesion requires further evaluation with CT or MR
  - NECT
    - Solid mass with macroscopic fat (< 20 HU)
    - Hemorrhage may be present in large (> 4 cm) AMLs
    - Mass will have claw sign to indicate renal parenchymal origin
  - MR
    - Heterogeneous signal intensity (components of fat, muscle, vessels)
    - Macroscopic fat
      - T1WI, T2WI: High signal intensity
      - Loss of signal on fat-suppressed (frequency selective) images
      - T1WI opposed-phase imaging: Signal loss at water-fat boundary ("India ink" artifact)
  - Minimal fat (fat-poor) AML
    - 5% of AML
    - Difficult to distinguish from RCC
    - CT: Often hyperattenuating on NECT
    - MR: Loss of signal on T1WI opposed-phase imaging
      - Clear cell RCC may also present with loss of signal on T1WI opposed-phase images

  - Small size and hypointensity on T2WI favor minimal fat AML over clear cell RCC
- **Wilms Tumor**
  - Always consider Wilms in child with fat-containing mass
  - Wilms tumor may have multiple morphologic features, including cystic, fat-containing, etc.
  - Check other imaging tests for signs of tuberous sclerosis
    - These or signs of multiple fat-containing masses in child would indicate AML

Helpful Clues for Less Common Diagnoses

- **Fat in Renal Scar**
  - Following partial nephrectomy
  - Surgeons may place perirenal fat into surgical defect to prevent leak of blood or urine
  - Appearance can be identical to AML
    - Look for surgical clips in or near defect
- **Renal Junction Line**
  - Also called junctional parenchymal defect
  - Normal variant of no clinical significance
    - Infolding of capsule and perirenal fat or outward bulging of renal sinus fat
    - Similar fat density or echogenicity as renal sinus
    - May have triangular shape
    - Often at junction of upper and middle third of kidney
- **Renal Cell Carcinoma**
  - Presence of fat in RCC is rare, and it may be related to
    - Large tumor invading and engulfing renal sinus or perirenal fat
    - Lipid-producing tumoral necrosis
    - Bone metaplasia
  - Look for other signs of RCC
    - Invasion of renal vein
    - Lymphadenopathy
    - Thoracic or osseous metastases
- **Retroperitoneal Liposarcoma (Mimic)**
  - Large liposarcoma may displace and compress kidney
  - Findings suggesting liposarcoma and not AML
    - Liposarcoma will not have claw sign
    - Liposarcoma is not vascular (few or no visible vessels on imaging)
- **Adrenal Myelolipoma (Mimic)**
  - Suprarenal; it may displace kidney
    - Absence of claw sign
- **Xanthogranulomatous Pyelonephritis (Mimic)**
  - Chronic renal infection with destruction of renal parenchyma and accumulation of lipid-laden macrophages (xanthoma cells)
    - Multiple low-attenuation renal lesions
      - Typically just below water density (but is solid, not fluid consistency)
  - Other signs of xanthogranulomatous pyelonephritis (XGP)
    - Enlarged kidney
    - Obstructing calculus, often large
    - Lack of function of obstructed part of kidney
    - Infiltration and proliferation of fat in perirenal space
    - Invasion of posterior abdominal wall (psoas, quadratus lumborum muscles)

- Clinical presentation
  - Dull flank pain, fever, palpable mass
  - More frequent in women
- **Renal Lipomatosis**
  - In response to chronic inflammation &/or obstruction
    - Renal calculi present in 70% (often staghorn)
  - Deposition of fat and inflammatory tissue in renal hilum and perirenal space
    - Analogous to "creeping," proliferating mesenteric fat in Crohn disease
    - Response to chronic inflammation
  - Outer contours and volume of kidney may be normal, decreased, or even increased
    - Functioning renal tissue is decreased or even absent
  - Some degree of renal sinus lipomatosis is considered normal in elderly and obese patients
    - Usually no clinical relevance in this setting
  - In advanced stages, very similar to XGP
    - Both may have infection, sinus tracts, or fistulas
    - Only replacement fibrolipomatosis has true fat

- XGP: Lipid-laden macrophages infiltrate renal parenchyma (interstitium)
- Lipomatosis: True fat and macrophages in renal sinus and perirenal space, adjacent to parenchyma
- **Renal Oncocytoma**
  - Rarely contains fat; would be indistinguishable from AML on imaging

Renal Angiomyolipoma

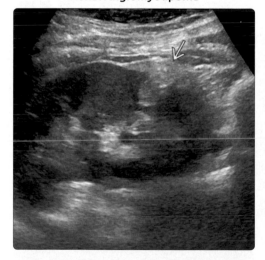

Renal Angiomyolipoma

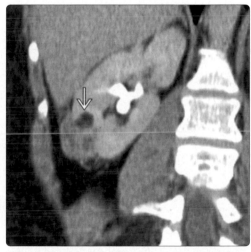

(Left) *Longitudinal ultrasound through the lower pole of the right kidney shows a hyperechoic and partially exophytic lesion ➡. The detection of a hyperechoic lesion on ultrasound requires further investigation with contrast-enhanced CT or MR because up to 30% of small renal cell carcinomas may appear as hyperechoic.* **(Right)** *Coronal CECT of the right kidney in the same patient confirms the presence of macroscopic fat ➡ within the lesion in keeping with diagnosis of angiomyolipoma (AML).*

Renal Angiomyolipoma

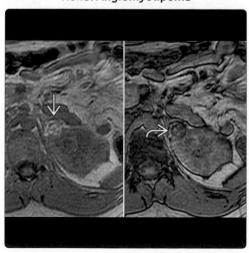

Renal Angiomyolipoma

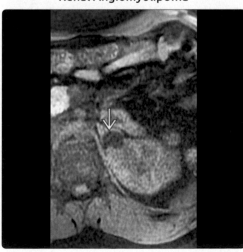

(Left) *Axial T1WI in-phase (left) and opposed-phase (right) in a 25-year-old woman with history of tuberous sclerosis show a left renal AML. The AML appears hyperintense ➡ on the in-phase T1WI and shows a hypointense border ("India ink") ➡ on the opposed-phase T1WI.* **(Right)** *Axial fat-suppressed T1WI in the same patient shows the AML as hypointense ➡ given the presence of macroscopic fat within the lesion.*

(Left) *Axial NECT shows a small focus of fat ➡ within a larger mass ⇒ that is slightly hyperdense to the kidney on this NECT. Minimal fat (fat-poor) AMLs are often hyperdense to the kidney on NECT.* (Right) *Axial NECT shows extensive perirenal hemorrhage ➡ and a fat-containing AML ➡ that was the source of bleeding. Note the prominent blood vessels within the AML.*

Renal Angiomyolipoma

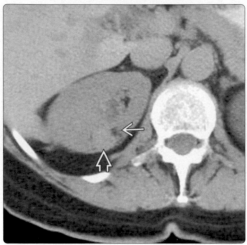

Renal Angiomyolipoma

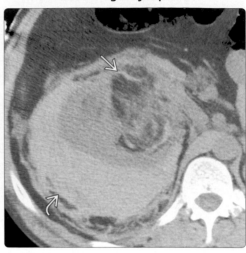

(Left) *Axial CECT shows a large heterogeneous fat density mass ➡ arising from the kidney. The prominent vascularity ➡ helps to identify it as an AML, rather than a retroperitoneal liposarcoma.* (Right) *Sagittal CECT shows a large heterogeneous fat density mass ➡ with a subtle claw sign ⇒, identifying it as an AML of renal origin.*

Renal Angiomyolipoma

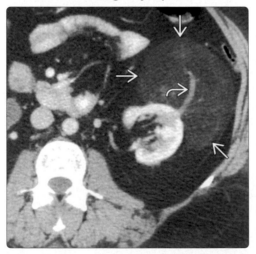

Renal Angiomyolipoma

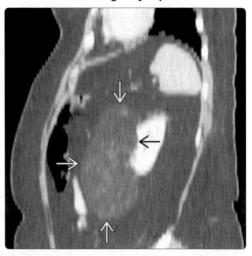

(Left) *Axial CECT shows a small focus of fat ➡ that was placed in the kidney at the site of resection of a small renal carcinoma. Note the surgical clips ➡.* (Right) *Sagittal ultrasound shows an echogenic focus ➡ in the renal cortex at the junction of the upper and middle thirds of the right kidney. This is contiguous with and of similar appearance to the renal sinus fat ➡, an appearance compatible with a renal junction line.*

Fat in Renal Scar

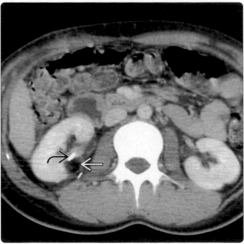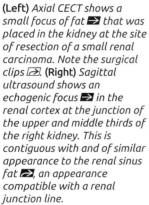

Renal Junction Line

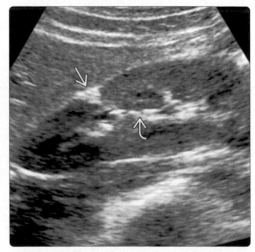

Renal Cell Carcinoma

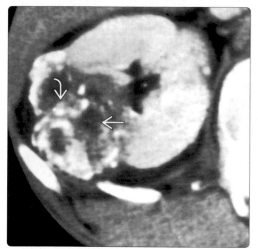

Retroperitoneal Liposarcoma (Mimic)

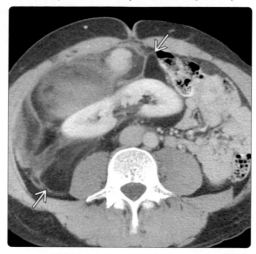

(Left) *Axial CECT shows a complex renal mass with foci of calcification ➘ and other areas that are less than water attenuation ➙. Lipid-producing necrosis or osseous metaplasia may account for the fat/calcification that rarely occurs within renal cell carcinoma.* (Right) *Axial CECT shows displacement and deformation of the kidney by a mass ➘ that has mixed fat and soft tissue density. The absence of a claw sign helps to identify this as a primary retroperitoneal liposarcoma rather than an AML.*

Adrenal Myelolipoma (Mimic)

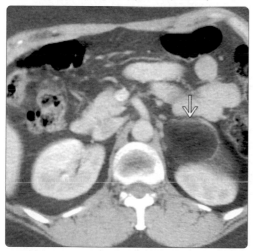

Xanthogranulomatous Pyelonephritis (Mimic)

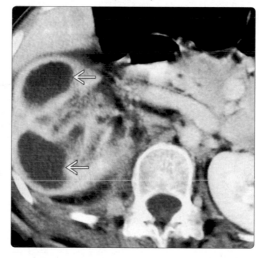

(Left) *Axial CECT shows a predominantly fat density left suprarenal mass ➘ compatible with an adrenal myelolipoma. The absence of a claw sign helps to exclude a renal origin of the mass.* (Right) *Axial CECT shows a deformed, nonfunctional right kidney with a large obstructing staghorn calculous (lower section). The low-density xanthomatous debris ➘ might be mistaken for a fat density AML.*

Renal Lipomatosis

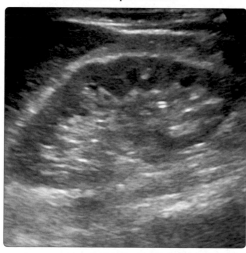

Renal Lipomatosis

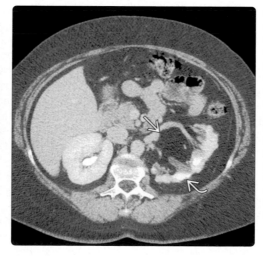

(Left) *Longitudinal ultrasound of the right kidney of a diabetic male patient with renal insufficiency shows proliferation of sinus fat, an appearance compatible with renal sinus lipomatosis.* (Right) *Axial CECT in a patient with renal replacement lipomatosis shows expansion of the left renal hilum with fibrolipomatous tissue ➘ and dilated calices ➘ with urine-contrast levels. Findings were due to a chronically obstructing left renal pelvis calculus.*

DIFFERENTIAL DIAGNOSIS

Common

- Urolithiasis (Renal Calculi)
- Renal Artery Calcification
- Nephrocalcinosis
- Medullary Sponge Kidney

Less Common

- Renal Cyst
- Autosomal Dominant Polycystic Disease, Kidney
- AIDS, Opportunistic Infection
- Renal Papillary Necrosis
- Calyceal Diverticulum
- Chronic Glomerulonephritis
- Chronic Pyelonephritis
- Renal Cell Carcinoma
- Transitional Cell Carcinoma
- Renal Tuberculosis

ESSENTIAL INFORMATION

Key Differential Diagnosis Issues

- Size, shape, number, and distribution of calcifications are important
- Association with soft tissue mass is important

Helpful Clues for Common Diagnoses

- **Urolithiasis (Renal Calculi)**
  - Often small, multiple
  - All renal calculi are opaque on CT except for indinavir-induced stones (in patients with HIV/AIDS)
  - Renal calculi may not cause signs of obstruction but may cause symptoms including hematuria and intermittent flank pain
    - Pain may be due to intermittent obstruction at ureteropelvic junction
- **Renal Artery Calcification**
  - Linear, parallel, branching pattern
    - Pattern depends on whether CT section is along long or short axis of vessel
  - Eggshell, curvilinear = renal artery aneurysm
  - Lumen enhancement variable
    - May enhance completely, partially, or not at all
- **Nephrocalcinosis**
  - May be either cortical or medullary
  - Cortical nephrocalcinosis
    - Causes
      □ Acute cortical necrosis
      □ Alport syndrome
      □ Oxalosis
      □ Chronic glomerulonephritis
      □ Sickle cell disease
    - Small kidneys with irregular cortical calcification
    - Often impaired renal function
  - Medullary nephrocalcinosis
    - Causes
      □ Hyperparathyroidism (40%)
      □ Renal tubular acidosis type 1 (20%)
      □ Medullary sponge kidney (20%)
    - Punctate calcifications localized to renal pyramids

- May also have calculi within collecting system
- Kidneys usually have normal size and function
- **Medullary Sponge Kidney**
  - Multiple tiny calculi within dilated tubules in papillae &/or calices
  - Generally bilateral but may be unilateral or asymmetric
  - Dilated tubules are best seen in pyelographic phase (either excretory or CT urography)
  - Renal pyramids appear hyperechoic on ultrasound
    - Tiny calculi may not cause posterior acoustic shadowing

Helpful Clues for Less Common Diagnoses

- **Renal Cyst**
  - Usually curvilinear or eggshell calcification, rather than small, punctate calcification
  - 1-2% of benign cysts have peripheral calcifications
    - CECT important to rule out cystic renal cell carcinoma
    - Look for areas of enhancement or nodularity within wall
  - Hyperdense cyst may be greater than renal attenuation, but rarely of calcific density
- **Autosomal Dominant Polycystic Disease, Kidney**
  - Usually curvilinear or eggshell calcification of cyst walls
    - Generally occurs after prior intracyst bleeding
  - Typically multiple cysts of varying size
  - Kidneys may become grossly enlarged
  - Patients often have end-stage renal disease
    - Heavy arterial atherosclerosis is another source of intrarenal calcification
  - May develop renal calculi
    - May be source of pain and acute renal dysfunction
- **AIDS, Opportunistic Infection**
  - Multiple causative organisms
    - Pneumocystis carinii
    - Mycobacterial infection
    - Cytomegalovirus
  - Often multiple, small, cortical calcifications
  - This represents healed phase of disease
    - During active infection, foci are hypodense to renal parenchyma (definitely on CECT, possibly on NECT)
- **Renal Papillary Necrosis**
  - Curvilinear, ring-shaped, or triangular calcifications in sloughed papillae
  - Calcifications arranged in arc conforming to position of papillary tips
  - Associated with clubbed and irregular calices
  - Often encountered in patients with history of chronic analgesic use/abuse
- **Calyceal Diverticulum**
  - Usually 1-3 cm in diameter
  - May be filled with milk of calcium or small stones
  - Contrast fills diverticulum on delayed images (either CT or urography)
- **Chronic Glomerulonephritis and Pyelonephritis**
  - Small scarred kidneys ± small focal calcifications
  - Chronic pyelonephritis is often associated with cystourethral reflux
  - May be unilateral or bilateral
- **Renal Cell Carcinoma**

- Foci of calcification in ~ 10%
  - Amorphous central calcification (most common)
  - Curvilinear (peripheral or central)
  - Dense or diffuse calcification
  - Osseous metaplasia may occur in large tumor
- If renal mass in adult patient has both calcification and fat density, it is probably renal cell carcinoma, not angiomyolipoma (AML)
  - In child with similar findings, it is probably Wilms tumor, not AML
- **Transitional Cell Carcinoma**
  - Small flecks of calcium within soft tissue mass in renal pelvis or parenchyma
  - On NECT, transitional cell carcinoma is often hyperdense to renal parenchyma, but not due to calcification
- **Renal Tuberculosis**
  - Calcifications common and variable in appearance
    - Punctate (healed granulomata) to diffuse
  - Amorphous calcification within atrophic kidney most common presentation

  - Often associated with low-density or cavitary lesions within kidney
  - Can progress to putty kidney (heavily calcified caseous mass replacing renal parenchyma)
- May see calcified sloughed papillae from papillary necrosis

SELECTED REFERENCES

1. Fabris A et al: Medullary sponge kidney: state of the art. Nephrol Dial Transplant. 28(5):1111-9, 2013
2. Eisner BH et al: Nephrolithiasis: what surgeons need to know. AJR Am J Roentgenol. 196(6):1274-8, 2011
3. Katabathina VS et al: Adult renal cystic disease: a genetic, biological, and developmental primer. Radiographics. 30(6):1509-23, 2010
4. Dyer RB et al: Abnormal calcifications in the urinary tract. Radiographics. 18(6):1405-24, 1998

Urolithiasis (Renal Calculi)

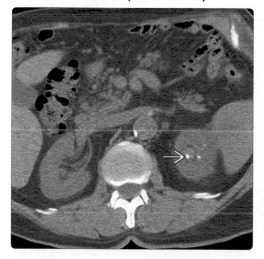

Urolithiasis (Renal Calculi)

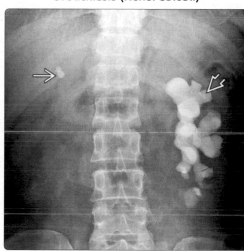

(Left) *Axial NECT shows small stones* ➡️ *in the left kidney, without evidence of ureteral obstruction.* (Right) *Anteroposterior radiograph shows a small opaque stone in the upper pole of the right kidney* ➡️ *and a staghorn calculus* ➡️ *in the left (conforming to the collecting system).*

Renal Artery Calcification

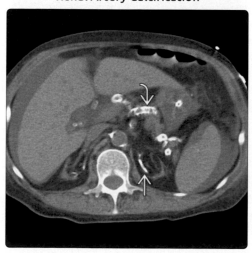

Nephrocalcinosis

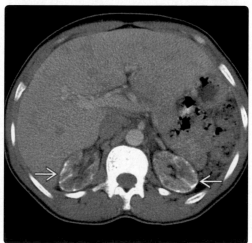

(Left) *Axial NECT shows extensive arterial calcification in this patient with diabetes, including the splenic* ➡️ *and renal* ➡️ *arteries. Note end-stage renal failure.* (Right) *Axial NECT through the kidneys shows calcifications in the renal cortex* ➡️ *in this patient with sickle cell anemia and cortical nephrocalcinosis.*

Nephrocalcinosis

Nephrocalcinosis

(Left) *Longitudinal ultrasound of the left kidney shows echogenic and shadowing medullae* ➡ *compatible with medullary nephrocalcinosis.* (Right) *Coronal NECT in the same patient shows calcifications distributed in the medullae of both kidneys, compatible with medullary nephrocalcinosis.*

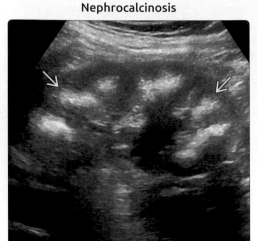

Nephrocalcinosis

Medullary Sponge Kidney

(Left) *Anteroposterior radiograph shows medullary nephrocalcinosis, with the calcifications* ➡ *located deep within the kidney, rather than in the cortex.* (Right) *Anteroposterior radiograph shows multiple renal calculi* ➡ *in a patient with medullary sponge kidney (renal tubular ectasia).*

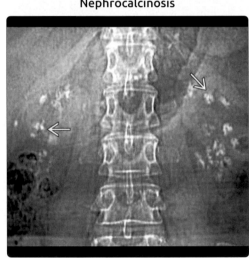
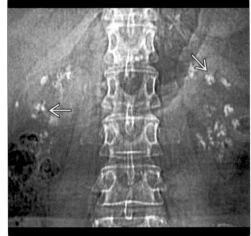

Medullary Sponge Kidney

Autosomal Dominant Polycystic Disease, Kidney

(Left) *Axial NECT shows innumerable tiny calculi,* ➡ *located within the renal pyramids. These were obscured within the opacified tubules on pyelographic-phase CECT.* (Right) *Axial NECT shows enlarged polycystic kidneys in a patient on dialysis for end-stage renal disease. Note calcifications in one of the cyst walls* ➡ *and in renal arteries* ➡.

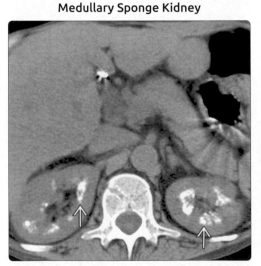
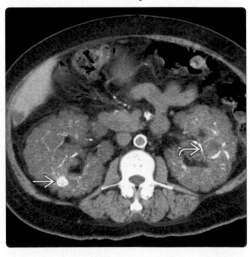

AIDS, Opportunistic Infection

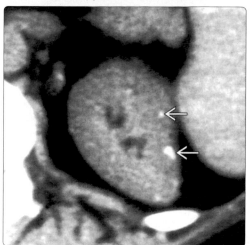

Renal Papillary Necrosis

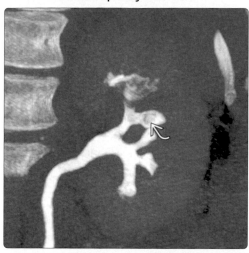

(Left) Axial NECT shows multiple punctate calcifications ➡ in the left kidney in a patient with extrapulmonary Pneumocystis carinii infection. Other opportunistic renal infections (mycobacterial, fungal, etc.) may have a similar appearance. (Right) Coronal CECT shows a sloughed papilla ➡ within a deformed calyx. Amorphous debris is present within the upper pole calices, and all calices are clubbed. The sloughed papillae may calcify.

Calyceal Diverticulum

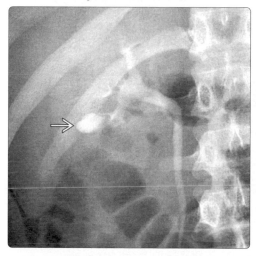

Chronic Pyelonephritis

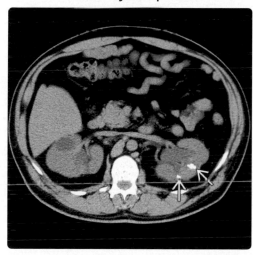

(Left) Anteroposterior IVP shows a typical calyceal diverticulum ➡ that was filled with small calculi or milk of calcium on the plain radiograph and NECT. (Right) Axial NECT shows focal calcifications ➡ in the left kidney with atrophy of the overlying cortex, characteristic findings of chronic pyelonephritis due to reflux. The calices are also dilated in this patient who was born with extrophy of the bladder, repaired in infancy.

Renal Cell Carcinoma

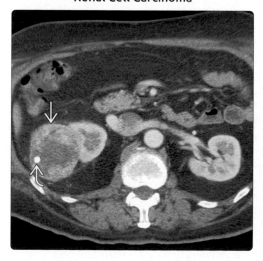

Renal Tuberculosis

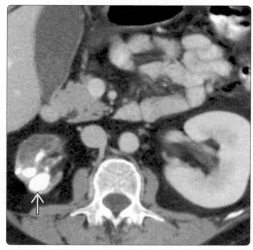

(Left) Axial CECT shows a heterogeneous, enhancing, exophytic right renal mass ➡, with a focus of calcification ➡. (Right) Axial CECT shows a small, nonfunctional, right kidney with focal, but amorphous, calcification ➡ of the parenchyma.

DIFFERENTIAL DIAGNOSIS

Common

- Urolithiasis
- Renal Sinus Cysts
- Renal Sinus Lipomatosis
  - Renal Replacement Lipomatosis
- Renal Trauma
- Urothelial Carcinoma
- Vascular Lesions
  - Renal Artery Aneurysm/Pseudoaneurysm
  - Arteriovenous Malformation
  - Renal Hilar Varices
- Coagulopathic Hemorrhage

Less Common

- Xanthogranulomatous Pyelonephritis
- Lymphoma
- Other Renal Tumors
  - Multilocular Cystic Nephroma
  - Renal Cell Carcinoma
  - Squamous Cell Carcinoma
  - Mesenchymal Renal Tumors
  - Neurogenic Tumors
- Fungal Infection

ESSENTIAL INFORMATION

Key Differential Diagnosis Issues

- Renal sinus is extension of perirenal space
  - Contains multiple structures, any one of which can give rise to mass lesion
    - Pelvocalyceal system (e.g., urothelial carcinoma, blood clot, fungus ball, stone)
    - Vessels [e.g., renal artery aneurysm, arteriovenous malformation (AVM), varices]
    - Lymphatics (e.g., lymphoma, lymph node metastases)
    - Nerves (e.g., neurogenic tumor)
  - CT, MR, and US easily distinguish many lesions that have similar appearance on IV urography
  - Urography or pyelography may still be best means of studying lesions within renal pelvis (such as urothelial cancer)

Helpful Clues for Common Diagnoses

- **Urolithiasis**
  - Most calculi are very dense and easily detectable on CT
    - Rare drug-induced calculi (such as ones induced by Indinavir, ciprofloxacin, sulfa medications, triamterene, etc.) and matrix calculi may be radiolucent on CT
  - Uric acid and xanthine stones are lucent on radiography
    - May appear as lucent filling defects within contrast-opacified renal pelvis on urography
- **Renal Sinus Cysts**
  - Peripelvic
    - Multiple confluent, noncommunicating cysts originating from lymphatics
    - Often bilateral and multiple
    - Surround and compress calices, displace blood vessels

- Easily confused with hydronephrosis on US and NECT
- Contrast-enhanced CT/MR during excretory phase helps to differentiate from hydronephrosis
  - Parapelvic
    - Renal cyst protruding into renal sinus fat
    - Usually solitary, unilateral, and spherical
    - Often found with other simple cortical cysts
- **Renal Sinus Lipomatosis**
  - Proliferation of renal sinus fat; usually age related but can be seen in obesity and with hypersteroidism
  - Increases gradually with aging, obesity, and loss of parenchyma due to disease
  - **Renal replacement lipomatosis**
    - Extreme proliferation of renal sinus fat replacing renal parenchyma
    - Sequela of severe atrophy or inflammation, usually due to chronic obstruction
    - Proliferation of fibrofatty tissue may expand renal sinus
      - May displace calyces, vessels in hilum
    - Some degree of renal sinus fibrolipomatosis is found in all causes of renal parenchymal atrophy
- **Renal Trauma**
  - Seen in setting of penetrating and high-impact blunt types of injuries
    - Consider iatrogenic trauma as well (e.g., extracorporeal or percutaneous lithotripsy)
  - May result in clot in renal pelvis, renal hilar hematoma, or urinoma
    - Excretory-phase CECT helps to detect urinary injury and urinoma
- **Urothelial Carcinoma**
  - Irregular filling defect in renal pelvis/calyx ± infiltration of renal parenchyma
    - Low-grade (superficial, sessile/polypoid) and invasive types
  - Often isodense to slightly hyperdense on NECT
  - Variable enhancement pattern depending on grade and growth pattern
    - Enhances moderately with IV contrast administration
    - May amputate (prevents filling of) calyces on IVU
  - Difficult to distinguish from squamous cell or mesenchymal tumors of renal pelvis
  - Higher incidence in patients who have had urothelial cancer of bladder or ureter previously
- **Vascular Lesions**
  - Renal artery aneurysm/pseudoaneurysm, AVM, arteriovenous fistula (AVF), renal varices
    - Aneurysm: Look for calcification in arterial wall
    - Pseudoaneurysm and dissection usually occur in setting of trauma
      - May be seen with vasculitides and spontaneous arterial mediolysis
    - AVM/AVF
      - Look for turbulent flow on color Doppler US, premature filling of renal vein on CECT and angiography
      - AVF is usually sequela of trauma or iatrogenic injury (biopsy)

– Renal varices: Seen in patients with cirrhosis and portal hypertension

- **Coagulopathic Hemorrhage**
  o Spontaneous coagulopathic bleeding may rarely be limited to renal pelvis
  o Blood will have attenuation of 45-65 HU on NECT; no enhancement
  o Follow-up imaging is required to document resolution and to exclude underlying mass lesion

Helpful Clues for Less Common Diagnoses

- **Xanthogranulomatous Pyelonephritis**
  o Low-density fluid-filled areas in affected parenchyma (lipid-laden macrophages)
  o Kidney, or affected portion, is usually nonfunctional and obstructed by large staghorn calculous
  o Overlapping features with renal replacement fibrolipomatosis

- **Lymphoma**
  o Infiltration of renal sinus ± renal parenchyma with preservation of renal shape
  o Homogeneous, showing mild enhancement (10-20 HU)
  o May simulate urothelial cancer, although latter is usually more heterogeneous and poorly circumscribed
  o Presence of regional hilar and retroperitoneal lymphadenopathy, bilaterality, and extension to perirenal space are helpful clues
  o Lymphoid hyperplasia
    – Extremely rare entity, a.k.a. pseudolymphoma, presenting as nonspecific soft tissue

- **Other Renal Tumors**
  o **Multilocular cystic nephroma**
    – Encapsulated multiseptate cystic mass in young boy or middle-aged woman
    – Arises in cortex but usually herniates into and distorts renal sinus
    – Differentiation from cystic renal cell carcinoma (RCC) may be difficult
      □ Latter has enhancing nodule and seen in different population (older male patient)

  o **Renal cell carcinoma**
    – Arises in cortex but may extend into renal sinus
    – More vascular and exophytic than urothelial cancer
      □ Papillary type is hypovascular
    – May invade renal vein and inferior vena cava
  o **Rare renal tumors**
    – Have overlapping features with RCC, lymphoma, and urothelial cancer
    – Usually cannot be diagnosed confidently by imaging alone
    – Primary renal sarcoma: Rare; patients often develop metastasis before initial presentation
      □ Usually large (> 10 cm) when discovered
      □ Imaging findings are variable
    – Renal sinus plasmacytoma: Rare tumor seen in patients with history of plasma cell dyscrasia
      □ Well circumscribed or infiltrative solitary lesion; imaging features similar to lymphoma and urothelial cancer
    – Renal sinus angiomyolipoma: Ones composed mainly of fat may blend with renal sinus fat or may mimic lipomatosis

- **Fungal Infections**
  o Usually in debilitated patients
  o May form fungus ball in renal pelvis
  o Diagnosis made by obtaining tissue and culture from urine and urothelium

SELECTED REFERENCES

1. Nikolaidis P et al: Computed tomography and magnetic resonance imaging features of lesions of the renal medulla and sinus. Curr Probl Diagn Radiol. 37(6):262-78, 2008
2. Sheth S et al: Imaging of renal lymphoma: patterns of disease with pathologic correlation. Radiographics. 26(4):1151-68, 2006
3. Rha SE et al: The renal sinus: pathologic spectrum and multimodality imaging approach. Radiographics. 24 Suppl 1:S117-31. Review, 2004
4. Pickhardt PJ et al: From the archives of the AFIP. Infiltrative renal lesions: radiologic-pathologic correlation. Armed Forces Institute of Pathology. Radiographics. 20(1):215-43, 2000
5. Amis ES Jr et al: The renal sinus: an imaging review and proposed nomenclature for sinus cysts. J Urol. 139(6):1151-9, 1988

Renal Sinus Cysts

Renal Sinus Cysts

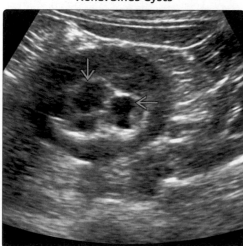

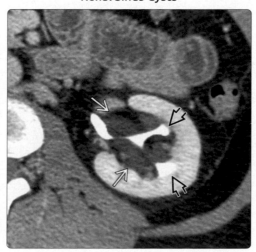

(Left) *Transverse ultrasound of the left kidney shows cystic dilatation in the renal pelvis* ⇒. *The ureter was not however dilated.* (Right) *Axial CECT obtained during the excretory phase in the same patient demonstrates peripelvic cysts* ⇒ *displacing the enhanced renal collecting system* ⇒. *Excretory phase of contrast-enhanced CT or MR helps in differentiating cysts from hydronephrosis.*

Renal Sinus Lipomatosis

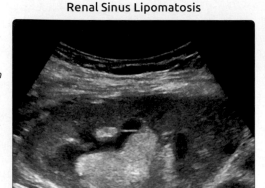

Renal Sinus Lipomatosis

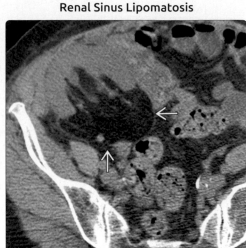

(Left) *Longitudinal US image through renal allograft, in 74-year-old woman with history of renal transplantation 15 years earlier, shows expansion of renal sinus fat with mild displacement of renal calyces.* (Right) *Unenhanced axial CT through renal allograft, in 74-year-old woman, shows renal sinus lipomatosis ➡ with marked expansion of renal sinus.*

Renal Sinus Lipomatosis

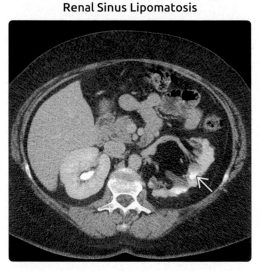

Renal Trauma

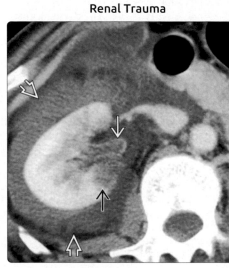

(Left) *Axial CECT shows mass-like expansion of the left renal sinus with fibrolipomatous tissue and dilated calices ➡ due to a chronic partial obstruction of the left ureteropelvic junction by calculi.* (Right) *Axial CECT shows a renal parenchymal laceration ➡ from blunt trauma. Note perirenal hemorrhage ➡ and clot in the renal pelvis ➡.*

Urothelial Carcinoma

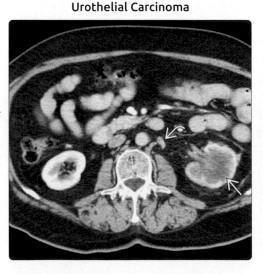

Urothelial Carcinoma

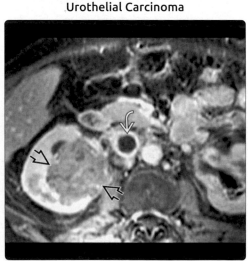

(Left) *Axial CECT shows infiltration of the renal parenchyma ➡ by an aggressive transitional cell carcinoma (TCC) from an inferior pole calyx that was amputated on pyelographic-phase images. Renal contour is preserved. Nodal metastases ➡ were better shown on adjacent images.* (Right) *Axial T1 C+ FS MR shows a tumor arising from the renal pelvis ➡ and infiltrating the renal parenchyma, without altering the renal contour. Note the thrombus in the inferior vena cava (IVC) ➡.*

Urothelial Carcinoma

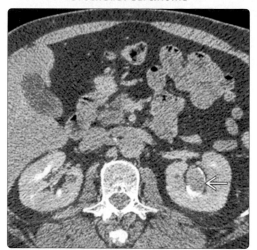

Urothelial Carcinoma

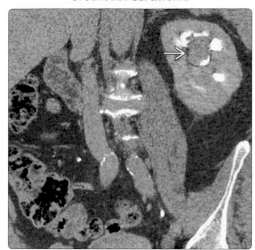

(Left) *Axial CECT shows a soft tissue density filling defect ➡ within an upper pole infundibulum on this excretory (pyelographic) phase CECT.* **(Right)** *Coronal CECT in the same patient shows the polypoid mass ➡ within the upper pole infundibulum. The patient had a history of remote bladder cancer.*

Urothelial Carcinoma

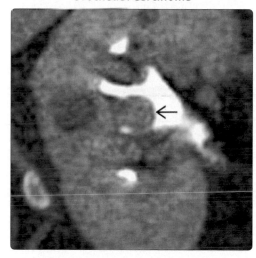

Arteriovenous Malformation

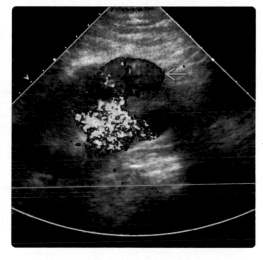

(Left) *Coronal CECT, obtained during excretory phase, shows amputation and distortion of calices and a filling defect ➡ in the renal pelvis compatible with urothelial carcinoma.* **(Right)** *Color Doppler ultrasound shows classic color aliasing and swirling within a renal hilar AVM ➡ in a 59-year-old man.*

Arteriovenous Malformation

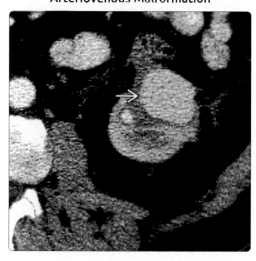

Arteriovenous Malformation

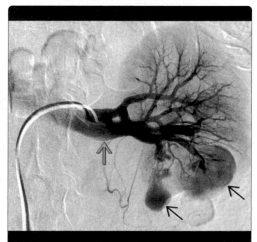

(Left) *Axial CECT shows a spherical mass ➡ that is isodense to blood vessels and represents an arteriovenous malformation, which was further confirmed on Doppler US, in this 59-year-old man.* **(Right)** *Frontal catheter angiography in the same patient shows large arteriovenous malformations ➡ with early filling of the left renal vein ➡.*

Renal Hilar Varices

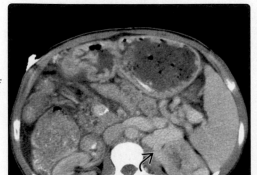

Coagulopathic Hemorrhage

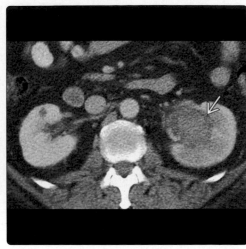

(Left) *Axial CECT shows large varices ⇨ near the left renal hilum and a spontaneous splenorenal shunt in this patient with cirrhosis and portal hypertension.* **(Right)** *Axial CECT shows distention of the left renal pelvis with blood ⇨. The patient was receiving heparin therapy and had spontaneous renal bleeding.*

Xanthogranulomatous Pyelonephritis

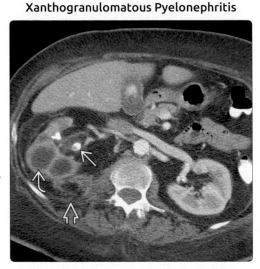

Lymphoma

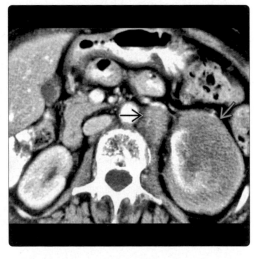

(Left) *Axial CECT shows decreased function or nonfunction of the right kidney with low-density material ⇨ representing destroyed parenchyma filled with lipid-laden macrophages. Note the obstructing renal calculi ⇨ and inflammation extending into the perirenal space ⇨.* **(Right)** *Axial CECT shows ill-defined tumor ⇨ infiltrating the perirenal space and extending into the renal sinus and renal parenchyma. An adjacent retroperitoneal node ⇨ is enlarged. Pathology revealed non-Hodgkin lymphoma.*

Lymphoma

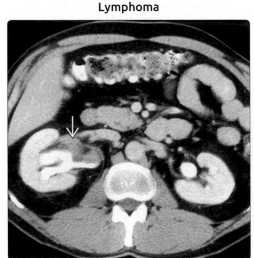

Lymphoma

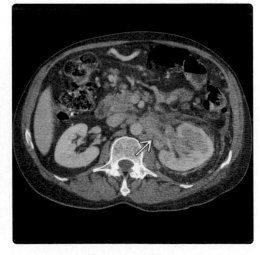

(Left) *Axial CECT shows a soft tissue density mass ⇨ arising from the renal pelvis; a rare case of lymphoma of the ureteropelvic junction, this is indistinguishable from TCC.* **(Right)** *Axial CECT shows extensive retroperitoneal lymphadenopathy, including the renal hilum ⇨, resulting in partial obstruction of the right ureter and a delayed nephrogram.*

Multilocular Cystic Nephroma

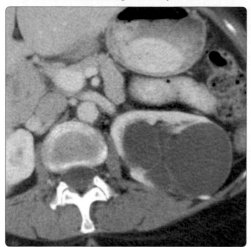

Multilocular Cystic Nephroma

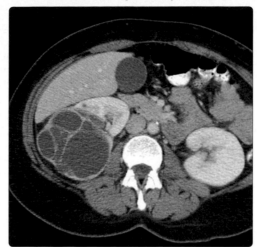

(Left) *Axial CECT shows a multiseptate renal mass that herniates into the renal sinus.* (Right) *Axial CECT shows a multiseptate mass that invaginates the renal sinus, a classic multilocular cystic nephroma in a 48-year-old woman.*

Renal Cell Carcinoma

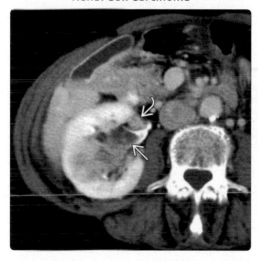

Renal Cell Carcinoma

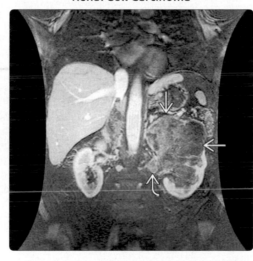

(Left) *Axial CECT of a 77-year-old woman shows the renal parenchymal tumor extending directly into the renal pelvis ➡. Also note adenopathy ➡ in the renal hilum.* (Right) *Coronal T1 C+ MR shows a large infiltrative and exophytic mass ➡ that invades the renal sinus ➡, filling both the renal pelvis and the renal vein.*

Mesenchymal Renal Tumors

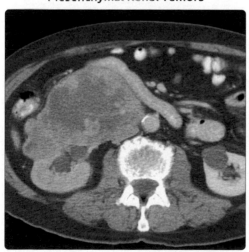

Neurogenic Tumors

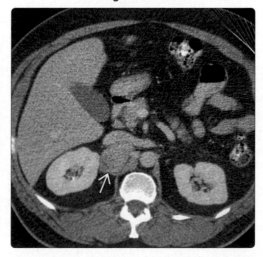

(Left) *Axial CECT shows a large heterogeneous mass arising from the right kidney. The renal pelvis is dilated due to extrinsic invasion of the proximal ureter; this is leiomyosarcoma of the kidney.* (Right) *Axial CECT shows a soft tissue density mass ➡ near the right renal hilum that displaces the IVC and renal vein; this is ganglioneuroma in a 50-year-old man. Neurogenic tumors commonly arise along the retroperitoneal path of the sympathetic ganglia.*

DIFFERENTIAL DIAGNOSIS

Common

- Emphysematous Pyelonephritis
- Renal Abscess
- Emphysematous Pyelitis
- Renal Infarction
- Instrumentation
- Postoperative State, Kidney

Less Common

- Extrarenal Sources
  - Duodenum: Ulcer; perforation; laceration
  - Pancreas: Infected necrotizing fluid collections
  - Barotrauma
- Pyonephrosis
- Xanthogranulomatous Pyelonephritis

ESSENTIAL INFORMATION

Key Differential Diagnosis Issues

- Always check for recent instrumentation, surgery, angiography for iatrogenic cause

Helpful Clues for Common Diagnoses

- **Emphysematous Pyelonephritis**
  - Necrotizing, gas-forming renal infection
    - Risk factors: Diabetes; urinary tract obstruction
  - CT: Gas in renal parenchyma
    - ± extension of gas into perirenal and pararenal space
    - ± renal or perirenal abscess
  - Ultrasound: Echogenic foci in the nondependent portion of renal parenchyma associated with "dirty shadowing"
  - Prognosis/treatment: Life-threatening infection that may require nephrectomy
- **Renal Abscess**
  - Gas within spherical collection of pus
  - CECT: Thick wall and rim-enhancing low-attenuation collection within kidney ± extension into perirenal space
  - Treatment: Usually antibiotics and percutaneous catheter drainage

- **Emphysematous Pyelitis**
  - Gas from infection of urine; limited to bladder, ureters, renal collecting system
    - No gas in renal parenchyma
  - Prognosis/treatment: Better prognosis than emphysematous pyelonephritis; usually managed with antibiotics
- **Renal Infarction**
  - Sudden death of renal tissue from arterial occlusion or avulsion can release intracellular gas from infarcted tissue
    - Examples: Traumatic renal artery occlusion; renal artery embolization; radiofrequency or cryoablation
  - Does not imply infection, but clinical symptoms are similar
- **Instrumentation**
  - Ureteral stent, nephrostomy, cystoscopy
  - Often introduces air into collecting system, ureters

Helpful Clues for Less Common Diagnoses

- **Extrarenal Sources**
  - Retroperitoneal gas from duodenum or pancreas can extend to para- and perirenal space, preferably on right
  - Duodenum: Ulcer; perforation; laceration
  - Pancreas: Infected necrotizing pancreatic or peripancreatic collections
  - Barotrauma
- **Pyonephrosis**
  - Infected, obstructed, and dilated renal collecting system
  - Dilated renal collecting system
    - Fluid attenuation may be higher than water for presence of debris/pus
    - ± gas

(Left) Sagittal ultrasound of the right kidney in a patient with emphysematous pyelonephritis shows the intraparenchymal gas ➡ as nondependent echoes associated with "dirty shadowing" ⇨. (Right) Axial NECT through the right kidney in the same patient confirms the presence of intraparenchymal gas ➡. Emphysematous pyelonephritis is a life-threatening infection with overall mortality ranging from 11-50%.

Emphysematous Pyelonephritis

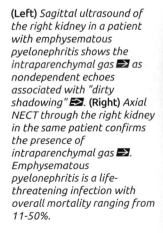
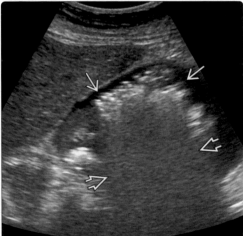

Emphysematous Pyelonephritis

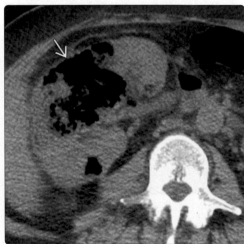

Renal Abscess

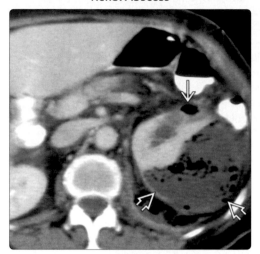

Emphysematous Pyelitis

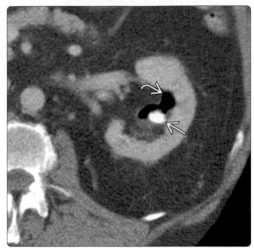

(Left) *Axial CECT shows gas* ➡ *and fluid within the kidney and a large perirenal fluid and gas collection* ➡ *compatible with abscess.* (Right) *Axial CECT shows gas* ➡ *and a calculous* ➡ *in the renal pelvis but no gas in the renal parenchyma. The infection cleared with removal of the stone and antibiotic therapy.*

Renal Infarction

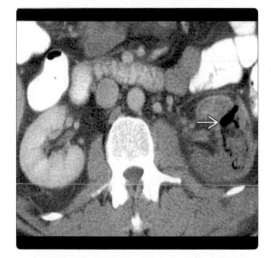

Instrumentation

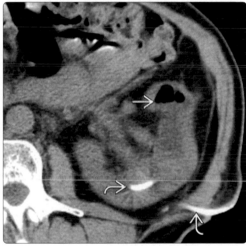

(Left) *Axial CECT shows a lack of enhancement of the left kidney and parenchymal gas* ➡. *Infarction followed attempted partial nephrectomy, complicated by renal arterial occlusion.* (Right) *Axial NECT shows a percutaneous nephrostomy catheter* ➡ *that had been placed to decompress an obstructed kidney. Gas within the nondependent calices* ➡ *is due to the catheter, not infection or infarction.*

Postoperative State, Kidney

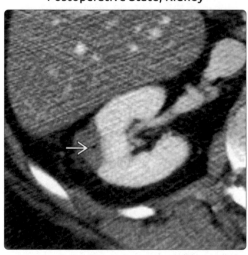

Extrarenal Sources

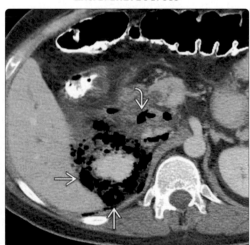

(Left) *Axial CECT shows a small bubble of gas* ➡ *within a necrotic renal mass as the result of percutaneous cryoablation therapy for a small renal cell carcinoma. There was no infection.* (Right) *Axial CECT shows gas in the right pararenal and perirenal space* ➡ *originating from a perforated ulcer* ➡ *in the second portion of the duodenum.*

DIFFERENTIAL DIAGNOSIS

Common

- Urinary Obstruction
  - Obstructing Calculus
  - Obstructing Tumor
    - Urothelial Carcinoma
    - Transitional Cell Carcinoma
    - Renal Cell Carcinoma
    - Retroperitoneal Metastases
    - Colorectal Carcinoma
    - Pelvic Malignancies
    - Retroperitoneal Lymphoma
  - Obstructing Clot
  - Ureteral Stricture
  - Retroperitoneal Fibrosis
- Renal Artery Stenosis
- Renal Vein Stenosis/Thrombosis
- Acute Tubular Necrosis
- Contrast-Induced Nephropathy
- Hypotension
- Pyelonephritis

Less Common

- Multiple Myeloma
- Rhabdomyolysis
- Leukemia
- Renal Papillary Necrosis

ESSENTIAL INFORMATION

Key Differential Diagnosis Issues

- Definition: Nephrogram that persists for > 30 min or becomes more dense after 5 min, following IV or intraarterial contrast administration
- Pathophysiology: (1) impaired renal perfusion; (2) impaired urine excretion and tubular transit
  - Slow inflow
    - Renal arterial stenosis (RAS), hypotension, ↓ tissue compliance (hydronephrosis, pyelonephritis, acute tubular necrosis, rejection)
  - Slow outflow
    - Renal vein thrombosis, renal vein obstruction
  - Slow urinary excretion/clearance
    - Urinary obstruction, nephron dysfunction
- Causes of unilateral delayed nephrogram
  - Renal artery/vein compromise (RAS, renal vein thrombosis), pyelonephritis, urinary obstruction
- Causes of segmental delayed nephrogram
  - Pyelonephritis, calyceal obstruction (stone, tumor, clot), focal injury to renal vessels, and parenchyma (contusion)

Helpful Clues for Common Diagnoses

- **Urinary Obstruction**
  - **Obstructing calculus**
    - Usually ureteral
      - Ureterovesical or ureteropelvic junction or at crossing of iliac vessels
    - Stone is almost always evident on CT as hyperdense focus with dilated ureter
    - Pelvocaliectasis ± perirenal stranding

- Obstructing tumor
  - **Urothelial carcinoma**
    - May obstruct renal pelvis &/or ureter
    - Dilated collecting system upstream
    - Soft tissue density mass in wall and lumen of collecting system
    - More common in elderly and in patients with history of bladder cancer (metachronous/synchronous lesion)
  - **Renal cell carcinoma**
    - May extend into renal pelvis, causing obstruction
    - Bleeding from tumor may cause obstruction of renal pelvis
    - Renal vein invasion may slow renal venous outflow
  - **Retroperitoneal metastases**
    - Enlarged metastatic retroperitoneal lymph nodes may displace and obstruct ureters
    - Bulky retroperitoneal nodal metastases are more common with GU/GYN malignancies
    - Metastases may be to ureteral wall itself
  - **Pelvic malignancies**
    - May encase and obstruct intrapelvic ureters (e.g., rectal or endometrial carcinoma)
  - **Retroperitoneal lymphoma**
    - Soft and bulky tumor; usually displaces ureters but may obstruct renal pelvis or ureter
- **Obstructing clot**
  - Blood clot may obstruct renal pelvis or ureter
  - Usually occurs following trauma or biopsy; also seen with tumors
- **Ureteral stricture**
  - Iatrogenic stricture is most common etiology
    - Lithotomy, ureteroscopy, ureteral catheterization, or radiation therapy
    - Also can be seen as complication of surgery to adjacent organs
  - May follow infection or inflammation of ureter itself
    - Rarely seen as sequela of adjacent inflammatory conditions (e.g., Crohn disease, diverticulitis)
- **Retroperitoneal fibrosis**
  - Mantle of soft tissue that encases aorta and inferior vena cava
    - Irregular margins
    - Extending from renal vessels down to iliac bifurcation
  - Draws ureters in toward midline and encases them with fibrous tissue
  - Unilateral or bilateral ureteral obstruction
  - 2/3 are idiopathic (primary type)
  - 1/3 are secondary: Medications, neoplasms
- **Renal Artery Stenosis**
  - Atherosclerosis, fibromuscular dysplasia, arteritis, dissection, embolism
  - Delayed "inflow" causes decreased and delayed nephrogram
  - Usually affected kidney is relatively small
- **Renal Vein Stenosis/Thrombosis**
  - "Outflow" obstruction can cause decreased and delayed nephrogram
  - Can be unilateral or bilateral

- o Etiology: Dehydration (most common cause in pediatric population), nephrotic syndrome (most common cause in adults), hypercoagulable state, tumoral vascular invasion (renal cell carcinoma)
  - o Intraluminal thrombus itself may be visualized on imaging
- **Acute Tubular Necrosis**
  - o Usually causes bilateral persistent nephrograms (and acute renal failure)
  - o Follows shock, placental abruption, nephrotoxic drugs
- **Contrast-Induced Nephropathy**
  - o Much more common after arterial rather than IV administration of contrast
  - o Risk factors include
    - – Prior renal insufficiency, dehydration, hypertension, diabetes, heart failure, advanced age, large doses of contrast media
- **Pyelonephritis**
  - o Diminished perfusion from ↓ tissue compliance (results of tissue edema) and ↓ renal function contribute to delayed nephrogram
  - o Leukocytes and bacteria (pus) may plug renal tubules
  - o Usually unilateral

Helpful Clues for Less Common Diagnoses

- **Multiple Myeloma**
  - o Renal tubules can become obstructed by myeloma protein
- **Rhabdomyolysis**
  - o Death of muscle tissue may release myoglobin into circulation
  - o Renal tubules can become blocked by protein plugs
- **Leukemia**
  - o Massive tumor necrosis from chemotherapy may release uric acid into circulation
    - – Can lead to calculi or plugging of tubules by uric acid
  - o Masses of leukemic tissue (chloroma) may directly obstruct ureters
- **Renal Papillary Necrosis**

- o Sloughed papilla may obstruct ureteropelvic junction or ureter
- o Characteristic deformities of calices on urography

Alternative Differential Approaches

- Unilateral persistent nephrogram
  - o Obstructed ureter (stone > tumor > other)
  - o Renal artery stenosis
  - o Renal vein stenosis/thrombosis
  - o Unilateral decreased nephron function (usually pyelonephritis)
- Bilateral persistent nephrogram
  - o Hypotension, shock
  - o Acute tubular necrosis
  - o Bilateral ureteral stenosis (tumor, retroperitoneal fibrosis)
  - o Bilateral arterial stenosis
  - o Bilateral venous stenosis or thrombosis

SELECTED REFERENCES

1. Wolin EA et al: Nephrographic and pyelographic analysis of CT urography: differential diagnosis. AJR Am J Roentgenol. 200(6):1197-203, 2013
2. Wolin EA et al: Nephrographic and pyelographic analysis of CT urography: principles, patterns, and pathophysiology. AJR Am J Roentgenol. 200(6):1210-4, 2013
3. Sidhu R et al: Imaging of renovascular disease. Semin Ultrasound CT MR. 30(4):271-88, 2009
4. Craig WD et al: Pyelonephritis: radiologic-pathologic review. Radiographics. 28(1):255-77; quiz 327-8, 2008
5. Jung DC et al: Renal papillary necrosis: review and comparison of findings at multi-detector row CT and intravenous urography. Radiographics. 26(6):1827-36, 2006
6. Tumlin J et al: Pathophysiology of contrast-induced nephropathy. Am J Cardiol. 98(6A):14K-20K, 2006
7. Kawashima A et al: Renal inflammatory disease: the current role of CT. Crit Rev Diagn Imaging. 38(5):369-415, 1997
8. Walker CP et al: Case report: rhabdomyolysis following grand mal seizures presenting as a delayed and increasingly dense nephrogram. Clin Radiol. 47(2):139-40, 1993
9. Dyer RB et al: The abnormal nephrogram. Radiographics. 6(6):1039-63, 1986

Obstructing Calculus

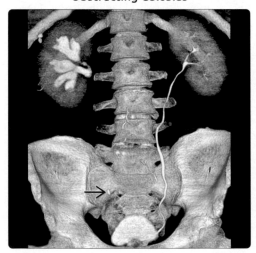

Obstructing Calculus

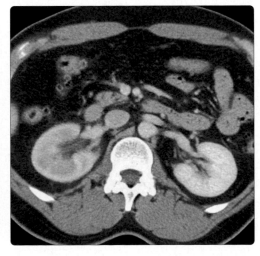

(Left) *Coronal volume-rendered reformat from delayed-phase CECT shows prompt concentration and excretion of urine from the left kidney, while the right kidney has a delayed nephrogram/pyelogram and dilated calices due to an obstructing ureteral stone ➡.* (Right) *Axial CECT in patient with obstructing right distal ureteral calculus shows a delayed right nephrogram. The right kidney is in the corticomedullary phase, while the left is in nephrographic phase of enhancement.*

(Left) *Axial CECT shows infiltrating hypovascular mass ➡ within the left kidney and renal pelvis, which was proven to be urothelial carcinoma. Note the delayed left nephrogram: The unaffected left kidney is still in a corticomedullary phase, while the right kidney is in a nephrographic phase.* **(Right)** *Coronal T1 C+ MR shows a large renal mass ➡ invading into the left renal vein and inferior vena cava (IVC) ⇨. Note the delayed left nephrogram ⇨.*

Transitional Cell Carcinoma

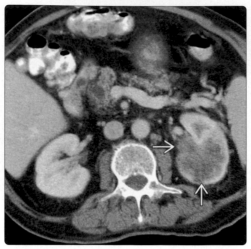

Renal Cell Carcinoma

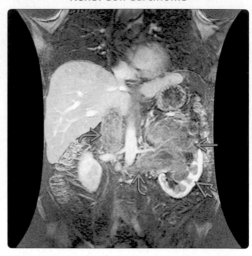

(Left) *Axial CECT of a female patient with a history of ovarian carcinoma shows bilateral hydronephrosis and bilateral, right > left, delayed nephrograms due to extensive retroperitoneal lymph node metastases ⇨.* **(Right)** *Axial CECT shows a delayed left nephrogram due to extensive retroperitoneal lymphadenopathy ⇨ that compressed the left renal vein and left ureter. Nodal biopsy showed non-Hodgkin lymphoma.*

Retroperitoneal Metastases

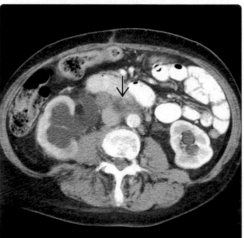

Retroperitoneal Lymphoma

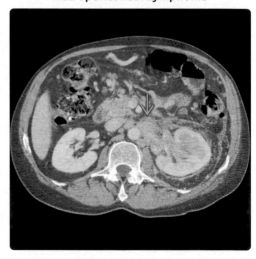

(Left) *Axial CECT of an 82-year-old woman with a history of sigmoid cancer shows left-sided hydronephrosis and a delayed left nephrogram. More inferior images demonstrated invasion of tumor into the left ureter (not shown).* **(Right)** *Axial CECT of a patient with a history of retroperitoneal fibrosis shows encasement and narrowing of the left renal artery ➡ and vein ⇨ by the fibrotic mass. The unilateral delayed nephrogram is due to a combination of renal vein, artery encasement, and ureteral obstruction.*

Ureteral Stricture

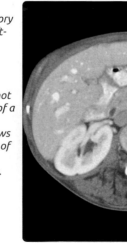

Retroperitoneal Fibrosis

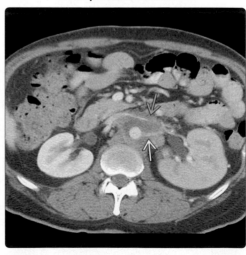

Renal Vein Stenosis/Thrombosis

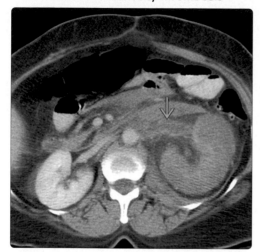

Renal Vein Stenosis/Thrombosis

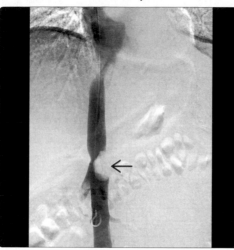

(Left) *Axial CECT in 56-year-old woman with history of blunt trauma to the flank shows marked enlargement and decreased enhancement of the left kidney secondary to presumed traumatic thrombosis of the left renal vein* ➡. **(Right)** *Coronal projection from cavogram, which was performed for IVC filter placement, in the same patient shows extension of left renal thrombus into the IVC* ➡.

Renal Artery Stenosis

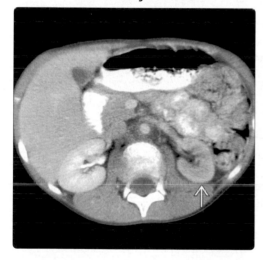

Contrast-Induced Nephropathy

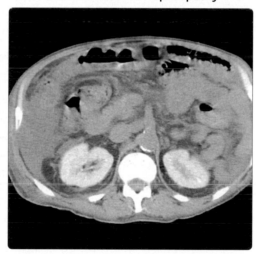

(Left) *Axial CECT shows a delayed nephrogram and decreased size of the left kidney* ➡ *in a 10-year-old boy, who subsequently was diagnosed with Takayasu arteritis.* **(Right)** *Axial NECT shows dense bilateral delayed nephrograms 1 day following coronary angiography in an elderly patient with congestive heart failure.*

Hypotension

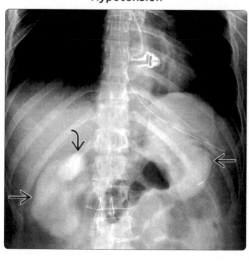

Pyelonephritis

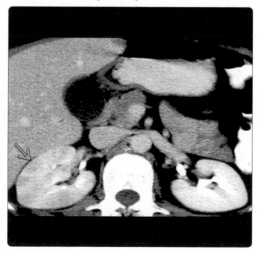

(Left) *Frontal radiograph shows dense persistent nephrograms* ➡ *and opacified bile in the gallbladder* ➡ *(due to vicarious excretion). This 33-year-old patient had been in shock due to blunt trauma and had a CECT the previous day.* **(Right)** *Axial CECT shows a delayed right nephrogram with patchy striation and wedge-shaped defects* ➡. *Signs of sepsis, pyuria, and flank pain helped to confirm the diagnosis of acute pyelonephritis.*

DIFFERENTIAL DIAGNOSIS

Common

- Acute Pyelonephritis
- Renal Trauma
- Renal Infarction
- Acute Ureteral Obstruction
- Medullary Sponge Kidney

Less Common

- Vasculitis, Abdominal Manifestations
- Multiple Myeloma
- Rhabdomyolysis
- Renal Cell Carcinoma
- Metastases and Lymphoma, Renal
- Radiation Nephritis
- Renal Vein Thrombosis
- IgG4-Related Kidney Disease
- Autosomal Recessive Polycystic Disease

ESSENTIAL INFORMATION

Key Differential Diagnosis Issues

- Acute renal inflammatory, traumatic, infectious, or vascular diseases
  - Tend to manifest as wedge-shaped &/or striated areas of diminished enhancement on CECT or CEMR, reflecting lobular architecture of kidney and presence of collecting tubules that comprise renal medulla
- Striated pattern
  - Alternating bands of high and low density/attenuation with radial distribution
  - Renal tubules plugged with casts of
    - White blood cells: Acute pyelonephritis
    - Red blood cells: Trauma
    - Protein: Multiple myeloma, rhabdomyolysis
- Wedge-shaped pattern
  - More potential etiologies
  - Anything that can injure or replace portion of kidney
- Straight-line demarcation between normal and abnormal kidney
  - Usually has vascular etiology
  - Ischemia or infarction most common cause

Helpful Clues for Common Diagnoses

- Acute Pyelonephritis
  - Kidney swollen with striated and wedge defects
  - Infiltration of perirenal fat ± abscess
  - Typical clinical setting
    - Acute flank pain, dysuria, high fever
    - More common in young women
- Renal Trauma
  - Contusion and renal hematoma may cause striated and wedge defects, respectively
  - Traumatic renal arterial injury can cause similar appearance but different mechanism
    - Stretched intima may tear and dissect
    - Platelet emboli cause scattered zones of decreased renal perfusion
  - Typical clinical setting: Blunt injury due to motor vehicle crash
    - Renal arterial injury usually follows rapid deceleration injury (fall or high-speed motor vehicle crash)
- Renal Infarction
  - Arterial dissection or emboli may result in wedge-shaped parenchymal defects
    - Cortical scarring and volume loss over time
  - Straight line demarcation of normal/abnormal kidney indicates vascular etiology
  - Cortical rim sign
    - Preserved perfusion of subcapsular rim of tissue
    - Seen in 50% of cases; 6-8 hours after infarction
  - Typical clinical settings
    - Embolic: Cardiac valve vegetations; prior myocardial infarction; atrial fibrillation
    - Thrombotic: Aortic &/or renal artery dissection; atherosclerosis
- Acute Ureteral Obstruction
  - Usually causes delayed nephrogram
  - Nephrogram may be heterogeneous, even striated, with infectious complication
- Medullary Sponge Kidney
  - Renal tubules are dilated; tiny calculi in pyramids and calyces
  - Tends to impart more of a striated appearance only of medulla (not cortex)
    - Most evident on pyelographic phase of urography (excretory or CTU)
  - Typical clinical setting: Intermittent episodes of flank pain due to ureteral obstruction by small calculi originating in dilated tubules

Helpful Clues for Less Common Diagnoses

- Vasculitis, Abdominal Manifestations
  - Polyarteritis, lupus, etc.
  - Striated and wedge-shaped lesions indistinguishable from acute pyelonephritis on imaging
  - Clinical setting: Patient with known autoimmune (collagen vascular) disease
    - Episodes of symptoms referable to visceral ischemia or spontaneous hemorrhage
- Multiple Myeloma
  - Collecting tubules may be plugged with excreted myeloma protein
  - Imaging findings similar to acute pyelonephritis
    - But clinical presentation is very different (no fever; known or easily confirmed myeloma)
- Rhabdomyolysis
  - Release of massive amounts of myoglobin into serum from damaged skeletal muscle may block renal tubules
    - Clinical: May cause acute renal failure
    - Imaging: Decreased or striated nephrogram, usually bilateral
  - Clinical setting: Crush injury, muscle trauma, certain drug effects
    - Especially drug overdose with prolonged muscle hypoxia
- Renal Cell Carcinoma
  - Or other tumors (metastases, lymphoma)
  - May have wedge shape but are usually spherical
    - Do not expect striated nephrogram

- o Clinical setting: Incidental discovery (renal cell carcinoma) or flank pain, hematuria
- **Metastases and Lymphoma, Renal**
  - o Primary tumor is usually known
  - o Extrarenal tumor is usually evident
- **Radiation Nephritis**
  - o Wedge shape correlates with field of external beam
    - – Radiation therapy to midline structures (e.g., nodal or spine metastases) may injure medial portions of kidneys
    - – Clinical setting: Should be able to elicit or deduce history of prior radiation therapy
  - o Often does not correspond to the expected wedge shape of renal lobules
- **Renal Vein Thrombosis**
  - o Acute renal vein thrombosis may cause striated or wedge-shaped defects
  - o Kidney usually swollen, may have delayed nephrogram
  - o Clinical setting: Nephrotic syndrome, hypercoagulable condition
    - – Acute flank pain

- **IgG4-Related Kidney Disease**
  - o Kidneys involved in 1/3 of cases of autoimmune pancreatitis
  - o Bilateral hypoenhancing renal lesions (lymphoplasmacytic infiltrate) with wedge or round shape
- **Autosomal Recessive Polycystic Disease**
  - o Usually manifest and diagnosed in childhood
  - o Striated enhancement due to accumulation of contrast in dilated tubules in excretory phase

Acute Pyelonephritis

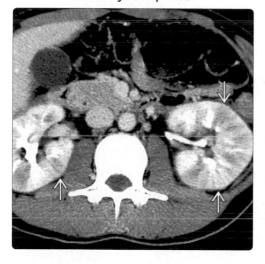

Acute Pyelonephritis

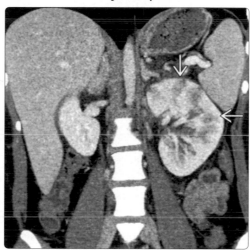

(Left) Axial CECT shows bilateral wedge-shaped areas of renal parenchymal hypoenhancement (striated nephrograms) from pyelonephritis ➡. (Right) Coronal CECT in a 19-year-old woman presenting with weakness and nausea while in treatment for UTI reveals radiating hypoenhancing bands ➡ of the left kidney, typical of striated nephrogram and compatible with acute pyelonephritis. The enhancement of the right kidney is normal, suggesting a unilateral process.

Acute Pyelonephritis

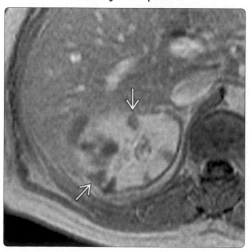

Acute Pyelonephritis

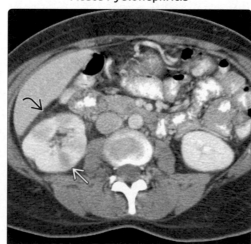

(Left) Axial T1WI C+ FS MR shows multiple wedge-shaped areas of hypoenhancement ➡ in the right kidney compatible with acute pyelonephritis. (Right) Axial CECT shows swelling of the right kidney with wedge-shaped zones of decreased enhancement ➡. Also note infiltration of the perirenal fat ➡.

Wedge-Shaped or Striated Nephrogram

Renal Trauma

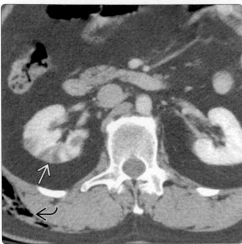

Renal Trauma

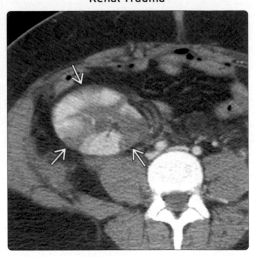

(Left) *Axial CECT shows wedge-shaped zones of decreased enhancement ➡ in the right kidney due to renal arterial injury with dissection. Note subcutaneous gas from a chest injury ➡ in this 34-year-old man post motor vehicle accident.* **(Right)** *Axial CECT obtained post blunt abdominal trauma reveals striated nephrogram ➡ of right lower quadrant renal allograft from multiple infarcts/contusions.*

Renal Infarction

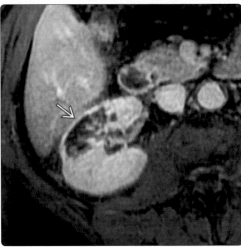

Renal Infarction

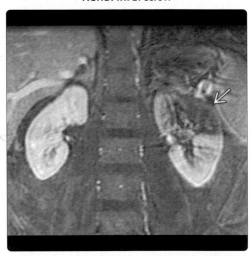

(Left) *Axial T1WI C+ FS MR in a 55-year-old woman with atrial fibrillation shows a wedge-shaped area of nonenhancement in the right kidney ➡ with cortical rim of enhancement compatible with a subacute infarction.* **(Right)** *Coronal T1WI C+ FS MR shows a large, wedge-shaped zone of decreased cortical and medullary enhancement ➡ of the left kidney due to renal infarction.*

Vasculitis, Abdominal Manifestations

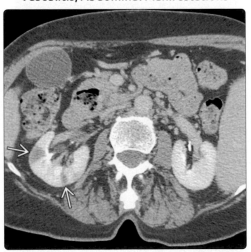

Vasculitis, Abdominal Manifestations

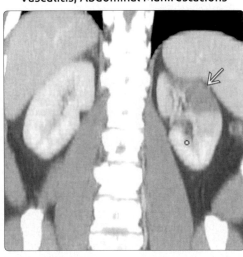

(Left) *Axial CECT in a 70-year-old woman with Wegener granulomatosis (vasculitis) shows multiple wedge-shaped areas of parenchymal hypoenhancement ➡ in the right kidney due to renal ischemic injury.* **(Right)** *Coronal CECT shows a wedge-shaped zone of decreased enhancement ➡ due to vasculitis and renal ischemia in this 40-year-old man. Note the straight-line demarcation sign of a vascular injury.*

Radiation Nephritis

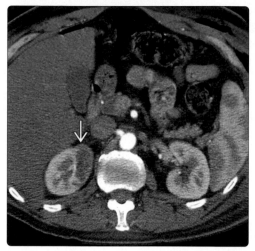

Radiation Nephritis

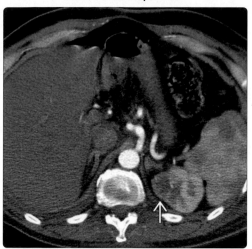

(Left) Axial CECT shows decreased parenchymal enhancement of the medial half of the right kidney ➡ due to radiation nephritis that followed therapy for vertebral metastasis. The left kidney was involved at a different level with the same features. (Right) Axial CECT shows decreased parenchymal enhancement and subtle volume loss in the medial half of the left kidney ➡ due to radiation nephritis that followed treatment for vertebral metastasis.

Medullary Sponge Kidney

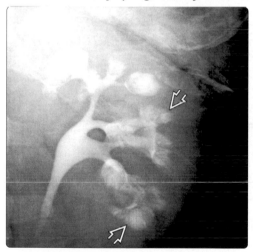

Metastases and Lymphoma, Renal

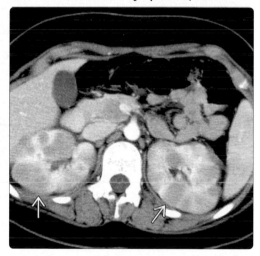

(Left) Frontal excretory urography shows a classic paint brush appearance of dilated, contrast-opacified, dilated tubules ➡ in the renal pyramids, giving a striated appearance to the renal medulla. (Right) Axial CECT shows a mottled appearance of both kidneys due to parenchymal deposits of lymphoma ➡. Most of the lesions have a spherical, rather than wedge, shape.

Renal Vein Thrombosis

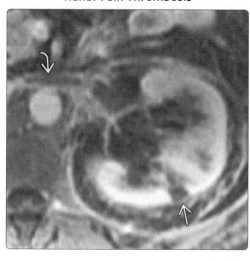

IgG4-Related Kidney Disease

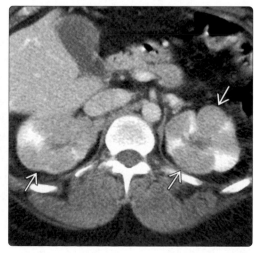

(Left) Axial T1WI C+ FS MR shows heterogeneous and focal decreased renal parenchymal enhancement ➡ due to renal vein thrombosis ➡ in this patient with nephrotic syndrome. (Right) Axial CECT shows multiple wedge-shaped, hypoenhancing lesions ➡ in both kidneys, biopsy-proven IgG4-related sclerosing disease.

DIFFERENTIAL DIAGNOSIS

Common

- Hydronephrosis
- Acute Pyelonephritis
- Primary Renal Tumors
  - Benign and Malignant
- Compensatory Renal Hypertrophy
- Duplex Kidney
- Renal Parenchymal Diseases
  - Acute Glomerulonephritis, Lupus Nephritis, Diabetic Nephropathy, Acute Tubular Necrosis
- Renal Vascular Diseases
  - Acute Renal Vein Thrombosis, Acute Renal Infarction, Acute Cortical Necrosis
- Renal Abscess
- Pyonephrosis
- Perinephric Fluid Collections
- Renal Trauma

Less Common

- HIV Nephropathy
- Autosomal Dominant Polycystic Kidney Disease
- Multicystic Dysplastic Kidney
- Horseshoe Kidney
- Crossed Fused Renal Ectopia

Rare but Important

- Autosomal Recessive Polycystic Kidney Disease
- Renal Lymphoma
- Renal Leukemia
- Xanthogranulomatous Pyelonephritis
- Renal Amyloidosis
- Renal Tuberculosis
- Exercise-Induced Nonmyoglobinuric Acute Renal Failure

ESSENTIAL INFORMATION

Key Differential Diagnosis Issues

- Establish if renal enlargement is unilateral or bilateral and if enlargement is focal or diffuse
- Acute causes: Obstruction, infection, inflammation
- Chronic causes: Cellular hypertrophy, abnormal protein deposition, malignancies, infection, glomerular or microvascular proliferation

Helpful Clues for Common Diagnoses

- **Hydronephrosis**
  - Splitting of central renal echocomplex by branching fluid-filled pelvis
  - Dilated calyces may be variable in size
  - Cortical thinning in chronic hydronephrosis
  - Look for dilated ureter and determine if simply dilated or truly obstructed (VCUG/MAG 3 renogram)
  - Gross hydronephrosis may mimic multicystic dysplastic kidney, ovarian or mesenteric cyst (in infants), or large collection
  - Causes include stones, tumors, congenital malformations, clot, infection, extrinsic compression, bladder outlet obstruction, and vesico ureteral reflux
- **Acute Pyelonephritis**
  - Normal renal size or diffuse enlargement
    - Echogenicity variable: Decreased or increased
  - Focal pyelonephritis
    - Focal alteration of cortical echogenicity
    - Wedge shaped, triangular, or round
    - May produce focal external cortical bulge
    - Wedge-shaped perfusion defect extending from papilla on color and power Doppler or contrast-enhanced ultrasound
      - Cortical vascularity decreased secondary to cortical vasoconstriction and edema
- **Primary Renal Tumors**
  - **Renal cell carcinoma**
    - Varied size and appearance
    - Exophytic echogenic renal mass when large
    - Hypoechoic rim, cystic change from necrosis, calcification
    - Diffuse infiltration is less common
  - **Upper tract urothelial carcinoma**
    - Hydronephrosis and dilated calyces secondary to pelvic or ureteral tumor
    - Infiltrating soft tissue mass in renal pelvis or pelvic wall thickening
  - **Renal angiomyolipoma**
    - Echogenic mass with posterior shadowing, single or multiple
    - Variable size and lipid content
      - Lipid poor are less echogenic
      - Usually require confirmation with CT or MR
    - Large angiomyolipoma may be indistinguishable from other renal solid tumors
  - **Multilocular cystic nephroma**
    - Multilocular encapsulated cystic lesion, which may herniate into renal pelvis
  - **Mesoblastic nephroma**
    - Typically solid unilateral mass in neonate or fetus
- **Compensatory Renal Hypertrophy**
  - Enlarged, otherwise unremarkable kidney
  - Occurs with contralateral renal disease, aplasia/dysplasia, or nephrectomy
- **Duplex Kidney**
  - Splitting of central echogenic renal sinus into upper and lower pole moieties
  - 2 distinct draining ureters may be seen if they are dilated
- **Renal Parenchymal Diseases**
  - **Acute glomerulonephritis**
    - Bilateral enlarged kidneys with hyperechoic cortex and prominent pyramids
  - **Lupus nephritis**
    - Acute: Normal or increased size bilaterally; cortical echogenicity increased or normal
    - May also have multiple focal infarcts
  - **Diabetic nephropathy**
    - Bilateral enlarged bright kidneys in early stage
  - **Acute tubular necrosis**
    - Normal or diffuse bilateral renal swelling
    - Prominent pyramids due to edema
- **Renal Vascular Diseases**
  - **Acute renal vein thrombosis**
    - Common in membranous glomerulonephritis

- Nonneoplastic causes: Dehydration and fever in children; hypercoagulability and nephrotic syndrome in adults
- Renal enlargement with ↓ echogenicity, renal vein thrombus ± collaterals
- Unilateral > bilateral
- **Acute renal infarction**
  - Embolic or traumatic arterial occlusion
  - Unilateral flank pain
  - Normal or enlarged kidneys with wedge-shaped defect on color Doppler
- **Acute cortical necrosis**
  - Caused by abruptio placentae, postpartum hemorrhage, shock, sepsis, and toxins
  - Results from microvascular thrombosis with cortical ischemia
  - Bilateral enlarged echogenic kidneys with hypoechoic subcapsular rim
- **Renal Abscess**
  - Solitary or multiple thick-walled intrarenal cystic lesions in setting of infection
  - More common in patients with diabetes mellitus, drug abuse, vesicoureteral reflux, renal calculi
- **Pyonephrosis**
  - Swollen obstructed kidney with debris or dependent echoes in collecting system
- **Perinephric Fluid Collections**
  - May represent abscess, blood, urine, and lymph
  - May mimic large renal mass or compress kidney, causing "page kidney"
- **Renal Trauma**
  - Perirenal and renal hematomas, renal fracture, contusion

Helpful Clues for Less Common Diagnoses

- **HIV Nephropathy**
  - Normal or enlarged kidneys
  - Typically increased echogenicity with decreased corticomedullary differentiation
  - Later small
- **Autosomal Dominant Polycystic Kidney Disease**
  - Usually presents in adulthood
  - Bilateral large kidneys with innumerable cysts of varying sizes that distort normal renal architecture
- **Multicystic Dysplastic Kidney**
  - Multiple noncommunicating renal cysts of varying size with echogenic intervening parenchyma
  - Initially enlarged kidney, later atrophy
  - Association with contralateral renal disease common
- **Horseshoe Kidney**
  - Lower poles joined by isthmus of functioning renal tissue or fibrous band
  - Lower in position with medially deviated lower poles
- **Crossed Fused Renal Ectopia**
  - Enlarged kidney with malrotation
  - Absence of contralateral kidney

Helpful Clues for Rare Diagnoses

- **Autosomal Recessive Polycystic Kidney Disease**
  - Detected in utero or in infancy
  - Bilaterally enlarged kidneys with increased echogenicity and multiple tiny cysts
- **Renal Lymphoma**
  - Focal or diffuse renal enlargement: Unilateral or bilateral
  - Infiltrative: Diffuse renal enlargement with disruption of internal architecture
  - Perirenal soft tissue rind
- **Renal Leukemia**
  - Gross renal involvement uncommon
  - Symmetrically enlarged kidneys with distorted central sinus and ↓ corticomedullary differentiation
- **Xanthogranulomatous Pyelonephritis**
  - Pelvicalyceal obstruction by stone (usually staghorn)
  - Diffuse unilateral renal enlargement with echogenic debris in dilated calyces and cortical thinning
  - Diabetes, recurrent urinary tract infections, immunocompromise
- **Renal Amyloidosis**
  - Abnormal protein deposition in kidneys
- **Renal Tuberculosis**
  - Dilated calyces and granulomatous abscesses

Hydronephrosis

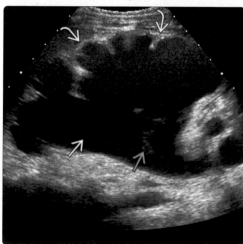

Acute Pyelonephritis

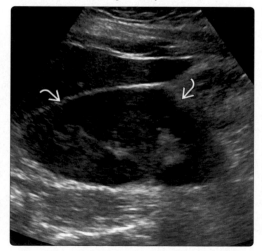

(Left) Longitudinal ultrasound shows a markedly enlarged right kidney with severe hydronephrosis ➡, hydroureter and cortical thinning ➡ in a patient with a history of posterior urethral valves and severe reflux. Renal pelvis echoes ➡ could represent infection, blood, or cellular debris. (Right) Longitudinal ultrasound in a patient with acute pyelonephritis and diabetes shows an enlarged hypoechoic right kidney ➡ with loss of corticomedullary differentiation.

(Left) *Longitudinal transabdominal ultrasound shows focal acute pyelonephritis in a pregnant woman. There is a wedge-shaped area of increased echogenicity* ➡ *in the upper pole.* (Right) *Longitudinal ultrasound shows an enlarged kidney* ➡ *with a large solid mass in the lower pole* ➡. *Given the size of this mass, renal cell carcinoma was suspected, but it was an oncocytoma at surgery.*

Acute Pyelonephritis

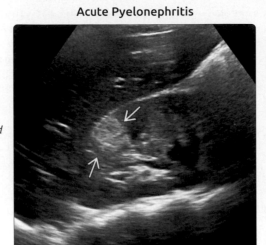

Primary Renal Tumors

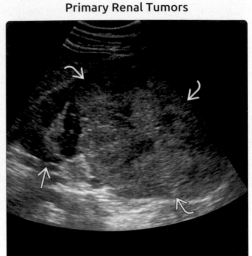

(Left) *Longitudinal ultrasound shows an enlarged kidney measuring 14 cm. The kidney is increased in echogenicity with increased prominence of the pyramids* ➡ *in this patient with a contralateral, severely hydronephrotic, poorly functioning kidney.* (Right) *Longitudinal ultrasound shows a nonobstructed duplex kidney with splitting of central sinus echoes by a hypoechoic band of tissue* ➡. *Duplex kidneys are normal variants, which are longer than normal kidneys.*

Compensatory Renal Hypertrophy

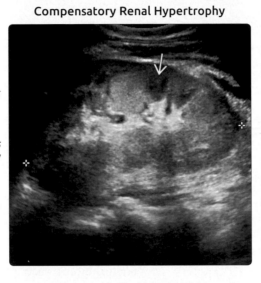

Duplex Kidney

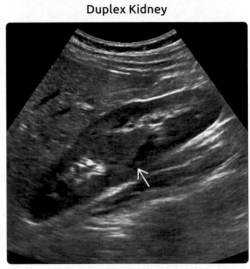

(Left) *Longitudinal ultrasound shows an enlarged (14 cm), hyperechoic kidney in a diabetic patient with fever, flank pain, and positive blood cultures. There is a large renal abscess* ➡ *with acoustic enhancement.* (Right) *Longitudinal ultrasound shows the right kidney in a patient with lupus nephritis, fever, and bacteriuria. There is severe hydronephrosis and cortical thinning* ➡. *The calyces are filled with low-level echoes representing pus* ➡.

Renal Abscess

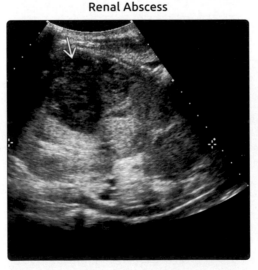

Pyonephrosis

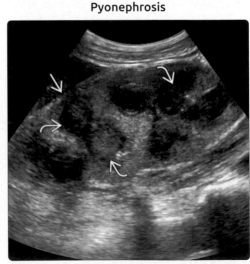

Perinephric Fluid Collections

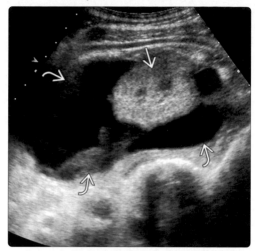

HIV Nephropathy

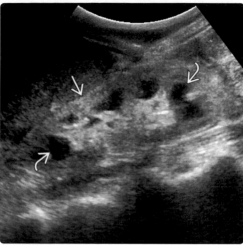

(Left) *Transverse ultrasound shows the right renal lower pole ➡, which is surrounded by a perinephric collection ➡ containing debris. Differential diagnosis includes hematoma, seroma, urinoma, or lymphocele.* (Right) *Longitudinal ultrasound shows a large right kidney with echogenic cortex ➡ and prominent pyramids ➡ in a patient with HIV nephropathy. Many pathologic processes cause increased cortical echogenicity.*

Autosomal Dominant Polycystic Kidney Disease

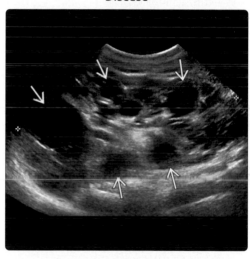

Multicystic Dysplastic Kidney

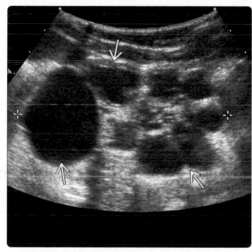

(Left) *Longitudinal ultrasound shows an enlarged left kidney (16 cm) with multiple cysts ➡ of varying sizes. There is no normal intervening parenchyma. The right kidney was similar. Liver cysts were also present.* (Right) *Longitudinal ultrasound of an infant with multicystic dysplastic kidney shows an enlarged left kidney with multiple noncommunicating cysts of varying sizes ➡ with no normal cortex. This was a nonfunctioning kidney.*

Crossed Fused Renal Ectopia

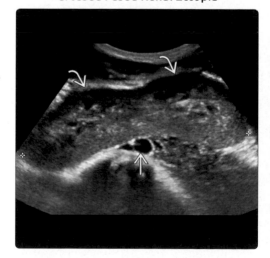

Autosomal Recessive Polycystic Kidney Disease

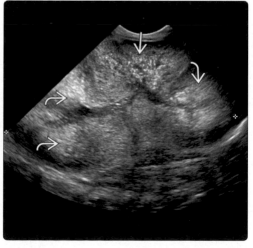

(Left) *Transverse oblique ultrasound shows a crossed fused ectopia with the 2 renal moieties ➡ fused in the upper pelvis anterior to the aorta ➡.* (Right) *Longitudinal ultrasound shows the right kidney in a neonate with abnormal kidneys detected in utero. The kidney is large (10.1 cm) and echogenic with innumerable tiny cysts ➡. These produce areas of increased reflectivity ➡ when too small to be resolved.*

DIFFERENTIAL DIAGNOSIS

Common

- Chronic Diabetic Nephropathy
- Chronic Glomerulonephritis
- Chronic Hypertensive Nephropathy
- Chronic Lupus Nephritis
- Chronic Reflux Nephropathy
- Postobstructive Atrophy
- Partial Nephrectomy/Post Ablative Therapy/Post Surgery
- Chronic Renal Allograft Rejection/Chronic Allograft Nephropathy

Less Common

- Chronic HIV Nephropathy
- Multicystic Dysplastic Kidney
- Recurrent Infection
- Chronic Renal Artery Stenosis
- Chronic Renal Infarction
- Chronic Vascular Injury
- Posttraumatic Renal Atrophy
- Following Acute Cortical Necrosis or Acute Tubular Necrosis
- Post Chemotherapy

Rare but Important

- Chronic Radiation Nephropathy
- Chronic Nephritis (Alport Syndrome)
- Renal Cystic Dysplasia
- Medullary Cystic Disease Complex
- Tuberculous Autonephrectomy
- Renal Hypoplasia
- Supernumerary Kidney
- Chronic Lead Poisoning

ESSENTIAL INFORMATION

Key Differential Diagnosis Issues

- Renal atrophy is end result of many pathologic processes
- Causes of loss of renal parenchyma include
  - Acquired: Infection, inflammation, obstruction, reflux, trauma, necrosis/ischemia, fibrosis, surgical intervention
  - Congenital: Hypoplasia, dysplasia
- Ultrasound findings are not specific for cause
- Renal size and cortical thickness are useful in differentiating acute from chronic kidney disease
- Determine if abnormality is unilateral or bilateral, global or focal/multifocal
- Hydronephrosis suggests ureteral obstruction or vesicoureteral reflux
- Renal echogenicity is variable but commonly increased in medical renal renal disease
- Usually not possible to determine cause of small echogenic scarred kidney
- Clinical history is essential for diagnosis
- Biopsy usually not indicated if kidneys are small

Helpful Clues for Common Diagnoses

- **Chronic Diabetic Nephropathy**
  - Small kidneys + ↑ cortical echogenicity
  - Corticomedullary differentiation (CMD) usually preserved, unless patient is in overt renal failure

- **Chronic Glomerulonephritis**
  - Small kidneys + smooth renal outline
  - Parenchyma remains echogenic
- **Chronic Hypertensive Nephropathy**
  - Due to progressive nephrosclerosis
  - Small kidneys + irregular cortical thinning
  - ↓ cortical vascularity due to arteriolar fibrosis and hyaline degeneration
- **Chronic Lupus Nephritis**
  - Small kidneys
  - Variable renal echogenicity and CMD
- **Chronic Reflux Nephropathy**
  - Unilateral or bilateral vesicoureteral reflux in childhood
  - May cause focal/diffuse renal scarring and atrophy
  - Cortical scars are common in upper and lower pole
  - Dilated calyces next to scar suggest diagnosis
  - Calyces and pelvis may be dilated initially but shrink as kidney atrophies
  - Focal areas of compensatory hypertrophy seen adjacent to cortical scars
  - Small kidneys + irregular renal outline
- **Postobstructive Atrophy**
  - Caused by longstanding ureteropelvic junction (UPJ), ureteric, or bladder outlet obstruction
  - Results in progressive decrease in renal blood flow and glomerular filtration
  - Small kidney with cortical thinning and variable hydronephrosis
- **Partial Nephrectomy/Post Ablative Therapy/Post Surgery**
  - Small residual kidney with preserved CMD
  - Compensatory hypertrophy of contralateral kidney may be evident
  - History is essential
- **Chronic Renal Allograft Rejection/Chronic Allograft Nephropathy**
  - Irreversible cause of renal allograft dysfunction
  - Small transplant kidney with cortical thinning and increased cortical echogenicity
  - Decreased color Doppler flow
  - Decreased arterial diastolic flow

Helpful Clues for Less Common Diagnoses

- **Chronic HIV Nephropathy**
  - Normal or enlarged kidneys becoming small with progressive renal failure
  - Increased cortical echogenicity, loss of CMD and sinus fat
  - Thickened urothelium
- **Multicystic Dysplastic Kidney**
  - Initially unilateral enlarged kidney replaced by noncommunicating cysts of varying sizes
  - Undergoes partial or complete involution in infancy
  - Later appears small and echogenic ± cysts
  - Contralateral diseases common such as vesicoureteric reflux, UPJ obstruction, and ureteric stenosis
- **Recurrent Infection**
  - Risk factors: Calculi, urinary tract obstruction, neurogenic bladder, and urinary diversion
  - Small kidney, parenchymal scarring
  - Focal cortical thinning causing irregular outline

- o Pseudotumors from adjacent hypertrophy
- **Chronic Renal Artery Stenosis**
  - o Mostly atherosclerosis affects main, interlobar, or interlobular renal arteries or arterioles
  - o Progressive generalized reduction in kidney size caused by ischemia
  - o Produces renal atrophy or collateralization
  - o Smooth contour
- **Chronic Renal Infarction**
  - o Renal atrophy after acute renal infarction caused by embolism or thrombosis
  - o Atrophy may be focal (segmental) or global
  - o Parenchymal loss depends on distribution of occluded artery
  - o Infarcted area may be contracted, producing renal scar
  - o More common in transplanted than native kidneys
- **Chronic Vascular Injury**
  - o Sequela of vasculitides such as polyarteritis nodosa or ischemia from fibromuscular dysplasia
  - o End result of nonspecific small echogenic kidneys
- **Posttraumatic Renal Atrophy**
  - o Caused by segmental renal infarction due to renal artery thrombosis after blunt renal trauma or after embolization for bleeding
  - o Contracted kidney + irregular outline
  - o Collateralization may be demonstrated
- **Following Acute Cortical Necrosis or Acute Tubular Necrosis**
  - o May be associated with cortical or medullary calcification
- **Post Chemotherapy**
  - o Scarring after therapy for renal lymphoma, leukemia, or metastases

Helpful Clues for Rare Diagnoses

- **Chronic Radiation Nephropathy**
  - o Occurs after renal irradiation for bone marrow transplantation
  - o Begins months to years after irradiation
  - o Areas of diminished perfusion may be seen
  - o Small kidneys with increased renal echogenicity

- **Chronic Nephritis (Alport Syndrome)**
  - o Chronic hereditary nephritis
  - o Small kidneys + smooth renal outline
  - o ↑ cortical echogenicity due to cortical nephrocalcinosis
- **Renal Cystic Dysplasia**
  - o May be bilateral
  - o Associated with posterior urethral valve, renal duplication, crossed-fused ectopia, horseshoe and pelvic kidneys
  - o Unilateral small kidney with increased echogenicity and small cortical cysts
- **Medullary Cystic Disease Complex**
  - o Inherited cystic renal disease
  - o Progressive tubular atrophy with glomerulosclerosis
  - o Echogenic kidneys with progressive decrease in size
  - o Multiple small medullary cysts
- **Tuberculous Autonephrectomy**
  - o Calcified caseous pyonephrosis with UPJ fibrosis
  - o Shrunken kidney + extensive calcification
  - o Dilated calyces
- **Renal Hypoplasia**
  - o At least 50% smaller than normal
  - o Has fewer calyces and papillae
  - o Renal function normal for its size
  - o Usually unilateral
  - o Differentiation from obstruction, chronic pyelonephritis, and ischemia difficult
- **Supernumerary Kidney**
  - o Extremely rare, hypoplastic 3rd kidney
  - o Connected to dominant kidney either completely or by loose areolar connective tissue
  - o Most are caudal to orthotopic kidney
- **Chronic Lead Poisoning**
  - o Bilateral small kidneys
  - o Indistinguishable sonographically from other causes of renal atrophy
  - o Blood level of lead useful for diagnosis

Chronic Diabetic Nephropathy

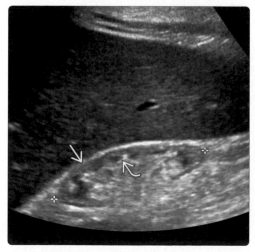

Chronic Glomerulonephritis

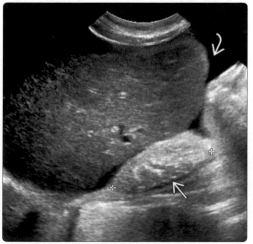

(Left) Longitudinal ultrasound of the right kidney in end-stage renal disease and diabetes shows diffuse cortical thinning ➡ with increased echogenicity and preserved corticomedullary differentiation ➔. (Right) Longitudinal ultrasound shows the right kidney in end-stage renal disease and cirrhosis. The kidney ➡ is small (8 cm) with increased echogenicity and loss of corticomedullary differentiation. Ascites and nodular liver contour ➔ are present.

Chronic Hypertensive Nephropathy

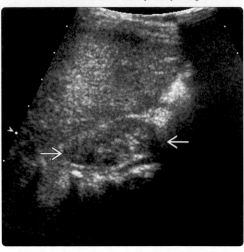

Chronic Reflux Nephropathy

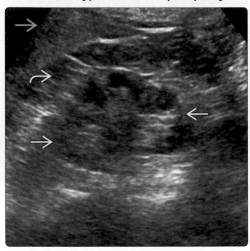

(Left) *Longitudinal ultrasound shows the right kidney in end-stage renal disease. The kidney ➡ is small and lobulated, a nonspecific appearance, which can be the end result of many disorders. Note the prominent perinephric fat ➡ between the liver ➡ and kidney. **(Right)** Longitudinal ultrasound of the right kidney in a 1 year old with a history of grade III-IV reflux on the right shows an atrophic kidney ➡ with no hydronephrosis. No focal scars were detected.*

Chronic Reflux Nephropathy

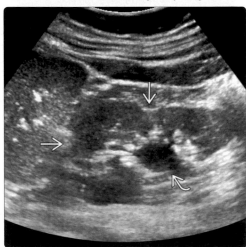

Chronic Reflux Nephropathy

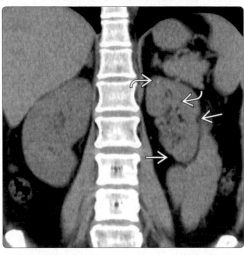

(Left) *Longitudinal ultrasound of the left kidney shows a lobulated contour with cortical loss ➡ in the upper and mid to lower poles. There is mild pelvic dilatation ➡. **(Right)** NECT of the same patient confirms the atrophy of the left kidney with cortical loss ➡. A few tiny calcifications ➡ were noted, not seen on the ultrasound.*

Chronic Reflux Nephropathy

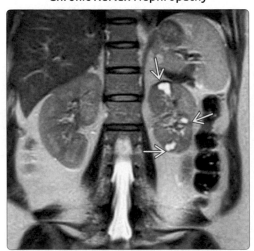

Chronic HIV Nephropathy

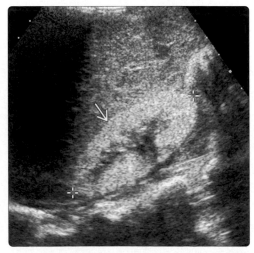

(Left) *T2 HASTE MR of the same patient performed for gallbladder disease shows calyceal dilatation under areas of cortical loss ➡. MR has superior contrast resolution to CT and is less affected by body habitus than ultrasound. **(Right)** Longitudinal ultrasound srhows the right kidney in a patient with established HIV nephropathy. The renal cortex is markedly echogenic ➡ and small with loss of sinus fat.*

Postobstructive Atrophy

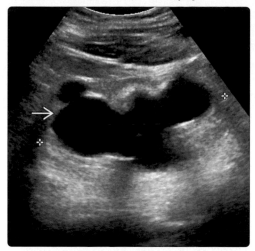

Postobstructive Atrophy

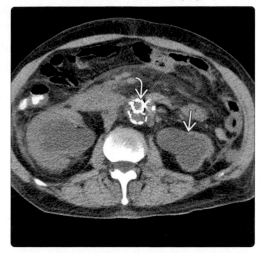

(Left) *Longitudinal ultrasound of the left kidney shows severe hydronephrosis* ➡ *and cortical thinning, which was secondary to chronic ureteral obstruction. However, severe reflux can also produce this appearance.* (Right) *Axial NECT of the same patient shows bilateral hydronephrosis with more atrophy on the left* ➡ *and an aortic stent graft* ➡. *Renal failure precluded the use of intravenous contrast.*

Partial Nephrectomy/Post Ablative Therapy/Post Surgery

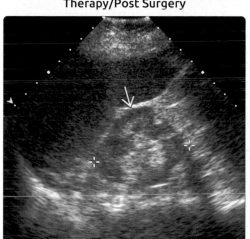

Partial Nephrectomy/Post Ablative Therapy/Post Surgery

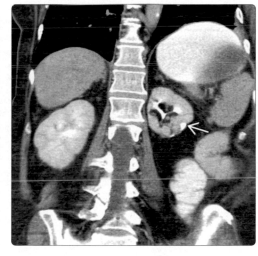

(Left) *Longitudinal ultrasound shows a left kidney* ➡ *post partial nephrectomy 20 years prior. The kidney is small (6 cm) with preserved corticomedullary differentiation.* (Right) *CECT of the same patient shows loss of cortex overlying mid pole calyces* ➡ *status post lower pole resection.*

Partial Nephrectomy/Post Ablative Therapy/Post Surgery

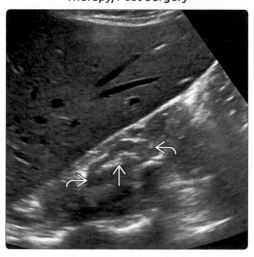

Chronic Renal Infarction

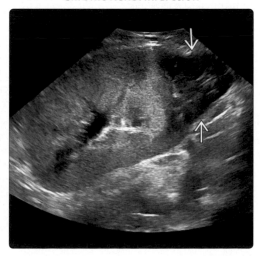

(Left) *Longitudinal ultrasound shows the liver and atrophic right kidney in a patient with testicular cancer post retroperitoneal lymph node dissection. The right kidney* ➡ *is very small with global cortical thinning. Renal sinus fat* ➡ *is preserved* (Right) *Longitudinal ultrasound shows a renal transplant with scarring of the lower pole* ➡, *a sequela of thrombosis of a lower pole accessory artery.*

DIFFERENTIAL DIAGNOSIS

Common

- Acute Pyelonephritis
- Severe Fatty Liver (Mimic)
- Renal Parenchymal Disease

Less Common

- Perinephric Hematoma or Other Fluid Collection
- Acute Renal Transplant Rejection
- Acute Renal Vein Thrombosis
- Acute Renal Artery Thrombosis
- Renal Cell Carcinoma
- Upper Tract Urothelial Carcinoma
- Multiple Myeloma
- Renal Leukemia
- Renal Lymphoma
- Hypoechoic Renal Fat With Atrophic Kidneys

Rare but Important

- Acute Amyloidosis
- Acute Cortical Necrosis
- Xanthogranulomatous Pyelonephritis

ESSENTIAL INFORMATION

Key Differential Diagnosis Issues

- Determine if there is diffuse hypoechogenicity or focal hypoechoic lesion
  - Assess if distortion of normal architecture by infiltration
- Use color Doppler to look for vascular flow or distortion of normal vessels
- Most commonly related to nonneoplastic conditions
  - Infection
  - Inflammation
  - Vascular thrombosis or arteritis
  - Deposition of abnormal proteins
- Neoplasms
  - Typically of infiltrative type
    - Renal lymphoma, leukemia and multiple myeloma
  - Less commonly renal cell or urothelial carcinoma
    - May be large and infiltrative
    - Tend to be more heterogeneous

Helpful Clues for Common Diagnoses

- **Acute Pyelonephritis**
  - Ascending bacterial infection
  - Manifestations include
    - Diffuse hypoechoic renal parenchyma
    - Focal hypoechoic or hyperechoic round or wedge-shaped lesions
    - May progress to thick-walled abscesses
    - Urothelial thickening
    - Decreased color Doppler flow secondary to vasoconstriction
- **Severe Fatty Liver (Mimic)**
  - Highly attenuating fatty liver may cause spurious decreased echogenicity of kidney
  - Attempt ultrasound imaging directly and posteriorly
- **Renal Parenchymal Disease**
  - Acute forms of glomerulonephritis and lupus nephritis

  - May cause enlarged hypoechoic kidney but typically hyperechoic
  - Diseases affecting tubules and interstitium tend to increase cortical echogenicity

Helpful Clues for Less Common Diagnoses

- **Perinephric Hematoma or Other Fluid Collection**
  - May occur spontaneously in patients with coagulopathy
    - Or after spontaneous forniceal rupture in acute ureteral obstruction
  - Also after trauma, surgery, interventional procedure
  - May compress kidney and cause renal dysfunction
  - Perirenal or subcapsular collection of blood, urine, lymphatic or serous fluid
  - Hematomas have variable echogenicity
  - Other collections are hypoechoic to anechoic
  - Color/power Doppler helpful to identify kidney
- **Acute Renal Transplant Rejection**
  - Swollen and hypoechoic kidney
  - Urothelial thickening
  - Resistive index may be elevated
  - Color perfusion may be decreased
  - Diagnosis requires biopsy
- **Acute Renal Vein Thrombosis**
  - Enlarged and relatively hypoechoic native or transplant kidney
  - Usually segmental or subsegmental venous thrombus
  - Abnormally high resistive index with reversal of arterial flow in diastole
  - Absence of venous flow, complete or partial
  - Secondary to hypercoagulability
    - Direct tumor invasion from renal or adrenal carcinoma
    - Nephrotic syndrome
    - Dehydration and sepsis in children particularly
  - After renal transplantation
    - May be iatrogenic from surgical injury or technical difficulties
    - May be due to fluid collections or compartment syndrome
- **Acute Renal Artery Thrombosis**
  - May affect main or segmental artery of native or transplant renal artery
  - Main renal artery embolism results in swollen kidney with decreased renal echogenicity
  - Absence of color flow may be segmental or total
  - Secondary to dissection, trauma, embolism, hypotension
  - After renal transplantation
    - Etiologic factors as above
    - Additionally associated with severe acute or chronic rejection
- **Renal Cell Carcinoma**
  - Variable size and echogenicity
  - Large tumors tend to be hypoechoic and can be necrotic
  - Smaller tumors are more echogenic
- **Upper Tract Urothelial Carcinoma**
  - Typically soft tissue mass in renal pelvis
  - Causes obstruction, resulting in hydronephrosis
  - Aggressive tumors can diffusely infiltrate kidney with preservation of renal contour
- **Multiple Myeloma**

- Bilateral nephromegaly
- Decreased echogenicity
- Nephrocalcinosis or urate calculi may be present
- **Renal Leukemia**
  - Leukemia may cause diffuse hypoechoic enlargement or focal masses
- **Renal Lymphoma**
  - Hypoechoic enlarged kidneys represent one phenotype of renal lymphoma
  - Associated with lymphadenopathy and perirenal rind
  - Rarely confined to kidneys
- **Hypoechoic Renal Fat With Atrophic Kidneys**
  - Prominent hypoechoic perirenal fat may be mistaken for kidneys when kidneys are atrophic and indistinct

Helpful Clues for Rare Diagnoses

- **Acute Amyloidosis**
  - Uncommon disease
  - Amyloid deposition is common in kidneys, particularly glomeruli
  - Amyloid nephropathy associated with proteinuria and renal insufficiency
  - Enlarged hypoechoic kidney due to deposition of amyloid fibrils
  - Later, kidneys may be echogenic and small
- **Acute Cortical Necrosis**
  - Hypoechoic cortex
  - Loss of corticomedullary differentiation
  - May subsequently become calcified
- **Xanthogranulomatous Pyelonephritis**
  - Enlarged kidney with dilated calyces
  - Staghorn calculus, perinephric collection
  - Hypoechoic/anechoic round collections
  - Chronic obstruction secondary to calculus with infection and development of cystic spaces

SELECTED REFERENCES

1. Hammond NA et al: Imaging of adrenal and renal hemorrhage. Abdom Imaging. 40(7):2747-60, 2015
2. Rodgers SK et al: Ultrasonographic evaluation of the renal transplant. Radiol Clin North Am. 52(6):1307-24, 2014
3. Dedekam E et al: Primary renal lymphoma mimicking a subcapsular hematoma: a case report. J Radiol Case Rep. 7(8):18-26, 2013
4. Bach AG et al: Prevalence and patterns of renal involvement in imaging of malignant lymphoproliferative diseases. Acta Radiol. 53(3):343-8, 2012
5. Herts BR: Renal lymphoma presenting as an incidental renal mass. J Urol. 188(1):271-3, 2012
6. Le O et al: Common and uncommon adult unilateral renal masses other than renal cell carcinoma. Cancer Imaging. 12:194-204, 2012
7. Piscaglia F et al: The EFSUMB Guidelines and Recommendations on the Clinical Practice of Contrast Enhanced Ultrasound (CEUS): update 2011 on non-hepatic applications. Ultraschall Med. 33(1):33-59, 2012
8. Raman SP et al: Beyond renal cell carcinoma: rare and unusual renal masses. Abdom Imaging. 37(5):873-84, 2012
9. Roy A et al: Common and uncommon bilateral adult renal masses. Cancer Imaging. 12:205-11, 2012
10. Smith AD et al: Bosniak category IIF and III cystic renal lesions: outcomes and associations. Radiology. 262(1):152-60, 2012
11. Taneja R et al: Common and less-common renal masses and masslike conditions. Radiol Clin North Am. 50(2):245-57, v-vi, 2012
12. Elsayes KM et al: Imaging of renal transplant: utility and spectrum of diagnostic findings. Curr Probl Diagn Radiol. 40(3):127-39, 2011
13. Israel GM et al: The incidental renal mass. Radiol Clin North Am. 49(2):369-83, 2011
14. Kitazono MT et al: CT of unusual renal masses invading the pelvicaliceal system: potential mimics of upper tract transitional cell carcinoma. Clin Imaging. 35(1):77-80, 2011

Acute Pyelonephritis

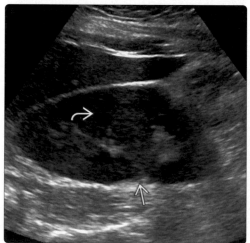

Severe Fatty Liver (Mimic)

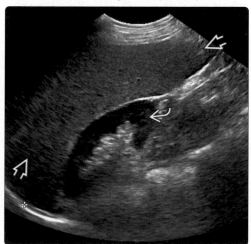

(Left) Longitudinal ultrasound of the right kidney in acute uncomplicated pyelonephritis shows an enlarged hypoechoic kidney ➡ with loss of corticomedullary differentiation ➡. (Right) Longitudinal ultrasound shows a large fatty liver ➡ causing the normal right kidney to appear hypoechoic ➡.

(Left) *Longitudinal ultrasound of the right kidney in a patient with sepsis, liver disease, and acute kidney injury shows loss of corticomedullary differentiation and a perirenal rind of fluid* ➡ *in addition to ascites* ➡. **(Right)** *Longitudinal ultrasound of a renal transplant with delayed graft function from acute tubular necrosis shows loss of corticomedullary differentiation* ➡.

Renal Parenchymal Disease

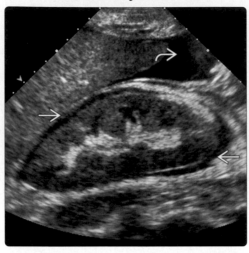

Renal Parenchymal Disease

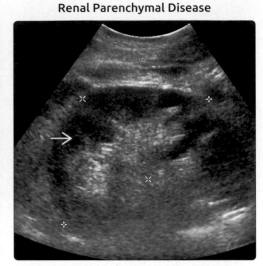

(Left) *Longitudinal ultrasound of the right renal fossa shows a hypoechoic reniform structure* ➡ *with some posterior acoustic enhancement* ➡. *Normal kidney could not be seen.* **(Right)** *Axial T2 HASTE MR in the same patient shows a large subcapsular collection* ➡ *compressing the kidney* ➡. *Drainage of the collection revealed abscess.*

Perinephric Hematoma or Other Fluid Collection

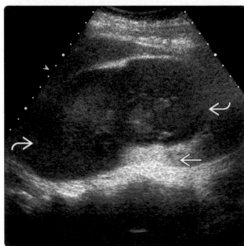

Perinephric Hematoma or Other Fluid Collection

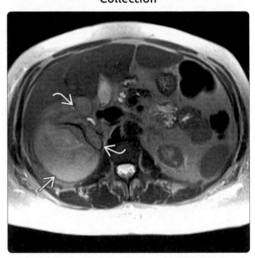

(Left) *Longitudinal ultrasound of a renal transplant with acute renal vein thrombosis shows renal edema* ➡ *and urothelial thickening* ➡. *Percutaneous ultrasound-guided biopsy showed cell-mediated rejection.* **(Right)** *Longitudinal power Doppler ultrasound of a renal transplant shows almost complete absence of intrarenal flow with a patent segmental artery* ➡. *The kidney is swollen and hypoechoic.*

Acute Renal Transplant Rejection

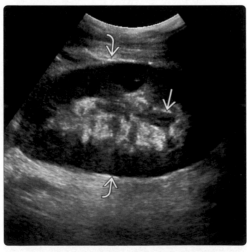

Acute Renal Vein Thrombosis

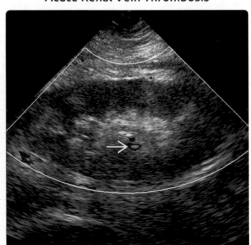

Acute Renal Artery Thrombosis

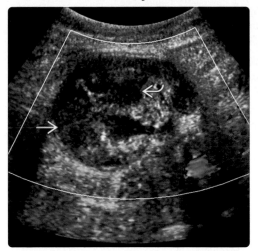

Renal Cell Carcinoma

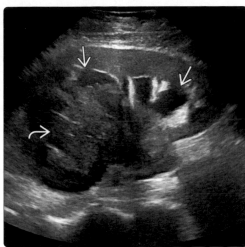

(Left) *Transverse color Doppler ultrasound of a renal transplant shows complete absence of intrarenal color flow secondary to renal artery thrombosis. The cortex ➡ and pyramids ➡ are hypoechoic.* (Right) *Longitudinal ultrasound of the right kidney shows an isoechoic solid mass in the upper to mid pole ➡ extending into the sinus and causing hydronephrosis ➡. Top differential diagnoses are renal cell and urothelial carcinoma. Biopsy showed renal cell carcinoma.*

Upper Tract Urothelial Carcinoma

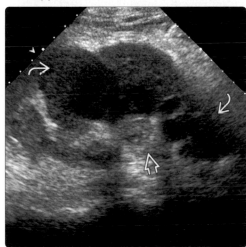

Renal Leukemia

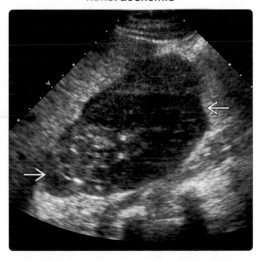

(Left) *Longitudinal ultrasound of the left kidney shows hydronephrosis and cortical thinning ➡. The obstruction was caused by a solid mass in the renal pelvis ➡ representing urothelial cancer.* (Right) *Longitudinal oblique ultrasound shows an enlarged hypoechoic kidney ➡ with loss of corticomedullary differentiation and sinus echogenicity. Biopsy showed acute myeloid leukemia.*

Renal Lymphoma

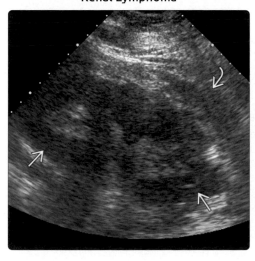

Xanthogranulomatous Pyelonephritis

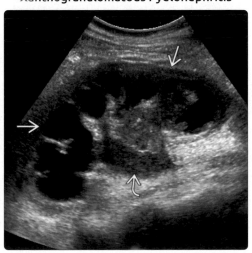

(Left) *Longitudinal ultrasound of the left kidney ➡ shows an enlarged (14 cm) hypoechoic kidney secondary to infiltrating lymphoma. Note the perirenal soft tissue rind ➡.* (Right) *Longitudinal ultrasound of the kidney shows hydronephrosis and cortical atrophy ➡ with avascular soft tissue ➡ in the renal pelvis. There were stones as well. These findings are indistinguishable from pelvic urothelial carcinoma and further evaluation is needed.*

DIFFERENTIAL DIAGNOSIS

Common

- Diabetic Nephropathy
- Chronic Glomerular Diseases
- Hypertensive Nephrosclerosis
- Acute Interstitial Nephritis
- Acute Tubular Necrosis
- Medullary Nephrocalcinosis
- Cortical Nephrocalcinosis
- Acute Pyelonephritis
- Reflux Nephropathy

Less Common

- Vasculitis
- Ischemia
- Lupus Nephritis
- Chronic Renal Transplant Rejection/Chronic Allograft Nephropathy
- Sarcoidosis
- Multicystic Dysplastic Kidney
- HIV Nephropathy
- Acute Cortical Necrosis

Rare but Important

- Emphysematous Pyelonephritis
- Autosomal Recessive Polycystic Kidney Disease
- Oxalosis
- Alport Syndrome
- Renal Amyloidosis
- Renal Tuberculosis
- Lithium Nephropathy
- Renal Cystic Dysplasia

ESSENTIAL INFORMATION

Key Differential Diagnosis Issues

- Increased renal echogenicity is most commonly diffuse and secondary to medical renal disease
- Cortical echogenicity greater than liver is abnormal
- Progresses through loss of corticomedullary differentiation (CMD)
- Pyramids may be dark, later bright
- Cortical echogenicity equal to sinus fat is markedly abnormal
- Secondary to multiple diseases
  - Tubular, glomerular or interstitial intrinsic renal disease
  - End result of obstruction, ischemia
  - Calcification: Cortical, medullary, interstitial, vascular
- Increased renal echogenicity indicates abnormal kidneys but not any particular cause
- Echogenicity correlates well with interstitial disease but not with glomerular disease
- Degree of echogenicity correlates poorly with severity of renal impairment
- Renal biopsy indispensable in diagnosis of renal parenchymal disease
- Role of ultrasound
  - Determine renal size and cortical thickness
    - Differentiating acute from chronic renal insufficiency
  - Exclude ureteral obstruction

- Large, hyperechoic kidneys: Diabetes, HIV, acute inflammation
- Small, hyperechoic kidneys nonspecific
- Differentiate from focal areas of increased echogenicity, e.g., medullary, cortical, or lesional

Helpful Clues for Common Diagnoses

- **Diabetic Nephropathy**
  - Single most important cause of renal failure in adults
  - Diabetes involves glomerulus, interstitium and vessels
  - Early: Normal or enlarged kidneys with preserved cortical thickness
  - Chronic: Small, echogenic kidney with thin cortex and variable CMD
  - ↑ resistive index (RI) on Doppler studies with ↑ cortical echogenicity
- **Chronic Glomerular Diseases**
  - Multiple pathologic entities and multiple diseases
    - Immunoglobulin A (IgA) disease most common type of idiopathic glomerulonephritis (GN)
    - Focal segmental glomerulosclerosis may be idiopathic or secondary to hypertension or reflux nephropathy
    - Membranous nephropathy most common cause of idiopathic nephrotic syndrome in Caucasians
  - Acute: Normal/enlarged kidney with normal or ↑ renal echogenicity
  - CMD disappears with chronic disease: Small echogenic kidney
- **Hypertensive Nephrosclerosis**
  - 25% of end-stage renal disease
  - Renal echogenicity depends on chronicity
  - ↑ RI with ↑ cortical echogenicity
- **Acute Interstitial Nephritis**
  - Hypersensitivity reaction to drug or infective antigen
  - Mimics acute tubular necrosis clinically
  - Kidney size may be normal or enlarged
  - Cortical echogenicity may be increased depending on severity of reaction
- **Acute Tubular Necrosis**
  - May be normal or increased in echogenicity
- **Medullary Nephrocalcinosis**
  - Cause: Hyperparathyroidism, renal tubular acidosis, medullary sponge kidney, vitamin D excess, gout, sarcoidosis, bone metastases
  - ↑ echogenicity of renal medullae compared to hypoechoic cortex, reversal of normal
  - Acoustic shadowing
- **Cortical Nephrocalcinosis**
  - Focal: Caused by trauma, infarction, or infection
  - Diffuse: Due to renal cortical necrosis, kidney transplant rejection, chronic GN, Alport syndrome
  - Characterized by peripheral parenchymal calcifications and ↑ cortical echogenicity
- **Acute Pyelonephritis**
  - Normal/swollen kidney with typically decreased echogenicity and loss of normal CMD
  - Focal areas of increased echogenicity may be seen but more commonly hypoechoic
  - Thickened urothelium and mild hydronephrosis
- **Reflux Nephropathy**
  - Secondary to interstitial nephritis caused by reflux

o Echogenic cortex, dilated calyces with overlying cortical scarring

Helpful Clues for Less Common Diagnoses

- **Vasculitis**
  o Polyarteritis nodosa, Wegener granulomatosis
  o Small kidneys with ↑ cortical echogenicity
  o May have focal scarring and fibrosis
- **Ischemia**
  o Renal artery stenosis or fibromuscular dysplasia
    - Low intrarenal RI, tardus parvus waveform
  o Renal vein thrombosis
    - Absent venous flow, reversal of arterial diastolic flow
  o Renal artery thrombosis
    - Global or segmental loss of arterial flow
  o Asymmetrical, initially enlarged and hypoechoic
  o Later, small and hyperechoic with global decreased perfusion
  o May have segmental wedge-shaped areas of scarring and decreased perfusion
- **Lupus Nephritis**
  o Acute: Renal echogenicity and size are nonspecific
  o Chronic: Small and echogenic kidney
- **Chronic Renal Transplant Rejection/Chronic Allograft Nephropathy**
  o End result of rejection and other insults
  o Occurs months to years after transplantation
  o Results in interstitial fibrosis
  o Echogenic kidney with decrease in size and perfusion ± calcifications
- **Multicystic Dysplastic Kidney**
  o Initially unilateral multicystic lesion with hyperechoic dysplastic renal parenchyma
  o Later cysts shrink and parenchyma remains echogenic
- **HIV Nephropathy**
  o Occurs almost exclusively in African American descent
  o Present with nephrotic syndrome and may progress rapidly to end-stage renal disease
  o Typically **large** echogenic kidneys with preserved CMD
  o Later sinus blends with cortex and kidneys become small

- **Acute Cortical Necrosis**
  o Subcapsular area spared, hypoechoic rim initially
  o Rapid cortical calcification may ensue: Curvilinear/shadowing
  o Diffuse ↑ parenchymal echogenicity

Helpful Clues for Rare Diagnoses

- **Emphysematous Pyelonephritis**
  o Diabetes, immunocompromise, clinical picture of sepsis
  o Gas-forming necrotizing renal infection
  o Diffuse or segmental
  o Bright echoes with posterior dirty shadowing
- **Autosomal Recessive Polycystic Kidney Disease**
  o Detected prenatally by ultrasound
  o Symmetrically enlarged echogenic kidneys
  o Innumerable small cysts
  o Echogenicity increased due to multiple reflections from small cyst walls
- **Oxalosis**
  o Characterized by combined cortical and medullary nephrocalcinosis
  o Hyperechoic kidneys; absent CMD
- **Alport Syndrome**
  o Inherited disease with hematuria, proteinuria, hypertension, and deafness
  o Initially normal kidneys, later small and echogenic
- **Renal Amyloidosis**
  o Enlarged kidneys in acute phase, ↓ cortical echogenicity
  o Chronic: ↓ renal size and ↑ echogenicity
- **Renal Tuberculosis**
  o Chronic parenchymal atrophy, hydronephrosis, calcifications
  o Calcified small kidney "autonephrectomy"
- **Lithium Nephropathy**
  o Innumerable tiny cysts in cortex and medulla of **normal-sized** kidneys
  o Cysts produce bright punctate echoes

Diabetic Nephropathy

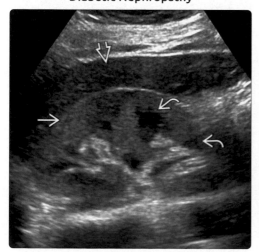

Chronic Glomerular Diseases

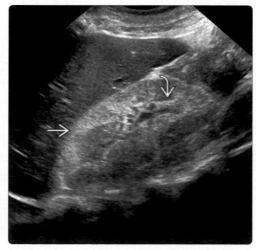

(Left) Longitudinal ultrasound of a normal-sized right kidney in early chronic kidney disease is shown. The renal cortex ➡ is isoechoic to slightly hyperechoic to the liver ➡. Pyramids ➡ are prominent. These findings are common in medical renal disease and not specific as to cause. (Right) Longitudinal ultrasound of a normal-sized right kidney with diffuse increase in cortical echogenicity ➡ is shown. Pyramids are not conspicuous. The renal sinus ➡ is barely seen.

(Left) *Longitudinal ultrasound shows increased cortical and medullary echogenicity ➡, equal to sinus fat in an enlarged kidney. There is perinephric fluid ➡ in a patient with nephrotic syndrome and HIV. Biopsy showed focal glomerulosclerosis.* (Right) *Longitudinal ultrasound of a small right kidney ➡ with diffuse increase in cortical echogenicity is shown. The cortex is thin and slightly lobulated ➡. This is compatible with established renal failure.*

Chronic Glomerular Diseases

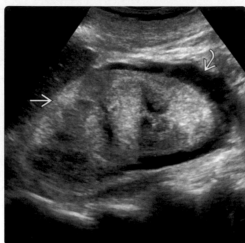

Hypertensive Nephrosclerosis

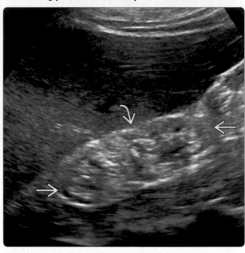

(Left) *Longitudinal ultrasound shows hyperechoic pyramids ➡ with some shadowing ➡. The cortex ➡ is less echogenic than the pyramids in medullary sponge kidney.* (Right) *Longitudinal ultrasound of the right kidney in a patient with end-stage renal failure and ascites ➡ is shown. There is calcification of the renal cortex ➡ causing significant shadowing ➡.*

Medullary Nephrocalcinosis

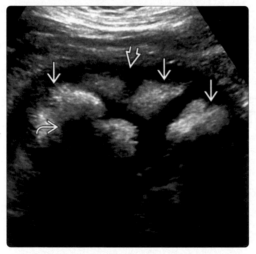

Cortical Nephrocalcinosis

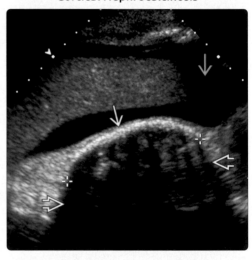

(Left) *Longitudinal ultrasound of a failed renal transplant shows a small kidney with cortical ➡ and diffuse parenchymal calcifications ➡. It is important not to confuse this for a calcified tumor.* (Right) *Axial NECT of the same patient shows the atrophic transplant kidney with coarse ➡ and peripheral ➡ calcifications.*

Chronic Renal Transplant Rejection/Chronic Allograft Nephropathy

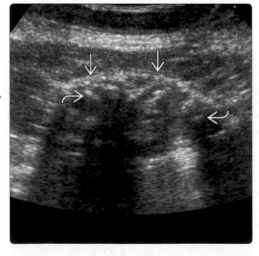

Chronic Renal Transplant Rejection/Chronic Allograft Nephropathy

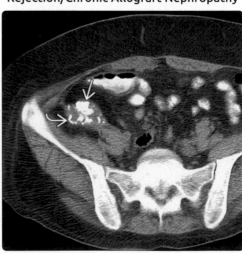

Chronic Glomerular Diseases

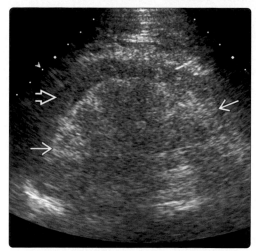

HIV Nephropathy

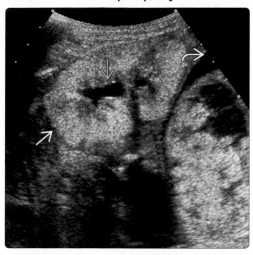

(Left) *Longitudinal ultrasound after biopsy of the kidney is shown. There is a very echogenic kidney* ➡ *with a hypoechoic perinephric hematoma* ➡, *which was managed conservatively. Biopsy revealed focal glomerulosclerosis. The noisy image results from diffuse edema/nephrotic syndrome.* (Right) *Longitudinal US of the left kidney in a patient with AIDS & renal failure is shown. The left kidney* ➡ *is small and markedly increased in echogenicity with pelviectasis* ➡. *There is a small amount of ascites* ➡.

Emphysematous Pyelonephritis

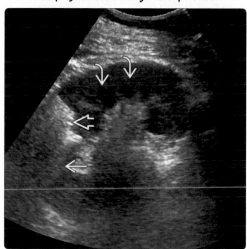

Autosomal Recessive Polycystic Kidney Disease

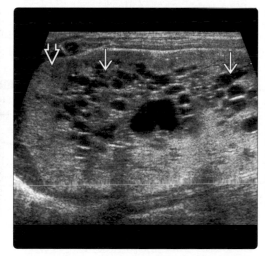

(Left) *Longitudinal ultrasound of a renal transplant shows normal pyramids* ➡ *in the lower pole. In the upper pole, there is an area of increased echogenicity* ➡ *with shadowing* ➡ *representing gas from segmental emphysematous pyelonephritis.* (Right) *Longitudinal ultrasound of the kidney in a neonate shows an enlarged hyperechoic kidney* ➡ *with innumerable tiny cysts* ➡. *The other kidney was the same.*

Lithium Nephropathy

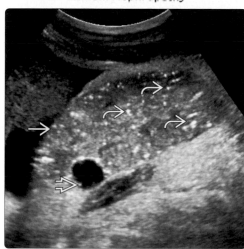

Ischemia

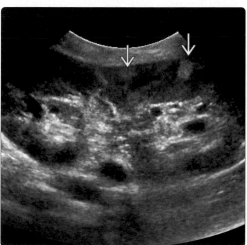

(Left) *Longitudinal ultrasound shows a hyperechoic right kidney* ➡ *with innumerable tiny echogenic nonshadowing foci* ➡ *representing microcysts. A larger cyst* ➡ *was also present.* (Right) *Longitudinal ultrasound of a renal transplant shows hyperechoic wedge-shaped cortical lesions* ➡. *Multiple cortical infarcts were found on biopsy.*

DIFFERENTIAL DIAGNOSIS

Common

- Column of Bertin
- Renal Junction Line, Junctional Parenchymal Defect
- Fetal Lobulation
- Dromedary Hump
- Hypertrophy Next to Scar
- Focal Pyelonephritis/Abscess

Less Common

- Crossed Fused Ectopia
- Hematoma
- Arteriovenous Malformation
- Focal Xanthogranulomatous Pyelonephritis
- Extramedullary Hematopoiesis
- Splenorenal Fusion

ESSENTIAL INFORMATION

Key Differential Diagnosis Issues

- Differentiate pseudotumors composed of normal variants from nonneoplastic lesions mimicking renal masses
- Note typical locations of normal variant pseudotumors
- Rare to have mass effect or distortion of normal architecture/vessels

Helpful Clues for Common Diagnoses

- **Column of Bertin**
  - Isoechoic, continuous with renal cortex, normal renal outline
  - No abnormal vascularity on color Doppler
  - Junction of upper and middle 1/3 of kidney
  - Changing sonographic window may clarify nature
- **Renal Junction Line, Junctional Parenchymal Defect**
  - Echogenic line at anterosuperior aspect of kidney without disruption of renal contour or cortical loss
  - Junction of upper and middle 1/3 of kidney and right side most common location
  - Junctional parenchymal defect: Triangular echogenic defect in renal cortex, upper to mid 1/3

  - Cine clips are helpful for confirmation
- **Fetal Lobulation**
  - Multiple indentations in renal outline, between renal pyramids or calyces; preserved cortical thickness
  - Distinguished from scars of pyelonephritis, which are directly over calyces with thinned cortex
- **Dromedary Hump**
  - Only occurs in left kidney: "Splenic hump"
  - Focal bulge in lateral border of midpole of left kidney with similar echogenicity as rest of kidney
  - Calyces extend laterally into hump, which contains normal vessels, unlike tumor
- **Hypertrophy Next to Scar**
  - Hypertrophied normal renal tissue adjacent to area of cortical loss
  - Similar echogenicity to normal parenchyma without vascular distortion
- **Focal Pyelonephritis/Abscess**
  - Pyelonephritis: Cortical hypo-/hyperechoic lesion with decreased color Doppler flow, lacking external bulge
  - Abscess: Thick-walled cystic lesion, clinical correlation essential, may need aspiration

Helpful Clues for Less Common Diagnoses

- **Crossed Fused Ectopia**
  - Kidney-like morphology, absence of contralateral kidney
- **Hematoma**
  - Echogenicity varies with age, avascular
- **Arteriovenous Malformation**
  - Tubular, internal color flow
- **Focal Xanthogranulomatous Pyelonephritis**
  - Hypoechoic lesion with calculi
- **Extramedullary Hematopoiesis**
  - Single or multiple lesions in patients with hematolologic disease, may require biopsy for diagnosis

Alternative Differential Approaches

- Consider CECT, CEUS, or CEMR if ultrasound is nondiagnostic
- Clinical correlation is essential

Column of Bertin

Column of Bertin

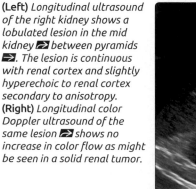

(Left) Longitudinal ultrasound of the right kidney shows a lobulated lesion in the mid kidney ⬈ between pyramids ⬈. The lesion is continuous with renal cortex and slightly hyperechoic to renal cortex secondary to anisotropy. (Right) Longitudinal color Doppler ultrasound of the same lesion ⬈ shows no increase in color flow as might be seen in a solid renal tumor.

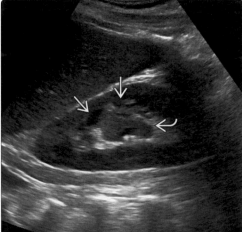

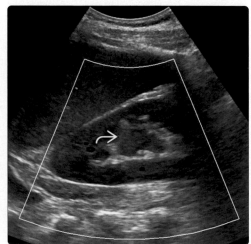

Column of Bertin

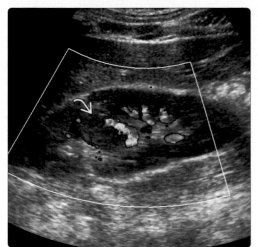

Column of Bertin

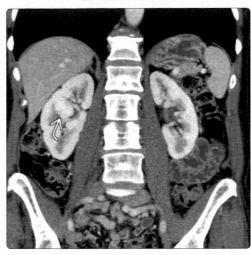

(Left) *Longitudinal color Doppler ultrasound of the right kidney shows a lesion* ➔ *that is isoechoic to cortex with no internal color flow.* (Right) *Coronal CECT of the same patient confirms that the lesion* ➔ *represents cortical tissue as it was isodense to cortex on all phases of the multiphasic CECT.*

Fetal Lobulation

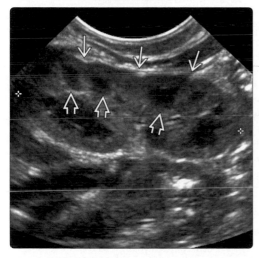

Focal Pyelonephritis/Abscess

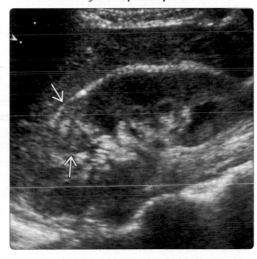

(Left) *Longitudinal ultrasound of the left kidney in a neonate shows fetal lobulation. The cortical indentations* ➔ *are located between pyramids* ➔*.* (Right) *Longitudinal ultrasound of right kidney shows a focal wedge-shaped area of increased cortical echogenicity* ➔ *in a patient with fever and pain from acute pyelonephritis.*

Dromedary Hump

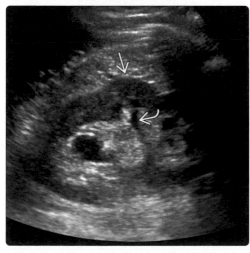

Dromedary Hump

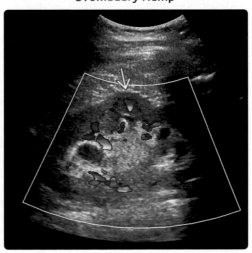

(Left) *Longitudinal ultrasound of the left kidney shows an exophytic hump on the anterior mid pole* ➔*. There is mild hydronephrosis with a calyx* ➔ *extending into the hump.* (Right) *Longitudinal color Doppler ultrasound of the same kidney shows no distortion of vascular supply in the dromedary hump* ➔*.*

DIFFERENTIAL DIAGNOSIS

Common

- Obstructed Renal Pelvis
- Reflux Into Dilated Renal Pelvis
- Extrarenal Pelvis
- Physiologic Distention of Renal Pelvis
- Parapelvic Cyst
- Prominent Renal Vessel
- Urothelial Carcinoma

Less Common

- Pyonephrosis
- Hemonephrosis
- Renal Sinus Hemorrhage
- Pararenal Fluid Collections
- Peripelvic Cyst
- Intrarenal Abscess
- Calyceal Diverticulum
- Acute Renal Vein Thrombosis

Rare but Important

- Pyelogenic Cyst
- Multilocular Cystic Nephroma
- Lucent Sinus Lipomatosis
- Renal Lymphoma
- Retroperitoneal Lymphoma
- Renal Artery Aneurysm
- Arteriovenous Malformation
- Intrarenal Varices
- Renal Lymphangiomatosis

ESSENTIAL INFORMATION

Key Differential Diagnosis Issues

- Important to differentiate between obstruction and nonobstruction
  - Follow ureter to level of obstruction to determine cause
- Ultrasound is 1st-line modality for detection but other modalities such as CT, MR, VCUG, and retrograde pyelography may be required for definitive diagnosis
- Nuclear scintigraphy differentiates obstruction from nonobstructive dilatation

Helpful Clues for Common Diagnoses

- **Obstructed Renal Pelvis**
  - Isolated dilatation of renal pelvis is uncommon
  - Dilatation elsewhere in GU tract determined by level of obstruction
    - For example, ureteropelvic junction obstruction manifests with pelvic dilatation and (to lesser degree) calyceal dilatation
    - Ureterovesical junction obstruction presents with hydroureter as well as pelvicalyceal dilatation
  - Determine if unilateral or bilateral
  - Level of obstruction helps narrow differential diagnosis
  - Most common cause of unilateral obstruction is stone disease
  - Other causes include bladder, ureteral or other pelvic mass, retroperitoneal mass or hemorrhage, aortic aneurysm, retroperitoneal fibrosis, iatrogenic injury
- **Reflux Into Dilated Renal Pelvis**

- Hydroureter may be present in addition to renal pelvic dilatation
  - VCUG essential in determining reflux
    - In future, contrast-enhanced voiding urosonography may be used in place of VCUG to evaluate for reflux without use of ionizing radiation
- **Extrarenal Pelvis**
  - Common finding in neonates and often incidentally noted in other age groups
    - Renal pelvis projects medial to renal sinus
  - Appearance may simulate early obstruction, but calyces are not dilated
- **Physiologic Distension of Renal Pelvis**
  - Commonly noted when bladder is distended
    - Frequent in pregnant patients, most commonly in 3rd trimester; R > L
    - Fetal pyelectasis can result in mild pelvic dilatation in neonates, which subsequently resolves
- **Parapelvic Cyst**
  - 1-3% of renal parenchymal cysts; usually solitary
  - May be mixed picture, as parapelvic cysts can compress collecting system resulting in true dilatation
- **Prominent Renal Vessel**
  - May mimic pelvic dilatation, but color Doppler denotes flow
    - Protocol advice: Always remember to use color Doppler when concerned about pelvic dilatation or cystic lesion to distinguish from vessel
- **Urothelial Carcinoma**
  - Hypoechoic mass in dilated pelvis, though usually slightly hyperechoic to renal parenchyma
  - Can mimic hemorrhage or pus
  - On color Doppler, note internal vascularity within urothelial carcinoma

Helpful Clues for Less Common Diagnoses

- **Pyonephrosis**
  - Debris (pus) in dilated pelvicalyceal system
  - Look for presence of urothelial thickening and cause such as stone
- **Hemonephrosis**
  - Blood within dilated pelvicalyceal system ± blood in bladder
  - Echogenicity variable depending upon age of blood products
- **Renal Sinus Hemorrhage**
  - In absence of trauma, most often secondary to anticoagulation, but can be secondary to occult neoplasm, vasculitis, or blood dyscrasia
  - Cystic lesion of variable echogenicity disrupting normal central echocomplex, with mass effect upon renal pelvis and tension upon infundibula
  - Should spontaneously resolve in 3-4 weeks
- **Pararenal Fluid Collections**
  - May occur in setting of infection, obstruction, or transplantation; include urinoma, hematoma, abscess, and lymphocele near renal hilum
- **Peripelvic Cyst**
  - Lymphatic collection in renal sinus, distinct from parapelvic cyst, which is intraparenchymal
  - Often multiple and bilateral (unlike parapelvic cyst)

- **Intrarenal Abscess**
  - Hypoechoic parenchymal lesion, which may mimic collecting system dilatation
  - May also be associated with hydronephrosis and urothelial thickening
  - Most often secondary to acute pyelonephritis, but relatively rare
- **Calyceal Diverticulum**
  - Typically upper pole, connects with calyx
    - Lined with transitional cell epithelium
  - May appear like simple cyst or dilated calyx
  - Prone to calculus formation and infection: Containing milk of calcium and debris
  - On excretory phase CT/ MR, VCUG, or retrograde pyelography, diagnostic filling of diverticulum with contrast
- **Acute Renal Vein Thrombosis**
  - Dilated vein with hypoechoic thrombus
    - Chronic thrombosis often demonstrates greater internal echogenicity and organized clot along walls
  - Absent venous color Doppler flow

Helpful Clues for Rare Diagnoses

- **Pyelogenic Cyst**
  - Similar to calyceal diverticulum but communicates with pelvis rather than calyx
- **Multilocular Cystic Nephroma**
  - Encapsulated multilocular cystic renal lesion with internal septa
    - On MR/CT, note enhancement of septa
  - May herniate into renal pelvis, mimicking pelviectasis, or may cause hydronephrosis
- **Lucent Sinus Lipomatosis**
  - Very rarely, renal sinus fat may appear less echogenic than normal and mimic hydronephrosis or hypoechoic mass
    - Secondary to chronic steroid use, obesity, diabetes, renal atrophy, and inflammation
  - More evident when there is chronic kidney disease and hyperechoic kidneys

- **Renal Lymphoma**
  - Multiple forms, including hypoechoic infiltration of renal sinus
    - May mimic dilated renal pelvis or cause hydronephrosis
- **Retroperitoneal Lymphoma**
  - Retroperitoneal adenopathy may demonstrate contiguous extension into renal pelvis, mimicking dilatation of collecting system
  - Distinct from renal lymphoma
- **Renal Artery Aneurysm**
  - Pulsatile fluid-filled structure with diagnostic color/power Doppler
  - Typically small (< 2 cm) and saccular
  - Located at bifurcation of main renal artery
- **Arteriovenous Malformation**
  - Congenital malformation which appears hypoechoic on grayscale ultrasound
  - Color Doppler flow reveals hypervascular mass with aliasing
- **Intrarenal Varices**
  - May present as cystic renal mass
  - May mimic hydronephrosis
  - Associated with arteriovenous malformation
- **Renal Lymphangiomatosis**
  - Multiple cystic lesions in both parapelvic and perirenal areas
  - Related to lymphatic obstruction

SELECTED REFERENCES

1. Ma TL et al: Parapelvic cyst misdiagnosed as hydronephrosis. Clin Kidney J. 6(2):238-9, 2013
2. Darge K et al: Pediatric uroradiology: state of the art. Pediatr Radiol. 41(1):82-91, 2011
3. Sheth S et al: Imaging of renal lymphoma: patterns of disease with pathologic correlation. Radiographics. 26(4):1151-68, 2006
4. Browne RF et al: Transitional cell carcinoma of the upper urinary tract: spectrum of imaging findings. Radiographics. 25(6):1609-27, 2005
5. Rha SE et al: The renal sinus: pathologic spectrum and multimodality imaging approach. Radiographics. 24 Suppl 1:S117-31. Review, 2004
6. Nahm AM et al: The renal sinus cyst-the great imitator. Nephrol Dial Transplant. 15(6):913-4, 2000

Obstructed Renal Pelvis

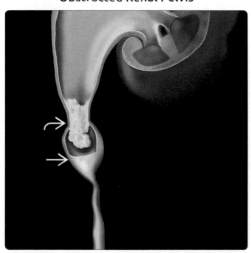

Obstructed Renal Pelvis

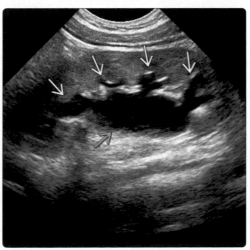

(Left) *Graphic shows an obstructing polypoid tumor ➡ at the ureteropelvic junction. The proximal ureter is dilated around the tumor, producing the goblet sign ➡. (Right) Longitudinal ultrasound demonstrates hydronephrosis, with pelvic dilatation ➡ to a greater degree than calyceal dilatation ➡, consistent with UPJ obstruction.*

Reflux Into Dilated Renal Pelvis

Reflux Into Dilated Renal Pelvis

(**Left**) *Longitudinal ultrasound of the left kidney demonstrates pelvic* ⇨ *and calyceal* ⇥ *dilatation.* (**Right**) *VCUG evaluation in the same patient reveals left grade 4 reflux.*

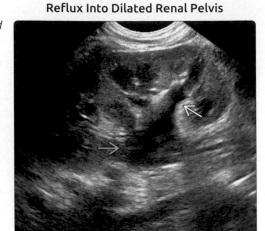

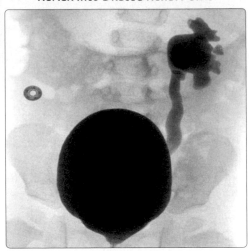

Extrarenal Pelvis

Extrarenal Pelvis

(**Left**) *Longitudinal color Doppler ultrasound demonstrates an anechoic central structure in the left kidney without flow* ⇨ *distinct from the central sinus fat* ⇥*, representing extrarenal pelvis.* (**Right**) *Axial contrast-enhanced CT obtained in the same patient demonstrates left extrarenal pelvis* ⇨*.*

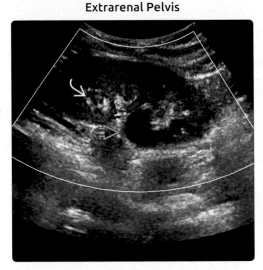

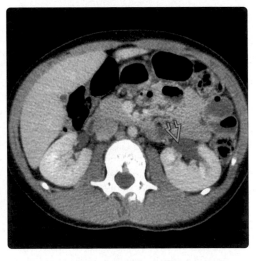

Parapelvic Cyst

Parapelvic Cyst

(**Left**) *On longitudinal ultrasound, note large anechoic structure in the upper pole and interpolar region* ⇨*.* (**Right**) *Coronal contrast-enhanced CT in the same patient reveals a discrete cyst in the upper pole of the left kidney* ⇨ *approaching the pelvis, representing parapelvic cyst.*

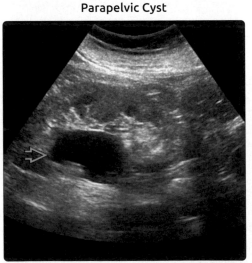

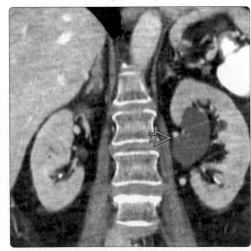

Pyonephrosis

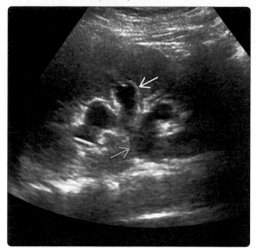

Pyonephrosis

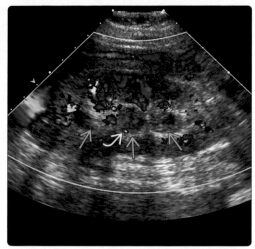

(Left) *Longitudinal ultrasound of the right kidney demonstrates low-level echoes in the dilated renal pelvis ⇨ representing pyonephrosis. Note urothelial thickening ➨, an ancillary finding of urinary tract infection.* (Right) *Longitudinal color Doppler ultrasound shows hypoechoic tissue filling the dilated renal collecting system ⇨ with internal color flow ➨ distinguishing this material as neoplasm rather than avascular pus or clot.*

Calyceal Diverticulum

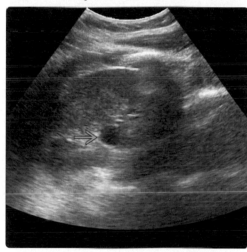

Calyceal Diverticulum

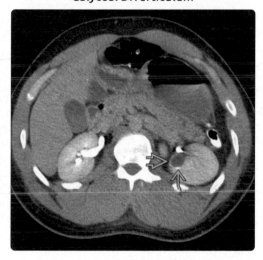

(Left) *Longitudinal ultrasound demonstrates an anechoic structure in the interpolar region of the left kidney ⇨. Given this image alone, one might suspect pelviectasis or a simple cyst.* (Right) *In this CT obtained in the same patient, however, one can appreciate a small amount of layering contrast ⇨ within the lesion ⇨ on excretory phase imaging, confirming calyceal diverticulum.*

Multilocular Cystic Nephroma

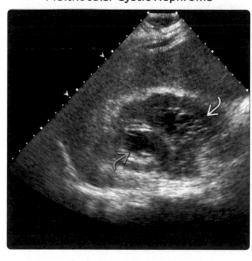

Multilocular Cystic Nephroma

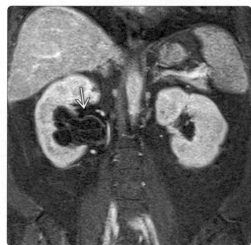

(Left) *Longitudinal ultrasound demonstrates dilatation of the renal pelvis ⇨, which contains a cystic mass with thin internal septa ➨.* (Right) *Coronal contrast-enhanced T1-weighted MR in the same patient shows a mass demonstrating septal enhancement ➨ entering the renal pelvis. Histopathology revealed multilocular cystic nephroma.*

DIFFERENTIAL DIAGNOSIS

Common

- Renal Angiomyolipoma
- Renal Cell Carcinoma

Less Common

- Fat in Renal Scar
- Renal Junctional Line/Cortical Parenchymal Defect
- Renal Calculi
- Medullary Sponge Kidney
- Column of Bertin
- Renal Papillary Necrosis
- Complex Cyst/Milk of Calcium Cyst
- Emphysematous Pyelonephritis
- Renal Metastases
- Wilms Tumor

Rare but Important

- Focal Bacterial Nephritis
- Xanthogranulomatous Pyelonephritis
- Tuberculosis, Urinary Tract
- Renal Oncocytoma
- Renal Trauma

ESSENTIAL INFORMATION

Key Differential Diagnosis Issues

- Same lesions that cause fat-attenuation (intensity) lesions on CT and MR usually cause echogenic lesion on US
  - However, echogenicity alone is not reliable indication of fat content
  - Other sources of renal echogenicity include calcification and gas
  - Lesions with calcification: Milk of calcium cyst, complex renal cysts, renal cell carcinoma (RCC), Wilms tumor
  - Lesions with gas: Renal abscess, emphysematous pyelonephritis

Helpful Clues for Common Diagnoses

- **Renal Angiomyolipoma**
  - Well-defined hyperechoic mass, echogenicity similar to renal sinus
  - Echogenicity created by high fat content and multiple vessel-tissue interfaces
  - May have posterior shadowing: Not typically seen with other masses
  - Echogenicity of small renal angiomyolipoma (AMLs) relative to size typically > small RCCs
  - Larger tumors usually have prominent vascularity, evident on color Doppler
  - May have central necrosis simulating malignant lesion
  - US alone is not reliable in diagnosing AML; significant overlap with RCC
    - Limited met analysis: All noncalcified echogenic renal lesions detected with ultrasound need CT to rule out RCC
    - Recent retrospective review though has called into question utility of follow-up CT (or MR) for echogenic lesions < 1 cm
      - □ < 1-cm echogenic lesions almost invariably benign

- Renal MR (with chemical shift, fat-saturation sequences) also useful to differentiate fat containing AML from RCC
- **Renal Cell Carcinoma**
  - 30% of small RCCs appear as hyperechoic masses, may mimic AML
    - Presence of necrosis in mass, cystic components, or anechoic rim favors RCC but large overlap
  - Larger RCC may have foci of calcification (also echogenic), rarely fat
  - Mass with calcification and fat in adult = RCC, not AML

Helpful Clues for Less Common Diagnoses

- **Fat in Renal Scar**
  - Example: Following partial nephrectomy
    - Fat may be placed into cortical defect
    - Ablation zone post RFA/cryoablation may appear echogenic (fat-halo sign)
- Complex cyst/milk of calcium cyst
  - Bright echogenic reflectors with ring down artifact may be seen within septa of minimally complex renal cysts: May be ignored
  - Milk of calcium cyst: Layering calcification may create fluid/debris level
- **Renal Junctional Line/Cortical Parenchymal Defect**
  - Echogenic line at anterosuperior aspect, upper pole of right kidney, lower pole of left kidney
    - Infolding of renal capsule and fat creates hyperechoic line or mass
  - Also can see extension of renal sinus fat into same location
  - Less commonly appears as triangular focus known as parenchymal defect
- **Renal Calculi**
  - Highly echogenic with sharp posterior shadowing
  - Calculi or milk of calcium may form within calyceal diverticulum, mimic hyperechoic mass
  - Most stones show color and power Doppler twinkling artifacts
    - Useful ancillary finding in equivocal cases (though twinkling may be seen without underlying stone)
- **Medullary Sponge Kidney**
  - Correlate at ultrasound: Echogenic medullary rings
  - Highly echogenic renal medulla: May simulate echogenic mass
- **Column of Bertin**
  - Renal cortex protruding into renal sinus: Between upper and mid calyces
  - Typically isoechoic to cortex, though alterations in tissue orientation change acoustic reflectivity
  - Column may be echogenic when seen en face
    - Power Doppler may confirm cortex origin; CECT for problematic cases
- **Renal Papillary Necrosis**
  - Early stage: Echogenic ring in medulla = necrotic papillae, surrounded by rim of fluid
  - Late stage: Multiple cystic cavities in medullary pyramids ± nonshadowing echogenic sloughed papillae
  - Calcified sloughed papilla with strong acoustic shadowing simulates stone, may cause obstructive hydronephrosis
- **Emphysematous Pyelonephritis**

- Gas within infarcted, infected parenchyma is echogenic
  - Nondependent linear echogenic lines with strong distal posterior acoustic shadowing
- Clinically, extremely ill patient with fever, flank pain, and electrolyte imbalance
- Different from emphysematous pyelitis where gas is limited to renal pelvis and calyces (less serious diagnosis)
- **Renal Metastases**
  - Variable echogenicity, typically hypoperfused masses
  - Look for metastases in other organs
  - Most common primary tumors include lung carcinoma, breast carcinoma, contralateral RCC
- **Wilms Tumor**
  - Highly variable morphology, including echogenic foci (fat &/or calcification)
  - Heterogeneous echotexture with areas of necrosis or hemorrhage
  - Consider Wilms for any renal mass in child (most present before age 5)
  - Most common abdominal malignancy
    - Assess contralateral kidney for synchronous tumor
    - Evaluate renal vein and cava: Tumor thrombus

Helpful Clues for Rare Diagnoses

- **Focal Bacterial Nephritis**
  - Increased echogenicity may be related to hemorrhage
  - Usually wedge-shaped, poorly defined margin, ↓ focal vascularity on power Doppler
  - Can be hypoechoic, related to liquefaction and abscess formation
  - Can be multiple lesions with patchy heterogeneous renal parenchyma
  - Other associated features of renal inflammation: Renal enlargement, urothelial thickening of renal pelvis
- **Xanthogranulomatous Pyelonephritis**
  - Highly reflective central echo complex with strong shadowing corresponding to large staghorn stone
  - Echogenicity depends on amount of debris and necrosis within masses
- **Tuberculosis, Urinary Tract**

- Active stage: Papillary destruction with echogenic masses near calyces
- Late stage: Calcified granuloma or dense dystrophic calcification associated with shrunken kidneys
- **Renal Oncocytoma**
  - Cannot be differentiated from RCC on imaging
  - Variable in echogenicity, may contain central scar, central necrosis, or calcification
- **Renal Trauma**
  - Hematoma can be hyperechoic or heterogeneous during acute phase
  - Regional distortion of corticomedullary differentiation

SELECTED REFERENCES

1. Itani M et al: Sonographically identified echogenic renal masses Up to 1 cm in size are so rarely malignant they can be safely ignored. J Ultrasound Med. 35(2):323-8, 2016
2. Sidhar K et al: Renal cell carcinomas: sonographic appearance depending on size and histologic type. J Ultrasound Med. 35(2):311-20, 2016
3. Bradley AJ et al: Imaging features, follow-up, and management of incidentally detected renal lesions. Clin Radiol. 66(12):1129-39, 2011
4. Craig WD et al: Pyelonephritis: radiologic-pathologic review. Radiographics. 28(1):255-77; quiz 327-8, 2008
5. Farrelly C et al: Do all non-calcified echogenic renal lesions found on ultrasound need further evaluation with CT? Abdom Imaging. 33(1):44-7, 2008
6. Vijayaraghavan SB et al: Sonographic features of necrosed renal papillae causing hydronephrosis. J Ultrasound Med. 22(9):951-6; quiz 957-8, 2003
7. Siegel CL et al: Angiomyolipoma and renal cell carcinoma: US differentiation. Radiology. 198(3):789-93, 1996
8. Yamashita Y et al: Hyperechoic renal tumors: anechoic rim and intratumoral cysts in US differentiation of renal cell carcinoma from angiomyolipoma. Radiology. 188(1):179-82, 1993
9. Yeh HC et al: Junctional parenchyma: revised definition of hypertrophic column of Bertin. Radiology. 185(3):725-32, 1992
10. Yeh HC et al: Milk of calcium in renal cysts: new sonographic features. J Ultrasound Med. 11(5):195-203, 1992

Renal Cell Carcinoma

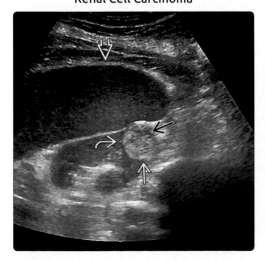

Renal Angiomyolipoma

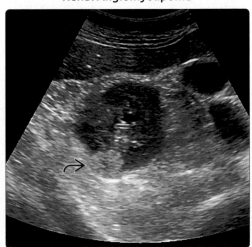

(Left) *Surveillance ultrasound performed on a patient with cirrhosis and splenomegaly ⇶ shows an echogenic left renal lesion ➡. Sonographic features that suggest renal cell carcinoma (RCC) include a hypoechoic halo ⬈ and tiny cystic spaces ➨. Biopsy confirmed clear cell RCC.* (Right) *Ultrasound shows a 1.3-cm uniform, highly echogenic lesion ➨. Although small, highly echogenic, renal lesions are likely AMLs (as in this case), renal CT confirmation is typically recommended to exclude a small RCC.*

Renal Cell Carcinoma

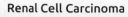

(Left) *Ultrasound of a 55-year-old woman with flank pain shows an echogenic right interpolar renal lesion* ➡. *Note cystic spaces* ➡ *and a halo* ➡. *Partial nephrectomy performed after staging CT confirmed clear cell RCC.*
(Right) *Ultrasound-guided biopsy performed on this echogenic renal lesion* ➡ *prior to cryoablation confirmed clear cell RCC. Large biopsy series have shown that a small minority of echogenic renal lesions that do not contain macroscopic fat at CT still prove to be benign, nonfat-containing AMLs.*

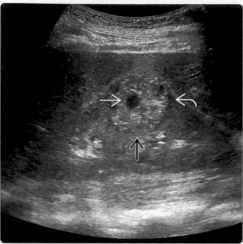

Renal Cell Carcinoma

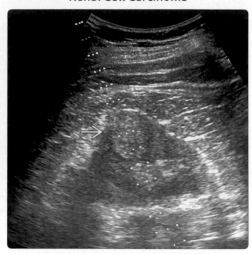

Renal Angiomyolipoma

(Left) *Sagittal and transverse ultrasound of the right kidney shows a < 1-cm, highly echogenic renal lesion* ➡. *Echogenicity is greater than sinus fat. Recent work has suggested that these tiny lesions may be ignored, but current dogma is that targeted NECT confirmation of fat, or ultrasound follow-up are needed.* **(Right)** *Sagittal ultrasound shows many small echogenic angiomyelolipomas* ➡ *in a patient with tuberous sclerosis.*

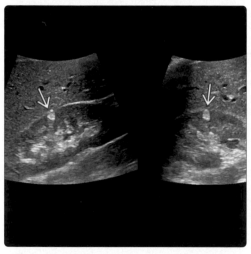

Renal Angiomyolipoma

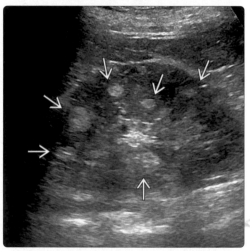

Renal Angiomyolipoma

(Left) *Ultrasound shows a huge, weakly shadowing, echogenic lower pole AML* ➡. *Shadowing* ➡ *is likely due to interspersed fat and soft tissue components. Large AMLs may hemorrhage.* **(Right)** *Oblique transabdominal ultrasound shows that this Wilms tumor* ➡ *is heterogeneous and mildly hyperechoic compared to displaced, but normal renal parenchyma* ➡. *Wilms tumor is the most common pediatric intraabdominal malignancy.*

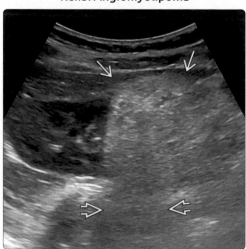

Wilms Tumor

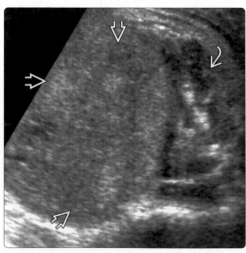

Fat in Renal Scar

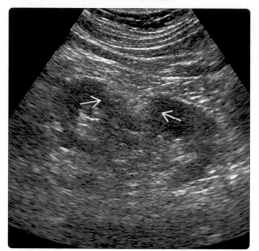

Fat in Renal Scar

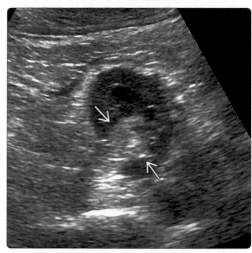

(Left) *Sagittal ultrasound of a patient with atherosclerosis and renal insufficiency shows an echogenic interpolar lesion ➡. Real-time ultrasound examination and coronal CT confirmed an old renal infarct and invaginating retroperitoneal fat within a renal scar.* (Right) *Ultrasound shows a lower pole echogenic lesion ➡ in a patient post partial nephrectomy. Fat packing within the resection site mimics an AML.*

Renal Junctional Line/Cortical Parenchymal Defect

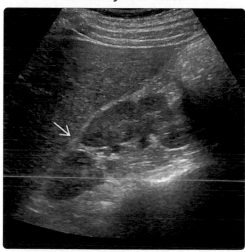

Column of Bertin

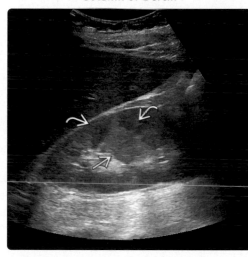

(Left) *Ultrasound of a young male patient with right upper quadrant pain shows a junctional cortical defect ➡. This line occurs at a plane of embryologic fusion of renunculi (embryologic elements forming kidneys) and is typically seen at the upper and middle 1/3 of the kidney.* (Right) *Ultrasound shows a band of cortical tissue ➡ separating pyramids ➡ of renal medulla, a column of Bertin. When viewed en face, columns may appear echogenic. Color Doppler or CECT may confirm normal invaginating cortex.*

Renal Calculi

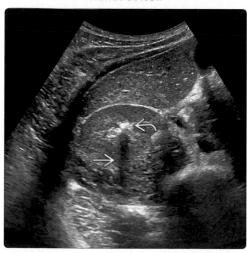

Medullary Sponge Kidney

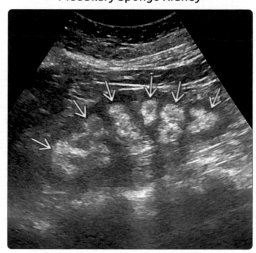

(Left) *Ultrasound shows a highly reflective renal calculus ➡. Posterior shadowing ➡ is the ultrasound hallmark of renal calculi. Technique (depth, focal zone, fundamental imaging) should be optimized to confirm shadowing.* (Right) *Sagittal ultrasound of a patient with hematuria shows highly echogenic renal medulla ➡. These medullary rings are thought to be due to the dilated collecting tubules of medullary sponge kidney. When viewed transverse, echogenic medulla may simulate a mass.*

(Left) *Ultrasound shows an echogenic right renal lesion ➡. Acute pyelonephritis is typically a clinical diagnosis, and ultrasound is utilized to assess complications (abscess) and causes (obstruction). Uncomplicated pyelonephritis is usually sonographically occult, though findings may include renal enlargement, urothelial thickening, and regions of altered echogenicity.* (Right) *Corresponding power Doppler image shows a lower pole perfusion defect ➡. (Courtesy R. Brooke Jeffrey, MD).*

Focal Bacterial Nephritis

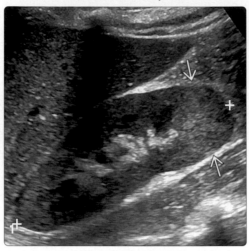

Focal Bacterial Nephritis

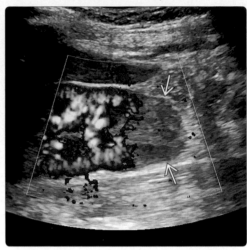

(Left) *Ultrasound of a diabetic, septic female patient shows that most of the right kidney is replaced by amorphous echogenicity ➡. Dirty posterior shadowing ➡ is due to the gas of emphysematous pyelonephritis, a life-threatening infection.* (Right) *Renal transplant ultrasound shows subtle lower pole echogenicity ➡. The corresponding power Doppler image demonstrates a perfusion defect ➡, the color Doppler equivalent of a CECT striated nephrogram. Urine analysis confirmed Escherichia coli pyelonephritis.*

Emphysematous Pyelonephritis

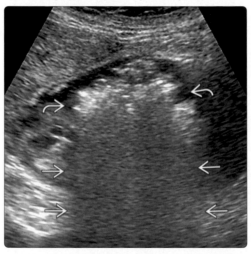

Focal Bacterial Nephritis

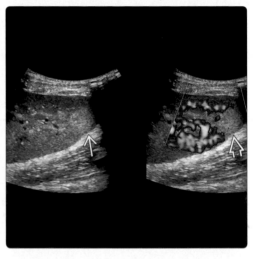

(Left) *Ultrasound shows a slightly complex exophytic renal cyst with a highly echogenic plug ➡. Note the posterior comet-tail artifact ➡. This appearance may be due to crystals within the wall or septa of cysts.* (Right) *Sagittal ultrasound shows a necrotic papilla appearing as an echogenic focus ➡ with ring calcification in the medullary pyramid. It is surrounded by a rim of fluid from the dilated and clubbed calyces ➡.*

Complex Cyst/Milk of Calcium Cyst

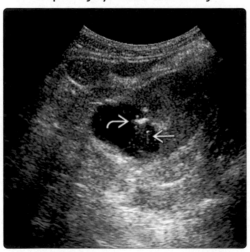

Renal Papillary Necrosis

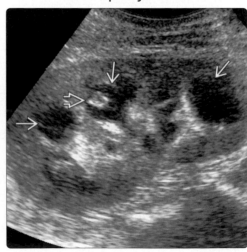

Complex Cyst/Milk of Calcium Cyst

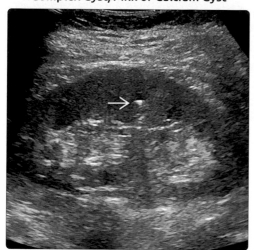

Xanthogranulomatous Pyelonephritis

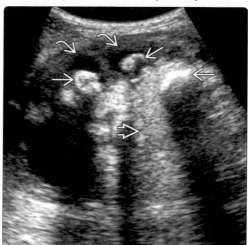

(Left) *Ultrasound of a patient with flank pain shows punctate echogenicity and a subtle posterior comet-tail artifact within the back wall of a tiny cyst ➡. Layering crystals (mild of calcium) within cysts or calyceal diverticula may be confused with calculi, though note the absence of shadowing.* (Right) *Sagittal ultrasound shows extensive peripelvic fat infiltration ➡ secondary to xanthogranulomatous pyelonephritis. Multiple echogenic calculi ➡ are associated with hydrocalycosis ➡.*

Tuberculosis, Urinary Tract

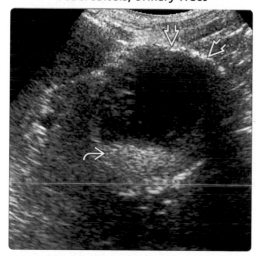

Renal Oncocytoma

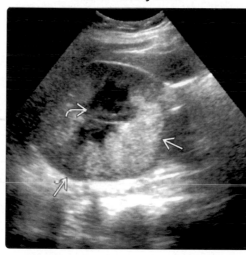

(Left) *Transverse ultrasound shows a renal TB abscess with a calcified wall ➡ and internal echogenic debris ➡. Abscess formation is secondary to stricture at the calyceal infundibulum.* (Right) *Longitudinal ultrasound shows a large, mildly hyperechoic mass ➡ within the right kidney. It has a spiculated, central hypoechoic scar ➡, which is suggestive of an oncocytoma; however, a renal cell carcinoma cannot be excluded, and excision is required.*

Renal Trauma

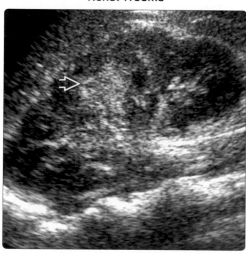

Renal Trauma

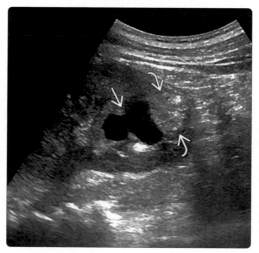

(Left) *Longitudinal ultrasound shows a focal, poorly defined area of hyperechogenicity ➡ in the midpole of the right kidney compatible with a contusion. Note there is loss of corticomedullary differentiation at the midpole when compared with the lower pole.* (Right) *Ultrasound of a patient with hematuria post trauma shows adherent, echogenic clot ➡ within a deformed lower pole cyst ➡. The appearance may simulate a cystic renal cell carcinoma; follow-up sonography confirmed clot resolution.*

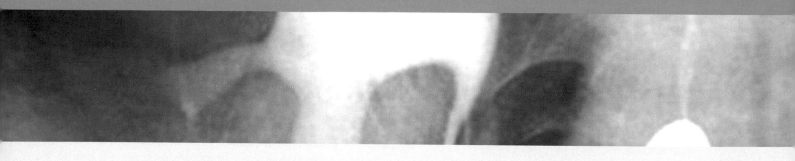

SECTION 16
Collecting System

DIFFERENTIAL DIAGNOSIS

Common

- Ureteral Obstruction
  - Ureteral Stone
  - Transitional Cell Carcinoma
  - Periureteral Metastases
  - Retroperitoneal Fibrosis
  - Primary Pelvic Malignancy
    - Prostate Carcinoma
    - Rectal Carcinoma
    - Cervical and Endometrial Carcinoma
- Ureterectasis of Pregnancy
- Ureteral Duplication
- Distended Urinary Bladder
- Overhydration, Diuresis
- Vesicoureteral Reflux
- Prominent Extrarenal Pelvis (Mimic)
- Renal Sinus Cysts (Mimic)
- Renal Sinus Blood Vessels (Mimic)
- Ureteropelvic Junction Obstruction
- Pyonephrosis

Less Common

- Renal Papillary Necrosis
- Renal Tuberculosis
- Pyelonephritis, Xanthogranulomatous
- Megacalyces, Megaureter
- Calyceal Diverticulum
- Renal Cysts (Mimic)
- Autosomal Dominant Polycystic Disease, Kidney
- Renal Metastases and Lymphoma
- Blood-Filled Renal Pelvis

ESSENTIAL INFORMATION

Key Differential Diagnosis Issues

- Determine if all calices are dilated and in communication with dilated renal pelvis and ureter
- CT and MR are complementary to US
  - Include pyelographic (delayed)-phase enhanced images

Helpful Clues for Common Diagnoses

- **Ureteral Obstruction**
  - Most common cause with several specific etiologies (calculi, tumor, etc.)
  - CT and MR better than US at showing etiology of ureteral obstruction
  - **Ureteral stone**
    - Dilated ureter ends at high-density intraluminal focus
  - **Transitional cell carcinoma**
    - Small soft tissue density mass within lumen or wall of ureter
    - May see goblet sign; dilation of ureteral lumen proximal and distal to obstructing tumor
  - **Retroperitoneal fibrosis**
    - Encases and obstructs ureters through lumbar region
    - Mantle of soft tissue surrounds aorta and inferior vena cava
    - Retroperitoneal nodal metastases may have similar appearance and may rarely cause ureteral obstruction

- Periureteral metastases
  - Clinical history crucial
  - Typical primaris: Breast lymphoma, melanoma
- **Primary pelvic malignancy**
  - Dilated ureter ends in soft tissue density mass or retroperitoneal nodes that encase ureter
- **Ureterectasis of Pregnancy**
  - Due to hormonal influence plus mass effect of gravid uterus
  - Affects right kidney more than left
  - May persist after pregnancy
  - Rarely associated with rupture of collecting system (usually with underlying renal disease, such as infection)
- **Ureteral Duplication**
  - Upper pole ureter is more often ectopic in insertion and dilated
  - Look for 2 ureters on 1 side; upper pole ureter will have delayed concentration and excretion of contrast medium if it is obstructed
  - Either ureter can be obstructed by calculi and other etiologies
- **Distended Urinary Bladder**
  - May cause back pressure and dilation of ureters and calices
  - Re-image after emptying bladder
    - Should return to normal caliber
- **Vesicoureteral Reflux**
  - Acute or chronic dilation of ureter and calices; scarred parenchyma
- **Prominent Extrarenal Pelvis (Mimic)**
  - Calices and ureter not dilated
  - Common and asymptomatic
- **Renal Sinus Cysts (Mimic)**
  - Diagnosis is based on demonstration of lack of communication of cysts with renal pelvis and proximal ureter
  - Delayed imaging on CECT often necessary to distinguish renal sinus cysts from hydronephrosis
    - Contrast-opacified urine distinguished from water-density peripelvic cysts
    - Coronal reformations are also helpful
- **Renal Sinus Blood Vessels (Mimic)**
  - Sonolucent, but show flow on Doppler
  - May also be mimic of hydronephrosis on black blood MR sequences
    - Usually not problem on CT
    - Even on NECT, blood vessels are different attenuation than calices
- **Ureteropelvic Junction Obstruction**
  - Relatively common congenital narrowing at ureteropelvic junction (UPJ) that often results in striking dilation of pelvis and calices, especially with fluid or diuretic challenge
  - May be due to crossing vessel that compresses UPJ
- **Pyonephrosis**
  - Hydronephrosis plus infected urine = urgent need for drainage
  - Fluid may be higher than water density on CT; diffusely mildly echogenic

○ Consider pelvic inflammatory conditions that may involve ureter (e.g., diverticulitis, Crohn disease, gynecologic infections)

Helpful Clues for Less Common Diagnoses

- **Renal Papillary Necrosis**
  ○ Calices may appear blunted and dilated due to sloughed papillae
- **Renal Tuberculosis**
  ○ May cause stricture of infundibula and focal hydronephrosis
  ○ Caseous infection of parenchyma may mimic caliectasis
- **Pyelonephritis, Xanthogranulomatous**
  ○ Underlying calculi may cause hydro- or pyonephrosis
  ○ Xanthomatous replacement of parenchyma may be low density, mimicking caliectasis
- **Megacalyces, Megaureter**
  ○ Rare congenital anomalies
  ○ Renal function may remain normal
- **Calyceal Diverticulum**
  ○ Outpouching from calyx may simulate focal caliectasis

- **Renal Cysts (Mimic)**
  ○ Multiple simple cysts or polycystic disease
  ○ If numerous, may simulate dilated calices
  ○ Usually spherical
- **Renal Metastases and Lymphoma**
  ○ Transitional cell carcinoma, metastases, lymphoma may infiltrate pelvis; cause or simulate hydronephrosis
  ○ Lymphoma is especially likely to be homogeneous and hypodense (CT), and hypoechoic (US)
- **Blood-Filled Renal Pelvis**
  ○ Trauma or coagulopathic hemorrhage may distend renal pelvis and calices with blood

SELECTED REFERENCES

1. Nikolaidis P et al: Computed tomography and magnetic resonance imaging features of lesions of the renal medulla and sinus. Curr Probl Diagn Radiol. 37(6):262-78, 2008
2. Browne RF et al: Transitional cell carcinoma of the upper urinary tract: spectrum of imaging findings. Radiographics. 25(6):1609-27, 2005
3. Rha SE et al: The renal sinus: pathologic spectrum and multimodality imaging approach. Radiographics. 24 Suppl 1:S117-31. Review, 2004
4. Zinn HL et al: Peripelvic cysts simulating hydronephrosis. Abdom Imaging. 22(3):346 7, 1997

Ureteral Stone

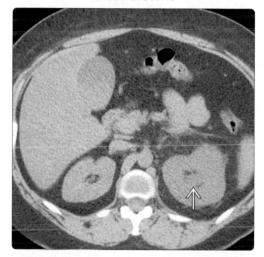

Ureteral Stone

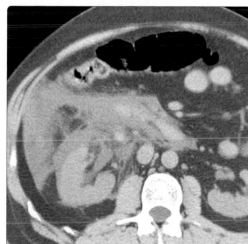

(Left) *Axial CECT shows left-sided hydronephrosis ➡, renal enlargement, and perinephric stranding, due to a distal ureteral stone.* **(Right)** *Axial NECT shows right-sided hydronephrosis and extensive infiltration of the perirenal space, due to forniceal rupture, caused by a small stone at the ureterovesical junction.*

Ureteral Stone

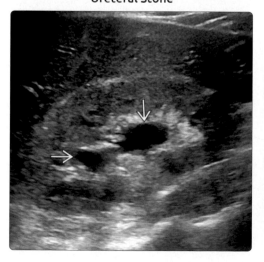

Ureteral Stone

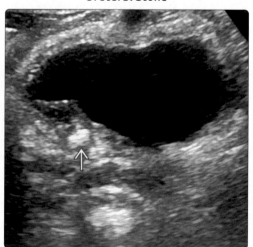

(Left) *Longitudinal ultrasound of the right kidney shows mild hydronephrosis ➡ in a patient presenting with right flank pain. (From DI: Genitourinary, 3e.)* **(Right)** *Transverse ultrasound of the pelvis in the same patient shows an echogenic stone ➡ impacted at the right ureterovesical junction causing obstructive hydronephrosis.*

Transitional Cell Carcinoma

Transitional Cell Carcinoma

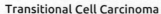

(Left) *Axial CECT shows dilated renal pelvis ➡ and calices ➡ in the right kidney, due to a transitional cell carcinoma of the distal ureter.* (Right) *Axial CECT in the same patient shows a soft tissue mass ➡ in the distal right ureter, a primary transitional cell carcinoma, causing ureteral obstruction.*

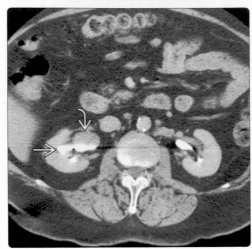

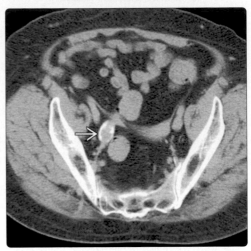

Periureteral Metastases

Periureteral Metastases

(Left) *Axial CECT in patient with lymphoma shows a soft tissue mass ➡ within the lumen or wall of the renal pelvis with dilated calices.* (Right) *Axial CECT shows soft tissue mass ➡ within the wall of the proximal ureter in this case of lymphoma. The ureteral lumen ➡ is aneurysmally dilated.*

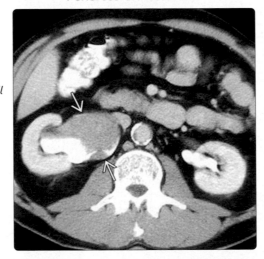

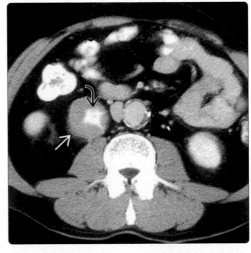

Retroperitoneal Fibrosis

Vesicoureteral Reflux

(Left) *Axial CECT shows a ureteral stent ➡ that was placed to decompress an obstructed left ureter. Mantle of soft tissue ➡ around the aorta is classic for retroperitoneal fibrosis.* (Right) *Axial NECT shows dilated calices ➡ bilaterally due to chronic reflux. Note the cortical calcifications ➡ associated with the cortical scarring.*

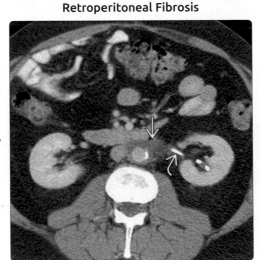

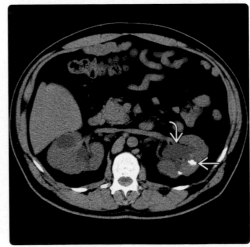

Distended Urinary Bladder

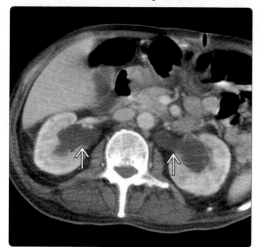

Distended Urinary Bladder

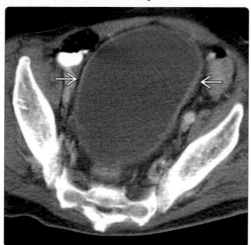

(Left) *Axial CECT shows bilateral dilation of the calices and ureters* ➡ *in an 80-year-old man with prostatism and a distended urinary bladder. These findings resolved after catheterization of the bladder.* (Right) *Axial CECT in the same patient shows distention of the urinary bladder* ➡ *due to prostatic hypertrophy.*

Prominent Extrarenal Pelvis (Mimic)

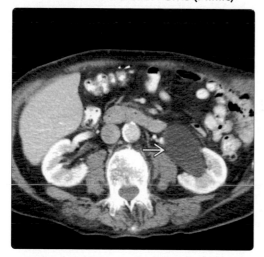

Prominent Extrarenal Pelvis (Mimic)

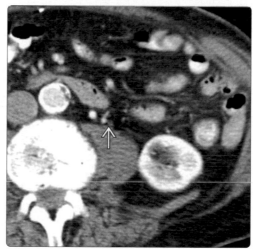

(Left) *Axial CECT shows a dilated left renal pelvis* ➡ *but no caliectasis, delayed nephrogram, or renal scarring, in this 83-year-old man.* (Right) *Axial CECT in the same patient shows a normal-caliber left ureter* ➡.

Renal Sinus Cysts (Mimic)

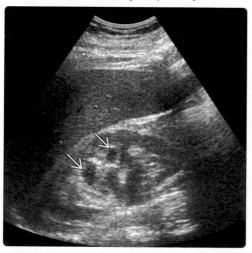

Renal Sinus Cysts (Mimic)

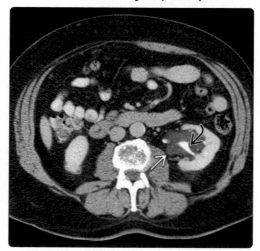

(Left) *Sagittal oblique ultrasound shows anechoic cysts* ➡ *in the renal sinus simulating dilated calices.* (Right) *Axial CECT shows renal sinus (peripelvic) cysts* ➡ *that are distinguished from hydronephrosis on this pyelographic-phase CECT by contrast-opacified urine* ➡ *in the collecting system.*

DIFFERENTIAL DIAGNOSIS

Common

- Urolithiasis
- Blood Clot
  - Trauma
  - Coagulopathic Hemorrhage
  - Tumor
- Fungus Ball
- Transitional Cell Carcinoma
- Gas in Collecting System
  - Emphysematous Pyelitis/Pyelonephritis
  - Instrumentation of Kidney
- Renal Papillary Necrosis

Less Common

- Renal Cell Carcinoma
- Foreign Bodies
- Papilloma
- Metastases and Lymphoma

ESSENTIAL INFORMATION

Key Differential Diagnosis Issues

- Usually easier to characterize attenuation of filling defects by CT; urography (excretory, retrograde, or CT) best for complete evaluation

Helpful Clues for Common Diagnoses

- **Urolithiasis**
  - Many calculi (especially uric acid and xanthine) are radiolucent by radiography but very dense on CT and are easy to distinguish from other etiologies
  - Indinavir stones are lucent on CT
- **Blood Clot**
  - History of trauma, anticoagulation, stone, and hematuria are helpful
  - Should lyse and dissolve within days
  - Look for underlying tumor if unexplained etiology
- **Fungus Ball**
  - Seen in setting of **candidiasis** and **aspergillosis**

- Usually seen in debilitated, elderly patients
- Usually have other findings of opportunistic renal infection, such as abscess/microabscesses and papillary necrosis
- **Transitional Cell Carcinoma**
  - Irregular filing defect; "amputates" calices
  - 8% of urothelial cancers occur in renal pelvis
    - Most are low grade
  - Usually seen in older men; history of smoking, analgesic abuse, or exposure to chemical or cyclophosphamide
- **Gas in Collecting System**
  - Iatrogenic: Ureteral stent, nephrostomy
  - Emphysematous pyelitis: Gas, infection limited to urine
- **Renal Papillary Necrosis**
  - Sloughed papilla with cavitation of adjacent calyx; club-shaped calices
  - Associated with analgesic abuse; also seen with opportunistic infections and TB

Helpful Clues for Less Common Diagnoses

- **Renal Cell Carcinoma**
  - May protrude into pelvis or cause hemorrhage as filling defect
  - Expansile vascular mass evident on CT
- **Foreign Bodies**
  - Pieces of nephrostomy or ureteral stent
  - Usually radiopaque
- **Papilloma**
  - Benign soft tissue, uroepithelial neoplasm
  - No renal parenchymal mass
  - Other rare tumors may have similar appearance
    - Fibroepithelial polyp, lipoma, fibroma

SELECTED REFERENCES

1. Gayer G et al: The renal sinus–transitional cell carcinoma and its mimickers on computed tomography. Semin Ultrasound CT MR. 35(3):308-19, 2014
2. Rosa M et al: Recent finding and new technologies in nephrolitiasis: a review of the recent literature. BMC Urol. 13:10, 2013
3. Sadegi BJ et al: Primary renal candidiasis: importance of imaging and clinical history in diagnosis and management. J Ultrasound Med. 28(4):507-14, 2009

Urolithiasis

Blood Clot

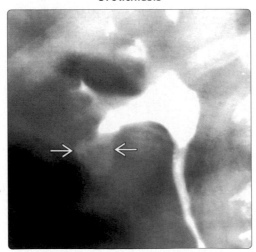

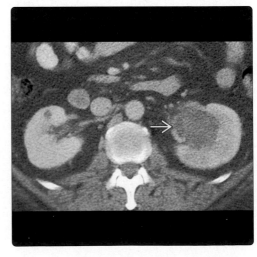

(Left) *Excretory urography in a 35-year-old man with microhematuria and hyperuricemia shows a radiolucent filling defect ➡ in the lower pole calix and infundibulum. CT showed this as a uric acid stone.* (Right) *Axial CECT in a patient with a history of hematuria on anticoagulation shows heterogeneous, slightly hyperdense blood filling the left renal pelvis ➡. Also note a delayed left nephrogram due to obstruction.*

Transitional Cell Carcinoma

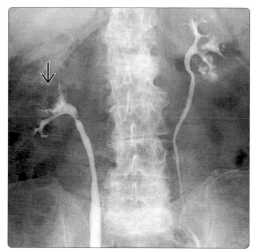

Transitional Cell Carcinoma

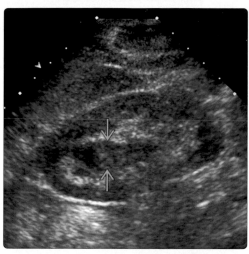

(Left) Frontal projection excretory phase IVU in an 81-year-old woman with a history of hematuria shows distortion of a right upper pole calyx and a radiolucent filling defect ➡. *(Right)* Corresponding ultrasound in the same patient shows an echogenic filling defect ➡ in an upper pole calyx, which was proved to be invasive urothelial carcinoma.

Emphysematous Pyelitis/Pyelonephritis

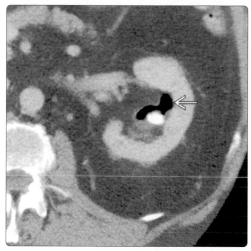

Renal Papillary Necrosis

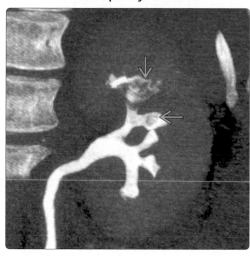

(Left) Axial CECT in an elderly man with signs and symptoms of a urinary tract infection shows gas within the renal pelvis ➡ without parenchymal gas, an appearance consistent with emphysematous pyelitis. *(Right)* Coronal MIP CECT shows filling defects ➡ within the upper pole calices, representing sloughed papillae (and, possibly, hemorrhage) in this patient with a history of papillary necrosis in the setting of sickle cell disease.

Renal Cell Carcinoma

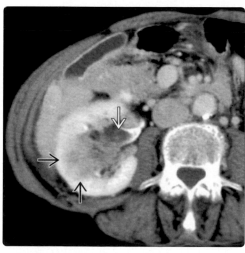

Papilloma

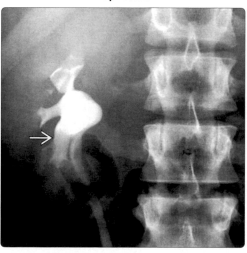

(Left) Axial CECT shows a heterogeneous hypervascular mass ➡ that extends into the renal pelvis ➡. It is difficult to differentiate this lesion from urothelial carcinoma based on its imaging appearance, but this lesion showed extension into the renal vein, which would favor renal cell carcinoma. *(Right)* Excretory urography shows a subtle, but persistent, filling defect ➡ in the lower pole infundibulum in a 21-year-old man with hematuria. The mass was resected and was compatible with a benign papilloma.

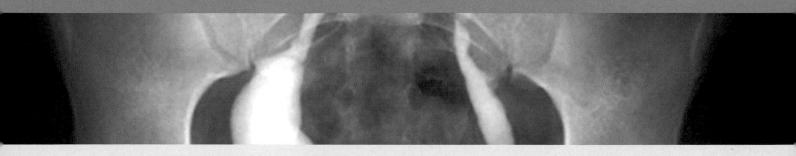

SECTION 17
Ureter

Generic Imaging Patterns

DIFFERENTIAL DIAGNOSIS

Common

- Urolithiasis
- Ureteral Blood Clot
- Ureteral Air Bubbles
- Urothelial Carcinoma (Transitional Cell Carcinoma)
- Iatrogenic and Postoperative Stricture

Less Common

- Extrinsic Compression
  - Diverticulitis
  - Crohn Disease
  - Endometriosis
  - Vascular Impression
- Sloughed Papilla
- Infectious Ureteritis
- Ureteral Metastases or Direct Invasion
- Retroperitoneal Fibrosis
- Congenital Ureteral Stricture
- Vasculitis
- Ureteritis Cystica
- Malakoplakia
- Ureteral Papilloma
- Ureteral Fibroepithelial Polyp
- Mesenchymal Tumor
- Ureteral Valves

ESSENTIAL INFORMATION

Key Differential Diagnosis Issues

- In order of frequency: Stones > clot > gas bubbles > tumor
  - Most have characteristic features that allow identification
  - Clinical information is key
    - e.g., known or prior history of urothelial malignancy (high risk of synchronous or metachronous ureteral cancer)
    - Check for recent instrumentation (may explain gas bubbles or blood clot within ureter)
    - Acute pain (suggestive of stone or obstructing clot)
  - CT gives best information about extrinsic processes that may involve ureters
    - e.g., pelvic tumors or inflammatory processes
    - CT also definitive for ureteral calculi (isodense/hypodense indinavir related or matrix stones are extremely rare)
    - CT urography has replaced IV urography ("IVP") for almost all indications
  - Retrograde pyelography still essential for best depiction of intraluminal and mucosal ureteral pathologies
    - Applying supraphysiologic pressure results in superior distention of ureteral lumen
    - Offers better spatial resolution as well
    - Allows brush biopsy of urothelial tumors
    - Essential for placement of ureteral stents for therapy

Helpful Clues for Common Diagnoses

- **Urolithiasis**
  - CT: Hyperdense (> 200 HU) focus with hydronephrosis/hydroureter and perinephric stranding

- Radiopacity: Calcium oxalate/phosphate > cystine > struvite > uric acid
  - Rim sign: Ureteral wall edema creates soft tissue rim around stone
    - Helps to differentiate from phlebolith
    - May not be present with large stones (wall is stretched too thin)
  - Stone may appear hypodense relative to contrast-opacified urine
    - On IV urography, retrograde, or antegrade pyelography
- **Ureteral Blood Clot**
  - 50-90 HU, no enhancement
  - Stipple sign on pyelogram
  - Resolves on follow-up studies
- **Ureteral Air Bubbles**
  - Mobile, usually multiple, do not elevate epithelium
  - Commonly seen on retrograde or antegrade pyelograms (due to instrumentation)
    - e.g., patient with nephrostomy catheter or ureteral stent
- **Urothelial Carcinoma (Transitional Cell Carcinoma)**
  - Soft tissue density (30-60 HU) on unenhanced CT; variable degrees of enhancement
  - Circumferential or eccentric wall thickening
  - More common in distal ureter (70%), presumably due to stasis
  - Fixation of ureter with irregular narrowing of lumen, nontapering margins
  - Smooth or frond-like surface (stipple sign)
  - Goblet or champagne glass sign
    - Dilatation of ureteral lumen at level of tumor
      - Implies distention and partial obstruction of ureteral lumen by mass
- **Iatrogenic & Postoperative Stricture**
  - Seen after lithotomy, ureteroscopy, ureteral catheterization
  - Most common site of postoperative stricture is at site of anastomosis of ureter to bladder, neobladder, or ileal conduit
  - Also seen following nonurologic abdominal surgeries
    - Often result of ischemic injury

Helpful Clues for Less Common Diagnoses

- **Extrinsic Compression**
  - CT is most useful modality for detection and differentiation of these entities
  - **Diverticulitis**
    - Inflammatory process may cause spasm, stricture, or even coloureteral fistula
    - Patients may present with pyuria and flank pain more than typical symptoms of diverticulitis
  - **Crohn disease**
    - Inflammation may extend to ureter with stricture or spasm
    - Right ureter affected more commonly due to its proximity to terminal ileum
  - **Endometriosis**
    - Involves ureter below pelvic brim
    - Compression from adjacent disease (80%), involvement of ureter wall or lumen (20%)

- History and patient's demographics are helpful clues
  - **Vascular impression**
    - By artery, vein, or lymphatic
    - Look for aneurysm, collateral vessels
    - Vascular impressions are common in renal anomalies, such as ectopic or horseshoe kidney
      - Supernumerary vessels often cross and may obstruct collecting system
- **Ureteral Metastases or Direct Invasion**
  - Direct invasion by adjacent tumor is more common
    - Colon and cervical carcinoma most common
  - Hematogenous metastases generally appear as intramural masses
    - Primary sites include lung, breast, and GI tract
  - Consider lymphoma if there is smooth circumferential wall thickening
    - Often see adenopathy elsewhere
- **Sloughed Papilla**
  - Seen in setting of renal papillary necrosis
    - Sequela of interstitial nephritis or ischemia
    - Caused by analgesic nephropathy, diabetes, sickle cell disease, UTI, TB, obstruction, etc.
  - Usually multiple, triangular-shaped
    - May have ring calcification
    - Nonenhancing
    - Noncontiguous with ureteral wall
- **Infectious Ureteritis**
  - TB causes multiple findings including irregularity, intraluminal filling defects, ulcerations, and strictures ("chronic granulomatous ureteritis")
    - Kidney and renal pelvis also generally involved
  - Schistosomiasis more often involves distal ureter and bladder
    - Calcifications common
- **Retroperitoneal Fibrosis**
  - Encases, obstructs, and medially displaces ureters
  - CT shows Mantle of soft tissue encasing aorta and inferior vena cava through lumbar region
- **Ureteritis Cystica**

- Reactive proliferative changes of urothelium with formation of multiple small, subepithelial cysts
  - Inflammatory stimulation → proliferation of urothelium → invaginating of urothelial cells → ureteritis glandularis et cystica
- Multiple subepithelial cysts in ureter wall
- Usually in proximal 1/3 of ureter
- Smooth small nodular filling defects (< 5 mm)
- **Malakoplakia**
  - Rare chronic granulomatous condition, thought to be due to altered host response and defective phagocytosis
  - Variable appearance ranging from flat plaques to nodules and masses ± ulceration
  - Imaging findings overlap with urothelial cancer
- **Ureteral Fibroepithelial Polyp**
  - Usually seen in children and young adults
  - Thick core of loose fibrous tissue beneath normal urothelium
  - May appear as long pedunculated filling defect

SELECTED REFERENCES

1. Hilton S et al: Recent advances in imaging cancer of the kidney and urinary tract. Surg Oncol Clin N Am. 23(4):863-910, 2014
2. Rosa M et al: Recent finding and new technologies in nephrolitiasis: a review of the recent literature. BMC Urol. 13:10, 2013
3. Rothschild JG et al: Ureteritis cystica: a radiologic pathologic correlation. J Clin Imaging Sci. 1:23, 2011
4. Wang ZJ et al: Ureteral fibroepithelial polyp. J Ultrasound Med. 27(11):1647-9, 2008
5. Jung DC et al: Renal papillary necrosis: review and comparison of findings at multi-detector row CT and intravenous urography. Radiographics. 26(6):1827-36, 2006
6. Menendez V et al: Cystic pyeloureteritis: review of 34 cases. Radiologic aspects and differential diagnosis. Urology. 50(1):31-7, 1997
7. Baumgartner BR et al: Malakoplakia of the ureter and bladder. Urol Radiol. 12(3):157-9, 1990

Urolithiasis

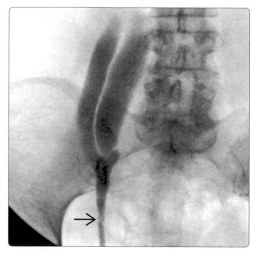

Ureteral Air Bubbles

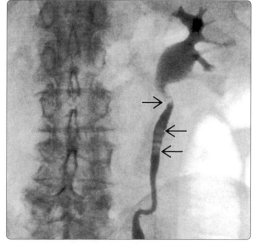

(Left) *Retrograde pyelogram shows a filling defect (stone) ➲ causing obstruction of the ureter. The ureter is bifid (duplicated) above the point of obstruction with dilation of both components.* **(Right)** *Retrograde pyelogram shows multiple mobile round filling defects ➲ in the ureter. These are usually easy to recognize at fluoroscopy but may be more difficult to distinguish from other filling defects on static films.*

Urothelial Carcinoma (Transitional Cell Carcinoma)

(Left) *Coronal MIP from CT urography in a 63-year-old man with history of hematuria shows a soft tissue density mass* ➡ *that expands and partially obstructs the ureteral lumen (goblet sign).* (Right) *Axial CECT in the same patient shows the irregular soft tissue density intraluminal mass that expands and partially obstructs the distal ureter* ➡.

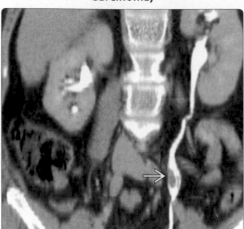

Urothelial Carcinoma (Transitional Cell Carcinoma)

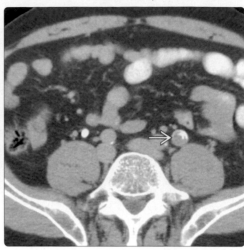

(Left) *Retrograde pyelogram shows partial obstruction of the ureteral lumen by a mass* ➡ *that has both smooth and irregular surface components. Brush biopsy revealed transitional cell carcinoma.* (Right) *Axial NECT in a 47-year-old woman with history of diverticulitis shows gas bubbles* ➡ *within a dilated ureter and renal pelvis, due to coloureteral fistula.*

Urothelial Carcinoma (Transitional Cell Carcinoma)

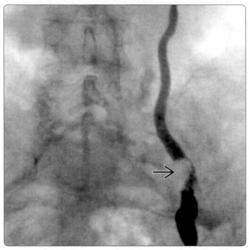

Diverticulitis

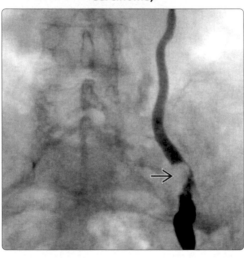

(Left) *Excretory urography in a young woman with known endometriosis shows irregular narrowing of the distal right ureter* ➡ *and impression on the dome of the bladder* ➡. *This tight stricture caused hydronephrosis. The distal ureter was resected, and endometriosis was confirmed at histology.* (Right) *Axial CECT in a patient with history of non-Hodgkin lymphoma shows marked circumferential thickening of the left ureter* ➡ *with resultant delayed nephrogram.*

Endometriosis

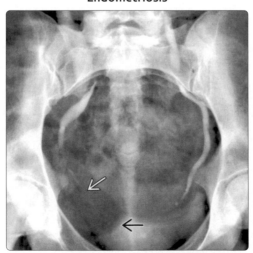

Ureteral Metastases or Direct Invasion

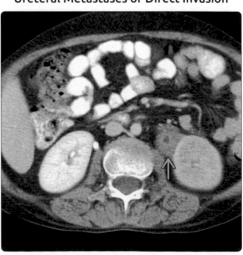

Ureteral Metastases or Direct Invasion

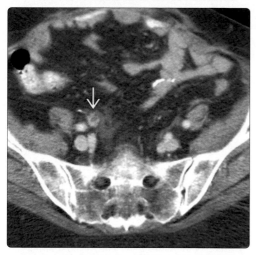

Ureteral Metastases or Direct Invasion

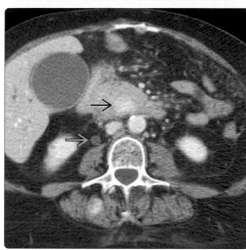

(Left) *Axial CECT in 61-year-old woman with a history of metastatic breast cancer shows circumferential wall thickening and enhancement ➡ of the right ureter, which was due to a metastasis.* (Right) *Axial CT through the upper abdomen in the same patient shows dilatation of right ureter ➡ secondary to the obstructing ureteral metastasis. Also note the hypervascular pancreatic metastasis ➡. Ureteral metastases are usually seen in patients with widespread metastatic disease.*

Ureteritis Cystica

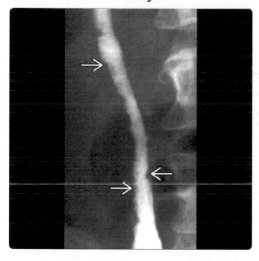

Malakoplakia

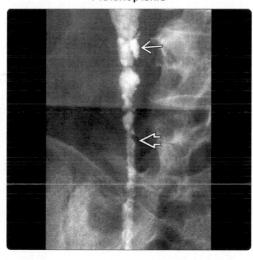

(Left) *Retrograde pyelogram shows a bubbly appearance of the ureter with multiple, small, smooth filling defects indenting the lumen ➡.* (Right) *Coned-down view of the right ureter in a case of malakoplakia shows diffuse irregularity with small plaques ➡ and ulcerations ➡. Urinary tract involvement can be quite variable from a focal lesion to diffuse abnormality.*

Ureteral Fibroepithelial Polyp

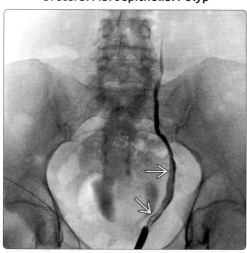

Ureteral Fibroepithelial Polyp

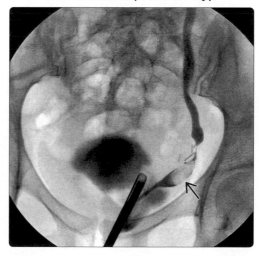

(Left) *AP retrograde urogram shows a well-delineated, elongated intraluminal filling defect in the distal left ureter ➡. Cystoscopy showed a polypoid lesion with a long stalk, which intermittently protruded through the ureteral orifice.* (Right) *AP retrograde urography shows a well-delineated intraluminal filling defect in the distal left ureter ➡. Pathology was consistent with a fibroepithelial polyp. The surgical clips in the left pelvis are related to a prior hysterectomy.*

DIFFERENTIAL DIAGNOSIS

Common

- Ureteral Obstruction
  - Stone, Tumor, Stricture
- Ureterocele
- Ectopic Ureter

Less Common

- Bladder Diverticulum (Mimic)
- Periureteral Cystic Lesions (Mimic)
- Congenital Megaureter

ESSENTIAL INFORMATION

Helpful Clues for Common Diagnoses

- **Ureteral Obstruction**
  - Obstructing distal ureteral lesions may result in acquired cystic dilatation of terminal ureter (pseudoureterocele)
    - Cobra-head appearance on IVP or VCUG; halo around cobra head is thicker and indistinct
  - Urolithiasis > bladder tumor > ureteral tumor
  - CT and MR superior to US
  - Detection of ureteral jet on US helps to exclude obstructive pathology
- **Ureterocele**
  - Several classification schemes exist; more widely accepted scheme divides ureteroceles between intravesical and ectopic subtypes
    - **Intravesical**: Ureterocele is entirely in bladder
      - Cobra-head or spring-onion deformity of distal ureter with surrounding radiolucent halo
    - **Ectopic**: Insertion at bladder neck or in posterior urethra
      - Smooth, radiolucent intravesicular mass near bladder base
      - 80% seen in association with duplicated collecting system
  - Excretory-phase CT or MR urography are preferred imaging tools
- **Ectopic Ureter**
  - Inserts along developing mesonephric duct (precursor of trigone, epididymis, vas deferens, ejaculatory ducts, and seminal vesicles)
  - Mostly inserts outside bladder
    - Always above external sphincter in males
      - Prostatic urethra most common insertion site in male patients
    - Insertion is usually below sphincter in female patients, resulting in urinary incontinence
      - Urethra or vestibule most common insertion site in female patients
  - 75-90% occur in setting of duplication

Helpful Clues for Less Common Diagnoses

- **Bladder Diverticulum (Mimic)**
  - Usually multiple; may contain stones, debris, or tumor
  - Diverticula near ureterovesical junction may mimic ureteral dilatation
  - Color jet connecting to bladder very useful to distinguish diverticulum from other paravesical masses and from dilated ureter
- **Periureteral Cystic Lesions (Mimic)**
  - Seminal vesicle cyst and Gartner duct cyst may occasionally be confused with ureterocele
  - Knowing classic location of these cysts is helpful for differentiation: MR is helpful in selected cases to better delineate anatomy
- **Congenital Megaureter**
  - Rare congenital anomaly caused by aperistaltic distal ureter (functional obstruction)
  - Favors dilation of distal ureter

SELECTED REFERENCES

1. Adeb M et al: Magnetic resonance urography in evaluation of duplicated renal collecting systems. Magn Reson Imaging Clin N Am. 21(4):717-30, 2013
2. Shebel HM et al: Cysts of the lower male genitourinary tract: embryologic and anatomic considerations and differential diagnosis. Radiographics. 33(4):1125-43, 2013
3. Shokeir AA et al: Primary megaureter: current trends in diagnosis and treatment. BJU Int. 86(7):861-8, 2000

Stone, Tumor, Stricture

Stone, Tumor, Stricture

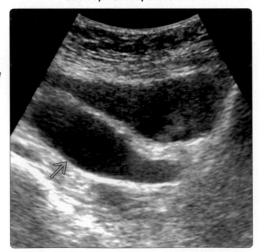

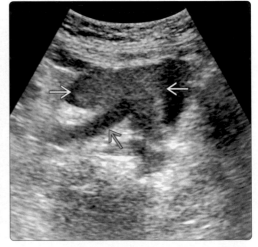

(Left) *Sagittal US shows dilation of the distal right ureter ➡, due to bladder carcinoma, in a 65-year-old woman.* **(Right)** *Axial US in the same patient shows a mass ➡ within the bladder that straddles the ureterovesical junction and obstructs the ureter ➡.*

Cystic Dilation of Distal Ureter

Stone, Tumor, Stricture

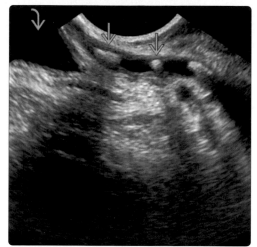

Ureterocele

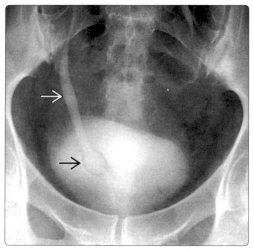

(Left) *Longitudinal transvaginal US of a 40-year-old woman with a history of groin pain shows mild dilatation of the distal left ureter and numerous shadowing calculi ➡. Note the bladder ➡.* (Right) *Frontal excretory urography shows a right-sided intravesical ureterocele ➡ with associated dilation of the ureter ➡. Note the thin radiolucent halo.*

Ureterocele

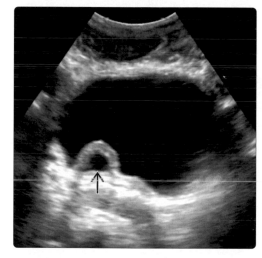

Ureterocele

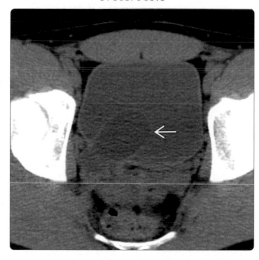

(Left) *Transverse US in a 23-year-old man shows cystic dilatation of distal left ureter ➡ protruding into the bladder base.* (Right) *Axial NECT in the same patient shows a large intravesical ("orthotopic") ureterocele ➡.*

Bladder Diverticulum (Mimic)

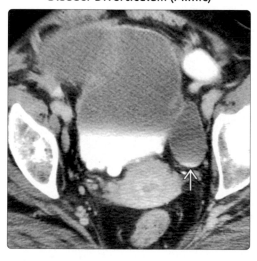

Congenital Megaureter

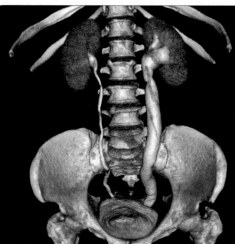

(Left) *Axial CECT shows a bladder diverticulum ➡ near the uterovesical junction with delayed partial opacification. This might be confused with a dilated ureter or even a cystic pelvic mass.* (Right) *Coronal CECT shows diffuse dilation of the left ureter and calices in a 55-year-old woman with repeated urinary tract infections and with no evidence of reflux. Note the absence of renal scarring or decreased function.*

SECTION 18
Bladder

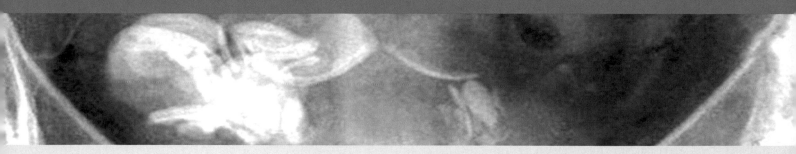

Generic Imaging Patterns

Filling Defect in Urinary Bladder

DIFFERENTIAL DIAGNOSIS

Common

- Bladder Carcinoma
- Bladder Calculi
- Blood Clot
- Ureterocele
- Diverticulitis
- Bladder Fistulas
- Foreign Body
- Extravesical Pelvic Mass
  - Benign Prostatic Hypertrophy
  - Prostate Carcinoma
  - Rectal Carcinoma
  - Cervical Carcinoma
  - Endometrioma
- Postoperative State
- Cystitis
  - Emphysematous Cystitis
  - Schistosomiasis

Less Common

- Urachal Carcinoma
- Inverted Papilloma
- Inflammatory Pseudotumor
- Mesenchymal Neoplasms
- Lymphoma and Metastasis

ESSENTIAL INFORMATION

Key Differential Diagnosis Issues

- Mobility, location, and shape of lesion suggest diagnosis or limit differential
  - Enhancement of lesion = neoplastic or inflammatory
    - Excludes calculi, blood clot, debris
  - Chronic inflammation of bladder leads to clinical and imaging features that are difficult to distinguish from neoplastic disease
  - Cystoscopy and biopsy often necessary to differentiate neoplastic and inflammatory lesions

Helpful Clues for Common Diagnoses

- **Bladder Carcinoma**
  - Types: Urothelial carcinoma (most common), squamous cell carcinoma, adenocarcinoma
  - Sessile or pedunculated soft tissue mass projecting into lumen
  - Similar density to bladder wall on CECT
  - Can never exclude cancer by imaging
    - Cystoscopy is gold standard for evaluation of lower urinary tract; all patients with unexplained hematuria require cystoscopy
- **Bladder Calculi**
  - Smooth round or ovoid; can be spiculated ("jack stone"), laminated, or faceted
  - US: Mobile, echogenic, shadowing foci
  - All radiopaque on CT; most radiopaque on plain films
- **Blood Clot**
  - US: Mobile mass, does not cast acoustic shadow, no internal vascularity
  - Attenuation value 50-60 HU; no enhancement on CECT

- **Ureterocele**
  - Intravesical: Ureterocele is entirely in bladder
    - Cobra-head or spring-onion deformity of distal ureter with surrounding radiolucent halo
  - Ectopic: Insertion at bladder neck or in posterior urethra
    - Smooth, radiolucent intravesicular mass near bladder base
  - High association with duplicated renal collecting system
- **Diverticulitis**
  - Commonly causes inflammatory thickening of adjacent wall of bladder
  - Abscess arising from sigmoid diverticulitis especially prone to involve bladder
  - May give rise to colovesical fistula (most common cause in industrialized countries)
- **Bladder Fistulas**
  - Gas in bladder, bladder wall thickening
  - Enterovesical: Diverticulitis most common cause
    - Other causes include Crohn disease, radiation (cystitis &/or enteritis), carcinomas of bladder, bowel, or other pelvic viscera
  - Vesicovaginal: Patient has persistent vaginal discharge
    - Cystography or delayed-phase CECT are preferred modalities to show communication
- **Foreign Body**
  - Bladder catheter (Foley) is extremely common in hospitalized patients
  - Next most common cause is introduction during autoeroticism or child abuse
    - Pieces of catheters, hair, sutures, and other objects are recognized
  - Can become nidus for calcification
- **Extravesical Pelvic Mass**
  - Any neoplastic (or inflammatory) process arising in pelvis can indent or invade bladder
    - Neoplastic: Carcinoma of prostate, rectum, cervix
    - Inflammatory: Endometriosis, pelvic abscess
  - Benign prostatic hypertrophy (BPH)
    - Displaces floor of bladder cephalad
    - Classic finding on urography is upward deviation of distal ureters
      - J-shaped ureters
    - Often accompanied by clinical symptoms of dysuria and hematuria, raising concern for bladder cancer
      - Trabeculation of bladder wall from chronic outlet obstruction may also simulate signs of bladder cancer
      - Cystoscopy usually necessary for definitive diagnosis
  - Prostate carcinoma
    - Mass effect of tumor may indent bladder floor similar to BPH
    - Tumor may invade bladder, causing intramural or even intraluminal mass
  - Endometrioma
    - Direct implantation of endometrium, typically in uterovesical pouch
    - Contains areas of hemorrhage (inherent T1 hyperintensity on MR) and shows avid enhancement
- **Postoperative State**

- Surgeries such as segmental cystectomy, bladder augmentation, and psoas-hitch ureterocystostomy result in distortion of normal bladder anatomy and apparent filling defects
- Teflon injection for treatment of vesiculoureteric reflux [subureteric Teflon injection (STING)] or incontinence
  - High-density, intramural and extravesical "mass"
- **Cystitis**
  - Many causes
    - Infectious: Bacterial, viral, fungal, parasites (*Schistosoma hematobium*)
    - Medication induced: Chemotherapy, especially with cyclophosphamide (Cytoxan); antibiotics
    - Interstitial (idiopathic); urine is sterile
    - Eosinophilic: May cause pseudotumoral cystitis, especially in children
    - Radiation therapy
  - Emphysematous cystitis
    - Most commonly seen in patients with longstanding and poorly controlled diabetes mellitus
    - Caused by bacterial fermentation of glucose in urine or urothelium
      - Can release gas (carbon dioxide) within bladder lumen &/or wall
      - Gas limited to lumen is difficult to recognize on radiography, and cause is more often iatrogenic (catheterization)
  - Schistosomiasis
    - Endemic in Middle East, Africa, and South America; extremely rare in USA
    - Causes nodular bladder wall thickening and calcification

Helpful Clues for Less Common Diagnoses

- **Urachal Carcinoma**
  - Mass ± calcification extending up from dome of bladder toward umbilicus
  - Infected urachal cyst may have similar appearance
- **Inverted Papilloma**
  - May arise in bladder (or ureter or renal pelvis)

- Usually small sessile or pedunculated mass
- **Inflammatory Pseudotumor**
  - Polypoid mass caused by nonneoplastic proliferation of myofibroblasts in inflammatory cells
  - a.k.a. myofibroblastic tumor, pseudosarcomatous fibromyxoid tumor, plasma cell granuloma
  - Usual appearance is vascular, bulky mass in patient with gross hematuria
- **Mesenchymal Neoplasms**
  - Primary neoplasms of bladder deriving from nonepithelial elements
    - Leiomyoma, paraganglioma, fibroma, hemangioma, neurofibroma, plasmacytoma
  - Rare; altogether account for < 5% of bladder tumors; malignant counterparts (sarcomas) are exceedingly rare
  - Mesenchymal tumors are intramural and overlying urothelium is intact
  - Imaging features of mesenchymal tumors and papillary urothelial carcinoma overlap
  - Several mesenchymal tumors have quasi-characteristic features on MR
    - ↑ T1 signal in paraganglioma; ↓ T2 in leiomyoma; target sign in neurofibroma

SELECTED REFERENCES

1. Mouli S et al: Imaging features of common and uncommon bladder neoplasms. Radiol Clin North Am. 50(2):301-16, vi, 2012
2. Philippou P et al: The management of bladder lithiasis in the modern era of endourology. Urology. 79(5):980-6, 2012
3. Sudakoff GS et al: CT urography of urinary diversions with enhanced CT digital radiography: preliminary experience. AJR 184: 131-138; 2005
4. Yu NC et al: Fistulas of the genitourinary tract: a radiologic review. Radiographics. 24(5):1331-52, 2004

Bladder Carcinoma

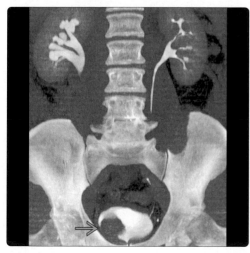

Bladder Carcinoma

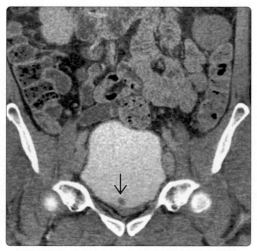

(Left) Coronal MIP reformat from delayed-phase CECT in a 69-year-old man shows a large intravesical filling defect ⇥ near the trigone (biopsy-proven invasive urothelial carcinoma). Note right-sided hydronephrosis due to obstruction at the right ureterovesical junction. (Right) Coronal delayed-phase CECT through the bladder shows a small polypoid filling defect ⇥ in the right bladder base. The lesion was resected during cystoscopy, and pathology showed low-grade urothelial carcinoma.

Filling Defect in Urinary Bladder

Bladder Calculi

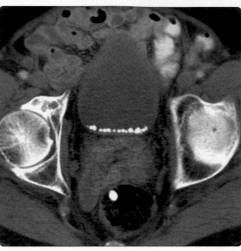

Bladder Calculi

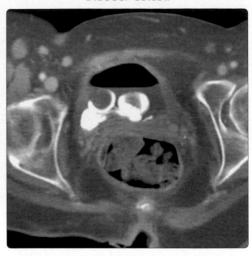

(Left) *Axial CECT through the urinary bladder shows multiple rounded, calcified stones layering in the dependent portion of the bladder. The patient had longstanding urinary obstruction in the setting of benign prostatic hypertrophy.* (Right) *Axial CECT shows multiple calcified stones and gas within the urinary bladder. Repeated urinary infections are a predisposing cause for calculi.*

Blood Clot

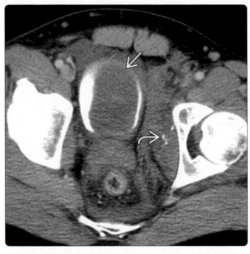

Ureterocele

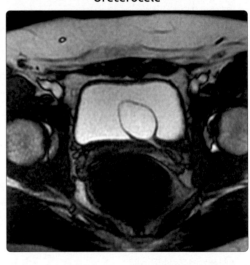

(Left) *Axial CECT shows a large filling defect ➡ within the bladder that represents blood clot, following a gunshot wound to the pelvis. Note the bone fragments ➡ and extraperitoneal pelvic sidewall hemorrhage.* (Right) *Axial steady-state free precession (FIESTA) image through the bladder shows a classic cobra-head appearance of an intravesical ("orthotopic") ureterocele with a thin wall.*

Diverticulitis

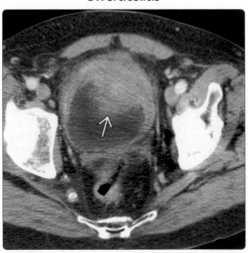

Diverticulitis

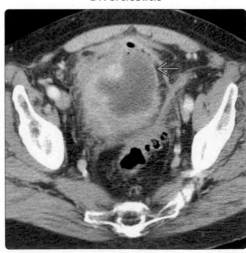

(Left) *Axial CECT shows marked asymmetric thickening of the bladder wall ➡ adjacent to sigmoid diverticulitis with a pericolic and perivesical abscess, causing inflammation of the bladder wall. The inflammatory mass may be complicated by a colovesical fistula.* (Right) *Axial CECT shows a large abscess ➡ arising from perforated sigmoid diverticulitis that abutted the dome of the bladder and led to marked bladder wall thickening simulating a bladder wall mass.*

Bladder Fistulas

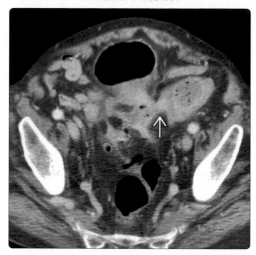

Bladder Fistulas

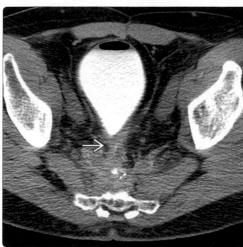

(Left) *Axial CECT shows intraluminal gas within the urinary bladder, as well as the fistulous tract* ➡ *between the sigmoid colon and bladder, due to diverticulitis in an 80-year-old man.* (Right) *Axial NECT shows a deformed bladder with gas and a soft tissue density tract* ➡ *extending toward the rectum. This colovesical fistula was due to rectal cancer that had been treated with low anterior resection and radiation therapy.*

Foreign Body

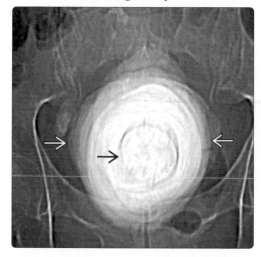

Foreign Body

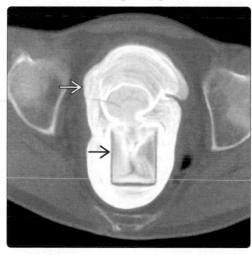

(Left) *Frontal radiograph shows a large, heavily calcified mass* ➡ *surrounding a foreign body* ➡, *a glass bottle that had been inserted into the vagina months before. The foreign body eroded into the bladder and lead to chronic urinary tract infections.* (Right) *Axial NECT in the same patient shows heavy calcification* ➡ *surrounding a foreign body (glass bottle)* ➡ *in the vagina that had eroded into the bladder and caused chronic urinary infection.*

Benign Prostatic Hypertrophy

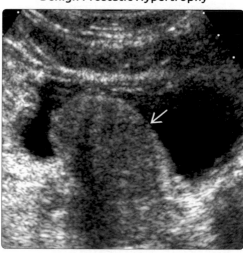

Benign Prostatic Hypertrophy

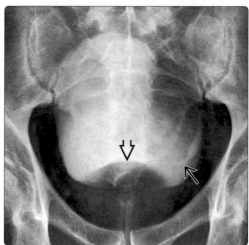

(Left) *Transverse grayscale ultrasound in an 82-year-old man presenting with symptoms of bladder outlet obstruction reveals marked distortion and indentation of the bladder base* ➡ *due to benign prostatic hypertrophy.* (Right) *Frontal projection from IVP in the same patient shows an extrinsic impression* ➡ *on the base of the bladder with fish-hooking or J-shaped appearance of the left ureter* ➡.

(Left) *Axial CECT shows an eccentric mass* ➡ *arising from the prostate. This unusually advanced and locally invasive prostate cancer indents and invades the bladder.* **(Right)** *Sagittal T2WI MR in a patient with history of cervical cancer shows a bulky cervical mass of intermediate signal intensity* ⬅ *that indents the posterior wall of the bladder.*

Prostate Carcinoma

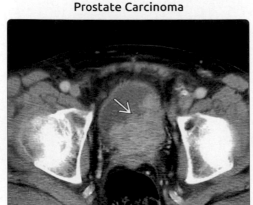

Cervical Carcinoma

(Left) *Longitudinal color Doppler US in a young female patient with history of pelvic pain shows an intramural mass* ➡ *centered within the ureterovesical recess that protrudes into the bladder lumen. The mass forms obtuse angles with the bladder wall. The mass was confirmed to be an endometrioma.* **(Right)** *Coronal CT in a patient with history of neurogenic bladder shows distortion of normal bladder anatomy following bladder augmentation using a segment of ileum. Note the submucosal fat deposition in the ileal segment* ➡.

Endometrioma

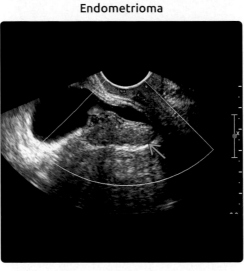

Postoperative State

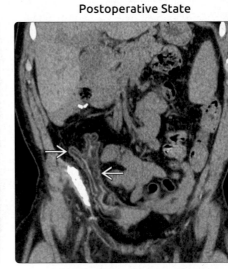

(Left) *Axial CECT shows marked bladder wall thickening* ➡ *due to chemotherapy-induced cystitis. A Foley catheter is in place.* **(Right)** *Axial NECT in an 80-year-old man with history of diabetes and emphysematous cystitis shows gas within the bladder lumen* ➡ *and bladder wall* ⬅.

Cystitis

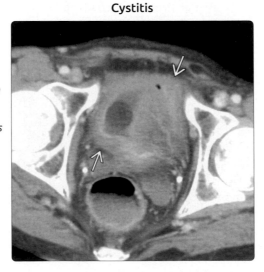

Emphysematous Cystitis

Urachal Carcinoma

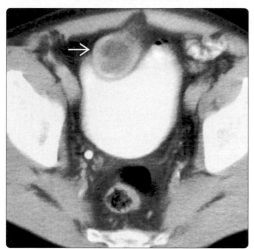

Urachal Carcinoma

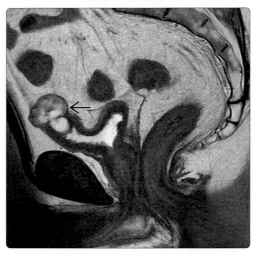

(Left) *Axial CECT shows a heterogeneous, near-midline mass* ➡ *that indents the dome of the bladder. The lesion was surgically resected and pathology showed adenocarcinoma arising in a urachal remnant.* **(Right)** *Sagittal T2 SSFSE MR demonstrates a complex solid/cystic mass* ➡ *in the bladder dome. The patient underwent partial cystectomy, and pathology was consistent with urachal adenocarcinoma.*

Inverted Papilloma

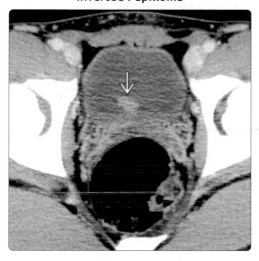

Inflammatory Pseudotumor

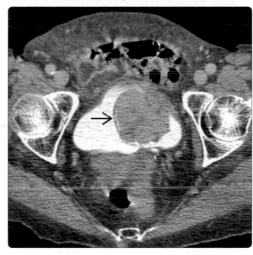

(Left) *Axial CECT in an 18-year-old man with history of gross hematuria shows a small polypoid mass* ➡ *arising from the posterior bladder wall. The lesion was resected during cystoscopy and was confirmed to be an inverted papilloma.* **(Right)** *Axial CECT in a 76-year-old woman shows a large, enhancing intraluminal bladder mass* ➡ *with surface calcification. At surgery, the mass was vascular and extremely firm and was consistent with an inflammatory pseudotumor.*

Mesenchymal Neoplasms

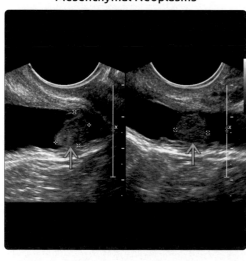

Mesenchymal Neoplasms

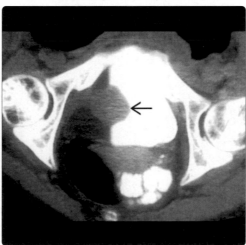

(Left) *Transverse and longitudinal US images through the bladder in a 66-year-old woman show a polypoid lesion* ➡ *at the inferior aspect of the bladder. Pathology was consistent with a bladder paraganglioma.* **(Right)** *Axial CECT shows a soft tissue density mass* ➡ *in the wall of the urinary bladder. This patient had symptoms of excess catecholamine release with bladder voiding.*

DIFFERENTIAL DIAGNOSIS

Common

- Bladder Diverticulum
- Bladder Fistulas
- Neurogenic Bladder
- Bladder Trauma
- Bladder Herniation

Less Common

- Urachal Remnant
- Bladder Augmentation Surgery
- Everted Ureterocele
- Iatrogenic

ESSENTIAL INFORMATION

Helpful Clues for Common Diagnoses

- **Bladder Diverticulum**
  - Most are acquired & secondary to bladder outlet obstruction
  - Congenital form, known as Hutch diverticulum, is rare
    - Caused by congenital weakness in detrusor muscle anterolateral to ureteral orifice
  - Usually near ureterovesical junction; can be multiple & large
  - More common in patients with bladder outlet obstruction or neurogenic bladder
- **Bladder Fistulas**
  - To bowel, colon, vagina, skin
  - Secondary to inflammatory or neoplastic processes in bladder or adjacent organs
  - Look for gas in bladder, thick wall, perivesical inflammatory changes
- **Neurogenic Bladder**
  - Suprasacral type (injury above S2-4 level) results in detrusor hyperreflexia & detrusor-sphincter dyssynergia
    - Christmas tree or pine cone shape
    - Elongated & pointed bladder with pseudodiverticula

  - Patient with suprasacral spinal injury (trauma, spinal tumor, multiple sclerosis)
- **Bladder Trauma**
  - Intraperitoneal rupture of dome: Surgical emergency
  - Extraperitoneal: Flame-shaped collection of extravasated urine
    - May extend beyond perivesical space (scrotum, thigh, retroperitoneum, etc.)
- **Bladder Herniation**
  - May herniate into inguinal, femoral, or obturator canals

Helpful Clues for Less Common Diagnoses

- **Urachal Remnant**
  - Incomplete obliteration of embryonic connection between bladder dome & allantoic duct
  - Midline cystic collection opening into bladder dome
- **Bladder Augmentation Surgery**
  - For patient with decreased bladder capacity or decreased detrusor compliance (e.g., neurogenic)
  - Isolated loop of ileum &/or segment of colon is used to augment bladder
    - Attached to superior surface of bladder
- **Everted Ureterocele**
  - Ureterocele may temporarily evert during voiding & mimic diverticula
  - Continuous with ureter
  - If seen during VCUG, check initial images & look for intravesical ureterocele
- **Iatrogenic**
  - Site of prior suprapubic catheterization

SELECTED REFERENCES

1. Jung JH et al: Establishment of the novel cystoscopic classification for bladder trabeculation of neurogenic bladder. Urology. 84(3):515-9, 2014
2. Alexander RE et al: Bladder diverticulum: clinicopathologic spectrum in pediatric patients. Pediatr Dev Pathol. 15(4):281-5, 2012
3. Tang YZ et al: Imaging features of colovesical fistulae on MRI. Br J Radiol. 85(1018):1371-5, 2012
4. Berrocal T et al: Anomalies of the distal ureter, bladder, and urethra in children: Embryologic, radiologic, and pathologic features. RadioGraphics 22: 1139-1164; 2002

Bladder Diverticulum

Bladder Diverticulum

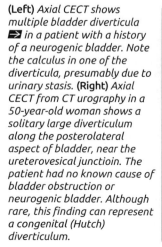
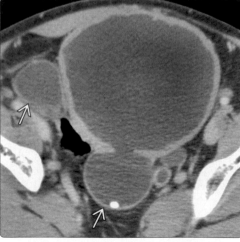
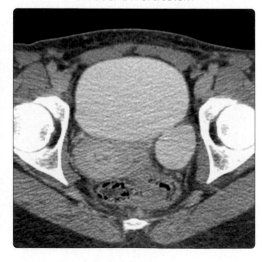

(Left) Axial CECT shows multiple bladder diverticula ➡ in a patient with a history of a neurogenic bladder. Note the calculus in one of the diverticula, presumably due to urinary stasis. (Right) Axial CECT from CT urography in a 50-year-old woman shows a solitary large diverticulum along the posterolateral aspect of bladder, near the ureterovesical junctioin. The patient had no known cause of bladder obstruction or neurogenic bladder. Although rare, this finding can represent a congenital (Hutch) diverticulum.

Bladder Fistulas

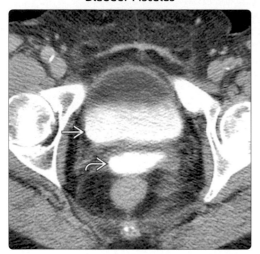

Neurogenic Bladder

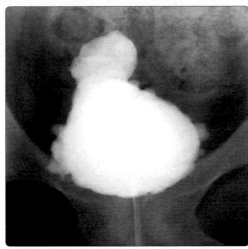

(Left) *Axial CECT in a 71-year-old woman with history of vesicovaginal fistula following hysterectomy shows extension of contrast-opacified urine from the bladder ➡ into the vagina ➡. (Right) Frontal cystogram shows a classic pine cone or Christmas tree appearance of a neurogenic bladder in 20-year-old man with spina bifida.*

Bladder Trauma

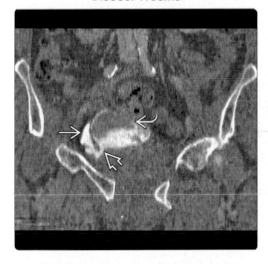

Urachal Remnant

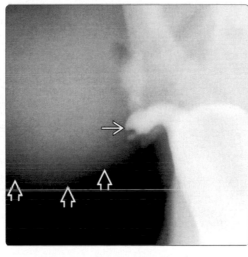

(Left) *Coronal CECT in 63-year-old man with a history of pelvic trauma shows a perivesical collection of extraluminal contrast ➡. Note the site of rupture ➡ and blood clot ➡ in the bladder. (Right) Lateral projection from voiding cystourethrogram shows an outpouching at the dome of the bladder ➡ that extends toward the umbilicus in this 8-year-old boy with an unrepaired omphalocele ➡ and other congenital anomalies.*

Bladder Augmentation Surgery

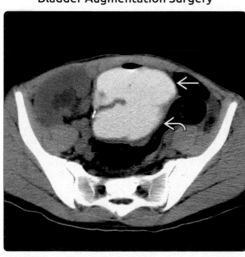

Everted Ureterocele

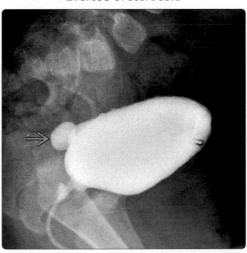

(Left) *Axial CECT shows augmentation of the bladder in a 20-year-old man with a neurogenic bladder and renal transplantation. The anastomosed pouch of bowel ➡ lies along the ventral surface of the bladder ➡. (Right) Anterior oblique projection from a VCUG in a male toddler shows bladder outpouching ➡ at the UVJ. The patient had a ureterocele in this area earlier during the procedure, which everted to outside of bladder upon further distention.*

DIFFERENTIAL DIAGNOSIS

Common

- Iatrogenic
- Bladder Fistulas
- Cystitis

Less Common

- Emphysematous Cystitis

ESSENTIAL INFORMATION

Key Differential Diagnosis Issues

- Gas in bladder should not be automatically attributed to catheterization
  - Confirm history of recent catheterization
  - Look for evidence of bladder fistula
- Evaluate medical record for clinical signs and symptoms of infected urine or fistula
  - Dysuria, pneumaturia, heavy growth of multiple coliform bacteria from urine

Helpful Clues for Common Diagnoses

- **Iatrogenic**
  - Most common cause of bladder gas
  - Check for history of recent instrumentation
    - Foley catheter, suprapubic bladder catheter
    - Cystoscopy
  - Usually not large volume of gas
  - Gas bubbles suspended within urine is suggestive of complex urine consistency and should raise possibility of infection &/or fistula
- **Bladder Fistulas**
  - Secondary to inflammatory or neoplastic process in bladder or adjacent organs
    - Colovesical fistula
      - Diverticulitis (most common cause: 80% of cases)
      - Look for signs of diverticulitis: Colonic wall thickening, diverticula, abscess adjacent to bladder, loss of fat plane between bowel and bladder
    - Enterovesical fistula

- Crohn disease is most common cause
    - Vesicocutaneous fistula
      - Usually due to surgical complication or trauma
    - Vesicovaginal fistula
      - Gynecologic surgery is most common cause
  - Cystography and enema can identify fistula in < 50% of cases; CT has much higher sensitivity for detection of fistula itself and secondary signs
- **Cystitis**
  - Bladder wall thickening ± mural hypodensity (edema) ± perivesical inflammatory changes
  - Hypoechoic bladder wall on US
  - Usually involves entire bladder wall

Helpful Clues for Less Common Diagnoses

- **Emphysematous Cystitis**
  - Most commonly seen in patients with longstanding and poorly controlled diabetes mellitus and patients on immunosuppression
  - Due to bacterial fermentation of excessive glucose within urothelium and urine
  - Gas in bladder wall &/or lumen
  - Responsible organisms are: *Escherichia coli*, *Klebsiella pneumoniae*, *Aerobacter aerogenes*, *Candida albicans*
  - Usually treated with medical therapy (parenteral antibiotics) alone; rarely bladder irrigation or debridement might be necessary

SELECTED REFERENCES

1. Yu M et al: Complicated genitourinary tract infections and mimics. Curr Probl Diagn Radiol. ePub, 2016
2. Yu NC et al: Fistulas of the genitourinary tract: a radiologic review. Radiographics. 24(5):1331-52, 2004
3. Grayson DE et al: Emphysematous infections of the abdomen and pelvis: a pictorial review. Radiographics. 22(3):543-61, 2002
4. Joseph RC et al: Genitourinary tract gas: imaging evaluation. Radiographics. 16(2):295-308, 1996

Iatrogenic

Bladder Fistulas

(Left) *Axial NECT shows gas* ➡ *within the bladder due to placement of a bladder (Foley) catheter* ➡. *The catheter bulb is spherical and usually has water density fluid and a gas bubble within it.* (Right) *Axial CECT in an 80-year-old man shows a large volume of gas* ➡ *within the bladder and a fistulous tract* ➡ *to the sigmoid colon that showed extensive signs of diverticulitis.*

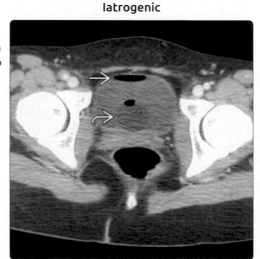
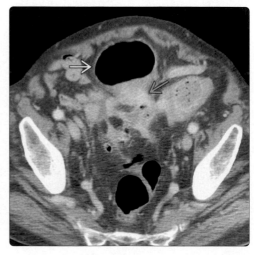

Bladder Fistulas

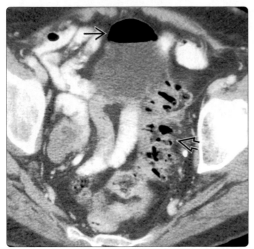

Bladder Fistulas

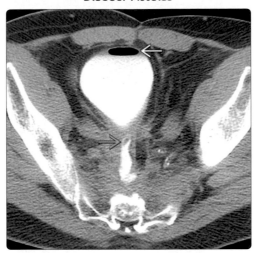

(Left) Axial CECT shows gas ➡ within the bladder due to a fistulous connection to the sigmoid colon. Note extensive diverticular disease ➡. (Right) Axial CT cystogram shows contrast-opacified urine extending from the bladder through a fistulous tract ➡ into the rectosigmoid colon. The patient had prior low anterior resection and radiation therapy for rectal cancer. Note gas ➡ in bladder.

Bladder Fistulas

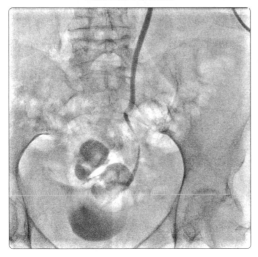

Emphysematous Cystitis

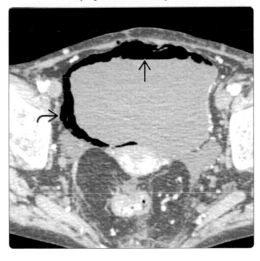

(Left) Frontal view from an antegrade ureterogram (performed during nephrostomy tube exchange) shows opacification of urinary bladder and sigmoid colon. The patient had extensive bowel surgeries complicated by multiple fistulas. (Right) Axial CECT shows gas within the lumen ➡ and wall ➡ of the bladder in a 33-year-old woman with a urinary infection and a prior small bowel transplantation. The infection and gas collections cleared with antibiotic therapy.

Emphysematous Cystitis

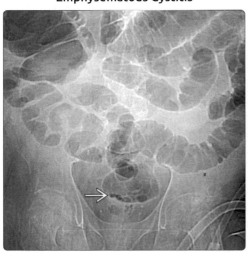

Emphysematous Cystitis

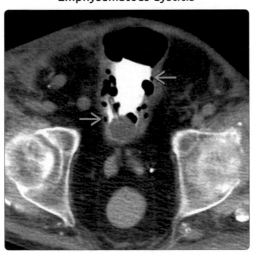

(Left) AP scout view in 55-year-old woman with a history of renal transplantation shows intravesical air as well as air locules ➡ in the expected location of the bladder wall. (Right) Axial CT cystogram in same patient who presented with abdominal pain and hypotension shows a large volume of intravesical air as well as intramural gas locules ➡ compatible with emphysematous cystitis.

DIFFERENTIAL DIAGNOSIS

Common

- Underfilled/Underdistended Bladder
- Normal Trigone
- Bacterial Cystitis
- Chronic Cystitis
- Neurogenic Bladder
- Chronic Bladder Outlet Obstruction
- Bladder Carcinoma
- Invasion by Pelvic Neoplasm

Less Common

- Fungal Cystitis
- Tuberculous Cystitis
- Bladder Schistosomiasis
- Emphysematous Cystitis
- Invasion by Pelvic Inflammatory Disease

ESSENTIAL INFORMATION

Key Differential Diagnosis Issues

- Bladder wall thickness should be commented on optimally distended bladder
- Be aware of sites of normal thickening near trigone
- Classify bladder wall thickening as focal or diffuse pattern
  - Focal suspicious for neoplastic process
- Color Doppler (including power Doppler) helps to identify intralesional vascularity in malignant conditions
- Check kidneys and ureters for hydronephrosis, other clues of infectious causes, such as TB and schistosomiasis
- Bladder echoes and debris often seen with cystitis

Helpful Clues for Common Diagnoses

- **Underfilled/Underdistended Bladder**
  - Common cause for pseudothickening of bladder wall
    - Rescan with optimal distension
- **Normal Trigone**
  - Normal mild thickening between ureteral orifices (interureteric ridge)
  - May pose diagnostic challenge in patients with prostatomegaly
- **Bacterial Cystitis**
  - Most common etiology: *Escherichia coli*
    - Transurethral invasion of bladder by perineal flora in women
    - Bladder outlet obstruction and urinary stasis in men
  - Usually smooth diffuse bladder wall thickening
  - Recurrent bacterial infection: Malakoplakia
    - Granulomatous inflammatory process
    - Associated with *E. coli*
- **Chronic Cystitis**
  - Associated with vesicoureteric reflux
  - Associated with decreased bladder capacity
  - Other complications associated with chronic cystitis
    - Hyperplastic uroepithelial cell clusters (Brunn nests) form in bladder submucosa
    - Cystitis cystica
      - Fluid accumulation → pseudocysts
      - Malignant potential
    - Cystitis glandularis

- Transformation into glands
  - Radiation cystitis: Sequelae of radiation therapy for pelvic malignant neoplasm (uterine, cervical, prostate, and rectal carcinoma)
    - Small-volume bladder with diffuse irregular wall thickening
    - May be associated with obstructive hydronephrosis
    - May have fistulous communication with adjacent viscera secondary to necrosis (from obliterative endarteritis)
  - Chemotherapeutic agents induced cystitis, often causing hemorrhagic cystitis
    - Common agents: Cyclophosphamide (cytoxan), ifosfamide, bacillus Calmette-Guérin (BCG) instillation for Ca bladder
- **Neurogenic Bladder**
  - Dysfunctional bladder secondary to neural injury regulating bladder
  - Diffuse bladder thickening ± trabeculations
    - Muscular hypertrophy leading to irregular outline of inner bladder wall
  - Typical Christmas tree-shaped bladder
  - Detrusor hyperreflexia
    - Gross trabeculation and abnormal shape
- **Chronic Bladder Outlet Obstruction**
  - Usually in males secondary to benign prostatic hypertrophy
  - Diffuse bladder wall thickening with trabeculations
  - ± focal pseudopolyps, which are indistinguishable from tumor
- **Bladder Carcinoma**
  - Commonly appears as focal bladder wall thickening
    - Polypoidal or broad-based most common
    - May see frond-like projections
  - Best diagnostic clue
    - Focal immobile mass with mixed echogenicity arising from bladder wall
      - Scan patient in decubitus position to differentiate from mobile blood clot or debris
    - Absent posterior acoustic shadowing
  - Color Doppler shows increased vascularity in most large tumors
  - Reported sensitivity for bladder tumor detection by US range from 50-95%
  - US may be useful in detecting tumor in bladder diverticulum, often inaccessible by cystoscopy
  - Tumor near bladder base in male may be confused with prostatic enlargement
    - Transrectal US differentiates bladder tumors from prostatic lesions
    - Bladder tumors and prostatic enlargement often coexist
    - Bladder tumors may invade prostate
- **Invasion by Pelvic Neoplasm**
  - Common tumors
    - Male
      - Rectal carcinoma
      - Prostate carcinoma
    - Female
      - Cervical carcinoma

□ Uterine carcinoma
□ Vaginal carcinoma
□ Ovarian carcinoma
o Loss of fat plane between bladder wall and adjacent pelvic neoplasm
o May have direct intramural and intralesional extension
– May be associated with fistulous communication
o Color Doppler
– Vascularity of tumor outside bladder cavity may be demonstrated

Helpful Clues for Less Common Diagnoses

- **Fungal Cystitis**
  o *Candida albicans* is most common organism
  o May be associated with fungal ball within bladder
- **Tuberculous Cystitis**
  o Hematogenous spread of primary tubercular infection, usually lungs (caused by *Mycobacterium tuberculosis*)
  o Secondary to renal ± ureteric involvement
  o Earliest form of bladder tuberculous cystitis starts around ureteral orifice
  o Typically low-volume bladder with diffuse wall thickening ("thimble bladder") ± wall calcification
  o Fibrotic changes near ureteric orifice result in vesicoureteric reflux
  o Associated with localized or generalized pyonephrosis
- **Bladder Schistosomiasis**
  o a.k.a. bilharziasis of bladder
  o Infection of urinary system by parasite *Schistosoma hematobium*
  o Thick-walled fibrotic bladder
  o Echogenic calcification within bladder wall
  o Small capacity bladder with inability to completely empty
  o ± hydronephrosis and hydroureter due to distal ureteric stricture
  o Late complication
  – Squamous cell carcinoma of bladder
  o Often difficult to differentiate from tuberculosis based on imaging
- **Emphysematous Cystitis**

o Infection of bladder wall by gas-forming bacterial or fungal organism
– *E. coli, Enterobacter aerogenes, Klebsiella pneumonia, Proteus mirabilis*
o Echogenic foci within area of bladder wall thickening with ring-down artifact
o Plain radiograph or CT for confirmation
- **Invasion by Pelvic Inflammatory Disease**
  o Crohn disease: Inflamed bowel or fistula formation
  o Sigmoid colonic diverticulitis
  o Endometriotic pelvic implants
  – Diffuse of focal bladder wall thickening, surrounding inflammatory changes
  – Increased vascularity in inflammatory tissue

SELECTED REFERENCES

1. Lee G et al: Cystitis: from urothelial cell biology to clinical applications. Biomed Res Int. 2014:473536, 2014
2. Manack A et al: Epidemiology and healthcare utilization of neurogenic bladder patients in a US claims database. Neurourol Urodyn. 30(3):395-401, 2011
3. Manikandan R et al: Hemorrhagic cystitis: A challenge to the urologist. Indian J Urol. 26(2).159-66, 2010
4. Vikram R et al: Imaging and staging of transitional cell carcinoma: part 1, lower urinary tract. AJR Am J Roentgenol. 192(6):1481-7, 2009
5. Figueiredo AA et al: Urogenital tuberculosis: update and review of 8961 cases from the world literature. Rev Urol. 10(3):207-17, 2008
6. Thomas AA et al: Emphysematous cystitis: a review of 135 cases. BJU Int. 100(1):17-20, 2007
7. Wein AJ et al: Overactive bladder: a better understanding of pathophysiology, diagnosis and management. J Urol. 175(3 Pt 2):S5-10, 2006
8. Wong-You-Cheong JJ et al: From the archives of the AFIP: Inflammatory and nonneoplastic bladder masses: radiologic-pathologic correlation. Radiographics. 26(6):1847-68, 2006
9. Abrams P: Bladder outlet obstruction index, bladder contractility index and bladder voiding efficiency: three simple indices to define bladder voiding function. BJU Int. 84(1):14-5, 1999

Underfilled/Underdistended Bladder

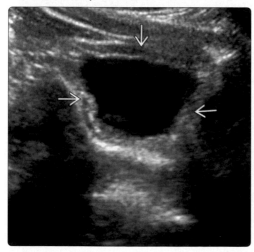

Normal Trigone

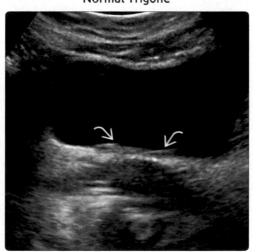

(Left) *Transverse transabdominal ultrasound shows an apparent uniformly thickened wall of an underdistended bladder ➡. The bladder wall was normal after optimal distension.* **(Right)** *Transverse transabdominal ultrasound shows a focal thickening ➡ at the interureteric ridge (trigone), a normal finding.*

(Left) *Transverse transabdominal ultrasound shows diffuse bladder wall thickening ➡ with internal debris ➡ and echoes ➡ in a patient with a urinary tract infection, with positive bacterial growth on urine culture.* **(Right)** *Transverse transabdominal ultrasound of the urinary bladder shows multiple large stones ➡ with diffuse wall thickening ➡, suggesting chronic cystitis.*

Bacterial Cystitis

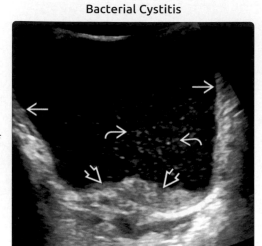

Chronic Cystitis

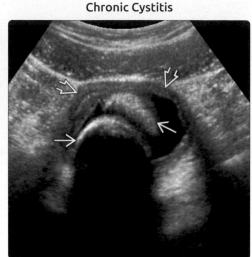

(Left) *Transverse transabdominal ultrasound shows a small-capacity bladder with wall thickening and an irregular inner bladder surface (trabeculations) ➡ in a neurogenic bladder.* **(Right)** *Longitudinal transabdominal ultrasound shows diffuse bladder wall thickening ➡ secondary to benign prostatic hyperplasia ➡ with a lobulated contour, indenting the bladder base. This is a common cause of chronic bladder outlet obstruction in elderly male patients.*

Neurogenic Bladder

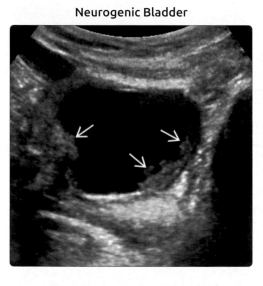

Chronic Bladder Outlet Obstruction

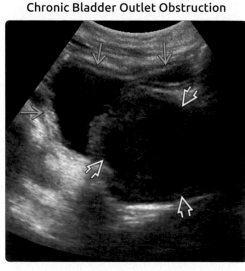

(Left) *Longitudinal color Doppler ultrasound of the bladder shows multiple solid masses ➡ arising from the posterior wall of the bladder with internal vascularity consistent with transitional cell carcinoma of the bladder. Note the echogenic debris ➡ within the bladder caused by associated hematuria.* **(Right)** *Transverse color Doppler image shows the bladder shows an irregular echogenic mass ➡ arising from the posterior wall of the bladder with internal vascularity ➡ consistent with bladder carcinoma.*

Bladder Carcinoma

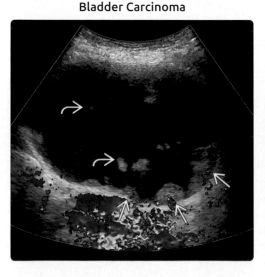

Bladder Carcinoma

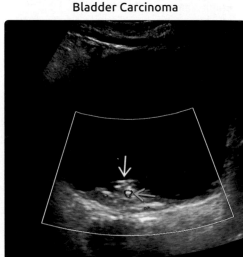

Invasion by Pelvic Neoplasm

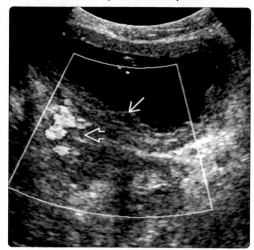

Tuberculous Cystitis

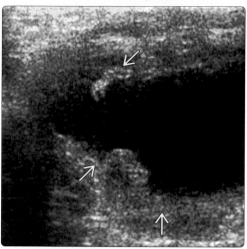

(Left) Longitudinal color Doppler ultrasound shows bladder wall thickening ➡ due to local invasion by uterine cancer. Increased vascularity is present in the tumor tissue ➡. (Right) Transverse transabdominal ultrasound shows a bladder infected by TB with an irregularly thickened bladder wall ➡. Tuberculous cystitis may be indistinguishable from other forms of bacterial cystitis.

Emphysematous Cystitis

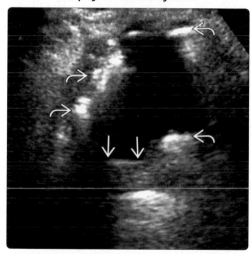

Emphysematous Cystitis

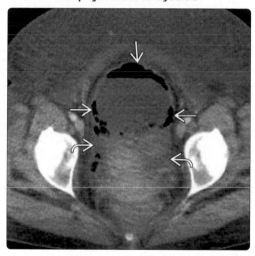

(Left) Transverse transabdominal ultrasound of the bladder shows diffuse wall thickening with several echogenic foci in the bladder wall (dependent and nondependent) ➡ with debris ➡ suggesting emphysematous cystitis. (Right) Axial contrast-enhanced CT through the pelvis shows gas within the bladder wall with ➡ perivesical/pelvic stranding ➡ (emphysematous cystitis).

Invasion by Pelvic Inflammatory Disease

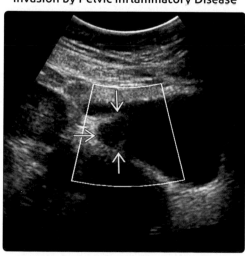

Invasion by Pelvic Inflammatory Disease

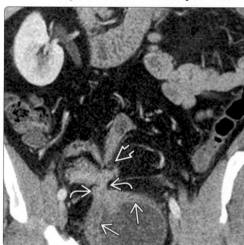

(Left) Transverse oblique transabdominal ultrasound shows a focal hypoechoic mass in the right bladder wall ➡ confirmed as endometriotic implant. (Right) Coronal reformat CECT in this patient with known Crohn disease shows asymmetric right bladder wall thickening ➡ secondary to fistulous communication ➡ with small bowel loops ➡ (enterovesical fistula).

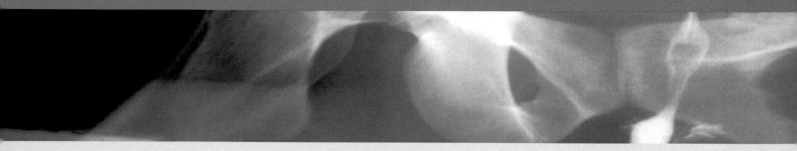

SECTION 19
Urethra

Generic Imaging Patterns

DIFFERENTIAL DIAGNOSIS

Common

- Infectious Stricture, Urethra
- Iatrogenic Stricture, Urethra
- Urethral Trauma
- Extrinsic Tumor Invasion

Less Common

- Urethral Carcinoma
- Reiter Syndrome
- Malakoplakia/Leukoplakia
- Cowper Gland Adenocarcinoma

Rare but Important

- Nonepithelial Neoplasms

ESSENTIAL INFORMATION

Key Differential Diagnosis Issues

- Presence and cause of stricture are usually evident to urologist performing cystoscopy

Helpful Clues for Common Diagnoses

- **Infectious Stricture, Urethra**
  - Filling of glands of Littré is highly suggestive of infectious process
  - Gonorrhea: Multifocal strictures
  - Nongonococcal: *Escherichia coli, Chlamydia, Mycoplasma,* herpes simplex virus, cytomegalovirus
  - Tuberculosis is rare, causes multiple fistulas ("watering can" perineum)
- **Iatrogenic Stricture, Urethra**
  - Mostly at penoscrotal junction, membranous portion, other narrow sites (bladder neck, meatus)
  - Secondary to passage of instruments, open surgery, indwelling catheter
  - Can be due to radiation therapy (for prostate cancer), periurethral Teflon injection (for incontinence)
- **Urethral Trauma**
  - Secondary to partial or complete urethral tears

  - – ± extravasation from partial or complete tear
  - Most often at membranous urethra
  - Solitary short segment stricture
- **Extrinsic Tumor Invasion**
  - Prostate, bladder, penile carcinoma

Helpful Clues for Less Common Diagnoses

- **Urethral Carcinoma**
  - Long, irregular narrowing ± fistula
  - Squamous cell carcinoma > transitional cell carcinoma > adenocarcinoma
  - 60% in bulbomembranous urethra
- **Reiter Syndrome**
  - Urethritis, balanitis, conjunctivitis, arthritis
  - 5x more common in men than in women
  - Involves entire penile urethra
- **Malakoplakia/Leukoplakia**
  - Malakoplakia: Rare granulomatous inflammation, mostly in females
  - Leukoplakia: Squamous metaplasia
- **Cowper Gland Adenocarcinoma**
  - Arises from bulbourethral glands in males
  - PSA(+)

Helpful Clues for Rare Diagnoses

- **Nonepithelial Neoplasms**
  - Extremely rare
  - Rhabdomyosarcoma (children) and leiomyosarcoma (adult) are most common

SELECTED REFERENCES

1. Angermeier KW et al: SIU/ICUD Consultation on urethral strictures: evaluation and follow-up. Urology. 83(3 Suppl):S8-17, 2014
2. Song L et al: Imaging techniques for the diagnosis of male traumatic urethral strictures. J Xray Sci Technol. 21(1):111-23, 2013
3. Kim B et al: Imaging of the male urethra. Semin Ultrasound CT MR. 28(4):258-73, 2007
4. Kawashima A et al: Imaging of urethral disease: a pictorial review. Radiographics. 24 Suppl 1:S195-216, 2004
5. Gallentine ML et al: Imaging of the male urethra for stricture disease. Urol Clin North Am. 29(2):361-72, 2002

Infectious Stricture, Urethra

Infectious Stricture, Urethra

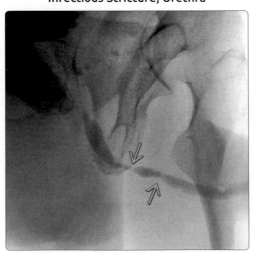

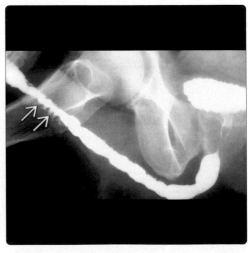

(Left) Retrograde urethrogram in a patient with gonococcal urethritis shows luminal irregularity of the urethra and multiple segments of mild stricturing ➡. (Right) Oblique retrograde urethrogram shows a long segment irregular narrowing of the penile and bulbous urethra with filling of the glands of Littré ➡. Filling of these small submucosal mucus-secreting glands is highly associated with an infectious process.

Urethral Stricture

Iatrogenic Stricture, Urethra

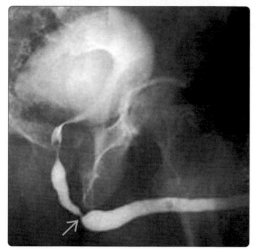

Iatrogenic Stricture, Urethra

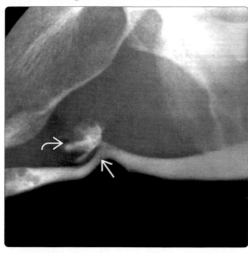

(Left) Retrograde urethrogram shows a focal stricture ➡ in the membranous portion of the urethra in a patient who had a prior history of cystoscopies. (Right) Oblique retrograde urethrogram shows a smooth stricture ➡ of the urethra and contrast filling of a cavity ➡ in the penis due to the passage of an instrument through the wall of the urethra.

Urethral Trauma

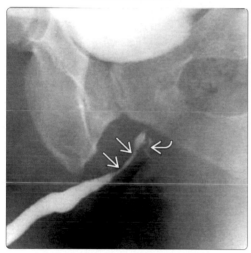

Urethral Trauma

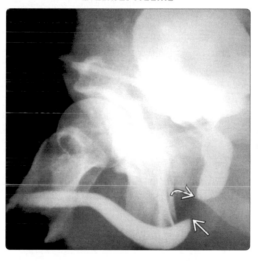

(Left) Oblique retrograde urethrogram shows a long, smooth urethral stricture ➡ in a man with a prior history of pelvic trauma. Note filling of the Cowper duct ➡. (Right) Simultaneous suprapubic and retrograde urethrogram shows a posttraumatic stricture extending from the prostatic ➡ to the bulbous ➡ urethra. This is the area of the urogenital diaphragm, which is the most common site of injury in blunt pelvic trauma.

Urethral Carcinoma

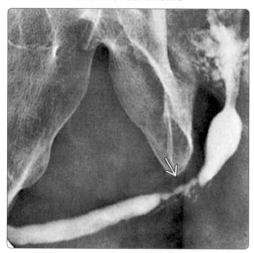

Urethral Carcinoma

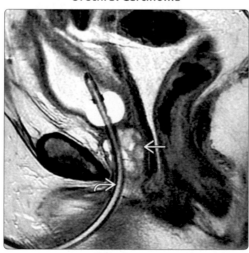

(Left) Retrograde urethrogram shows an irregular segment of stricture ➡ in the bulbous portion of the urethra due to transitional cell carcinoma. Unlike most iatrogenic strictures, malignant strictures have an irregular appearance. (Right) Coronal T2WI MR shows a heterogeneous mass ➡ arising from the urethra in a 63-year-old woman. This had caused bladder outlet obstruction and dysuria; note the bladder catheter ➡.

SECTION 20
Scrotum

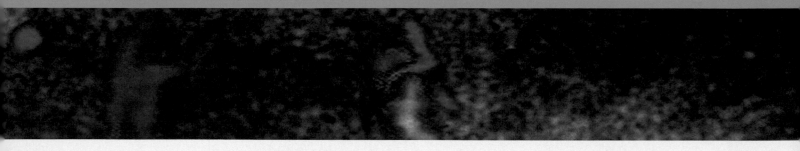

Generic Imaging Patterns

DIFFERENTIAL DIAGNOSIS

Common

- Testicular Carcinoma: Germ Cell Tumor
- Testicular Hematoma
- Epididymitis/Orchitis
- Testicular Torsion/Segmental Infarction

Less Common

- Testicular Abscess
- Testicular Lymphoma and Metastases
- Testicular Leukemia
- Gonadal Stromal Tumors, Testis
- Testicular Epidermoid Cyst

Rare but Important

- Granulomatous Orchitis
- Adrenal Rests

ESSENTIAL INFORMATION

Key Differential Diagnosis Issues

- Age, clinical presentation, color Doppler exam
  - Trauma and avascular testicular mass: Consider hematoma
  - Young male patient, acute scrotal pain, ↑ color Doppler flow within epididymis and adjacent testis: Epididymoorchitis
  - Acute scrotal pain, heterogeneous (or normal) testis with no or relatively ↓ Doppler flow: Testicular torsion
  - Young male patient with slowly growing palpable hypoechoic testicular mass: Seminoma or mixed germ cell tumor
  - Testicular mass and endocrinopathy: Gonadal stromal tumor
  - Elderly man, HIV(+), and bilateral hyperemic testicular masses: Lymphoma
- Sonographic findings are key (but overlap among various tumors)
  - Histopathological correlation is needed

Helpful Clues for Common Diagnoses

- **Testicular Carcinoma: Germ Cell Tumors**
  - Most common neoplasm in males aged 15-34 years
  - Vast majority are seminomas and mixed germ cell tumors
  - Seminoma: Typically solitary, homogeneous testicular mass
    - Rarely multifocal or partially cystic if necrotic
  - Other germ cell tumors: Teratoma, teratocarcinoma, embryonal cell carcinoma, yolk sac tumor, choriocarcinoma
    - Mixed echogenicity, heterogeneous masses often with cystic components, calcification
    - Imaging overlap precludes imaging diagnosis
    - Tumor markers and demographics (beta hCG, AFP, LDH) may suggest nonseminomatous component
      □ Endodermal sinus tumor/teratoma: 1st decade
    - Assess retroperitoneum if identify intratesticular mass
    - CECT is imaging modality of choice though for preoperative staging of nodal chains, lung metastases
- **Testicular Hematoma**

- Typically focal, elongated avascular intratesticular "mass" and history of trauma
- Echogenicity depends upon hematoma age
  - Acute hematoma may be relatively echogenic
- Critical additional findings at scrotal sonography
  - Tunica integrity and surrounding testicular viability (assessed by color Doppler)
  - Viable testis may allow for tunica repair, hematocele evacuation of testicular salvage
- Small, contained intratesticular hematomas: Ultrasound follow-up needed to ensure resolution (and to exclude underlying neoplasm)
- **Epididymitis/Orchitis**
  - Most common cause for acute scrotal pain in adolescent boys and adults
  - Epididymis primarily involved: 20-40% with secondary orchitis due to contiguous spread of infection
  - Ill-defined focal testicular echogenicity or diffusely enlarged, heterogeneous testis
  - Relatively increased Doppler flow
    - Mimic: Torsion-detorsion
  - Primary Mumps orchitis: Uni- or bilateral
    - Enlarged, heterogeneous, hyperemic testis (also mimics torsion-detorsion)
- **Testicular Torsion/Segmental Infarction**
  - Torsion: Grayscale appearance depends upon time course
    - Acute setting: Enlarged, heterogeneous testis with absent or relatively decreased Doppler flow
    - Chronic: Small testis, central hypoechogenicity with preserved peripheral testicular flow
  - Spiral twist of spermatic cord cranial to testis (whirlpool sign)
  - Color Doppler critical for diagnosis
    - 80-90% sensitivity for acute (complete) torsion
    - Partial torsion may have normal or nearly normal exam
    - Optimize technique for slow flow: Low pulse repetition frequency, low wall filter
  - Segmental infarction
    - Elongated, geographic hypoechogenicity: MR for confirmation
    - Rare cause for acute scrotum
    - Predisposing history: Vasculitis, sickle cell disease, hypercoagulable states

Helpful Clues for Less Common Diagnoses

- **Testicular Abscess**
  - Clinical history critical: Poorly or untreated epididymoorchitis
  - Avascular, mixed cystic and solid intratesticular mass, surrounding pyocele
- **Testicular Lymphoma and Metastases**
  - Lymphoma
    - Most common testicular tumor in men > 60 years, multiple lesions; 50% of cases are bilateral
    - Often large in size at time of diagnosis, commonly occurs in association with disseminated disease
    - Ill-defined, predominantly hypoechoic lesions: Increased flow at color Doppler interrogation

- o Metastases are rare; most common sites include prostate, lung, and GI tract
- **Testicular Leukemia**
  - o Appearance similar to lymphoma: Uni- or bilateral testicular masses/enlargement
  - o Blood-testis barrier limits chemotherapeutic effect in patients with acute leukemia: Testis acts as harbor for leukemic cells
- **Gonadal Stromal Tumors, Testis**
  - o Majority are benign but are indistinguishable from germ cell tumors
  - o Clinical history (endocrinopathy secondary to ↑ estrogen or testosterone by tumor) may be suggestive
    - Children: Precocious puberty/gynecomastia
    - Adults: Impotence, ↓ libido
- **Testicular Epidermoid Cyst**
  - o Benign tumor: Likely monodermal teratoma composed entirely of ectoderm
  - o 4 ultrasound appearances
    - Type 1: Classic onion skin appearance due to alternating layers of keratin and desquamated squamous cells
    - Type 2: Densely calcified echogenic mass with posterior shadowing
    - Type 3: Target/bull's-eye appearance (cystic appearing with echogenic center secondary to compact keratin)
    - Type 4: Mixed pattern
  - o Classic appearance may prompt enucleation rather than orchiectomy

Helpful Clues for Rare Diagnoses

- **Granulomatous Orchitis**
  - o Ill-defined hypoechoic mass: Mycobacterium infection or idiopathic
  - o Multiple hypoechoic masses in appropriate population (young black males); consider testicular sarcoidosis
- **Adrenal Rests**
  - o Clinical history (congenital adrenal hyperplasia) suggests diagnosis

- Aberrant adrenal rests trapped within developing gonad: Without stimulation typically < 5 mm
- If exposed to ↑ ACTH, they enlarge and become palpable masses
- May result in testicular structure damage, spermatogenesis disorder, infertility
- Glucocorticoid replacement therapy may stabilize or cause regression of masses
  - o Bilateral, often weakly shadowing testicular lesions

SELECTED REFERENCES

1. Shiraj S et al: Segmental testicular infarction, an underdiagnosed entity: case report with histopathologic correlation and review of the diagnostic features. Case Rep Radiol. 2016:8741632, 2016
2. Bertolotto M et al: Grayscale and color Doppler features of testicular lymphoma. J Ultrasound Med. 34(6):1139-45, 2015
3. Sommers DN et al: Sonographic findings of typical and atypical scrotal trauma. Ultrasound Q. 31(2):99-108, 2015
4. Yannes M et al: Testicular adrenal rests in congenital adrenal hyperplasia: a rare presentation of testicular masses. Ultrasound Q. ePub, 2015
5. Sommers D et al: Ultrasonography evaluation of scrotal masses. Radiol Clin North Am. 52(6):1265-81, 2014
6. Remer EM et al: ACR Appropriateness Criteria ® acute onset of scrotal pain–without trauma, without antecedent mass. Ultrasound Q. 28(1):47-51, 2012
7. Saxon P et al: Segmental testicular infarction: report of seven new cases and literature review. Emerg Radiol. 19(3):217-23, 2012
8. Sung EK et al: Sonography of the pediatric scrotum: emphasis on the Ts–torsion, trauma, and tumors. AJR Am J Roentgenol. 198(5):996-1003, 2012
9. Wasnik AP et al: Scrotal pearls and pitfalls: ultrasound findings of benign scrotal lesions. Ultrasound Q. 28(4):281-91, 2012
10. Bhatt S et al: Imaging of non-neoplastic intratesticular masses. Diagn Interv Radiol. 2011 Mar;17(1):52-63. Epub 2010 Jun 30. Review. Erratum in: Diagn Interv Radiol. 17(4):388, 2011
11. Dogra V et al: Acute painful scrotum. Radiol Clin North Am. 42(2):349-63, 2004
12. Woodward PJ et al: From the archives of the AFIP: tumors and tumorlike lesions of the testis: radiologic-pathologic correlation. Radiographics. 22(1):189-216, 2002

Testicular Carcinoma: Germ Cell Tumor

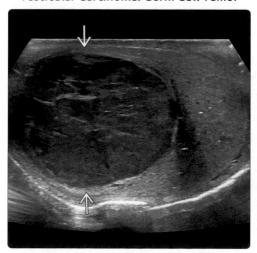

Testicular Carcinoma: Germ Cell Tumor

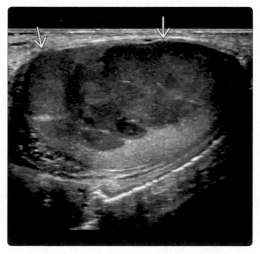

(Left) *Scrotal US in a 23-year-old man with a palpable mass shows a well-circumscribed, solid, hypoechoic testicular mass ➡. The vast majority of solid testicular masses in this age group are either seminomas or mixed germ cell tumors. Orchiectomy confirmed seminoma.* **(Right)** *Scrotal ultrasound shows a lobulated hypoechoic mass ➡ in this young male patient with brain, liver metastases, and retroperitoneal adenopathy. Increased LDH and β-hCG suggested a mixed germ cell tumor, which was identified at orchiectomy.*

Intratesticular Mass

Testicular Carcinoma: Germ Cell Tumor

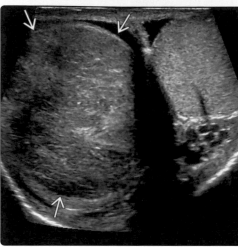

Testicular Hematoma

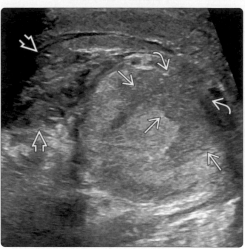

(Left) *Scrotal ultrasound of a young male patient shows almost complete replacement and enlargement of the right testis by a solid mass ➡. Ultrasound performed in the same setting demonstrated interaortocaval adenopathy (confirmed by staging CT). A seminoma was identified at orchiectomy.* **(Right)** *Scrotal ultrasound performed after blunt trauma shows an elongated testicular hematoma/laceration ➡, tunica disruption ➡, and an adjacent hematocele ➡.*

Testicular Hematoma

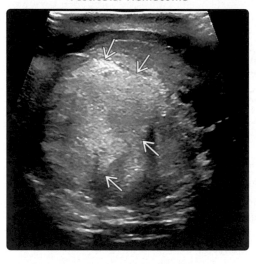

Epididymitis/Orchitis

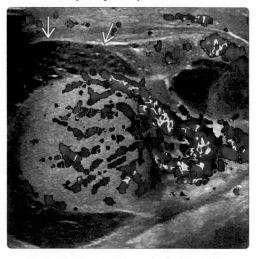

(Left) *Scrotal ultrasound post trauma shows an echogenic clot ➡ within a fractured testis. The testis was entirely necrotic despite emergent exploration and an orchiectomy was performed. Acute clot may rarely appear echogenic.* **(Right)** *Color Doppler ultrasound of a male patient with acute scrotal pain shows epididymal/adjacent testicular hyperemia and a surrounding pyocele ➡. Elongated testicular hypoechogenicity is typically the only grayscale manifestation of secondary orchitis.*

Epididymitis/Orchitis

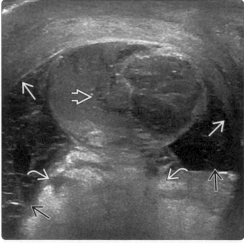

Testicular Torsion/Segmental Infarction

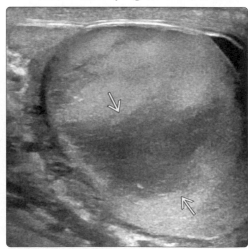

(Left) *Ultrasound performed for evaluation of persistent pain after antibiotic treatment for epididymitis shows focal orchitis ➡, paratesticular ➡ and scrotal wall edema ➡, and a pyocele ➡. Orchiectomy was eventually performed for a testicular abscess/necrosis.* **(Right)** *Ultrasound performed for evaluation of acute scrotal pain shows triangular hypoechogenicity ➡, an appearance suggestive of segmental infarction. Symptoms and hypoechogenicity resolved after steroid treatment of drug-induced vasculitis.*

Testicular Torsion/Segmental Infarction

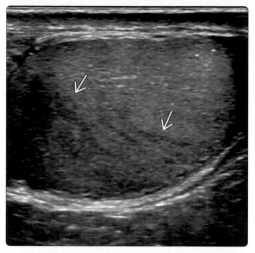

Testicular Torsion/Segmental Infarction

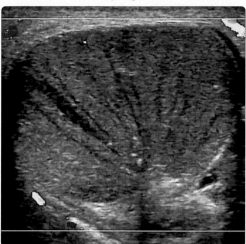

(Left) *Ultrasound performed after rapid resolution of acute scrotal pain shows focally prominent, hypoechoic septa* ➡. *Color Doppler (not shown) demonstrated corresponding hyperemia. The appearance might suggest primary (mumps) orchitis, but clinical history indicates detorsion, and hypoechogenicity resolved at follow-up.* (Right) *Color Doppler ultrasound performed after herniorrhaphy shows no flow within an enlarged, heterogeneous, hypoechoic, infarcted testis. Note the prominent septal pattern.*

Testicular Lymphoma and Metastases

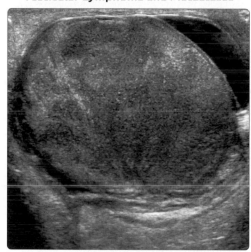

Testicular Epidermoid Cyst

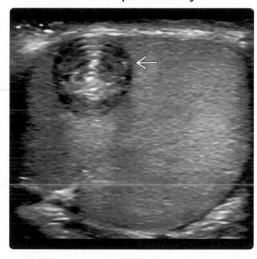

(Left) *US of an 83-year-old man with a scrotal mass shows an enlarged, heterogeneous testis. Retroperitoneal adenopathy was identified in the same setting. The age of the patient and US findings suggested lymphoma; B-cell lymphoma was identified at orchiectomy.* (Right) *Ultrasound of a young male patient shows a well-circumscribed, hypoechoic testicular mass* ➡. *Its characteristic onion skin appearance is almost pathognomic of an epidermoid cyst, which was successfully enucleated.*

Granulomatous Orchitis

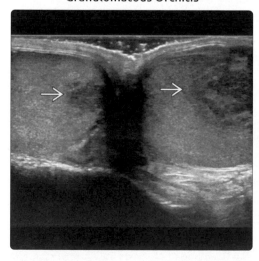

Adrenal Rests

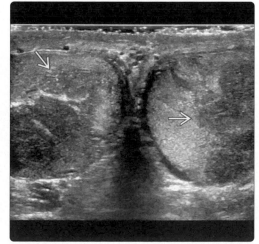

(Left) *Scrotal ultrasound performed on a black male patient with scrotal discomfort shows bilateral hypoechoic lesions* ➡. *Bilaterality might suggest multifocal germ cell tumor or lymphoma, but demographics and a clinical history of longstanding sarcoidosis indicate granulomatous orchitis (subsequently biopsy confirmed).* (Right) *Ultrasound of an infertile 35-year-old man with a history of congenital adrenal hyperplasia shows large bilateral adrenal rests* ➡.

DIFFERENTIAL DIAGNOSIS

Common

- Nonseminomatous Germ Cell Tumor
- Intratesticular Cyst
- Tubular Ectasia of Rete Testis
- Tunica Albuginea Cyst
- Testicular Abscess

Less Common

- Tunica Vaginalis Cyst
- Necrosis or Hemorrhage in Tumor
- Epidermoid Cyst
- Intratesticular Varicocele

ESSENTIAL INFORMATION

Key Differential Diagnosis Issues

- Testicular cysts are common (8-10% of men)
- Most cystic neoplasms have complex features
  - Mural nodularity, hemorrhage, or necrosis
  - Flow on color Doppler imaging

Helpful Clues for Common Diagnoses

- **Nonseminomatous Germ Cell Tumor**
  - Teratomas are usually well-defined complex masses
    - Cysts are common feature and may be anechoic or complex, depending on cyst contents
  - Cystic necrosis of tumor is not uncommon in other nonseminomatous germ cell tumors
- **Intratesticular Cyst**
  - Simple cyst: No septation
  - 2- to 18-mm diameter
  - Near mediastinum testis
- **Tubular Ectasia of Rete Testis**
  - Variably sized cystic lesions near mediastinum testis
    - Turn transducer to elongate into tubular channels
  - No flow on color Doppler
  - May be bilateral, asymmetrical
  - Often with associated spermatocele

- Typically in men > 55 yr
- **Tunica Albuginea Cyst**
  - Within tunica surrounding testis
  - Usually solitary, 2- to 3-mm diameter, can be septate
  - Gel pad and patient-targeted ultrasound of palpable mass aids ultrasound localization
- **Testicular Abscess**
  - Usually complication of epididymo-orchitis
  - Enlarged testis with hypoechoic or mixed pattern
  - Imaging alone cannot distinguish from tumor

Helpful Clues for Less Common Diagnoses

- **Tunica Vaginalis Cyst**
  - Rare, arises from visceral or parietal layer of tunica vaginalis
  - Usually anechoic; may have septations or may contain echoes due to hemorrhage
- **Necrosis or Hemmorrhage in Tumor**
  - Complex mixed cystic solid mass
    - Clinical history/close ultrasound follow-up helpful
- **Epidermoid Cyst**
  - Contents are cheesy keratin
  - Occasionally anechoic, but layered keratin often creates lamellated, onion skin appearance
  - May have calcified capsule
  - Presents as painless nodule in young man
- **Intratesticular Varicocele**
  - May mimic tubular ectasia: Color Doppler confirms venous flow
  - Often without extratesticular varicocele component

SELECTED REFERENCES

1. Garriga V et al: US of the tunica vaginalis testis: anatomic relationships and pathologic conditions. Radiographics. 29(7):2017-32, 2009
2. Bhatt S et al: Sonography of benign intrascrotal lesions. Ultrasound Q. 22(2):121-36, 2006
3. Dogra VS et al: Benign intratesticular cystic lesions: US features. Radiographics. 21 Spec No:S273-81, 2001
4. Langer JE et al: Epidermoid cysts of the testicle: sonographic and MR imaging features. AJR Am J Roentgenol. 173(5):1295-9, 1999
5. Martínez-Berganza MT et al: Cysts of the tunica albuginea: sonographic appearance. AJR Am J Roentgenol. 170(1):183-5, 1998

Nonseminomatous Germ Cell Tumor

Intratesticular Cyst

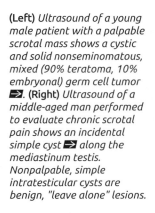

(Left) Ultrasound of a young male patient with a palpable scrotal mass shows a cystic and solid nonseminomatous, mixed (90% teratoma, 10% embryonal) germ cell tumor ➡. (Right) Ultrasound of a middle-aged man performed to evaluate chronic scrotal pain shows an incidental simple cyst ➡ along the mediastinum testis. Nonpalpable, simple intratesticular cysts are benign, "leave alone" lesions.

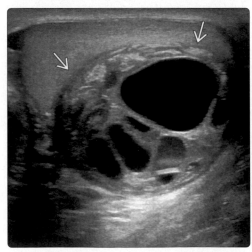

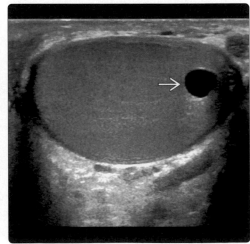

Tunica Albuginea Cyst

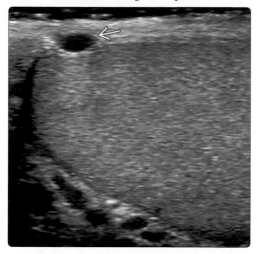

Tubular Ectasia of Rete Testis

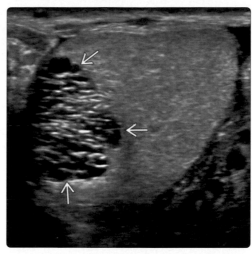

(Left) *Ultrasound of a young male patient with a palpable lesion shows a classic tunica albuginea cyst* ➡. *Copious gel and patient-directed ultrasound aids identification of these small, superficial benign cysts.* (Right) *Transverse ultrasound of an elderly man with epididymal cysts (not shown) shows a complex cystic mass* ➡ *along the mediastinum testis. Longitudinal imaging confirmed tubular ectasia. Location, patient age, and ultrasound features distinguish this benign entity from cystic testicular tumors.*

Necrosis or Hemorrhage in Tumor

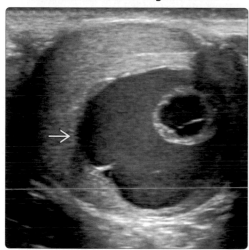

Testicular Abscess

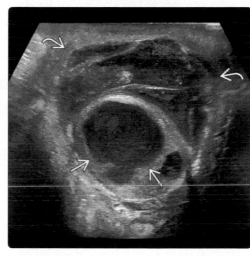

(Left) *US of a young male patient with persistent scrotal pain 3 weeks after mild trauma shows a complex cystic testicular mass* ➡. *Configuration and clinical history suggested intratumoral hemorrhage rather than testicular trauma. Hemorrhage within a mixed germ cell tumor was confirmed at orchiectomy.* (Right) *US performed on a male patient with profound mental retardation, scrotal pain, fever, and leukocytosis shows a large intratesticular abscess* ➡ *and a complex surrounding pyocele* ➡.

Intratesticular Varicocele

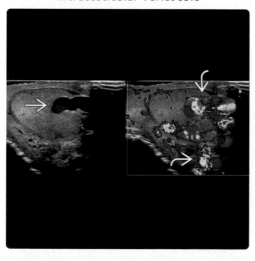

Epidermoid Cyst

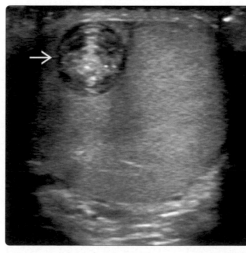

(Left) *Ultrasound of an elderly man with ischemic cardiomyopathy shows a tubular, cystic lesion* ➡ *within the mediastinum testis. Simultaneous color Doppler confirms a combined intra- and extratesticular varicocele* ➡. (Right) *This palpable scrotal mass* ➡ *has the characteristic onion skin appearance of a benign epidermoid cyst. Such an ultrasound appearance may prompt testis-sparing resection (as in this case).*

DIFFERENTIAL DIAGNOSIS

Common

- Hydrocele
- Spermatocele/Epididymal Cyst
- Pyocele
- Hematocele
- Varicocele

Less Common

- Scrotal Wall Fluid Collection
- Epididymal Papillary Cystadenoma

ESSENTIAL INFORMATION

Helpful Clues for Common Diagnoses

- **Hydrocele**
  - Serous fluid contained within layers of tunical vaginalis
    - Congenital: Communicating hydrocele secondary to failure of processus vaginalis to close
    - Secondary: e.g., due to epididymitis, varicocelectomy
  - Envelopes testis except for "bare area" where tunica vaginalis is deficient
  - Chronic hydroceles contain low-level echoes
- **Spermatocele/Epididymal Cyst**
  - Differentiated by contents (simple fluid within epididymal cyst, milky fluid containing spermatozoa within spermatocele)
  - Location within head suggests spermatocele
  - Epididymal cysts occur throughout epididymis
  - Septation, debris may suggest spermatocele, but imaging differentiation ultimately irrelevant: Both are benign lesions
  - Epididymal cysts associated with dilatation of rete testis
- **Pyocele**
  - Complex fluid collection containing septations, low-level echoes within layers of tunica vaginalis
  - Color Doppler
    - Testicular/epididymal hyperemia
  - Complication of epididymoorchitis

- **Hematocele**
  - Blood within tunica vaginalis potential space
  - Post trauma (assess testicle flow, tunica disruption)
  - Echogenicity depends upon age of blood; acute clot may appear echogenic
- **Varicocele**
  - Dilation of veins of pampiniform plexus > 2-3 mm in diameter due to retrograde flow in gonadal (testicular) vein
  - Dilated serpiginous veins behind superior pole of testis on color Doppler US, best imaging tool
  - Enlarge with Valsalva maneuver
  - Majority left sided: Consider retroperitoneal tumor if right sided

Helpful Clues for Less Common Diagnoses

- **Scrotal Wall Fluid Collections**
  - Clinical context key (e.g., trauma: Consider hematoma/fever, leukocytosis: consider abscess)
  - Slowly growing complex scrotal wall mass in pediatric population: Consider cystic lymphangioma
- **Papillary Cystadenoma of Epididymis**
  - Rare benign neoplasm, typically in young adult male patients
  - Associated with von Hippel-Lindau disease
  - Pathology (cystic spaces, intracystic papillary projections lined by clear cells) mimics renal cell carcinoma

SELECTED REFERENCES

1. Park SH et al: Sonographic findings in a case of scrotal lymphangioma. J Clin Ultrasound. 42(4):234-6, 2014
2. Toutziaris C et al: Papillary cystadenoma of epididymis: is there a need for further investigation in unilateral cases? Int J Surg Case Rep. 4(7):616-8, 2013
3. Aganovic L et al: Imaging of the scrotum. Radiol Clin North Am. 50(6):1145-65, 2012
4. Lee JC et al: Imaging of the epididymis. Ultrasound Q. 24(1):3-16, 2008
5. Smart JM et al: Ultrasound findings of masses of the paratesticular space. Clin Radiol. 63(8):929-38, 2008
6. Woodward PJ et al: From the archives of the AFIP: extratesticular scrotal masses: radiologic-pathologic correlation. Radiographics. 23 (1):215-40, 2003

Hydrocele

Spermatocele/Epididymal Cyst

(Left) Ultrasound shows a large simple hydrocele that expands the potential space between visceral and parietal layers of the tunica vaginalis. The hydrocele surrounds the entire testis, with the exception of the "bare area" . *(Right) Scrotal ultrasound shows a simple paratesticular cyst* ➡. *Differentiation between large epididymal cysts/spermatoceles and complex hydroceles may be difficult, but cysts displace, rather than envelop, the testis. Dilated rete testis* ➡ *are frequently associated with epididymal cysts.*

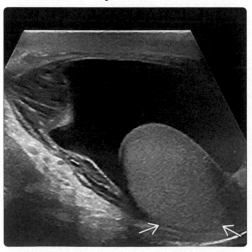

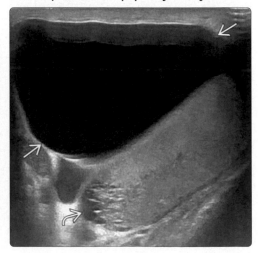

Hydrocele

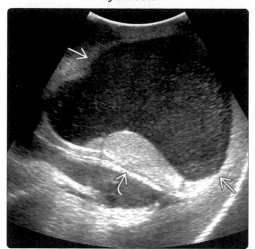

Spermatocele/Epididymal Cyst

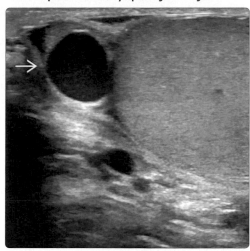

(Left) *Ultrasound of a middle-aged man with longstanding scrotal swelling shows a huge hydrocele* ➡ *containing low-level echoes. The hydrocele envelopes and compresses the testis* ➡. *Low-level echoes are frequently shown in large, chronic hydroceles.* (Right) *Ultrasound of a young male patient with a palpable mass shows a simple cyst within the head of the epididymis* ➡. *Location within the head might suggest a spermatocele, but differentiation between spermatoceles and epididymal cysts is typically not clinically important.*

Pyocele

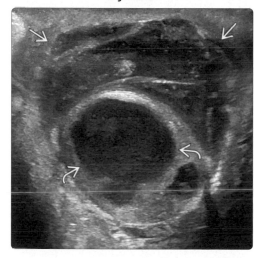

Hematocele

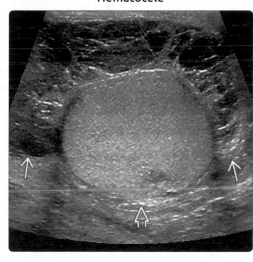

(Left) *Ultrasound of an institutionalized male patient with scrotal pain, ↑ WBC, and fever shows a testicular abscess* ➡ *and a surrounding pyocele* ➡ *containing low-level echoes and septations.* (Right) *Ultrasound performed 1 month post hernia repair shows a subacute hematocele* ➡ *containing multiple septations. Note how the collection surrounds the testis* ➡. *The herniorrhaphy was complicated by hemorrhage that extended along the inguinal ring. The echo pattern of hematoceles depends upon the age of the clot.*

Varicocele

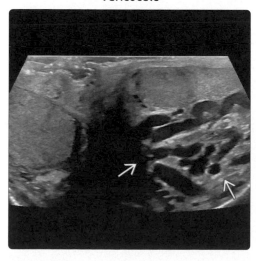

Epididymal Papillary Cystadenoma

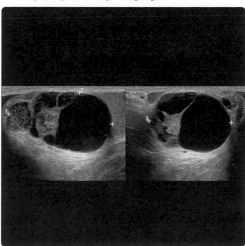

(Left) *Ultrasound of a young male patient with a left scrotal "mass" shows a large left varicocele* ➡. *Color Doppler (not shown) performed during a Valsalva confirmed flow within dilated peritesticular veins.* (Right) *Sagittal and transverse scrotal sonography shows a complex mixed cystic and solid epididymal head mass. Increased flow was shown at color Doppler. A patient history of von Hippel-Lindau suggested an epididymal papillary cystadenoma, a rare benign epididymal lesion. (Courtesy of T. Desser, MD.)*

DIFFERENTIAL DIAGNOSIS

Common

- Epididymitis
- Hematocele
- Inguinal Hernia
- Scrotal Pearl
- Adenomatoid Tumor
- Fibrous Pseudotumor

Less Common

- Mesenchymal Tumors, Scrotum
- Papillary Cystadenoma, Epididymis
- Polyorchidism

ESSENTIAL INFORMATION

Key Differential Diagnosis Issues

- Clinical presentation + US findings key

Helpful Clues for Common Diagnoses

- **Epididymitis**
  - Increase or decrease in echogenicity depending upon acute or chronic stage
  - Enlarged, hyperemic epididymis &/or testis on color Doppler US
  - Compare with contralateral side
- **Hematocele (Chronic)**
  - Associated with trauma, torsion, infarct
  - Complex echogenic fluid
    - May be chronic and fibrotic, appearing as solid mass
  - No intrinsic vascularity demonstrable
  - Ipsilateral testis should be separately identified to exclude injury
- **Inguinal Hernia**
  - Inguinoscrotal hernia; indirect type
  - Bowel or echogenic omental fat seen within scrotum
    - Important to identify vascularity of bowel to exclude strangulation
- **Scrotal Pearl**

- Detached and calcified testicular appendages postinflammatory or secondary to prior torsion
- **Adenomatoid Tumor**
  - Most common epididymal tumor
    - 30% of all extratesticular neoplasms
  - Well-defined, solid, hypoechoic mass
  - Peripheral vascularity on color Doppler
- **Fibrous Pseudotumor**
  - Reactive fibrous proliferation, usually associated with tunica albuginea
  - Generally hypoechoic with strong posterior shadowing
  - Can be as large as 8 cm in diameter

Helpful Clues for Less Common Diagnoses

- **Mesenchymal Tumors, Scrotum**
  - Lipoma most common benign neoplasm
    - Often appear hypoechoic
  - Most common malignant tumors include rhabdomyosarcoma and liposarcoma
    - Large, irregular, heterogeneous masses
- **Papillary Cystadenoma, Epididymis**
  - Epididymal component of von Hippel-Lindau syndrome (VHL)
    - Seen in 65% of patients with VHL
  - Often bilateral; found in young adults
  - Ill-defined solid mass with scattered cysts
- **Polyorchidism**
  - Extremely rare congenital disorder
  - Extratesticular mass with similar echo pattern as adjacent testis: MR for confirmation
  - Classified based upon presence or absence of epididymis/vas deferens
  - Mimic: Splenogonadal fusion

SELECTED REFERENCES

1. Mukherjee S et al: Clinico-radiological and pathological evaluation of extra testicular scrotal lesions. J Cytol. 30(1):27-32, 2013
2. Park SB et al: Imaging features of benign solid testicular and paratesticular lesions. Eur Radiol. 21(10):2226-34, 2011
3. Kim W et al: US MR imaging correlation in pathologic conditions of the scrotum. Radiographics. 27(5):1239-53, 2007

Epididymitis

Hematocele

(Left) *Ultrasound of a young man with acute onset of scrotal pain shows an enlarged and heterogeneous epididymal head ➡. Note the slightly complex hydrocele ➡. The epididymis is hyperemic at color Doppler exam ➡.* **(Right)** *Ultrasound performed post scrotal trauma shows a huge, complex hematocele ➡. A fracture line is shown within the testis ➡. Chronic hematoceles may occur post trauma and inguinal herniorrhaphy.*

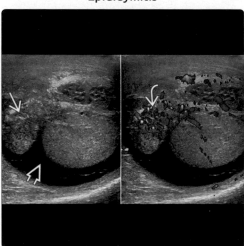

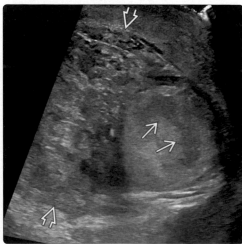

Inguinal Hernia

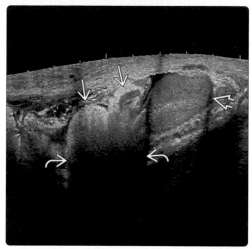

Adenomatoid Tumor

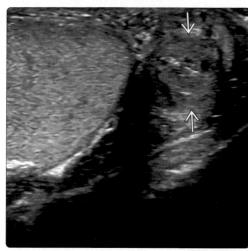

(Left) *Extended field-of-view ultrasound shows a huge inguinal hernia that displaces the testis ➡. "Dirty shadowing" ➡ is shown posterior to the gas-containing bowel ➡. Nonperistalsing echogenicity within hernias may suggest omentum or mesentery.* (Right) *Ultrasound performed to evaluate a slowly growing scrotal mass shows a hypoechoic, solid epididymal tail lesion ➡. An adenomatoid tumor, a benign, mesenchymal epididymal tumor, was resected.*

Scrotal Pearl

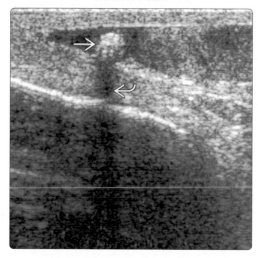

Papillary Cystadenoma, Epididymis

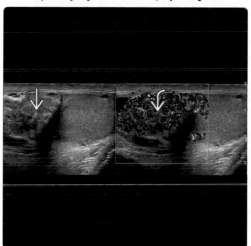

(Left) *Oblique US shows a small intrascrotal (extratesticular) calcified body ➡ causing posterior acoustic shadowing ➡. This is typical of a scrotal pearl (scrotolith).* (Right) *US of a young male patient with von Hippel-Lindau (VHL) syndrome to assess growing bilateral extratesticular lesions shows an enlarged, heterogeneous right epididymis ➡; it is hyperemic at color Doppler ➡. The left was similar appearing. Papillary cystadenomas of epididymis are rare; benign lesions are strongly associated with VHL.*

Polyorchidism

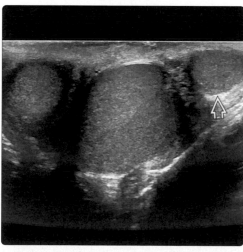

Mesenchymal Tumors, Scrotum

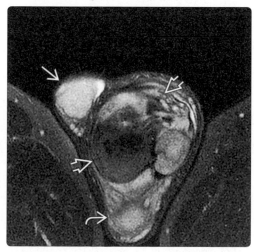

(Left) *Ultrasound to evaluate a palpable scrotal mass shows a supernumerary testis ➡. Polyorchidism is an extremely rare, typically inconsequential, congenital disorder, although ↑ cancer risk has been suggested.* (Right) *T2WI MR of an elderly man performed to evaluate a growing extratesticular mass shows a mixed signal mass ➡, which displaces right ➡ and left ➡ testes. A spermatic cord liposarcoma was resected. MR is particularly helpful for evaluating large, extratesticular masses.*

DIFFERENTIAL DIAGNOSIS

Common

- Orchitis
- Testicular Torsion/Infarction
- Testicular Carcinoma
- Scrotal Trauma

Less Common

- Testicular Lymphoma
- Testicular Metastases
- Testicular Cyst

ESSENTIAL INFORMATION

Key Differential Diagnosis Issues

- Diagnosis depends, not on sonographic appearances alone, but on combination of clinical and ultrasound features

Helpful Clues for Common Diagnoses

- **Orchitis**
  - Characterized by edema of testes contained within rigid tunica albuginea
  - Heterogeneous parenchymal echogenicity and septal accentuation, seen as hypoechoic bands
  - Diffuse increase in testicular parenchymal vascularity on color Doppler ultrasound
- **Testicular Torsion/Infarction**
  - Acute infarction: Diffusely enlarged hypoechoic testis
  - Chronic infarction: Small, shrunken, heterogeneous testis
  - "Whirlpool" or "torsion knot" at level of spermatic cord; dampened or absent vascularity in testis
- **Testicular Carcinoma**
  - Discrete hypoechoic or mixed echogenic testicular mass ± vascularity
  - Although seminomas are usually discrete hypoechoic lesions, they may cause diffuse enlargement of involved testis
- **Scrotal Trauma**
  - History of scrotal trauma

- Focal hypoechoic area, discrete linear/irregular fracture plane within testis, tunica albuginea rupture, hematocele
- Abnormal testicular parenchymal echogenicity, avascular mass; echogenicity of hematoma depends on its age

Helpful Clues for Less Common Diagnoses

- **Testicular Lymphoma and Metastases**
  - Multiple > > solitary lesion(s); 50% of cases bilateral
  - Metastases are rare; most common sites include prostate, lung, and GI tract
  - Often large in size at time of diagnosis; associated with disseminated disease
    - Ill-defined, mostly hypoechoic lesions
- **Testicular Cyst**
  - Intratesticular cysts are usually simple cysts located near mediastinum testis
  - Need to differentiate them from cystic neoplasms
    - Search carefully for solid components and internal vascularity

SELECTED REFERENCES

1. Coursey Moreno C et al: Testicular tumors: what radiologists need to know—differential diagnosis, staging, and management. Radiographics. 35(2):400-15, 2015
2. Nicola R et al: Imaging of traumatic injuries to the scrotum and penis. AJR Am J Roentgenol. 202(6):W512-20, 2014
3. Bhatt S et al: Imaging of non-neoplastic intratesticular masses. Diagn Interv Radiol. 2011 Mar;17(1):52-63, 2010. Erratum in: Diagn Interv Radiol. 17(4):388, 2011
4. Loberant N et al: Striated appearance of the testes. Ultrasound Q. 26(1):37-44, 2010
5. Bhatt S et al: Role of US in testicular and scrotal trauma. Radiographics. 28(6):1617-29, 2008
6. Dogra VS et al: Torsion and beyond: new twists in spectral Doppler evaluation of the scrotum. J Ultrasound Med. 23(8):1077-85, 2004
7. Dogra V et al: Acute painful scrotum. Radiol Clin North Am. 42 (2): 349-63, 2004
8. Dogra VS et al: Sonography of the scrotum. Radiology. 227(1):18-36, 2003
9. Dogra VS et al: Benign intratesticular cystic lesions: US features. Radiographics. 21 Spec No:S273-81, 2001
10. Subramanyam BR et al: Diffuse testicular disease: sonographic features and significance. AJR Am J Roentgenol. 145(6):1221-4, 1985

Orchitis

Orchitis

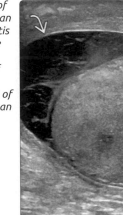

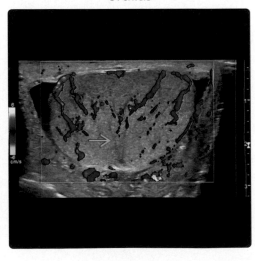

(Left) Sagittal grayscale US of the left testis demonstrates an enlarged heterogeneous testis ➡ with surrounding pyocele ⬈ and overlying skin thickening ➡, suggestive of acute orchitis. (Right) Transverse color Doppler US of the left testis demonstrates an enlarged, heterogeneous testis with a striated ➡ pattern and increased vascularity, suggestive of acute orchitis.

Testicular Torsion/Infarction

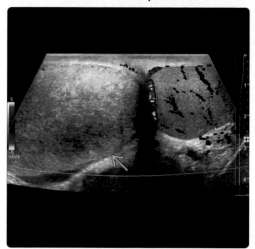

Testicular Carcinoma

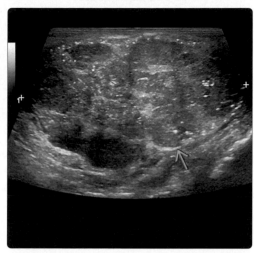

(Left) *Transverse color Doppler US of bilateral testes demonstrates an enlarged heterogeneous right testis* ➡ *with complete absence of blood flow, suggestive of acute testicular torsion with infarction.* (Right) *Sagittal grayscale US of the right testis demonstrates an enlarged heterogeneous testis* ➡ *with multiple hypoechoic masses in the background of testicular microlithiasis pathologically confirmed to be testicular seminoma.*

Scrotal Trauma

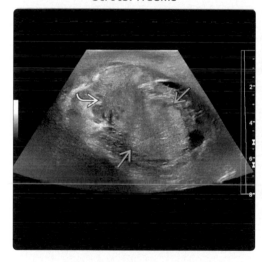

Testicular Lymphoma

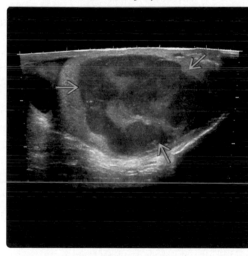

(Left) *Sagittal grayscale US of the left testis in a young man recently involved in a motor vehicle accident demonstrates an enlarged heterogeneous irregular testis* ➡ *with contour abnormality* ➡, *suggestive of testicular rupture.* (Right) *Sagittal grayscale US of the left testis demonstrates an enlarged heterogeneous testis with a large hypoechoic mass* ➡ *that was pathologically confirmed to be testicular lymphoma.*

Testicular Metastases

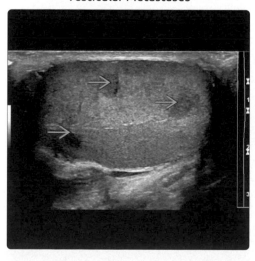

Testicular Cyst

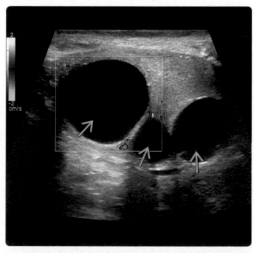

(Left) *Transverse grayscale US of the right testis in a young man with history of rhabdomyosarcoma demonstrates an enlarged testis with multiple hypoechoic masses* ➡ *that were pathologically confirmed to be metastases from rhabdomyosarcoma.* (Right) *Transverse color Doppler US demonstrates an enlarged left testis with multiple anechoic structures* ➡ *without internal blood flow or solid components, compatible with testicular cysts.*

DIFFERENTIAL DIAGNOSIS

Common

- Testicular Infarction
- Scrotal Trauma
- Chronic Mass Effect
- Undescended Testis

Rare but Important

- Hypogonadism
- Polyorchidism

ESSENTIAL INFORMATION

Key Differential Diagnosis Issues

- Consider testicular atrophy if combined axis measurements of testes differ by ≥ 10 mm, or if testicular size < 4 x 2 cm
- Reduction in size considered significant if volume of affected testis reduced to 50% of unaffected testis
- Critical to identify viability of testis to determine whether orchiopexy or orchiectomy is needed

Helpful Clues for Common Diagnoses

- **Testicular Infarction**
  - Ischemic orchitis is known complication of inguinal hernia surgery
  - Epididymoorchitis may result from severe inflammation/induration of cord
    - Venous infarction is rare complication of orchitis
  - Missed torsion: In utero cord torsion (45%), or may present later in life
  - Uniformly hypoechoic or focal mixed echogenicity of testis (or striated appearance) with absence of flow are features of diffuse or focal infarction, respectively
    - Reduced echogenicity is sensitive marker of poor outcome compared to clinical parameters
- **Scrotal Trauma**
  - Acute testicular hematoma may lead to ischemia/infarction of viable parenchyma due to raised intratesticular pressure

- Resorption of nonviable testicular tissue leads to atrophy or scarring
- **Chronic Mass Effect**
  - Longstanding extratesticular mass or hydrocele may compromise testicular blood flow and result in atrophy
- **Undescended Testis**
  - Exhibits different degrees of atrophy with altered parenchymal echogenicity
    - Less echogenic and smaller than normally descended testis
  - Testes < 1 cm often not detected by US

Helpful Clues for Rare Diagnoses

- **Hypogonadism**
  - Pituitary neoplasm, Kallmann syndrome, hypogonadotrophic hypogonadism
  - Diffuse heterogeneous echogenicity
- **Polyorchidism**
  - Supernumerary or duplicated testis
    - Tunica albuginea surrounds and separates bifid testis
    - Epididymis may also duplicate
    - Homogeneously echogenic oval structure with echogenicity identical to that of normal testis, but smaller in size

SELECTED REFERENCES

1. Loberant N et al: Striated appearance of the testes. Ultrasound Q. 26(1):37-44, 2010
2. Patel SR et al: Prevalence of testicular size discrepancy in infertile men with and without varicoceles. Urology. 75(3):566-8, 2010
3. Chu L et al: Testicular infarction as a sequela of inguinal hernia repair. Can J Urol. 16(6):4953-4, 2009
4. Bhatt S et al: Role of US in testicular and scrotal trauma. Radiographics. 28(6):1617-29, 2008
5. Pinto KJ et al: Varicocele related testicular atrophy and its predictive effect upon fertility. J Urol. 152(2 Pt 2):788-90, 1994
6. Desai KM et al: Fate of the testis following epididymitis: a clinical and ultrasound study. J R Soc Med. 79(9):515-9, 1986

Testicular Infarction

Undescended Testis

(Left) Transverse color and spectral Doppler view of bilateral testes shows the right testicle ➡ is atrophic and hypoechoic compared to the left testicle in a 35-year-old man with prior history of right epididymoorchitis. (Right) Sagittal color Doppler ultrasound in an 8-year-old boy with tenderness in his right suprapubic region demonstrates an avascular hypoechoic small undescended testis ➡. Patients who have an undescended testis have an increased risk of development of seminoma.

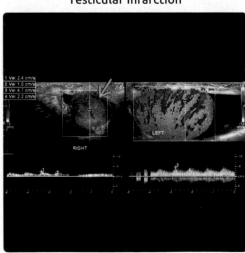

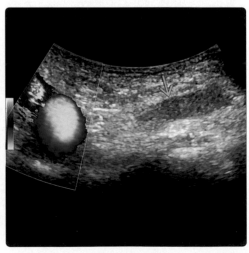

Testicular Infarction

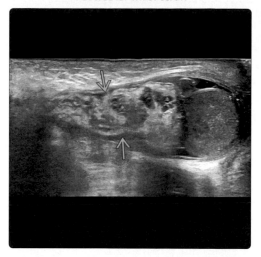

Testicular Infarction

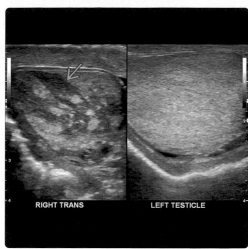

(Left) Sagittal grayscale US of the right scrotum in a 42-year-old man with recent history of right inguinal hernia surgery who presented with worsening right scrotal pain is shown. Color Doppler US demonstrates complete absence of flow in the testis and an edematous cord ⮕. (Right) Transverse grayscale US image of bilateral testes shows an atrophic right testis with a striated pattern ⮕. Patient had a remote history of right-sided epididymoorchitis.

Chronic Mass Effect

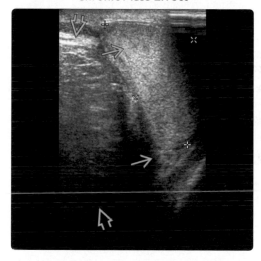

Chronic Mass Effect

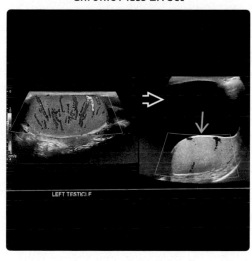

(Left) Sagittal grayscale US of the left scrotum shows a small left testis ⮕ pushed to one side by the large echogenic "mass" confirmed to be an omental inguinal hernia ⮕. (Right) Sagittal color Doppler US images of bilateral testis show an atrophic right testis ⮕, secondary to a large hydrocele ⮕.

Testicular Infarction

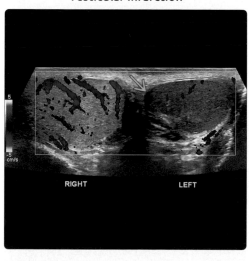

Testicular Infarction

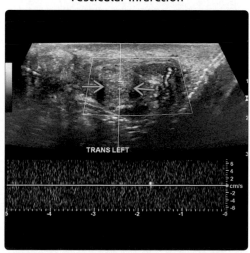

(Left) Transverse color Doppler view of bilateral testicles shows that the left testis is atrophic ⮕ with reduced vascularity. The patient had a prior history of mumps orchitis. (Right) Follow-up power Doppler image of a 50-year-old patient with prior history of orchitis demonstrates a severely atrophic and avascular left testis ⮕, consistent with infarction, a rare complication of orchitis.

DIFFERENTIAL DIAGNOSIS

Common

- Testicular Microlithiasis
- Nonseminomatous Germ Cell Tumor
- Sertoli Cell Tumor

Less Common

- Scrotal Trauma
- Scrotal Pearl
- Epidermoid Cyst
- Scrotal Abscess or Epididymoorchitis
- Calcified Tunica Albuginea Cyst

ESSENTIAL INFORMATION

Key Differential Diagnosis Issues

- Correlation between clinical and sonographic features essential
  - Incidental finding: Testicular microlithiasis, scrotal pearl
  - History of pain: Abscess, chronic infections, tumors
  - Mass with intrinsic calcification: Testicular tumors, epidermoid cyst
  - Associated with trauma: Testicular hematoma, hematocele

Helpful Clues for Common Diagnoses

- **Testicular Microlithiasis**
  - Multiple small (2-3 mm), discrete, nonshadowing, echogenic intratesticular foci
  - Unilateral or bilateral involvement
  - Concurrent germ cell tumor in up to 40%
- **Nonseminomatous Germ Cell Tumor**
  - Complex solid-cystic testicular mass
  - Heterogeneous echogenic foci due to calcification ± fibrosis, along with retroperitoneal lymphadenopathy can be seen with burnt out testicular tumor
  - Calcifications more common in tumors that contain teratomatous components
- **Sertoli Cell Tumor**
  - Small, hypoechoic, solid-cystic mass

- Punctate calcification may be present
- Occasionally, tumoral calcification may form large calcified mass, known as large calcifying Sertoli cell tumor

Helpful Clues for Less Common Diagnoses

- **Scrotal Trauma**
  - Chronic hematocele
    - Complex echogenic fluid
    - If chronic, appears as heterogeneous echogenic mass, ± calcification
    - No intrinsic vascularity on Doppler
- **Scrotal Pearl**
  - Calcification of detached testicular epididymal appendages due to previous inflammation or torsion of appendages
  - Solitary, discrete, echogenic focus in tunica vaginalis
- **Epidermoid Cyst**
  - Lamellated appearance on ultrasound
  - May have peripheral calcified rim
- **Scrotal Abscess or Epididymoorchitis**
  - Tuberculous infections may produce intrascrotal calcifications, scrotal sinuses
  - Granulomas appear as small echogenic foci, ± calcification
- **Calcified Tunica Albuginea Cyst**
  - Typically located at anterosuperior aspect of testis
  - Within tunica albuginea; may cause mass effect on testicular parenchyma if large
  - Avascular

SELECTED REFERENCES

1. Richenberg J et al: Testicular microlithiasis imaging and follow-up: guidelines of the ESUR scrotal imaging subcommittee. Eur Radiol. 25(2):323-30, 2015
2. Alvarez DM et al: Sonographic spectrum of tunica albuginea cyst. J Clin Imaging Sci. 1:5, 2011
3. Woodward PJ et al: From the archives of the AFIP: tumours and tumorlike lesions of the testis:radiologic-pathologic correlation. Radiographics. 22(1):189-216, 2002
4. Taghizadeh AK et al: Calcified epidermoid cyst in the testis: an unusual finding on ultrasound. Eur J Ultrasound. 11(3):199-200, 2000

Testicular Microlithiasis

Nonseminomatous Germ Cell Tumor

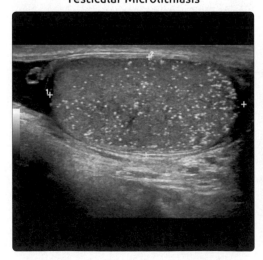
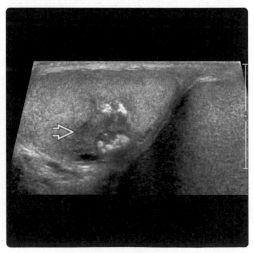

(Left) Sagittal grayscale ultrasound of the right testis demonstrates multiple tiny calcific foci consistent with testicular microlithiasis. (Right) Transverse grayscale ultrasound of the right testis demonstrates a partially calcified heterogeneous mass ➡. Pathology confirmed a mixed germ cell tumor with 75% embryonal cell, 15% teratoma, and 10% yolk cell components.

Sertoli Cell Tumor

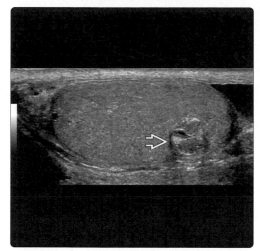

Scrotal Trauma

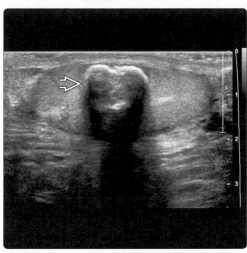

(Left) *Sagittal grayscale ultrasound of the right testis demonstrates a partially calcified mass ⇒. Pathology confirmed Sertoli cell tumor.* **(Right)** *Sagittal grayscale ultrasound of the right testis demonstrates a densely calcified mass ⇒. Pathology confirmed fibrosis with heterotopic ossification likely secondary to prior traumatic injury.*

Scrotal Pearl

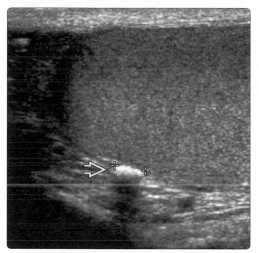

Epidermoid Cyst

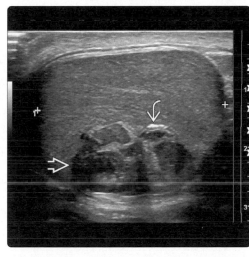

(Left) *Sagittal grayscale ultrasound of the superior pole of the right testis demonstrates a small extratesticular calcific focus ⇒. This is suggestive of a scrotal pearl or scrotolith.* **(Right)** *Transverse grayscale ultrasound of the left testis demonstrates a heterogeneous complex cystic mass ⇒ with areas of calcification ⇒. Pathology confirmed epidermoid cyst.*

Scrotal Abscess or Epididymoorchitis

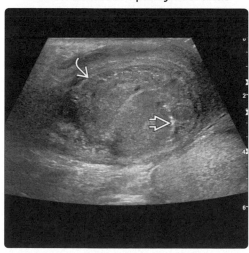

Calcified Tunica Albuginea Cyst

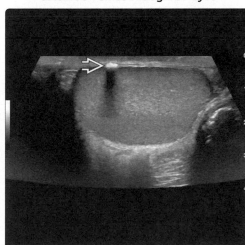

(Left) *Sagittal grayscale ultrasound of the right testis demonstrates a heterogeneous left testis ⇒ with calcification ⇒. Findings represent sequela of prior epididymoorchitis.* **(Right)** *Sagittal grayscale ultrasound of the right testis demonstrates a calcified lesion in the tunica albuginea ⇒. Findings represent a calcified tunica albuginea cyst.*

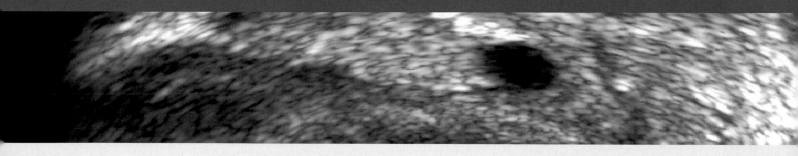

SECTION 21
Prostate and Seminal Vesicles

Generic Imaging Patterns

DIFFERENTIAL DIAGNOSIS

Common

- Benign Prostatic Hyperplasia Nodules
- Prostatic Calcification
- Prostatic Carcinoma
- Retention Cyst
- Prostatic Utricle Cyst
- Müllerian Duct Cyst

Less Common

- Prostatitis, Focal
- Prostatic Abscess
- Seminal Vesicle Cyst or Ductal Ectasia
- Ejaculatory Duct Cyst or Diverticulum
- Metastases and Lymphoma, Prostate

Rare but Important

- Prostatic Carcinoma, Cystic
- Multilocular Prostatic Cystadenoma
- Prostatic Urethral Diverticulum
- Prostatic Stromal Tumors

ESSENTIAL INFORMATION

Key Differential Diagnosis Issues

- Focal lesion might be discovered by palpation (digital rectal exam), as incidental finding, or part of screening exam
- Clinical information helpful to order differential diagnosis
  - Symptoms and signs: Fever, pain, dysuria, hemospermia, painful ejaculation
  - PSA level
  - History of biopsy; cancer treatment
- Helpful imaging features
  - Location
    - Intraprostatic [peripheral zone (PZ); transition zone (TZ); central zone (CZ)]
    - Periprostatic (e.g., seminal vesicles)
  - Cystic vs. solid

Helpful Clues for Common Diagnoses

- **Benign Prostatic Hyperplasia Nodules**
  - Enlarged prostate secondary to stromal and glandular hyperplasia
    - Nodular hypertrophy in transition/periurethral zone
  - Ultrasound
    - Typically hypoechoic nodular enlargement of TZ and periurethral zone
    - 10-20% of hyperplastic nodules are isoechoic or echogenic
  - T2WI MR: Enlarged TZ with multiple nodules; signal of nodule depends on histologic composition
    - ↑ signal intensity: Prevalent glandular proliferation (± secretion and cystic ectasia)
      - Cystic degeneration of benign prostatic hyperplasia (BPH) nodule is most common cystic prostatic lesion
    - ↓ signal intensity: Prevalent proliferation of stromal elements

- Differentiation of stromal BPH nodule from cancer originating from TZ is challenging and is mainly based on morphology features: Presence of capsule and round shape favors BPH nodule
- **Prostatic Calcification**
  - Common feature of chronic prostatitis
    - Caused by calcium precipitation inside acini whose ducts are obstructed by inflammation
  - Intraglandular or periurethral
    - Typically between TZ and PZ
    - In young patients, calcifications are usually periurethral
  - Ultrasound: Echogenic foci associated with shadowing
  - MR: ↓ signal intensity on T2WI and apparent diffusion coefficient (ADC) map
  - NECT: Hyperdense foci
- **Prostatic Carcinoma**
  - > 95% of tumors are adenocarcinoma
  - Location
    - 70-75%, PZ; 20-30%, TZ; < 5%, CZ
  - Ultrasound
    - > 90% are hypoechoic (less commonly iso- or hyperechoic)
    - Up to 30% of tumors are not evident on ultrasound
      - Indistinguishable from hyperplastic nodules in the TZ
  - Multiparametric MR (mpMR)
    - T2WI
      - PZ: ↓ signal intensity lesion ± extraprostatic extension
      - TZ: Ill-defined, lenticular shape, ↓ signal intensity lesion ± invasion of anterior fibromuscular stroma
    - DWI: ↑ signal intensity on high b-value image (b > 800-1000 s/mm²) and ↓ signal intensity on ADC map
    - T1WI C+: Early washin ± rapid washout
- **Retention Cyst**
  - Results from obstructed glandular acinus
  - Unilocular with smooth walls
  - Location variable; size ~ 1-2 cm
  - May be indistinguishable from glandular BPH nodule with cystic ectasia
- **Prostatic Utricle Cyst**
  - Cystic dilatation of prostatic utricle, acquired or congenital
    - Congenital results from abnormality in regression of müllerian duct system
  - Intraprostatic, midline, arises from verumontanum
  - Usually small, tubular, or pear-shaped
  - Normally communicates with urethra
  - Associated with hypospadias, undescended testes, and unilateral renal agenesis
- **Müllerian Duct Cyst**
  - Originates from remnant of müllerian duct
  - Extraprostatic, midline
    - Differentiation from utricle cyst is difficult
  - Usually large, extends above prostatic base
  - Oval/teardrop-shaped, rarely communicates with urethra
  - Though rare, may contain calculi

Helpful Clues for Less Common Diagnoses

- **Prostatitis, Focal**
  - Clinical history is helpful for differential diagnosis, e.g., urinary symptoms; gland tender at palpation
  - Ultrasound
    - Acute: Size may be normal but often enlarged; ill-defined margin; hypoechoic areas with ↑ vascularity
    - Chronic: Normal-sized gland; heterogeneous echo pattern ± calculi
  - mpMR
    - PZ; wedge shape
    - Commonly alteration of signal intensity affects gland diffusely; when focal it simulates cancer
    - ↓ signal intensity on T2WI and ADC map; ↑ signal intensity on DWI; ↑ enhancement on T1WI C+
- **Prostatic Abscess**
  - Complication of prostatitis
    - Fever, chills, urinary symptoms
  - 1/multiple prostatic rim-enhancing cystic lesions ± septa ± gas
  - More common in periphery of gland
    - ± extension into periprostatic space
- **Seminal Vesicle Cyst or Ductal Ectasia**
  - Variable in size
    - Rarely bilateral
  - Unilocular or multilocular
  - Associated with renal agenesis/dysgenesis
  - Ductal ectasia caused by ejaculatory duct or vas deferens obstruction
- **Ejaculatory Duct Cyst or Diverticulum**
  - Rare; intraprostatic, along ejaculatory duct
  - Paramedian at base, midline at verumontanum
  - Normally communicates with urethra
  - Intracystic calculi are common
- **Metastases and Lymphoma, Prostate**
  - Metastases: Most frequent from direct extension from carcinoma of rectum, bladder, seminal vesicle
  - Lymphoma: Usually part of disseminated disease

Helpful Clues for Rare Diagnoses

- **Prostatic Carcinoma, Cystic**
  - Complex cyst contains solid and cystic components
  - Predominantly peripheral in location
- **Multilocular Prostatic Cystadenoma**
  - Rare benign prostatic tumor
  - Can enlarge to cause urinary obstruction
- **Prostatic Urethral Diverticulum**
  - Anterior: Commonly due to instrumentation trauma or infection
  - Posterior: Commonly related to rupture of prostatic abscess
- **Prostatic Stromal Tumors**
  - Prostatic stromal sarcoma
    - Heterogeneous, enhancing solid tumor
  - Prostatic stromal tumor of uncertain malignant potential
    - Cystic or mixed solid and cystic mass; ↑ signal intensity on T2WI

Alternative Differential Approaches

- **Cystic lesion**
  - Midline: Utricle cyst, müllerian duct cyst, prostatic urethral diverticulum, ejaculatory duct cyst, or diverticulum
  - Paramedian: Vas deferens cyst, ejaculatory duct cyst, or diverticulum
  - Lateral: Seminal vesicle cyst, BPH cystic degeneration (TZ)
  - Variable: Retention cyst, abscess

SELECTED REFERENCES

1. Kitzing YX et al: Benign conditions that mimic prostate carcinoma: MR imaging features with histopathologic correlation. Radiographics. 36(1):162-75, 2016
2. Weinreb JC et al: PI-RADS prostate imaging - reporting and data system: 2015, version 2. Eur Urol. 69(1):16-40, 2016
3. Chu LC et al: Prostatic stromal neoplasms: differential diagnosis of cystic and solid prostatic and periprostatic masses. AJR Am J Roentgenol. 200(6):W571-80, 2013
4. Curran S et al: Endorectal MRI of prostatic and periprostatic cystic lesions and their mimics. AJR Am J Roentgenol. 188(5):1373-9, 2007

Benign Prostatic Hyperplasia Nodules

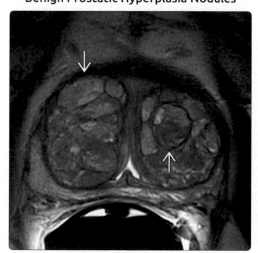

Benign Prostatic Hyperplasia Nodules

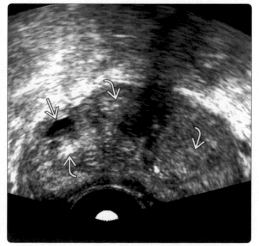

(Left) Axial T2WI MR of the prostate shows a hypertrophic transition zone with multiple well-defined nodules ➡ of various signal intensity. The signal intensity of benign prostatic hyperplasia (BPH) nodules depends on the histologic composition. (Right) Coronal transrectal ultrasound of the prostate shows BPH with multiple echogenic nodules ➡ in the transition zone. Note that one is anechoic, indicating cystic degeneration ➡.

Benign Prostatic Hyperplasia Nodules

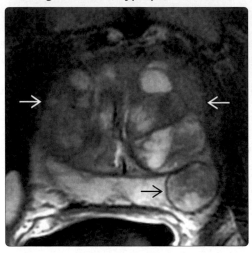

Prostatic Calcification

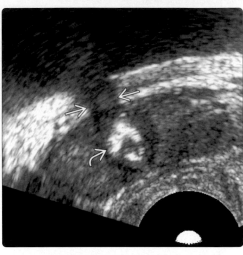

(Left) Axial T2WI MR of the prostate shows BPH ➡ and a well-defined, encapsulated nodule ⇥ in the peripheral zone of the left midgland. The heterogeneous signal intensity of the nodule and the presence of a capsule strongly suggest an exophytic BPH nodule over carcinoma. (Right) Coronal transrectal ultrasound of the prostate shows dense periurethral calcifications ➦ with characteristic shadowing ➡. This feature is common in young patients with chronic prostatitis due to calcium precipitation in obstructed acini.

Prostatic Carcinoma

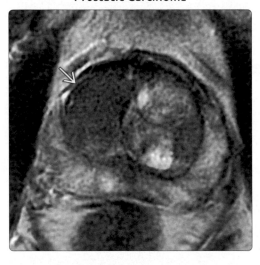

Prostatic Carcinoma

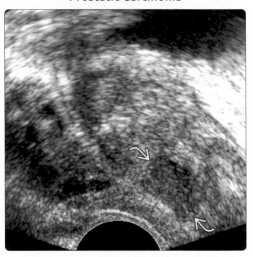

(Left) Axial T2WI MR of the prostate performed for increased PSA shows a nodule ➡ in the transition zone of the midgland with homogeneous low signal intensity and ill-defined margins. Target biopsy revealed adenocarcinoma (Gleason score, 7). (Right) Longitudinal transrectal ultrasound of the prostate shows an irregular hypoechoic lesion ➦ in the peripheral zone, suspicious for prostatic carcinoma (CA). Over 90% of prostatic CAs are hypoechoic, and about 70-75% are in the peripheral zone.

Prostatic Carcinoma

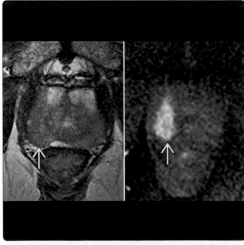

Prostatic Carcinoma

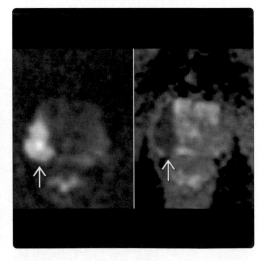

(Left) Axial T2WI (left) and T1WI C+ (right) MR show the prostate. In the peripheral zone of the right apex, there is a lesion ➡ hypointense on T2WI with early hyperenhancement postcontrast administration compatible with prostatic carcinoma. (Right) Axial DWI MR (left) and apparent diffusion coefficient (ADC) map (right) in the same patient show restricted diffusion (i.e., ↑ signal intensity on DWI and ↓ signal intensity on ADC) corresponding to the lesion ➡ in the right peripheral zone.

Müllerian Duct Cyst

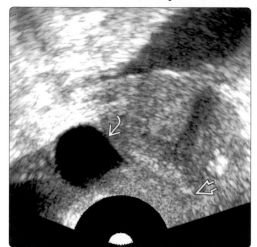

Müllerian Duct Cyst

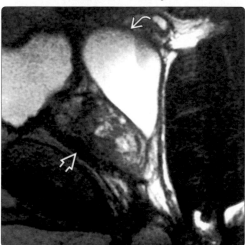

(Left) Longitudinal transrectal ultrasound of the prostate shows a teardrop-shaped cystic lesion ➔ typical of a müllerian duct cyst lying posterior to the verumontanum ➔. (Right) Sagittal T2WI MR shows the same teardrop-shaped cyst ➔ extending cephalad to the prostate gland ➔. Müllerian duct cysts are typically midline and large, extending above the base of the prostate, and only rarely communicate with the urethra. This patient presented with acute pain from the intracystic hemorrhage.

Prostatitis, Focal

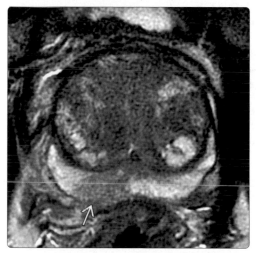

Prostatic Abscess

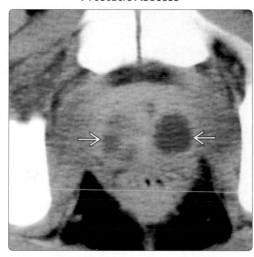

(Left) Axial T2WI MR of the prostate in a patient with elevated PSA and history of recurrent prostatitis shows a wedge-shaped, hypointense lesion ➔ in the peripheral zone of the right midgland. Target biopsy revealed chronic inflammation and lack of cancer. (Right) Axial CECT shows 2 foci of low attenuation ➔ within the prostate in a 62-year-old man with prostatic abscess following inadequately treated bacterial prostatitis.

Seminal Vesicle Cyst or Ductal Ectasia

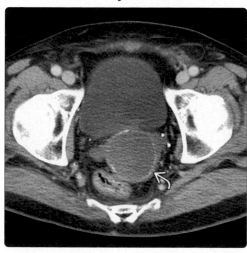

Ejaculatory Duct Cyst or Diverticulum

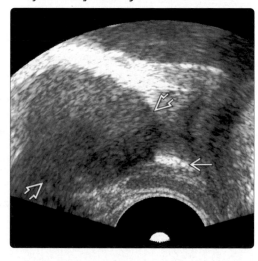

(Left) Axial CECT in a patient with a history of left renal agenesis shows a large, rim-calcified, left seminal vesicle cyst ➔. (Right) Longitudinal transrectal ultrasound of the prostate shows a large cyst ➔ in a patient complaining of hemospermia. The cyst is seen arising from the ejaculatory duct ➔ and extending beyond the prostatic base. The aspirate contained spermatozoa, confirming it to be an ejaculatory duct cyst.

DIFFERENTIAL DIAGNOSIS

Common

- Benign Prostatic Hyperplasia

Less Common

- Prostatic Adenocarcinoma
- Prostatitis ± Abscess
- Prostatic Cyst
- Secondary Involvement of Periprostatic Tumors

Rare but Important

- Other Primary Prostatic Tumors
  - Benign and Malignant

ESSENTIAL INFORMATION

Helpful Clues for Common Diagnoses

- **Benign Prostatic Hyperplasia**
  - By far, most common cause of prostatomegaly
  - Epithelial and stromal hyperplasia in transition zone (TZ) and periurethral glands
  - Heterogeneously enlarged TZ compressing peripheral and central zones

Helpful Clues for Less Common Diagnoses

- **Prostatic Adenocarcinoma**
  - Most cases of prostate cancer do not cause global enlargement
- **Prostatitis ± Abscess**
  - Prostatitis: Diffusely enlarged prostate (but may be normal in size), global vs. focal hypoechogenicity, ↑ glandular or perilesional vascularity
    - Often coexists with urinary tract infection
  - Prostatic abscess: Uni- or multilocular cyst with thick walls/septa and peripheral hyperemia
    - More common in elderly, diabetic, or immunocompromised patients
- **Prostatic Cyst**
  - Large müllerian duct cysts often extend above base
- **Secondary Involvement of Periprostatic Tumors**

- Urothelial carcinoma of bladder is most common tumor to secondarily infiltrate prostate
- Colorectal carcinoma and gastrointestinal stromal tumor may also secondarily invade prostate

Helpful Clues for Rare Diagnoses

- **Other Primary Prostatic Tumors**
  - **(Giant) multilocular prostatic cystadenoma**
    - Large multiseptated cystic pelvic mass
    - Evidence of local invasion excludes this diagnosis
    - Can regenerate and cause recurrent symptoms if incomplete resection
  - **Prostatic phyllodes tumor**
    - Large, well-circumscribed mass with variable amounts of cystic and solid components
    - Despite aggressive resection, up to 65% locally recur
    - Up to 39% undergo sarcomatous transformation and may spread to contiguous organs (bladder, colon)
  - **Small cell and squamous cell carcinomas**
    - Both are very aggressive and do not change serum prostate specific antigen; usually already advanced at time of diagnosis
  - **Prostate sarcomas**
    - Most common type in children: Rhabdomyosarcoma
    - Most common type in adults: Leiomyosarcoma
    - Predominantly solid, heterogeneous, vascular mass; high-grade tumors show tumor necrosis; occurs more often in younger men (between ages of 35-60)
  - **Prostate lymphoma**
    - Usually secondary prostate involvement
      □ Most reported is chronic lymphocytic leukemia or small lymphocytic lymphoma
    - Primary prostate lymphomas even more rare

SELECTED REFERENCES

1. Warrick JI et al: Diffuse large B-cell lymphoma of the prostate. Arch Pathol Lab Med. 138(10):1286-9, 2014
2. Chu LC et al: Prostatic stromal neoplasms: differential diagnosis of cystic and solid prostatic and periprostatic masses. AJR Am J Roentgenol. 200(6):W571-80, 2013
3. Rusch D et al: Giant multilocular cystadenoma of the prostate. AJR Am J Roentgenol. 179(6):1477-9, 2002

Benign Prostatic Hyperplasia

Benign Prostatic Hyperplasia

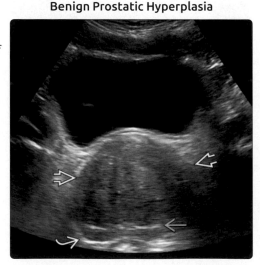
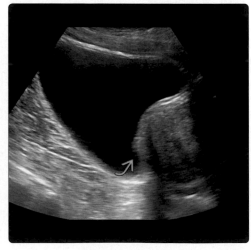

(Left) Transverse transabdominal sonogram shows marked enlargement of the transition zone (TZ) ⇒ causing compression of the peripheral zone (PZ) ⇒. Echogenic line represents the pseudocapsule ⇒ separating the TZ from PZ. (Right) Sagittal ultrasound from the same patient shows elevation of the bladder base ⇒ by the enlarged TZ.

Benign Prostatic Hyperplasia

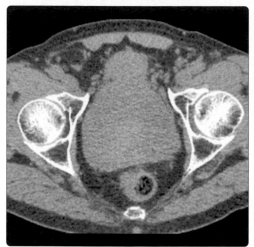

Benign Prostatic Hyperplasia

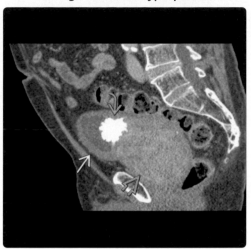

(Left) *Axial NECT shows a markedly enlarged prostate, which is homogeneous with well-defined margins.* (Right) *Sagittal CT in the same patient shows mildly heterogeneous enhancement of the markedly enlarged TZ ➡. Associated severe bladder wall trabeculation ➡ is consistent with bladder outlet obstruction. Presence of a large jackstone ➡ within the bladder indicates bladder decompensation.*

Benign Prostatic Hyperplasia

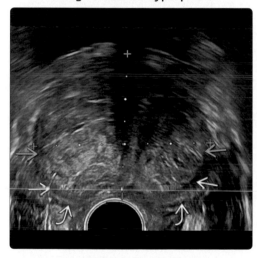

Prostatic Adenocarcinoma

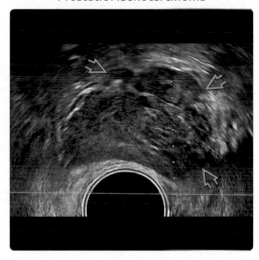

(Left) *Transverse transrectal ultrasound (TRUS) shows heterogeneous enlargement of both lobes of the TZ ➡. The peripheral zone is severely compressed ➡. Hypoechoic line represents the pseudocapsule ➡.* (Right) *Transverse TRUS at the level of the apex shows a slightly hypoechoic mass causing asymmetric, nodular enlargement of the left 1/2 of the prostate ➡. Targeted MR-US fusion biopsy of this mass revealed Gleason 4+5 prostate adenocarcinoma.*

Prostatic Adenocarcinoma

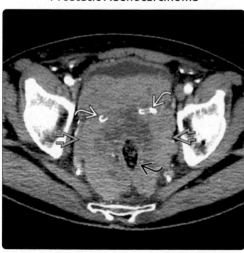

Other Primary Prostatic Tumors

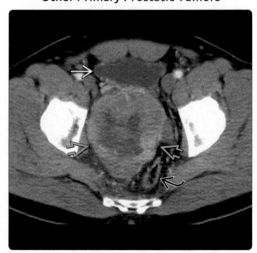

(Left) *Large, centrally necrotic pelvic mass ➡ encases the rectum ➡ and calcified vas deferens ➡. Pathology from TRUS-guided biopsy showed Gleason 5+5 adenocarcinoma.* (Right) *Centrally necrotic, enhancing pelvic mass ➡ arising from the prostate anteriorly displaces the bladder ➡. The rectum ➡ is separate. Surgical pathology from surgical resection revealed prostate sarcoma, not otherwise specified.*

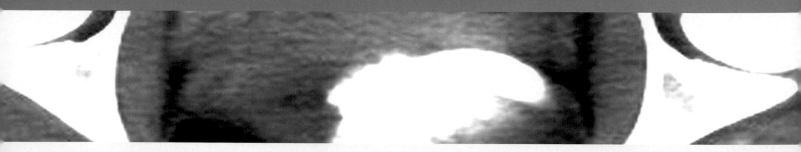

SECTION 22
Female Pelvis

Generic Imaging Patterns

Clinically Based Differentials

DIFFERENTIAL DIAGNOSIS

Common

- Physiologic Fluid
- Ruptured Hemorrhagic Cyst
- Disrupted Ectopic Pregnancy

Less Common

- Peritoneal Inclusion Cysts
- Pelvic Inflammatory Disease
- Pelvic Abscess Due To Bowel Disease
  - Appendicitis
  - Other Bowel-Related Abscess
- Ascites
- Endometriosis

Rare but Important

- Ovarian Torsion
- Ovarian Cancer
- Ovarian Metastases
- Ovarian Hyperstimulation Syndrome

ESSENTIAL INFORMATION

Key Differential Diagnosis Issues

- Simple fluid
  - Anechoic at US, fluid attenuation at CT, and fluid signal intensity at MR
  - Small amount of simple fluid in asymptomatic woman is likely physiologic
  - Small amount of simple fluid in patient with acute pelvic pain
    - Ruptured hemorrhagic cyst
    - Disrupted ectopic pregnancy
    - Pelvic inflammatory disease (PID)
    - Ovarian torsion
    - Ovarian hyperstimulation syndrome
  - Large amount of simple fluid likely ascites
  - If signs of metastatic disease, check ovaries
- Fluid with debris in cul-de-sac
  - Blood: Patient may be hemodynamically unstable
    - Ruptured hemorrhagic cyst
      - Variable amount of pelvic blood
      - Blood can extend along paracolic gutter and to subdiaphragmatic spaces
    - Disrupted ectopic pregnancy
    - Endometriosis
  - Pus: Patient acutely ill with elevated white blood cell count and fever
    - PID
    - Pelvic abscess due to bowel disease
  - Cells: Metastatic disease
- Fluid with septations
  - Peritoneal inclusion cysts
  - Endometriosis

Helpful Clues for Common Diagnoses

- **Physiologic Fluid**
  - Small amount of simple fluid may be seen during all phases of menstrual cycle
  - Should not be seen in postmenopausal women

- **Ruptured Hemorrhagic Cyst**
  - Hematocrit may initially be normal if patient has not had time to hemodilute after rehydration
  - Check for fluid by kidneys and around liver in cases of massive hemoperitoneum
    - Sentinel clot sign
      - Blood closest to rupture site has more time to retract, forming higher attenuation clotted blood and pinpoint origin of hemoperitoneum
  - Characteristic imaging appearance of hemorrhagic cyst
    - US: Different patterns may be seen
      - Echogenic, avascular, homogeneous, or heterogeneous nonshadowing in early stage
      - Retracted clot
      - Avascular, mass-like structure within anechoic cyst with characteristic concave contour
      - May jiggle with transducer ballottement
      - Reticular, lacy, fishnet, or spongy pattern
    - CT
      - Usually single unilocular cyst containing high-attenuation homogeneous fluid (around 50 HU)
    - MR
      - Usually single unilocular cyst
      - High signal intensity on T1WI
      - Signal intensity remains high on T1WI FS
      - Hyperintense or hypointense on T2WI
      - No T2 dark spots
      - Pelvic blood usually has high signal intensity on T1WI

- **Disrupted Ectopic Pregnancy**
  - Positive pregnancy test
  - Fluid is usually echogenic and may contain particulate matter
    - Pelvic hemorrhage is specific finding of ectopic pregnancy, with 86-93% positive predictive value when β-hCG levels are abnormal
  - Adnexal mass separate from ovary may be seen
    - May see tubal ring ± yolk sac and embryonic pole
  - Hematocrit may initially be normal if patient has not had time to hemodilute after rehydration

Helpful Clues for Less Common Diagnoses

- **Peritoneal Inclusion Cysts**
  - History of prior surgery or pelvic inflammatory conditions (e.g., Crohn disease)
  - Fluid usually simple at imaging
  - Multilocular cystic lesion surrounding ovary
  - Loculi separated by thin septa
  - No mass effect on pelvic structures
    - Cyst insinuates itself between pelvic structures rather than displace them
- **Pelvic Inflammatory Disease**
  - Adnexal cystic mass with irregular thick wall in case of tuboovarian abscess
  - Fluid-filled fallopian tubes in case of pyosalpinx
  - May be associated with peritoneal thickening because of associated peritonitis
  - Associated stranding of pelvic fat
- **Pelvic Abscess Due to Bowel Disease**
  - Patient acutely tender in region of complex fluid collection

- o May see abnormal loop of bowel/appendix in region
- **Ascites**
  - o Many causes include liver cirrhosis, heart failure, hypoproteinemia, etc.
  - o Usually simple-appearing fluid
  - o Ascites may also be seen in Meigs syndrome
    - Triad of ascites, pleural effusion, and benign ovarian tumor (fibroma, Brenner tumor, and, occasionally, granulosa cell tumor)
- **Endometriosis**
  - o Women with endometriosis have larger than normal amount of peritoneal fluid volume
  - o Usually small amount of fluid
  - o Fluid may be simple or hemorrhagic
  - o Evidence of peritoneal adhesions with obliteration of cul-de-sac may be found
    - Negative sliding sign
      - □ Gentle pressure by transvaginal probe to assess whether rectum glides freely across posterior vaginal wall and whether rectosigmoid glides freely over uterus
    - Kissing ovaries
      - □ Ovaries are adherent to each other behind uterus due to pelvic adhesions
  - o Peritoneal endometriotic implants or areas of fibrosis may be seen on MR

Helpful Clues for Rare Diagnoses

- **Ovarian Torsion**
  - o Small amount of fluid usually surrounding torsed ovary or within cul-de-sac
    - In up to 87% of cases of ovarian torsion
  - o Unilateral enlarged ovary (> 4 cm)
    - Multiple small, uniform cysts aligned in periphery of engorged ovary
      - □ String of pearls sign
    - Twisted vascular pedicle
    - ± mass within twisted ovary
    - Usually located in midline and superior to fundus of uterus

- **Ovarian Cancer**
  - o Pelvic ascites ± soft tissue nodules on surface of pelvic organs
- **Ovarian Metastases**
  - o Usually bilateral
  - o Known abdominal primary tumor, usually from gastrointestinal source
  - o Always check appendix for neoplasm, if no known primary tumor
- **Ovarian Hyperstimulation Syndrome**
  - o Enlarged ovaries containing numerous simple cysts
  - o Pelvic fluid in severe cases

SELECTED REFERENCES

1. Reid S et al: Prediction of pouch of Douglas obliteration in women with suspected endometriosis using a new real-time dynamic transvaginal ultrasound technique: the sliding sign. Ultrasound Obstet Gynecol. 41(6):685-91, 2013
2. Chang HC et al: Pearls and pitfalls in diagnosis of ovarian torsion. Radiographics. 28(5):1355-68, 2008
3. Lin EP et al: Diagnostic clues to ectopic pregnancy. Radiographics. 28(6):1661-71, 2008
4. Ghezzi F et al: "Kissing ovaries": a sonographic sign of moderate to severe endometriosis. Fertil Steril. 83(1):143-7, 2005
5. Bedaiwy MA et al: Peritoneal fluid environment in endometriosis. Clinicopathological implications. Minerva Ginecol. 55(4):333-45, 2003
6. Davis JA et al: Fluid in the female pelvis: cyclic patterns. J Ultrasound Med. 5(2):75-9, 1986

Physiologic Fluid

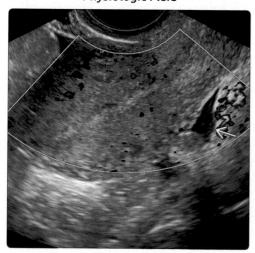

Ruptured Hemorrhagic Cyst

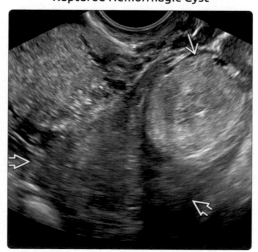

(Left) *Transvaginal color Doppler ultrasound shows a small amount of simple fluid ➡ posterior to the uterus within the cul-de-sac. A small amount of simple free fluid within the pelvis in a premenopausal woman is a common finding that may be seen in all phases of the menstrual cycle.* (Right) *Transvaginal ultrasound shows an echogenic left ovarian lesion ➡ representing hemorrhagic cyst with large amount of echogenic pelvic fluid ➡.*

Ruptured Hemorrhagic Cyst

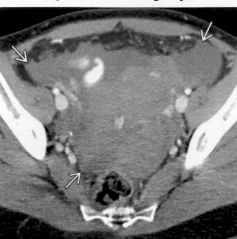

Ruptured Hemorrhagic Cyst

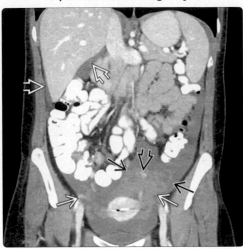

(Left) Axial CECT in the same patient shows a large amount of high-attenuation fluid ➡ filling the pelvis. The CT appearance is concerning and can be confused with carcinomatosis. (Right) Coronal CECT in the same patient shows high-attenuation fluid ➡ filling the pelvis and extending along the paracolic gutters to the perihepatic region ➡. The fluid has high attenuation with the highest attenuation present around the left ovary (sentinel clot sign) ➡. A small area of active extravasation ➡ is also seen.

Disrupted Ectopic Pregnancy

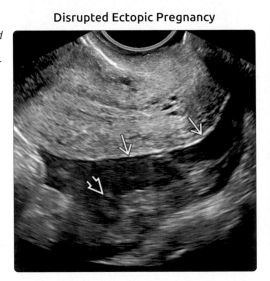

Disrupted Ectopic Pregnancy

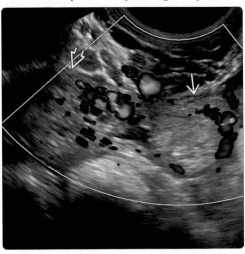

(Left) Transvaginal ultrasound shows large amount of echogenic fluid within the cul-de-sac ➡ with retracted clot ➡ due to hemoperitoneum. (Right) Transvaginal color Doppler ultrasound in the same patient shows an adnexal mass ➡, separate from the ovary ➡, and displaying peripheral ring of increased vascularity.

Peritoneal Inclusion Cysts

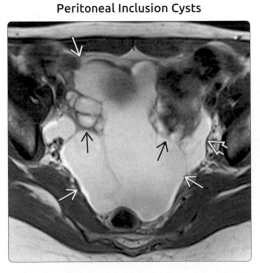

Peritoneal Inclusion Cysts

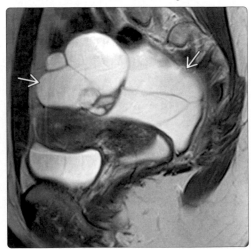

(Left) Axial T2WI MR in a patient with history of multiple pelvic surgeries shows a multilocular cystic lesion ➡ occupying much of the pelvic cavity. The lesion surrounds both ovaries ➡ and insinuates itself between pelvic structures ➡ without significant mass effect. (Right) Sagittal T2WI MR in the same patient shows a multilocular cystic mass ➡ superior to the uterus. The mass is composed of multiple loculi separated by thin septa.

Pelvic Inflammatory Disease

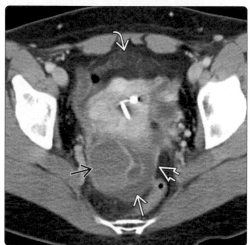

Pelvic Inflammatory Disease

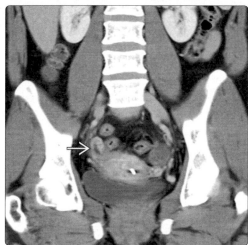

(Left) *Axial CECT shows a small amount of pelvic fluid ➡. The peritoneum of the cul-de-sac is slightly thickened and enhancing ➡. There is stranding of the pelvic fat ➡. High-attenuation right ovarian lesion ➡ is present and was found to represent an abscess.* **(Right)** *Coronal CECT in the same patient shows thickening and enhancement of the right fallopian tube ➡.*

Endometriosis

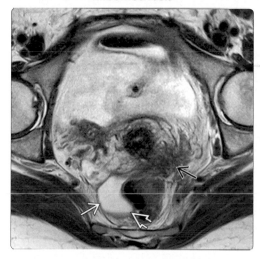

Endometriosis

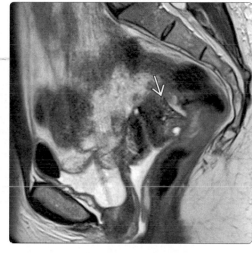

(Left) *Axial oblique T2WI MR shows a small amount of free pelvic fluid ➡ with a fluid level ➡ and an ill-defined, infiltrative mass-like structure of low signal intensity ➡ obliterating the left side of the cul-de-sac and containing small foci of high signal intensity.* **(Right)** *Sagittal T2 MR in the same patient shows the ill-defined, infiltrative mass-like structure of low signal intensity ➡ containing small foci of high signal intensity representing endometrial glands in a patient with pelvic endometriosis.*

Ovarian Torsion

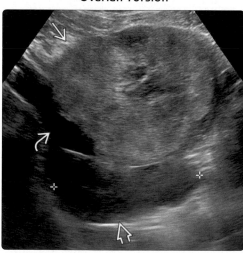

Ovarian Torsion

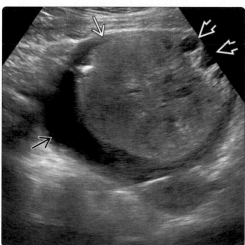

(Left) *Transabdominal pelvic ultrasound shows an enlarged ovary ➡ located anterior to the uterus ➡. A small amount of fluid is present around the enlarged ovary ➡.* **(Right)** *Transabdominal pelvic ultrasound in the same patient shows an enlarged ovary ➡ containing multiple peripheral follicles ➡ and surrounded by a small amount of fluid ➡.*

DIFFERENTIAL DIAGNOSIS

Common

- Nabothian Cyst
- Skene Gland Cyst
- Bartholin Gland Cyst
- Gartner Duct Cyst
- Urethral Diverticulum
- Cystocele

Less Common

- Epidermal Inclusion Cyst

Rare but Important

- Endometrioma of Rectovaginal Septum
- Subpubic Cartilaginous Cyst
- Endocervicosis

ESSENTIAL INFORMATION

Key Differential Diagnosis Issues

- Relation to level of perineal membrane and symphysis pubis
  - Above
    - Gartner duct cyst
    - Endometrioma of rectovaginal septum
    - Urethral diverticulum
    - Nabothian cyst
    - Cystocele
    - Endocervicosis
  - Below
    - Skene gland cyst
    - Bartholin gland cyst
    - Epidermal inclusion cyst
    - Subpubic cartilaginous cyst

Helpful Clues for Common Diagnoses

- **Nabothian Cyst**
  - Located within uterine cervix
    - Single cyst or as multiple cystic lesions in fibrous cervical stroma
  - Few mm in diameter but may reach 4 cm or more
  - Intermediate or slightly high signal intensity on T1WI and prominent high signal intensity on T2WI
  - Purely cystic without solid component
    - Distinguish nabothian cysts from malignant adenoma malignum
- **Skene Gland Cyst**
  - Rounded or ovoid cyst located lateral to external urethral orifice
  - Inferior to symphysis pubis and below level of perineal membrane
  - US
    - Anechoic or low-level echoes
  - CT
    - Fluid attenuation
  - MR
    - Variable T1 and T2 signal intensity depending on presence of hemorrhage &/or proteinaceous material
      - Usually hyperintense on T2W MR when uncomplicated

- **Bartholin Gland Cyst**
  - Located at posterolateral vaginal introitus
    - At or below level of symphysis pubis, inferior to perineal membrane
  - US
    - Anechoic or low-level echoes
  - CT
    - Fluid attenuation
  - MR
    - Variable T1 and T2 signal intensity depending on presence of hemorrhage &/or proteinaceous material
      - Usually hyperintense on T2W MR when uncomplicated
  - Thin wall without significant enhancement in absence of complication
    - Bartholin abscess will show thickened and irregular rim enhancement with adjacent inflammatory stranding
- **Gartner Duct Cyst**
  - Classically located in anterolateral wall of upper vagina
    - Above level of perineal membrane and symphysis pubis
    - Commonly arising from upper vaginal wall (though may be located distally as well)
  - US
    - Anechoic or low-level echoes
  - CT
    - Fluid attenuation
  - MR
    - Variable T1 and T2 signal intensity depending on presence of hemorrhage &/or proteinaceous material
      - Usually hyperintense on T2W MR when uncomplicated
  - May be associated with other congenital urogenital abnormalities, such as ectopic ureteral insertion and unilateral renal agenesis/hypoplasia
- **Urethral Diverticulum**
  - Round, oval, crescentic, horseshoe- or saddlebag-shaped, or circumferential periurethral cystic lesions
  - Located at posterolateral aspect of mid to distal urethra
    - Above level of perineal membrane and symphysis pubis
  - Direct urethral communication may be seen
    - High-resolution, fat-saturated, post contrast FSE T1WI are extremely useful in identification of diverticular neck
  - Anechoic on US, fluid attenuation on CT, and hyperintense on T2W MR when uncomplicated
  - Stones within diverticula may be seen in up to 5-10% of cases
- **Cystocele**
  - Defined as abnormal descent of bladder neck inferior to pubococcygeal line (PCL) on midline sagittal image, either at rest or upon stress
    - PCL is line drawn from inferior aspect of pubic bone to last coccygeal joint
  - Often associated with additional pelvic organ prolapse or pelvic floor laxity
  - Small cystocele may simulate pelvic floor cystic lesion on axial imaging

o Diagnosis is made upon recognizing clear communication with bladder lumen

Helpful Clues for Less Common Diagnoses

- **Epidermal Inclusion Cyst**
  - o Located at sites of prior trauma or surgery around vaginal introitus
  - o Commonly at posterior or lateral vaginal walls
    - − Episiotomy is common cause
  - o US
    - − Hypoechoic mass with variable echogenic foci without color Doppler signals
  - o CT
    - − Homogeneous well-defined lesion with attenuation higher than simple fluid
      - □ Can be mistaken for solid mass

Helpful Clues for Rare Diagnoses

- **Endometrioma of Rectovaginal Septum**
  - o Centered in rectovaginal region between rectum posteriorly and posterior vaginal wall anteriorly
  - o Cyst with homogenous low-level internal echoes on US
  - o Homogeneous well-defined structure on CT with attenuation higher than simple fluid
    - − Around 40 HU
  - o Hemorrhagic cyst with characteristic T1 hyperintensity and T2 shading on MR
- **Subpubic Cartilaginous Cyst**
  - o Midline, rounded, cystic mass
  - o Located anterosuperior to urethra and posteroinferior to pubic symphysis
  - o Sclerotic &/or erosive changes may be seen in symphysis pubis on CT and plain radiography
  - o Hypointense relative to muscle on T1WI and heterogeneously hyperintense on T2WI
  - o Thin enhancing wall with no internal enhancement
  - o MR may show direct communication between cyst and pubic symphysis
- **Endocervicosis**
  - o Closely clustered cysts of various sizes surrounding proximal 1/3 of urethra and may extend into bladder

o Usually low signal intensity on T1WI and high signal intensity on T2WI

o No solid elements and no enhancement with gadolinium

SELECTED REFERENCES

1. Silva PD et al: Large epidermal inclusion cyst presenting as a pelvic mass. WMJ. 113(6):239-41, 2014
2. Tubay M et al: Resident and fellow education feature: what is that cyst? Common cystic lesions of the female lower genitourinary tract. Radiographics. 34(2):427-8, 2014
3. Surabhi VR et al: Magnetic resonance imaging of female urethral and periurethral disorders. Radiol Clin North Am 51(6):941-53, 2013
4. Eskridge MR et al: MRI of endocervicosis: an unusual cause of clustered periurethral cystic masses involving the bladder. AJR Am J Roentgenol. 188(2):W147-9, 2007
5. Kim CE et al: MRI diagnosis of subpubic cartilaginous cyst. AJR Am J Roentgenol. 182(1):144-6, 2004

Nabothian Cyst

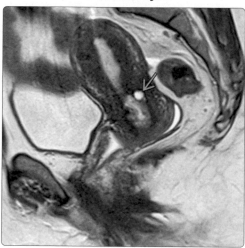

Nabothian Cyst

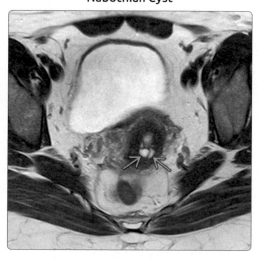

(Left) Sagittal T2WI MR shows a hyperintense cystic lesion ⮕ within the cervical dark stroma. (Right) Axial T2WI MR in the same patient shows hyperintense cystic lesions ⮕ within the cervical dark stroma.

Nabothian Cyst

Nabothian Cyst

(Left) *Sagittal transabdominal pelvic ultrasound shows 2 simple-appearing cystic lesions* ➡ *within the uterine cervix.* (Right) *Sagittal T2WI MR shows multiple small cervical cysts* ➡ *representing nabothian cysts. Note also the presence of urethral diverticulum* ➡ *and a Bartholin gland cyst* ➡.

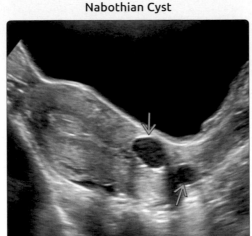

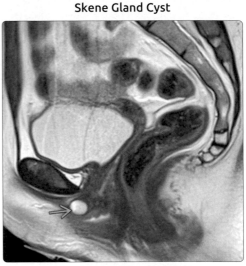

Skene Gland Cyst

Skene Gland Cyst

(Left) *Axial T2WI MR shows a well-defined oval cystic structure* ➡, *adjacent to the urethral meatus* ➡, *demonstrating homogeneous high signal intensity.* (Right) *Sagittal T2WI MR shows a well-defined oval structure* ➡ *demonstrating homogeneous high signal intensity adjacent to the urethral meatus. The cyst is located below the level of the symphysis pubis.*

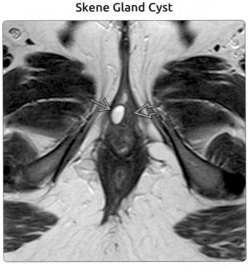

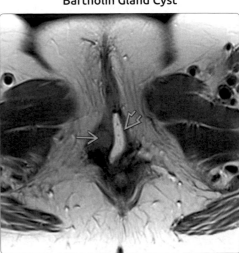

Bartholin Gland Cyst

Bartholin Gland Cyst

(Left) *Axial T2WI MR shows an oval structure* ➡ *at the right side of the vaginal introitus. The lesion shows high signal intensity characteristic of uncomplicated cyst.* (Right) *Axial T2WI MR in a patient who presented with vaginal pain shows an oval structure* ➡ *at the right side of the vaginal introitus* ➡. *The lesion shows signal intensity that is lower than gel within the vaginal introitus and slightly higher than signal intensity of pelvic muscles.*

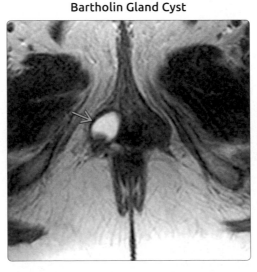

Bartholin Gland Cyst

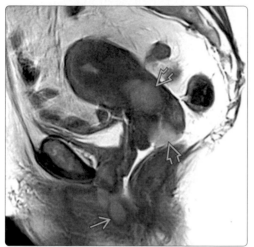

Bartholin Gland Cyst

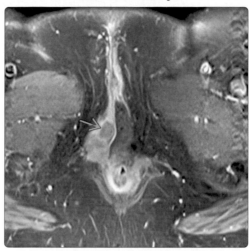

(Left) Sagittal T2WI MR in the same patient shows an oval structure ⇒ at the vaginal introitus, below the level of the symphysis pubis. The lesion shows intermediate signal intensity. Note also the presence of unrelated cervical masses ⇒. (Right) Axial T1 C+ FS MR in the same patient shows a structure ⇒ on the right side of the vaginal introitus. The lesion shows a thin enhancing wall and no enhancement of its content. Pus was aspirated from the cyst, consistent with Bartholin abscess.

Gartner Duct Cyst

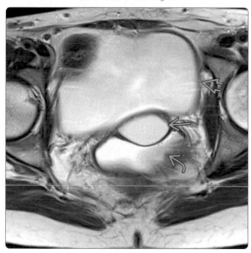

Gartner Duct Cyst

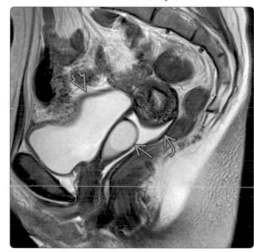

(Left) Axial T2WI MR shows a lesion ⇒ between the urinary bladder anteriorly ⇒ and the gel-filled vagina ⇒ posteriorly. The lesion shows homogeneous high signal intensity. (Right) Sagittal T2WI shows a lesion ⇒ between the urinary bladder anteriorly ⇒ and the gel-filled vagina ⇒ posteriorly. The lesion shows homogeneous high signal intensity.

Urethral Diverticulum

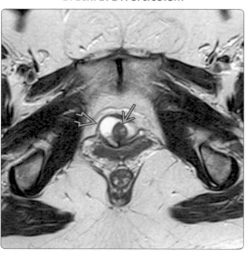

Urethral Diverticulum

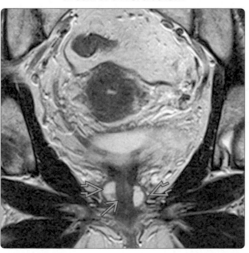

(Left) Axial T2WI MR shows a horseshoe-shaped T2 high signal intensity lesion ⇒ surrounding the urethra ⇒. (Right) Coronal T2WI MR shows a lesion with T2 high signal intensity ⇒ on both sides of the urethra ⇒.

Cystocele

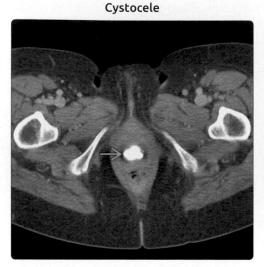

Cystocele

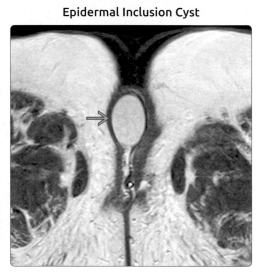

(Left) *Axial NECT shows a rounded lesion ➡ at about the level of the vaginal introitus that is now filled with contrast.* (Right) *Sagittal CECT shows downward extension of the urinary bladder ➡ far below a line drawn from the lower border of the symphysis pubis to the last coccygeal joint.*

Epidermal Inclusion Cyst

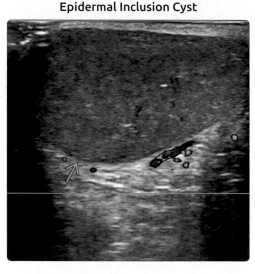

Epidermal Inclusion Cyst

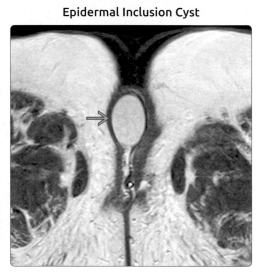

(Left) *Transvaginal ultrasound shows a right labia majora lesion ➡. The mass is hypoechoic with posterior acoustic enhancement. There is no blood flow within the mass, confirming its cystic nature despite its solid appearance.* (Right) *Axial T2WI MR in the same patient shows a well-defined lesion ➡ within the right labia majora. The lesion demonstrates high T2 signal intensity.*

Epidermal Inclusion Cyst

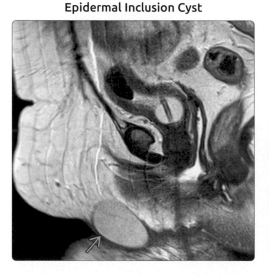

Epidermal Inclusion Cyst

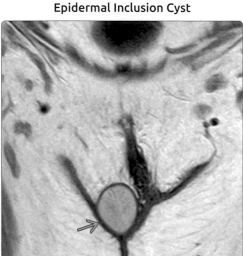

(Left) *Sagittal T2WI MR in the same patient shows a well-defined lesion ➡ within the right labia majora. The lesion demonstrates high T2 signal intensity and is located immediately under the skin.* (Right) *Coronal T2WI MR in the same patient shows a well-defined lesion ➡ within the right labia majora. The lesion demonstrates high T2 signal intensity.*

Endometrioma of Rectovaginal Septum

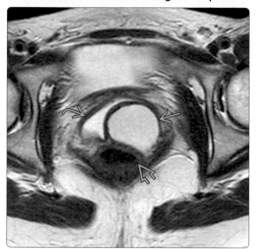

Endometrioma of Rectovaginal Septum

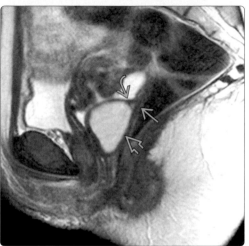

(**Left**) *Axial T2WI MR shows a lesion ➡ between the rectum ⇨ and the gel-filled vagina ➡. The lesion shows homogeneous high signal intensity.* (**Right**) *Sagittal T2WI MR in the same patient shows a T2 high signal intensity lesion ➡ between the anterior wall of the rectum ➡ and posterior wall of the vagina ➡.*

Endocervicosis

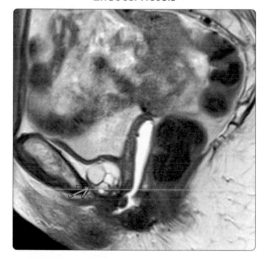

Endocervicosis

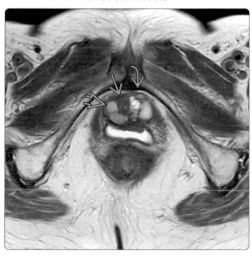

(**Left**) *Sagittal T2WI MR shows a cluster of periurethral cysts ➡.* (**Right**) *Axial T2WI MR shows a cluster of periurethral cysts ➡ surrounding the upper urethra ➡. Some cysts ➡ show signal intensity less than simple fluid, likely due to hemorrhage.*

Endocervicosis

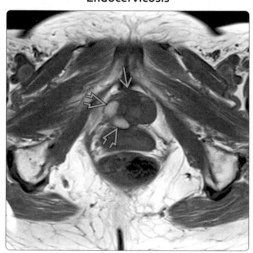

Endocervicosis

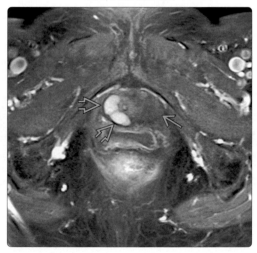

(**Left**) *Axial T1WI MR shows a cluster of periurethral cysts ➡. Some cysts ➡ show high signal intensity, likely due to hemorrhage.* (**Right**) *Axial T1 C+ FS MR shows a cluster of periurethral cysts ➡. Some cysts ➡ show high signal intensity, likely due to hemorrhage. There was no enhancement following contrast injection.*

DIFFERENTIAL DIAGNOSIS

Common

- Tubal
  - Tubal Ectopic Pregnancy
  - Hydrosalpinx
  - Pyosalpinx
  - Hematosalpinx
  - Primary Fallopian Tube Carcinoma
  - Tubal Leiomyoma
  - Fimbrial Cyst
- Gynecologic (Not Tubal)
  - Endometriosis
    - Endometrioma
    - Endometrial Implant
  - Subserosal Leiomyoma
  - Paraovarian/Paratubal Cysts
  - Exophytic Ovarian Mass

Less Common

- Peritoneal Inclusion Cyst
- Lymphocele
- GI Related
  - Bowel Loop
  - Bowel Obstruction
  - Sigmoid Diverticulitis
  - Appendicitis
  - Appendiceal Mucocele
  - Meckel Diverticulitis
  - GI Duplication Cyst
- GU Related
  - Hydroureter
  - Bladder Diverticulum
  - Renal Ectopia (Pelvic Kidney)
- Tarlov Cyst
- Pelvic Varices

Rare but Important

- Wolffian Duct Remnant
- Particle Disease Related to Hip Prosthesis
- Tubal Torsion
- Heterotopic Pregnancy
- Tubal Carcinoma
- Nerve Sheath Tumor
- Sarcoma
  - Ovarian Vein Leiomyosarcoma
  - Extraperitoneal Sarcoma

ESSENTIAL INFORMATION

Key Differential Diagnosis Issues

- Is patient pregnant?
  - Ectopic pregnancy, tubal
  - Ectopic pregnancy, heterotopic
- Is patient febrile with elevated white blood cell count?
  - Pelvic inflammatory disease (salpingitis, pyosalpinx)
  - Appendicitis
  - Diverticulitis
- Is mass tubular?
  - Fallopian tube DDx

- GI (bowel obstruction, mucocele)
- GU (hydroureter)
- Vascular (varices, aneurysm, venous leiomyosarcoma)
- Is mass intimately associated with ovary?
  - If adherent to ovary, may be exophytic ovarian mass
  - Tubal lesions may compress ovary and appear to arise from ovary
  - Pelvic inflammatory disease (tuboovarian abscess)
- Is mass related to uterus?
  - Leiomyomas may show broad base of attachment to uterus
  - Leiomyomas may show blood flow from uterus

Helpful Clues for Common Diagnoses

- **Tubal**
  - **Tubal ectopic pregnancy**
    - Pain &/or bleeding in 1st trimester
    - Echogenic, ring-like mass separate from ovary
    - May see yolk sac or embryo
    - Free fluid with debris is blood
  - **Hydrosalpinx**
    - Tubular anechoic mass, incomplete septations
    - Separate from ovary
    - Prior pelvic inflammatory disease or endometriosis
  - **Pyosalpinx**
    - Tubular hypoechoic mass, incomplete septations
    - Separate from ovary
    - Internal debris, ± fluid level
    - Irregular margins, thick wall
    - Free fluid
    - Clinical findings of infection
      - □ Pain
      - □ Fever
      - □ Elevated white blood cell count
      - □ Vaginal discharge
      - □ Cervical motion tenderness
  - **Hematosalpinx**
    - Associated with tubal ectopic pregnancy or endometriosis
    - Distended fallopian tube with fluid and debris
    - Rarely due to fallopian tube carcinoma
- **Gynecologic (Not Tubal)**
  - **Endometriosis**
    - Endometrioma ("chocolate" cyst) with diffuse, homogeneous, low-level, internal echoes
      - □ ± layering debris
      - □ Thick wall
      - □ May have punctate calcifications in wall of cyst
      - □ May have septations with blood flow
    - May also see endometrial implants and fibrotic plaques
    - Cyclic pelvic pain
  - **Subserosal leiomyoma**
    - Fibrous appearance with shadowing
    - Separate from ovary
    - Connection to uterus may be visualized
    - Blood flow from uterus may be present (bridging vessel sign)
    - MR helpful in establishing diagnosis
  - **Paraovarian/paratubal cysts**

– Separate from ovary
– Thin walled
– Anechoic
– Tend not to change in size over time
– Most commonly arise from peritoneal mesothelium of broad ligament or less commonly from fimbrial of fallopian tube

Helpful Clues for Less Common Diagnoses

- **Peritoneal Inclusion Cyst**
  o History of prior surgery
  o Cystic mass surrounding ovarian tissue
  o Conforms to shape of pelvic space as allowed by adjacent organs
  o Septations with blood flow can simulate malignancy
- **Lymphocele**
  o Septated cystic mass resulting from disrupting lymphatics following surgery
  o Not associated with ovaries or uterus
- **GI Related**
  o **Bowel loop**
    – Assess for peristalsis
    – Change in appearance over time
  o **Appendicitis**
    – Rebound tenderness to scanning in right lower quadrant
    – Dilated, tubular, blind-ending structure in region of patient's pain
    – Tubular structure noncompressible
    – ± adjacent fluid or appendicolith
    – Clinical signs of infection
- **GU Related**
  o **Renal ectopia (pelvic kidney)**
    – Reniform shape of mass
    – Collecting system
    – Absent kidney in ipsilateral renal fossa

Helpful Clues for Rare Diagnoses

- **Tubal Torsion**
  o Acute, colicky pain

o Associated with tubal mass or paraovarian cyst
o Elongated cystic mass that tapers near cornua
- **Heterotopic Pregnancy**
  o Intrauterine and extrauterine pregnancy
  o Common in patients undergoing assisted fertilization
  o Check for ovary separate from mass
- **Tubal Carcinoma**
  o Seen between and separate from uterus and ovary
  o Tube may be dilated: Hydrosalpinx with mural nodules
  o Tube may be enlarged with tubular solid mass
- **Sarcoma**
  o Leiomyosarcoma may begin in wall of ovarian vein and extend into inferior vena cava

Alternative Differential Approaches

- Acute pelvic pain, no signs of infection
  o Endometriosis
  o Bowel obstruction
  o Hydroureter
  o Tubal torsion
- Acute pelvic pain with signs of infection
  o Pelvic inflammatory disease (salpingitis, pyosalpinx, tuboovarian abscess)
  o Diverticulitis (sigmoid or Meckel)
  o Appendicitis
- Acute pelvic pain with positive pregnancy test
  o Ectopic pregnancy (tubal, heterotopic)
- Asymptomatic/incidental mass
  o Hydrosalpinx
  o Leiomyoma (tubal, subserosal uterine)
  o Cyst (paraovarian, paratubal, fimbrial, peritoneal inclusion cyst, GI duplication, bladder diverticulum, Tarlov)
  o Endometriosis
  o Mucocele
  o Lymphocele
  o Malignancy (tubal, sarcoma, nerve sheath)
  o Wolffian duct remnant
  o Particle disease of hip prosthesis

Hydrosalpinx

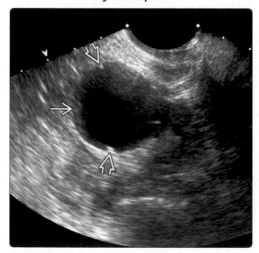

Hydrosalpinx

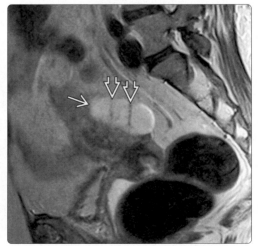

(Left) Transvaginal sonogram shows a cystic adnexal mass ➡ with multiple tiny, echogenic mural nodules ➡. The structure is tubular and separate from the ovary (not shown). This is hydrosalpinx with the "mural nodules" representing the longitudinal folds of the fallopian tube. (Right) Sagittal T2WI shows a tubular adnexal mass ➡ separate from the ovary. Note the incomplete septations ➡. Signal characteristics are hyperintense on T2WI, hypointense on T1WI, with no enhancement consistent with hydrosalpinx.

Pyosalpinx

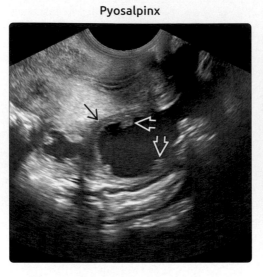

Pyosalpinx

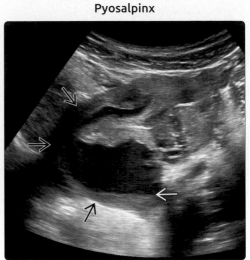

(Left) *Transvaginal sonogram shows a complex cystic adnexal mass* ⮕ *separate from the ovary. The thickened wall and nodular projections* ⮕ *give the appearance of a cogwheel consistent with pyosalpinx.* **(Right)** *Transabdominal sonogram in the same patient shows the complex cystic adnexal mass* ⮕ *is tubular. Note the thickened wall and the fluid-debris level* ⮕. *The ipsilateral ovary is separate.*

Hematosalpinx

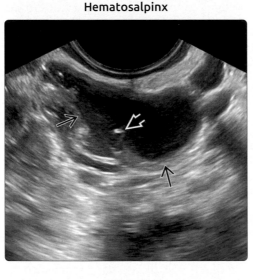

Hematosalpinx

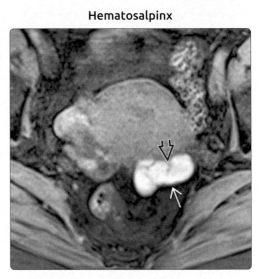

(Left) *Transvaginal sonogram shows an adnexal mass* ⮕ *with low-level internal echoes, a thick wall, and incomplete septations* ⮕. *The ovary is not shown but separate. The tubular shape and incomplete septations suggest a fallopian tube. Internal echoes and thick wall can be seen with pyosalpinx or hematosalpinx.* **(Right)** *Axial T1WI FS in the same patient shows a tubular hyperintense left adnexal mass* ⮕ *with incomplete septations* ⮕ *compatible with hematosalpinx. In this nonpregnant patient, this is consistent with endometriosis.*

Fimbrial Cyst

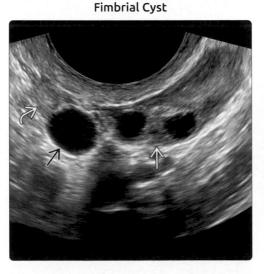

Fimbrial Cyst

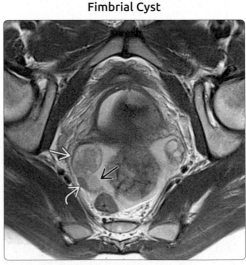

(Left) *Transvaginal sonogram shows a simple cyst* ⮕ *adjacent to, but separate from, the ovary* ⮕. *Better seen real time is tubular soft tissue* ⮕ *extending to the cyst.* **(Right)** *Axial oblique T2WI in the same patient shows the right fallopian tube* ⮕ *extending to a simple cyst* ⮕, *which is separate from the right ovary* ⮕. *This is consistent with a fimbrial cyst.*

Endometrial Implant

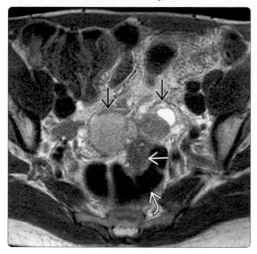

Endometrial Implant

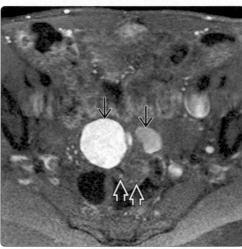

(Left) *Axial T2WI shows bilateral ovaries ⇨ with endometriomas. There is an extraovarian adnexal mass ➡ adjacent to the ovaries and intimately associated with the sigmoid colon ⮡. The ill-defined margins and T2 bright foci in the mass are compatible with an endometrial implant.* (Right) *Axial T1WI FS in the same patient shows the hyperintense endometriomas ⇨. The endometrial implant contains hyperintense foci ⮞ compatible with hemorrhagic glands.*

Subserosal Leiomyoma

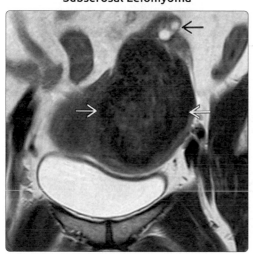

Subserosal Leiomyoma

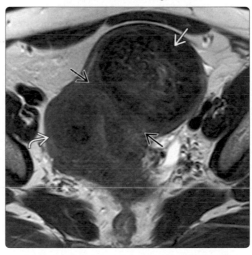

(Left) *Coronal T2WI shows the normal left ovary ⇨ with an adjacent, circumscribed, hypointense mass ⮞.* (Right) *Axial T2WI in the same patient shows the hypointense mass ➡ has a broad-based attachment ⇨ to the uterus ⮞ consistent with a subserosal leiomyoma. MR can be very helpful in localizing an adnexal mass due to its multiplanar capability and soft tissue contrast.*

Paraovarian/Paratubal Cysts

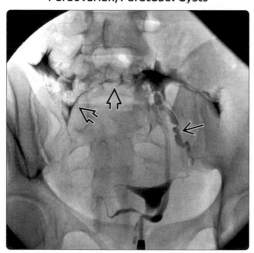

Paraovarian/Paratubal Cysts

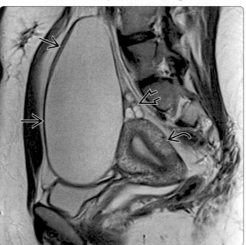

(Left) *Hysterosalpingography shows peritoneal contrast ⮞ being displaced by a large central pelvic mass. The left fallopian tube ⇨ is also stretched around the mass.* (Right) *Sagittal T2WI in the same patient shows a large simple cyst ⇨ separate from the ovary ⮞ and uterus ⮞. This was a large paratubal cyst.*

Peritoneal Inclusion Cyst

Peritoneal Inclusion Cyst

(Left) *Longitudinal transabdominal ultrasound of the pelvis shows the left ovary ➡ with associated loculated fluid ➡ and posterior acoustic enhancement.* (Right) *Axial T2WI in the same patient shows loculated fluid ➡ in the pelvic peritoneal cavity surrounding the left ovary ➡. There is no mass effect on adjacent structures; rather, the fluid fills the space provided. This is characteristic of a peritoneal inclusion cyst.*

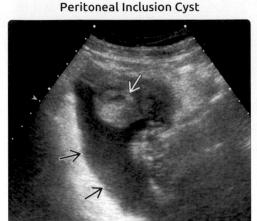

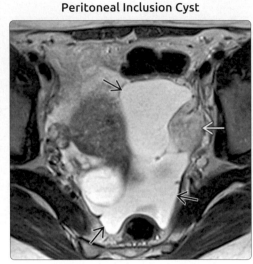

Lymphocele

Lymphocele

(Left) *Transverse transabdominal ultrasound of pelvis shows the uterus ➡ and a right adnexal hypoechoic mass ➡ with internal septations and posterior acoustic enhancement.* (Right) *Coronal oblique T2WI in the same patient shows the cystic mass ➡ along the right pelvic sidewall displacing the urinary bladder ➡. The uterus and right ovary ➡ are separate and displaced superolaterally. This was a lymphocele related to renal transplant surgery. Note the mass is not between the uterus and ovary as with most tubal pathologies.*

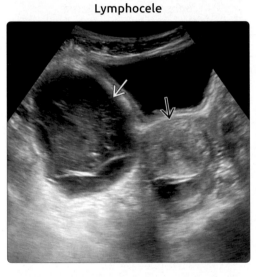

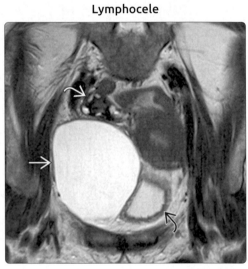

Sigmoid Diverticulitis

Sigmoid Diverticulitis

(Left) *Transabdominal ultrasound shows a bowel loop ➡ with surrounding echogenic inflammation ➡. This was separate from the ovary.* (Right) *Coronal CECT in the same patient shows focal fat stranding and inflammation ➡ surrounding a thick-walled diverticulum ➡ arising from the sigmoid colon ➡.*

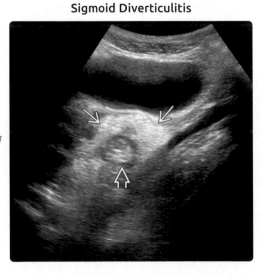

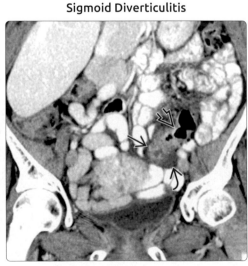

Appendicitis

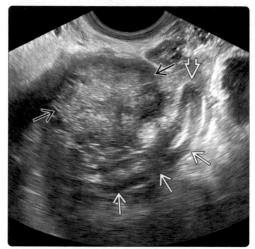

Appendicitis

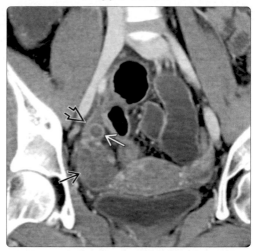

(Left) *Transvaginal ultrasound of the right ovary ⟶ shows an adjacent tubular ⟶, blind-ending ⟶ structure with bowel signature.* (Right) *Coronal CECT in the same patient confirms appendicitis with a dilated, hyperenhancing appendix ⟶ adjacent to the right ovary ⟶. Note the periappendiceal fluid and peritoneal enhancement ⟶.*

Appendiceal Mucocele

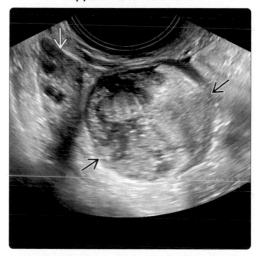

Appendiceal Mucocele

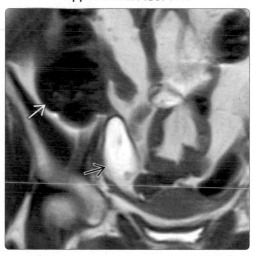

(Left) *Transvaginal ultrasound shows a normal right ovary ⟶ and an adjacent, but separate, echogenic mass ⟶. The mass is tubular (not evident on this image).* (Right) *Coronal T2WI in the same patent shows the tubular cystic structure ⟶ extending from the tip of the cecum ⟶, consistent with a dilated appendix. There is no surrounding inflammation, consistent with an appendiceal mucocele.*

Sarcoma

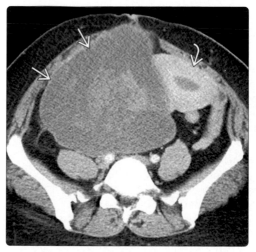

Sarcoma

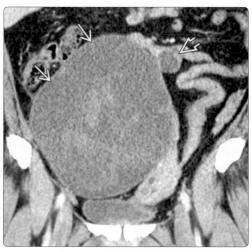

(Left) *Axial CECT shows a large solid and cystic right adnexal mass ⟶ displacing the uterus ⟶ to the left.* (Right) *Coronal CECT in the same patient shows the right adnexal mass ⟶ displacing the right ovary ⟶ superiorly and the fallopian tube (not shown) stretched around the mass. Surgical resection revealed spindle cell sarcoma of the mesosalpinx.*

DIFFERENTIAL DIAGNOSIS

Common
- Ovarian Follicular Cyst
- Ovarian Corpus Luteum
- Ovarian Hemorrhagic Cyst
- Pelvic Inflammatory Disease

Less Common
- Endometrioma
- Ovarian Torsion
- Complicated Paraovarian Cyst

Rare but Important
- Complications of Uterine Leiomyomas
- Complications of Mature Cystic Teratoma
- Ovarian Hyperstimulation Syndrome
- Hematosalpinx
- Ovarian Abscess Due to Diverticulitis
- Cervical Stenosis

ESSENTIAL INFORMATION

Key Differential Diagnosis Issues
- Ovarian abnormalities
  - Ovarian follicular cyst
  - Ovarian corpus luteum
  - Ovarian hemorrhagic cyst
  - Pelvic inflammatory disease
  - Ovarian endometrioma
  - Ovarian torsion
  - Ovarian abscess due to diverticulitis
  - Complications of mature cystic teratoma
  - Ovarian hyperstimulation syndrome
- Adnexal abnormalities
  - Pelvic inflammatory disease
  - Complicated paraovarian cyst
  - Hydrosalpinx
  - Hematosalpinx
- Uterine abnormalities
  - Pelvic inflammatory disease
  - Complications of uterine leiomyomas
  - Cervical stenosis

Helpful Clues for Common Diagnoses
- **Ovarian Follicular Cyst**
  - Physiologic cysts seen only in premenopausal women
  - Follicular cysts causing pain are often large, measuring 3-8 cm
  - Thin-walled simple cyst
  - Curvilinear septations may be seen (i.e., cumulus oöphorus)
  - Resolve on follow-up examinations
- **Ovarian Corpus Luteum**
  - Postovulatory corpus luteum measures up to 3 cm
  - Thick-walled cyst with crenulated margin
    - May appear completely solid on US with peripheral increased vascularity
  - Doppler US demonstrates prominent peripheral blood flow with low-resistance waveform

---

  - Irregular collapsed cyst with peripheral enhancement at CT and MR
- **Ovarian Hemorrhagic Cyst**
  - Different sonographic patterns depending on chronicity
    - Acute hemorrhage is echogenic, avascular, homogeneous, or heterogeneous nonshadowing in early stage
    - Diffuse pattern of low-level echoes
    - Retracted clot
      - Avascular, mass-like structure within anechoic cyst
      - Has characteristic concave contour
      - May jiggle with transducer ballottement
    - Reticular, lacy, fishnet, or spongy pattern
      - Irregular fine lines that typically do not completely traverse cyst
    - Color Doppler imaging shows characteristic peripheral vascularity within cyst wall with low-impedance flow on spectral Doppler imaging
  - MR appearance
    - Usually single unilocular cyst
      - High signal intensity on T1WI, remains high on T1WI FS
      - May be hypointense on T2WI (more commonly hyperintense)
      - No T2 shading or T2 dark spots
- **Pelvic Inflammatory Disease**
  - Pain in both lower quadrants
  - Cervical motion tenderness
  - Elevated white blood cell count
  - Normal imaging early in course
  - Swollen tubes with thickened endosalpingeal folds (cogwheel sign)
  - Tubal obstruction and dilatation with complex fluid or fluid-pus level (pyosalpinx)
    - Waist sign: Best to discriminate hydrosalpinx from other masses
  - Endometrial thickening/fluid (endometritis)
  - Complex adnexal mass comprised of adhesed ovary and tube (tuboovarian abscess)
  - Echogenic fluid (pus) in cul-de-sac

Helpful Clues for Less Common Diagnoses
- **Endometrioma**
  - US
    - Well-defined, smooth-walled unilocular cyst(s)
    - Contains homogeneous low-level echoes → characteristic ground-glass appearance
    - Small echogenic mural foci occur in 35% of endometriomas
  - MR
    - High signal intensity on T1WI
    - Signal intensity remains high on FS T1WI
    - T2 shading (signal loss on T2WI in ovarian cyst that appears hyperintense on T1WI)
    - T2 dark spots (discrete, markedly hypointense foci within cyst on T2WI ± T2 shading)
  - Rupture of endometrioma is rare complication most commonly occurs during pregnancy
    - May be associated hemoperitoneum
- **Ovarian Torsion**
  - Pain is usually localized to pelvis on side of torsion

- o Most common imaging finding is enlarged ovary or ovarian mass complex, although ovarian architecture is variable
  - – Heterogeneous appearance of enlarged ovary may be present, which correlates with intraovarian hemorrhage
  - – Peripherally placed follicles and homogeneous appearance centrally, consistent with diffuse stromal edema, may be seen within enlarged ovaries
- o Doppler flow patterns are variable (depending on degree of torsion and its chronicity)
  - – Lack of arterial and venous Doppler flow is helpful
  - – Ovarian arterial or venous color Doppler signal can be seen in cases of ovarian torsion
- **Complicated Paraovarian Cyst**
  - o May cause pain due to rupture or torsion
  - o Well-defined, unilocular, contain simple fluid and separate from ovary

Helpful Clues for Rare Diagnoses

- **Complications of Uterine Leiomyomas**
  - o Red degeneration (hemorrhagic necrosis)
    - – MR appearance
      - □ Peripheral or diffuse high signal intensity on T1WI (due to methemoglobin or proteinaceous content of blood)
      - □ Variable signal intensity on T2WI
  - o Torsion
    - – Change in location of pedunculated fibroid
    - – May demonstrate twisted vascular pedicle
    - – Hypoenhancement/nonenhancement due to infarction
    - – Normal ovaries distinguished separately
- **Complications of Mature Cystic Teratoma**
  - o May be lead point for torsion
  - o Rupture is rare complication
    - – Free-floating abdominal fat, fat-fluid level
    - – Discontinuity of the cyst wall
    - – Infiltration of surrounding fat suggesting inflammation

- **Ovarian Hyperstimulation Syndrome**
  - o History of ovulation induction therapy
  - o Massively enlarged ovaries, multicystic ovaries
  - o Ascites, as well as pleural or pericardial effusions in severe cases
- **Hematosalpinx**
  - o May occur in setting of tubal endometriosis, ectopic pregnancy, tumor, and torsion
  - o Hypoechoic with internal echoes on US and no internal blood flow on Doppler evaluation
  - o Hyperattenuating tubular adnexal mass separate from ovary on CT
  - o MR imaging shows hyperintense distention of fallopian tube on fat-saturated T1- and T2-weighted images ± T2 shading
- **Ovarian Abscess Due to Diverticulitis**
  - o Complex air and fluid-containing adnexal mass
  - o Tethering of adnexal structures to adjacent inflamed bowel
  - o Loss of fat plane between ovary and inflamed colon
- **Cervical Stenosis**
  - o Commonly caused by endometrial atrophy in postmenopausal women
    - – May also be caused by tumors, trauma, and instrumentation
  - o Results in accumulation of fluid within endometrial cavity
  - o At imaging, appears as distended uterine cavity filled with fluid (hydrometra) or blood (hematometra)

Other Diagnoses to Consider

- Ectopic pregnancy
  - o Should always be considered in premenopausal woman with positive pregnancy test
- Nongynecologic causes of pelvic pain should also be considered
  - o GI causes
    - – e.g., appendicitis, diverticulitis, Crohn disease, etc.
  - o Urinary causes
    - – e.g., urolithiasis, cystitis, etc.

Ovarian Follicular Cyst

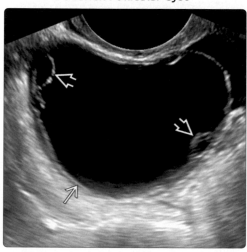

Ovarian Corpus Luteum

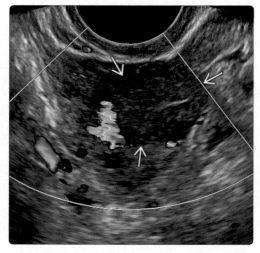

(Left) Transvaginal ultrasound shows a unilocular ovarian cyst ➡ measuring ~ 8 cm with peripheral curvilinear septations ➡ representing the cumulus oophorus. Follow-up ultrasound in 4 weeks revealed complete resolution. (Right) Transvaginal color Doppler ultrasound shows a slightly hypoechoic avascular ovarian structure ➡ with peripherally increased vascularity. Follow-up ultrasound in 4 weeks revealed complete resolution.

(Left) *Axial CECT shows large amount of high-attenuation pelvic fluid* ➡ *surrounding the uterus* ➡. **(Right)** *Axial CECT in the same patient shows large high-attenuation pelvic fluid* ➡ *and a right ovarian lesion* ➡ *that is predominantly cystic with a high-attenuation nodular structure* ➡ *representing a hemorrhagic cyst with retracted clot. Hemoperitoneum is the result of rupture of the hemorrhagic cyst.*

Ovarian Hemorrhagic Cyst

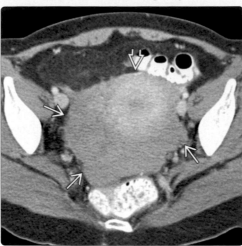

Ovarian Hemorrhagic Cyst

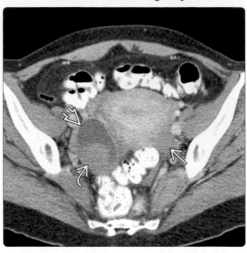

(Left) *Axial T2 MR shows a left adnexal fluid-containing lesion* ➡ *with thick wall and fluid level.* **(Right)** *Coronal T1 C+ FS MR in the same patient shows the left adnexal lesion* ➡ *with a thick uniformly enhancing wall due to tuboovarian abscess.*

Pelvic Inflammatory Disease

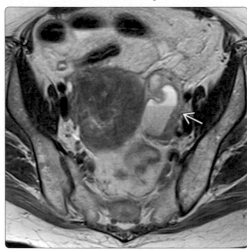

Pelvic Inflammatory Disease

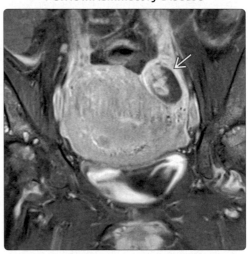

(Left) *Axial CECT shows a large-volume ascites indenting the liver* ➡ *and extending into a ventral hernia* ➡. *Ascitic fluid has high attenuation value of 50 HU, consistent with hemoperitoneum.* **(Right)** *Axial CECT in the same patient shows 2 cystic ovarian masses* ➡ *surrounded with ascitic fluid. The presence of ascites and cystic ovarian lesions suggested a cystic epithelial ovarian neoplasm. Surgery confirmed hemoperitoneum due to ruptured ovarian endometrioma.*

Endometrioma

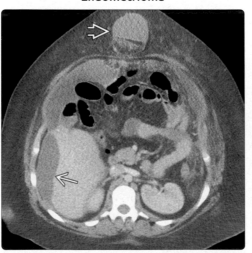

Endometrioma

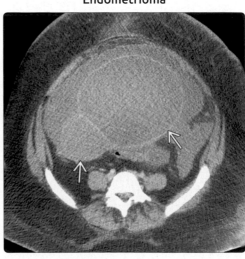

Endometrioma

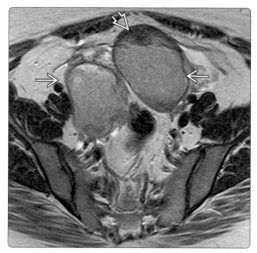

Endometrioma

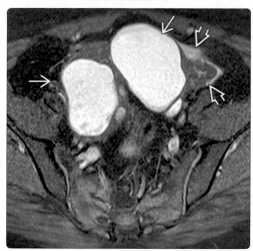

(**Left**) *Axial T2WI shows bilateral adnexal masses ➡ demonstrating high signal intensity with areas of very low signal intensity ➡. (**Right**) Axial T1 FS MR in the same patient shows bilateral adnexal masses ➡ demonstrating high signal intensity. Adjacent to the left lesion there is free fluid of high signal intensity ➡ due to hemoperitoneum resulting from rupture of endometrioma.*

Ovarian Torsion

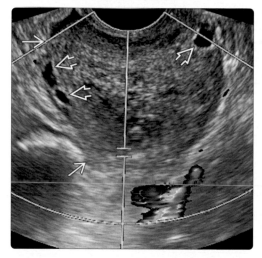

Ovarian Torsion

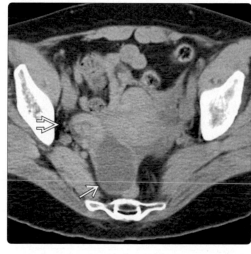

(**Left**) *Color Doppler ultrasound shows an enlarged right ovary ➡ (~ 6 cm) with absent flow. Small follicles ➡ are seen at the periphery. (**Right**) Axial NECT in the same patient shows an enlarged nonenhanced ovary ➡ and twisting of the vascular pedicle ➡.*

Complications of Uterine Leiomyomas

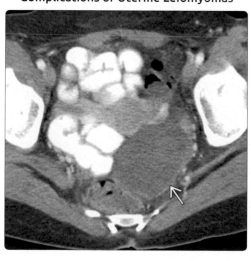

Complications of Uterine Leiomyomas

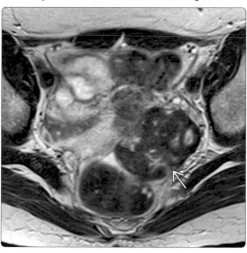

(**Left**) *Axial CECT shows a poorly enhancing left adnexal mass ➡. (**Right**) Axial T2WI in the same patient shows a left adnexal mass ➡. The mass was separate from the ovary and demonstrated low signal intensity with small areas of high signal intensity.*

Complications of Uterine Leiomyomas

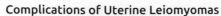

Complications of Uterine Leiomyomas

(Left) *Axial T1WI in the same patient shows a left adnexal mass ⮕ with intermediate signal intensity similar to that of the uterus ⮕. (Right) Axial T1 C+ FS MR in the same patient shows a left adnexal mass ⮕. The mass shows no enhancement following contrast administration. Comparison with prior imaging showed change in the location of the mass relative to the uterus. The imaging features are consistent with torsion of an exophytic uterine leiomyoma.*

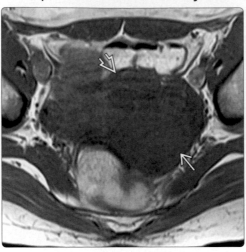

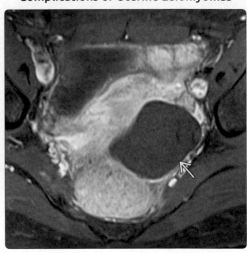

Complications of Uterine Leiomyomas

Complications of Uterine Leiomyomas

(Left) *Axial T2WI in a 37-year-old woman on oral contraceptive pills with pelvic pain and vaginal bleeding demonstrates a single pedunculated fundal fibroid ⮕. The fibroid shows central area of high signal intensity ⮕ surrounded by a thick rind of low signal intensity. (Right) Sagittal T2WI in the same patient demonstrates a single dominant exophytic fundal fibroid ⮕.*

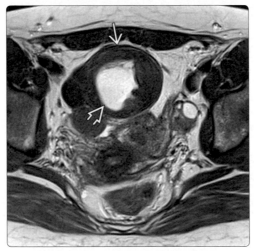

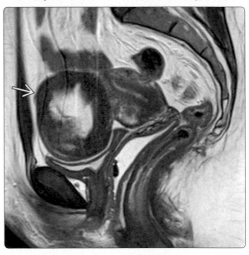

Complications of Uterine Leiomyomas

Complications of Uterine Leiomyomas

(Left) *Axial T1 FS MR in the same patient demonstrates marked T1 hyperintensity indicative of blood products. (Right) Axial T1 C+ FS MR in the same patient demonstrates absent enhancement of the central portion of the mass due to complete infarction of the fibroid with evidence of hemorrhagic or red degeneration.*

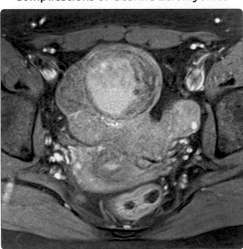

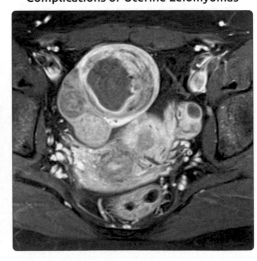

Hematosalpinx

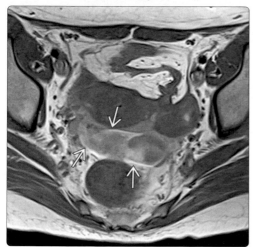

Hematosalpinx

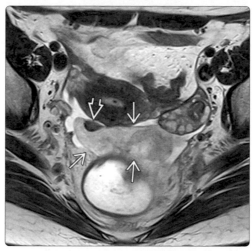

(Left) *Axial T1 MR shows a distended tubular structure ➡ posterior to the uterus showing heterogenous predominantly high signal intensity.* **(Right)** *Axial T2 MR in the same patient shows a distended tubular structure ➡ demonstrating high signal intensity due to blood-filled fallopian tube (hematosalpinx). This is caused by endometrial implant ➡.*

Ovarian Abscess Due to Diverticulitis

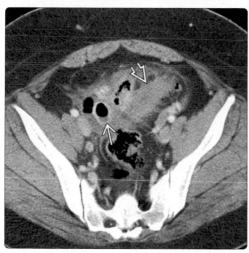

Ovarian Abscess Due to Diverticulitis

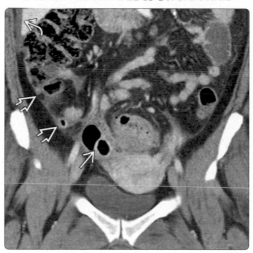

(Left) *Axial CECT shows a right air- and fluid-filled adnexal cavity ➡ adjacent to an inflamed sigmoid colon ➡.* **(Right)** *Coronal CECT shows a right air- and fluid-filled adnexal cavity ➡. Note the extension of inflammatory changes along the right paracolic gutter ➡ to the perihepatic region ➡.*

Cervical Stenosis

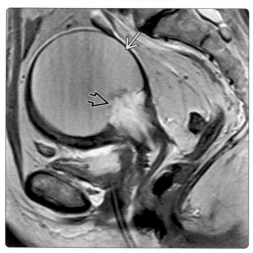

Cervical Stenosis

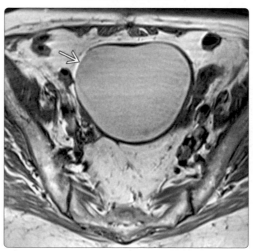

(Left) *Sagittal T2 MR shows distended uterine cavity ➡ filled with high signal intensity fluid due to an obstructing cervical mass ➡.* **(Right)** *Axial T1 MR in the same patient shows distension of the uterine cavity ➡. The cavity is filled with blood exhibiting high signal intensity (hematometra).*

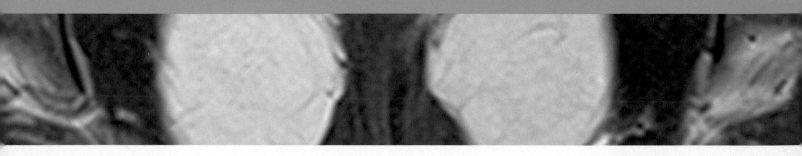

Generic Imaging Patterns

Clinically Based Differentials

DIFFERENTIAL DIAGNOSIS

Common

- Leiomyoma
- Adenomyosis
- Post Partum
  - Normal Post Partum
  - Endometritis

Less Common

- Endometrial Cancer

Rare but Important

- Uterine Leiomyosarcoma
- Cervical Lesion
  - Cervical Cancer
  - Cervical Stenosis
  - Cervical Leiomyoma

ESSENTIAL INFORMATION

Key Differential Diagnosis Issues

- Enlarged uterus without focal mass
  - Diffuse adenomyosis
  - Postpartum uterus
  - Endometrial cancer
- Enlarged uterus with focal mass
  - Multiple, round, well-defined masses
    - Intramural leiomyomas
  - Single, ill-defined mass
    - Focal adenomyosis
    - Endometrial cancer
- Fluid in endometrial cavity causing uterine enlargement
  - Cervical stenosis
  - Cervical cancer
- Lesion centered in cervix
  - Cervical leiomyoma
  - Cervical cancer
- MR can differentiate various etiologies of enlarged uterus

Helpful Clues for Common Diagnoses

- **Leiomyoma**
  - Focal, well-defined masses
  - Lobulated external contour of uterus
  - MR is diagnostic
    - Well-defined T2 hypointense masses
- **Adenomyosis**
  - Asymmetric myometrial thickening
  - Cystic spaces in endometrium
  - Alternating bands of increased through transmission and shadowing
  - Uterus may be tender during examination
  - MR is diagnostic
    - Thickened junctional zone ≥ 12 mm
    - T1 and T2 hyperintense foci

Helpful Clues for Less Common Diagnoses

- **Endometrial Cancer**
  - Typically postmenopausal woman with bleeding
  - Diffuse uterine enlargement
  - Ill-defined endometrium

Helpful Clues for Rare Diagnoses

- **Cervical Lesion**
  - MR best modality for visualization and differentiation of cervical abnormalities
  - Cervical cancer
    - US: Hypoechoic, ill-defined lesion
    - MR: T2 hyperintense cervical mass
    - ± hydronephrosis
    - ± fluid in endometrial cavity
  - Cervical leiomyoma
    - US: Well-defined, shadowing, hypoechoic lesion
    - MR: Well-defined T2 hypointense mass
    - Typically will not obstruct endocervical canal
  - Cervical stenosis
    - No identifiable mass
    - Fluid distention of endometrial cavity
    - Thin surrounding endometrium
    - History of curettage or childbearing

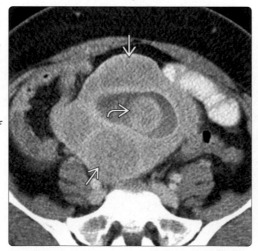
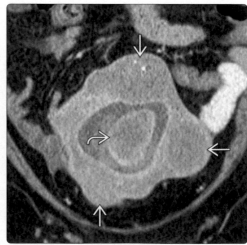

Leiomyoma   **Leiomyoma**

(Left) Axial CECT of the pelvis shows an enlarged uterus with multiple masses, both intramural ➡ and submucosal ➡. (Right) Coronal CECT in the same patient shows the uterus is enlarged with multiple intramural ➡ and submucosal ➡ masses. Note the lobular external contour of the uterus typically seen with leiomyomatosis. Adenomyosis and endometrial cancer cause uterine enlargement, while the normal smooth external contour is maintained.

Leiomyoma

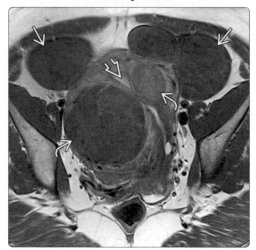

Leiomyoma

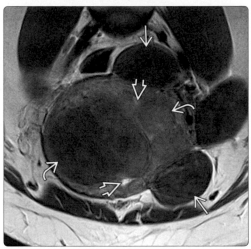

(Left) Axial oblique T2 FSE image in another patient shows enlargement of the uterus and distortion of the endometrial stripe ➡ by well-defined hypointense intramural ➡ and subserosal ➡ masses. MR is helpful for diagnosis and mapping of leiomyomas prior to treatment. (Right) Coronal oblique T2 FSE image in the same patient shows marked distortion of the endometrial stripe ➡ by multiple intramural leiomyomas ➡. Note the lobular external uterine contour due to subserosal leiomyomas ➡.

Leiomyoma

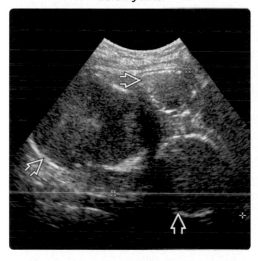

Uterine Leiomyosarcoma

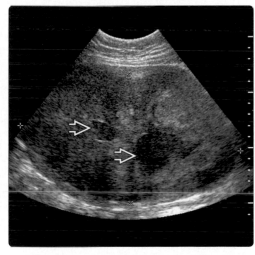

(Left) Longitudinal transabdominal ultrasound shows an enlarged uterus (over 20 cm in length) with multiple masses ➡ surrounded by calcific rims that is consistent with degenerated leiomyomas. (Right) Longitudinal transabdominal ultrasound shows an enlarged uterus with a hypoechoic mass (calipers) with areas of necrosis ➡. The uterus had rapidly increased in size since a study 3 months before, raising the likelihood of malignancy.

Adenomyosis

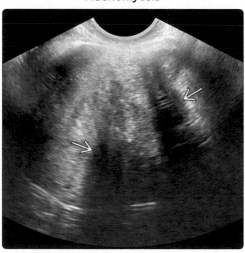

Adenomyosis

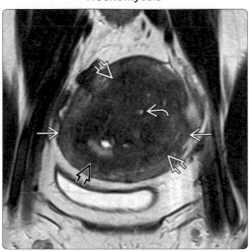

(Left) Transverse transvaginal ultrasound of the pelvis shows an enlarged uterus with ill-defined, shadowy ➡ hypoechoic areas. (Right) Coronal oblique T2 FSE image in the same patient shows enlargement of the uterus ➡ by focal hypointense thickening ➡ of the posterior junctional zone with foci of T2 hyperintensity ➡. Note the normal thin junctional zone anteriorly ➡. Adenomyomas are typically contiguous with the junctional zone and may have functional endometrial glands, as in this case.

Adenomyosis

Adenomyosis

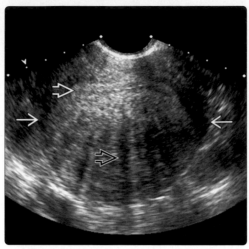

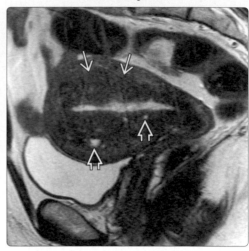

(Left) *Transverse transvaginal ultrasound shows an enlarged uterus ➡ with asymmetric thickening of the posterior wall & alternating echogenic and hypoechoic striations ➡ emanating from the junctional zone. Note the normal endometrial echo complex ➡.* (Right) *Sagittal T2 FSE image shows enlargement of the uterus ➡ with diffuse thickening of the junctional zone. Hyperintense foci ➡ in the thickened junctional zone are typical of adenomyosis and represent endometrial glands. The external contour of the uterus is smooth.*

Endometritis

Endometritis

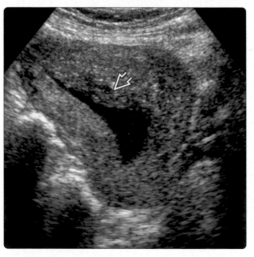

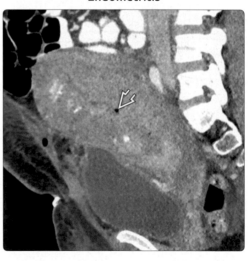

(Left) *Longitudinal transabdominal ultrasound shows an enlarged uterus with endometrial fluid and a shaggy irregular appearance to the endometrium anteriorly ➡.* (Right) *Sagittal CECT of the pelvis in a postpartum patient with fever shows enlargement of the uterus with foci of gas ➡ in the endometrial cavity. These can be normal postpartum findings, and the clinical history of fever and pain should be used to help make the diagnosis of endometritis, as in this case.*

Endometrial Cancer

Endometrial Cancer

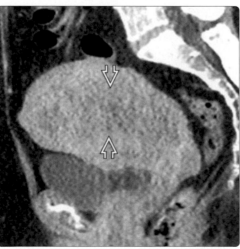

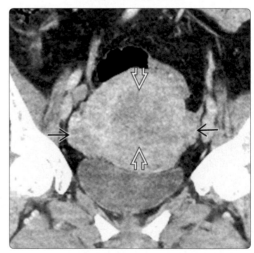

(Left) *Sagittal CECT of the pelvis shows an enlarged uterus with ill-defined central hypodensity ➡. The overall shape of the uterus is preserved with a smooth external contour.* (Right) *Coronal CECT in the same patient again shows the enlarged uterus with a normal external contour and central ill-defined hypodensity ➡. The ill-defined endometrial mass fills and distends the endometrial cavity, resulting in uterine enlargement. Biopsy confirmed endometrial cancer. Note the ovaries ➡.*

Cervical Cancer

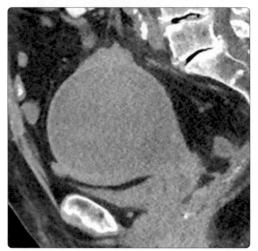

Cervical Cancer

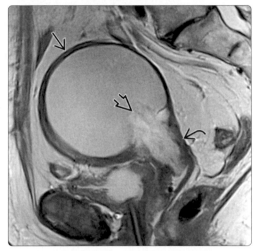

(Left) Sagittal NECT of the pelvis shows an enlarged uterus. There is suggestion of hypodense distention of the uterine cavity and thinning of the surrounding myometrium. (Right) Sagittal T2 FSE image in the same patient shows the uterus ⊟ is enlarged due to fluid-filled distention of the uterine cavity. The cervical obstruction is due to a hyperintense mass ⊟. There is preservation of an outer rim of low signal cervical stroma ⊟, confirming the absence of parametrial invasion. Biopsy confirmed adenocarcinoma.

Cervical Cancer

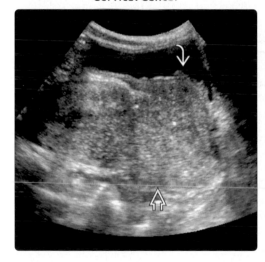

Cervical Stenosis

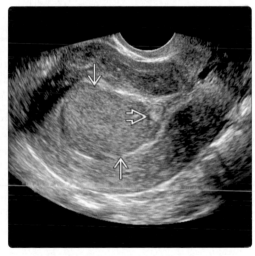

(Left) Longitudinal transabdominal ultrasound shows a large, irregular, hypoechoic mass in the region of the cervix ⊟. The mass invades the bladder ⊟. (Right) Longitudinal transvaginal ultrasound in a woman after endometrial ablation shows that the endometrial cavity is filled with complex fluid ⊟ with some echogenic debris ⊟. The surrounding endometrium is thin.

Cervical Leiomyoma

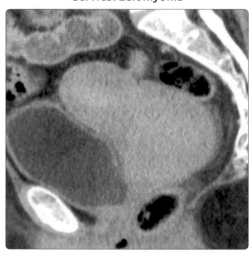

Cervical Leiomyoma

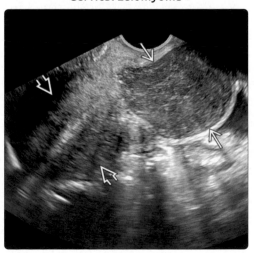

(Left) Sagittal NECT shows enlargement of the cervix with homogeneous density and smooth external margins. (Right) Longitudinal transvaginal ultrasound in the same patient shows a well-defined homogeneously hypoechoic mass ⊟ in the cervix. Note the normal uterine body ⊟ and lack of distention of the uterine cavity.

DIFFERENTIAL DIAGNOSIS

Common

- Secretory-Phase Endometrium
- Endometrial Polyps
- Leiomyoma
- Diffuse Adenomyosis
- Early Pregnancy

Less Common

- Endometrial Hyperplasia
- Endometrial Cancer
- Tamoxifen-Induced Changes
- Retained Products of Conception
- Hematometra

Rare but Important

- Endometritis
- Molar Pregnancy
- Unopposed Estrogen
- Metastatic Disease

ESSENTIAL INFORMATION

Key Differential Diagnosis Issues

- Diffuse endometrial thickening
  - Normal secretory-phase endometrium
  - Endometrial hyperplasia
  - Endometrial cancer
  - Diffuse adenomyosis
  - Hematometra
  - Focal endometrial lesions can also mimic diffuse thickening
    - Techniques that may be helpful for identifying the focal abnormality
      - □ Color Doppler
      - □ 3D ultrasound
      - □ Phase of menstruation
- Focal endometrial thickening
  - Endometrial polyp
  - Endometrial cancer
  - Submucosal leiomyoma
- Postpartum patient
  - Endometritis
  - Retained products of conception
- Indistinct endometrial-myometrial interface
  - Endometrial cancer
  - Adenomyosis
  - Submucosal leiomyoma

Helpful Clues for Common Diagnoses

- **Secretory-Phase Endometrium**
  - In last 1/2 of menstrual cycle, endometrium can be thick, heterogeneous, and echogenic
  - Follow-up early in subsequent menstrual cycle will show thin endometrium
- **Endometrial Polyps**
  - Focal endometrial lesion
  - Typically more echogenic than surrounding endometrium
  - May have cysts

- Stalk with flow
- May have broad base
- Frequently multiple
- Smooth margins
- May have surrounding thin endometrium
- **Leiomyoma**
  - Submucosal leiomyoma is > 50% within endometrium
  - Intramural leiomyoma can cause appearance of endometrial thickening
  - Iso- or hypoechoic lesion
  - Posterior acoustic shadowing
  - Can be confirmed with MR
    - Well-defined T2 hypointense myometrial mass
- **Diffuse Adenomyosis**
  - Endometrial pseudowidening
  - Enlarged globular uterus
  - Indistinct endometrial-myometrial interface
  - Can be confirmed with MR
    - Thickened junctional zone (JZ) ≥ 12 mm
    - High SI foci in JZ on T1WI and T2WI
- **Early Pregnancy**
  - Positive urine/serum human chorionic gonadotropin
    - Normal early pregnancy
    - Miscarriage
    - Ectopic pregnancy
    - Hydatiform mole, complete mole
    - Hydatiform mole, partial mole

Helpful Clues for Less Common Diagnoses

- **Endometrial Hyperplasia**
  - Typically diffuse endometrial thickening but may be focal
  - ± cystic spaces
  - Well-defined endometrial-myometrial interface
  - Risk factors
    - Nulliparity
    - Obesity
    - Age > 70
    - Hypertension
    - Diabetes mellitus
    - Tamoxifen
- **Endometrial Cancer**
  - Irregular endometrial thickening ± mass
  - Heterogeneous endometrium with areas of hypoechogenicity
  - Ill-defined margins, indistinct endometrial-myometrial interface
  - Myometrial invasion is diagnostic
  - Typically postmenopausal woman with abnormal bleeding
- **Tamoxifen-Induced Changes**
  - ↑ incidence with ↑ dose and time of treatment
  - Reactivation of foci of adenomyosis
  - Due to estrogenic effect in endometrium, can lead to polyps, hyperplasia, and carcinoma
  - Endometrial cancer in patients taking tamoxifen is frequently in endometrial polyps
- **Retained Products of Conception**
  - Focal endometrial lesion
  - May have calcifications

○ May have blood flow, but lack of flow does not exclude diagnosis

- **Hematometra**
  ○ Echogenic fluid in endometrial cavity
    – Mobile debris
    – No flow on Doppler
  ○ Look for underlying cause of obstruction
    – Uterine duplication anomaly
    – Leiomyoma
    – Endometrial cancer
    – Cervical cancer
    – If thin surrounding endometrium and no obstructing lesion, cervical stenosis is diagnosis of exclusion

Helpful Clues for Rare Diagnoses

- **Endometritis**
  ○ In postpartum patient, painful enlarged uterus
  ○ In nonpregnant patient, associated with pelvic inflammatory disease
  ○ Clinical diagnosis, imaging is nonspecific
  ○ Elevated white blood cell count
- **Molar Pregnancy**
  ○ Most common type of gestational trophoblastic disease
  ○ Hyperechoic early in pregnancy with classic grape-like appearance developing as pregnancy advances
- **Unopposed Estrogen**
  ○ Can result in endometrial polyps, hyperplasia, and carcinoma
  ○ Estrogen use without progesterone
  ○ Due to chronic anovulatory states (i.e., polycystic ovary syndrome), exogenous estrogen exposure, tamoxifen, obesity, estrogen-secreting ovarian tumors (i.e., thecoma, granulosa cell tumor)
- **Metastatic Disease**
  ○ Ovarian primary with metastasis to endometrium
  ○ Cervical primary with direct extension to endometrium
    – MR helpful for cervical cancer staging, local extent of disease, and to differentiate cervical from endometrial primary when both are involved by tumor

○ Distant primary with hematogenous metastasis to endometrium

Other Essential Information

- Use transvaginal scanning for best evaluation of endometrium
- Sonohysterography can differentiate focal and diffuse endometrial abnormalities to determine best sampling technique
  ○ Diffuse thickening can be sampled with blind biopsy
  ○ Focal mass best assessed with hysteroscopic biopsy
- Sonohysterography helpful if endometrium is not adequately visualized by transvaginal ultrasound in symptomatic patient
- In uterine duplication anomalies, must evaluate each endometrium separately
  ○ 3D ultrasound and MR can be helpful for further evaluation

Alternative Differential Approaches

- Solid or complex ovarian lesion in association with endometrial lesion
  ○ Estrogenic effect from granulosa cell tumor produces endometrial lesion
  ○ Estrogen secretion from thecoma produces endometrial lesion
  ○ Concordant ovarian and endometrial carcinoma
  ○ Endometrioid tumor
  ○ Metastatic disease

SELECTED REFERENCES

1. Benacerraf BR et al: Which patients benefit from a 3D reconstructed coronal view of the uterus added to standard routine 2D pelvic sonography? AJR Am J Roentgenol. 190(3):626-9, 2008
2. Barwick TD et al: Imaging of endometrial adenocarcinoma. Clin Radiol. 61(7):545-55, 2006
3. Cohen I: Endometrial pathologies associated with postmenopausal tamoxifen treatment. Gynecol Oncol. 94(2):256-66, 2004
4. Smith-Bindman R et al: How thick is too thick? When endometrial thickness should prompt biopsy in postmenopausal women without vaginal bleeding. Ultrasound Obstet Gynecol. 24(5):558-65, 2004
5. Davis PC et al: Sonohysterographic findings of endometrial and subendometrial conditions. Radiographics. 22:803-16, 2002

Secretory-Phase Endometrium

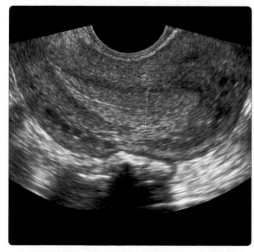

Early Pregnancy

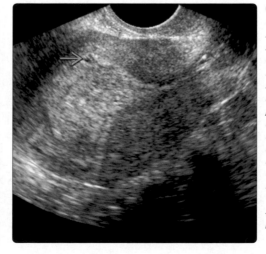

(Left) *Longitudinal transvaginal US of the uterus shows a homogeneous symmetric endometrial echo complex that measures 11 mm, which is normal in the secretory phase of the menstrual cycle. There is no focal thickening, heterogeneity, or abnormal blood flow.* (Right) *Longitudinal transvaginal US in a woman with bleeding in the 1st trimester shows a heterogeneous endometrium with small cysts ➡. Follow-up showed a normal early pregnancy.*

Endometrial Polyps

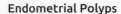

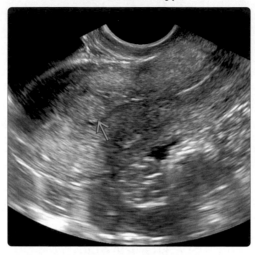

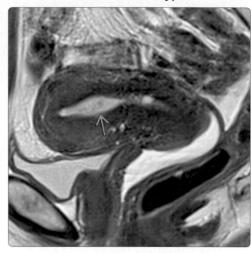

(Left) *Longitudinal transvaginal US of the uterus shows focal echogenic thickening ⇨ of the fundal endometrium. Note the normal thin endometrium of the lower uterine segment.* **(Right)** *Sagittal T2 FS MR of the uterus in the same patient shows focal endometrial ⇨ thickening and mild heterogeneity in this area. Small endometrial polyps can be difficult to see on MR, and focal thickening of the stripe can be a clue, as in this case.*

Endometrial Polyps

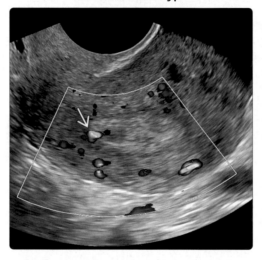

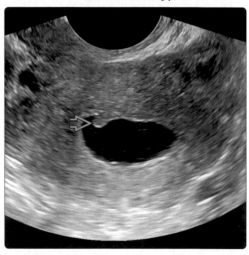

(Left) *Longitudinal color Doppler US of the uterus shows diffuse endometrial thickening. No focal abnormality could be identified on grayscale imaging, but Doppler shows focal flow ➡ extending into endometrium.* **(Right)** *Saline-infused sonohysterogram in the same patient shows a small echogenic endometrial lesion ⇨. This was removed and confirmed to be an endometrial polyp. Doppler imaging can help indicate a focal lesion when grayscale imaging only shows diffuse endometrial thickening.*

Endometrial Polyps

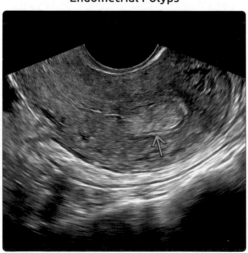

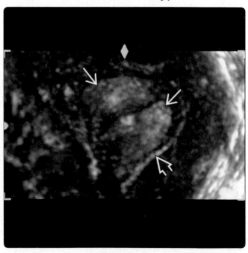

(Left) *Longitudinal transvaginal US of the uterus shows focal hyperechoic thickening ⇨ of the endometrial echo complex.* **(Right)** *3D coronal view of the uterus in the same patient shows 2 echogenic endometrial masses consistent with polyps ➡. The surrounding normal thin echogenic endometrium ➡ is well seen. 3D ultrasound has been shown to be helpful in identifying focal endometrial abnormalities when the endometrium appears thick on 2D imaging.*

Leiomyoma

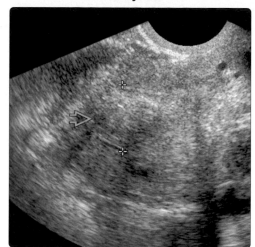

Leiomyoma

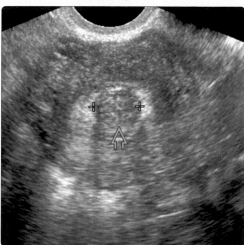

(Left) *Longitudinal transvaginal US shows a hypoechoic mass* ⇨ *projecting into the endometrial cavity with the appearance of a thick endometrium (calipers).* (Right) *Transverse transvaginal US in the same patient, during the secretory phase, shows how the leiomyoma (⇨, calipers) is now more apparent when surrounded by the echogenic endometrium.*

Leiomyoma

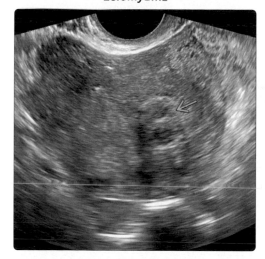

Leiomyoma

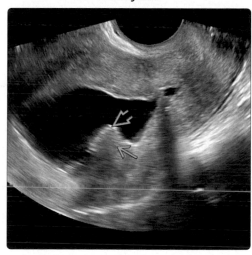

(Left) *Transvaginal US of the uterus shows a hypoechoic shadowing mass* ⇨ *centrally in the uterus. The normal endometrial echo complex is obscured. The differential diagnosis for hypoechoic masses in this location includes submucosa leiomyoma or endometrial cancer.* (Right) *Saline-infused sonography (same patient) shows the hypoechoic shadowing mass* ⇨*. The echogenic endometrial lining* ⇨ *overlying the lesion is thin and intact, confirming a submucosal leiomyoma and not endometrial lesion.*

Leiomyoma

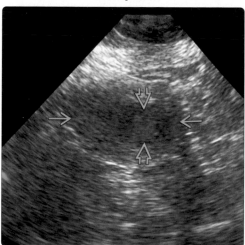

Leiomyoma

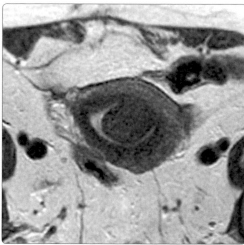

(Left) *Transverse transvaginal US of the uterus* ⇨ *shows a subtle hypoechoic lesion* ⇨ *centrally in the uterus.* (Right) *Axial T2 FSE MR of the pelvis shows the uterus in short axis. There is a well-defined homogeneously hypointense mass projecting into the endometrial cavity, compatible with a submucosal leiomyoma. MR is helpful for characterization of endometrial abnormalities when a leiomyoma is suspected on a challenging ultrasound.*

Diffuse Adenomyosis

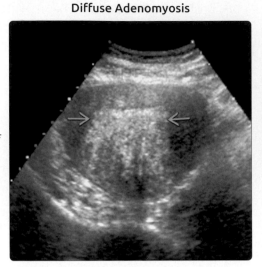

Endometrial Hyperplasia

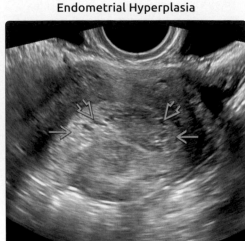

(Left) *Transabdominal US of uterus shows ill-defined thickening of endometrial echo complex ➡. There is asymmetric thickening of posterior uterine wall with echogenic and hypoechoic striations emanating from endometrial-myometrial interface. This constellation of findings indicates that appearance of endometrial thickening is due to diffuse adenomyosis.* **(Right)** *Transvaginal US of the uterus shows diffuse thickening of the endometrial echo complex ➡ with foci of cystic change ➡.*

Endometrial Cancer

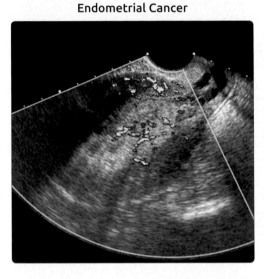

Endometrial Cancer

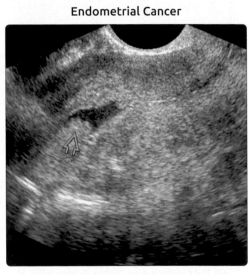

(Left) *Longitudinal color Doppler US shows increased flow within the irregular thickened endometrium. Although the differential is wide for this appearance, cancer should always be excluded, particularly in a postmenopausal woman with bleeding. This was confirmed to be endometrial cancer on biopsy and hysterectomy.* **(Right)** *Longitudinal transvaginal US shows fluid in the endometrial cavity with a focal area of endometrial thickening ➡ in the fundal region.*

Tamoxifen-Induced Changes

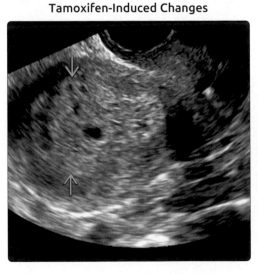

Metastatic Disease

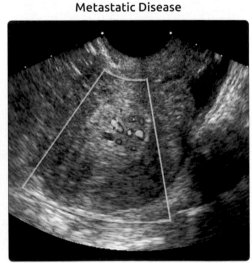

(Left) *Longitudinal transvaginal US in a 76-year-old woman taking tamoxifen shows a thickened heterogeneous endometrium ➡ with multiple cysts.* **(Right)** *Longitudinal transvaginal US of the uterus with color Doppler shows blood flow within the thickened heterogeneous endometrium. In this patient with breast cancer, tamoxifen change and metastatic disease were thought to be most likely. Biopsy showed metastatic disease from breast primary.*

Thickened Endometrium

Retained Products of Conception

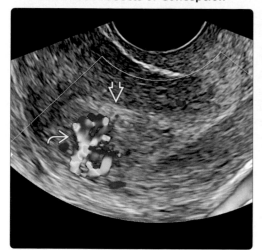

Retained Products of Conception

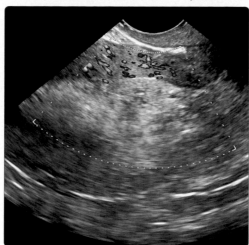

(Left) *Color Doppler US shows a thickened heterogeneous endometrium ⇨ with feeding vessels ⇨ to the region of retained placental tissue. Histology showed partially necrotic decidua with the hemorrhage.* (Right) *Color Doppler US of the uterus (same patient) demonstrates no blood flow within the thickened endometrium. When there is blood flow, it is helpful to confirm retained products of conception; however, its absence does not exclude this diagnosis, which was confirmed with dilation and curettage.*

Molar Pregnancy

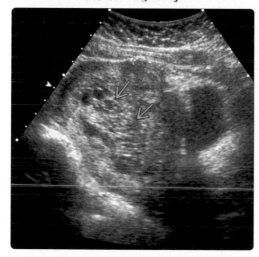

Molar Pregnancy

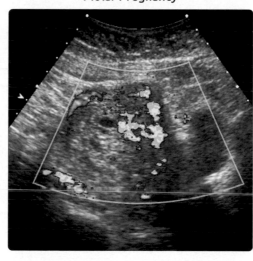

(Left) *Longitudinal transabdominal US of the uterus shows cystic thickening ⇨ of the endometrial echo complex.* (Right) *Color Doppler US of the uterus in the same patient shows increased flow within the cystic mass. The grape-like appearance of the cystic mass and the patient's markedly elevated β-HCG are consistent with a molar pregnancy.*

Unopposed Estrogen

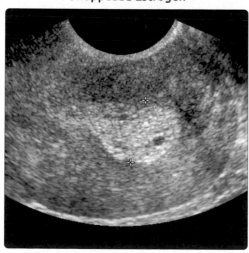

Unopposed Estrogen

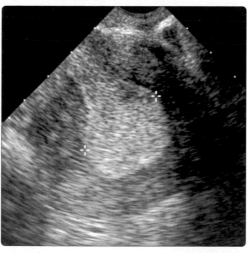

(Left) *Transvaginal US in patient with a giant cell tumor of the ovary shows a 15-mm thickened endometrium (calipers) with multiple cysts. In the setting of ovarian mass, endometrial abnormalities may be due to an estrogen secretion by the tumor.* (Right) *Transvaginal US in a patient with oligomenorrhea and PCOS shows a thickened 23-mm endometrium (calipers). Chronic anovulation and unopposed estrogen result in chronic stimulation of endometrium and an increased risk of endometrial hyperplasia or, rarely, cancer.*

DIFFERENTIAL DIAGNOSIS

Common

- Anovulatory Bleeding
- Endometrial Polyp
- Endometrial Atrophy
- Leiomyoma
- Pregnancy and Complications
  - Subchorionic Hematoma
  - Tubal Ectopic Pregnancy
  - Hydatiform Mole

Less Common

- Adenomyosis
- C-Section Defect
- Endometrial Hyperplasia
- Endometrial Cancer
- Cervical Cancer
- Endometritis
- Retained Products of Conception

Rare but Important

- Uterine Leiomyosarcoma
- Vulva Carcinoma
- Vaginal Carcinoma
- Intrauterine Device Perforation
- Estrogen-Producing Tumor of Ovary
  - Granulosa Cell Tumor
  - Fibrothecoma, Ovary
- Ovarian Carcinoma
- Bleeding From GI or GU Tract

ESSENTIAL INFORMATION

Key Differential Diagnosis Issues

- Is patient premenopausal?
  - Anovulatory bleeding (most common)
  - Pregnancy and complications
  - Endometrial polyp
  - Leiomyoma, submucosal
  - Endometrial hyperplasia
  - Malignancy (uterine, endometrial, cervical)
  - Nongynecologic sources of bleeding: GI or urinary tract
- Is patient postmenopausal?
  - Bleeding due to hormone use
    - Hormones can affect endometrial thickness
  - Endometrial atrophy (most common)
  - Endometrial polyp
  - Endometrial cancer
    - Over 90% present with bleeding in postmenopausal woman, therefore if endometrium is not adequately seen on US, further imaging with SIS or MR must be recommended
  - Leiomyoma
  - Malignancy (uterine, endometrial, cervical)
  - Nongynecologic sources of bleeding: GI or urinary tract
- Is there focal thickening of endometrium?
  - Endometrial polyps (most common)
  - Submucosal leiomyoma
  - Endometrial hyperplasia, rarely focal
  - Endometrial cancer

- Is endometrial-myometrial interface obscured?
  - Leiomyoma, submucosal
  - Endometrial cancer
  - Adenomyosis
- Is patient pregnant?
  - Normal pregnancy
  - Subchorionic hematoma
  - Tubal ectopic pregnancy
  - Hydatiform mole
- Is patient peripartum?
  - Retained products of conception
  - Endometritis

Helpful Clues for Common Diagnoses

- **Endometrial Polyp**
  - Focal endometrial lesion
  - Echogenic ± cystic change
  - Smooth margins
  - ± vascular stalk
- **Endometrial Atrophy**
  - 50-75% of postmenopausal bleeding attributed to atrophy
  - Sonographic appearance of thin endometrium < 5-mm double-layer thickness
- **Leiomyoma**
  - Shadowing
  - Iso- or hypoechoic
  - Submucosal leiomyomas most likely associated with bleeding
  - If > 50%, leiomyoma projects into endometrial cavity, can be removed hysteroscopically
  - MR is diagnostic and helpful for treatment planning
    - Circumscribed hypointense mass on T2WI
- **Pregnancy and Complications**
  - Positive urine/serum human chorionic gonadotropin
  - If intrauterine pregnancy
    - Normal pregnancy
    - Normal or abnormal intrauterine pregnancy with subchorionic hematoma
    - Miscarriage
    - Hydatidiform mole
    - Consider heterotopic pregnancy with ectopic if fertility treatment
  - If no intrauterine pregnancy visualized
    - Ectopic pregnancy
    - Normal pregnancy, too early to visualize
    - Miscarriage

Helpful Clues for Less Common Diagnoses

- **Adenomyosis**
  - Diffuse or asymmetric enlargement
  - ± tender uterus
  - ± small myometrial cysts
  - MR is diagnostic
- **C-Section Defect**
  - Triangular collection anterior lower uterine segment
  - Acts as reservoir for blood products, leading to intermenstrual bleeding
- **Endometrial Hyperplasia**
  - Diffuse thickening most common, but also can be focal

- ○ ± cystic spaces
- **Endometrial Cancer**
  - ○ Poor definition of endometrium
  - ○ Irregular, thickened, heterogeneous endometrium
  - ○ Loss of endometrial-myometrial interface
  - ○ Most commonly presents with abnormal bleeding in postmenopausal woman
  - ○ Risk factors: Recurrent bleeding, estrogen hormone replacement therapy, obesity, polycystic ovary syndrome, chronic anovulation, hypertension, diabetes mellitus
- **Cervical Cancer**
  - ○ May be missed by ultrasound when small
  - ○ MR used for staging

Other Essential Information

- Use transvaginal scanning for best evaluation of endometrium
- Measure greatest double-layer endometrial thickness in sagittal plane
- Sonohysterography helpful to distinguish focal and diffuse endometrial abnormality
  - ○ Diffuse thickening can be sampled with blind biopsy
  - ○ Focal mass best assessed with hysteroscopic biopsy
- Sonohysterography helpful if endometrium is not adequately visualized with transvaginal ultrasound
- In uterine duplication anomalies, must evaluate each endometrium separately
- Tamoxifen use leads to polyps, hyperplasia, and carcinoma, as well as reactivation of foci of adenomyosis
  - ○ Number of endometrial lesions related to cumulative dose
  - ○ Endometrial cancer in patients taking tamoxifen frequently arises in endometrial polyps
- Postmenopausal patients with bleeding
  - ○ If endometrium is not visualized adequately in its entirety, must further evaluate another imaging modality, biopsy, or direct visualization
  - ○ < 5 mm likely atrophy, no need to biopsy

- ○ Society of Radiologists in Ultrasound consensus: Double-layer endometrial thickness > 5 mm is abnormal
  - – 96% sensitivity for endometrial cancer
- ○ Recommend biopsy for diffuse thickening
- ○ Recommend biopsy for any focal abnormality
- ○ Use of HRT increases false-positive rate

Alternative Differential Approaches

- Enlarged uterus
  - ○ Leiomyoma
  - ○ Adenomyosis
  - ○ Cervical stenosis with uterus distended with debris
  - ○ Endometrial carcinoma
- Solid or complex ovarian lesion in association with endometrial lesion
  - ○ Estrogenic effect from granulosa cell tumor leading to endometrial lesion
  - ○ Estrogen secretion from thecoma leading to endometrial lesion
  - ○ Concordant ovarian and endometrial carcinoma
  - ○ Endometrioid tumor
  - ○ Metastatic disease

SELECTED REFERENCES

1. Goldstein SR: Sonography in postmenopausal bleeding. J Ultrasound Med. 31(2):333-6, 2012
2. American College of Obstetricians and Gynecologists: ACOG Committee Opinion No. 426: The role of transvaginal ultrasonography in the evaluation of postmenopausal bleeding. Obstet Gynecol. 113(2 Pt 1):462-4, 2009
3. de Kroon CD et al: Saline contrast hysterosonography in abnormal uterine bleeding: a systematic review and meta-analysis. BJOG. 110(10):938-47, 2003
4. Kazandi M et al: Transvaginal sonography combined with saline contrast sonohysterography to evaluate the uterine cavity in patients with abnormal uterine bleeding and postmenopausal endometrium more than 5 mm. Eur J Gynaecol Oncol. 24(2):185-90, 2003
5. Davis PC et al: Sonohysterographic findings of endometrial and subendometrial conditions. Radiographics. 22:803-16, 2002
6. Goldstein RB et al: Evaluation of the woman with postmenopausal bleeding: Society of Radiologists in Ultrasound-Sponsored Consensus Conference statement. J Ultrasound Med. 20(10):1025-36, 2001
7. Nalaboff KM et al: Imaging the endometrium: disease and normal variants. Radiographics. 21:1409-24, 2001
8. Ascher SM et al: Tamoxifen-induced uterine abnormalities: The role of imaging. Radiology. 214:29-38, 2000

Endometrial Polyp

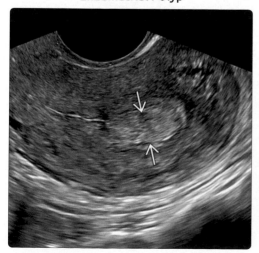

Endometrial Polyp

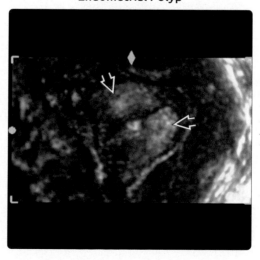

(Left) *Longitudinal transvaginal ultrasound of the uterus shows focal hyperechoic thickening ➡ of the endometrial echo complex.* (Right) *3D ultrasound in the same patient shows to better advantage 2 endometrial polyps ➡ resulting in the focal endometrial thickening seen on 2D images. 3D ultrasound is helpful in clarifying focal abnormalities that may not be evident with 2D technique.*

Endometrial Polyp

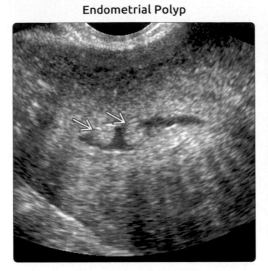

Endometrial Polyp

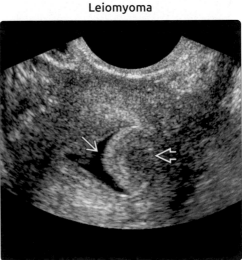

(Left) *Transverse hysterosonogram shows multiple small echogenic masses ➡ arising from the endometrium.* **(Right)** *Longitudinal transvaginal ultrasound shows a well-defined, oblong, soft tissue echogenicity mass ➡ in the endocervical canal.*

Endometrial Polyp

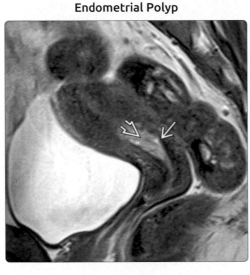

Endometrial Polyp

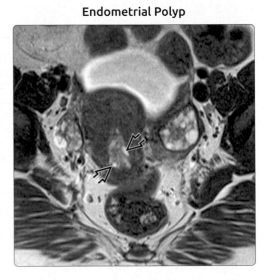

(Left) *Sagittal T2WI MR shows focal endometrial thickening ➡ in the lower uterine segment extending through the internal cervical os ➡.* **(Right)** *Axial T2WI MR in the same patient shows small cystic spaces ➡ in the focal endometrial thickening. This pedunculated polyp extends into the endocervical canal (seen best on the prior sagittal image). Endometrial polyps tend to be isointense to normal endometrium and are seen on MR due to focal thickening and internal cystic spaces.*

Endometrial Atrophy

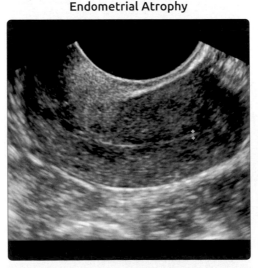

Leiomyoma

(Left) *Longitudinal transvaginal ultrasound shows a retroflexed uterus with a thin atrophic endometrium (calipers).* **(Right)** *Oblique transvaginal ultrasound shows a hypoechoic mass ➡ projecting into the endometrial cavity, with a small amount of endometrial fluid ➡. Note that more than 50% of the leiomyoma projects into the endometrial cavity. This will allow for hysteroscopic removal of the leiomyoma.*

Leiomyoma

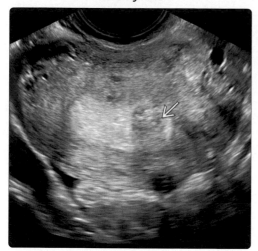

Leiomyoma

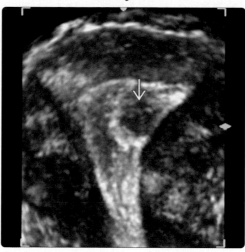

(Left) *Transverse transvaginal ultrasound of the uterus shows a hypoechoic shadowing mass ➡ in the endometrium.* (Right) *Coronal 3D image in the same patient shows the hypoechoic mass ➡ projecting into the endometrium.*

Leiomyoma

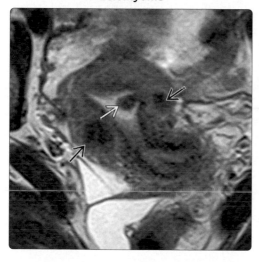

Leiomyoma

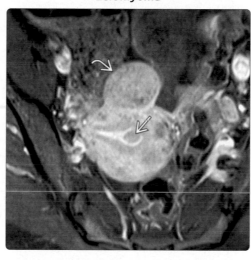

(Left) *Coronal oblique T2WI MR in the same patient shows a pedunculated circumscribed hypoechoic mass consistent with a submucosal leiomyoma ➡. Note also intramural leiomyomas ➡. MR is ideal for definitive diagnosis of leiomyomas.* (Right) *Axial T1WI C+ FS MR in the same patient shows the pedunculated submucosal leiomyoma ➡. Despite its hypointensity relative to the surrounding endometrium, the leiomyoma is enhancing and is therefore viable. Also note the larger viable subserosal leiomyoma ➡ anteriorly.*

Pregnancy and Complications

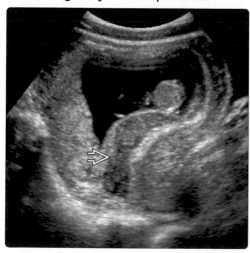

Pregnancy and Complications

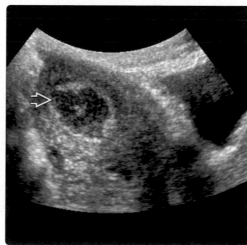

(Left) *Oblique transabdominal ultrasound shows a marginal subchorionic hematoma ➡ in a patient 13 weeks' pregnant with pain and bleeding.* (Right) *Longitudinal transabdominal ultrasound shows a complex fluid collection ➡ in the endometrial cavity in a woman with an ectopic pregnancy. This finding is consistent with a pseudosac.*

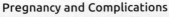

Pregnancy and Complications

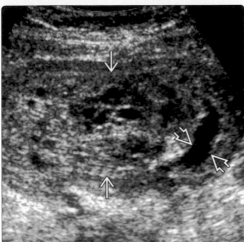

Adenomyosis

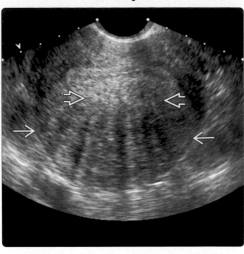

(Left) *Transverse ultrasound shows a typical complete hydatidiform mole with the uterus filled by a complex cystic mass ➡. The fluid collection adjacent to the mass is hemorrhage ➡.* (Right) *Transverse transvaginal ultrasound of the uterus shows asymmetric thickening of the posterior uterine wall ➡ as well as echogenic and hypoechoic striations emanating from the ill-defined posterior endometrial-myometrial interface ➡.*

Adenomyosis

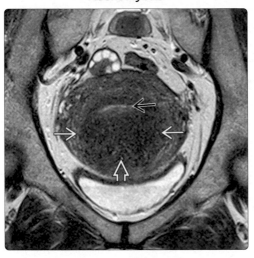

C-Section Defect

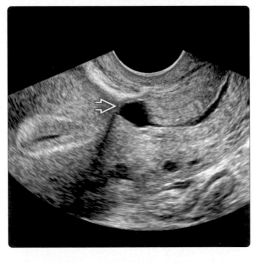

(Left) *Coronal oblique T2WI MR shows thickening of junctional zone ➡ anteriorly with numerous punctate T2 hyperintense foci ➡. Cystic foci represent endometrial glands. Note normal thickness of the endometrium ➡ and junctional zone posteriorly.* (Right) *Longitudinal transvaginal ultrasound shows focal myometrial thinning in the anterior lower uterine segment consistent with C-section scar. There is a fluid collection ➡ in the scar. This C-section defect can act as a reservoir for midcycle bleeding.*

C-Section Defect

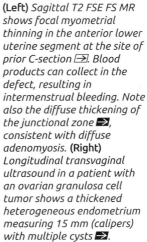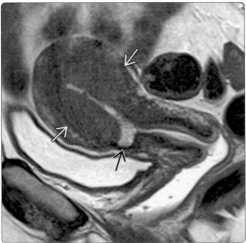

Endometrial Hyperplasia

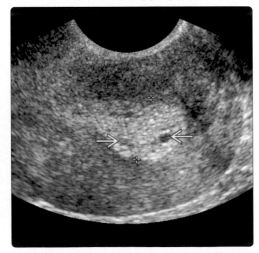

(Left) *Sagittal T2 FSE FS MR shows focal myometrial thinning in the anterior lower uterine segment at the site of prior C-section ➡. Blood products can collect in the defect, resulting in intermenstrual bleeding. Note also the diffuse thickening of the junctional zone ➡, consistent with diffuse adenomyosis.* (Right) *Longitudinal transvaginal ultrasound in a patient with an ovarian granulosa cell tumor shows a thickened heterogeneous endometrium measuring 15 mm (calipers) with multiple cysts ➡.*

Endometrial Cancer

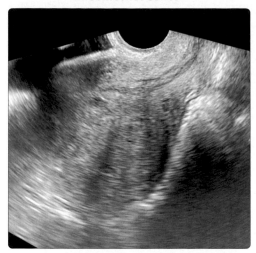

Endometrial Cancer

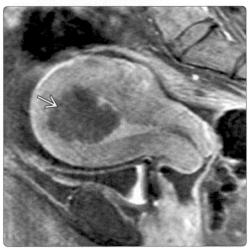

(Left) *Longitudinal transvaginal ultrasound shows an enlarged uterus without a normal endometrial echo complex. MR was recommended to determine if the ill-defined stripe is due to body habitus or pathology.* (Right) *Sagittal T1 C+ FS MR in the same patient shows an endometrial mass ➡ arising from the fundus with less than 50% invasion of the myometrial thickness. MR can be helpful when suspecting adenomyosis or fibroids, or to exclude a large endometrial mass, particularly when US is limited by patient factors.*

Endometrial Cancer

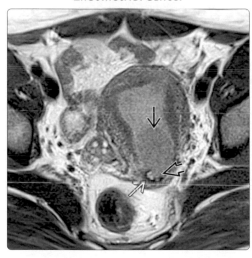

Endometrial Cancer

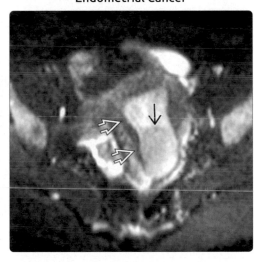

(Left) *Axial T2 FS MR shows an endometrial mass ➡ in the lower uterine segment. There is invasion ➡ of the low signal cervical stroma ➡. MR can be helpful for staging endometrial cancer due to the superior soft tissue contrast allowing visualization of tumor and its depth of invasion.* (Right) *Axial DWI MR (same patient) with endometrial cancer ➡ shows the utility of DWI in assessing the depth of myometrial invasion. Junctional zone ➡ is particularly well seen on DWI, and, when intact, excludes deep myometrial invasion.*

Endometrial Cancer

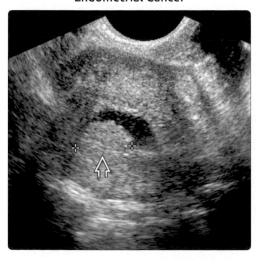

Cervical Cancer

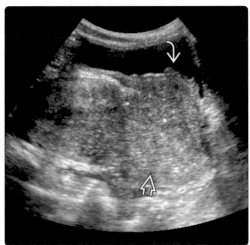

(Left) *Transverse transvaginal ultrasound shows fluid in the endometrial cavity with a focal broad-based mass (calipers) in the posterior endometrium ➡.* (Right) *Longitudinal transabdominal ultrasound shows a large, irregular, hypoechoic mass in the region of the cervix ➡. The mass invades the bladder ➡.*

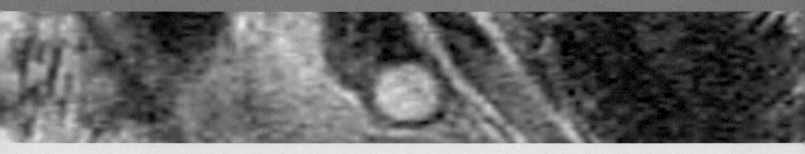

Generic Imaging Patterns

Modality-Specific Imaging Findings

MAGNETIC RESONANCE IMAGING

DIFFERENTIAL DIAGNOSIS

Common

- Mucinous Cystadenoma
- Serous Cystadenoma
- Polycystic Ovarian Syndrome
- Endometriomas
- Tuboovarian Abscess

Less Common

- Theca Lutein Cysts
- Cystadenofibroma
- Malignant Ovarian Epithelial Neoplasms
    - Serous Cystadenocarcinoma
    - Mucinous Cystadenocarcinoma
    - Endometrioid Carcinoma
    - Clear Cell Carcinoma
    - Transitional Cell Carcinoma
- Metastases

Rare but Important

- Brenner Tumor
- Struma Ovarii
- Ovarian Hyperstimulation Syndrome
- Granulosa Cell Tumor
- Yolk Sac Tumor

ESSENTIAL INFORMATION

Key Differential Diagnosis Issues

- Imaging Pattern
    - Multilocular cystic mass without solid component
        - Mucinous cystadenoma
        - Tuboovarian abscess
        - Borderline ovarian epithelial neoplasms
        - Serous cystadenoma
        - Granulosa cell tumor
    - Multilocular cystic mass + solid component
        - Tuboovarian abscess
        - Serous cystadenoma
        - Mucinous cystadenoma
        - Cystadenofibroma
        - Brenner tumor
        - Malignant ovarian epithelial neoplasms
        - Struma ovarii
        - Yolk sac tumor
        - Granulosa cell tumor
    - Enlarged ovary with multiple cysts
        - Endometriomas
        - Polycystic ovarian syndrome
        - Ovarian hyperstimulation syndrome
        - Theca lutein cysts
- Ovarian cystic lesions associated with endometrial pathology
    - Endometrioid carcinoma
    - Granulosa cell tumor
    - Theca lutein cysts

Helpful Clues for Common Diagnoses

- **Mucinous Cystadenoma**
    - Almost always multilocular and may be quite large

- MR, CT, and US appearance of individual locules may vary as result of differences in degree of hemorrhage or protein content
- **Serous Cystadenoma**
    - Occasionally multilocular (more commonly unilocular)
    - Thin wall and thin septa
    - Usually anechoic on ultrasound, fluid attenuation on CT, and fluid signal intensity on MR
    - Occasionally contain small papillary projections
- **Polycystic Ovarian Syndrome**
    - Characterized clinically by menstrual irregularities, hirsutism, and obesity
    - Enlarged ovaries (volume > 10 cm^3)
    - Presence of > 26 follicles per ovary
    - Individual follicles are generally similar in size and measure 2-9 mm in diameter
    - Peripheral distribution of follicles → string of pearls appearance
- **Endometriomas**
    - Usually unilocular but presence of multiple endometriomas gives ovary multicystic appearance
    - Characteristic sonographic features include
        - Homogeneous low-level echoes
        - Echogenic mural foci
    - Characteristic MR features include
        - T2 shading
        - T2 dark spots
- **Tuboovarian Abscess**
    - Complex multilocular cystic mass ± solid component
    - ± fluid-debris level
    - ± intracystic air
    - Surrounding inflammation, which may be seen as increased echogenicity of pelvic fat, or infiltration and enhancement of surrounding fat on CT and MR
    - Enhancement of wall and septa on CECT and MR
    - Thick-walled adnexal mass with low signal intensity contents on T1WI and high signal intensity on T2WI

Helpful Clues for Less Common Diagnoses

- **Theca Lutein Cysts**
    - Bilateral enlarged, multicystic ovaries, similar to ovarian hyperstimulation syndrome
    - Occurs in setting of gestational trophoblastic disease or multiple gestations
- **Cystadenofibroma**
    - Rims, plaques, or nodules of low signal intensity on T2WI
    - Locules show fluid characteristics on imaging in cases of serous cystadenofibroma
        - MR, CT, and US appearance of individual locules may vary as result of differences in degree of hemorrhage or protein content in cases of mucinous cystadenofibroma
- **Malignant Ovarian Epithelial Neoplasms**
    - Elevated CA-125
    - Mixed solid and cystic ovarian mass
    - Thick irregular septa and large vascular solid components
    - Invasion of surrounding structures
    - Ascites, peritoneal caking, and nodal metastases in advanced disease
- **Metastases**

- Commonly occur in setting of known gastrointestinal tract malignant tumor
- Unilateral or bilateral
- Mixed solid and cystic or solid with cystic areas due to necrosis

Helpful Clues for Rare Diagnoses

- **Brenner Tumor**
  - Solid component in multilocular cystic mass may exhibit amorphous calcifications
  - Low signal intensity of solid component on T2WI
- **Struma Ovarii**
  - Multilocular cystic mass with solid components (solid masses, thick wall, and septa)
  - Cyst fluid is anechogenic or of low-level echogenicity on US
    - Cysts contain 1 or more vascularized, well-circumscribed, roundish echogenic structures with smooth contours (struma pearls)
  - Cystic spaces demonstrate high attenuation on CT
    - Due to presence of thyroglobulin
  - ± calcifications in solid component
  - Cystic spaces demonstrate locules of low intensity on T2WI and punctuate foci of high intensity on T1WI
  - May be associated with, or part of, mature cystic teratoma
    - Characteristic imaging features of mature cystic teratoma because of presence of fat
- **Ovarian Hyperstimulation Syndrome**
  - History of ovulation induction therapy
  - Massively enlarged ovaries, multicystic ovaries
  - Ascites, as well as pleural or pericardial effusions in severe cases
  - Empty uterus
- **Granulosa Cell Tumor**
  - Multilocular ± solid component
  - Cysts typically contain large numbers of small locules (> 10)
  - Variable appearance of cyst content on imaging due to presence of hemorrhage

- Papillary projections may be found
- Most common estrogen-producing ovarian tumor
  - May be associated with endometrial hyperplasia, polyps, or carcinoma
- **Yolk Sac Tumor**
  - Elevated level of α-fetoprotein in young patient with pelvic mass
  - Mixed solid and cystic mass with hemorrhagic portion
  - Bright dot sign is common finding seen at contrast-enhanced CT and MR imaging as enhancing foci in wall or solid components
    - Due to dilated vessels in these highly vascular tumors
  - Capsular tears may be observed on imaging

SELECTED REFERENCES

1. Choi JI et al: Imaging features of complex solid and multicystic ovarian lesions: proposed algorithm for differential diagnosis. Clin Imaging. 40(1):46-56, 2016
2. Shaaban AM et al: Ovarian malignant germ cell tumors: cellular classification and clinical and imaging features. Radiographics. 34(3):777-801, 2014
3. Lujan ME et al: Updated ultrasound criteria for polycystic ovary syndrome: reliable thresholds for elevated follicle population and ovarian volume. Hum Reprod. 28(5).1361-8, 2013
4. Van Holsbeke C et al: Imaging of gynecological disease (3): clinical and ultrasound characteristics of granulosa cell tumors of the ovary. Ultrasound Obstet Gynecol. 31(1):450-6, 2008
5. Jung SE et al: CT and MR imaging of ovarian tumors with emphasis on differential diagnosis. Radiographics. 22(6):1305-25, 2002

Mucinous Cystadenoma

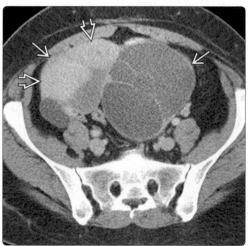

Serous Cystadenoma

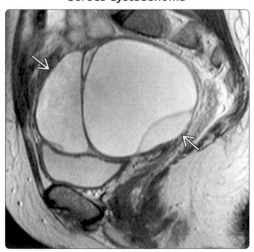

(Left) *Axial CECT shows bilateral multilocular cystic ovarian masses* ➡. *Some of the locules within the right ovarian lesion contain high-attenuation material* ➡ *due to hemorrhage or high protein content.* (Right) *Sagittal T2WI MR shows a large multilocular cystic ovarian mass* ➡. *The lesion is composed of multiple locules separated by thin smooth septa.*

Polycystic Ovarian Syndrome

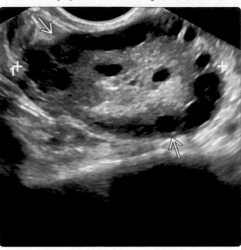

Polycystic Ovarian Syndrome

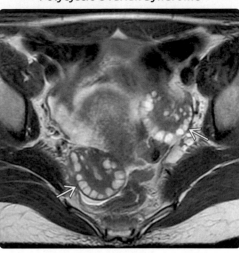

(Left) *Transvaginal ultrasound shows enlarged ovary* ➡ *composed of numerous discrete uniform small ovarian cysts. Note the peripheral location of follicles, which results in a string of pearls appearance.* (Right) *Axial T2WI MR shows enlarged ovaries* ➡ *with numerous discrete small ovarian cysts. Note the peripheral location of follicles, which results in a string of pearls appearance.*

Endometriomas

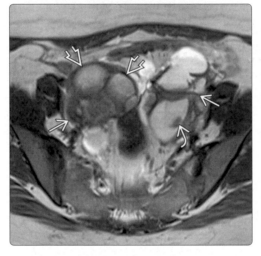

Endometriomas

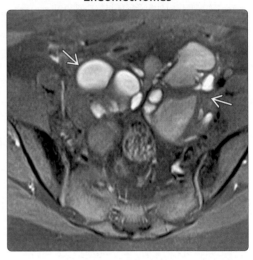

(Left) *Axial T2WI MR shows bilateral enlarged ovaries* ➡, *each containing multiple discrete high T2 signal lesions. Some of the lesions show T2 shading* ➡. *A left ovarian lesion shows a T2 dark spot* ➡. (Right) *Axial T1 FS MR shows bilateral ovarian enlargement* ➡. *Both ovaries contain multiple lesions displaying high signal intensity.*

Tuboovarian Abscess

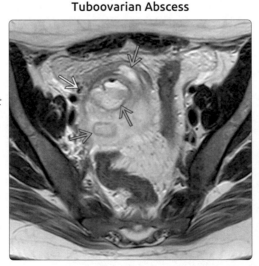

Tuboovarian Abscess

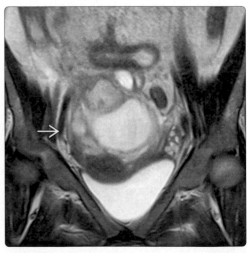

(Left) *Axial T2WI MR shows a right ovarian mass* ➡ *composed of multiple cystic loculi* ➡ *and a thick rind of high T2 signal intensity.* (Right) *Coronal T2WI MR in the same patient shows a right ovarian mass* ➡ *composed of multiple cystic loculi. Note the difference in signal intensity within various loculi.*

Tuboovarian Abscess

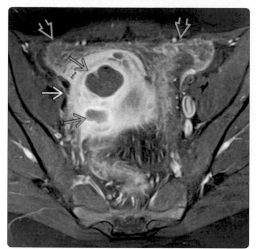

Tuboovarian Abscess

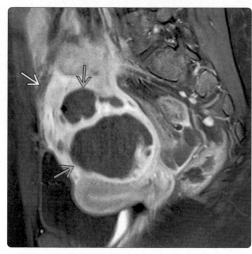

(Left) *Axial T1 C+ FS MR shows a right ovarian mass ➡️ composed of multiple cystic loculi ➡️ and a thick enhancing rind. Note enhancement of the pelvic fat ➡️.* **(Right)** *Sagittal T1 C+ FS MR shows a right ovarian mass ➡️ composed of multiple cystic loculi ➡️ and a thick enhancing rind. Individual loculi tend to be irregular in shape with irregular contour.*

Theca Lutein Cysts

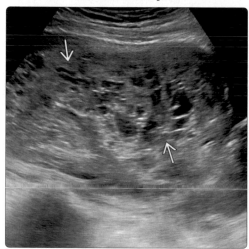

Theca Lutein Cysts

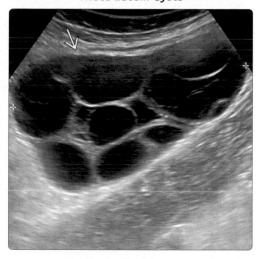

(Left) *Axial transabdominal ultrasound in a patient with a high level of hCG shows a heterogeneous mass ➡️ filling the uterine cavity due to hydatidiform mole.* **(Right)** *Transvaginal ultrasound in the same patient shows an enlarged ovary ➡️ composed of numerous discrete cysts. The other ovary was similarly enlarged.*

Cystadenofibroma

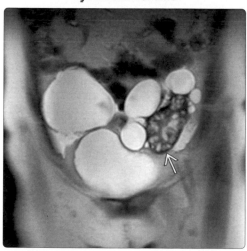

Malignant Ovarian Epithelial Neoplasms

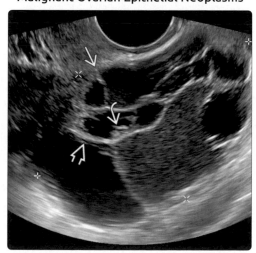

(Left) *Coronal T2WI MR shows an enlarged left ovary ➡️ with numerous intraovarian and exophytic cysts. Note the diffuse low signal intensity of the ovarian parenchyma in between the small parenchymal cysts.* **(Right)** *Transvaginal ultrasound shows a multilocular cystic ovarian mass ➡️ composed of multiple locules displaying variable echogenicity. The septa are thick and irregular ➡️ and show small papillary projections ➡️.*

Malignant Ovarian Epithelial Neoplasms

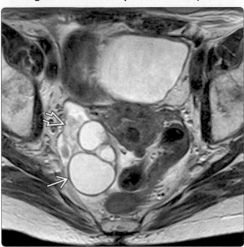

Malignant Ovarian Epithelial Neoplasms

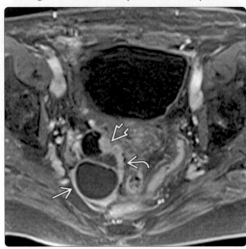

(Left) *Axial T2WI MR shows a multilocular cystic ovarian mass ➡ with a peripheral solid component ➡. (Right) Axial T1 C+ FS MR in the same patient shows a multilocular ovarian mass ➡ with a enhancing solid component ➡ and thick enhancing wall ➡. Pathological examination revealed serous cystadenocarcinoma.*

Malignant Ovarian Epithelial Neoplasms

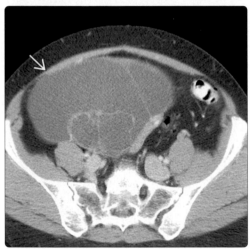

Metastases

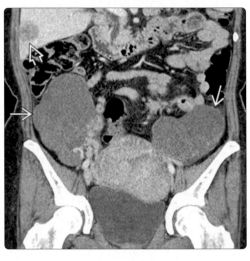

(Left) *Axial CECT shows a multilocular cystic ovarian mass ➡. Pathological examination revealed mucinous cystadenocarcinoma. (Right) Coronal CECT in a patient with history of colonic carcinoma shows bilateral enlarged cystic ovaries ➡ and a right lobe liver mass ➡ due to metastatic disease.*

Struma Ovarii

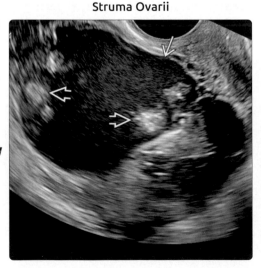

Struma Ovarii

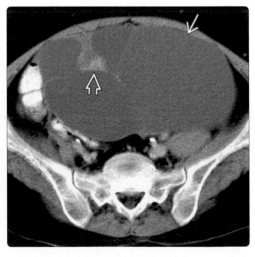

(Left) *Transvaginal ultrasound shows a multilocular cystic ovarian mass ➡ containing multiple rounded echogenic structures (strumal pearls) ➡. (Right) Axial CECT shows a large pelvic mass ➡ composed of large loculi separated by thin enhancing septa. There is an intensely enhancing solid component ➡ in the center of the mass.*

Struma Ovarii

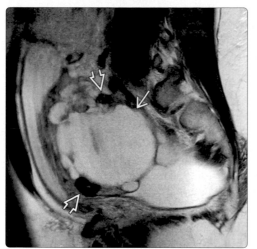

Ovarian Hyperstimulation Syndrome

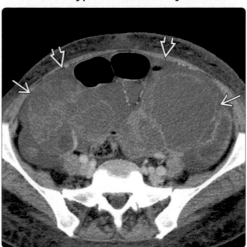

(Left) *Sagittal T2WI MR shows a multilocular cystic mass ➡ composed of numerous locules filling the pelvic cavity. Note that some locules ➡ demonstrate very low signal intensity, a characteristic feature of struma ovarii.* **(Right)** *Axial CECT in a patient receiving ovarian induction therapy for in vitro fertilization shows bilateral enlarged multicystic ovaries ➡ and small volume ascites ➡. Note also diffuse subcutaneous edema resulting from increased capillary permeability.*

Granulosa Cell Tumor

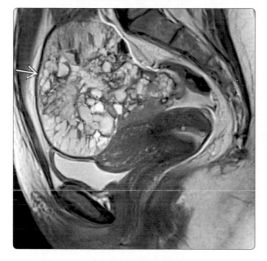

Granulosa Cell Tumor

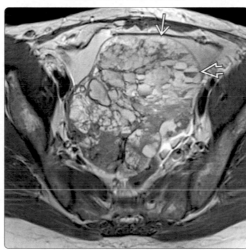

(Left) *Sagittal T2WI MR shows a large ovarian multilocular cystic mass ➡ composed of numerous small cystic spaces.* **(Right)** *Axial T2WI MR shows a large ovarian multilocular cystic mass ➡ composed of numerous small cystic spaces. Some of the locules show fluid level ➡ due to intracystic hemorrhage.*

Granulosa Cell Tumor

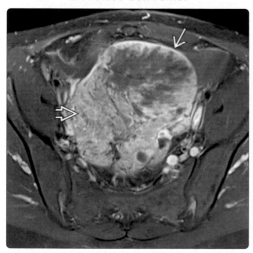

Yolk Sac Tumor

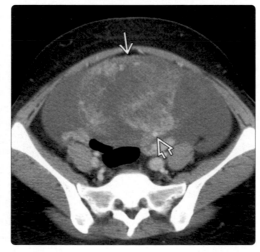

(Left) *Axial T1 C+ FS MR shows a large ovarian multilocular cystic mass ➡ composed of numerous small cystic spaces and enhancing solid component ➡.* **(Right)** *Axial CECT shows a mixed solid and multilocular cystic mass ➡. The bright dot sign ➡ represents aneurysmally dilated vascular structures and is commonly seen in yolk sac tumors due to its high vascularity.*

DIFFERENTIAL DIAGNOSIS

Common

- Physiologic Follicles
- Corpus Luteum
- Hemorrhagic Cyst
- Mature Cystic Teratoma
- Endometrioma
- Postmenopausal Cyst

Less Common

- Tuboovarian Abscess
- Serous Cystadenoma
- Mucinous Cystadenoma
- Serous Cystadenocarcinoma
- Mucinous Cystadenocarcinoma
- Cystadenofibroma

Rare but Important

- Granulosa Cell Tumor

ESSENTIAL INFORMATION

Key Differential Diagnosis Issues

- Complexity
  - Simple cyst (round or oval with smooth, thin walls, no solid component or septation); anechoic with posterior acoustic enhancement on US, no internal flow at color Doppler US, fluid attenuation at CT, and homogeneous fluid signal intensity on MR
    - Physiologic follicles
    - Cystadenoma (serous and mucinous)
    - Cystadenofibroma
  - Complex cysts
    - Corpus luteum
    - Endometrioma
    - Hemorrhagic cyst
    - Dermoid cyst
  - Cysts with solid component
    - Dermoid cyst
    - Endometrioma
    - Cystadenoma (serous and mucinous)
    - Cystadenocarcinoma (serous and mucinous)
    - Granulosa cell tumor

Helpful Clues for Common Diagnoses

- **Physiologic Follicles**
  - Premenopausal woman
  - Thin-walled, round to oval, avascular simple cyst
    - May reach diameter up to 3 cm
    - When ovulation fails to occur → follicle continues to enlarge → functional follicle
      - Remains simple in appearance
  - Curvilinear septation may be seen within dominant preovulatory follicle
    - Represents oocyte and its supporting structures (i.e., cumulus oöphorus)
- **Corpus Luteum**
  - Postovulatory corpus luteum measures up to 3 cm
  - Thick-walled cyst with crenulated margin

  - Cyst appears collapsed, giving it relatively solid appearance
  - Doppler US demonstrates prominent peripheral blood flow with low-resistance waveform
  - Irregular collapsed cyst with peripheral enhancement
- **Hemorrhagic Cyst**
  - Resolve on follow-up examinations
  - US: Different patterns may be seen
    - Echogenic, avascular, homogeneous, or heterogeneous nonshadowing in early stage
    - Retracted clot
      - Avascular mass-like structure within anechoic cyst with characteristic concave contour
      - May jiggle with transducer ballottement
    - Reticular, lacy, fishnet, or spongy pattern
  - MR
    - Usually single unilocular cyst
    - High signal intensity on T1WI
      - Signal intensity remains high on T1WI FS
    - Hyperintense or hypointense on T2WI
    - No T2 dark spots
- **Mature Cystic Teratoma**
  - US
    - Focal high echogenic nodules
    - Heterogeneous internal echoes ± acoustic shadows
    - Multiple hyperechoic fine lines and dots
    - Atypical features include fluid-fluid level, anechoic cyst, and multiple floating globules
  - CT and MR
    - Presence of fat is characteristic
      - Fat attenuation on CT
      - High signal intensity on T1WI MR and low signal intensity on fat-suppressed T1WI
- **Endometrioma**
  - US
    - Well-defined, smooth-walled cyst(s)
    - Contains homogeneous low-level echoes → characteristic ground-glass appearance
    - Small echogenic mural foci
    - Mural irregularities: Usually avascular (likely due to adherent mural clot or fibrin)
    - ± flow due to presence of endometrial tissue
  - MR
    - Single or multiple
    - High signal intensity on T1WI, remains high on FS T1WI
      - To differentiate from fat-containing dermoid cyst
    - T2 shading (signal loss on T2WI in cyst that appears hyperintense on T1WI)
    - T2 dark spots (hypointense foci within cyst on T2WI)
- **Postmenopausal Cyst**
  - Simple cyst in postmenopausal woman
  - Hemorrhagic cyst should not occur in late menopause
  - Normal CA-125

Helpful Clues for Less Common Diagnoses

- **Tuboovarian Abscess**
  - Occasionally presents as unilocular cystic mass ± irregular wall and mural irregularity
- **Cystadenoma (Serous and Mucinous)**
  - Simple cyst with thin wall

- Persistent on follow-up examinations
- Features suggestive of benignity include
  - Entirely cystic with diameter < 4 cm
    - ± small papillary projections
  - Thin wall < 3 mm
  - Lack of internal structure
  - Absence of both ascites and invasive features such as peritoneal disease or adenopathy
- **Cystadenocarcinoma (Serous and Mucinous)**
  - Elevated CA-125
  - Features suggestive of malignancy include
    - Thick, irregular wall, thick septa, papillary projections, and large soft tissue component with necrosis
- **Cystadenofibroma**
  - Simple cyst with smooth wall of low signal intensity

Helpful Clues for Rare Diagnoses

- **Granulosa Cell Tumor**
  - Rare presentation
  - Hyperestrogenemia → endometrial pathology
  - Unilocular cyst with thick solid rind

Management of Simple Ovarian Cyst

- In women of reproductive age
  - Cyst size ≤ 3 cm
    - Normal physiologic finding
    - May or may not be described in imaging report
    - Does not need follow-up
  - Cyst size > 3 and ≤ 5 cm
    - Should be described in imaging report with statement they are almost certainly benign
    - Do not need follow-up
  - Cyst size > 5 and ≤ 7 cm
    - Should be described in imaging report with statement they are almost certainly benign
    - Yearly US follow-up
  - Cyst size > 7 cm
    - May be difficult to assess completely with US, further imaging with MR or surgical evaluation should be considered

- In postmenopausal women
  - Cyst size ≤ 1 cm
    - Clinically inconsequential
    - May or may not be described in imaging report
    - Does not need follow-up
  - Cyst size > 1 and ≤ 7 cm
    - Should be described in imaging report with statement they are almost certainly benign
    - Yearly US follow-up, at least initially
      - Continue follow-up annually; decrease frequency of follow-up once stability or decrease in size has been confirmed
      - Cysts in larger end of this range should be followed on regular basis
  - Cyst size > 7 cm
    - Further imaging with MR or surgical evaluation should be considered

Management of Hemorrhagic Ovarian Cyst

- In women of reproductive age
  - Cyst size ≤ 3 cm
    - May or may not be described in imaging report
    - Does not need follow-up
  - Cyst size > 3 and ≤ 5 cm
    - Should be described in imaging report
    - Does not need follow-up
  - Cyst size > 5 cm
    - Should be described in imaging report
    - Short interval sonographic follow up (6-12 weeks) to ensure resolution
- In postmenopausal women
  - Early postmenopause
    - May occasionally ovulate
    - Cyst should be described in imaging report
    - Short interval (6-12 weeks) US follow-up is recommended to ensure resolution
  - Late postmenopause
    - Hemorrhagic cysts should be considered neoplastic and surgically evaluated

Physiologic Follicles

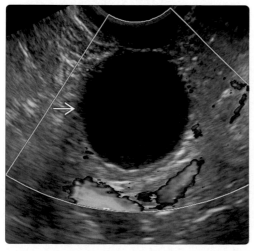

Physiologic Follicles

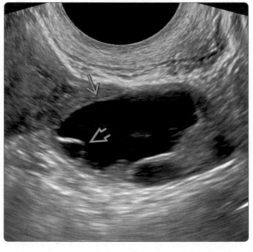

(Left) Transvaginal color Doppler ultrasound in a 23-year-old woman shows a single unilocular simple cyst measuring 28 mm ➡. The finding of such a cyst in a premenopausal woman woman does not require follow-up. (Right) Transvaginal ultrasound in a 28-year-old woman shows a single unilocular ➡ cyst measuring 25 mm. There is a curvilinear peripheral septation ➡, which indicates that the ovum is surrounded by a cumulus oöphorus within the mature follicle.

(Left) *Transvaginal color Doppler ultrasound shows an isoechoic ovarian lesion ➡ with peripheral vascularity, surrounded by normal ovarian tissue ⇥. **(Right)** Transvaginal color Doppler ultrasound shows a hypoechoic ovarian lesion ➡ with irregular internal avascular septa, giving the lesion a lacy or fishnet appearance.*

Corpus Luteum

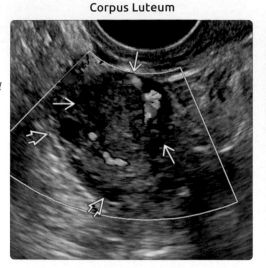

Hemorrhagic Cyst

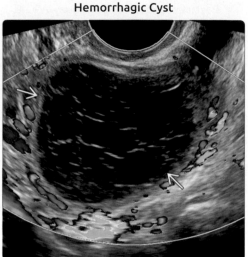

(Left) *Transvaginal ultrasound shows a unilocular cyst ➡ containing homogeneous low-level echoes, initially thought to represent an endometrioma. **(Right)** Axial T2 MR in the same patient shows a left ovarian lesion ➡. The lesion displays high signal intensity with a fluid level ⇥. The floating part has slightly higher signal intensity than the dependent part.*

Mature Cystic Teratoma

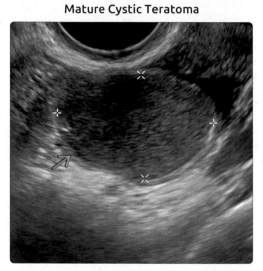

Mature Cystic Teratoma

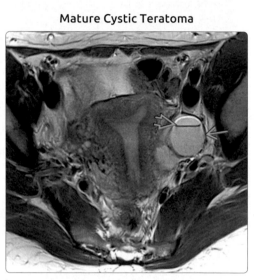

(Left) *Axial T1 MR in the same patient shows a left ovarian lesion ➡. The lesion demonstrates a fluid level ⇥. The floating part has high signal intensity, similar to that of subcutaneous fat, while the dependent part has low signal intensity similar to that of simple fluid. **(Right)** Axial T1 FS MR in the same patient shows a left ovarian mass ➡, with suppression of the T1 high signal intensity of the floating part ➡ (due to its fatty nature), on this fat-suppressed sequence*

Mature Cystic Teratoma

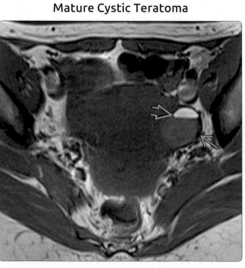

Mature Cystic Teratoma

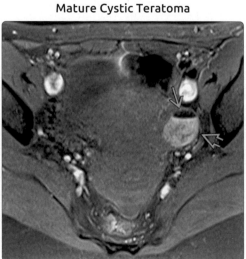

Endometrioma

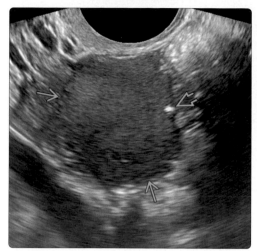

Endometrioma

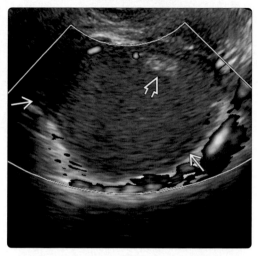

(Left) *Transvaginal ultrasound shows a hypoechoic ovarian lesion ➡ with uniform low-level echoes and a mural echogenic focus ➡, a characteristic feature of endometriomas.* **(Right)** *Transvaginal color Doppler ultrasound shows an endometrioma ➡ with an avascular echogenic mural nodule ➡. The presence of a mural nodule does not necessarily mean malignant transformation, as nodules may develop as a result of retracted clot or nonmalignant changes of the endometrial tissue.*

Endometrioma

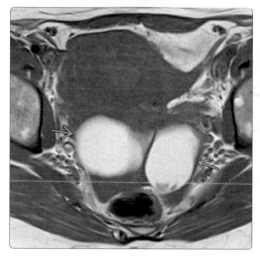

Endometrioma

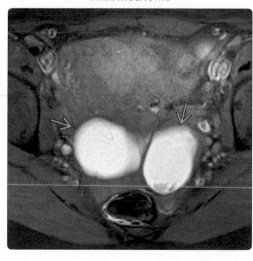

(Left) *Axial T1WI MR shows bilateral ovarian endometriomas ➡ demonstrating high signal intensity.* **(Right)** *Axial T1WI FS MR in the same patient shows bilateral ovarian endometriomas ➡ displaying high signal intensity. Persistent high signal intensity on fat-suppressed T1WI differentiates endometriomas, and hemorrhagic cysts, from dermoid cysts, which lose signal on fat-suppressed T1WI.*

Endometrioma

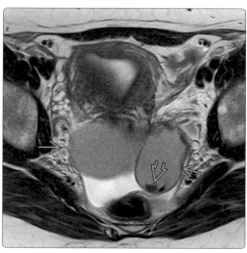

Endometrioma

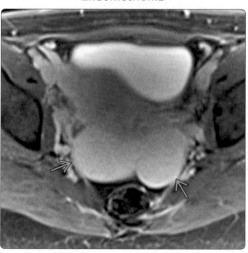

(Left) *Axial T2WI MR in the same patient shows bilateral ovarian endometriomas ➡ displaying T2 shading (signal loss on T2WI in a cyst that appears hyperintense on T1WI). Note also the T2 dark spots ➡ (hypointense foci within cyst on T2WI).* **(Right)** *Axial T1 C+ FS MR in the same patient shows bilateral ovarian endometriomas ➡ displaying high signal intensity without enhancement.*

Tuboovarian Abscess

Tuboovarian Abscess

(Left) *Axial T2 MR shows a left ovarian lesion ⇨ with fluid-fluid level. The dependent portion has lower signal intensity than simple fluid.* (Right) *Axial T1 MR in the same patient shows enlargement of the left ovary ⇨. There is stranding of the fat surrounding the pelvis and left ovary ⇨.*

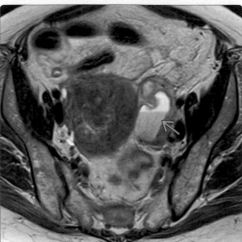

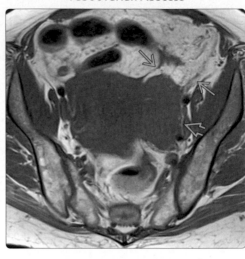

Tuboovarian Abscess

Tuboovarian Abscess

(Left) *Axial T1 C+ FS MR in the same patient shows a left ovarian lesion ⇨ with enhancing rind surrounding unilocular low signal center. Note stranding of the pelvic fat ⇨.* (Right) *Axial DWI (with a b factor of 800) in the same patient shows high signal intensity of the content of the lesion due to diffusion restriction.*

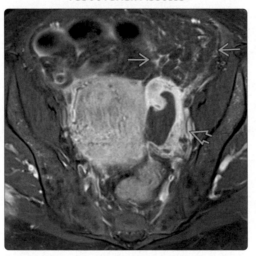

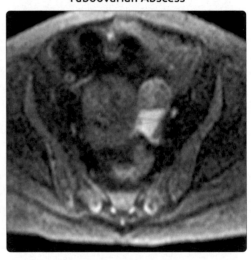

Postmenopausal Cyst

Serous Cystadenocarcinoma

(Left) *Transvaginal ultrasound in a 58-year-old woman shows a simple-appearing ovarian cyst ⇨. CA-125 was normal, and the cyst has been stable for 3 years.* (Right) *Transabdominal ultrasound shows a unilocular cyst ⇨ with mural nodules ⇨. Pathological examination revealed serous cystadenocarcinoma.*

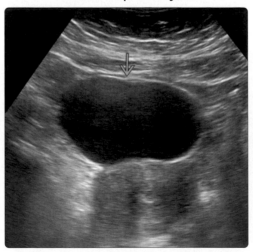

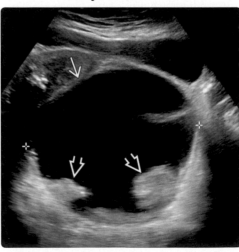

Mucinous Cystadenoma

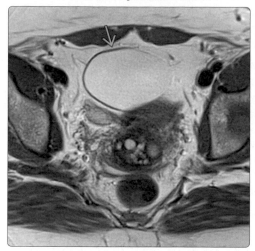

Mucinous Cystadenoma

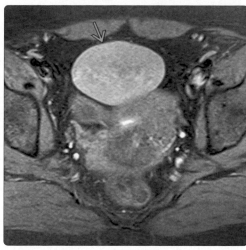

(Left) *Axial T2 MR shows a simple-appearing unilocular ovarian lesion ➡ displaying high signal intensity.* (Right) *Axial T1 FS MR in the same patient shows a unilocular ovarian lesion ➡ displaying high signal intensity. Mucinous cystadenomas may show locules of high T1 signal intensity because of their mucin contents.*

Serous Cystadenoma

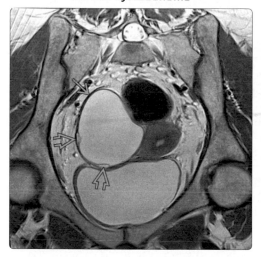

Serous Cystadenoma

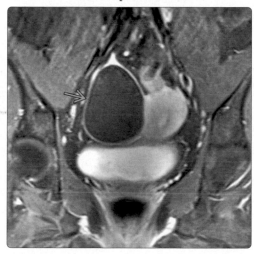

(Left) *Coronal T2WI MR shows a right ovarian simple cystic lesion ➡ measuring 7 cm and displaying homogeneous high signal intensity. Ovarian follicles ➡ are seen stretched around the cyst.* (Right) *Coronal T1 C+ FS MR in the same patient shows a right ovarian low signal intensity lesion ➡ with a uniformly thin enhancing wall. Pathological examination revealed an ovarian serous cystadenoma.*

Cystadenofibroma

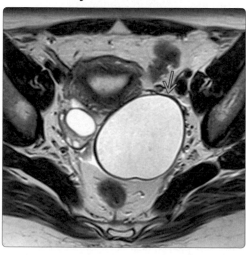

Granulosa Cell Tumor

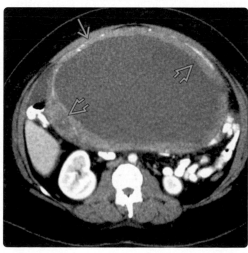

(Left) *Axial T2 MR shows a left ovarian cyst ➡ with a smooth, fine T2 low signal intensity wall.* (Right) *Axial CECT shows a large, predominantly unilocular cystic mass ➡ with a thick rind of soft tissue attenuation ➡. Pathological evaluation revealed granulosa cell tumor.*

DIFFERENTIAL DIAGNOSIS

Common

- Malignant Serous Epithelial Tumors
- Torsion and Massive Ovarian Edema
- Fibroma/Fibrothecoma/Thecoma

Less Common

- Krukenberg Tumors
- Brenner Tumor
- Granulosa Cell Tumor

Rare but Important

- Dysgerminoma
- Immature Teratoma
- Yolk Sac Tumor
- Sertoli-Leydig Cell Tumors
- Carcinoid
- Choriocarcinoma
- Lymphoma
- Leukemia
- Leiomyoma
- Hyperthecosis
- Fibromatosis
- Sarcoma
  - Chondrosarcomas, Fibrosarcomas, Endometrial Stromal Sarcomas, Angiosarcomas, Rhabdomyosarcomas, and Leiomyosarcomas

ESSENTIAL INFORMATION

Key Differential Diagnosis Issues

- Hormone and tumor marker-producing tumors
  - Granulosa cell tumors → hyperestrogenism
  - Thecoma/fibrothecoma → hyperestrogenism
  - Carcinoid → carcinoid syndrome
  - Choriocarcinoma → β-hCG
  - Yolk sac tumor → α-fetoprotein
  - Sertoli-Leydig cell tumors → hyperandrogenism
  - Dysgerminoma → β-hCG (only 5% of cases)
  - Hyperthecosis → hyperandrogenism
- Calcifications
  - Malignant serous epithelial tumors
  - Brenner tumor
  - Dysgerminoma (speckled pattern)
  - Leiomyoma
  - Immature teratoma
- Low signal on T2WI MR
  - Brenner tumor
  - Fibroma
  - Fibromatosis
  - Leiomyoma
  - Krukenberg tumor
  - Adenofibroma
- Bilateral
  - Malignant serous epithelial tumors
  - Krukenberg tumors
  - Lymphoma
  - Dysgerminoma (6.5-10.0% of cases)
  - Hyperthecosis

- Preservation of normal follicles
  - Torsion and massive ovarian edema
  - Fibromatosis
  - Lymphoma
  - Leukemia (granulocytic sarcoma)

Helpful Clues for Common Diagnoses

- **Malignant Serous Epithelial Tumors**
  - ↑ serum CA-125 level
  - Extensive peritoneal carcinomatosis ± calcifications
  - Tumor invasion of pelvic organs
  - Pelvic and retroperitoneal adenopathy
- **Torsion and Massive Ovarian Edema**
  - Diffuse ovarian enlargement (massive enlargement with massive ovarian edema) with preserved ovarian shape
  - Edematous ovarian stroma with peripheral follicles
  - Decreased vascular flow on Doppler studies (variable)
  - No enhancement with contrast-enhanced studies
  - Whirlpool sign: Twisted vascular pedicle
    - Highly sensitive (87%) and specific (88%)
  - Pelvic free fluid (nonspecific)
  - Displacement of adnexal structures/uterus
- **Fibroma/Fibrothecoma/Thecoma**
  - Can be associated with ascites and pleural effusions in classic Meigs syndrome
  - Fibrothecomas may manifest with hyperestrogenism
    - Endometrial polyps, hyperplasia, or carcinoma
  - US
    - Round, oval, or slightly lobulated tumors
    - Most are hypoechoic and solid, with homogeneous internal echogenicity
    - Dramatic sound attenuation resulting in posterior acoustic shadowing
    - Minimal to moderate vascularization on color Doppler images
  - MR
    - Hypo- to isointense to pelvic muscles on T1WI and low signal intensity on T2WI
    - T1WI C+: Mild enhancement

Helpful Clues for Less Common Diagnoses

- **Krukenberg Tumors**
  - Known primary tumors commonly originating from gastrointestinal tract
  - Bilateral in 60-80% of patients
  - MR
    - Intratumoral cysts within solid component
    - Predominantly hyperintense with variable hypointensity on T2WI due to presence of metastatic mucin-filled signet ring cells in ovarian stroma and abundant collagen formation
    - Moderate to marked enhancement of solid component
- **Brenner Tumor**
  - US
    - Minimal flow on color Doppler ultrasound
    - Hypoechoic with posterior shadowing due to presence of calcifications
  - CT
    - Soft tissue attenuation ± calcifications (83% of cases)
  - MR

- – Very low T2 signal intensity and low T1 signal intensity due to presence of fibrous elements
- – At least moderate enhancement after contrast material administration
- **Granulosa Cell Tumor**
  - Hyperestrinism is common → endometrial hyperplasia, polyps, or carcinoma
  - US
    - – Solid tumors with homogeneous or heterogeneous echogenicity
      - □ Heterogeneity results from intratumoral bleeding, infarcts, and fibrous degeneration
    - – Increased vascularity is demonstrated on Doppler
  - CT and MR
    - – Solid granulosa cell tumor has no specific features to suggest diagnosis

Helpful Clues for Rare Diagnoses
- **Dysgerminoma**
  - Most cases occur in adolescence and early adulthood
  - Tumor divided into component lobules by vascularized enhancing septa
    - – Septa are usually hypo- or isointense on T2WI and are difficult to appreciate on T1WI
- **Immature Teratoma**
  - Peak incidence between 15-19 years of age; rarely seen in menopause
  - Predominantly solid mass with interspersed small foci of fatty elements, coarse irregular calcifications, and numerous cysts of variable sizes
- **Yolk Sac Tumor**
  - Most common in 2nd and 3rd decades; rare in women > 40 years old
  - Bright dot sign
    - – Enhancing foci in wall or solid components attributed to dilated vessels
  - Capsular tears
  - Very rapid rate of growth
- **Sertoli-Leydig Cell Tumors**
  - Hyperandrogenism

- Small (almost always < 3 cm) unilateral, solid nodule
- Hemorrhage, necrosis, and large size are suggestive of malignancy
- Variable intensity on T2WI
- Intense enhancement with contrast
- **Carcinoid**
  - May be associated with carcinoid syndrome
    - – Even in absence of metastases, as ovarian veins drain directly into systemic circulation
- **Choriocarcinoma**
  - ↑ β-hCG level
    - – Presence of adnexal mass with ↑ β-hCG level → erroneous diagnosis of ectopic pregnancy
  - Solid or mixed solid and cystic adnexal mass
  - Strong enhancement of solid component
- **Lymphoma**
  - Solid homogenous large ovarian mass or bilateral ovarian involvement is seen in absence of ascites
  - Usually maintains normal ovarian structure and shows no invasion of surrounding structures
- **Hyperthecosis**
  - Hyperandrogenism
  - Bilateral symmetric ovarian enlargement
  - Mostly postmenopausal
  - Homogeneous low echogenicity on US and low signal intensity on T2WI with few, if any, follicles
- **Fibromatosis**
  - Enlargement of ovary + low T2 signal of ovarian parenchyma and multiple small follicles

SELECTED REFERENCES

1. Salem U et al: Hematopoietic tumors of the female genital system: imaging features with pathologic correlation. Abdom Imaging. 39(4):922-34, 2014
2. Shaaban AM et al: Ovarian malignant germ cell tumors: cellular classification and clinical and imaging features. Radiographics. 34(3):777-801, 2014
3. Van Holsbeke C et al: Imaging of gynecological disease (3): clinical and ultrasound characteristics of granulosa cell tumors of the ovary. Ultrasound Obstet Gynecol. 31(4):450-6, 2008
4. Jung SE et al: CT and MR imaging of ovarian tumors with emphasis on differential diagnosis. Radiographics. 22(6):1305-25, 2002

Malignant Serous Epithelial Tumors

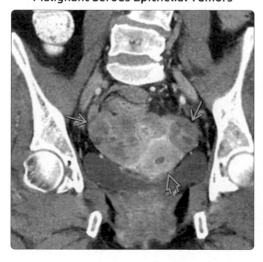

Krukenberg Tumors

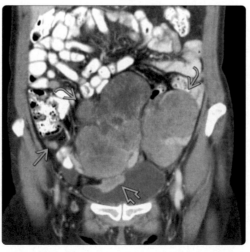

(Left) Coronal CECT shows bilateral, predominantly solid masses ➡ abutting the uterus ➡. Both masses are solid with small cystic areas. (Right) Coronal CECT shows bilateral heterogeneous ovarian masses ➡. The primary tumor was identified as appendiceal carcinoma ➡. Also note the peritoneal metastasis invading into the urinary bladder ➡.

Torsion and Massive Ovarian Edema

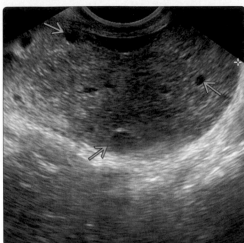

Torsion and Massive Ovarian Edema

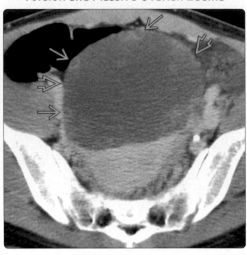

(Left) *Transvaginal ultrasound shows an enlarged ovary demonstrating heterogeneous echogenicity and scattered multiple follicles ➡.* (Right) *Axial CECT in a 23-year-old woman presenting with acute pelvic pain shows an enlarged left ovary ➡ with multiple preserved ovarian follicles ➡ that are predominantly at the periphery of the enlarged ovary.*

Fibroma/Fibrothecoma/Thecoma

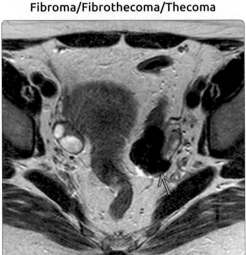

Fibroma/Fibrothecoma/Thecoma

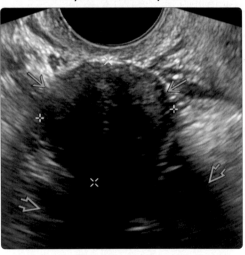

(Left) *Axial T2WI MR shows a well-defined left ovarian mass ➡. The mass demonstrates homogeneous low signal intensity relative to pelvic muscles.* (Right) *Transvaginal ultrasound shows an ovarian mass ➡. The mass shows low echogenicity with dramatic sound attenuation resulting in posterior acoustic shadowing ➡.*

Brenner Tumor

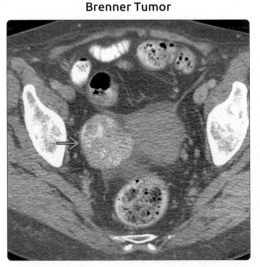

Granulosa Cell Tumor

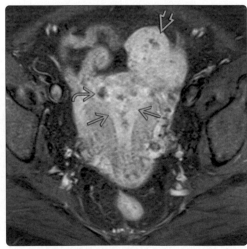

(Left) *Axial CECT shows a right ovarian mass ➡ that has diffuse amorphous calcifications.* (Right) *Axial T1 C+ FS MR shows an enhancing solid left ovarian mass ➡ in a 45-year-old woman with vaginal bleeding. Note the thickened enhancing endometrium ➡ with cystic changes ➡. An endometrial biopsy revealed endometrial hyperplasia.*

Dysgerminoma

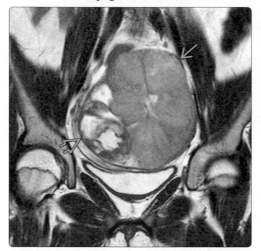

Immature Teratoma

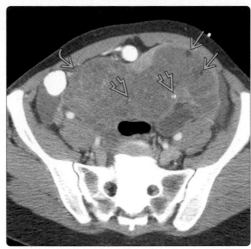

(Left) *Coronal T2WI MR shows a multilobulated right ovarian mass ➡. The mass is hyperintense relative to muscle with hypointense septa separating the mass into multiple lobules. An associated mature cystic teratoma ➡ is also present.* **(Right)** *Axial CECT shows a large pelvic mass ➡ demonstrating heterogeneous attenuation with small foci of fat ➡ and calcifications ➡.*

Yolk Sac Tumor

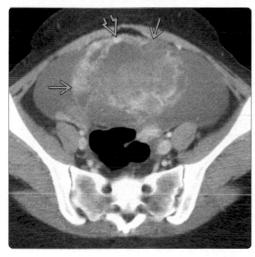

Sertoli-Leydig Cell Tumors

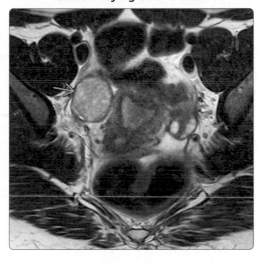

(Left) *Axial CECT shows a large abdominal mixed solid and cystic mass ➡ with small foci of enhancement ➡, a finding known as the bright dot sign that indicates increased tumor vascularity.* **(Right)** *Axial T2WI MR in a 17-year-old girl with virilism shows a right ovarian mass ➡. The mass demonstrates high signal intensity relative to pelvic muscles.*

Lymphoma

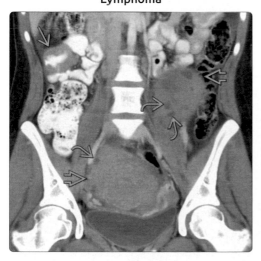

Hyperthecosis

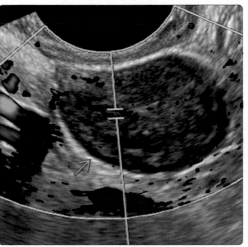

(Left) *Coronal CECT shows bilateral ovarian masses ➡ with preserved follicles ➡ within both the ovarian masses. Note also the circumferential thickening of the wall of the terminal ileum ➡ in this patient with Burkitt lymphoma.* **(Right)** *Transvaginal Doppler ultrasound in a 68-year-old woman who presented with virilism shows an enlarged ovary ➡ (with a volume of 12 cm³). The other ovary was similarly enlarged. Both ovaries showed homogeneous low echogenicity without discernible masses.*

DIFFERENTIAL DIAGNOSIS

Common

- Mature Cystic Teratoma (Dermoid Cyst)
- Mucinous Ovarian Neoplasms
- Serous Ovarian Neoplasms
- Leiomyoma (Mimic)

Less Common

- Fibroma
- Brenner Tumor
- Cystadenofibroma

Rare but Important

- Immature Teratoma
- Dysgerminoma

ESSENTIAL INFORMATION

Key Differential Diagnosis Issues

- Associated with fat
  - Mature cystic teratoma (dermoid cyst)
  - Immature teratoma
- Not associated with fat
  - Mucinous ovarian neoplasms
  - Serous ovarian neoplasms
  - Fibroma
  - Cystadenofibroma
  - Brenner tumor
  - Dysgerminoma

Helpful Clues for Common Diagnoses

- **Mature Cystic Teratoma (Dermoid Cyst)**
  - Calcifications in form of tooth, coarse calcifications in Rokitansky nodule, or mural calcifications
  - Fat attenuation on CT
- **Mucinous Ovarian Neoplasms**
  - Calcifications in 34.1% of mucinous cystic tumors on CT
  - Patterns of calcifications
    - Fine sand-like intacystic calcifications located in necrotic material within cystic structures

- □ More common in malignant tumors
- Mural curvilinear calcification pattern
  - □ More common in benign tumors
- **Serous Ovarian Neoplasms**
  - Calcifications in 4.7% of serous cystic tumors on CT
  - Calcifications may be seen in peritoneal and nodal metastases
  - Calcifications appear to be more common in low-grade serous carcinoma
- **Leiomyoma (Mimic)**
  - Calcified exophytic uterine leiomyoma can be mistaken for ovarian mass
  - Careful evaluation of relation of mass to uterus can establish its uterine origin
    - Bridging vascular sign

Helpful Clues for Less Common Diagnoses

- **Fibroma**
  - < 10% of fibromas calcify
  - Solid mass with calcifications
- **Brenner Tumor**
  - Solid or mixed solid and cystic mass with calcifications in 83% of cases
  - Calcifications are frequently extensive and amorphous
- **Cystadenofibroma**
  - Calcifications may occur in solid component or even extend beyond mass into pelvis

Helpful Clues for Rare Diagnoses

- **Immature Teratoma**
  - Peak incidence 15-19 years of age
  - Solid mass with interspersed small foci of fat, calcifications, and numerous cysts of variable sizes
  - Coarse, irregular calcifications within solid component or mural calcifications in walls of cysts
- **Dysgerminoma**
  - Most cases occur in adolescence and early adulthood
  - Calcification may be present in speckled pattern
  - Multilobulated solid masses with prominent fibrovascular septa

---

Mature Cystic Teratoma (Dermoid Cyst)

Mature Cystic Teratoma (Dermoid Cyst)

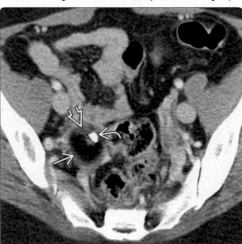
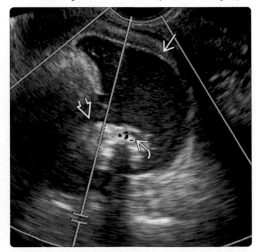

(Left) Axial CECT shows a right ovarian mass ➡ of predominantly fatty attenuation with a mural nodule of soft tissue attenuation (Rokitansky nodule) ➡ containing coarse calcifications ➡. (Right) Transvaginal color Doppler ultrasound shows a cystic ovarian lesion ➡ with echogenic mural nodule ➡ containing densely echogenic structure ➡ with posterior shadowing.

Mature Cystic Teratoma (Dermoid Cyst)

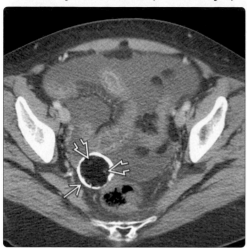

Mature Cystic Teratoma (Dermoid Cyst)

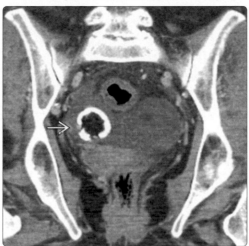

(Left) *Axial CECT shows a fat attenuation right ovarian lesion* ➡ *with surrounding thick rim of irregular calcifications. Small foci of soft tissue attenuation* ➡ *are present within the fatty mass.* (Right) *Coronal CECT in the same patient shows a fat attenuation right ovarian lesion* ➡ *with surrounding thick interrupted rim of irregular calcifications.*

Mucinous Ovarian Neoplasms

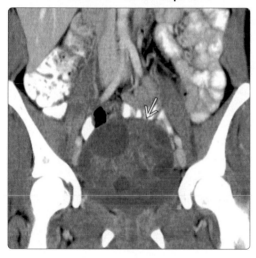

Mucinous Ovarian Neoplasms

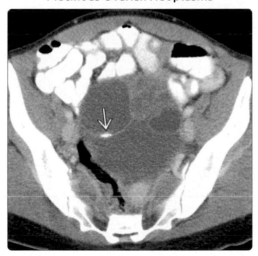

(Left) *Coronal CECT shows a well-defined, predominantly solid pelvic mass* ➡ *with multiple well-defined, cystic spaces.* (Right) *Axial CECT in the same patient shows curvilinear calcifications* ➡ *in the wall of 1 of the cysts. Pathology revealed borderline mucinous tumor.*

Serous Ovarian Neoplasms

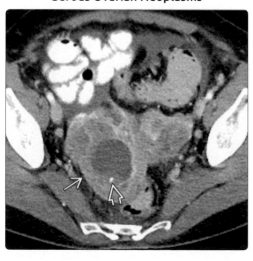

Serous Ovarian Neoplasms

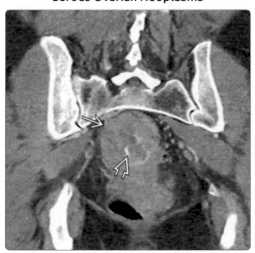

(Left) *Axial CECT shows a mixed solid and cystic right ovarian mass* ➡ *with a small area of calcifications* ➡. (Right) *Coronal CECT in the same patient shows a right ovarian mass* ➡ *with a small area of calcifications* ➡. *Pathological evaluation revealed low-grade serous carcinoma.*

Serous Ovarian Neoplasms

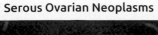

(Left) *Axial CECT shows a cystic right ovarian mass ➜ with soft tissue attenuation mural nodules ➜ containing foci of calcifications ➜. (Right) Coronal CECT in the same patient shows extensive peritoneal metastases ➜ with small calcific focus ➜ within the peritoneal implants.*

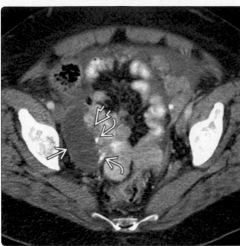

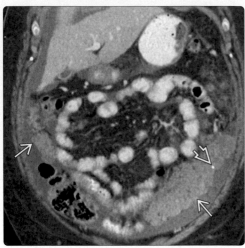

Leiomyoma (Mimic)

(Left) *Axial CECT shows a solid right adnexal mass ➜ with scattered foci of calcifications. Enhancing vessels ➜ are seen bridging from the uterus to the mass (bridging vascular sign), which help establish the uterine origin of the mass. (Right) Coronal CECT in the same patient shows the calcified right ovarian mass ➜ separate from the right ovary ➜.*

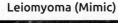

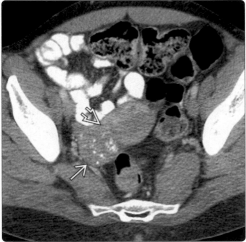

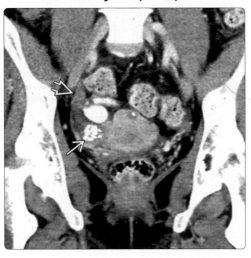

Fibroma

(Left) *Axial CECT shows a large pelvic mass ➜ with homogeneous attenuation, a large chunk of irregular calcifications ➜, and curvilinear calcifications of the wall ➜. (Right) Coronal CECT in the same patient shows a homogeneous soft tissue attenuation mass ➜ with peripheral curvilinear calcifications ➜.*

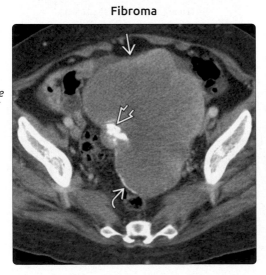

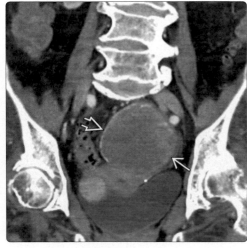

Brenner Tumor

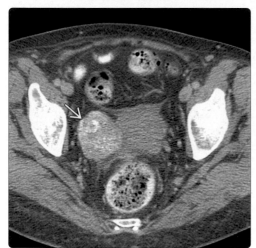

Brenner Tumor

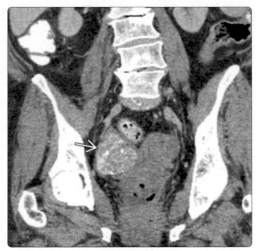

(Left) Axial CECT shows a solid right ovarian mass ➡ with extensive amorphous calcifications. (Right) Coronal CECT in the same patient shows a solid right ovarian mass ➡ with extensive amorphous calcifications. Pathological evaluation revealed benign Brenner tumor.

Cystadenofibroma

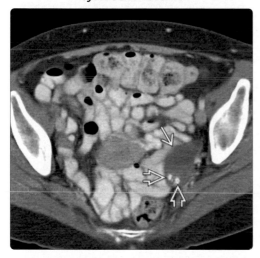

Cystadenofibroma

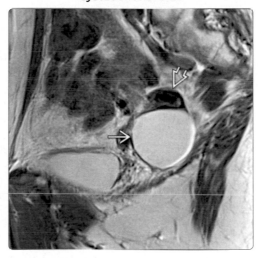

(Left) Axial CECT shows a left ovarian mass ➡ with foci of coarse calcifications ⇨. (Right) Sagittal T2 MR shows a left ovarian mass composed of cystic ➡ and solid ➡ components. The solid component demonstrates very low signal intensity due to fibrous tissue. Pathological evaluation revealed serous cystadenofibroma.

Immature Teratoma

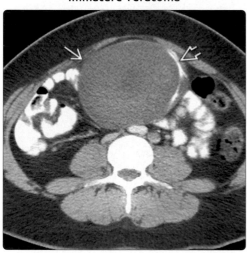

Immature Teratoma

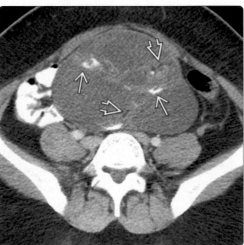

(Left) Axial CECT shows a fluid attenuation lesion ➡ with peripheral curvilinear calcifications ⇨. (Right) Axial CECT in the same patient shows a multilobular mass with irregular linear calcifications ➡ and small foci of fat attenuation ➡.

DIFFERENTIAL DIAGNOSIS

Common

- Endometrioma
- Hemorrhagic Cyst
- Fibroma/Fibrothecoma

Less Common

- Krukenberg Tumor
- Adenofibroma/Cystadenofibroma

Rare but Important

- Brenner Tumor
- Struma Ovarii
- Fibromatosis

ESSENTIAL INFORMATION

Key Differential Diagnosis Issues

- T2 signal intensity relative to pelvic muscles
  - T2 isointense relative to muscles
    - Endometrioma
    - Fibroma/fibrothecoma
    - Cystadenofibroma
    - Struma ovarii
  - T2 hypointense relative to muscles
    - Hemorrhagic cyst
    - Krukenberg tumor
    - Mucinous cystic neoplasm
- Solid vs. cystic
  - Solid
    - Fibroma/fibrothecoma
    - Krukenberg tumor
    - Adenofibroma
  - Cystic
    - Endometrioma
    - Hemorrhagic cyst
    - Mucinous cystic neoplasm
  - Cystic and solid
    - Cystadenofibroma
    - Struma ovarii

Helpful Clues for Common Diagnoses

- **Endometrioma**
  - US
    - Well-defined, smooth-walled, uni- or multilocular cyst(s)
    - Contains homogeneous low-level echoes → characteristic ground-glass appearance
    - Small echogenic foci occur in 35% of endometrioma walls
      - ↑ likelihood that cystic mass is endometrioma
    - Atypical features that may be seen (15% of cases)
      - Mural irregularities: Usually avascular (likely due to adherent mural clot or fibrin)
      - Flow due to presence of endometrial tissue
      - Malignant transformation to endometrioid or clear cell carcinoma
  - MR
    - Single or multiple, uni- or multilocular cyst
    - High signal intensity on T1WI

- Signal intensity remains high on FS T1WI (to differentiate from fat-containing mature cystic teratoma)
    - T2 shading (signal loss on T2WI in ovarian cyst that appears hyperintense on T1WI)
    - T2 dark spots (discrete, markedly hypointense foci within cyst on T2WI ± T2 shading)
- **Hemorrhagic Cyst**
  - Physiologic cysts seen only in premenopausal women
  - Resolve on follow-up examinations
  - US: Different patterns may be seen
    - Echogenic, avascular, homogeneous, or heterogeneous nonshadowing in early stage
    - Retracted clot
      - Avascular mass-like structure within anechoic cyst
      - Has characteristic concave contour
      - May jiggle with transducer ballottement
    - Reticular, lacy, fishnet, or spongy pattern
      - Irregular fine lines that typically do not completely traverse cyst
  - MR
    - Usually single unilocular cyst
    - High signal intensity on T1WI
      - Signal intensity remains high on T1WI FS (to differentiate from fat-containing mature cystic teratoma)
    - May be hypointense on T2WI (more commonly hyperintense)
      - No T2 shading
      - No T2 dark spots
- **Fibroma/Fibrothecoma**
  - Fibromas can be associated with ascites and pleural effusions in classic Meigs syndrome
  - Fibrothecomas may manifest with hyperestrogenism
    - Endometrial polyps, hyperplasia, or carcinoma
  - US
    - Round, oval, or slightly lobulated tumors
    - Most are hypoechoic and solid, with regular or slightly irregular internal echogenicity
      - Some contain cystic spaces
    - Dramatic sound attenuation resulting in posterior acoustic shadowing
    - Minimal to moderate vascularization on color Doppler images
  - MR
    - T1WI: Hypo- to isointense to pelvic muscles
    - T2WI: Low signal intensity
      - Allows differentiation from other solid ovarian masses
    - T1WI C+: Mild enhancement

Helpful Clues for Less Common Diagnoses

- **Krukenberg Tumor**
  - Known primary tumors commonly originating from stomach (70% of cases), followed by breast, colon, and appendix
  - Bilateral in 60-80% of patients
  - MR
    - Heterogeneous solid and cystic masses with intratumoral cysts within solid component

- Variable hypointensity on T2WI due to presence of metastatic mucin-filled signet ring cells in ovarian stroma and abundant collagen formation
- Moderate to marked enhancement of solid component
- **Adenofibroma/Cystadenofibroma**
  - US
    - Primarily solid (adenofibromas)
      - Resemble ovarian fibromas
    - Primarily cystic (cystadenofibromas)
      - Predominantly cystic
      - Irregular thick wall or septa (possibly > 3 mm) in 30-67% of cases
      - Solid component or papillary projections
  - MR
    - Uni- or multilocular cystic mass, with solid fibrous component that demonstrates low signal intensity on T2WI
    - Primarily solid (adenofibromas)
      - Resemble ovarian fibromas with small foci of high signal cystic spaces
    - Primarily cystic (cystadenofibromas)
      - Solid low signal fibrous component may result in irregular wall or septal thickening (possibly > 3 mm)

Helpful Clues for Rare Diagnoses

- **Brenner Tumor**
  - US
    - Most Brenner tumors contain solid components
      - Purely solid
      - Uni- or multilocular cystic with solid component
    - Cystic content is anechoic or of low echogenicity
    - Minimal flow on color Doppler ultrasound
    - Calcifications in majority of cases (best seen on CT)
  - MR
    - Very low T2 signal intensity and low T1 signal intensity due to presence of fibrous elements ± calcifications
      - Imaging finding overlaps with those of fibrothecomas

- Solid component demonstrating low T2 signal intensity in mixed solid and cystic lesions
- Typically demonstrates at least moderate enhancement after contrast material administration
  - Helps differentiate Brenner tumor from fibrothecomas, which are typically hypovascular
- Presence of calcification and coexisting epithelial neoplasms favors diagnosis of Brenner tumor over fibrothecoma
- **Struma Ovarii**
  - US
    - Solid and cystic appearance
    - May be associated with mature cystic teratoma
    - May show rounded or oval echogenic nodules (stromal pearls)
  - MR
    - Hyperthyroidism in ~ 5% of patients
    - ± mature cystic teratoma with its characteristic appearance due to fat contents
    - Loculated cystic mass with variable signal characteristics
      - Some locules may show marked hypointensity at T2WI and intermediate signal intensity at T1WI due to thick, gelatinous colloid
    - Strong enhancement of solid components on postcontrast T1WI
- **Fibromatosis**
  - Enlarged ovary with preserved ovarian shape
  - Preserved ovarian follicles

SELECTED REFERENCES

1. Corwin MT et al: Differentiation of ovarian endometriomas from hemorrhagic cysts at MR imaging: utility of the T2 dark spot sign. Radiology. 271(1):126-32, 2014
2. Khashper A et al: T2-hypointense adnexal lesions: an imaging algorithm Radiographics. 32(4):1047-64, 2012
3. Paladini D et al. Imaging in gynecological disease (5): clinical and ultrasound characteristics in fibroma and fibrothecoma of the ovary. Ultrasound Obstet Gynecol. 34(2):188-95, 2009
4. Savelli L et al: Imaging of gynecological disease (4): clinical and ultrasound characteristics of struma ovarii. Ultrasound Obstet Gynecol. 32(2):210-9, 2008

Endometrioma

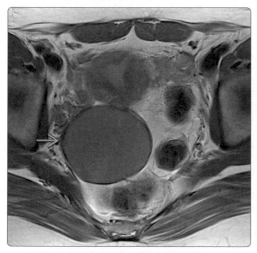

Endometrioma

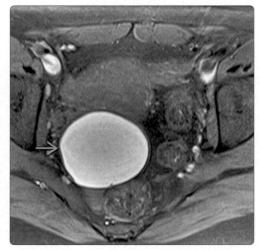

(Left) *Axial T2WI MR shows a right ovarian lesion ➡. The lesion shows homogeneous signal intensity similar to that of pelvic muscles.* **(Right)** *Axial T1WI MR shows a right ovarian mass ➡. The mass demonstrates high signal intensity. This is an example of T2 shading (signal loss on T2WI in an ovarian cyst that appears hyperintense on T1WI).*

Endometrioma

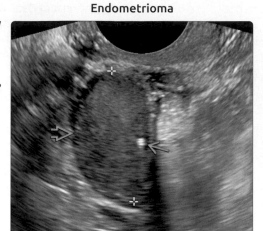

Endometrioma

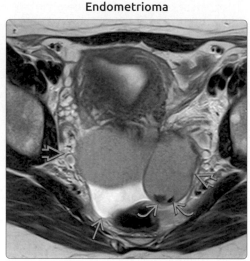

(Left) *Transvaginal ultrasound shows a hypoechoic ovarian lesion* ⇒ *with homogeneous low-level echoes and a small echogenic mural focus* ⇒*.* (Right) *Axial T2WI MR shows 2 endometriomas* ⇒*. Both endometriomas show signal intensity that is lower than that of simple fluid* ⇒*. Multiple T2 dark spots* ⇒ *are present within the left endometrioma.*

Hemorrhagic Cyst

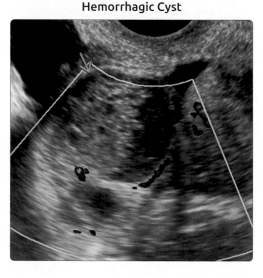

Hemorrhagic Cyst

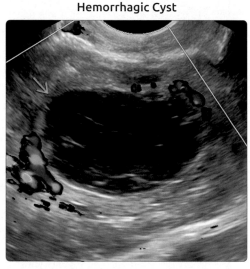

(Left) *Transvaginal color Doppler ultrasound shows an ovarian lesion* ⇒ *with an avascular, heterogeneous hyperechoic pattern.* (Right) *Transvaginal color Doppler ultrasound shows an ovarian lesion* ⇒ *with irregular fine lines that do not completely traverse the cyst, a pattern that has been described as cobweb, reticular, lacy, fishnet, or spongy.*

Hemorrhagic Cyst

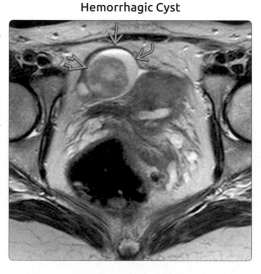

Hemorrhagic Cyst

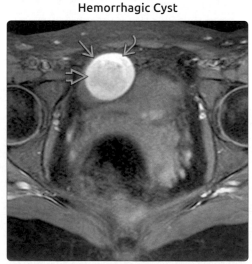

(Left) *Axial T2 MR shows a right ovarian hemorrhagic cyst* ⇒ *with a retracted clot pattern. An eccentric low signal intensity blood clot* ⇒ *is present within the high signal intensity component* ⇒*.* (Right) *Axial T1 FS MR shows a right ovarian hemorrhagic cyst* ⇒ *with a retracted clot pattern. An eccentric high signal intensity blood clot* ⇒ *is present within the higher signal intensity component* ⇒*.*

Fibroma/Fibrothecoma

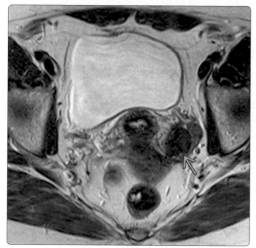

Fibroma/Fibrothecoma

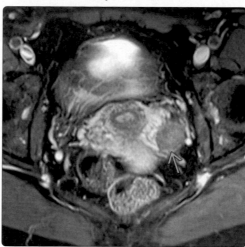

(Left) *Axial T2WI shows a left ovarian mass* ➡. *The mass demonstrates homogeneous low signal intensity.* **(Right)** *Axial T1 C+ FS MR shows poor enhancement of the left ovarian mass* ➡.

Fibroma/Fibrothecoma

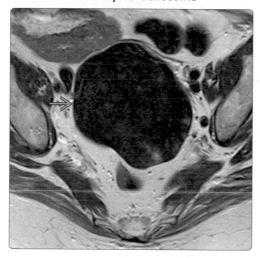

Fibroma/Fibrothecoma

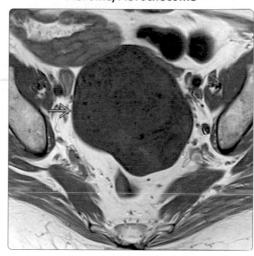

(Left) *Axial T2WI shows a well-defined ovarian mass* ➡ *demonstrating homogeneously low signal intensity.* **(Right)** *Axial T1WI in the same patient shows a well-defined ovarian mass* ➡ *demonstrating homogeneously low signal intensity.*

Fibroma/Fibrothecoma

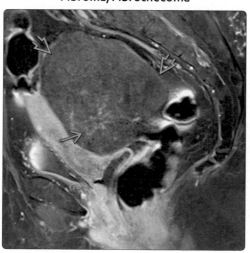

Fibroma/Fibrothecoma

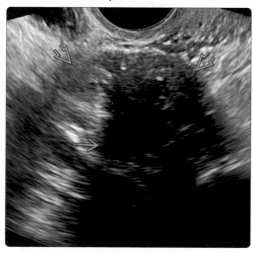

(Left) *Sagittal T1WI C+ FS in the same patient shows a well-defined ovarian mass* ➡ *demonstrating minimal enhancement* ➡. **(Right)** *Transvaginal ultrasound in the same patient shows a well-defined hypoechoic ovarian lesion* ➡ *with marked attenuation of the sound waves, resulting in posterior acoustic shadowing* ➡.

Ovarian Lesions With Low T2 Signal Intensity

Krukenberg Tumor

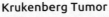

Krukenberg Tumor

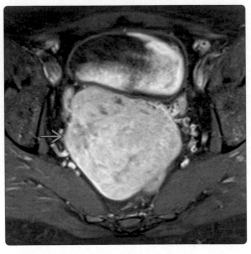

(Left) *Axial T2WI MR in a patient with a history of gastric carcinoma shows a heterogeneous right ovarian mass ➡ with areas of low signal intensity that is similar to pelvic muscles.* **(Right)** *Axial T1 C+ FS MR in the same patient shows heterogeneous intense enhancement of a right ovarian mass ➡.*

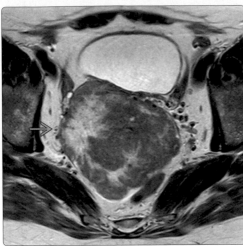

Adenofibroma/Cystadenofibroma

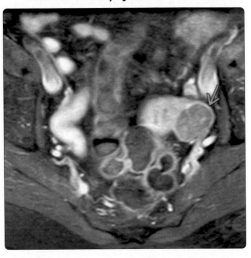

Adenofibroma/Cystadenofibroma

(Left) *Axial T2WI shows a well-defined, predominantly solid left ovarian mass of low signal intensity ➡ and a small central area of high signal intensity ➡.* **(Right)** *Axial T1WI C+ FS shows a well-defined, predominantly solid left ovarian mass ➡ demonstrating mild homogeneous enhancement.*

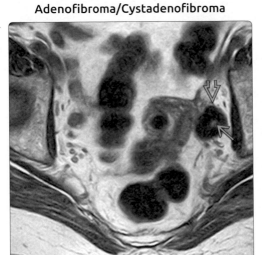

Adenofibroma/Cystadenofibroma

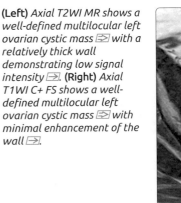

Adenofibroma/Cystadenofibroma

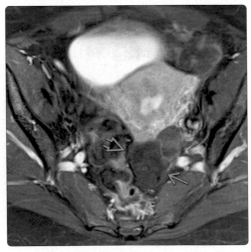

(Left) *Axial T2WI MR shows a well-defined multilocular left ovarian cystic mass ➡ with a relatively thick wall demonstrating low signal intensity ➡.* **(Right)** *Axial T1WI C+ FS shows a well-defined multilocular left ovarian cystic mass ➡ with minimal enhancement of the wall ➡.*

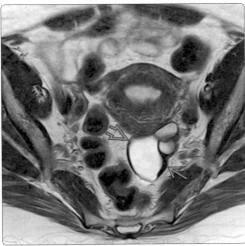

Brenner Tumor

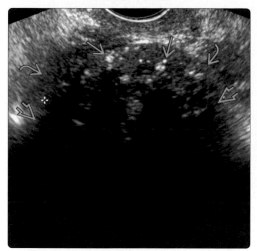

Brenner Tumor

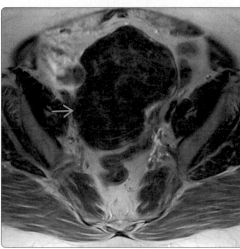

(Left) *Transvaginal ultrasound shows a solid ovarian mass ⊿ with foci of increased echogenicity ⊿ due to calcifications. There is marked attenuation of the sound waves resulting in posterior shadowing ⊿.* (Right) *Axial T2 MR shows a pelvic mass ⊿ with relatively homogeneous low signal intensity. It is difficult to appreciate calcifications on MR images.*

Struma Ovarii

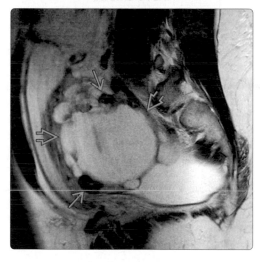

Struma Ovarii

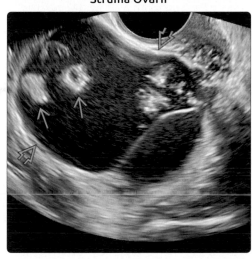

(Left) *Sagittal T2WI MR in a 24 year old shows a multilocular cystic mass ⊿. Most of the loculi demonstrate high signal intensity; few ⊿ demonstrate very low signal intensity.* (Right) *Transvaginal ultrasound shows a multilocular cystic ovarian mass ⊿ with multiple, echogenic, rounded intracystic stroma pearls ⊿, a characteristic sonographic feature of struma ovarii.*

Fibromatosis

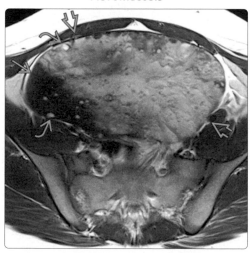

Fibromatosis

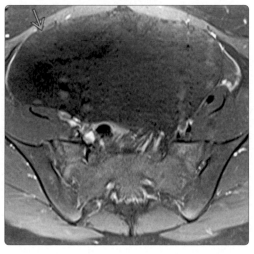

(Left) *Axial T2WI MR in a 13-year-old girl with repeated episodes of severe pelvic pain shows a massively enlarged left ovary ⊿. The enlarged ovary demonstrates increased signal intensity except for a segmental area of very low signal ⊿ at the periphery. Note the preserved ovarian follicles ⊿ throughout the ovary.* (Right) *Axial T1 C+ FS MR in the same patient shows no significant enhancement of the enlarged ovary ⊿. This case demonstrates the development of ovarian fibromatosis in massive ovarian edema.*

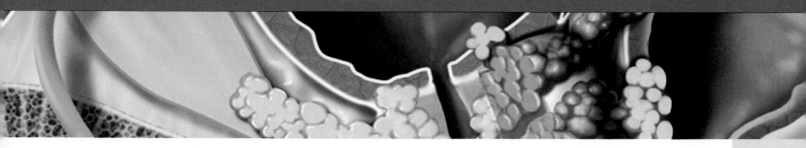

INDEX

A

INDEX

INDEX

INDEX

G

INDEX

O

INDEX

INDEX

INDEX

INDEX

INDEX